ENCYCLOPAEDIA

of

FOOD SCIENCE
FOOD TECHNOLOGY

and

NUTRITION

ENCYCLOPAEDIA

of

FOOD SCIENCE
FOOD TECHNOLOGY
and
NUTRITION

Volume Two

Catering–Down's Syndrome

Edited by

R. Macrae
University of Hull, Hull, UK

R. K. Robinson
University of Reading, Reading, UK

M. J. Sadler
Consultant Nutritionist, Ashford, UK

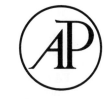

ACADEMIC PRESS

Harcourt Brace Jovanovich, Publishers
London   San Diego   New York
Boston   Sydney   Tokyo   Toronto

ACADEMIC PRESS LIMITED
24/28 Oval Road
LONDON NW1 7DX

United States Edition published by
ACADEMIC PRESS INC.
San Diego, CA 92101

A catalogue record for this book is available from the British Library

Library of Congress Cataloging-in-Publication Data

Encyclopaedia of food science, food technology, and nutrition/edited
   by R. Macrae, R. K. Robinson, M. J. Sadler.
      p.   cm.
   1. Food—Encyclopedias.   2. Food industry and trade—
—Encyclopedias.   3. Nutrition—Encyclopedias.   I. Macrae, R.
II. Robinson, R. K. (Richard Kenneth).   III. Sadler, M. J. (Michèle
J.)
   TX349.E47   1993
   664′.003—dc20   92-15557
                                                                                         CIP

ISBN   Volume 1 0-12-226851-2   Volume 5 0-12-226855-5
         Volume 2 0-12-226852-0   Volume 6 0-12-226856-3
         Volume 3 0-12-226853-9   Volume 7 0-12-226857-1
         Volume 4 0-12-226854-7   Volume 8 0-12-226858-X

ISBN Set 0-12-226850-4

EDITORIAL STAFF

Managing Editor
Gina Fullerlove

Assistant Editor
Sarah Robertson

Production Editors
David Atkins
Sara Hackwood

Production Controller
Anne Doris

Editorial Assistants
Jill Farrow
Lara King
Martina Tuohy

Copy Editors
Len Cegielka
Rich Cutler
Alison Walsh

Cross-referencer
Jane Wells

Proof Reader
Alison Woodhouse

Indexer
Merral-Ross International

Editorial and Technical Support Manager
Christopher Gibson

Head of Book Production
Helen Whitehorn

Typeset by The Alden Press, Oxford
Printed in Great Britain by Butler and Tanner Ltd, Frome, Somerset, UK

D. B. Emmons
Food Research Centre, Ottawa, Canada

O. R. Fennema
University of Wisconsin-Madison, Madison, USA

D. L. Georgala
AFRC Institute of Food Research, Reading, UK

M. J. Gibney
Trinity College Medical School, Dublin, Eire

C. Gopalan
The Nutrition Foundation of India, New Delhi, India

P. Gray
Commission of the European Communities, Bruxelles, Belgium

M. S. Y. Hadaddin
University of Jordan, Amman, Jordan

B. Hallgren
Swedish Nutrition Foundation, Goteborg, Sweden

J. M. Hutchinson
FAO, Rome, Italy

B. Jarvis
HP Bulmer Ltd, Hereford, UK

M. E. Knowles
MAFF, London, UK

J. A. Kurmann
Institut Agricole de Fribourg, Posieux, Switzerland

R. A. Lawrie
University of Nottingham, Loughborough, UK

F. A. Lee
Cornell University, New York, USA

D. X. Lin
Wuxi Institute of Light Industry, Wuxi, People's Republic of China

V. Loureiro
Technical University of Lisbon, Lisbon, Portugal

P. Lunven
FAO, Rome, Italy

E. J. Mann
International Dairy Federation, Reading, UK

V. Marks
University of Surrey, Guildford, UK

H. E. Nursten
University of Reading, Reading, UK

R. Paoletti
Universita di Milano, Milan, Italy

K. L. Parkin
University of Wisconsin-Madison, Madison, USA

G. T. Prance
Royal Botanic Gardens, Kew, UK

A. Reps
Institute of Food Biotechnology, Kortowo, Poland

D. R. Richardson
Nestle, Croydon, UK

P. Richmond
AFRC Institute of Food Research, Norwich, UK

A. Rougerea
Robert Debre Hospital, Amboise, France

J. D. Schofield
Kings College, University of London, UK

N. E. Schwartz
National Centre for Nutrition and Dietetics, Chicago, USA

R. L. Sellars
Chr. Hansen's Laboratory Inc., Wisconsin, USA

J. Solms
Swiss Federal Institute of Technology, Zurich, Switzerland

D. A. T. Southgate
AFRC Institute of Food Research, Norwich, UK

K. R. Spurgeon
South Dakota State University, South Dakota, USA

M. Stasse-Wolthuis
Netherlands Nutrition Foundation, Wageningen, The Netherlands

P. S. Steyn
National Food Research Institute, Pretoria, South Africa

P. Trayhurn
Rowett Research Institute, Aberdeen, UK

A. S. Truswell
University of Sydney, Sydney, Australia

G. Varela
Universidad Complutense de Madrid, Madrid, Spain

J. V. Wheelock
University of Bradford, Bradford, UK

E. M. Widdowson
Addenbrooke's Hospital, Cambridge, UK

R. B. Wills
Food Industry Development Centre, Kensington, Australia

GUIDE TO USE OF THE ENCYCLOPAEDIA

Structure of the Encyclopaedia

The material in the Encyclopaedia is arranged as a series of entries in alphabetical order. Some entries comprise a single article, whilst entries on more diverse subjects consist of several articles that deal with various aspects of the topic. In the latter case the articles are arranged in a logical sequence within an entry.

To help you realize the full potential of the material in the Encyclopaedia we have provided three features to help you find the topic of your choice.

Contents Lists

Your first point of reference will probably be the contents list. The complete contents list appearing in Volume 8 will provide you with both the volume number and the page number of the entry. Additionally each volume has a list of entries and articles to be found within that particular volume, which allows you to locate material within the volume without having to return to the complete contents list each time a new topic is required. On the opening page of an entry a contents list is provided so that the full details of the articles within the entry are immediately available.

Alternatively you may choose to browse through a volume using the alphabetical order of the entries as your guide. To assist you in identifying your location within the Encyclopaedia a running headline indicates the current entry and a running footer indicates the current article within that entry.

You will find 'Dummy Entries' where obvious synonyms exist for entries or where we have grouped together related analytical techniques or commodities. Dummy entries appear in both the contents list and the body of the text. For example, a Dummy Entry appears for Vitamin C which directs you to Ascorbic Acid, where the material is located.

Example

If you were attempting to locate material on Oranges via the Contents List.

Volume 5

Then once you have been directed to the correct location in the contents list this would then provide the page number.

If you were trying to locate the material by browsing through the text and you looked up Oranges then the following is the information you would be provided.

ORANGES

See Citrus Fruits

Alternatively, if you were looking up Citrus Fruits the following information would be provided.

CITRUS FRUITS

Contents

Types on the Market
Composition and Characterization
Oranges
Processed and Derived Products
  of Oranges

Lemons
Grapefruits
Limes

Cross References

All of the articles in the Encyclopaedia have been extensively cross referenced.

The cross references, which appear at the end of a paragraph, have been provided at three levels:

1. To indicate if a topic is discussed in greater detail elsewhere.

     Groups at Risk of Vitamin C Deficiency (Scurvy)
     The major determinant of vitamin C intake is the consumption of fruit and vegetables, and the range of intakes in healthy adults in Britain reflects this. The 2·5 percentile intake is 19 mg per day (men) and 14 mg per day (women), while the 97·5 percentile intake is 170 mg per day (men) and 160 mg per day (women). Deficiency is likely in people whose habitual intake of fruit and vegetables is very low. Smokers may be more at risk of deficiency; there is some evidence that the rate of ascorbate catabolism is two-fold higher in smokers than

in non-smokers. Clinical signs of deficiency are rarely seen in developed countries. *See* Scurvy

2. To draw the reader's attention to parallel discussions in other articles.

    Fruit Morphology

    Grapefruit is composed of three distinctly different morphological parts. The epicarp consists of the coloured portion of the peel and is known as the flavedo. In the flavedo are cells containing the carotenoids which give the characteristic colour to the fruit. The oil glands, also found in the flavedo, are the raised structures in the skin of the fruit that contain the essential oil, naringin, characteristics of the grapefruit. *See* Citrus Fruits, Oranges; Citrus fruits, Lemons

3. To indicate material that broadens the discussion.

    Plasma Concentration of Ascorbate

    At intakes below 30 mg per day the plasma concentration of ascorbate is extremely low, and does not reflect increasing intake to any significant extent. As the intake rises, so the plasma concentration begins to increase sharply, reaching a plateau of 55–85 μmol l^{-1} at intakes between 70 and 100 mg per day, when the renal threshold is reached and the vitamin is excreted quantitatively with increasing intake. *See* Dietary Reference Values

Index

The index will provide you with the volume number and page number of where the material is to be located, and the index entries differentiate between material that is a whole article, is part of an article or is data presented in a table. On the opening page of the index detailed notes are provided.

Colour Plates

The colour figures for each volume have been grouped together in a plate section. The location of this section is cited both in the contents list and on the opening page of the pertinent articles.

Contributors and Referees

A full list of contributors and a full list of referees appears in Volume 8.

CONTENTS

Colour Plate Section appears between pages 1146 and 1147

CATERING

Contents

Catering Systems

This article reviews the three main catering systems (cook–serve, cook–freeze and cook–chill) and their variations; it includes the methods and equipment used, and aspects of food quality and food control.

The Catering Industry

The catering industry is very diverse in size, market and technology, ranging from small cafés using domestic cooking techniques to large centralized kitchens which in some respects resemble food factories. In general, the industry is composed of small units, often producing a wide range of food items. Traditional quality control and quality assurance are less evident than in the food manufacturing industry, although current legislation and other factors are likely to bring about change. *See* Quality Assurance and Quality Control

Cook–Serve System

Most catering establishments cook and serve the food on a single site. In addition to the long established methods of cooking food by contact with hot fluids (air, water, steam, and oil), metals, and electromagnetic radiation (microwave and infrared), a number of newer methods, or variations of the old ones, have been developed. These include induction heating, ohmic heating, short- ($< 1 \cdot 25$ μm) and long-wave ($> 1 \cdot 25$ μm) infrared heaters, and jet impingement ovens in which air jets are directed onto the food surface at about 15 m s^{-1}. Developments in traditional equipment include the use of heat foils and heat pipes in griddles. Many of these changes are designed to lead to faster and more controlled heating.

In the fast food industry this trend is coupled with the development of homogeneous food products of standardized composition, size and shape, e.g. the standard beefburger. The cooking is therefore highly controlled and microbiological safety is high.

Another trend is the use of continuous cookers instead of batch cookers in some large kitchens. Examples of batch cookers include steamers, deep-fat fryers, ovens, boilers, grills, microwave ovens, and jet impingement ovens. The amount of cooking received by the product is controlled by varying the temperature of the cooking medium and the speed of the conveyor belt.

The desirable minimum temperature attained by food during cooking has been a matter of recent debate. Current UK legislation embodied in the Food Hygiene (General) Regulations of 1970 stipulates 63°C for foods of greatest potential danger, such as meat and poultry, although the 1989 guidelines for cook–chill and cook–freeze catering recommend 70°C for 2 min, which has been claimed to give a 10^6 reduction in numbers of *Listeria monocytogenes*. *See Listeria*, Properties and Occurrence

Hot-holding of food between cooking and service can be considerable in some large-scale operations, owing to the problems of cooking in large batches and feeding large numbers of people. Hot-holding above 63°C generally reduces the bacterial load, but can also impair the sensory quality, and lead to a loss of heat-labile nutrients such as vitamin C and thiamin, and these effects generally increase with increasing temperature. For example, potatoes have been found to become unacceptable in flavour after 3 h at 60°C, whereas a similar change takes only 1·5 h at 90°C. *See* Ascorbic Acid, Properties and Determination; Thiamin, Properties and Determination

If cooking is to be controlled, it must be quantifiable. This can be done by means of the cook value, which is equivalent to the time required to cook isothermally at 100°C. This is analogous to the F_0 value, used to quantify the extent of heat sterilization. The other factor needed to quantify the extent of temperature–time on cooking is the Zc factor, which is the temperature change required to alter the time of cooking by a factor of 10. Sensory work on potatoes has produced a cook value of 6·0 min and a Zc value of 17°C using texture as the criteria. These data transcribe into isothermal cooking times of 6 min at 100°C and 0·6 min at 117°C. This approach can be used to measure the degree of cooking achieved by different heating regimes, and can include hot-holding and preblanching.

The question of energy utilization during cooking is important because of cost, overheating of kitchen environment by surplus heat, and the general need for energy conservation. Heat balance experiments have shown that for a range of products and cooking methods the heat absorbed by the food during cooking is usually between 0·5 and 1·0 MJ per kg of food, and is equal to the sum of the sensible heat and latent heat of water evaporation. By contrast, the amount of energy used in a typical kitchen is usually between 10·0 and 21·5 MJ per kg according to a 1983 survey. The efficiency can sometimes be increased by better equipment design, and especially by better catering practice.

Cook–Freeze System

The traditional cook–serve system has a number of drawbacks. Hot-holding is often excessive and working schedules can be uneven, with high work inputs often necessary near to the time of service. This led to the development of the cook–freeze system, in which precooked frozen food is produced in large central production units (CPUs) and then transferred to small satellite kitchens where the frozen food is reheated immediately prior to service. In this way the production and service of the meals are separated in time. Work in a CPU can carry on smoothly around the clock with potential financial saving. Many CPUs resemble small food factories and this can make it easier to operate good systems of quality control and quality assurance.

Cook–freeze operators in the UK are strongly advised to follow the UK Department of Health Publication, *Guidelines on Cook–Chill and Cook–Freeze Catering Systems*, of 1989 (henceforth referred to as the DoH Guidelines).

Prime cooking is usually carried out according to conventional methods and recipes, although products sensitive to textural damage during freezing, including batters and starch-based sauces, are often modified. In addition, products which are easily overcooked, including some fish and vegetables, may have to be lightly cooked initially in order to compensate for the extra degree of cooking achieved during regeneration.

After cooking to at least 70°C for 2 min, the food can be weighed out in multiple or single portions into metal or plastic containers. Freezing should commence within 30 min of leaving the cooker and the temperature should be reduced to at least −5°C within 90 min, and subsequently taken to −18°C for storage and transportation. Most operations use blast freezers or occasionally cryogenic freezers. After freezing the packs can be transferred to thin plastic bags and sealed. The temperature should be maintained throughout storage and transportation from CPU to satellite kitchens. Transportation vehicles are fitted with refrigeration systems in which a cold gas (carbon dioxide, nitrogen or air) is circulated. *See* Freezing, Blast and Plate Freezing; Freezing, Cryogenic Freezing; Freezing, Freezing Operations; Freezing, Principles

During regeneration, the food is usually heated in metal containers directly from the frozen state to at least 70°C for 2 min or more. Some establishments use forced-convection ovens designed to heat rapidly and evenly when fully loaded; these ovens should maintain a uniform air temperature and air velocity. Other regeneration methods used include fryers, infrared ovens, boiling water, steam, and microwave ovens designed for frozen food. Ideally, the regeneration method should be matched to suit each particular food, although some establishments, for logistic reasons, tailor their systems so that all food is regenerated by the same method. *See* Freezing, Storage of Frozen Foods Freezing, Structural and Flavour Changes

Cook–Chill System

Many of the developments in cook–freeze catering came in the late 1960s and 1970s. However, the 1980s saw a marked shift in interest towards the use of precooked chilled food (cook–chill). The reasons include a variety of factors, including the need to conserve energy, and the public image of chilled or 'fresh', in contrast to the perception of frozen food as 'processed'.

In common with cook–freeze catering, the cook–chill system separates meal production from service, with a potential reduction in labour arising from large-scale central production. One of the main differences is the shelf life; chilled foods usually have a maximum shelf life of only 5 days when stored at 3°C, compared with a month or more for frozen foods. A great deal of quantitative data on vitamin C losses, costs, energy utilization, sensory properties and microbiological counts have been produced on cook–chill and cook–freeze operations. Unfortunately, it is difficult to carry out a comparative evaluation of the two types of operation from these data because there are so many variable factors.

In the cook–chill system cooked food is chilled, usually in mechanical air-blast chillers, then stored at low temperatures for up to 5 days and subsequently reheated prior to service.

Although there is at present no specific legislation, operators in the UK are strongly urged to adopt the 1989 DoH Guidelines. The main DoH recommendations are as follows:

1. Food should be cooked to an internal temperature of not less than 70°C for at least 2 min.
2. Chilling should commence within 30 min of leaving the cooker, and the food should be chilled to between 0°C and 3°C within a further 90 min, except for joints of meat which should not exceed 2·5 kg in weight and should be chilled to 10°C or less within 2·5 h after removal from the cooker.
3. Food should be stored for a maximum of 5 days,

including the day of production, at 0–3°C with a 2°C tolerance.

4. Food should be reheated immediately after removal from chilled storage and reach a temperature of at least 70°C for not less than 2 min.

These guidelines are based on epidemiological studies that clearly show the relationship between inadequate temperature–time control and the risk of food poisoning.

Precooked chilled foods covering a wide range of commodities, including meat, fish, vegetables, pasta and desserts, are manufactured for use in the retail as well as the catering markets. Discussions of the safety of the cook–chill system usually focus on the feasibility of achieving the recommended temperature–time conditions. The most difficult stage is to chill a 50-mm-thick pack of food from 70°C to between 3°C and 0°C within 90 min. The time taken depends on the thermal diffusivity of the food, and on the air temperature and heat transfer coefficient of the blast chiller. In practice, air velocities of about 5 m s^{-1} and air temperatures of around −5°C are often used. If the required performance is not achieved, it is necessary to reduce the depth of the food. As alternatives to mechanical blast chillers, cryogenic equipment using nitrogen, or immersion in chilled water can be used. Systems using liquid nitrogen can quickly restore the fluid temperature to −5°C after hot food is introduced, and water has a higher heat transfer coefficient than gas cooling systems.

Various regeneration methods are used. One example which is part of the integrated Regethermic Cook–Chill system is an infrared oven with a removable shelf system. After loading with chilled food, this is fitted into the heating chamber so as to constitute the oven end. Precooked chilled food is also widely reheated with forced-convection ovens or microwave ovens.

The effect of the cook–chill process on the microbiological and sensory quality has been recently reviewed. There is support for the microbiological safety of food processed according to the DoH Guidelines. However, changes in texture and flavour, including oxidative rancidity, can occur within the recommended 5 days' storage. This has prompted experimental trials using storage in modified atmospheres of nitrogen and carbon dioxide. This retards the development of rancidity in roast pork and also reduces the development of bacterial counts. *See* Chilled Storage, Effect of Modified Atmosphere Packaging on Food Quality; Chilled Storage, Use of Modified Atmosphere Packaging

Variations on Cook–Freeze and Cook–Chill Systems

Sous-vide System

A development on the cook–chill theme, developed in the 1980s through the work of the French chef Georges Pralos, is based on vacuum or *sous-vide* (without air) cooking. After preparation the food is vacuum-sealed in plastic pouches. It is then prime-cooked to give an adequate pasteurization, chilled by air or nitrogen in a blast chiller or by iced water, stored between 0°C and 3°C, and finally regenerated, either in the sealed bag or after removal. *See* Chilled Storage, Packaging Under Vacuum

Vacuum cooking has a number of potential advantages over atmospheric cooking. Flavour and juices are likely to be better retained, and shrinkage and weight loss from meat reduced. Especially important, there is no actual handling of food after the initial vacuum packing, until the final regeneration. Furthermore, the elimination of air can reduce oxidation during storage and extend the organoleptic shelf life. This method has been used with hotel kitchens or small factories as the CPUs. There is great potential for extending the microbiological and sensory shelf life, although this can only be carried out safely through good control based on sound scientific information.

The Capkold System

Another cook–chill variation employing high-temperature controlled cooking and minimum handling, was developed by the Groen and WR Grace companies in the USA. There are two methods of cooking for liquid and solid foods respectively.

Liquid and semiliquid foods, e.g. stews, casseroles and soups, are cooked in a large kettle and then pumped at 83°C into a plastic casing, which is then sealed by clip, and tumble-chilled in ice water prior to storage.

Bulk solid foods, including joints of meat, poultry and fish, are placed into a plastic casing before cooking. The sealed casings are steam-heated in a cooking tank, after which the hot water is replaced by chilled water to bring the product temperature down to about 2°C. The system is based on controlled temperature thoughout, and a shelf life of 45 days is claimed.

Cook–Freeze–Thaw

The basic cook–freeze system involves direct regeneration from the frozen state. In the cook–freeze–thaw modification the food is thawed under controlled conditions, e.g. using high-speed air preferably at a temperature between 0°C and 5°C. The food can then be used alongside cook–chill items using similar regeneration methods. This enables the caterer to obtain the advantages of cook–freeze (long shelf life), whilst operating at the satellite kitchens alongside a cook–chill system.

Control of Catering Systems

Good manufacturing practice, widely practised in the food industry, has been adapted to the catering industry under the general term 'good catering practice' (GCP), which has two integrated components:

1. An effective system of meal production and service.
2. An effective system of food control.

A small survey indicated that those units which operated cook–freeze or cook–chill systems had a greater degree of control than cook–serve units. Overall, there are many units that do not adhere strictly to precise dish specifications, and do not keep records of temperatures, times and other key data. In view of changes in technology and problems of food poisoning, there is a necessity for hazard analysis critical control points (HACCP). This method, which is described fully elsewhere is a systematic procedure which (1) identifies and assesses the severity of risks and hazards, (2) determines the critical control points at which a hazard may be controlled, and (3) establishes control and monitoring procedures to control such hazards. The hazard analysis of a particular product, e.g. fried battered fish, would include raw materials (fish, flour, seasoning, salt, etc.), processing operations (evisceration, washing, seasoning, breading, frying, hot-holding, etc.) and present the relevant information on a flow chart, on which critical control points are marked. These could include potentially hazardous foods, employee practices, time–temperature combinations, procedures, and environmental conditions. *See* Hazard Analysis Critical Control Point

Good catering practice also pays attention to other quality features, including sensory quality and nutrient content, as well as portion control, and could help to minimize overproduction and food waste. *See* Wastage of Food

Bibliography

Collison R (1991) *Advances in Catering Technology – 4*. Bradford: Horton Publishing.

Department of Health (1989) *Guidelines on Cook–Chill and Cook–Freeze Catering Systems*. London: Her Majesty's Stationery Office.

Glew G (1980) *Advances in Catering Technology*. Essex: Elsevier Science Publishers.

Glew G (1985) *Advances in Catering Technology – 3*. Essex: Elsevier Science Publishers.

Robson CP and Collison R (1989) Pre-cooked chilled foods. *Catering and Health* 1: 151–163.

R. Collison
The Polytechnic, Huddersfield, UK

Nutritional Implications

Definition of Catering

Whilst there is no precise definition of what is meant by the catering industry, here it is taken to include the provision of food and drink away from home and, as such, it covers both food consumed on the premises of the caterer and also food bought from the caterer but consumed off the premises.

However, within this definition, there are several grey areas. Thus the term 'catering' is normally extended to include food consumed in the home as part of a 'take-away' or 'home delivered' service. It also covers the 'meals-on-wheels' service in situations where the food is produced in a catering establishment. On the other hand, some food consumed away from home is not considered to come under the definition of catering. For example, many retail food stores sell prepared sandwiches and snacks for consumption away from home.

Food Consumption Data

The significance of the contribution of food eaten in catering establishments to the nutritional status of individuals depends on a number of factors, the most significant of which is the proportion of the total food consumption which comes from a catering establishment.

Official statistics for the UK show that the proportion of food expenditure on food away from home continues to increase as shown in Table 1. These figures are broadly in line with those for Western Europe. The equivalent figure for the USA is of the order of 35–40%. Whilst these figures cannot be directly related to food consumption figures, they do demonstrate an increase in the proportion of food consumed away from home, an increase in the number of meal occasions taking place outside the home (Table 2) and an increase in the proportion of food energy resulting from eating out (Table 3). Recent surveys have shown that, on average, men consumed 34% of their total energy (including alcohol) away from home, compared with a figure of 24% for women. However, the proportion of fibre, protein, minerals and vitamins contained in food eaten away from home was less than the above figures for total

Table 1. UK household expenditure on food per household per week

	1978		1983		1988	
	(£)	(%)	(£)	(%)	(£)	(%)
Household food	16·3	(84·5)	24·55	(83·1)	30·30	(79·2)
Meals away from home	3·0	(15·5)	5·01	(16·9)	7·98	(20·8)

Source: Ministry of Agriculture, Fisheries and Food (MAFF) (1990) *Household Food Consumption and Expenditure 1989*. London: Her Majesty's Stationery Office (HMSO).

Table 2. Number of meals per person per week eaten outside the home where the food is not from the household supply (UK)

	1986	1987	1988	1989
Midday meals	1·73	1·84	1·85	1·89
All meals out	3·37	3·54	3·69	3·84

Source: MAFF (1990) *Household Food Consumption and Expenditure 1989*. London: HMSO.

Table 3. Food energy (%) derived from eating out (UK)

	Age (years)			
	16–24	25–34	35–49	50–64
Male	41·4	37·7	30·0	24·8
Female	36·1	27·9	24·0	18·1

Source: Office of Population Census and Surveys (OPCS) (1990) *The Dietary and Nutritional Survey of British Adults*. London: HMSO

energy. Within these overall figures, some groups consume a greater proportion of their food in catering establishments. In particular, the number of meals consumed away from home varies with age and socio-economic group. For example, the 15–35 age group eat more meals away from home, as do professional and managerial groups.

Another factor which must be taken into account when looking at food consumption data is that, in general, the catering industry produces higher levels of food waste than is the case for domestic consumption. Surveys of industrial, hospital, school meals and commercial catering have shown overall wastage levels of 11·4%. The figures are significantly higher in commercial operations such as restaurants, hotels and pubs, where total waste can be as high as 18·2%, kitchen waste 5·8%, service waste 4·5%, and customer waste 7·9% (Collison R and Colwill JS (1986)). *See* Wastage of Food

Nutritional Considerations

The contribution that caterers make to the nutritional intake of individuals is, as previously discussed, highly dependent on the proportion of food eaten outside of the home. However, the contribution that caterers might be expected to make to the achievement of *good* nutrition depends upon the nature of the catering unit under consideration.

Commercial caterers primarily respond to consumer demands. Changes in the types of foods offered within this sector are particularly dependent on changes in consumer tastes, which in turn may be influenced by nutrition education. The fast food sector is one of the most buoyant in the hotel and catering industry. The nutritional profile of the products offered is not always in line with nutritional recommendations. However, in the face of healthy eating trends this sector has increased its offerings to include healthier items such as pizzas, baked potatoes, baked products with higher fibre, and salads.

In the institutional sectors the nutritional quality of foods is likely to be viewed more positively since it influences performance of workers and schoolchildren, it speeds recovery of those who are ill, and prevents ill health in the elderly. Good nutrition can contribute indirectly to the goals of the organization and may form the basis upon which reputation is judged. On the other hand, issues of costs are frequently significant in this sector. Systems which maintain or improve quality and reduce costs are seen as highly desirable.

Nutritional Losses during Preparation and Storage

The nutritional content of foods consumed by clients in catering establishments depends upon the following factors:

1. the nature and quality of the starting materials used by the caterer to prepare menu items;
2. the ways in which those starting materials are transformed into menu items, i.e. recipe formulations, cooking methods and distribution systems;
3. the ways in which menu items are combined by either the caterer or the client, i.e. menu planning and choice;
4. the degree to which the food is consumed by the client.

The overall nutritional content of foods served in catering establishments probably owes as much to ingredient specifications and recipe formulation as it does to losses resulting from the effects of preparation and processing. This applies particularly to fat, sugar, salt, fibre, iron and calcium, but less so to vitamins.

Nutrient Content

Fat

The fat content of foods is highly variable both in terms of content and type. This applies to both commodity-type ingredients and convenience foods. Cooking is influential: for example, grilling reduces fat content, whilst deep fat frying has the opposite effect. Fast foods, particularly fried foods, frequently contain very high levels of fat. For example, the amount of fat, as a percentage of total energy of the meal, supplied by fish and chips is 50·2%, by chicken and chips 46·9%, by baked potato with cheese filling 45%, and by hamburger with French fries 44·2% (Pascoe JM *et al.* (1985)). *See* Cooking, Domestic Techniques; Fats, Digestion, Absorption and Transport

Fats are relatively stable during storage and processing. Oxidative rancidity is a possibility, particularly during lengthy storage of products such as frozen meat and potato crisps, but such changes have a detrimental effect on flavour and taste of the product. Essential fatty acids, whilst crucial for health, are not a prime consideration since deficiency could only occur on extremely low-fat diets. *See* Essential Fatty Acids, Physiology

Carbohydrate

The carbohydrate content of foods comprises sugar and starch. Sugar in excess is an undesirable constituent of the diet. Confectionery items, soft drinks, puddings, cakes and biscuits are major dietary sources of sucrose and such items frequently occur in the offerings of the caterer. Starch, on the other hand, is an important and desirable component of the diet. Neither sugars nor starches are affected by cooking, apart from some minor losses of reducing sugars in Maillard browning and a small amount of starch dextrinization during, for example, the grilling of bread. *See* Browning, Nonenzymatic; Starch, Structure, Properties and Determination; Sucrose, Properties and Determination

Fibre

Dietary fibre may be lost during preparation of foods prior to cooking. Activities such as peeling potatoes and other root vegetables, stripping green vegetables of their outer leaves, and the removal of pods all reduce fibre content. Fibre itself is not destroyed during cooking. Extra fibre can be included in meals by serving baked potatoes, wholemeal bread and high-bran breakfast cereals, and using wholewheat flour rather than white. High-fibre diets potentially increase demand for iron and calcium, but unrefined foods generally contain higher levels of these minerals than their refined equivalents. The practice of sprinkling refined fibre on foods essentially provides extra fibre with few extra bioavailable vitamins and minerals and is therefore not recommended. *See* Bioavailability of Nutrients; Dietary Fibre, Properties and Sources

Protein

Like sugars and starch, protein is not destroyed during cooking, apart from some loss of sulphur-containing amino acids, which are rendered unavailable during browning. Judicious combinations of vegetable proteins (such as sweetcorn and peas with rice, baked beans on toast, bread and cheese) can be as nutritious as the more expensive animal proteins. An understanding of protein complementation is useful in planning nutritious meals on a limited budget. *See* Protein, Food Sources

Vitamins

The most labile of the vitamins are ascorbic acid (vitamin C), thiamin (vitamin B_1) and folic acid. Deficiency of vitamin C is generally only seen in at-risk groups. However, its destruction is often used as an indicator of overall quality in catering operations. Vitamin C is destroyed by oxidation, enzymes, and leaching into cooking water. Significant losses may occur during the storage of fresh green vegetables particularly in conditions of elevated temperature and strong sunlight. Losses are also very significant during the warm holding of foods, particularly if the food is held, as it should be, at relatively high temperatures. Newer catering systems that avoid warm holding, e.g. cook–freeze and cook–chill, should conserve the vitamin, but significant losses of vitamin C can occur in these systems during reheating and during chilled storage. *Sous vide* catering, in so far as it eliminates oxygen during storage, also conserves ascorbic acid. Vitamin C retention in cabbage (as a percentage of freshly cooked) for conventional catering is 46%, for cook–freeze is 51%, and for cook–chill is 49% (Mottishaw J (1983)). *See* Ascorbic Acid, Physiology

The B vitamins particularly thiamin, riboflavin and folic acids are also labile. All may be leached out of foods during wet cooking and all are detroyed by heat, particularly in nonacid environments. In addition, riboflavin (vitamin B_2) is light-sensitive. Marginal folic acid status is seen in the UK in certain at-risk groups. Folic acid is destroyed during the pasteurization of milk, and when vegetables are cooked or processed. The provision of raw vegetables, e.g. in salads, the use of fresh rather than processed vegetables, and the consumption of liver are all ways to ensure improved intakes of folic acid. Systems such as cook–freeze and cook–chill generally conserve the B vitamins more efficiently than do traditional large-scale catering procedures. Vitamin B_1 retention in peas (as a percentage of fresh frozen) for conventional catering is 75%, for cook–freeze is 92%, and for cook–chill is 86% (after 3 h chilled storage) (Daly L (1977)). *See* Folic Acid, Properties and Determination; Riboflavin, Properties and Determination; Thiamin, Properties and Determination

The fat-soluble vitamins are generally more stable than those in the water-soluble group. Losses of vitamins A and D are only likely if the food becomes oxidized. A major problem with vitamin D is its restricted distribution in foods. For individuals who are rarely exposed to sunlight, dietary items such as oily fish, margarine, liver and eggs are essential, despite the fact that many of the foods listed are unpopular.

Similarly, vitamin E is prone to oxidation. A great deal of attention is currently being focused on vitamin E because of its role as an antioxidant in biological systems and the implications of deficiency of the vitamin for the incidence of heart disease. *See* Antioxidants, Natural Antioxidants; Cholecalciferol, Properties and Determination; Retinol, Properties and Determination; Tocopherols, Properties and Determination

Minerals

Excessive sodium intake is a major problem in many countries, leading to hypertension in susceptible individuals. Sodium content is generally low in fresh unprocessed foods, e.g. fresh fruit and vegetables, milk, eggs, fresh poultry and meat, and raw cereals. Processed foods, such as breakfast cereals, cheese, cured meats and condiment sauces, usually contain high levels of sodium. Where dishes are made from processed ingredients and/or include sauces such as soy sauce, a high sodium content typically results. This is particularly the case for ethnic fast foods. For example, compare the sodium contents (g per portion) of the following fast/take-away foods: Italian $1·68 \pm 0·63$; Chinese, $1·58 \pm 0·50$; Greek, $1·08 \pm 0·35$; fried chicken, $0·40 \pm 0·10$; chips, $0·14 \pm 0·11$ (Pascoe JM *et al.* (1985)). *See* Sodium, Physiology

Iron may be leached out of food during wet cooking or through losses in drip during thawing and cooking. The most significant influence on iron content of the diet is the level of consumption of red meat. For those who do not eat meat, nonanimal foods, such as green vegetables and whole cereals, are major sources. Efficient absorption of iron from nonmeat sources depends on adequate vitamin C in the diet. Calcium intakes are significantly influenced by consumption of dairy products. *See* Iron, Physiology

Menu Planning

Until recently, hospitals, school meals and similar institutional catering establishments were the only areas in which the caterer had a direct responsibility for the nutritional value of meals. In commercial areas, most caterers have seen their responsibility as being that of providing the choice of foods demanded by their customers whilst, at the same time, producing the food in such a way as to maximize the nutritional value. However, things have changed over the last few years and some caterers have taken a more proactive role.

In looking at the impact of nutrition on menu planning, we are involved in a spectrum of concerns from nutritional deficiencies in some groups of con-

sumers through to concerns about diet-related diseases, such as coronary heart disease, in other groups. In addition to this, some areas of the industry are concerned with catering for individuals with special dietary needs and diet-related illnesses such as diabetes and coeliac disease. *See* Coeliac Disease

School meals and hospital catering departments traditionally plan their menus to conform to Dietary Reference Values (DRVs) for the target population. Use of computers to analyse menus now makes this task easier. Attempts have been made to use the computer to plan (rather than simply analyse) menus in hospitals and school meals, but, in general, these have not proved successful. This is for two main reasons: (1) the difficulty of numerical optimization techniques where consumer choice was allowed; and (2) it has proved difficult to 'program' the complex skills of the dietitian. Therefore the major use of the computer has been to analyse the menu developed by the caterer or dietitian and to compare the results with DRVs. However, the development of more advanced computer systems, such as expert systems, may change this. *See* Dietary Requirements of Adults

Even within commercial catering, there has been an attempt to develop an awareness of healthy eating through the design of menus. Many of the new developments in cooking are projected as being more sound from a nutritional point of view. It is not true of all the new methods, where there is still often reliance on full-fat dairy products, sugars and refined foods. The ratio of meat products to vegetables is also often very high. Developments such as *nouvelle cuisine* have resulted in a reduction in the sizes of portions offered to customers, with the emphasis on concentrated flavours and attractive appearance, rather than quantity. Some of the newer developments encompass sound nutritional principles. This is true of developments such as *cuisine minceur* and *cuisine naturelle*, which require few oils, fats and sugars.

Similarly, there have been very interesting developments in school meal programmes and hospital catering in developing healthy diets, whilst at the same time taking a proactive and educational stance in promoting healthy choices. This approach is taken a stage further in some hospitals where, for example, the cardiac ward may educate patients in ways of improving their diet.

Despite these recent developments towards more consideration being given to nutritional aspects of the food, the hotel and catering industry still comes in for criticism for its failure to offer more healthy options in line with official recommendations, such as the UK Committee on Medical Aspects of Food Policy (COMA) reports (1984 and 1991). In general, the industry has been slow to develop new cooking methods with less reliance on cream, other saturated fats, sugar and refined carbohydrates.

Nutritional Implications

Cost

The proportion of food selling price which equates to food cost varies from one sector of the catering industry to another.

Obviously, in commercial restaurants and hotels there is an added cost, over and above the cost of food, which represents the value added through preparation, cooking and service, together with the cost of providing the decor and ambience of the eating environment. The food component of the selling price, which is usually referred to as the food cost percentage, varies between 30% and 50% of the selling price.

In industrial catering, which covers staff feeding in areas such as factories, offices, hospitals, schools and shops, practice varies from one organization to another. Surveys of industrial catering indicate that 59% of employers subsidize the price of meals, whilst 41% aim to break even or produce a gross profit on food and beverage sales (gross profit is the difference between the cost of the food and the selling price, expressed as a percentage of the food cost). Where gross profit is made, the contribution to labour costs is between 5% and 100% of the cost of labour.

Hygiene and Safety

The importance of food safety within the hotel and catering industry cannot be overemphasized. The results of a survey by the Audit Commission of Great Britain, published in 1990, showed that the least hygienic type of food premises were take-aways, with more than one in five judged to be a significant health risk by environmental health officers. The performance of restaurants was only slightly better. Hospitals, educational establishments and residential homes were judged as having least risk. The commonest risk factors identified were poor hygiene awareness by staff and management alike, lack of effective monitoring and control of temperature, inadequate hand-washing facilities, cross-contamination, and a low priority given to hygiene by management.

The issue of food safety has recently become prominent both within the UK and Europe. In the UK the Food Safety Act 1990 has highlighted and tackled the issue of the training of food handlers. Within the catering industry, high staff turnover, coupled with the seasonal nature of employment and the typical pattern of part-time employment, create a difficult environment within which to ensure that staff are properly trained, particularly in the commercial sector.

Traditionally, a number of foods such as poultry and eggs have been regarded as cheap alternatives to red meat, easy to eat, and generally well liked by most consumers. More recently, healthy eating trends have seen sales of poultry soar within both the grocery and catering sectors. Poultry and eggs, however, are relatively high-risk foods. A high percentage of poultry carcasses are contaminated with Salmonellae and the birds may also be carriers of *Listeria*. The importance of avoiding cross-contamination, and of temperature control during preparation, storage, cooking and subsequent storage, cannot be overemphasized. The practice of lightly cooking eggs or incorporating them raw into foods is unacceptable. Hygiene considerations must take precedence over all other aspects of food quality. *See Listeria*, Properties and Occurrence; Poultry, Chicken; Poultry, Ducks and Geese; Poultry, Turkey

The growth of sandwich bars and of the take-away trade in prepacked sandwiches highlights issues regarding the quality of both cooked and raw ingredients and the need for strict chilled temperature control. Many sandwiches include salad – a healthy ingredient but nevertheless a raw one. The other ingredients may provide an excellent medium for bacterial growth. Sandwiches which are put together by hand pose further potential risk.

Technological developments, such as cook–freeze, cook–chill and *sous vide* systems, may also pose risks. Many such developments arise out of a desire to improve upon the organoleptic quality of the food as served, whilst obtaining the efficiencies and productivity of long shelf-life and centralized factory-like production. In all these systems strict attention has to be paid to microbiological quality; the use of Hazard Analysis and Critical Control Point (HACCP) analysis is essential, as is the ability to monitor microbiological outcomes. *See* Hazard Analysis Critical Control Point

Sous vide poses particular risks in respect of anaerobes such as *Clostridium perfringens* and *C. botulinum*. A growing body of professional opinion holds that this technique should only be available to caterers that are licensed for the purpose. *See Clostridium*, Occurrence of *Clostridium Perfringens*; *Clostridium*, Occurrence of *Clostridium Botulinum*

In cook–chill systems, risks are posed by incorporating ready-cooked items into the system and by cooling cooked vegetables in chilled water. These are deviations from the standard method of production, incorporating potential hazards which must be subjected to standard HACCP techniques if safety is to be maintained.

In the fast food sector microwave regeneration is a problem. In one London survey, in 60% of regenerations the foods tested did not reach a safe internal temperature of 70°C for a minimum of 2 min. In response, some caterers claim that customers do not want their foods reheated to high internal temperatures as they are then too hot to hold and eat. This type of situation highlights some of the complex behavioural issues involved.

Nutritional Implications

Significance for Institutionalized Patients

The problem of minority 'at-risk groups' features in almost all developed countries. At-risk groups include the elderly, the poor, young children, addicts, and those suffering from disease. Members of all of these groups are likely to find themselves dependent on institutional care at some time or another. The impact on nutritional status of illness, addiction, old age and poverty is likely to require special consideration for the dietary needs of such groups.

More significantly for those with lowered resistance, any outbreak of food poisoning can prove fatal. Whilst standards of hygiene are generally highest in residential establishments, the explosion in the population of dependent elderly in the face of reduced welfare resourcing is something which requires attention and monitoring.

Within those groups for which the caterer is solely responsible for the nutritional intake of individuals, there is obviously a significant responsibility for providing a balanced diet. Surveys have shown that institutional diets often contain too many calories and are relatively deficient in vitamins and minerals. Reliance on catering as a source of food increases in the over 75s, amongst whom there is considerable dependence on meals-on-wheels, residential homes, nursing homes and hospitals. Diminished appetites and difficulties with both chewing and digesting food can lead to a consumption which is lower than planned.

The bulk of residential care caters for the elderly. In the UK the number of people aged 65 or over is projected to rise from 8·4 million in 1985 to 9·0 million in the year 2001, with greatest increase occurring in the over 75s, of whom nearly a million will be severely disabled. Currently over half a million elderly people live in residential accommodation, of which over 50% are resident in private homes.

In particular, the number of people aged 80 and over in the UK has increased by 50% between the years 1961 and 1990. Many of these groups are in hospitals and nursing homes, where all their meals are provided by the catering industry. Of those living at home, a large proportion have some of their meals in local authority or voluntary dining rooms, or have home delivery of meals-on-wheels. For example, in the UK 20% of people aged 85 and over use either the meals-on-wheels service, or a luncheon club.

Demographic trends are such that at the same time as those numbers dependent on residential care are increasing, the catering industry is faced with a shortage of manpower. Issues around technology, food safety and nutritional quality are likely to intensify.

Bibliography

BNF (1987) Nutrition in catering – the impact of nutrition and health concepts on catering practice. Proceedings of the 8th British Nutrition Foundation Annual Conference. Carnforth: Parthenon Publishing Group.

Collison R and Colwill JS (1986) The analysis of food waste results and related attributes of restaurants and public houses. *Journal of Foodservice Systems* 4: 17–30.

COMA (1984) *Diet and Cardiovascular Disease*. Report on Health and Social Subjects 28. London: Her Majesty's Stationery Office.

COMA (1991) *Dietary Reference Values for Food Energy and Nutrients for Groups of People in the United Kingdom*. Report on Health and Social Subjects 41. London: HMSO.

Daly L (1977) Thiamin content of frozen peas prepared by cook–freeze, cook–chill and conventional methods of catering. University of Leeds: Unpublished MSc thesis.

Drummond KE (1989) *Nutrition for Foodservice Professionals*. New York: Van Nostrand Reinhold.

Kinderlerer JL (ed.) (1989) *Food Safety – Salmonella and Listeria*. Bradford: MCB University Press.

Light N and Walker A (1990) *Cook-Chill Catering: Technology and Management*. London: Elsevier Applied Science.

Mottishaw J (1983) Ascorbic acid content of vegetables from a conventional catering system and from a cook–freeze–thaw catering hospital system. *Laboratory Report 180*. Huddersfield Polytechnic: Hotel and Catering Research Centre.

Pascoe JM, Dockerty J and Ryley J (1985) *Fast Foods*, chapter 5. Carnforth: Parthenon Publishing Group.

David Kirk
Queen Margaret College, Edinburgh, UK
Lorna Daly
Sheffield City Polytechnic, Sheffield, UK

CELLS

Structure and Function of Human and Animal Cells

The cell is the fundamental functional unit of life of all living organisms. Cellular processes are ultimately responsible for activities such as breathing, moving, combating infection, digesting food, thinking – in fact, all bodily functions. These functions require energy, and it is inside cells that fuels are used to produce the energy needed to drive these activities. This article examines the structure inside the cell and the combined activities of cells that make all of this possible.

Structure and Organization of Human and Animal Cells

Structure

Common to nearly all cells are three compartments, namely the cell (plasma) membrane, the cytoplasm, and the nucleus (mature, human red blood cells have no nucleus). This basic structure is evident in a wide variety of cells even though they may differ dramatically in size and shape (Fig. 1). The plasma membrane not only encloses the contents of the cell but performs many vital functions. The cytoplasm is that compartment between the nucleus and the cell membrane. It is composed of a soluble component (the cytosol) in which are immersed various microscopic components called organelles. Among the many important biochemical reactions that take place in the cytosol is glycolysis, an energy releasing process involving the breakdown of glucose to pyruvic acid. *See* Glucose, Function and Metabolism

The cellular organelles are a diverse group of structures that perform many different functions within the cell. The structure and function of these will be considered below under *Cellular Components*. The nucleus of the cell is a membrane-bound structure that contains within it the genetic material of the cell. It is here that the genes reside in the form of DNA (deoxyribonucleic acid) molecules grouped into structures called chromosomes.

Organization

In the body, cells often function in combination with other cells of the same type and are held together with varying degrees of tenacity and with varying amounts of extracellular material between them. Clusters of cells of the same type are called tissues. Four different types of tissues are recognized:

1. Epithelial tissue, in which the cells are held very tightly together and there is very little extracellular material between them. This tissue forms glands and the linings of the body cavities and surfaces.
2. Connective tissue, in which the cells are not bound closely to one another. There is much extracellular material in such tissue and the cells may be held rigidly in place by this material, as in the case of bone, or they may be freely moving, as in blood.

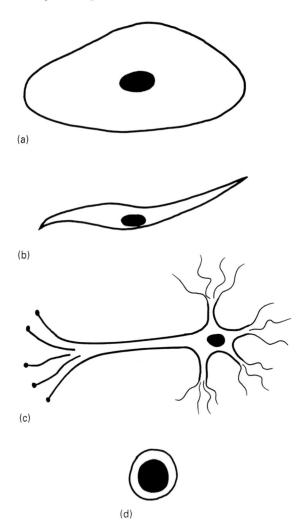

Fig. 1 Different shapes of cells. The nucleus is darkly shaded; the plasma membrane is represented by the outline of the cell; the cytoplasm is represented by the clear space between the plasma membrane and the nucleus. (a) Epithelial cell; (b) smooth muscle cell; (c) neuron; (d) lymphocyte.

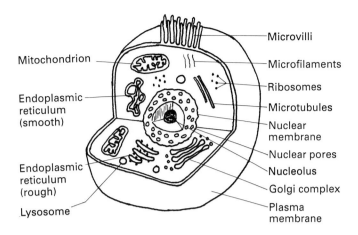

Fig. 2 Drawing of a 'generalized' cell showing many of the organelles found in human and animal cells.

3. Muscle tissue, in which the cells may be bound to each other, as in cardiac muscle and smooth muscle, or separate from each other but gathered into bundles by connective tissue, as in skeletal muscle. *See* Exercise, Muscle

4. Nervous tissue, which is composed of neurons (nerve cells) which conduct electrical impulses from one neuron to another. These cells are not physically coupled but are held in place by specialized connective tissue cells.

The organs of the body are in turn, composed of different types of tissues. For example, the heart is composed mainly of muscle tissue but also includes connective tissue, epithelial tissue and some nervous tissue.

Cellular Components

There are numerous chemical activities occurring simultaneously inside the cell. Eukaryotic cells (cells which have membrane-bound compartments) are able to minimize interference of one chemical reaction with another by confining certain chemical activities to specific membrane-bound components of the cell. This design also facilitates cellular specialization. Prokaryotic cells (cells which lack membrane-bound compartments) such as bacteria are disadvantaged in this regard. These membrane-bound components and other specific structures inside the cell are called organelles. Although some of these (e.g. the nucleus) can be seen under the light microscope, it has been necessary to employ electron microscopy to clearly visualize most of them. Not all of the organelles are found in every cell, and the relative abundance of a particular type of organelle varies from cell to cell depending on the activity of the cell. Figure 2 is a drawing of a generalized cell with various organelles represented.

Nuclear Components

The nucleus contains the chromosomes. In humans there are 46 chromosomes (23 pairs) and the number in other animals varies from species to species. The chromosomes are very long, thin strands of DNA. They also contain proteins called histones. They are not easily seen under the light microscope until just prior to cell division when they shorten and coil up, making them visible following appropriate staining. The nucleus also contains other structures called nucleoli. These are roughly spherical structures containing strands of RNA (ribonucleic acid) molecules, DNA, and proteins. The nucleoli are responsible for manufacturing rRNA (ribosomal RNA) of the ribosome. The nucleus is enclosed by a membrane which is perforated by holes (nuclear pores) that are big enough to allow large molecules, such as RNA, to pass through. This is important as the RNA is manufactured in the nucleus but needs to move out into the cytoplasm where it is needed for the manufacture of proteins. *See* Nucleic Acids, Physiology

Cytoplasmic Components

There are many organelles or structures within the cytoplasm that are involved with specific cell functions. These are listed below with a brief description of their structure and function.

Ribosomes

Ribosomes are tiny granules (about 25 nm in diameter) composed of rRNA and protein. A ribosome consists of two subunits, one about twice the size of the other. Ribosomes play an integral role in protein synthesis.

Endoplasmic Reticulum

The endoplasmic reticulum is actually a series of double-membrane channels distributed throughout the cyto-

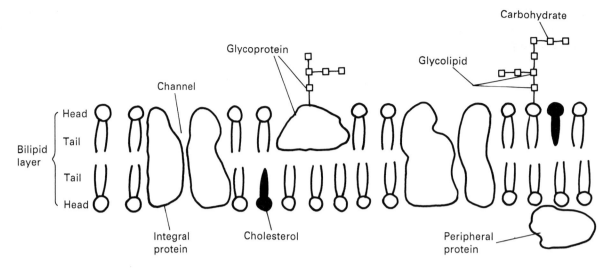

Fig. 3 The arrangement of molecules in the plasma membrane.

plasm. Ribosomes may be attached to the membranes and it is then referred to as rough endoplasmic reticulum. Without ribosomes attached it is called smooth endoplasmic reticulum. This organelle serves several important functions in the cell, among which are involvement in the synthesis and storage of molecules, providing a system of channels for distribution and transport of materials throughout the cell, release of calcium ions into the cytosol which initiate contraction in muscle cells, and providing some structural support for the cell.

Golgi Complex

The Golgi complex consists of flattened membranous sacs stacked upon each other with expanded areas at their ends. The main function of this organelle is in the sorting and packaging of various molecules, particularly proteins, for distribution to various parts of the cell. The Golgi complex is particularly extensive in cells with high secretory activities.

Mitochondria

Mitochondria are double-membrane-bound organelles that may have a variety of shapes. The inner of the two membranes is thrown into folds or plates called cristae. This arrangement provides a large surface area for chemical reactions to take place. Many enzymes involved in energy-releasing reactions are located on the cristae. These reactions are collectively known as cellular respiration and include the reactions of the tricarboxylic acid cycle and the electron transport chain. Since much of the cell's energy is produced through these reactions, mitochondria are sometimes called the 'powerhouses' of the cell. Cells that have a high energy expenditure, e.g. muscle, liver, and kidney tubule cells,

have large numbers of mitochondria. It has been speculated that mitochondria may have evolved from bacteria that were incorporated into the cell. Certainly, mitochondria have their own DNA and are capable of reproducing themselves.

Lysosomes

Lysosomes are membrane-bound, spherical structures containing powerful digestive enzymes. They are formed from vesicles budding off the Golgi complex. These enzymes are capable of digesting bacteria and other solid matter that may be engulfed by a cell. Leucocytes, specifically neutrophils and monocytes that engulf bacteria and other foreign particles (a process known as phagocytosis) contain large numbers of lysosomes.

The Cytoskeleton

Helping to maintain the shape of the cell and supporting various organelles within the cell is a scaffolding-like assembly of filaments and tubules called the cytoskeleton. The filaments and tubules are composed of proteins similar to those found in the contractile machinery of muscle. They are rod-shaped structures and vary in length and thickness. Microtubules average about 24 nm in diameter and may also provide channels for the transport of materials within the cell. Microfilaments are about 6 nm in diameter and may also play a special role in movement of cells, e.g. movement of phagocytes. Intermediate filaments, diameters ranging from 8 to 12 nm, have also been discovered inside cells.

The Plasma Membrane

The plasma membrane (Fig. 3) is composed mainly of lipid molecules. The lipid is arranged in two layers, the hydrophobic tail regions of the lipid molecules pointing to the inside of the bilipid layer and the hydrophobic heads of the lipid pointing to the outside. Proteins and carbohydrates float in this lipid membrane. The plasma membrane facilitates contact and communication with other cells, it mediates the entry and exit of materials into and out of the cell, and it is the site of many important biochemical reactions. *See* Lipids, Classification

The composition of the fluid inside the cell (intracellular fluid) is very different to that outside (extracellular fluid). This difference is largely due to the properties of the plasma membrane. Among the important differences that exist are that intracellular fluid has a high concentration of potassium ions, a low concentration of sodium ions, and a high concentration of proteins with respect to extracellular fluid.

The plasma membrane is selectively permeable – it will allow the transit of some substances but not of others, and furthermore, some substances are allowed across more readily than others (differentially permeable). It has specific channels for the passage of certain substances and it contains molecular 'pumps' which can move substances from one side to the other against their concentration gradient. These properties contribute not only to chemical differences between the inside and the outside of the cell but also to an electrical difference. A small voltage (of the order of tens of millivolts) can be measured across the plasma membrane. The inside of the cell is electrically negative with respect to the outside. This electrical difference, or membrane potential as it is called, is particularly important when considering the functions of neurons and muscle cells, both of which can conduct electrical impulses.

The cell membrane in some cells is thrown into many small folds which project from the bulk of the cell and are called microvilli. These greatly increase the surface area of the cell and provide a much larger surface for the absorption of materials across the cell membrane. Such specializations are seen in cells lining the small intestine and in tubule cells in the kidneys. In some cells similar types of projections of the plasma membrane are seen with underlying contractile machinery of the cytoplasm. These form cilia. The cilia move in unison, providing a sweeping motion which moves material over the surface of the cell. Cells bearing cilia line many of the larger respiratory passages, and the mucus produced here traps dust and foreign particles and is swept up to the throat region by this mucociliary escalator.

Requirement of Cells

For cells to properly carry out their normal functions certain conditions need to apply. For human and most animal cells, environmental conditions such as temperature, pH and ionic strength of solutions bathing the cell need to be kept fairly constant. Many of the body's mechanisms are geared towards this homeostatic control. Cells also need to be supplied with nutrients. They need the basic building blocks to manufacture complex organic molecules, such as amino acids for the synthesis of proteins. They need fuels to supply the substrates for generating energy, and oxygen to oxidize the fuels and allow energy to be released. The fuel requirements of some cells are very exacting. While several types of fuel molecules may be available to cells, neurons need to use glucose almost exclusively. If the glucose cannot be supplied to these cells then the brain will stop functioning properly. Such is the importance of glucose to neurons that many body mechanisms operate to maintain adequate levels of glucose in the blood at all times. Other fuels used by cells are fatty acids and, to a limited extent, proteins. When glucose is in short supply, many cells turn to a greater utilization of fatty acids to derive energy. *See* Fatty Acids, Metabolism; Protein, Synthesis and Turnover

Importance of Specialized Cells

While all cells are able to (and need to) carry out certain basic functions such as protein synthesis and energy metabolism, many cells develop special intracellular machinery to carry out specific functions. The complex behaviour of animals is possible only because of this cellular specialization. All somatic cells (body cells, as opposed to the gametes, or sex cells) contain the full complement of genetic information. With cellular specialization however, the plasticity to develop in a variety of ways is sacrificed. In some cases, cells become so constrained and devoted to their special task in the body that they even lose the ability to divide and provide more of the same type. Such is the case with neurons; these cells make up the main controlling and information transfer system of the body. They do this by detecting various environmental stimuli, interpreting this information and responding appropriately. All this is achieved by transmitting electrical signals around the body which ultimately determine the activity of muscles and glands. When neurons are injured and die they are not replaced. Muscle cells too are incapable of dividing. These cells devote their energies to building contractile machinery within them that when activated will bring about movement of various organs, limbs, etc., of the body. Adipocytes, or fat cells, are specialized to store large amounts of fat to such an extent that the nucleus of the cell becomes confined to a small part of the cell squashed against the cell membrane. It is thought that mature adipocytes do not divide. Erythrocytes are packed with the protein, haemoglobin, which is responsible for transporting the blood gases, particularly oxygen. It enhances the oxygen-carrying capacity of the blood about 60-fold. Human erythrocytes are peculiar cells in that they have no nucleus. They lose their nucleus during maturation. They have a limited lifespan of about 120 days. Under normal circumstances human erythrocytes are produced in the body at a rate of 2×10^6 per s. Hepatocytes are specialized cells of the liver. These cells contain large amounts of specific enzymes involved in the metabolism and detoxification of many different molecules in the body. These are just some of the many specialized cells in the body; there are numerous others, including osteocytes (bone cells), endocrine cells (hormone-producing cells), chondrocytes (cartilage cells). *See* Adipose Tissue, Structure and Function of White Adipose Tissue; Adipose Tissue, Structure and Function of Brown Adipose Tissue

Bibliography

de Duve C (1984) *A Guided Tour of the Living Cell* (vols 1 and 2). New York: Scientific American Library.

Fawcett DW (1981) *The Cell* 2nd edn. Philadelphia: WB Saunders.

Keeton WT and Gould JL (1986) *Biological Science* 4th edn. New York: WW Norton and Co.

Reid RA and Leech RM (1980) *Biochemistry and Structure of Cell Organelles*. Glasgow: Blackie.

Tortora GJ and Anagnostakis NP (1989) *Principles of Anatomy and Physiology* 6th edn. New York: Harper and Row.

Tribe MA, Morgan AJ and Whittaker PA (1981) *The Evolution of Eukaryotic Cells*. London: Edward Arnold.

Paul McGrath
University of Newcastle, New South Wales, Australia

CELLULOSE

Cellulose is the world's most abundant material. An estimated 10^{11} tonnes are produced annually, a daily production of about 50 kg per person. Because of its rigidity, cellulose provides structure to plants. It is almost always associated with other components as a composite material termed 'lignocellulose'. *See* Hemicelluloses; Lignin

The most studied celluloses are from cotton, ramie, *Valonia* algae and *Acetobacter xylinum* bacteria.

Structure

Polymer Structure

Cellulose is a polymer of the monomer glucose (see Fig. 1(a)). The free-aldehyde glucose conformation is very unstable, so it cyclizes into a six-membered pyranose ring. (In aqueous solutions at 25°C, only about 0·02% of the glucose is in the free aldehyde form.) The Cl hydroxyl of the cyclic ring can be in the equatorial β position or the axial α position. The β position is favoured thermodynamically and accounts for 62% of the glucose with the remaining 38% in the α position.

Cellulose is a linear, unbranched polymer of anhydroglucose joined with ether linkages between Cl and C4 (see Fig. 1(b)). Cellulose is polymerized from β-glucose, whereas starch (see Fig. 1(c)) is polymerized from α-glucose. In the rightward anhydroglucose unit, C1

retains its hydroxyl group so it may potentially form free-aldehyde glucose which has reducing power. Hence, this terminus is called the 'reducing end'.

β-Linked cellulose has dramatically different properties than α-linked starch. Starch is helical, water-soluble and easily hydrolysed by enzymes, whereas cellulose is planar, water-insoluble and difficult to hydrolyse. Whereas starch is a widely utilized animal food, cellulose is used only by a select few, ruminants being the most prominent example. In starch, the repeating unit is anhydroglucose. For cellulose, anhydrocellobiose is the repeating unit since adjacent anhydroglucoses are rotated 180° degrees with respect to their neighbours. This rotation causes cellulose to be highly symmetrical, since each side of the chain has an equal number of hydroxyl groups, while starch is unsymmetrical. The cellulose degree of polymerization (DP) ranges from 500 to 15 000. When fully stretched, a single cellulose molecule could extend as long as 7 μm. Amylose starch has a lower DP (100–3000) and could extend as long as 1 μm if fully stretched. Cellulose is completely unbranched whereas amylopectin starch has branches at C6. *See* Starch, Structure, Properties and Determination

Crystalline Structure

The cellulose hydrogen atoms are all in the axial position whereas the hydroxyl groups are all equatorial.

These equatorial hydroxyl groups can hydrogen bond with their nearest neighbours, allowing cellulose to crystallize. The monoclinic crystalline unit cell for cellulose I (native cellulose) is shown in Fig. 2. The hydrogen bonds run in the a direction and are medium-strength ($15\,kcal\,mol^{-1}$). In the c direction, the structure is held by weak van der Waals forces ($8\,kcal\,mol^{-1}$). Covalent bonds run in the b direction and give cellulose

its strength ($50\,kcal\,mol^{-1}$). A continuous cellulose strand is about four to five times stronger than steel with the same cross-section. Cellulose I is parallel; that is, all the cellulose molecules run in the same direction from nonreducing to reducing ends (see Fig. 3(a)).

Native cellulose (cellulose I) can be converted to other crystalline forms. Cellulose II is formed by (1) treating cellulose with sodium hydroxide (mercerization), (2)

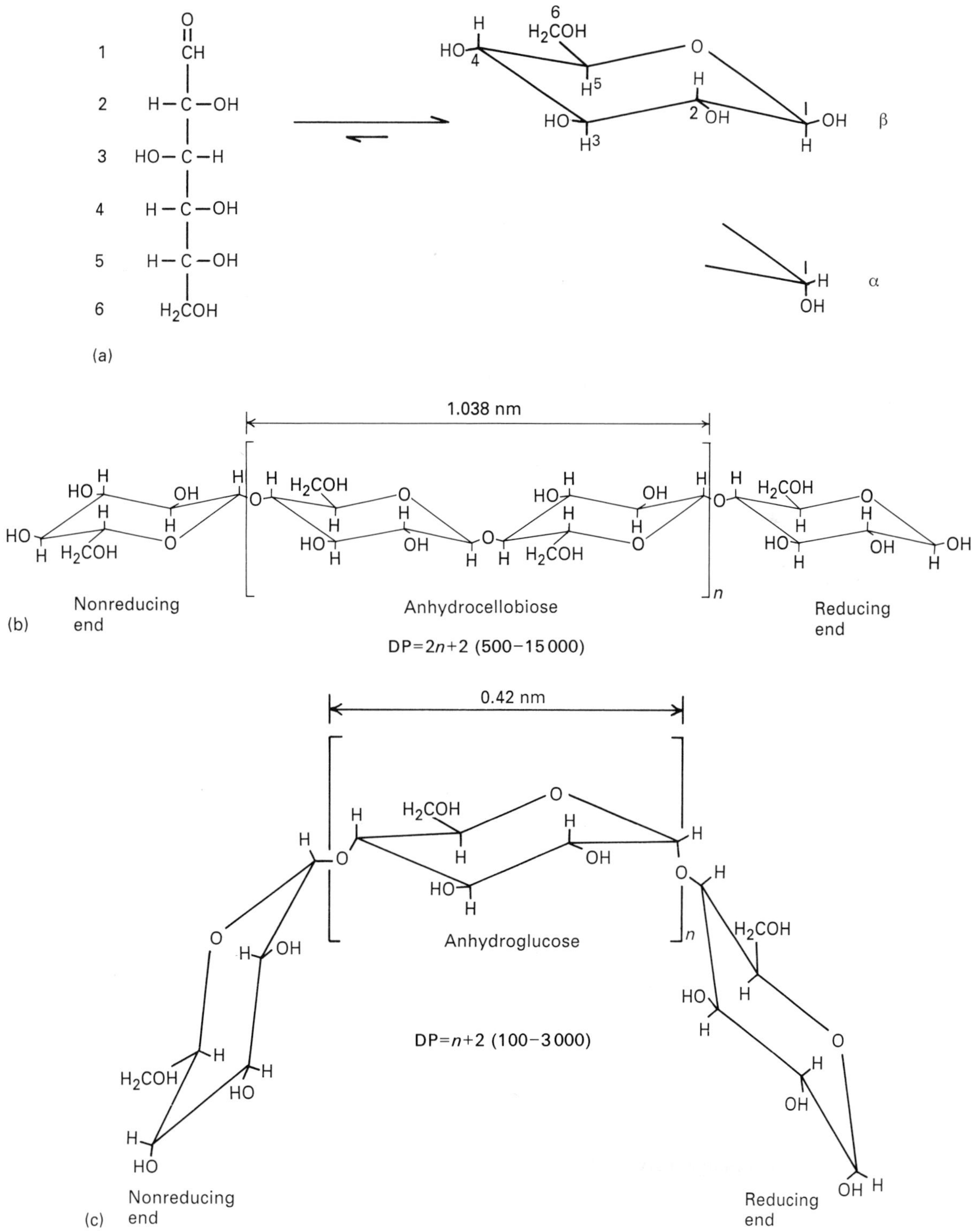

Fig. 1   (a) Glucose, (b) cellulose and (c) amylose starch.

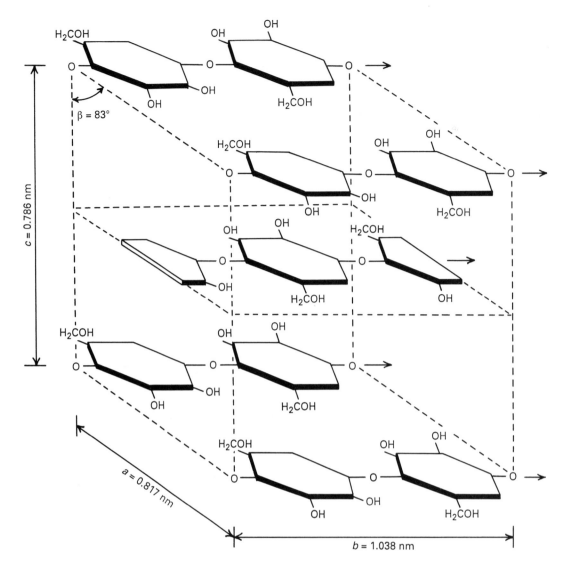

Fig. 2 Parallel cellulose I unit cell.

precipitating from solutions of alkali/salt (e.g. cuprammonium hydroxide) or (3) removing the added functional groups from cellulose derivatives (i.e. regenerated cellulose). Cellophane and rayon are both forms of cellulose II. Table 1 shows that the unit cell dimensions are slightly expanded in the c direction and compressed in the a direction. Of course, the b direction is essentially the same, since it is the covalent bond. Cellulose II is the most thermodynamically stable form of cellulose since it can always be produced from cellulose I, but not vice versa. The stability may result from hydrogen bonds extending in the c direction, which normally has only van der Waals bonds. There is general agreement that cellulose II is antiparallel (see Fig. 3(b)) with three to four anhydroglucose moieties required to make the bend. Precipitation of cellulose II from solution appears to favour the antiparallel conformation, as occurs with many synthetic polymers.

Cellulose III is formed by soaking cellulose in cold (about $-80°C$) liquid anhydrous ammonia, which is subsequently removed by evaporation. Cellulose I is transformed into cellulose III_1 and cellulose II is transformed into cellulose III_2. When rehydrated, cellulose III reverts back to its original form.

Cellulose IV is formed by soaking cellulose in hot (about $200°C$) glycerol, with subsequent removal by washing with 2-propanol and water. Cellulose I is transformed to cellulose IV_1 and cellulose II is transformed to cellulose IV_2.

Native cellulose (Fig. 3(a)) forms crystalline regions (40% bacteria, 60% cotton, 70% *Valonia*) interspersed with amorphous regions. The amorphous regions are more porous than the crystalline regions allowing water or dyes to penetrate, and increasing the reactivity to acid or enzymatic hydrolysis. When purified cellulose fibres are subjected to dilute acid hydrolysis, the amorphous

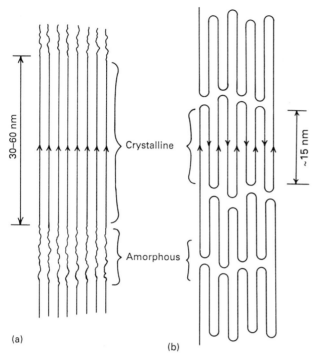

Fig. 3 (a) Cellulose I parallel and (b) cellulose II antiparallel structures.

Table 1. Unit cell dimensions of cellulose I and II

Cellulose	a (nm)	b (nm)	c (nm)	β (°)
I	0·817	1·038	0·786	83·0
II	0·801	1·036	0·904	62·9

Source: Blackwell J, Kurz D, Su M-Y and Lee DM (1987) X-ray studies of the structure of cellulose complexes. In: Atalla RH (ed.) *The Structures of Cellulose. ACS Symposium Series*, No. 340, pp 199–213. Washington, DC: American Chemical Society.

regions selectively hydrolyse, leaving the more resistant crystalline regions which have a 'levelling-off DP' of 100–300 in the case of cotton.

Cellular Structure

Young plant cells have only the primary wall to resist osmotic pressure. It is composed principally of hemicellulose and pectin with small amounts of cellulose and protein, and is flexible enough to accommodate cell growth. When cell growth ceases, the secondary wall is formed in three layers (S_1, S_2 and S_3) with S_2 the thickest (see Fig. 4). *See* Protein, Chemistry

All cell wall layers are composed of 7–30 nm diameter microfibrils which are visible using an electron micro-scope. In the primary cell wall, the fibrils are randomly oriented. In the S_1 layer, the microfibrils are oriented helically, with each successive layer alternating between right-handed and left-handed helices. In the S_2 layer which provides much of the plant strength, the microfibrils are arranged in steep right-handed helices nearly oriented along the cell axis. The S_3 layer is another shallow helix. All higher plants (softwoods, hardwoods, herbaceous) are thought to have cell structures similar to that shown in Fig. 4.

The plant cell diameters range from 15 to 80 μm, depending on the species and time of year. Spring cell diameters are larger than summer diameters, giving rise to the familiar growth rings in trees. The wall thickness is typically about 2–5 μm, with thicker walls formed in the summer. Softwood cells are about 3–4 mm long, which makes them particularly useful for paper pulp, while hardwood cells tend to be shorter (0·7–2 mm long). Cotton cells suitable for textiles are about 25 mm long.

Microfibrils are composed of elementary fibrils of pure cellulose embedded in a matrix of hemicellulose. The fringes of the elementary fibrils are paracrystalline and intermingle with tightly adsorbed hemicellulose. (An exception to this is cotton in which the fringes contain only cellulose.) In Fengel's model of the microfibril, the elementary fibrils are clustered into four 4×4 arrays. The lignification process occurs late in cell life, so lignin is located primarily on the microfibril exterior where it covalently bonds to the hemicellulose. Lignification is initiated in the middle lamella where lignin constitutes about 70% of the wall. The wall interior is less lignified with only about 15% lignin. The hemicellulose content is fairly constant (20–30%), with cellulose the remaining 10–50% of the wall. The cells in fruit pulp are composed mainly of primary walls containing approximately 34% pectin, 24% hemicellulose, 23% cellulose and 19% protein.

Properties

Physical

Table 2 shows the physical properties of cellulose and cellulosic materials. The listed heat of combustion is the 'higher heat' (i.e. the combustion water is 25°C liquid). Cellulose is stable up to 300°C.

The DP for various types of cellulose is shown in Table 3. For cotton, the DP may be as high as 15 000. Cellulose is insoluble in water because of the strong hydrogen bonding in its crystal lattice. However, it is soluble in a number of solvents, including concentrated acids (e.g. 85% phosphoric, 72% sulphuric and 40% hydrochloric acids) and inorganic salt solutions (e.g. cuprammonium hydroxide, cadoxen (i.e. cadmium ions

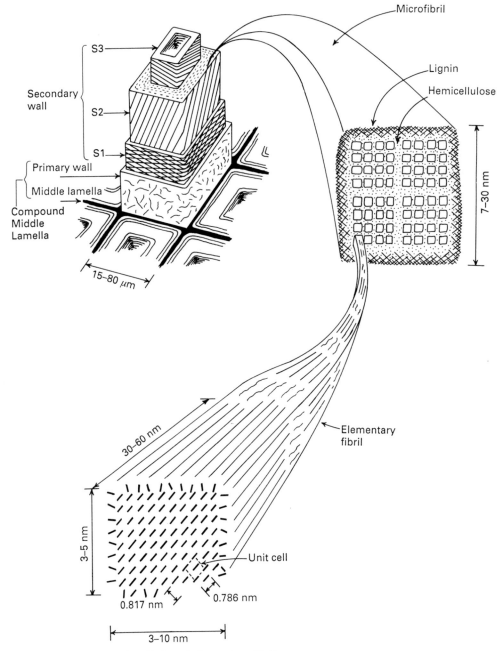

Fig. 4 Schematic of plant cell, microfibril and elementary fibril.

and ethylenediamine)). The viscosity of cellulose dissolved in salts is often used for molecular weight determinations.

Chemical

Cellulose may be hydrolysed to glucose by acids or enzymes. Acid hydrolysis produces a number of degradation products, such as 5-hydroxymethylfurfural, formic acid, laevulinic acid, formaldehyde, furfural and resins. Enzymatic glucose production requires a cellulase system containing *endo*-cellulase (to produce nonre-

ducing ends from the chain interior), *exo*-cellulase (to produce cellobiose from the nonreducing end) and cellobiase (to hydrolyse cellobiose to glucose). Up to about 10% of cellulose is enzymatically digested by microbes in the human large intestine, so it is not completely noncaloric.

Cellulose is fairly stable to base, provided oxygen is excluded. The reaction terminates after approximately 50 anhydroglucose units are 'peeled off' from the cellulose reducing end; D-glucoisosaccharinate is the soluble product. Under severe conditions (e.g. 1 M sodium hydroxide, 170°C), alkaline hydrolysis readily occurs.

Table 2. Physical properties of cellulose and cellulosic materials

Property	Compressed cellulose	Paper	Pine	Oak
Specific gravity[a]	1·47	0·70–1·15	0·43–0·67	0·64–0·87
Heat capacity (kJ kg^{-1} K^{-1})[b]	1·3	1·3	2·8	2·4
Heat of combustion (MJ kg^{-1})[b]	17·6	17·6	20·4	19·2
Thermal conductivity (W m^{-1} K^{-1})[b]				
With grain	—	0·13	0·35	—
Across grain	—	0·13	0·15	0·21
Tensile strength (MPa)[a]				
With grain	—	—	62	99
Across grain	—	—	2·8	5·5
Water diffusion constant (cm^2 s^{-1})[c]	—	—	$5·3 \times 10^{-7}$	$1·9 \times 10^{-7}$

Source:
[a] Baumeister T, Avallone EA and Baumeister III T (1978) *Mark's Standard Handbook for Mechanical Engineers*, 8th edn. New York: McGraw-Hill.
[b] Graboski M and Bain R (1981) Properties of biomass relevant to gasification. In: Reed TB (ed.) *Biomass Gasification: Principles and Technology*, pp 41–71. Park Ridge: Noyes Data.
[c] Summitt R and Sliker A (1980) *CRC Handbook of Materials Science: Wood*, vol. IV, pp 26–27. Boca Raton: CRC Press.

Table 3. Cellulose polymer length

Material	Degree of polymerization	Molecular weight
Native cellulose	3500–10 000	600 000–1 500 000
Chemical cottons	500–3000	80 000–500 000
Wood pulps	500–2100	80 000–340 000
Rayon filaments	350–450	57 000–73 000

Source: Hamilton JK and Mitchell RL (1964) Cellulose. In: Standen A (ed.) *Kirk-Othmer Encyclopedia of Chemical Technology*, 2nd edn, vol. 4, pp 593–616. New York: Wiley.

Cellulose is more stable to oxidants than lignin, a property exploited in pulp bleaching and analytical methods which selectively oxidize lignin. However, oxidants (e.g. chromic acid, permanganate and hypochlorite) can damage cellulose by cleaving the chain or by inserting carbonyl functional groups.

The three cellulose hydroxyl groups are very reactive, allowing ready formation of the cellulose derivatives described later.

Speciality Celluloses

Microcrystalline cellulose (Avicel, FMC Corporation) is prepared by acid hydrolysis of cellulose using 2 M hydrochloric acid at 105°C for 15 min. The highly reactive amorphous regions selectively hydrolyse, releasing the crystallites which are subsequently mechanically dispersed. Aqueous suspensions of microcrystalline cellulose have constant viscosities over a wide temperature range, are heat-stable and have good mouth feel properties. Avicel is used to extend starches, stabilize foams, and control ice crystal formation. Avicel has found widespread acceptance in the food industry for meringue, whipped toppings, confections and ice cream, and is also used as a binder in pharmaceutical tablets and in cosmetics.

Bacterial cellulose (Cellulon, Weyerhaeuser Co.) is produced by selected strains of *Acetobacter xylinum* which maintain their ability to produce cellulose in agitated submerged fermentors. The cellulose fibres are about 0·1 μm in diameter, which is substantially smaller than softwood pulp fibres (about 30 μm diameter). Cellulon is a potential noncaloric food thickener or texturizer.

Modified Celluloses

Alkali cellulose is prepared by soaking cellulose in concentrated sodium hydroxide (> 14%) in the 'mercerization' process invented by John Mercer in 1844. The sodium ions are incorporated into the cellulose structure according to the following reaction (1).

$$R_{cell}OH + NaOH \rightarrow R_{cell}ONa + H_2O \qquad (1)$$
$$\text{Alkali cellulose}$$

The cellulose structure swells, allowing easy penetration by dyes or reagents for the manufacture of cellulose derivatives.

Cellulose xanthate is formed by reacting alkali cellulose with carbon disulphide (eqn [2]).

$$R_{cell}ONa + CS_2 \rightarrow R_{cell}O\overset{\overset{\textstyle S}{\|}}{C}SNa \qquad (2)$$
$$\text{Cellulose xanthate}$$

Table 4.   Composition of cellulosic materials (g per 100 g of dry matter)

	Cellulose	Lignin	Hemicellulose	Pectin	Starch	Free sugars
Vegetables[a]						
Leafy						
Broccoli	7·2	0·26	24	—	1·7	15
Brussels sprouts	9·04	2·1	26	—	8·7	18
Cabbage	8·9	4·3	26	—	4·3	47·3
Cauliflower	13·4	Tr	13	—	5·0	29
Lettuce	20·6	Tr	9·2	—	0	17
Legumes						
Beans, haricot	5·3	0·9	22·0	—	51·3	—
Beans, runner	17	3	21	—	2·9	39·6
Peas	14	2	36	—	66	6·9
Root						
Carrot	12·9	Tr	19	—	0·9	24·8
Turnip	11	Tr	23	—	Tr	47·7
Fruiting vegetables						
Pepper	3·5	Tr	10	—	Tr	34·2
Tomato	9·1	5·3	11	—	Tr	46·4
Tuber						
Potato	1·2	Tr	9·2	—	84·6	1·5
Fruits[a]						
Apples	2·9	Tr	5·8	2·3	1·8	63·9
Apricots		—— 15 ——		3·3	0	56·6
Banana	1·3	0·93	3·83	—	10·4	55·8
Blackberries		—— 44 ——		1·9	0	34·1
Cherries, sweet	1·2	0·3	4·5	0·4	0	65·4
Grapefruit	0·6	0·9	4·9	—	0	67·7
Lemons		—— 35 ——		3·4	0	21·1
Oranges		—— 14 ——		3·3	0	59·6
Peaches	1·8	5·1	12·2	3·3	0	74
Pears	4·2	2·7	8·2	—	Tr	63·5
Pineapples		—— 7·64 ——		0·25	0	74·1
Strawberries	3·6	8·4	10	3·5	Tr	61·8
Seeds[b]						
Barley		—— 5·3 ——	—	—	64·1	—
Corn		—— 2·4 ——	—	—	71·8	1·9
Grain sorghum		—— 2·7 ——	2·5	—	70·2	1·4
Oats		—— 11·9 ——	—	—	60·6	—
Peanut		—— 2·8 ——	2·5	—	4·0	4·7
Wheat		—— 2·1 ——	—	—	74	—
Agricultural residues[c]						
Barley straw	44	7	27	—	—	—
Cottonseed hulls	59	13	15	—	—	—
Oat straw	41	11	16	—	—	—
Rice straw	33	7	26	—	—	—
Sorghum straw	31	11	30	—	—	—
Sugarcane bagasse	40	13	29	—	—	—
Wheat straw	39	10	36	—	—	—

continued

Table 4. *continued*

Trees[d]						
Hardwood						
Aspen	53·3	16·3	26·2	—	—	—
White birch	41·0	18·9	36·2	—	—	—
Red maple	44·1	24·0	29·2	—	—	—
Softwood						
Balsam fir	44·8	29·4	23·6	—	—	—
Jack pine	41·6	28·6	25·6	—	—	—
White spruce	44·8	27·1	26·1	—	—	—
Bast fibres[e]						
Flax	71·2	2·2	18·6	2·0	—	—
Leaf fibres[e]						
Manila hemp	70·2	5·7	21·8	0·6	—	—
Seed fibres[e]						
Crude cotton	95·3	0	0	1·0	—	—

Tr, trace.
Source:
[a] Southgate DAT (1976) *Determination of Food Carbohydrates*, pp 91–93. London: Applied Science.
[b] Zaborsky OR (1981) *CRC Handbook of Biosolar Resources*, vol. II. Boca Raton: CRC Press.
[c] Marsden WL (1986) *CRC Critical Reviews in Biotechnology*, vol. 3, issue 3, p 235. Boca Raton: CRC Press.
[d] Timell TE (1957) Carbohydrate composition of ten North American species of wood. *TAPPI* 40: 568.
[e] Turbank AF, Durso DF, Battista OA, Bolker HI, Colving JR, Eastman N, Kleinert TN, Krassig H and St John Manley R (1979) Cellulose. *Kirk-Othmer Encyclopedia of Chemical Technology*, 3rd edn, vol. 5. New York: Wiley.

Regenerated cellulose is made by dissolving cellulose xanthate in 4–7% sodium hydroxide and contacting with aqueous sulphuric acid. These steps convert the cellulose xanthate back into cellulose, which may be spun into viscose rayon or cast into films. The fibres are used in textiles (artificial silk), tyre cords, and V belts. The films are used in packaging (Cellophane) or sausage casings. Weiner casings (70% regenerated cellulose, 12% glycerol and 18% water) are peeled away after the meat emulsion is cooked. Hemp paper casings (23% paper, 46% regenerated cellulose, 21% glycerol and 10% water) are used in bologna, salami, pepperoni, summer sausage and liverwurst.

Cellulose hydroxyl moieties are highly reactive, allowing a variety of esters and ethers to be manufactured. Since each anhydroglucose has three hydroxyl groups, the maximum degree of substitution (DS) is three. Purified wood pulp or cotton linters (short fibres) are the industrial sources of 'chemical cellulose'.

Cellulose Ethers

Sodium carboxymethyl cellulose (CMC) is formed by reacting sodium chloroacetate with alkali cellulose (eqn [3]).

$$R_{cell}ONa + ClCH_2 \overset{O}{\overset{\|}{C}} ONa \rightarrow R_{cell}OCH_2 \overset{O}{\overset{\|}{C}} ONa + NaCl$$
$$\text{CMC} \tag{3}$$

Commercially available CMC has a DS range from 0·38 to 1·4 with 0·65–0·85 more common. The negatively charged carboxyl group makes CMC soluble in both hot and cold water. The solution viscosity decreases as the temperature increases. CMC is 'generally recognized as safe' (GRAS) and is used as a thickener in many foods such as cheese, frozen desserts, and salad dressings. It is not metabolized, so it is used in low-calorie foods.

Methyl cellulose is formed by reacting alkali cellulose with methyl chloride (eqn [4]).

$$R_{cell}ONa + ClCH_3 \rightarrow R_{cell}OCH_3 + NaCl \tag{4}$$
$$\text{Methyl cellulose}$$

Methyl cellulose (DS 1·8) solutions form a firm gel when heated to 50–55°C and return to solution when cooled. Methyl cellulose is added to salad dressings, jams and preserves, soda water and meat patties as a binder.

Ethyl cellulose is produced by reacting alkali cellulose with ethyl chloride. In commercial products the DS ranges from 2·0 to 2·6. It is water-insoluble and may be incorporated into inks used for marking foods and in vitamin tablet binders.

2-Hydroxypropyl methyl cellulose is formed by reacting alkali cellulose with mixtures of methyl chloride and 2-hydroxypropyl chloride. It forms gels like methyl cellulose, but has a higher gelation temperature. It may be used an emulsifier, film former, stabilizer or thickener in foods such as salad dressings, sherbet, pie fillings, fried foods, whipped toppings, breading batters, and baked goods.

2-Hydroxyethyl cellulose (HEC) is produced by reacting cellulose with ethylene oxide using a sodium hydroxide catalyst at 30–35°C for about 4 h (eqn [5]).

$$R_{cell}OH + CH_2\!\!-\!\!CH_2 \rightarrow R_{cell}OCH_2\!\!-\!\!CH_2OH \quad (5)$$
$$HEC$$

Since the side-chain also has a hydroxyl group, ethylene oxide can continue to react and form a side-chain with several units. HEC is soluble in both hot and cold water. The solution viscosity decreases as the temperature increases. HEC is not permitted as a direct food additive, but it may be used in food-packaging adhesives and coatings.

2-Hydroxypropyl cellulose is produced using propylene oxide, rather than the ethylene oxide used for HEC. It has a thermal gel point, like methyl cellulose, and is used in food coatings and glazings.

Cellulose Esters

Cellulose acetate is the most important cellulose ester. The cellulose is first 'activated' in aqueous acetic acid to ensure uniform acetylation. It is then dehydrated and reacted with acetic anhydride using a catalyst (e.g. sulphuric acid) in a solvent (e.g. anhydrous acetic acid) (eqn [6]).

$$R_{cell}OH + CH_3\overset{O}{\overset{\|}{C}}O\overset{O}{\overset{\|}{C}}CH_3 \rightarrow R_{cell}O\overset{O}{\overset{\|}{C}}CH_3 + CH_3\overset{O}{\overset{\|}{C}}OH$$
$$\text{Cellulose acetate}$$
$$(6)$$

The resulting cellulose triacetate (DS ~ 3) product may be subsequently acid hydrolysed to lower the DS. Cellulose triacetate is water-insoluble and hydrophobic whereas cellulose monoacetate is water-soluble. Cellulose acetate is used in fibres, plastics, photographic films, lacquers and reverse osmosis or dialysis membranes.

Other esters (e.g. cellulose formate, cellulose propionate, cellulose butyrate) may be formed, but they do not have the widespread commercial applications of cellulose acetate. Also, mixed esters (e.g. cellulose acetate propionate, cellulose acetate butyrate, cellulose acetate phthalate) may be produced.

Cellulose nitrate is made by reacting cellulose with nitric acid/sulphuric acid for 20–30 min. The acids are then removed by washing with water. The water must be removed with great care since dry cellulose nitrate is extremely explosive. It is often shipped wetted with water or alcohol. Highly nitrated (DS 2·4–2·6) forms are used as explosives (gun cotton). Less nitrated forms (DS 2·1–2·3) find applications in plastics, films and inks.

Composition of Cellulosic Materials

Table 4 shows the composition of many cellulosic materials. The cellulose content in vegetables ranges from 1 to 21%; fruits range from 0·6 to 4·2%; seeds range from about 2 to 12%; agricultural residues range from 31 to 59%; wood ranges from 41 to 53%; flax and hemp have about 70% cellulose; and cotton (the purest natural cellulose) has about 95% cellulose. The free sugars shown in Table 4 are the sum of glucose, fructose and sucrose. The 'crude fibre' is reported as the sum of cellulose and lignin in the case of the seeds. The indigestible portion of some fruits, called 'dietary fibre,' is reported as the sum of cellulose, lignin and hemicellulose. *See* Dietary Fibre, Properties and Sources; Fructose; Sucrose, Properties and Determination

Cellulose Isolation and Analysis

Gravimetric Methods

Van Soest Procedure

The raw plant material is contacted with dilute acid and washed with solvents to remove starch, pectin, hemicellulose, fats, oils, protein, free sugars, and soluble minerals. The residue, called 'acid detergent fibre,' contains cellulose, lignin and insoluble minerals (mainly silica).

Air-dried plant material (1 g), ground to particles of less than 1 mm, is placed in a beaker with 100 ml of acid-detergent solution (49 g l^{-1} H_2SO_4, 20 g l^{-1} cetyl trimethylammonium bromide). Decahydronaphthalene (2 ml) is added and the contents are slowly boiled for 1 h while the reflux condenser maintains a constant liquid volume in the beaker. Then, the beaker contents are filtered through a tared Gooch crucible, washed with boiling water, acetone and hexane (optional). The residual acid detergent fibre (ADF) is dried at 100°C and weighed.

The cellulose content in ADF can be measured by two methods: (1) cellulose removal with acid, or (2) lignin removal by oxidation.

Method 1. The ADF prepared above is placed in a tared Gooch crucible containing an equal volume of asbestos as a filter aid. The crucible contents are contacted with room temperature 72% sulphuric acid for 3 h and then thoroughly washed with hot water. The sample is dried at 100°C for 8 h and weighed. The weight loss corresponds to the cellulose content.

Method 2. The ADF (0·5–1·0 g) is placed in a tared Gooch crucible. A saturated potassium permanganate solution (50 g l^{-1} $KMnO_4$, 0·05 g l^{-1} $AgSO_4$) and buffer solution (6 g l^{-1} $Fe(NO_3)_3 \cdot 9H_2O$, 0·15 g l^{-1} $AgNO_3$, 500 ml l^{-1} glacial acetic acid, 5 g l^{-1} potassium acetate, 400 ml l^{-1} t-butyl alcohol) are mixed in a 2:1 ratio (by volume). This mixture (25 ml) is added to the crucible for 90 min at room temperature to oxidize the lignin in the ADF. The spent reagent is then removed by vacuum filtration. The crucible contents are soaked for 5 min in demineralizing solution (50 g l^{-1} oxalic acid dihydrate, 700 ml l^{-1} 95% ethanol, 50 ml l^{-1} 12 M HCl) which is then removed by filtration. The filter contents are washed with ethanol and acetone. The crucible is dried at 100°C for 8 h. The crucible contains cellulose and insoluble ash. The crucible may be placed in a 500°C oven for 3 h; the weight loss corresponds to the cellulose content.

A simpler approach to removing the lignin from the ADF has been described by C.S. Edwards. The ADF is soaked in activated trigol (i.e. 6·3 ml of 32% hydrochloric acid dissolved in 1 litre of pure triethylene glycol) in a 121°C autoclave for 60 min. The sample is then washed with 95% ethanol and acetone. The residue contains cellulose and insoluble ash.

Other Gravimetric Methods

Cross and Bevan cellulose is the lignocellulose portion remaining after removing hemicellulose with two boilings in NaOH and removing lignin with chlorine and bleach.

Monoethanolamine cellulose is the lignocellulose portion remaining after monoethanolamine treatment, chlorination and bleaching.

Norman–Jenkins cellulose is the lignocellulose portion remaining after sodium sulphite boiling, bleaching, and acid treatment.

α-Cellulose is the cellulose fraction insoluble in room temperature 17·5% sodium hydroxide wash water (DP > 90).

β-Cellulose is the cellulose fraction in the alkaline wash water which precipitates upon neutralization (15 < DP < 90).

γ-Cellulose is the cellulose fraction soluble in the neutralized alkaline wash water (DP < 15).

Holocellulose is the residue which remains after lignocellulose is defatted with hot, azeotropic benzene/ethanol and delignified with hot chlorous acid ($HClO_2$). Holocellulose contains the cellulose and hemicellulose of the original plant material.

Colorimetric Method

Hexosan assays may be used to measure cellulose, the dominant hexose polymer in starch-free plant materials (other than softwoods). Holtzapple describes an assay in which the hexosan sample is placed in a sealed test tube with 1530 g l^{-1} sulphuric acid and 20 g l^{-1} chromotropic acid and boiled for 1 h. Hexose C6 degrades to form formaldehyde, which reacts with the chromotropic acid to form a purple compound that is measured spectrophotometrically. There is minor interference by pentosans that may be reduced by lowering the chromotropic acid concentration to 1 g l^{-1} and shortening the reaction time to 20 min. There is also some interference with lignin, so the most accurate results are obtained with holocellulose, rather than the original lignocellulose. *See* Spectroscopy, Visible Spectroscopy and Colorimetry

Chromatographic Method

The cellulose content can be estimated from the glucose composition, since cellulose is the main source of glucose in plant materials (assuming free sugars and starch are not present). *See* Chromatography, Principles

Bibliography

Atalla RH (1987) *The Structures of Cellulose. ACS Symposium Series*, No. 340, Washington, DC: American Chemical Society.

Bogan RT, Kuo CM and Brewer RJ (1979) Cellulose derivatives, esters. *Kirk-Othmer Encyclopedia of Chemical Technology*, 3rd edn, vol. 5. New York: Wiley.

Edwards CS (1973) Determination of lignin and cellulose in forages by extraction with triethylene glycol. *Journal of the Science of Food and Agriculture* 24: 381–388.

Fengel D (1970) Ultrastructural behavior of cell wall polysaccharides. *Tappi* 53(3): 497–503.

Goering HK and Van Soest PJ (1970) *Forage Fiber Analysis. Agricultural Handbook*, No. 379, Jacket No. 387–598. Washington DC: US Department of Agriculture.

Greminger GK (1979) Cellulose derivatives, ethers. *Kirk-Othmer Encyclopedia of Chemical Technology*, 3rd edn, vol. 5. New York: Wiley.

Holtzapple MT and Humphrey AE (1983) Determination of soluble and insoluble glucose oligomers with chromotropic acid. *Analytical Chemistry* 55: 584–585.

Jayne G (1971) Cellulose and cellulose derivatives. In: Bikales NM and Segal L (eds) *High Polymers*, 2nd edn, vol. V, part IV. New York: Wiley Interscience.

Plunguian M (1943) *Cellulose Chemistry*. New York: Chemical Publishing.

Southgate DAT (1976) *Determination of Food Carbohydrates*. London: Applied Science.

Turbank AF, Durso DF, Battista OA, Bolker HI, Colving JR, Eastman N, Kleinert TN, Krassig H and St John Manley R (1979) Cellulose. *Kirk-Othmer Encyclopedia of Chemical Technology*, 3rd edn, vol. 5. New York: Wiley.

M. T. Holtzapple
Texas A&M University, College Station, USA

CEREALS

Contents

Contribution to the Diet

Cereals and the World's Food Supply

From the dawn of civilization and throughout history, cereal grains have been a major food source for mankind. The rise of human culture approximately 10 000 years ago was associated with the invention of plant cultivation, an innovation which was a precursor to the generation of permanent communities and the development of large-scale social structures. Primitive forms of wheat and rice were probably the first cultivated cereals, together with barley, sorghum, millet, oats, rye, and maize. There are several reasons for the fact that cereals have become the staple food of mankind: harvested cereal grains are dense and nutritious packages of food; they can be produced and traded economically in large quantities, and they can be easily stored for long periods if moisture and insect infestation are controlled. *See* Barley; Oats; Rice; Rye; Sorghum; Wheat

Today, approximately 50% of the world's total food energy and 45% of the dietary protein are supplied by the eight principal species of cereal grains. Wheat and rice together furnish approximately 40% of the total dietary energy and somewhat less of the protein. However, cereal grains are not merely an important source of dietary energy and protein, they also contribute to the intake of certain vitamins, mineral elements, and complex carbohydrates, including dietary fibre. Cereals are universally consumed in a wide variety of products both industrially processed and home-made. There are large variations, of both a quantitative and a qualitative nature, between the consumption of cereal grains of different nations. This results in large variations in the contribution of cereals to the diets of different peoples. While an increase in the consumption of cereals is a dietary goal in many industrial countries, the substitution of some of the cereals with foods of animal origin would improve the diets in many developing countries. *See* National Nutrition Policies

Most of the present production of maize and barley, as well as smaller fractions of other cereals, are used for animal feed, industrial purposes or beer making, and their contribution to man's diet is concomitantly smaller or indirect.

Potential of Cereals to Meet all Food Requirements

Cereal grains contain, on average, 75% carbohydrate, 10–15% protein, 2% fat, and 10–15% water. Cereals provide approximately 14–15 MJ per kg. The total recorded harvest of the eight cereal grains would suffice to supply 1 kg per day for each individual if they were evenly distributed between the world's population, and this would be more than adequate to meet the daily dietary energy requirement of an adult:

- Total harvest of cereal grains (as is basis): 1950×10^6 t per year.
- World human population: approximately 5300×10^6.
- Cereal grains per individual: approximately 365 kg per year, or 1 kg per day.
- Dietary energy provided by 1 kg of cereal on a dry-weight basis (dbw): 14 MJ.
- Dietary energy required by an adult person: 10 MJ.

No more than 30% of dietary energy in a properly balanced diet should come from fat. Another principle is that the intake of protein should be at least 60 g, and that 10–15% of the dietary energy should come from protein. The 10 MJ daily requirement of an average person should be made up as follows: fat, 80 g or less (providing <3 MJ); protein, 60 g or more (providing >1 MJ); with carbohydrates providing the rest (7 MJ). A comparison of the approximate composition of a diet based on these principles with an average composition of cereals indicates that cereals as sole source of food would provide more protein than required, whereas the fat intake on a pure cereal diet would be much lower than necessary or desirable. Most industrialized popula-

Table 1. A comparison of the approximate compositions of a recommended daily diet and 700 g of cereal, adequate to meet the daily energy requirement of an adult

	Provided by a recommended daily diet[a]	Provided by 700 g (dwb) of cereal[a]
Dietary energy (MJ)	10 (100%)	10 (100%)
Protein (g)	>60 (>10%)	80 (14%)
Fat (g)	<80 (<30%)	10 (4%)
Carbohydrate (g)	353 (60%)	482 (82%)

[a] Percentage of energy provided is shown in parenthesis.

tions tend to get more than 30% of their dietary energy from fat, so that cereals low in fat make a balancing contribution to the diet (Table 1). *See* Energy, Measurement of Food Energy

Cereals as an Energy and Protein Source

The yearly per capita consumption of cereal grains varies from 90 kg to more than 250 kg in different parts and societies of the world. There are areas in Asia and Africa where cereals may provide more than 70% of the energy in the diet (see Table 2). In most industrialized countries, the consumption of cereals has declined continuously in the twentieth century; today, cereals may provide less than 25% of daily energy. However, cereals still maintain their position as the most important single food source universally. Approximately 80% of the dietary energy content of cereals comes from carbohydrates, and more than 10% comes from protein. *See* Carbohydrates, Requirements and Dietary Importance; Fats, Requirements; Protein, Requirements

The role of cereals as a protein source follows their contribution to dietary energy. Cereals provide 20–70% of dietary protein, depending on the amount consumed. Table 2 shows the role of cereals in the supply of dietary energy and protein in various selected countries.

The biological value of cereal protein is lower than that of animal origin. This is mainly because of the relatively low lysine content of cereal proteins. However, several studies have shown that cereal protein contains an adequate amount of lysine and other amino acids to maintain a positive nitrogen balance in adults. In most diets, the somewhat lower biological value of cereal protein is virtually irrelevant, since foods of animal origin, or from the leguminous family, compensate for the low lysine content of cereals. In such situations, the contribution of cereals is to serve as an economical source of protein. *See* Amino Acids, Properties and Occurrence

Table 2. Consumption of cereal grains (average for the period 1984–1986) and their contribution to the estimated intake of dietary energy and protein in selected countries

Country	Total consumption of cereals (kg per person per year)[a]	Contribution of cereal grains to the intake of	
		Energy[b] (%)	Protein[b]
Australia	112·6	23	23
Bangladesh	237·7	83	78
Brazil	142·3	39	39
China	266·0	71	66
Czechoslovakia	146·2	30	31
Egypt	247·7	61	69
West Germany	98·1	21	23
India	180·1	63	61
Italy	162·5	32	33
Japan	167·7	43	26
Nigeria	114·2	42	52
Sweden	87·9	22	21
Turkey	203·5	51	58
UK	87·0	20	23
USA	94·3	19	19

[a] Unmilled grain.
[b] Derived by taking into account appropriate conversion factors.
Source: FAO (1991).

Mineral Elements and Vitamins

Cereal grains also contribute significantly to mineral and vitamin intakes. However, a diet based solely on cereals would be inadequate to meet the required intakes of several vitamins and minerals. This is illustrated in Fig. 1, which shows the nutrient density of wholemeal flour and white flour. The mineral element and vitamin content of cereal products depends upon the proportion of germ, bran and endosperm present in the particular product. A white flour consisting mainly of endosperm may contain less than one third of the particular mineral or vitamin found in whole grains. *See* Flour, Dietary Importance

Whole-grain products include every part of the grain and they provide significant amounts of the dietary supply of several mineral and trace elements such as iron, magnesium, calcium, manganese, zinc, etc. However, these may not be completely absorbed because of the presence of phytic acid, which forms insoluble phytates with divalent cations and reduces their bioavailability. Most of the phytate is removed along with bran in the flour milling process, and most of it is also degraded in a sourdough breadmaking process. Comparative studies have shown that the absolute quantity of most trace elements available from wholemeal pro-

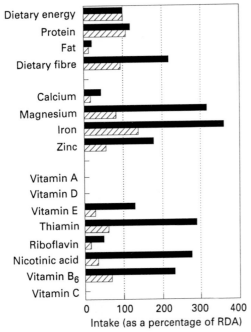

Fig. 1 Nutrient density of wholemeal wheat flour and white flour, as based on Recommended Dietary Allowances (RDAs) of an adult male and food composition data. Estimated daily dietary fibre requirement is 3 g per MJ. ■ Wholemeal; ▨ white flour.

for enrichment because there are virtually no major population subgroups which would not be able to use cereal grains, and because cereals are consumed by all socioeconomic subgroups. *See* Food Fortification

The bioavailability of the added minerals is higher than that of the minerals originally found in the bran. The contribution of cereal products to the intake of the vitamins and minerals is, to a great extent, dependent on whether or not the white flour is enriched. For example, in some countries up to 40% of the total iron intake comes from the iron fortification of white flour. *See* Bioavailability of Nutrients

Complex Carbohydrates and Dietary Fibre

Cereal grains are composed of up to 85% (dwb) of polysaccharides, mainly starch but also cellulose, arabinoxylans, mixed linked β-glucans, and other complex carbohydrates defined as dietary fibre. Cereals make a prominent contribution to the dietary fibre intake in most populations. In countries where whole-grain products, such as wholemeal bread, are popular, cereal products may contribute more than 40% of the average dietary fibre intake and be the most important source of dietary fibre in the diet. *See* Dietary Fibre, Properties and Sources

Whole-grain cereals contain up to 10% (dwb) dietary fibre. When wheat is milled into white flour, two thirds or more of the fibre is removed along with the bran. Wheat bran may contain more than 35% dietary fibre. It is one of the most effective faecal-bulking agents, and the consumption of wheat bran or wholemeal products makes a beneficial contribution to bowel function and alleviates constipation. There is evidence that bran and whole-grain products are protective with regard to different types of cancer, and by many different mechanisms. Wheat bran is chiefly composed of cellulose and other polysaccharides of the insoluble fibre fraction. Wheat bran does not appear to alter serum lipid levels. *See* Cancer, Diet in Cancer Prevention; Dietary Fibre, Physiological Effects

Soluble and viscous forms of dietary fibre are associated with a reduction in serum lipid levels, including cholesterol level. Examples of these fibres are guar gum and pectin, as well as the soluble dietary fibre fraction of oats and oat bran. Several studies have shown the efficacy of oat bran, when consumed in sufficient quantity, in reducing serum cholesterol level.

Dietary fibre present in cereal products may also contribute to the diet by affecting the satiety value of food, thus helping to control bodyweight.

Bread and Other Cereal Foods

Bread, pasta and noodles are among the major products made from wheat. Although in many countries there has

ducts is similar, or only marginally higher, than that from white wheat products. *See* Bread, Sourdough Bread; Phytic Acid, Nutritional Impact *See also* individual minerals

Whole cereal grains also contain significant amounts of B group vitamins, thiamin (B_1), riboflavin (B_2) and nicotinic acid. The germ contains considerable amounts of vitamin E. Cereal grains are deficient in vitamins A, C and D. The ascorbic acid that is customarily added to white flour to improve its baking properties has no nutritional significance. *See* individual vitamins

Wheat and rice are usually consumed as foods made from white flour or polished white rice. The white flour used for breadmaking, pasta and noodle production retains only 20–50% of the nutrients found in whole grains. An analogous change occurs when rice is husked and polished. However, the parboiling process, which involves soaking and steaming of the husked paddy rice, allows some of the water-soluble B group vitamins located in the bran to penetrate into the endosperm, and helps to retain 40–90% of the vitamins. In parts of the world where rice is the staple food, parboiling has been used as an effective measure against beriberi, a thiamin deficiency disorder.

In some countries, low-extraction (white) flours and other cereal products are enriched with certain minerals and vitamins, such as calcium, magnesium, iron, vitamins and B_1 and B_2, and nicotinic acid. Wheat flour and other common cereal products are very suitable vehicles been an increase in sales of brown bread containing some dark flour, most bread is made from white flour. Baking itself does not significantly affect the nutrient content of flour. However, regular soft bread contains more water (35–40%) than flour (13–15%) and the nutrients are diluted. In breadmaking, salt (sodium chloride) is added primarily for flavouring purposes, and this may multiply the sodium content more than 100-fold. The sodium chloride content of regular bread is 0·8–1·4% (as is basis). In many bread-eating populations, bread is the most prominent source of sodium, contributing more than 25% of the dietary sodium intake. *See* Sodium, Properties and Determination

Salt and yeast are virtually mandatory ingredients of bread. Optional customary ingredients, which are normally used in quantities less than 2–4%, are fat, sugar, nonfat dry milk, soya bean flour, malt flour, and others. Some of these ingredients may contribute significantly to the nutritional composition of the resulting bread.

The baking industry and the housewife also produce from flour a variety of sweet buns, cakes, confectionery, biscuits, etc. In many of these products, fat and sugar may literally predominate and the nutrients of the flour are accordingly diluted.

Bread itself is low in fat. However, a slice of bread often becomes a carrier of butter or margarine, cheese, salami, or other fat-containing foods, which significantly alter the nutritive balance of the entity (see Fig. 2). For example, if a slice of bread with butter and a slice of cheese or salami is added, the fat present in the resulting sandwich may easily provide up to 50% or more of the dietary energy, so that the sandwich becomes a fat-increasing food item in the diet.

Internationally, bread is made in hundreds and thousands of varieties. In addition to breadmaking, various cooking procedures are used to make cereal foods from milled grains and flours. Cooked rice, noodles, porridges, etc., are staples in Asia, Africa and elsewhere, and their contribution to the local diets may be estimated from food consumption data (cf. Table 2).

Dietary Guidelines and Cereal Products

Dietary goals, as defined in industrialized countries, place heavy emphasis on the consumption of cereals, breads, rice and pasta. Consumers are encouraged to choose a diet low in fat and with plenty of vegetables, fruits and cereal products. When put in practical terms, an ideal daily diet, composed according to the dietary guidelines, should include six to eight slices of bread, and alternatively some muesli, a breakfast cereal or pasta is recommended. In many industrialized countries this would require an increase of 10–30% in cereal grain consumption. Attention should be given, however, to the control of the amount of salt in bread, and to the

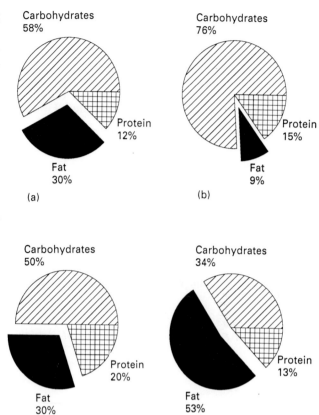

Fig. 2 Percentage of dietary energy derived from carbohydrates, protein and fat (a) in a balanced diet, (b) from bread, (c) from bread (25 g) and cheese (10 g), and (d) from bread and butter (3·3 g) with salami (10 g).

amount of fat-containing spreads on sandwiches; otherwise, bread could become a vehicle for excess salt and fat.

In conclusion, cereals are the most important sources of dietary energy and protein for the world's increasing population. Cereals contain complex carbohydrates, including dietary fibre, and they also contribute significantly to the intake of many essential vitamins and minerals. Cereals are consumed universally and in a measureless variety of versatile foods, which may originate from elaborated industrial processes, handicraft bakeries, or from the most rudimentary domestic kitchen. There are practically no major population subgroups unable to consume cereals. Enrichment of certain cereal foods is practised in some countries, and this measure adds to the value of cereal foods as sources of essential nutrients. The vital contribution of cereals in diets is recognized in the national guidelines, which encourage consumers to increase the use of cereals.

Bibliography

Betschart AA (1988) Nutritional quality of wheat and wheat foods. In: Pomeranz Y (ed.) *Wheat: Chemistry and Tech-*

nology 3rd edn, pp 91–130. St Paul, Minnesota: American Association of Cereal Chemists.

FAO (1991) *Food Balance Sheets*: 1984–86 average. Rome: Food and Agriculture Organization.

Holland B, Unwin ID and Buss DH (1988) *Cereals and Cereal Products*. Third supplement to *McCance and Widdowson's The Composition of Foods* 4th edn. London: The Royal Society of Chemistry, and Ministry of Agriculture, Fisheries and Food.

Juliano BO (ed.) (1985) *Rice Chemistry and Technology* 2nd edn, pp 1–16. St Paul, Minnesota: American Association of Cereal Chemists.

National Research Council (1989) *Recommended Dietary Allowances* 10th edn. Washington, DC: National Academy Press.

Passmore R and Eastwood MA (1986) *Human Nutrition and Dietetics* 8th edn. London: Churchill Livingstone.

US Department of Agriculture and US Department of Health and Human Services (1990) *Nutrition and Your Health: Dietary Guidelines for Americans*. Home and Garden Bulletin No. 232, 3rd edn. Washington DC: US Government Printing Office.

Hannu Salovaara
Department of Food Technology, University of Helsinki, Finland

Bulk Storage of Grain

General Considerations

Currently, world production of cereal grains is about 1500 million tonnes. This represents by far the greatest production of staple food material, the tuber-producing crops being far behind, with a total production of less than 100 million tonnes of edible dry matter. A very simple arithmetic calculation shows that cereal crops will be able to provide more than the 1·3 kg of bread or cooked rice per day to all of the 6000 million world population at the beginning of the 21st century.

Whatever the political problems and ethnic questions, two essential facts must be taken into account: cereals are produced in excess in only a limited number of countries of the world, and only during limited periods in the year. Good storage would allow consumption to be delayed and grain to be exported anywhere in the world throughout the year and is, therefore, of primary economic, political and social importance.

Existing Losses of Cereal Crops

It is difficult, if not impossible, to accurately calculate the postharvest losses resulting from poor storage conditions and inadequate practices. However, in 1976, it was estimated that losses of grains represented a commercial value of about US $4000 million.

The Food and Agriculture Organization (FAO) reports generally consider that percentage losses remain at rather low levels in industrialized countries, probably never more than 1 or 2%, whereas they can reach very high levels, maybe 50% or even more, in undeveloped countries where modern storage equipment is lacking. It is important, however, to realise that, in developed countries, low percentage levels of loss involve enormous quantities of grain, leading to problems of significant economical importance. By contrast, high levels of losses in developing areas apply in most cases to only limited quantities of stored cereals, raising questions of vital importance only for the populations concerned.

It must also be emphasized that losses in grain quality can occur without significant losses of dry matter, e.g. decreases of nutritional value, losses of vitamins or essential fatty acids, appearance of toxicity, off-flavours or discolorations and low insect pest infestation. The assessment of such losses remains quite impossible at the present time.

In every situation that can be encountered it is of primary importance to have the best understanding of local environmental, economic, climatic and ethnic conditions, and appreciation of possible causes of grain deterioration during storage, in order to minimize losses.

Some basic questions still lack satisfactory technical or economic answers but, usually, it can be said that postharvest losses are mostly due to lack of adequate training of the people who handle and store the grain. Most significant losses result generally from insect infestation or from the growth of microorganisms. To a lesser extent, biochemical changes in the grain itself can also be important.

The causes and extent of grain losses may differ widely from one place to another. They depend on many parameters but three major environmental factors determine the extent of damage in a given situation: the water content of the grain, the mean temperature of the bulk and the duration of storage. Of these factors, water is by far the most important and also the most interesting because it can be managed; it is very difficult to control temperature in practice. *See* Storage Stability, Mechanisms of Degradation; Storage Stability, Parameters Affecting Storage Stability

Main Biological Causes of Losses

Unless cereal grains are sufficiently dry at harvest, they must be considered as perishable biological products that will be damaged by microorganisms or insects, depending on the environmental conditions. Surprisingly, the major role played by microorganisms, and particularly by moulds, has been recognized only recently, but it is now understood that artificial drying of moist grains after harvest is essential for the avoidance of mould growth during storage, rather than for the prevention of development of insects or biochemical changes in the kernel itself. *See* Spoilage, Moulds in Food Spoilage

Respiration of grain is a secondary phenomenon in most situations, when germination is not taking place. Respiration of the germ seems to remain more or less constant and at a very low level, compatible with seed conservation, whatever the hydration or the gaseous environmental conditions.

To initiate germination of the grain, very large moisture contents, greater than 70–80% (wet basis), i.e. sufficient for the complete inbibition of the grain, are necessary. When much moisture migration occurs in metallic bins, intense condensation is produced, generally on the roof of silos, and grain sprouting at the top of farm silos or in railway wagons frequently occurs. *See* Water Activity, Effect on Food Stability

Role of Microorganisms in Grains

The microorganisms which make up the microflora of cereal grain and their products are now well known in regard to their ecological requirements and the damage they are able to produce during storage.

As soon as the relative humidity in equilibrium with the grain is sufficient for the growth of microorganisms (with freely available oxygen), the greater are the humidity and temperature, and the more intense and rapid the activity of microorganisms. Fortunately, there exists an absolute hydration limit below which microbial activity cannot take place. Expressed in terms of relative humidity of the air in equilibrium with the stored grain, this is about 65% for all cereal species of interest for humans. It corresponds to a moisture content of about 13% (wet basis) for wheat at 25°C. Below this limit, absolutely nothing of importance can occur in the kernel for many years with the exception of possible weak evolution of the lipids as explained below. Above this hydration limit, which is in fact very low, some mould species belonging to the genera *Aspergillus*, *Eurotium* (Fig. 1) and *Monascus*, among others, can develop. With extraordinary physiological abilities to grow in extremely dry conditions, these moulds invariably do develop unless additional 'barriers' such as cooling, antifungal agents or modified atmospheres are utilized. Such moulds contaminate cereal grains all over the world, but it must be emphasized that the growth of these so-called 'xerotolerant or xerophilic' species is very slow, and usually not accompanied by mycotoxin formation or significant deterioration of nutritional value. For their growth, moulds utilize lipids and carbohydrates from the grain (as do humans) and

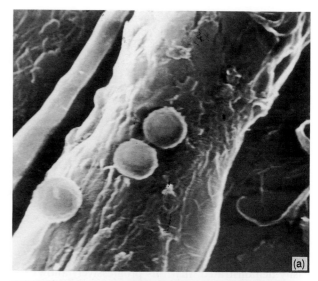
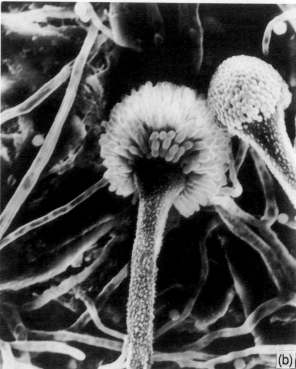

Fig. 1 Scanning electron micrographs of *Eurotium chevalieri*, a xerophilic species common on stored grains: (a) ×1400, round conidia on the surface of the kernel; (b) ×280, conidial heads, responsible for vegetative multiplication and dissemination). Courtesy of INRA, LMTC, Nantes.

produce carbon dioxide, water and heat in exchange, following the simplified scheme shown in eqn [1].

$$\text{Grain components} + \text{Oxygen from air} \atop \downarrow \atop CO_2 + H_2O + \text{Energy} + \text{Heat} \tag{1}$$

The main consequence is an increase in relative humidity and temperature and it is generally accepted, but not

Table 1. Microorganisms able to grow and approximate safe storage periods for various moisture contents of wheat

Moisture (% wet basis)	ERH	Microorganism	Safe storage period
12	50	None	Indefinite
14	65	*Aspergillus glaucus*	Years
15	68	*Aspergillus candidus*, *Penicillium* sp.	Years
16	75	*Aspergillus ochraceus*, most penicillia	Year
17	77	Most storage fungi	Months
18	80	Some yeasts, some lactic bacteria	Month
20	85	Most yeasts, most fungi	Week
30	95	Most fermentative bacteria	Days

Data mainly from the cited literature.

easily demonstrated, that this progressively allows the growth of moulds with greater requirements for water, such as *Penicillium* spp., other *Aspergillus* spp. or even *Fusarium* spp., these kinds of moulds being able to completely destroy the grains and to produce extremely dangerous mycotoxins, such as the hepatotoxic aflatoxin B_1 or the immunosuppressive T_2 toxin. *See* Mycotoxins, Occurrence and Determination

In practice, chiefly for economic reasons, grains are most often stored at moisture contents around 15–16% (wet basis), which allow storage without visible moulding for some months, as shown in Table 1, but also allows xerophilic species to develop slowly. At such hydration levels, only a slight increase in water content, due for example to water vapour migration or to insect respiration in a limited pocket, can be sufficient to cause a significant acceleration in microbiological activity, leading to formation of 'hot spots' in the bulk.

In 'hot spots', moulds grow actively, producing further heat and water, leading to moisture contents eventually sufficient to permit the growth of yeasts and bacteria. Grain dust and small particles accumulate at the centre of the pile of grain in bulk silos, because grain tends to separate into heavier and lighter components when poured into a bin. Such accumulations of dust and broken kernels greatly increase the risk of 'hot spot' formation by moulds and insects, because they reduce the circulation of dry or cool air through the grain and promote the accumulation of heat and moisture. In such situations, it becomes urgent to cool and dry the grain by forced ventilation in order to avoid further problems throughout the bulk of the silo. *See* Spoilage, Bacterial Spoilage; Spoilage, Yeasts in Food Spoilage

Role of Insects in Stored Grains

Among the animal pests (i.e. mites, insects, rodents and birds), insects cause by far the most damage to stored cereal. They are also the most feared because, even if they do not produce clearly toxic substances or strong off-flavours as do moulds, their presence depreciates the value of grain even in cases of light infestations. Insects secrete some metabolic residues like quinones or uric acid that produce objectionable smells and tastes. They may also transmit pathogenic bacteria to the grain or leave fragments (such as faeces) in flours and other cereal products. Most consumers have a strong repulsion towards this filth, and one can say that, due to their contamination, insects ruin much more grain than they consume. *See* Insect Pests, Insects and Related Pests; Insect Pests, Problems Caused by Insects and Mites

Infestation of grain by insects is still considered to be accidental, but most species are well adapted to the grain ecosystem. They exist permanently in machines and buildings for crop reception and must always be regarded as a permanent, potential pest danger.

Storage insects belong mainly to the orders Coleoptera and Lepidoptera. Most of them are adapted forms of crop-destroying species. The most injurious genera, *Sitophilus*, *Trogoderma*, *Cryptolestes*, *Sitotroga*, *Tribolium* and *Rhyzopertha*, are those which are very flexible and adaptable with only minimal nutritive requirements and tolerant, for example, to movements of grain during intersilo transfers or to temperature fluctuations induced by heating and ventilation. Most of the important species have a development cycle comparable to that of butterflies: the females lay fertilized eggs which lead to worm-like larvae, and then to adults through successive moultings and a final metamorphosis via a pupal stage.

Adults usually live for several months, sometimes for more than 1 year, depending on storage conditions. Insects do not like light or low temperatures and cannot survive subzero temperatures. For this reason, damage caused by insects is generally only a peripheral problem in cold or temperate climates.

Like moulds, insects are aerobic organisms, only able to 'burn' with oxygen the dry matter they eat, producing carbon dioxide, heat and water. They can initiate 'hot spots' in grains with moisture contents below 14%, but

Bulk Storage of Grain

such dry heating generally remains below 40°C, which is the lethal temperature for most grain-infesting insects. By contrast, heating due to aerobic microorganisms can exceed 65–70°C and can even lead to autocombustion, when the moisture content becomes sufficient for the development of thermophilic fermentative bacteria and, subsequently, occurrence of exothermic chemical reactions.

Despite their absolute requirement for oxygen, insects are able to stop breathing for several hours. However, they are also very sensitive to high concentrations of carbon dioxide and this is why it is possible to control insect infestations with efficiency by the use of modified atmospheres. *See* Controlled Atmosphere Storage, Applications for Bulk Storage of Foodstuffs

They are remarkably tolerant to dryness, and commonly develop in grains with 11–14% water content (wet basis). Several cereal weevils cannot multiply below 9% moisture content and adults cannot survive long in such dry grains. On the other hand, flour beetles seem to be able to develop in completely dry flour. At least some storage insects seem capable of reutilizing their own metabolic water (produced by respiration as with moulds) when surviving in extremely dry grains (below 6% moisture content).

Moisture Migration in Silos

In silos, elevators and other installations for storage and transportation, the temperature fluctuates as a consequence of solar heating and daily or seasonal fluctuations in ambient temperature. The outermost layers of grain are most affected by such temperature variations. In a dark-green metallic silo, the wall temperature on the sunny side can frequently change from 15 to 80°C on a sunny summer day in northern Europe. This produces measurable temperature changes in the outermost 30–40 cm of grain, and large oscillations occurring in the first 5–10 cm. Such fluctuations are less pronounced in concrete silos.

When heated, grain loses water vapour and dehydrates. Due to convective movements of the intergranular atmosphere, the lost water vapour is transported to the coldest zones in the bulk where it condenses, increasing the water content of the cold grain. The main consequence is always an increase in microbial activity.

In nonhermetic silos, when the intergranular atmosphere is not controlled, oxygen is always available, at least in the outer layers, for respiration of moulds, which in turn produce heat and moisture and an acceleration of microbial activity, which may cause carbon dioxide to accumulate deeper in the bulk. This chain reaction always occurs, everywhere in the world, under all climatic conditions. The main difference from one place to another is the speed and intensity of this general

phenomenon but, whatever the initial moisture content of the grain, sunshine will more or less rapidly destroy the stored cereals it previously helped to produce. *See* Oxidation of Food Components

The only way this process can be slowed is by removing heat and moisture using forced ventilation of the bulk, or by transfer of the grain from one bin to another to mix the hot and dry grain with cold and moist grain from other parts of the silo. Underground storage under airtight conditions, where temperature fluctuations and moisture migration are minimized, provides an interesting alternative to bin storage, especially when germinative capacity is not the main characteristic to be preserved.

Losses Due to Rodents

Many species of small rodents cause grain losses throughout the world. Rats and mice, which are found everywhere, are probably the most important, causing damage mainly at farms where grain is stored in loose structures. Control measures against rats and mice include traps, baits containing rodenticides, and fumigation similar to that used against insects. In many cases, it is important to know which kind of rodent is concerned in order to take its feeding preferences into account for poisoning, or to find the best way to trap it. Rodent control in larger grain stores requires a sound concrete construction that is able to resist rat gnawing, and the silo must be maintained in good condition. *See* Fumigants

Biochemical Changes During Storage

For dry grains, i.e. with moisture contents just permitting only very slow development of moulds, only slight changes in biochemical composition can be observed over several months. The lipid fraction of the grain deteriorates most rapidly during open air storage under the influence of microbial enzymes, leading to the accumulation of fatty acids. Unsaturated acids can be further oxidized by the oxygen in air to produce volatile compounds with rancid odours and off-flavours. When moisture contents exceed 15–16% (wet basis), amylases from both grain and microorganisms start to hydrolyse starch into dextrins and maltose, resulting in losses of dry matter and a deterioration in quality. Only very small changes seem to occur in the protein fraction of stored grains when moulds cannot develop significantly in a few months, i.e. below 15% moisture content. However, the aggregative properties of some proteins may be modified after several years of storage, leading to a decrease in the water-soluble fraction. This may result in slightly lowered digestibility or, for wheat, in losses in breadmaking value.

In order to verify good storage of cereal grains, several simple laboratory examinations can be performed. Arguably the most sensitive is the germinative capacity of the grain, which clearly indicates the presence or absence of mould growth during storage in the open air. Fat acidity is another excellent criterion which correlates very well with the metabolic activity of storage fungi and the quality of the grain after a long period of storage.

In practice, in many commercial situations, the most important criterion is to ensure the absence of any live insect. In most cases, whether screening is carried out by acoustic detection or a more traditional counting technique, it is often still necessary to fumigate the grains before dispatching from the elevator.

Bibliography

Christensen CM (ed.) (1982) *Storage of Cereal Grains and their Products*, 3rd edn. St Paul: American Association of Cereal Chemists.

Calderon M and Barkai-Golan R (eds) (1990) *Food Preservation by Modified Atmospheres*. Boca Raton: CRC Press.

Multon JL (ed.) (1988) *Preservation and Storage of Grains, Seeds and their By-Products* Paris: Lavoisier.

Richard-Molard D, Lesage L and Cahagnier B (1985) Effect of water activity on mold growth and mycotoxin formation. In: Simatos D (ed.) *Properties of Water in Foods*, pp 273–292. La Hague: Martinus Nijhof.

D. Richard-Molard
INRA, Nantes, France

Handling of Grain for Storage

Storage Facilities

Storage facilities may take many forms, from a simple pile of unprotected grain on the ground in a farm building to the most sophisticated terminal elevator designed to handle grain for long distance exportation. At the farm level, grain may be temporarily stored in small concrete or round steel bins of small capacity (25–100 tonnes) which receive the crop immediately after harvest and before transport to a better long-term storage facility or in order to wait for the best market situation.

Grain may also be taken from the farm directly to a collecting centre, a small storage installation with several small bins providing an average capacity of about 1000 tonnes. It is not generally equipped with machinery for grain cleaning or drying since the grain is most often soon transferred to a country elevator (Fig. 1).

Country elevators (5000–50 000 tonnes), so called because they are filled with grain elevated into them by rolling belts with buckets, receive grain from the individual producer or from the collecting centre. Their capacity is adapted to the seasonal production of the area and their main role is to keep crops in good condition before and during storage, and to reload it into trucks or rail cars for transportation to terminal silos or export elevators.

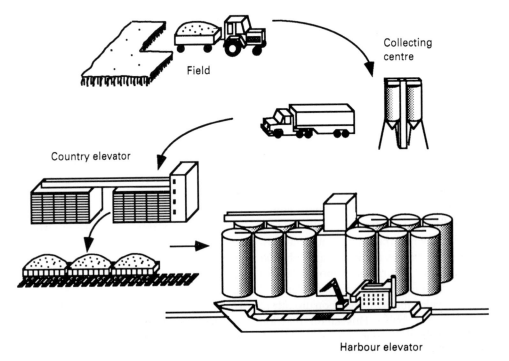

Fig. 1 Grain collection, from field to terminal elevator, a long trip for the grain.

Handling of Grain for Storage

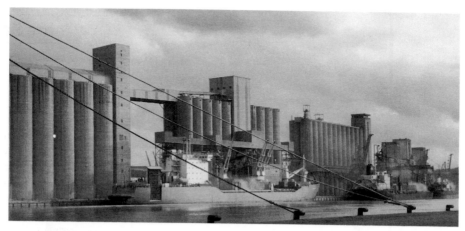

Fig. 2 The harbour elevator in Rouen, France, with a total storage capacity of 200 000 tonnes, is able to load grains into vessels at 2800 tonnes h^{-1} (Photo courtesy of H. Gomond).

There is no general rule for determining the best dimension of a farm bin or a country elevator. Usually the cost of storage increases sharply as the size of the silo decreases, so there is a tendency to build large structures. However, the management of grains is facilitated in multiple silos where grains of different grades or water contents can easily be separated.

The terminal elevators are generally located close to trade centres and/or transportation terminals, such as harbours (Fig. 2). Terminal elevators commonly offer storage capacities of 5000–500 000 tonnes in the USA or in northern Europe.

Equipment for grain handling and control is often basic at the farm level, with only very simple devices for grain elevation and ventilation. By contrast, country and terminal elevators have handling capacities adapted to their transportation facilities, and usually have sufficient capacity for peak load handling during the short period just following harvest. Most are today fully equipped with remote control and automation, so that grain can be automatically transferred from one silo to another or to ships and railway cars. Weighing, cleaning, sampling and even several tests of grain samples are now electronically controlled.

When possible, gravity discharge from grain bins is ideal, but the cost of the corresponding structures and equipment is high. As a consequence, flat storage of cereals is also commonly carried out in many situations, both at the farm level and at terminal elevators, to provide additional storage capacities when necessary. Such flat-bottomed silos are emptied through a central outlet where a rotating screw-conveyor draws the grain away beneath the floor. Many other sophisticated devices have been developed for moving the grain using air blown through metallic networks of ducts below the bins, or with suction blowers as back-up devices.

Quality Maintenance During Storage

When the farmer brings freshly harvested cereals to the elevator, several tests are performed to determine the appropriate treatment for safe storage, such as cleaning, dust removal to avoid very dangerous dust explosions, drying, cooling, chemical treatments against insects, etc.

As previously emphasized, the major parameter to be controlled is water content. Even with mature dry grain harvested at about 12–13% moisture content, serious problems will be encountered within a few months if moisture cannot be properly managed to prevent the heat and moisture transfer that can occur in bulk during storage and transportation. It is, therefore, important to store grains with a sufficiently low initial moisture content to prevent mould development and biochemical changes and to maintain it everywhere in the silo throughout the storage period. This can be achieved by artificially drying grains with excessive humidity at harvest, like maize in Europe, and by periodic forced ventilation during storage to remove excess water where condensation has occurred. *See* Storage Stability, Mechanisms of Degradation; Storage Stability, Parameters Affecting Storage Stability

Moisture Levels for Safe Storage

Determination of the correct moisture level for safe storage of a given crop in a given situation and for a given storage time is difficult. Very general and theoretical rules can be given, but it must never be forgotten that a large mass of cereal grain is never homogeneous in temperature, moisture, apparent density, thermal conductivity, etc., so that continuous monitoring with modern techniques, such as silothermometry, and perio-

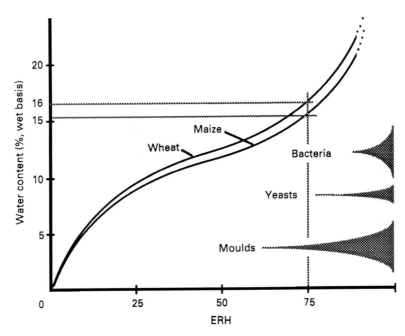

Fig. 3 Sorption isotherms for wheat and maize at 20°C and zones of activity for the main causes of grain degradation during storage (the wider the zone representing a cause of spoilage, the more intense and rapid the spoilage).

dical sample examination is highly recommended in every situation.

The availability of water in the grain is the most important physical parameter governing grain stability during storage, determining both biochemical changes and microbial growth. The availability can be estimated (and measured) by the relative humidity (ERH) of the intergranular air in equilibrium with the grain. A nonlinear relation relates ERH to moisture content as shown in Fig. 3 for wheat and maize. This curve is named a 'sorption isotherm' and depends on both the average temperature and biochemical composition of the grain. It differs from one cereal to another, but its relationship to the level of deterioration by different causes, such as microorganisms or enzymes, remains constant to a first approximation. Wheat stored at 16% moisture content is in equilibrium with a relative humidity of about 80% and will undergo the same kind of degradation at the same rate as maize with 15% moisture content which also has an ERH of 80% at the same temperature. As the temperature increases, the sorption isotherm is shifted to the left, i.e. at the same water content a higher ERH occurs and spoilage progresses faster. *See* Water Activity, Effect on Food Stability

Silothermometry is a sophisticated technique, utilizing thermocouples placed in the silo able to detect slight variations of the grain temperature, which indicate the beginning of deterioration through an aerobic process, resulting from a local elevation of the humidity. Modern sensors can detect temperature changes of less than 0·5°C in the surrounding 2–5 m. In most situations, this

gives sufficient sensitivity and overcomes the problem of the very low thermal conductivity of cereal grains which allows temperature differences to be transmitted only over short distances in the bulk. This method also permits determination of the best moment for applying drying, or ensures the completion of grain cooling by nocturnal ventilation.

Drying Methods and Alternatives

In any situation, the primary rule to respect in cereal storage is to fill the silo with dry or dried grains, with sufficient microbial and biochemical stability, as shown in Fig. 3. Many types of driers, such as full-bin driers, layer driers, continuous-flow driers, etc., are presently used on farms or at country elevators, but all utilize the same principle: heated dry air is blown through the grain to remove excess water. Figure 4 represents a farm bin equipped with a low-heat drier capable of drying grains with moisture contents of less than 20% (wet basis). *See* Drying, Theory of Air Drying

When large quantities of moist grain are to be rapidly dried, high-temperature drying is necessary. This gives a higher extractive capacity but can also cause thermal degradation of the grain, if used improperly, as often happens with maize, which is commonly harvested with a water content as high as 35% (wet basis). When dried with too hot air, the functional proteins are denatured and the value of the crop is decreased. On the other hand, high drying temperatures destroy all forms of insects in the bulk. *See* Drying, Hygiene

When possible, a combination of different drying and

Handling of Grain for Storage

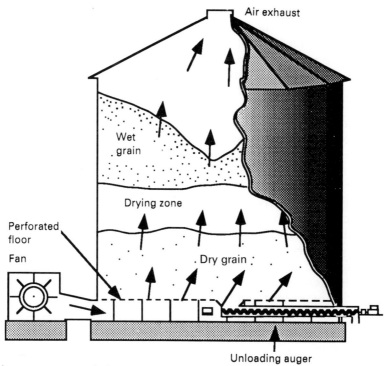

Air exhaust

Wet grain

Drying zone

Perforated floor

Fan

Dry grain

Unloading auger

Fig. 4 Farm bin for low-temperature drying.

cooling practices often gives the best technical and economic results. The essential principle is to decrease rapidly the moisture content to a level which allows only a slow development of moulds, i.e. to about 18% moisture in a first step, then to decrease the residual humidity to 15–16% by forced aeration when the ambient air is cool and dry enough to be efficient.

Natural Drying Methods

Alternative natural methods for grain drying have often been used, and at least two must be cited: the first one, used mostly for maize, utilizes gentle drying by the wind of cobs stored outside in cribs or other forms of mesh silos. This is satisfactory provided the temperature remains sufficiently low to inhibit the growth of such toxinogenic fungi as *Fusarium* species.

Solar driers have also been tested in efforts to save energy, but their use can only be recommended in regions where sufficient energy is provided by the sun to achieve drying in a time short enough to avoid spoilage by microorganisms. Unless drying to 80–82% ERH can be achieved in less than 7–10 days, the grain will certainly be damaged. *See* Drying, Drying Using Natural Radiation

Modified Atmosphere Storage

When cereals are not intended for uses requiring particular properties, such as high germination ability or functional properties of proteins for breadmaking, it is possible to store them with a greater water content than usual, provided the oxygen is removed from the system.

Underground storage and storage in anoxic atmospheres in hermetically sealed silos, or silos continuously flushed with nitrogen, for example, are quite possible. For example, it was recently shown that the nutritional value of wheat for animal feeding could be successfully maintained over several months by storing it, after grinding, in air-tight conditions at 21% water content and 15–20°C. Storing wet (35% water content or more) maize for pig feed in hermetic silos is now popular in several countries. Because of an important demand for intergranular oxygen at so high a humidity, through respiration of yeasts and lactic acid bacteria especially, the concentration of available oxygen remains extremely low in the silo. The growth of moulds is inhibited and, at least until the silos are nearly empty, that is to say, when free oxygen again appears and concentrations of carbon dioxide are decreasing, no mycotoxins can be produced. With such hermetic silos it is not necessary to grind the humid grain in order to produce silage, and the handling of the commodity is easier than with traditional practices. *See* Controlled Atmosphere Storage, Applications for Bulk Storage of Foodstuffs; Spoilage, Moulds in Food Spoilage

Control of Insects

Storing dry or wet grains under modified atmospheres is an excellent way to kill insects. Modern techniques for

Handling of Grain for Storage

storage of dry wheat under high concentrations of carbon dioxide have given very good results in Australia in recent years. Most often the obligation to kill all living insects forces the use of chemicals when infestations are detected in a silo or a ship. *See* Insect Pests, Insects and Related Pests; Insect Pests, Problems Caused by Insects and Mites

Now that use of organochlorine insecticides is forbidden, insecticides can be divided into two classes: contact insecticides, which kill insects and prevent reinfestation, and fumigants, which destroy insects without leaving significant residues.

In the first group are phosphoric esters, such as malathion, dichlorvos or methyl pirimifos, which are used at concentrations of about 4–8 g of active substance per ton of grain. They are very fast-acting and highly toxic by contact and ingestion. The main problem in using these products are their residues, which oblige careful consideration of the time of treatment, and also their relative inefficiency against the hidden forms of insect that live within the kernels. *See* Pesticides and Herbicides, Residue Determination

Fumigants, such as hydrogen phosphide are used to rapidly kill all live insect stages, including adults. They are employed in air-tight structures equipped with systems which allow the safe introduction and removal of the gas. *See* Fumigants

Apart from modified-atmosphere storage under nitrogen or carbon dioxide, only persistent insecticides can provide good long-term protection of grain. It is then of primary importance to ensure the absence of any residue in by-products like flour and brans used for human and animal food. At the present time, there is a general tendency to decrease concentrations of toxic substances used against insect infestations. A possible approach would be to combine the use of carbon dioxide with an active substance, such as methyl bromide or hydrogen phosphide, which would permit a considerable reduction in the dose of fumigant used because of synergism with carbon dioxide.

The Future

All over the world, safe storage of cereal grains is a vital but expensive activity. Many cereal grains are still utilized in the food industry despite the poor quality that results from inappropriate storage conditions. Current scientific and technical knowledge in this domain is sufficient to satisfactorily answer most questions on the handling and storage of grain. It is easy to test the quality of cereals discharged from silos. It now depends on the consumer's attitude if the best quality is to be obtained and systematically verified.

Bibliography

Christensen CM (ed.) (1982) *Storage of Cereal Grains and their Products*, 3rd edn. St Paul: American Association of Cereal Chemists.

Fleurat-Lessard F (1987) Control of storage insects by physical means and modified environment. Feasibility and applications. *Proceedings of the International Symposium on Stored Product Pest Control, BCPC, British Crop Protection Council Management*, No. 37, pp 209–218.

Multon JL (ed.) (1988) *Preservation and Storage of Grains, Seeds and their By-products*, Paris: Lavoisier.

Richard-Molard D (1990) Conservation of humid grains in controlled atmosphere storage. In: Calderon M and Barkai-Golan R (eds) *Food Preservation by Controlled Atmosphere*, pp 57–82., Boca Raton: CRC Press.

D. Richard-Molard
INRA, Nantes, France

Breakfast Cereals

The US breakfast cereals (BC) industry, in its history of about 100 years, has emerged as an important segment of the food industry, with annual sales of about 8×10^{12}. This remarkable progress has been achieved through a combination of knowledge gained in human nutrition, innovative progress in cereal processing technology, and imaginative marketing. The chief driving force has been the continued need for new, convenient, nutritions and fun foods for a discriminating, affluent and mobile society. Any large local grocery store in the USA, Canada or the UK is likely to stock about 100 different BC foods. In the UK, sales for the year ending March 1991 amounted to £792 × 10⁶. The low penetration of BC into other European and other developing countries is forecasted to increase over the next decades.

Breakfast cereals have been defined as processed grains for human consumption. The major grains used in the manufacturing of BC are corn, rice, wheat, oats and barley. The available products can be divided into ready-to-eat (RTE) and ready-to-cook or hot cereals (HC). The RTE cereal products are usually made from mixtures of several grain components; they require extensive processing, are often fortified with vitamins and minerals, and are specially packaged to protect their flavour, texture and nutrients during storage. The HC, on the other hand are primarily made from a single grain component by using relatively simple processing and packaging technologies. The difference between the RTE and HC products is reflected in the price at the consumer level. The typical single serving (28·35 g, or 1 oz) of RTE cereal costs about $0·22 (0·15–0·25) and represents about 90% of the business. The typical one serving of HC costs about five cent less. According to a survey of the US Department of Commerce in 1990, the per capita consumption of RTE cereal had increased from 3·76 to 5·26 kg (8·3 to 11·6 lb) per year from 1970 to 1987. The corresponding increase for HC was 1·09 to 1·63 kg (2·4 to 3·6 lb) per year. The latest per capita consumption in UK was 5·99 kg (13·2 lb) and 1 kg (2·2 lb) per year for RTE and HC respectively. *See* Barley; Oats; Rice; Wheat

Methods of Manufacture

Ready-to-eat Cereals

The RTE cereals are grain formulations, suitable for human consumption without further cooking. The manufacturing technology varies according to type of cereal.

Flaked Cereal

The flaked cereals can be divided into two groups: flakes made from whole grains or parts of the whole grains, and flakes made from finer flour materials, which must be extruded or agglomerated to produce appropriate size flakes. The whole grains (wheat and rice) or their special components (e.g. dehulled and degermed corn grits) are cooked with flavourings such as sugar, salt and malt; they are then dried to a firm but slightly plastic state, flaked by passing between rolls, and toasted or dried to a final specified moisture content. The cooking is usually done in batches of the traditional flakes made from grits or whole grains. Alternatively, cooking may be carried out as a continuous process by conveying the grain through a steam pressure vessel with pressure lock ports. The moisture content of the cooked mass at the end of cooking is usually 28%. The cooked material should not be mushy, soft and sticky. After cooking, the material is cooled and dried at about 121°C, with agitation to separate the particles and dry them to a final moisture content of 10–18%, depending upon the grains.

The dried, delumped and tempered material is then flaked. Tremendous pressures are necessary to flatten the prepared material into flakes, which are toasted by keeping them suspended in hot air between 270°C and 330°C for about 90 s. The properties of the finished flakes can be modified by heating or roasting steps immediately before flaking (e.g. rapid heating with minimum of drying before roasting will result in flakes which absorb liquid milk slower and are softer). Similarly, other properties, such as expansion, blistering colour, crispiness, tenderness, and flavour of the final product, are controlled during roasting. The moisture content of the finished product is about 1–3%.

Puffed Cereals

The predominant grains used for making puffed cereals are wheat and rice. The rice that is used for puffing is either short- or medium-grain white rice. Rice usually requires no pretreatment. Wheat, on the other hand, is either pretreated with concentrated brine solution, or its bran removed by pearling. In the pearling operation, the wheat is passed through a machine which contains a grindstone. Usually hard wheat, preferably durum, is used for puffing. During this operation the outside coat is removed. The grain flour mixture can also be formed into desired shapes for puffing by an appropriate extrusion process, and dried to a moisture content of 9–12%.

The puffing guns are vessels capable of holding very-high-temperature and high-pressure steam. The critical feature of a puffing gun is a quick opening lid which seals the vessel. The operation of the gun consists of placing the grain in the vessel, closing the lid and raising the pressure and temperature into the gun to about $1·38 \times 10^3$ kPa (200 psi). The quick-opening lid is activated, causing rapid pressure drop. The pressure drop instantaneously causes the moisture in the grain to 'flash off' as steam. The guns can be single-shot or multiple-shot automatic operations. Another group of cereals is made by oven-puffing. Specially prepared rice or corn grains or their mixtures are heated to 288–343°C in order to puff or precondition for further processing. Most puffed rice cereal sold in the USA is oven-puffed (e.g. Rice Krispies) and is prepared from short-grain rice. The puffed grains are then screened to remove any unpuffed kernels, loosened bran, fine dust and broken kernels. The product is heated to remove any additional moisture. Processes such as coating or vitamin enrichment can be carried out during the drying operation.

Shredded Cereals

Shredded wheat, one of the oldest mass-produced cereals, is still an important cereal. White wheat is the primary grain, because the finished product ends up with a golden colour. Other varieties of wheat, as well as other cereals such as rice, corn and oats, can also be incorporated to make shredded products. The grains are cleaned, cooked in boiling water, partially dried and tempered. The shredding operation consists of passing the tempered grain between two rollers. One roller is grooved and the other is smooth. Strong forces in the magnitude of $6·9 \times 10^3$ kPa (1000 psi) of roller length are often required to maintain the rollers in tight contact. The moist grain is plasticized, squeezed into the grooves of the roller and emerges as strands roughly 1 mm in diameter. These strands are removed, accumulated in multiple layers and formed into biscuits or bite-sized pieces. A refinement of the shred process is the use of a shred roller with added cross-grooves, which provide lateral strands that can tie the shreds together in a coherent sheet. Mixtures of other cereal products, along with sugar, salt, malt and flavouring, can also be cooked by extrusion or other devices, equilibrated and shredded.

The formed pieces are oven-dried and baked to desired colour, texture and moisture. The baking procedure is done in a highly specialized manner to impart fluffy texture, particularly in products containing rice and corn. Various flavourings, nutrients, antioxidants, etc. can also be used during drying and baking.

Granola Cereals

The main grain used to make granola cereals is either regular rolled oats or quick-cook oats. The cereal products are mixed with desired nut pieces, coconut, brown sugar, honey, malt extract, dried milk, dried fruits, water and vegetable oil. The liquid and dried ingredients are mixed separately, then mixed together, and spread in a uniform layer on the band of a continuous oven. The baking temperatures are in the range of 150–220°C, until the product is uniformly toasted to a light brown colour and the moisture is reduced to about 3%. After baking, the product is broken into small pieces and packaged.

Extruded Expanded Cereals

The successful application of extrusion technology for producing cereal products from grain flours or meal mixtures by continuous conditioning, cooking, formulating, has been an important achievement of the BC processing industry. The extruders can be single-screw, twin-screw, low-shear, high-shear, and combinations of these or other features. The extrusion technology was developed both to produce feed material and to produce flaked, puffed, shredded and expanded cereals. To produce extruded expanded cereals, the cereal flour mixtures having about 25–30% moisture are conditioned, cooked and extruded. The perforations in the die at the end of the extruder, as well as knife cutting, can control the shape, size and even texture. Sudden change from high-pressure and high-temperature to ambient conditions as the product exits the extruder imparts the necessary expansion, texture and other characteristics. The extruded products are coated with mixtures of sugar, lipid, vitamins, minerals, etc., and are then oven-dried to desired moisture levels.

Hot Cereals

Hot cereals are products of a single grain, or a simple mixture, that require cooking or heating in water before consumption. The main HC products are rolled oats, farina and corn grits.

The oat kernels are first dehulled by an impact process. The resulting groats are steamed to deactivate lipase, lipoxygenase and peroxidase enzymes, then flattened, dried and packaged. Quick-cook oats are made by steel cutting groats into three or four pieces before the steaming and flaking process. Instant oat flakes are made by subjecting groats to a special proprietary process, which results in rapid cooking of the flakes. Incorporation of 0·1–1·0% of an edible gum onto the oat surface during processing was reported to achieve this objective.

Instant products essentially require addition of boiling water and stirring to make the product ready for consumption. The industry has successfully incorporated dried fruits, nuts and other flavourings to make the instant oat products attractive to the consumers.

Wheat farina is another important hot cereal. In the USA, both farina and enriched farina have to meet legal standards of identity. Farina is basically wheat endosperm, preferably obtained from hard red spring or winter wheats, the granules of which stay intact during cooking at home. Farina is normally obtained by drawing off chunks of endosperm during milling of wheat into bread flour. The product is heated at around 60°C for 15 min or so to kill insects, etc., before packaging. Quick and instant products are prepared by the use of disodium phosphate, enzymes and other treatments. Similarly, wheat germ, bran, malted barley, cocoa and other flavourings are mixed into farina to enhance the consumer appeal.

Other important HC products are corn grits and wheat products such as bulgur wheat and cracked wheats. These products are generally used as a cereal accompaniment to other meal menu components, e.g. eggs, sausage, meat and related preparations. Corn grits are mostly used in southern parts of the USA and are usually garnished with butter and salt, not with sugar and milk as in traditional breakfast cereals. They are produced by regular dry milling of white degermed corn and can be fortified with vitamins and minerals. Bulgur or gelatinized wheat is one of the oldest cereal-based foods, which has been consumed for centuries in Turkey, Syria, Jordan, Lebanon and Egypt. To prepare bulgur wheat, the durum or other common hard, or even soft, wheat varieties are soaked in water and heated to about 90°C for 2–3 h to gelatinize the starch. During this operation, light foreign material floats on the surface and is removed. The cooked wheat is cooled, dried, moistened, peeled, redried, cleaned and sized. Peeling (optional) is done to remove the bran. The process can be performed on batches (as practised in homes or cottage industry) or in large-scale continuous operations, which exist in Syria, India and the USA. The usage of bulgur depends upon the particle size of the finished product. Coarse bulgur similar to rice is boiled or steamed with meats or vegetables. Fine bulgur (called smesma) is used in many other traditional dishes. These products have good shelf life because cooking destroys insects present in harvested crops.

There are a number of other special food products, such as corn soy milk, which have been developed either under the auspices of US Department of Agriculture (PL-480) or the United Nations (UN) to meet the unique nutritional needs of populations in developing countries. These foods are formulated by mixing gelatinized cereals, defatted oilseed, milk components, minerals and vitamins. These foods are used as gruel, weanling food and for supplementing other foods.

Significance in the Diet and Fortification

Breakfast cereals are one of the most highly fortified foods in both vitamins and minerals. One serving, typically can supply 25% of the Recommended Dietary Allowances (RDAs) of most vitamins and trace minerals. Some consumer groups have characterized them as nutritional supplements rather than as breakfast foods. The cereal industry, on the other hand, has justified these practices by claiming that they fulfil a genuine need to improve the overall nutritional need of the consumers: Nationwide Food Consumption surveys had shown that some of the US population had inadequate intakes of several vitamins and minerals; vitamin A, pyridoxine, calcium, iron, zinc and magnesium were often inadequately consumed by several groups. *See* Calcium, Physiology; Food Fortification; Iron, Physiology; Magnesium; Vitamin B$_6$, Properties and Determination; Retinol, Physiology; Zinc, Physiology

The practice of fortification of cereal foods started in 1941, when the Food and Drug Administration (FDA) established the standard of identity for enriched flour. These recommendations developed after extensive discussions of the various committees of the American Medical Association, hearings sponsored by the FDA, and the Food and Nutrition Board. As a result of these meetings, various guidelines were developed: (1) the intake of nutrient is below the desirable level in the diet of a significant number of people; (2) the food used to supply the nutrient is likely to be consumed in quantities that will make a significant contribution to the diet of the population in need; (3) the addition of nutrient is not likely to create imbalance of essential nutrients; (4) the nutrient added is stable under proper conditions of storage; (5) the nutrient is physiologically available from the food; and (6) there is reasonable assurance against excessive intake to a level of toxicity. Various studies have confirmed that fortification of BC food is appropriate and it has contributed significantly in improving overall nutrition.

Many nutritionists consider eating breakfast regularly as one of the important health habits associated with subsequent favourable health status and reduced mortality. Breakfast consumers were found to do significantly more work in the morning than those who did not. Children and the elderly (above 65 years old) are the largest consumers of BC. Half of the school-age children in the USA prepare their own breakfast because more than 60% of their mothers work outside their homes. These groups are more likely to skip breakfast. Studies have indeed confirmed that BC consumers are likely to skip fewer breakfasts and they obtained higher levels of vitamins and minerals than those who did not. Most BC also contain 2–5 g of fibre per serving. Some high-fibre products can provide 10 g or more of fibre and thus help the consumer to improve their fibre intake and to meet the recent recommendations of the National Cancer Institute. The high-fibre diet, of course, lowers the absorption of trace minerals. Cereals, with few exceptions, are not high in protein contents. In some cereals, such as puffed, flaked and toasted products, their proteins may have little or no biological values, due to excessive Maillard browning. Some RTE cereals may also be high in sugar, salt (sodium) and saturated fats. Nevertheless, BC with milk and fruit make an inexpensive, nutritious and easy-to-prepare breakfast. *See* Browning, Nonenzymatic; Dietary Fibre, Properties and Sources

Packaging, Storage and Spoilage

The BC industry, over the years, has developed efficient processing, packaging, storage and shipping technologies to supply consumers with cereal foods which routinely have 6 months or longer shelf life. It is indeed quite a feat to have such an array of vitamins and minerals, which often interact with each other, in a highly processed food and yet end up with a wholesome product with a desirable flavour and texture. In the process, industry has developed novel vitamin 'encapsulation' and techniques for the incorporation of antioxidants in the packaging material. The BC packages not only protect the product against moisture, oxygen and insects during shipping and storage but also provide attractive consumer appeal at the point of purchase. The industry has accomplished this by establishing effective Hazard Analysis Critical Control Points, following Good Manufacturing Practices and other quality control measures.

Novel and Unusual Products

Over the last decade or so, the BC industry has been dominated by the introduction of cereal products

Breakfast Cereals

containing fibre and oat components. These products account for most of the increase in BC consumption and popularity, but this trend appears to be levelling off. A recent study has concluded that high-fibre and low-fibre dietary grain supplements reduce serum cholesterol levels about equally, probably by replacing dietary fat. Although this study has been criticized for its poor design and its conclusions have been challenged, it may still be responsible for the decreased impetus to test-market new fibre-containing cereal products. The National Labeling and Education Act of 1990, which was signed into US law on 8 November 1990, probably also contributed to re-evaluation of product development, marketing and advertisement strategies by the BC industry.

It may be that the BC industry will now endeavour to develop new products made from whole grains which are also low in saturated fats, sugar and salts (sodium). It will be quite a challenge to develop new, tasty and long-shelf-life products without these additives. In the meantime, the BC industry will probably consolidate their existing products by modifying them as needed, to conform with new labelling law and health claim regulations.

Bibliography

Anonymous (1990) Cereals slow after oat bran flurry. *Milling and Baking News* 69(30): 37–44.
Fast RB and Caldwell EF (ed.) (1990) *Breakfast Cereals and How They Are Made*. St Paul, Minnesota: American Association of Cereal Chemists.
Leveille GA (1984) Food fortification – opportunities and pitfalls. *Food Technology* 38(1): 58–63.
Miller RC (1988) Continuous cooking of breakfast cereals. *Cereal Foods World* 33: 284–291.
Pomeranz Y (ed.) (1988) Wheat: Chemistry and Technology Volume I & II. St Paul, Minnesota: American Association of Cereal Chemists.

Ranjit S. Kadan
US Department of Agriculture, New Orleans, USA

Dietary Importance

Cereal-based foods are by far the major source of energy, protein, B vitamins and minerals for the world population. In many countries, diets have a single cereal as the primary staple. The most widely used cereals are rice, wheat and maize. These cereals constitute the main staple for Asia, Europe and America, respectively. In Africa and India, sorghum and millets are widely grown and consumed.

According to the Food and Agriculture Organization (FAO), the amount and proportion of food energy and protein provided by vegetables (mainly cereals) in human diets in 1986–1988 were 2253 cal per day (84·3%) and 45·8 g per day (65·4%), respectively. Cereal grains are considered primarily as caloric or starchy foods and, more recently, as an important source of dietary fibre. However, their protein quality, especially for infants, is marginal. In developing countries, cereals are usually consumed with legumes and pulses, thus significantly increasing protein intake and, more importantly, complementing the essential amino acid composition of cereals. Protein and/or calorie malnutrition (i.e. marasmus, kwashiorkor) is prevalent among groups of people who have inadequate food intake or rely solely upon cereals as their source of protein. *See* Energy, Measurement of Food Energy; Malnutrition, The Problem of Malnutrition

Cereal breeders have developed corn, sorghum and barley genotypes with high lysine which results in an improved protein quality and nutritional value. A high lysine and tryptophan corn, called quality protein maize, with satisfactory grain yield and structure, looks especially promising for commercial use. *See* individual cereals

Carbohydrates

Cereals provide about 50% of human caloric intake. Starch is the most abundant carbohydrate and the main contributor of calories (Table 1). It is composed of molecules of branched amylopectin and linear amylose. Most cereals contain 70–75% amylopectin. Waxy maize, rice and sorghum contain more than 95% amylopectin. Most food processes partially or totally gelatinize the starch granules, making the molecules more prone to amylase hydrolysis. *See* Starch, Structure, Properties and Determination

Starch is highly digestible by the human digestive system. Practically all starch disappears in the gastro-intestinal tract. A small portion of the starch (1–5%) resists enzymatic hydrolysis when cereal foods are thermically abused. This residual starch can be quantified in the soluble dietary fibre residue and is highly susceptible to fermentation in the large intestine. *See* Starch, Resistant Starch

Other factors that can decrease starch digestibility are excessive amounts of fibre and enzyme inhibitors (i.e. tannins). The digestible energy of cereals is negatively and positively related to the grain's fibre and lipid contents, respectively. Refined grains contain more digestible energy than whole products (Table 1). As a result of its high fat and low fibre content, maize contains high quantities of digestible energy.

Cereals contain small quantities of soluble carbohydrates (i.e. glucose, fructose, maltose); they are

Table 1. Nutrient composition of cereal grains[a]

Cereal	Proximate composition					Starch (%)	Digestible energy (kcal kg^{-1})	Dietary fibre	
	Protein (%)	Ether extract (%)	Crude fibre (%)	Ash (%)	NFE (%)			Total (%)	Soluble (%)
Wheat									
Hard	14·4	2·3	2·9	1·9	78·5	64·0	3865	12·1	1·7
	11·5–17·0	1·8–2·8	2·8–3·0	1·8–2·0	75·2–82·1				
Soft	9·9	2·8	2·7	1·7	82·9	69·0	3865	12·1	1·7
	8·0–12·0	2·6–2·9	2·5–2·8	1·8–1·9	80·4–85·1				
Durum	13·2	2·8	2·8	2·0	79·2	70·2	4056	12·1	1·7
	12·0–15·6	1·8–3·8	2·4–3·1	1·8–2·1	75·4–82.0				
Rice									
Paddy	7·5	2·4	10·2	4·7	75·2	—	2821	—	—
	6·7–9·0	1·7–2·7	8·4–12·1	3·4–6·0	70·2–79·8				
Brown	9·2	2·5	0·9	1·5	85·9	77·2	4321	3·7	0·9
	8·3–10·1	1·8–3·3	0·7–1·2	1·2–1·8	83·6–88·0				
Milled	7·8	0·5	0·4	0·6	90·7	90·2	3938	1·3	0·4
	7·3–8·3	0·3–0·6	0·2–0·6	0·3–0·9	89·6–91·9				
Maize									
Dent	9·1	4·4	3·0	1·7	81·8	71·8	4056	12·8	1·1
	8·1–11·5	3·9–5·8	2·4–3·5	1·4–2·0	77·2–84·2				
Flinty	11·1	4·9	2·2	1·7	80·1	—	4056	—	—
	9·5–12·8	4·0–5·8	1·6–2·8	1·4–2·0	76·6–83·5				
Popcorn	12·1	4·6	2·3	1·8	79·2	62·3	—	13·1	0·4
	11·0–13·2	4·0–5·3	2·2–2·4	1·6–1·9	77·2–81·2				
Sweet	13·2	4·6	2·7	2·3	77·0	54·1	4145	9·4	1·2
	12·1–14·2	3·7–9·0	2·2–3·2	2·0–2·7	70·9–80·1				
Barley	11·5	2·2	5·6	2·9	77·8	58·5	3543	15·4	3·9
	7·5–15·6	1·8–2·6	5·3–5·9	2·6–3·1	72·8–82·8				
Rye	13·4	1·8	2·1	2·0	80·7	68·3	3794	16·1	3·8
	12·6–14·5	1·6–2·2	1·6–2·6	1·7–2·2	78·5–82·5				
Oats									
Whole	17·1	6·4	11·3	3·2	62·0	52·8	3058	—	—
	12·4–24·4	4·5–10·3	10·4–14·3	2·9–3·4	47·6–69·8				
Groats	16·9	7·4	1·6	2·1	72·0	65·0	4316	12·5	6·6
	13·8–22·5	5·9–8·4	1·0–3·3	1·9–2·4	65·2–77·4				
Sorghum	11·0	3·2	2·7	1·8	81·3	73·8	3880	11·8	1·0
	7·3–15·6	0·5–5·2	1·2–6·6	1·1–4·5	68·1–89·9				
Millets									
Pearl	14·5	5·1	2·0	2·0	76·4	60·5	2822	—	—
	8·6–19·4	1·5–6·8	1·4–7·3	1·6–3·6	62·9–86·9				
Finger	8·0	1·5	3·0	3·0	84·5	59·0	—	—	—
	6·0–10·9	1·0–4·6	2·0–6·8	2·3–3·9	73·8–88·7				
Italian	11·7	3·9	7·0	3·0	74·2	59·1	3395	—	—
	6·0–14·0	1·2–5·2	2·6–8·6	1·5–3·6	68·3–88·7				
Proso	11·0	3·5	9·0	3·6	72·9	56·1	3636	—	—
	6·4–12·8	2·9–4·9	4·6–12·0	1·4–5·0	65·3–84·7				
Japanese	11·8	4·9	14·3	4·9	64·1	62·0	—	—	—
	11·2–12·7	2·5–6·3	13·9–14·7	4·7–5·0	61·3–68·0				
Fonio	8·7	2·8	8·0	3·8	76·6	—	—	—	—
	5·1–10·4	2·1–5·2	4·6–11·3	1·8–6·0	67·1–86·4				
Kodo	10·4	3·7	9·7	3·6	72·6	72·0	—	—	—
	6·2–13·1	3·2–4·9	8·4–11·0	3·0–4·1	66·9–79·2				
Teff	10·9	2·4	2·4	2·2	82·1	—	—	—	—
	7·9–12·6	2·3–2·5							

[a]All values are expressed on a dry matter basis. Protein conversion factors: for wheat, 5·7; rice, 5·95; other cereals, 6·25.
NFE = Nitrogen free extract.

Dietary Importance

therefore suitable foods for diabetics. Highly refined cereals have a higher glycaemic index than whole grain products. *See* Glucose, Glucose Tolerance and the Glycaemic Index

Whole cereal grains are considered a rich source of fibre (Table 1). However, foods from grains have marked differences in the amount and type of dietary fibre. Fibre components are concentrated in the outer tissues of the kernel (pericarp). The dietary fibre content in cereal-based foods varies greatly depending on the extent of milling. Refined flours lose most of their fibre during decortication and milling. All cereals are considered a rich source of insoluble dietary fibre (i.e. cellulose, insoluble hemicellulose). Insoluble fibre binds water, speeds up intestinal transit and binds some carcinogens. Epidemiological evidence has related a high-fibre diet to a lower incidence of diabetes, obesity and diverticular disease. A high dietary fibre consumption benefits diabetics because of the reduced diffusion of glucose in the intestinal mucosa and the diminished insulin secretion rate. *See* Dietary Fibre, Properties and Sources; Dietary Fibre, Determination; Dietary Fibre, Effects of Fibre on Absorption; Dietary Fibre, Fibre and Disease Prevention

Oats, barley and rye are considered good sources of soluble dietary fibre (i.e. pentosans, β-glucans, soluble hemicellulose) which has been associated with increased excretion of bile salts and dietary cholesterol, thus lowering blood cholesterol levels.

Proteins

Cereal grains provide about 50% of our total protein intake. Genotype, environment and growing conditions affect the amount of protein in the kernel. In general, brown rice and oats contain the lowest and highest protein content, respectively (Table 1). Protein quality is mostly dictated by the amino acid profile and digestibility (Table 2). The apparent protein digestibilities in cereals range from 80% to 90%. Sorghum (especially kernels with condensed tannins), whole barley, rye and oats are consistently lower in digestibility than other cereals. Milling, decortication, fermentation and germination all increase protein digestibilities because of the removal of fibre and the enzymatic breakdown of proteins. *See* Protein, Chemistry; Protein, Quality

The storage protein in cereals (prolamines) contains small amounts of essential amino acids. The albumins and globulins, mainly located in the germ, contain the best essential amino acid profile. High-lysine cultivars of maize, sorghum and barley are genetically modified to contain lower amounts of prolamines, and higher amounts of albumins and globulins. Thus they have a more balanced protein. *See* Amino Acids, Metabolism

For all cereals, the most limiting amino acid is lysine.

Oats, rice, rye, barley and the high-lysine cultivars contain a more favourable essential amino acid composition or amino acid score than the rest of the cereals (Table 2). Lysine deficiency is observed particularly in postweaned infants who rely on cereals and/or starchy tubers as the only food source. The supplementation of cereal-based foods with small quantities of legumes or animal foods drastically improves protein intake and protein quality. The next most limiting amino acids for maize and rest of the cereals are tryptophan and threonine, respectively.

Decortication or milling partially or totally removes the pericarp and germ tissues, therefore improving the digestibility and reducing the lysine level. Malting improves protein quality due to enzymatic degradation of proteins. Fermentation improves protein quality via improved digestibility and *de novo* synthesis of lysine by the fermenting bacteria.

Lipids

Lipids are relatively minor constituents in cereal grains (Table 1). However, cereal lipids are rich in the essential fatty acid, linoleic acid (18:2; 30–60% of total fatty acids), and practically devoid of saturated fatty acids. Cereals contain trace quantities of phytosterols; they do not have any cholesterol. Cereals with yellow endosperm (i.e. yellow corn, yellow sorghum, durum wheat) contain some provitamin A activity (carotenes). Various types of tocopherols are responsible for the vitamin E activity of cereal grains. Degermination of cereal grains greatly reduces the content of lipid and tocopherol. *See* Fatty Acids, Properties; Lipids, Occurrence

Minerals and Vitamins

The pericarp, germ and aleurone layer are rich in vitamins and minerals. Refined cereal products therefore lose part of these important nutrients. The enrichment of cereal-based foods is aimed toward the replacement of minerals (Fe) and vitamins (thiamin, riboflavin, pyridoxine) lost during milling. In some countries, the enrichment of cereal-based foods is required by law.

In general, cereals are a very poor source of calcium, except for finger millet and teff (Table 3). Some food processes, such as nixtamalization of maize for tortilla production, greatly increase calcium.

Phosphorus is the mineral found in greatest amounts (Table 3). Unfortunately, its availability is questionable because it is associated with phytic acid. The phytic acid has the property of binding strongly with cations, thus decreasing their bioavailability. Phytic acid decreases significantly during malting and fermentation due to

Table 2. Amino acid composition of cereal grains[a]

Amino acid (g per 100 g of protein)	Wheat		Maize		Rice		Sorghum		Barley
	Hard	Durum	Normal	High-lysine	Brown	Milled	Normal	High-lysine	
Essential									
Phenylalanine	4·6	4·1	4·8	4·3	5·2	5·2	5·1	4·9	5·2
Histidine	2·0	1·9	2·9	3·8	2·5	2·5	2·1	2·3	2·1
Isoleucine	3·0	3·6	3·6	3·4	4·1	4·5	4·1	3·9	3·6
Leucine	6·3	7·0	12·4	9·0	8·6	8·1	14·2	12·3	6·6
Lysine	2·3	2·2	2·7	4·3	4·1	3·9	2·1	3·0	3·5
Methionine	1·2	0·9	1·9	2·1	2·4	1·7	1·0	1·6	2·2
Threonine	2·4	2·9	3·5	3·9	4·0	3·7	3·3	3·3	3·2
Tryptophan	1·5	—	0·5	0·9	1·4	1·3	1·0	0·9	1·5
Valine	3·6	4·6	4·9	5·6	5·8	6·7	5·4	5·1	5·0
Nonessential									
Aspartic acid	4·7	4·7	6·4	7·7	9·3	9·8	6·4	7·5	6·0
Glutamic acid	30·3	32·3	19·2	17·1	17·3	19·3	20·6	20·1	25·5
Alanine	3·1	4·8	7·7	6·3	5·8	5·8	8·6	8·4	2·1
Arginine	4·0	3·5	4·8	6·9	9·5	8·8	3·5	4·5	4·6
Cysteine	2·8	—	1·4	—	2·3	2·2	1·6	1·5	1·8
Glycine	3·8	6·5	3·8	5·0	4·8	4·8	2·9	3·5	3·9
Proline	10·1	13·4	8·2	9·1	5·0	4·0	7·9	7·6	11·6
Serine	4·2	5·7	4·6	4·7	5·3	4·3	4·1	4·2	3·8
Tyrosine	2·7	2·0	4·2	3·5	4·2	5·0	3·2	4·2	2·8
Amino acid score (%)	42·3	40·4	49·6	79·0	75·4	71·7	38·6	55·1	64·3
Protein digestibility	89·8	87·9	88·2	88·9	88·5	89·0	85·9	88·9	84·9

	Rye	Oats	Groats	Millets						
				Pearl	Finger	Proso	Japanese	Italian	Kodo	Teff
Essential										
Phenylalanine	5·0	5·4	4·2	5·2	5·2	5·2	5·9	5·5	5·8	5·7
Histidine	2·4	2·4	2·2	2·2	2·2	2·2	1·9	2·9	1·8	3·2
Isoleucine	3·7	4·2	3·9	4·4	4·4	4·6	4·5	5·9	3·1	4·0
Leucine	6·4	7·5	7·4	11·0	9·5	12·9	11·5	14·1	8·6	8·5
Lysine	3·5	4·2	4·2	2·9	2·9	2·2	1·7	2·2	3·2	3·5
Methionine	1·6	2·3	2·5	2·0	3·1	2·0	1·8	2·6	1·7	4·1
Threonine	3·1	3·3	3·3	3·9	4·2	3·3	2·7	4·3	2·9	4·3
Tryptophan	0·8	—	1·3	2·3	1·5	0·9	1·0	1·4	0·8	1·4
Valine	4·9	5·8	5·3	5·7	6·6	5·1	6·1	5·1	4·2	5·5
Nonessential										
Aspartic acid	6·7	9·2	8·9	8·6	6·5	5·7	6·1	6·9	6·3	6·6
Glutamic acid	24·7	21·6	23·9	20·7	20·3	20·4	23·9	18·8	23·1	24·8
Alanine	2·4	5·1	5·0	8·5	6·2	10·7	9·3	8·9	5·5	5·7
Arginine	5·9	6·4	6·9	5·3	4·5	3·2	3·6	2·8	3·6	5·0
Cysteine	2·0	1·7	1·6	2·1	2·6	1·6	2·7	1·4	1·0	0·9
Glycine	4·0	5·1	4·9	3·3	4·0	2·2	2·3	2·9	3·8	3·8
Proline	9·1	5·7	4·7	6·6	7·0	7·2	10·1	10·6	7·2	5·5
Serine	4·1	4·0	4·2	4·9	5·1	6·3	5·6	5·8	4·1	5·2
Tyrosine	2·6	2·6	3·1	3·2	3·6	2·4	2·4	2·6	3·8	3·9
Amino acid score (%)	64·3	77·2	77·2	53·3	53·3	40·4	31·2	40·4	58·8	64·3
Protein digestibility	86·7	86·2	90·6	89·0	—	89·9	—	89·8	—	—

[a] Essential amino acid requirements for infants (g per 100 g of protein): lysine, 5·44; methionine and cysteine, 3·52; threonine, 4·0; isoleucine, 4·0; leucine, 7·04; phenylalanine and tyrosine, 6·08; histidine, 1·4; tryptophan, 0·96. Tyrosine and cysteine are not essential amino acids but they can spare the requirement for phenylalanine and methionine, respectively.

Table 3. Mineral and vitamin composition of cereal grains

Nutrient	Wheat Hard	Wheat Durum	Maize	Rice Brown	Rice Milled	Sorghum	Barley
Minerals							
Ca (%)	0·03	0·04	0·03	0·03	0·02	0·04	0·04
P (%)	0·35	0·51	0·29	0·25	0·12	0·35	0·56
Phytic acid (%)	0·97	—	0·71	0·56	—	0·77	1·06
K (%)	0·36	0·49	0·37	0·17	0·10	0·38	0·50
Na (%)	0·04	—	0·03	0·03	0·00	0·05	0·02
Mg (%)	0·14	0·17	0·14	0·19	0·03	0·19	0·14
Fe (ppm)	40·1	47·8	30·0	28·0	19·0	50·0	36·7
Co (ppm)	0·05	—	0·1	0·07	0·01	3·1	0·04
Cu (ppm)	4·9	5·6	4·0	4·2	2·0	10·8	15·1
Mn (ppm)	40·0	33·5	5·0	24·0	12·0	16·3	18·9
Zn (ppm)	30·9	41·0	20·0	18·0	10·0	15·4	23·6
Vitamins							
Thiamin (mg per 100 g)	0·57	0·67	0·38	0·34	0·07	0·46	0·44
Riboflavin (mg per 100 g)	0·12	0·11	0·14	0·09	0·03	0·15	0·15
Nicotinic acid (mg per 100 g)	7·40	11·10	2·80	4·62	1·60	4·84	7·20
Pyridoxine (mg per 100 g)	0·35	0·43	0·53	0·92	0·45	0·59	0·44
Pantothenic acid (mg per 100 g)	1·36	—	0·66	1·35	0·75	1·25	0·57
Biotin (mg per 100 g)	0·01	—	0·01	0·01	—	0·02	0·01
Folacin (mg per 100 g)	0·04	0·04	0·03	0·02	0·02	0·02	0·04
Carotenes (mg kg^{-1})	0·2	0·2	29·5	—	—	15·7	1·0
Vitamin E (mg kg^{-1})	12·8	28·0	24·0	1·7	0·14	13·8	24·8

				Millets Pearl	Millets Finger	Millets Proso	Millets Italian	Millets Kodo	Millets Teff	Millets Fonio
	Rye	Oats	Groats	Pearl	Finger	Proso	Italian	Kodo	Teff	Fonio
Minerals										
Ca (%)	0·05	0·11	0·08	0·01	0·33	0·01	0·01	0·01	0·17	0·03
P (%)	0·36	0·38	0·51	0·35	0·24	0·15	0·31	0·32	0·45	0·18
Phytic acid (%)	0·97	1·80	—	—	—	0·32	—	—	—	—
K (%)	0·47	0·47	0·44	0·44	0·43	0·21	0·27	0·17	0·31	0·16
Na (%)	0·01	0·02	—	0·01	0·02	0·01	0·01	0·01	0·02	0·02
Mg (%)	0·11	0·13	0·14	0·13	0·11	0·12	0·13	0·13	0·18	0·40
Fe (ppm)	38·0	62·0	47·2	74·9	46·0	33·1	32·6	7·0	14·9	36·0
Co (ppm)	—	0·05	—	0·50	0·10	—	—	—	0·06	3·30
Cu (ppm)	9·0	4·7	4·8	6·2	0·3	8·3	9·2	—	4·4	15·0
Mn (ppm)	58·4	45·0	46·0	18·0	7·5	18·1	21·9	—	2·5	30·0
Zn (ppm)	32·2	37·0	35·8	29·5	15·0	17·2	21·4	—	6·7	30·0
Vitamins										
Thiamin (mg per 100 g)	0·69	0·77	0·72	0·38	0·48	0·63	0·48	0·32	0·45	0·30
Riboflavin (mg per 100 g)	0·26	0·14	0·16	0·22	0·12	0·22	0·12	0·05	0·10	0·10
Nicotinic acid (mg per 100 g)	1·52	0·97	0·91	2·70	1·30	1·32	3·70	0·70	2·00	3·00
Pyridoxine (mg per 100 g)	0·34	0·12	0·21	—	—	—	—	—	—	—
Pantothenic acid (mg per 100 g)	0·73	1·36	1·23	1·09	—	1·10	0·82	—	—	—
Biotin (mg per 100 g)	0·01	0·02	—	—	—	—	—	—	—	—
Folacin (mg per 100 g)	0·05	0·06	—	—	—	—	0·02	—	—	—
Carotenes (mg kg^{-1})	—	—	—	5·4	—	—	—	—	—	—
Vitamin E (mg kg^{-1})	16·6	16·7	17·0	19·0	22·0	—	31·0	—	—	—

Dietary Importance

activation of phytases. These processes considerably improve the bioavailability of minerals.

Cereals are considered a good source of potassium and are practically devoid of sodium. Whole grains provide a significant source of magnesium, iron, zinc and copper, which is reduced by degermination, decortication and milling.

Cereals are also considered an important source of B vitamins, but dried-matured grains do not contain vitamin C. According to the FAO (1990), vegetable products (mainly cereal grains) provided 80·5%, 52·5% and 72% of the 1986–1988 world consumption of thiamin, riboflavin and nicotinic acid, respectively. The B vitamins are concentrated in the aleurone layer. Beriberi (a thiamin deficiency disease), endemic in eastern and southern Asia, is prevalent among people who consume milled rice. Milled rice contains about 10% of the thiamin of brown rice (Table 3).

Nicotinic acid is found in a free and bound form and can be synthesized from tryptophan. The alkali treatment of maize for tortilla production considerably improves nitotinic acid bioavailability because the glycosidic bond that renders it unavailable is alkali labile. Nicotinic acid deficiency produces pellagra, which causes dermatitis, diarrhoea and dementia and has been prevalent in regions of Southern Africa where people rely on maize as the main food source. *See* individual vitamins and minerals

Toxins and Contaminants

Naturally Occurring Toxins

All cereals contain relatively high levels of phytic acid which binds minerals (cations). Germination and/or fermentation improves mineral bioavailability due to the enzymatic activity of phytases and bacteria.

Brown sorghums contain condensed tannins in their testa. The brown sorghums are grown to avoid bird damage and grain deterioration due to sprouting and weathering. The tannins bind hydrophobically with, and precipitate, proteins in food systems, thus lowering digestibility. Germination and the treatment of grain with calcium oxide (CaO), potassium carbonate (K_2CO_3), ammonium bicarbonate ((NH_4)HCO_3) or sodium bicarbonate ($NaHCO_3$) detoxifies the grain and consequently improves its nutritional value. In Tanzania, Magadi soda is used to detoxify brown sorghum in small villages.

A higher incidence of goitre among pearl millet eaters in West Africa (Sudan) has been attributed to a goitrogenic compound. The goitrogen has been identified as a thioamide, mainly found in the bran and endosperm. Heat treatment (autoclaving) apparently detoxifies the grain. Trypsin inhibitors and saponins have been isolated in pearl millet. *See* Goitrogens and Antithyroid Compounds

Contaminants

Cereal grains are susceptible to mould attack, especially when storage conditions are inappropriate. Some moulds produce many toxic compounds that can severely affect human health or even cause death. The most important mycotoxin is the one produced by *Aspergillus flavus*. Aflatoxins have been found in most cereal grains, but they are most prevalent in maize. The toxin is a potent hepatocarcinogen at concentrations in parts per billion. The most prevalent aflatoxins in cereal grains are B_1 and B_2. For optimum growth and aflatoxin production, the mould requires a relative humidity of 85% and a temperature range of 27–30°C. The alkali treatment of maize for tortilla production significantly reduces the amount of aflatoxins. Most of the aflatoxins end up in the steep and wash waters. *See* Mycotoxins, Occurrence and Determination; Spoilage, Moulds in Food Spoilage

Ochratoxin is produced predominantly by the storage fungus *Aspergillus ochraceus*. Toxicity is characterized by nephropathy, mild degeneration of the liver, and enteritis in swine, poultry and humans.

Species of *Fusarium* produce toxins that affect humans and animals. An example is scab wheat and barley contaminated with *F. graminearum*. The preparation of bakery products with contaminated grain causes vomiting and inebriation in humans.

Zeralenone, another *Fusarium* toxin, is the most frequent mycotoxin in cereal grains. It is mainly found in maize. Zeralenone produces vomiting in monogastrics, and diarrhoea, haemorrhage, swelling of genitals and infertility in swine.

Ergot (*Claviceps purpurea*) is a fungus that infects rye and, less often, wheat, barley and oats. Honey disease of millet and sorghum is caused by ergot. The toxicity of ergot has been documented for several centuries. Epidemics of poisonings have occurred in North America, the UK, Europe, Russia and other places. Ergot toxicity produces a disease commonly called 'Saint Anthony's fire', which produces gangrenous necrosis, hallucinations and convulsions. The fungi produces toxicity via the formation of alkaloids (ergotamine, ergotoxine and ergometrine). Growth of the fungus is promoted by moist, warm climatic conditions.

Bibliography

FAO (1990) Production Yearbook. *FAO Statistics Series* no. 94, vol. 43. Rome: Food and Agriculture Organization.

Finley JW and Hopkins DT (1985) *Digestibility and Amino Acid Availability in Cereal and Oilseeds*. St Paul, Minnesota: American Association of Cereal Chemists.

Dietary Importance

Hulse JH, Laing EM and Pearson OE (1980) *Sorghum and the Millets: their Composition and Nutritive Value.* New York: Academic Press.

Lorenz KJ and Kulp K (1991) *Handbook of Cereal Science and Technology.* New York: Marcel Dekker.

Mirocha CJ and Christensen CM (1982) Mycotoxins. In: Christensen CM (ed.) *Storage of Cereal Grains and their* Products. St Paul, Minnesota: American Association of Cereal Chemists.

S.O. Serna-Saldivar
Texas A & M University, Texas, USA

CEREBRAL PALSY – NUTRITIONAL MANAGEMENT

Causation and Classification of Cerebral Palsy

Cerebral palsy may be briefly defined as a group of neurological disorders caused by defects or damage to the brain *in utero* or at birth, or via infection from a variety of causes. It is characterized by muscle paralysis, abnormal (dystonic) movements and altered muscle tone.

Cerebral palsy is further classified by the nature and distribution of the motor deficits or abnormality. Hitchcock (1978) described it as a condition showing the following features:

1. Spasticity (which affects 70% of cases) produces rigidity of the limbs and inability to relax muscles.
2. Athetosis (affects 10% of cases) interferes with normal body movements and is evident by slurred speech and writhing movements of the limbs.
3. Ataxia (affects 10% of cases) results in poor balance, unsteady gait, and poor hand–eye coordination.
4. Some patients (10% of cases) may show all these disorders.

Varying nutritional disorders are found in patients with cerebral palsy, ranging from gross obesity to chronic malnutrition. For this reason the nutritional assessment of patients with cerebral palsy should be considered on an individual basis, and suitable advice and nutrition regimens drawn up for each person.

When deciding on 'ideal' nutritional status the carer is faced with several problems. These include how best to measure nutritional status in physically misshapen people, and a lack of appropriate guidelines as to what is considered a normal range for this group (especially in the UK population). Until further work is published, the most appropriate action appears to be to use patients as their own controls. Initial comparisons with other groups can be useful before intervention begins. *See* Nutritional Status, Importance of Measuring Nutritional Status

Assessing Nutritional Status

Before any intervention is commenced, it is essential to assess the patient's nutritional status in order to decide on the most appropriate therapy. It is advisable to measure height and weight, to devise the body mass index (see below), to measure biceps, triceps, subscapular and suprailiac skin folds, and to determine percentage body fat. Subjective impressions should also be recorded (e.g. does the patient appear wasted, thin or lethargic?). *See* Nutritional Status, Anthropometry and Clinical Examination

Measurement techniques may have to be altered to ensure that all patients, however physically misshapen, are measured in the same way.

Height

It may be difficult to achieve an accurate measure of height owing to physical deformity. Experience has shown that where clients cannot stand against a height measuring stick, individual parts of the body should be measured (ankle–knee, knee–hip, hip–waist, etc.). If the patient has a spinal deformity it is best to measure the outside and inside of the curvature and take an average; some workers measure the curvature of the spine. These measures are crude but provide a basis from which to assess future changes following intervention. Most patients with cerebral palsy do not achieve 'normal' growth. This may be the result of poor nutrition in early life, or of genetic and other indirect developmental factors.

Weight

Weight may also be difficult to measure in patients who are unable to stand unaided. The use of sling scales should be encouraged for those who find sitting or standing difficult or impossible. There are no standard weight–height charts for this patient group, and it is more appropriate to use individual changes in weight, rather than single measurements, as a measure of the effectiveness of nutrition intervention.

Body Mass Index

Body mass index (BMI) is calculated from height and weight (bodyweight, in kg, divided by the square of height, in m). It must be used with discretion as the inaccuracies in measurement described above may affect the results.

Mid-upper Arm Circumference and Mid-upper-Arm Muscle Circumference

Mid-upper arm circumference and mid-upper-arm muscle circumference may be affected by muscle wasting resulting from decreased activity. However, it is important to collect this information because of the possible longitudinal changes brought about by nutrition intervention. *See* Obesity, Aetiology and Assessment

Percentage Body Fat

Percentage body fat is calculated from the four skin-fold measurements (biceps, triceps, subscapular and supra-iliac) and gives an accurate measure of fat stores. There may be some problems in taking the measurements, caused by physical deformity and abnormal distribution of fat in some individuals. Total percentage body fat stores should still be within the normal range for the general population, and this value may prove to be the most discriminating measure of nutritional status in the more physically handicapped patients since it is little affected by physical deformity. The triceps skin fold measured on its own is a useful and easily accessible measure of nutritional status. Further studies are needed to validate this simple measure in this group.

Physical handicaps, in particular neurological ones, may also have important effects on nutritional status. Physical handicap can affect the ability of patients to feed themselves and make them reliant on others. This can have a profound effect on nutrient intake. Patients may dislike being fed; they may dislike the person feeding them, or the way in which they are fed. If dexterity with cutlery and crockery is a problem, the patient is reliant on others to help with cutting of food.

The ratio of staff to patients may not be high enough, and mealtimes may be rushed in order to ensure that everyone is fed. Patients may feel rushed or unable to eat quickly enough. Staff may then feel they dislike the offered food and throw it away. All these factors play a part in the adequacy of nutritional intake.

Dentition can affect the ability to chew foods. The ability to chew affects the type of food eaten and the time taken to finish meals. If patients are edentulous, this obviously affects the texture of food which can be eaten, leading to an increased use of soft or liquidized foods with an attendant loss of some labile nutrients. The ability to swallow affects not only total intake but the texture and consistency of intake (fluids, liquidized meals, etc.).

A psychological assessment can give guidance in dealing with behaviour problems and eating disorders which may lead to nutritional problems, either increased intake leading to obesity, or reduced intake leading to undernutrition.

In addition to anthropometric measurements and clinical nutritional assessment, the patient's normal food and fluid intake should be considered. It may be helpful to carry out a 3- or 5-day weighed food intake, or carers may be asked to record the patient's intake of food and fluid for 3 days. This information may then be used to assess the patient's nutritional requirements or, perhaps, restrictions, including their ability to eat required amounts or their need for supplements, tube feeding or, in severe cases, gastrostomy. Other health care professionals can be approached for their opinions and a nutritional programme developed.

As many patients are dependent on carers for all their needs, it is important to realize that the carers themselves often require help and education to ensure that they are providing the correct nutritional support. Education should be a major consideration in induction courses for new staff, and should include information on general nutrition and special problems, with both obese and underweight patients.

Obesity

Less physically handicapped people with cerebral palsy may have increased food intakes along with low activity levels, and obesity is often the result. Obesity is a major factor in other health problems, such as diabetes, cardiac and respiratory illness. In an attempt to solve the problem of obesity through restricting energy intakes, vitamin and mineral intakes may be compromised. This in turn may result in other nutrition-related problems unless the weight reduction programme is carefully planned.

Some patients may have behaviour problems, and a strict reducing diet may be deleterious to their mental condition. A dietitian can help with the formulation of an individual nutrition plan designed to cater for each person's special needs. Exercise plays an important part in losing weight and a movement therapist or physiotherapist may often help in treatment, by designing a suitable exercise programme to suit the ability of each individual. Account should be taken of the degree of physical handicap and realistic targets established for weight loss. It is important to encourage continued weight loss and not accept that because the patient is 'handicapped' they can cheat by eating what they like or excuse themselves from exercise. Obesity and its obvious health-related problems should be uppermost in the minds of those carers who are involved in the nutritional intake of patients trying to lose weight. Gross obesity also has profound effects on the social aspects of the patient's quality of life (e.g. ability to take part in sports). *See* Obesity, Treatment

Undernutrition

For many years, carers of the profoundly handicapped cerebral palsy patient struggled valiantly to ensure adequate nutritional intakes. Where there were associated chewing and swallowing problems, the task was an extremely difficult and time-consuming one. For many patients this meant tiny, child-size portions and small quantities of fluids. Nutrient intake was further reduced by the use of liquidized, mashed or puréed foods. Profoundly handicapped cerebral palsy patients were therefore thin, short in stature and at high risk of infection because nutrient intakes were grossly under recommended amounts. *See* Malnutrition, Malnutrition in Developed Countries

The problems associated with feeding profoundly handicapped cerebral palsy patients have been widely documented. These include the problem of physically handling utensils, requiring either specially adapted feeding aids or assistance with cutting food and help with eating and drinking. The use of adaptations to normal crockery and cutlery should be considered early in the assessment of treatment. An occupational therapist should be actively involved in providing equipment which is tailor-made for the individual. On no account should the use of this equipment be jeopardized by the principles of 'normalization'. If patients need a special cup, plate or table mat to make feeding easier, they should automatically receive it, and should be encouraged to use it. Progress may be monitored by attempting to introduce normal items of cutlery, but it should not adversely affect nutrient intake which should always be paramount in the carer's mind.

Hypersensitivity around the facial and oral areas leads to grossly abnormal reflexes when food and fluids are brought close to the face. The added handicap of poor lip closure, tongue thrust, dental clearances or dental decay from drug therapies all lead to increased problems in eating adequate amounts of food. Swallowing problems which can now be demonstrated by videofluoroscopy, may include silent aspiration, lack of a gag or cough reflex, and an inability to handle the food

bolus appropriately. Swallowing problems are often associated with poor muscle tone, which in turn may be related to poor nutritional intake. As food intake improves, the swallow may also improve.

A primary objective of care should be to ensure an adequate intake of fluid. Hypernatraemic dehydration has been identified in a large hospital for the mentally handicapped. It is the patients most dependent on others (i.e. the more profoundly handicapped) who run the highest risk of being dehydrated. This life-threatening condition is best remedied by ensuring an adequate intake of fluids (up to 3 l each day) and by reducing (if they are used) the use of hypertonic enemas for constipation. Ambient temperatures in patients' accommodation should also be reviewed to ensure that they are within acceptable limits; if too high they should be reduced in order to reduce water loss.

Ideal fluid and food intakes can be difficult to achieve and help and advice should be sought from a speech therapist. They will advise on the texture and consistence of the most easily manageable foods and fluids and provide instruction on the use of desensitization and feeding programmes to help with swallowing problems. Thickeners may be used to make the fluid more manageable in the mouth, but these should only be used with the advice of a dietitian.

Energy Requirements

Energy requirements vary according to the type of cerebral palsy. A patient with severe athetoid movements or hyperkinesis requires more energy to maintain bodyweight than a nonambulant spastic quadriplegic. Feeding problems are usually more severe in the profoundly handicapped individual, and the problem may be twofold – feeding problems and increased energy requirements – in an athetoid or hyperkinetic client.

Supplementation

Mealtimes and eating play a major role in developing and maintaining social interaction skills, and many psychological implications must be considered before a decision is taken to stop normal food intake for whatever reason. If a patient finds eating difficult, it is still worthwhile to continue normal food or meals of modified texture and consistency, unless otherwise indicated. A speech therapist should assess physical problems and swallowing and decide on appropriate textures and consistencies. Patients at risk of aspiration should be examined. Videofluoroscopy may be recommended to assess the risk of aspiration and to check on progress once oral feeding programmes have been established.

When only small quantities of normal foods are consumed, inadequate nutrient intake may result. Adapting normal foods by modifying texture and consistency may help. When these measures are inadequate, individual assessment is required to decide on the type and amount of supplement required. The nutritional assessment should be carried out by a dietitian or nutritionist to determine which nutrients are lacking. Nutritional supplements may then be introduced to ensure optimum nutrition.

The use of nutritional supplements should be considered very early in treatment. These may take the form of special drinks or additions to normal food. They help to increase the nutritional density of food without increasing the bulk. Thus a considerable quantity of energy and nutrients can be added to relatively small portions of food.

Tube Feeding

If swallowing problems are extreme and fluid and food intakes are low, alternative forms of nutrient intake should be considered. This may take the form of a tube feed. It is important to use this type of intervention quickly before the patient's nutritional state deteriorates too far, as this can decrease the chances of infection caused by aspiration, chronic undernutrition, and dehydration.

If a risk of aspiration is apparent, then advising 'nil by mouth' must be considered. This is obviously abhorrent to most carers, and the life-threatening risks of aspiration must be weighed against the improvements in health brought about by allowing nothing orally. The decision to give nil by mouth can be reviewed at any time and altered as swallowing improves and the chances of chest infections decrease. If there is to be nil by mouth, the introduction of tube feeding is preferable to parenteral feeding.

Nasogastric tube feeding is the least invasive form of tube feeding but experience has shown that patients already hypersensitive around the facial area can quickly become more so with the introduction of a nasogastric tube. Nasogastric tube feeding should therefore be considered only in extremely acute cases where the tube feed will be used for a matter of days or weeks at the most.

There are well-documented risks associated with nasogastric feeding, including nasal irritation, associated risks of tube displacement in patients who aspirate, and a risk of reflux and hypersensitivity. Carers of cerebral palsy patients may also wish to consider the psychological effects of the nasogastric tube in place in the nose and the public's reaction to it.

An alternative form of tube feeding is by way of a percutaneous endoscopic gastrostomy (PEG) tube. The tube is surgically placed through an endoscope, under a local anaesthetic and valium sedation, directly into the stomach. There are still associated risks with this form of feeding. Chronic reflux may continue to be a problem and require conversion to a jejunostomy tube. There may be infection at the wound site, although this should not be a problem with correct care of the site. Tube displacement has been documented in the past, but this does not appear to be a problem with more recent tubes. The PEG tube can remain in place for up to a year, reducing the need for replacement, hospital admission and nursing, and medical time. There are many benefits to this system, including optimal patient nutrition. The tube is the only visible component and this is perhaps an important aesthetic consideration; no-one is aware of it unless the feed is being administered.

There are other physical benefits with an increased chance of desensitization around the face and oral area and possibility of the longer term reintroduction of oral feeding once the nutritional state improves.

The PEG tube may be removed if oral feeding is reestablished, or remain in place for use during times of emergency, e.g. illness.

Feeds should be established slowly and the advice of a dietitian who has experience of this method of feeding should always by sought. Many patients may not have been supplied with adequate nutrient and fluid intakes for many years and any regimen should be drawn up after careful individual assessment of nutritional needs. This should be altered frequently to suit the changing needs of the patient. Refeeding oedema should be noted in the profoundly undernourished patient, and care and time should be taken in reaching the patient's optimal intake (often many weeks or months may pass before an ideal intake can be achieved). Once target weight has been reached and oral feeding improved, the tube feed may be reduced if oral intake increases.

Outcome of Nutritional Support

Nutritional support has obvious benefits in the cerebral palsy population. More work is required to validate the full extent of the improvements noted to date. Physical and psychological improvements that are readily apparent include the following.

Bowel Habits

Carers of patients who may have required suppositories every third or fourth day from a very early age, to ensure that the bowel does not become impacted, find that once nutritional support is introduced, bowel habit improves dramatically and suppositories can be discontinued.

Behaviour Problems

Patients who are undernourished or slightly dehydrated are often misdiagnosed as having behaviour problems (including irritability, aggression, lethargy and apathy). Once nutritional support has commenced these problems often diminish or disappear.

Infections and Wound Healing

Hospital admissions for chest infections are reduced when the incidence of aspiration is reduced following the introduction of tube feeding. Wound healing is seen to improve when nutrition is optimal.

Costs

It obviously costs money to provide the necessary equipment and products for adequate nutritional support. The benefits and cost savings derived from improved nutrition far outweigh the initial outlay.

Involvement of Other Professions

Once nutrition is improved, general wellbeing improves and other professionals may become more actively involved with the patient. These include speech therapists to improve the ability to communicate, and physiotherapists to improve ability to flex limbs and exercise (patients may now join hydrotherapy sessions).

Team Approach to Care

The only way to improve the nutrition of the cerebral palsy patient is by the combined efforts of a multidisciplinary team of professional carers who can better understand the overall approach to eating. It may be best to have a core team of carers who are responsible for the day-to-day running of the service, and an extended team whose members can be called upon for specialist advice.

The *core team* may include dietitian, speech therapist, occupational therapist, physiotherapist, nurse, and doctor.

In the *extended team* there may be a physician, ENT (ear, nose and throat) surgeon, chest physician, psychologist, behaviour therapist, psychiatrist, dentist, movement therapist, and caterers.

Institutional Care

It is still the case and will be for many years to come that in the UK many cerebral palsy patients are cared for in large institutions. This in itself has many nutritional implications.

The Type of Catering Facilities

The kitchens and catering facilities of large Victorian institutions are often small, poorly equipped and inefficient to run. It is essential that nutritional intakes are monitored.

The Budget Allowance for Catering and Food

In the UK, large institutions for mental handicap have suffered for many years from inadequate funds to provide suitable food for specialized needs. Through current research, these needs are being identified and money is being made available to help alleviate the problems.

Restricted Choice of Menus

As more money becomes available, menu choices should improve. The dietitian and caterers should work closely together to produce suitable menus.

Standard Portion Sizes Available for Men and Women

In many institutions food is calculated in standard portions. As the requirements of men and women are different, the portion sizes provided should reflect these requirements more closely.

Nutritional Knowledge of Care Staff

A major consideration for the dietitian should be the nutritional knowledge of carers, as staff can have such a significant effect on the nutritional intake of patients. A nutrition education programme should be available for all new staff and ongoing in-service education should be available as required.

Staffing Levels

In large institutions staffing levels are often less than in small homes and the domestic environment. Research is needed to decide whether or not current staffing levels are appropriate, and to make recommendations to change them if necessary. Consideration must also be given to the motivation of staff to provide adequate nutrition for their charges, and assessment of staff should take place at regular intervals to ensure that motivation remains high.

Nutrition in Cerebral Palsy

As noted above, many factors influence the nutritional status of the patient with cerebral palsy. These must all be considered in preparing individual nutrition plans for each patient, with ongoing reviews in order to adapt care plans as patients' nutritional status improves.

The results of treating individual patients with cerebral palsy are particularly gratifying, not only in terms of their improved nutritional status but also in the improved quality of life which is exhibited in the psychological sequelae of chronic malnutrition. There is no doubt that this aspect of the care of the cerebral palsy patient has been neglected in the past and will receive increasing attention as its benefits become more widely recognized. The management of diet in cerebral palsy patients, as in all mentally handicapped people, presents formidable problems for carers, and few easy solutions.

Bibliography

American Dietetic Association (1985) A statement, infant and child nutrition: concerns regarding the developmentally disabled. *Journal of the American Dietetic Association* 78: 443–452.

Craft M, Bicknell J and Hollins S (eds) (1985) *Mental Handicap – A Multidisciplinary Approach*. London: Baillière Tindall.

Durnin JVGA and Womersley J (1974) Body fat assessed from total body density and its estimation from skinfold thickness: measurements on 481 men and women aged from 16 to 72 years. *British Journal of Nutrition* 32: 77–97.

Garn SM and Weir HF (Letter) (1971) Assessing the nutritional status of the mentally retarded. *American Journal of Clinical Nutrition* 24: 853–854.

Heilfrich-Miller KR, Rector KL and Straka JA (1986) Dysphagia: its treatment in the profoundly retarded patient with cerebral palsy. *Archives of Physiological and Medical Rehabilitation* 67: 520–525.

Hitchcock EF (1978) Stereotactic surgery for cerebral palsy. *Nursing Times* 74: 2064–2065.

Keyes A, Brozek J, Henschel A, Mickelsen O and Taylor HL (1950) *The Biology of Human Starvation*. Minneapolis: University of Minnesota Press.

MacDonald NJ, McConnel KN, Stephen MR and Dunnigan MG (1989) Hypernatraemic dehydration in a large hospital for the mentally handicapped. *British Medical Journal* 299(6713): 1426–1429.

Shanley E (ed.) (1986) *Mental Handicap – A Handbook of Care*. Edinburgh: Churchill Livingstone.

Sloan RF (1977) The cineofluorographic study of cerebral palsy deglutition patterns. *Journal of Osaka Dental University* 11(1): 58–73.

Sobsey RJ (1983) Nutrition of children with severely handicapping conditions. *Journal of the Association for Persons with Severe Handicap* 8: 14–17.

M. Kennedy and L. McCombie
Lennox Castle Hospital, Glasgow, UK

CHAPATIS AND RELATED PRODUCTS

The chapati, also known as the *roti*, is a flat unleavened baked product which forms the staple food of the majority of the population in the Indian subcontinent. The consumption of this traditional product is increasing, and has become popular even in areas where traditionally rice has been the staple diet. Chapatis are normally made and served hot at breakfast, lunch or dinner, and are eaten along with other adjuncts in households, restaurants and industrial canteens. There are several culinary variations of the chapati—the important ones being the *parotha*, stuffed *parotha*, *tandoori roti* and *phulka*.

Either whole-wheat flour, generally known as *atta*, obtained by grinding wheat in a plate/disc mill, or 'resultant *atta*', a by-product of the roller flour-milling industry, similar to whole-wheat flour, is used for the preparation of chapatis. Sometimes, whole-wheat flour is first sieved to remove 3–5% of the coarse bran, and then used for chapati making. The flour, after having been mixed with water to form the dough, is sheeted to a circular shape and baked on a heated iron plate or an electric hot-plate. The major differences between chapatis and similar products arise mainly from differences in processing conditions. *See* Flour, Roller Milling Operations; Wheat

Characteristics of Products

The chapati and its culinary variations come under the category of unfermented flat breads; consequently, they are dense in texture, comprising mostly crust with little or no crumb (Fig. 1). They are usually round, but are sometimes made triangular in shape. The diameter varies from 10 to 20 cm, and the thickness from 3 to 10 mm. Soft, smooth and pliable texture, light creamish brown colour, slight chewiness, and wheaty aroma are the characteristics mainly desired in this type of product. However, there are very few distinct differences in the product characteristics of the various forms of chapatis.

Chapati

The chapati is circular in shape, having a diameter of 10–15 cm and a thickness of 3–4 mm. The dough sheet is baked on a heated iron plate and puffed on a live coal-fire or flame. The thinner chapati with a thickness of 1–2 mm is known as *phulka*.

Complete and full puffing is one of the important quality attributes of a chapati, as it results in a soft and pliable texture. The chapati should have an attractive appearance without any cracks on the surface. The surface should have uniformly distributed light-brown spots. The texture should be soft, smooth and pliable, and these characteristics should be retained for at least 2–3 h.

The chapati should have a sweetish, wheaty taste, and a baked wheaty aroma, and it should not be perceived as being tough and leathery when chewed.

Parotha

Like the chapati, the *parotha* is also made from whole-wheat flour or resultant *atta*. However, in a very few cases, even refined wheat flour obtained from the roller flour-milling industry is also used. *Parotha* dough contains salt and fat. The dough is sheeted and laminated at least three times; oil is applied during lamination as well as during baking.

The major difference between the chapati and the *parotha* is that the latter contains four to eight discrete layers, and has a more pronounced taste and flavour of oil. In view of the presence of oil, its keeping quality is better than that of chapatis. The *parotha* is slightly thicker (4–6 mm) than the chapati, and is normally

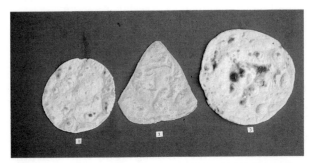

Fig. 1 Chapati and its culinary variations. (1) Chapati, (2) *parotha* and (3) *tandoori roti*.

triangular in shape. Its colour is creamish brown and it is slightly brittle on chewing. The *parotha* can be stuffed with cooked vegetables, e.g. potato.

Tandoori Roti

The *tandoori roti* is similar to the chapati in composition but it is somewhat thicker and larger in dimensions. It is made in restaurants and other road-side eating places known as *dhabas*. It is rarely made at home as it requires a special type of oven, called a *tandoor*, which is essentialy an enclosed cavity dug into a layer of soil and heated by live coal. In some urban areas, ovens of this type can be seen in centralized places; customers normally bring the dough sheet and get the *rotis* made and baked in the *tandoor* for a nominal charge. The thickness of a *tandoori roti* is greater than that of a chapati; it may be 8–10 mm thick, and its diameter may range between 15 and 20 cm. The crumb to crust ratio is greater than in a chapati. A *tandoori roti* is less pliable than a chapati; its surface is rough, and exhibits several large blisters. The moisture content of a *tandoori roti* is also lower.

Choice of Ingredients

Whole-wheat flour and water are the major ingredients used in the preparation of chapatis and other similar products. Salt and oil form the optional ingredients in products like chapatis and *tandoori rotis*, while they are essential in the preparation of *parothas* and stuffed *parothas*.

Wheat Flour

Whole-wheat flour obtained by grinding wheat in a plate/disc mill is preferred for the preparation of chapatis. The mill consists of two chilled-cast corrugated iron plates placed vertically. One of the plates is stationary while the other rotates. The wheat entering from the hopper is ground between the plates due to the shearing action as well as the friction. The particle size of the flour is adjusted by varying the clearance between the plates. It is desirable to grind wheat to a fine particle size, so that 80–90% can pass through a 60-mesh sieve. It is a normal practice in households to remove 3–5% of the coarse bran from whole-wheat flour by sieving through a 30-mesh sieve. Resultant *atta* is also used for chapati making, as it is available at a lower price, being the by-product of the roller flour-milling industry. There is not much difference in the composition of resultant *atta* and whole-wheat flour, except that the former has lower contents of ash and damaged starch,

Table 1. Characteristics of resultant *atta* and whole-wheat flour

Characteristics[a] (%)	Resultant *atta*	Whole-wheat flour
Ash	1·31	1·68
Protein	10·80	10·60
Dry gluten	9·90	9·90
Ether extractives	3·20	2·30
Crude fibre	2·09	2·24
Starch	52·20	54·50
Damaged starch	7·00	14·50
Water absorption capacity[b]	62·80	73·5

[a] Values are the average of 18 samples and are expressed on a 14% moisture basis.
[b] Required to prepare chapati dough of optimum consistency.

Table 2. Characteristics of whole-wheat (*aestivum*) flour suitable for chapati making

Characteristics	Level
Ash (%)	1·2–1·5
Protein (%)	9·0–10·5
Sedimentation value (ml)	25–35
Pelshenke value (ml)	120–150
Total sugars (%)	2·5–4·0
Diastatic activity (mg per 10 g flour)	250–375
Damaged starch (%)	14–15
Water absorption capacity (%)[a]	70–75

[a] Required to prepare dough of optimum consistency.

while its water absorption capacity is appreciably less (see Table 1).

The higher water absorption capacity of whole-wheat flour is attributed to its greater damaged starch content. Resultant atta has 1·5 times greater thiamin and riboflavin content, and twice as much niacin as that of whole wheat flour. *See* Niacin, Properties and Determination; Riboflavin, Properties and Determination; Starch, Structure, Properties and Determination; Thiamin, Properties and Determination

Whole-wheat flour, obtained from medium-hard aestivum wheat, and having the quality characteristics listed in Table 2, is suitable for chapati making.

The dough should show an alveograph stability value of 100–120 mm, strength of 15–20 cm^2 and extensibility of 20–27 cm.

Part of the whole-wheat flour can also be replaced by other (i.e. nonwheat) cereal flours and flours obtained from legumes or millets, either to improve the taste and texture, or the nutritional quality. Among the legume products used in this way the most common is Bengal gram flour, which is normally added at the 20–30% level; the chapati so made is locally known as a *mesi roti*. The other flours that are used or could be used in chapati making at levels ranging from 10 to 20% are defatted soya, groundnut or cottonseed flours, or refined flours from barley, bajra, sorghum, maize, cassava and sweet potato. Triticale, a man-made cereal, was not found suitable for chapati making, but it can be used after blending with wheat flour in a ratio of 1:1. Soft wheat, which is also not suitable for chapati making, can be improved by blending with hard wheat, or extra-hard durum wheat. *See* Barley; Cassava, Use as a Raw Material; Sorghum; Soya Beans, The Crop; Vegetables of Tropical Climates, Root Crops of Uplands

Salt

Salt is generally dispersed in water and added to the dough. Hence, edible common salt of any particle size can be used.

Oil

Refined oil is used during dough preparation and during rolling and lamination of the dough sheet in the process of *parotha* preparation. Solid fat (hydrogenated oil) can also be used, after it has been melted for easy application during lamination.

Water

There is no information on the type of water suitable for chapati making. Generally, any potable water, having medium hardness, and a pH value close to neutrality, is suitable.

Influence of Ingredients

Wheat Flour

Since whole-wheat flour is the major ingredient in the preparation of chapatis and other products, its quality has a considerable influence on the quality of the end-products. Whole-wheat flour obtained from medium-hard aestivum wheat is preferred, as it yields a chapati having the desired quality characteristics. Use of a strong wheat flour, with a protein content of more than 11·0%, results in a chapati having a tough and leathery texture, while a soft wheat, having less than 9% protein, yields a chapati with a stiff and brittle texture. Such chapatis also tend to become hard and brittle within an hour of storage.

The quality of a chapati also depends on the relative amounts of gliadin, glutenin and residue protein present in the flour. A flour having equal amounts of the above proteins gives fully puffed chapatis having a soft texture, while a flour that has more residue proteins, or gliadin, gives a stiff and leathery chapati. The presence of high amounts of polar lipids gives softer chapatis.

In addition to the type of wheat, the content of damaged starch, the diastatic activity, and the sugars present in the flour affect the quality of a chapati. The higher the damaged starch content, the higher will be the water absorption capacity; hence, the softer will be the texture of the chapati. A significant direct correlation exists between damaged starch content and water absorption ($r = 0.89$, $p < 0.001$) and soft texture of chapatis ($r = 0.56$, $p < 0.001$). A flour having high diastatic activity and sugar content yields a chapati with a sweetish taste.

The characteristics of chapati dough which are influenced by the quality of the flour affect the sensory quality of chapati. The sensory texture of a chapati is related significantly to farinograph consistency ($r = 0.47$, $p < 0.01$), extensograph extensibility ($r = -0.51$, $p < 0.01$), resistance to extension ($r = 0.52$, $p < 0.01$), and textureometer cohesiveness ($r = -0.57$, $p < 0.01$).

Wheat with low polyphenolase activity is desirable, to avoid an excessive brownish colour in the chapati. These enzymes are found to be low in indigenous wheat varieties, whereas the imported Mexican hybrid wheat varieties now grown in India have a high content of this enzyme. The adverse effect of enzymatic browning is greater when the chapati dough is rested for a longer period, or when the baked chapati is stored for a few hours.

Among the different *Triticum* species, the wheat, *T. aestivum*, which yields a nonsticky dough with good machinability, and a fully puffed chapati with soft and pliable texture, is most suitable for chapati preparation. When the species *T. durum* and *T. dicoccum* are used for chapati making, dry and hard-textured products result which are perceived to be leathery when chewed. They are also more sweet, due to the higher damaged starch content. In addition to the type and species of wheat, the severity of grinding and particle size of the flour play important roles in influencing the quality of chapatis. Among the different types of mills (plate mill, hammer mill, pin mill, roller mill, etc.) the flour obtained from plate mills has been found to be the best for chapati making. This is because of the greater severity of grinding which results in flour having a desirably high damaged starch content, and hence a higher water absorption, resulting in a soft and pliable chapati. These characteristics are retained for a long period on storage. The heat developed in such a mill during grinding tends to yield a chapati with better flavour. Among the plate mills, the power- or water-driven mills are found to be better than hand-driven mills, as the latter yield flour with a low maltose figure of 1.72–1.99%, and a water absorption capacity of just 66–69%, in contrast to the higher desired values of 2.6–4.65% for maltose content and 72–78% for water absorption.

A fine-ground flour is desirable for chapati making. The coarse flour, with more than 70–80% overtailing on a 10XX sieve, yields a chapati having a poor appearance and tough texture. The shear force required to cut such chapatis is related to the sensory texture ($r = 0.67$, $p < 0.001$), and is as high as 18–20 kg, compared to the force of 5–6 kg required for chapatis made from normal flour (20–30% overtailing). The quantity of water required to prepare the chapati dough of desired consistenccy is significantly related to the fraction passing through a 10XX sieve ($r = 0.89$, $p < 0.01$) and the protein content of the flour ($r = 0.53$, $p < 0.05$).

The extraction rate of flour used for chapati making has a considerable influence on the chapati quality. The quality of a chapati is not affected by removing 4–6% of the coarse bran by sieving (extraction rate 94–96%), as is the practice in households. However, removing higher amounts of bran particles by sieving, or using a flour of a lower extraction rate makes the chapati tough and leathery. Hence, to make good chapatis, a considerable amount of bran needs to be present in flour.

The chapati made from resultant *atta* is slightly tough, and has a bland flavour; the latter is attributed to a lower damaged starch content, as well as to the negligible heat developed during grinding. The temperature reached while grinding can be as low as 30–40°C, as against 90–95°C in a plate mill. The high temperature reached during the milling operation seems to favour the wheaty aroma in chapatis.

If wheat is infected by karnal bunt, at infection levels above 3%, chapatis will have a dark colour and an undesirable flavour. However, these adverse affects are minimized by soaking or washing the infected grains before grinding. Storing whole-wheat flour for more than 3 months at a high temperature adversely affects the quality of chapatis.

Salt

Incorporation of salt in the dough reduces the stickiness and, hence, improves the sheeting characteristics. The texture of the chapati is also slightly softened.

Oil

Incorporation of oil in the chapati dough improves the texture and pliability. It also keeps the chapati soft and pliable during storage. Puffing characteristics are also slightly improved on incorporation of very small amounts of oil in the dough. Higher levels of fat or shortening in the dough adversely affect the puffing quality of chapatis.

Discrete layers in a *parotha* are due to the application of oil during lamination. Oil is also used during the dough preparation to improve the rolling property.

Water

The amount of water required to prepare a dough of optimum consistency for chapati preparation ranges from 65 to 75%. The amount depends on several factors, such as the type of wheat, grinding method, extraction rate, particle size distribution, severity of grinding, etc. The higher the water requirement, the softer will be the texture of the chapati and the sweeter the taste. Such chapatis keep well on storage.

Additives

Incorporation of yeast (0·5%) or yoghurt (10%) softens the texture, which is also retained during storage. Emulsifiers or surfactants, such as glyceryl monostearate, sucrose esters and sodium stearoyl lactylate, and the enzyme α-amylase also improve the texture of a chapati as well as its keeping quality. *See* Emulsifiers, Organic Emulsifiers; Enzymes, Uses in Food Processing

Methods of Production

Chapatis and their culinary variations are generally freshly made and served, while still hot, in households, restaurants and industrial canteens. Fresh, hot chapatis are preferred, as they have a better flavour and soft texture. Consequently, chapatis produced on a large scale and marketed in unit packs have not become popular among consumers.

Chapati

The method of preparation of chapatis involves three important steps, viz. preparation of the dough, sheeting and baking-cum-puffing (Fig. 2).

The main ingredients used in chapatis are wholewheat flour, or resultant *atta*, and water. The water level varies from 65 to 75%, depending on the type of wheat and the milling method. In households, and even in restaurants, the dough is kneaded by hand to a consistency which is stiffer than bread dough, but enables easy sheeting without sticking to the base of the rolling pin. In large industrial canteens, however, either a planetary

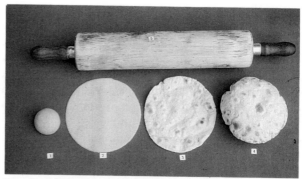

Fig. 2 Method of preparation of chapati. (1) Dough ball, (2) sheeted chapati, (3) partially-baked chapati, (4) puffed chapati and (5) rolling pin.

vertical mixer with a U-shaped blade, or a horizontal mixer similar to that used for bread dough, is used. The dough is mixed for 10–15 min, for complete development of the gluten, rested for a period ranging from 30 to 120 min, depending on the convenience. Normally, dough is rested for proper hydration and for stress relaxation, which enables easy sheeting without much stickiness. The optimum resting time is less (15–20 min) for a dough mixed in a mixer while the requirement is higher for hand-mixed dough (30–120 min).

The dough is divided into 35–40 g pieces, and then rounded between the palms. The rounded dough is sheeted using a rolling pin to a circular shape of about 15 cm diameter and 1·5–2·0 mm thickness. It is usual to dust with flour to reduce the stickiness. The rolled circular dough sheet is then baked on each side, on a heated shallow iron plate (200–220°C), for a total time of 1–2 min. At the final stages of baking on the second side, the surface of the chapati is gently pressed with a clean dry cloth for puffing. Alternately, puffing is also done by placing the baked chapati on a gas flame, or live, glowing coals for few seconds. The hot chapati is served either as such, or after smearing the surface with fat, preferably ghee or butter.

As yet, little work has been done on the mechanization of chapati production, particularly with respect to sheeting or baking. However, in some countries, the equipment generally used for the manufacture of tortillas is also used for chapati sheeting and baking. A few mechanized chapati-sheeting units have been developed and are being used in restaurants and industrial canteens. *See* Tortillas

Sheeting of dough using a rolling pin is time consuming and requires experienced persons to produce chapatis having a circular shape as well as uniform size and thickness.

Shaping by Pressing

Simple machines are now available to shape chapati dough. A 'Hilliff' chapati press with a capacity to produce 100–200 chapatis per hour is used in some households and restaurants for sheeting. It consists of two circular cast iron discs connected by a hinge. The contacting surfaces are covered with Teflon sheets. A lever-type handle is attached to the bottom disc. About 30–40 g of dough is placed at the centre of the bottom disc and covered by the top disc; pressure is applied to the top disc for few seconds with the help of the lever.

The pressed chapati is removed carefully and baked. Oil is applied to the surface of the disc to avoid sticking.

Another mechanical device available for flattening chapati dough is based on the principle of the can flanger, and consists of two discs, one of which is fixed, while the other is movable. A toggle mechanism is used to press the dough, which is placed in between the discs, as it develops a high pressure with little effort. The thickness of the chapati can be varied by adjusting the clearance between the discs. The bottom plate, on which 40–50 g of dough has been placed, is made to press onto the top disc, with the help of a pedal connected to the toggle. This machine has the capacity to produce 200–300 chapatis per hour. This device is either hand or foot operated.

Shaping by Sheeting

All the equipment described above is of the batch type. Hence, little effort has been made to develop continuous shaping machines for shaping by sheeting, which is accomplished by feeding the dough through a hopper and passing it through four sets of rollers to attain the desired thickness. The sheet then passes under a rubber-lined drum, and is cut (or stamped) with a Teflon-coated cutter of 18 cm diameter. The scrap dough is fed back to the hopper. The machine has the capacity to produce 1200–1800 chapatis per hour. Though some machines, based on continuous sheeting and rotary cutting, are now available for the shaping of chapati dough, suitable baking and puffing units have not been developed to match the capacity.

Parotha

The dough made by kneading whole-wheat flour, salt (1·0–2%), fat (2–5%) and water (65–70%) is divided into pieces of 35–45 g and sheeted, using a rolling pin, to a circular shape of 10 cm diameter. Then oil is applied to the top surface (1–2 g) and spread uniformly. The sheet is folded into a semicircle, and oil is again applied uniformly over the surface (0·5–1·0 g); the semicircle is then folded into a quarter circle. This laminated piece of dough is then sheeted (by rolling) into the shape of a triangle with a thickness of 2–3 mm, and sides of 15–18 cm in length. The sheeted dough is baked on an electric hot plate, or heated iron plate, for about 1–2 min

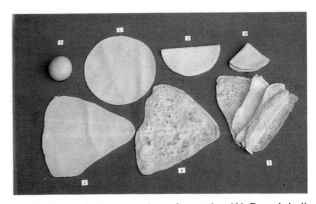

Fig. 3 Method of preparation of *parotha*. (1) Dough ball, (2) circular dough sheet, (3) first fold, (4) second fold, (5) sheeted *parotha*, (6) baked *parotha* and (7) different layers of *parotha*.

till the colour becomes light brown. Oil is applied to both sides (1–2 g) while baking (Fig. 3).

No attempt has so far been made to mechanize the sheeting and lamination processes in *parotha* making.

Stuffed Parotha

A *parotha* stuffed with vegetables and spices, so that it may be eaten as such, without any side dishes, is known as a stuffed *parotha*.

The dough for stuffed *parothas* is made in the same manner as that for *parothas*. A filling is prepared by adding chopped onion (25 g), salt (1 g) and chilli powder (0·5 g) to boiled, peeled and mashed potato (100 g), and mixing the ingredients well. A small portion of filling (about 20 g) is placed on the centre of the sheeted dough (5-cm diameter). The dough is folded over the filling to make a ball again. The dough is then rolled into a circular shape (12–15 cm) and baked on a hot plate by applying oil, or butter, to both sides.

The ingredients of the filling may be changed depending on the availability of vegetables and preferences of consumers. Stuffed *parothas* can be prepared using radish, cauliflower, fenugreek leaves, etc. Sometimes vegetables are mashed and mixed with dough and *parothas* prepared in the normal manner.

Tandoori Roti

The ingredients used are the same as those used for a chapati, except that salt (1·25–1·5%) is added sometimes. The quantity of dough used for a *tandoori roti* is higher (40–60 g) than for a chapati (35–40 g). The dough is flattened by beating and pressing between the hands to a thickness of 4–6 mm and a diameter of 15–18 mm. The sheeted dough is baked in an oval-shaped oven, the walls of which are plastered with clay (a *tandoor*). The oven is heated by burning wood or coal on the inside bottom. The sheeted dough is placed on a cloth pad, and pasted to the heated walls of the *tandoor*. Depending on the temperature of the *tandoor*, the *roti* is baked in 60–90 s. When a *roti* is baked properly, it falls from the side of the wall to the bottom surface. The baked *roti* is taken out using a long L-shaped iron rod. The major heat transfer in a *tandoor* oven is mainly by radiation, though some heating also occurs through conduction.

Handling, Storage and Distribution

As already mentioned, chapatis and other similar products are normally consumed fresh and hot. On storage they stale, becoming brittle and hard, and lose their typical flavour; hence they are not liked by consumers. The very short keeping quality of chapatis poses serious problems when they have to be served to a large number of consumers at one time, as in industrial canteens or in restaurants. It is expected that a good chapati should retain its soft, pliable texture for at least 2–3 h. No serious mechanization attempts were made to enable large-scale preparation of these products until recently. However, with the increase in demand for convenience foods, continuous efforts are now being made to commercialize the preparation and distribution of such products. Persistent research and development efforts are also being made in different parts of the world to improve upon the storage and distribution of chapatis.

The chapati, being a high-moisture product, containing 28–30% moisture, stales like bread or cake, becoming less acceptable on storage. Compared to other bakery products, a perceptible staling is observed on cooling. Further storage tends to make chapatis harder and brittle. In addition to these changes, mould growth also occurs after 3–4 days of storage.

Sorbic acid is normally used as an antifungal agent for preserving chapatis/parothas. The maximum level that could be incorporated without affecting the taste is 0·1%. The mould growth is delayed by 2–3 days at this level. However, use of a higher level of sorbic acid (0·3%) along with 1·5% salt, and packing in polythene (200 gauge), or in an aluminium foil/polythene laminate, can delay mould growth for as long as 180 days.

Sorbic acid is found to be a better preservative than its potassium salt. The level of sorbic acid could be reduced further either by including 0·4% citric acid, 3% sugar and 2·5% salt in the recipe, or by heating the packed chapatis for 2 h at 90°C. The chapatis made for defence personnel are preserved by in-pack heat sterilization after being packed in paper/foil/polylaminate. Such chapatis can be preserved for 180 days. Subjecting packed chapatis/*parothas* to γ radiation of 1 Mrad also delays the mould growth for 180 days. *Parothas* can be preserved well for 10 months by using 0·19% sorbic acid and 1·6% salt; the inner pack, made of MST cellophane, is repacked in paper/foil/polythene pouches. *See* Spoilage, Moulds in Food Spoilage

A shelf life of one year can be obtained for products such as chapatis/*parothas*/stuffed *parothas* by packing under a moderate vacuum of about 560 mmHg in sanitary cans, and heating in an oven at 115°–120°C for 1 h.

For civilian consumption, polypropylene or polyethylene metallized polyester laminate pouches are found to be quite adequate. Four chapatis are packed and sealed in each pouch. The individual packets are then packed in fibreboard boxes for transportation.

Bibliography

Arya SS, Vidyasagar K and Parihar DB (1977). Preservation of chapati. *Lebensmittel—Wissenschaft and Technologie* 10(4): 208–210.

Austin A and Ram A (1971) *Studies on Chapati Making Quality of Wheat. Technical Bulletin*, No. 31, New Delhi: Indian Council of Agricultural Research.

Faridi H (1988) Flat breads. In: Pomeranz Y (ed.) *Wheat: Chemistry Technology*, vol. II, pp 457–506. St Paul: American Association of Cereal Chemists.

Haridas Rao P (1982) *Studies on chapati and similar traditional foods.* PhD thesis, University of Mysore

Sidhu JS and Seibel W (1988) Effect of flour milling conditions on the quality of Indian unleavened flat bread (chapati) *Journal of Food Sciences* 53(5): 1563–1565.

P. Haridas Rao
Central Food Technological Research Institute, Mysore, India

CHEESES

Contents

Types of Cheese*

> Cheese is a fresh or matured product, obtained by the drainage of liquid after the coagulation of milk, cream, skimmed or partly skimmed milk or a combination thereof.

So reads the definition published in the *Code of Principles* issued by the Joint FAO/WHO (Food and Agricultural Organization, World Health Organization) Expert Committee, a subsidiary of the Codex Alimentarius Commission. The definition, however, did not include whey cheese, so a second sentence had to be added:

> Whey cheese is the product obtained by concentration of whey with or without the addition of milk or milk fat.

Cheesemaking is a way of preserving milk. In the old days, bacteria present in raw milk or the surrounding environment caused the milk to separate into curds and whey after a certain length of time. Nowadays, hygienic practices and large-scale production mean that specially prepared bacterial cultures must be added and a precisely controlled method followed. *See* Whey and Whey Powders, Production and Uses

Fermentation of the lactose in milk by lactic acid bacteria (LAB or 'starter') produces lactic acid and this gives the fresh acidic flavour. As well as acting as a preservative, the lactic acid helps to give the right texture to the curd formed when rennet is added to coagulate the milk protein. Living organisms remaining in the drained curd also affect the development of flavour in the finished cheese. *See* Lactic Acid Bacteria

After the milk has coagulated, the curd is cut into small pieces. Whey is released by the shrinkage of the coagulum – a process known as syneresis – and the remaining lactose is 'squeezed' out. The whey is then drained off and the curd moulded into the shape characteristic of the particular cheese being made.

---

* The colour plate section for this article appears between p. 1146 and p. 1147.

Combination of the amounts of starter culture and rennet used, the temperature and length of time they are left to develop, the required level of acidity and the way in which the curd is handled, together with the enzymatic action of additional bacterial or mould cultures necessary for certain types of cheese, lead to the development of a texture and flavour characteristic of each individual cheese. *See* Enzymes, Uses in Food Processing, Starter Cultures

Exacting procedures are followed so that the same conditions apply every time a particular cheese is made. Consistent ripening practices are equally important in the production of each specific variety.

The steps involved are as follows:

1. The cheese milk, raw or pasteurized, is warmed.
2. Starter cultures are added, followed by the rennet.
3. The coagulum formed is cut and stirred to release the whey and determine the moisture content of the curd.
4. The temperature of the mixture of curds and whey is raised, a process known as scalding.
5. The whey is drained off.
6. The curd is distributed into moulds and left to drain naturally or under pressure (hard-pressed) to reduce the residual moisture.
7. The demoulded cheeses are treated in specific ways which influence the final flavour characteristics (salted, waxed, pierced, smeared or mould-sprayed) and left to ripen – or mature – in controlled environments.

All cheese is salted at some stage of production, either before moulding, by placing in brine baths, or before being left to ripen, by rubbing the surface.

These procedures are carried out to varying degrees in the production of any cheese, the flavour and texture of the final cheese depending on the period and method of ripening, and any further microbial action, e.g. in the smear- or mould-ripened cheeses.

The length of time a cheese can be kept depends largely on its moisture content and this in turn is a result of the way the curd was handled during production. The very hard cheeses of Italy and Switzerland, e.g. Parmegianno Reggiano or Sbrinz, with moisture contents of the order of 30% (26–34%), continue to ripen and improve in flavour over periods of 1–2 years, even as long as 3 and 4 years. The hard pressed cheeses popular in the UK – Cheddar, Cheshire, Leicester, etc. – with around 40% (35–45%) moisture, keep and mature in flavour between 3 and 12 months or more, while the semihard or semisoft varieties favoured in mainland Europe (Gouda, Edam, Emmental types), with 45–50% moisture, are usually consumed after 2–3 months.

Soft mould-ripened cheeses, such as Brie and Camembert, with a maximum of 55% moisture, ripen within 8–12 weeks; the internally mould-ripened – the blue-vein cheeses, e.g. Gorgonzola, Roquefort, Stilton – take a little longer. Fresh cheeses (between 50% and 80% moisture) will keep for only for a few days.

A Gift from the Gods

The art of cheesemaking has evolved over the centuries, with recipes being handed down from mother to daughter, using the milk of domesticated animals to make a cheese with the keeping qualities needed to fit in with the lifestyle and taste of the local community. The science of many of the processes involved is only now being elucidated and much work still remains to identify the chemical changes behind the flavour and texture development that occurs during ripening.

Cheese, according to the ancient Greeks, was 'a gift from the Gods', and so it would have appeared as no-one understood the nature of the 'ferment' that was responsible for speeding the process of coagulation and preserving the milk.

There is evidence of cheesemaking long before the written records of the Greeks and the Romans; it probably dates back as long ago as Neolithic peoples first domesticated their animals. The Bible tells us that David was on his way to deliver cheese when he encountered Goliath. Archaeological surveys in the Middle Eastern region between the rivers Euphrates and Tigris, known as 'the cradle of civilization', indicate that cheese was being made from the milk of sheep and goats as far back as 6000 and 7000 BC. An early Sumerian frieze shows animals being milked and the milk curdled while remnants of material found in a tomb of 3000 BC have been identified as cheese.

According to legend, Aristaeus, the son of Apollo and the nymph Cyrene, was taught the art of cheesemaking by the centaur Chiron and this skill he passed on as a 'gift to mankind'.

In Homer's Odyssey, there is a description of Ulysses arriving in Sicily and watching Polyphemus milking his sheep and goats. The cyclops then drank half the milk with his evening meal and curdled the other half, placing the curds in specially woven baskets to drain. Baskets made from reeds or other stems are still in use to this day in parts of India for making certain types of curds. Impressions of similar baskets have also been found in the UK, in Dorset, dated to around 1800 BC, suggesting that cheese was being made there too, even before the Roman invasion. Earthenware bowls with a perforated base, presumed to be used for draining the cheese curds, have also been found in excavation sites in Europe and in Asia.

By the time Rome was founded, cheesemaking was well established in all regions of Italy and there are reports of a regular cheese market in the city. Soldiers in the Roman army received a daily ration of 27 g of cheese and, at the height of Roman splendour, recipes from a famed chef of the time showed that cheeses were to be found on all the most elegant tables in Europe. Furthermore, because the trade in cheese with overseas countries was becoming so extensive, the Emperor Diocletian (AD 284–305) was called on to fix maximum prices for the cheese and it was about that time that the first 'trade-marked' cheese was observed, on a cheese later to become Parmesan.

After the Roman conquest of Britain, Palladius wrote in his treatise, *Agriculture in Britain*, that cheese should best be made in the early summer, with milk curdled with rennet from the stomach of the kid, the calf or the lamb, or from the milk of the fig tree or the teasel flower, so demonstrating that the principles of cheesemaking were well understood even at that time.

Reports also have it that Attila the Hun was partial to a piece of cheese, and the Emperor Charlemagne requested that cheese from the village of Roquefort should be regularly dispatched to him at Aix-la-Chappelle.

As the centuries wore on, the spread and growing sophistication of cheese could be seen to be linked with geographical migrations and historical influence. The types of cheese associated with particular regions were as much the result of socioeconomic change as with gastronomic demand. Production tended to be centred on the monasteries or noble houses, or in remote farming areas where the secret was passed down within families. Now we are in a position where the history of the majority of cheeses developed in the past millenium has been lovingly documented, and still more are being developed for the gourmet market.

Types of Cheese

Cheese can be made from any milk. The milk varies in composition from animal to animal and from species to species, depending too on the time of the year, stage of lactation, climate, diet, etc. The cheese made depends on both the constituents of the milk (Table 1) and the microstructure of individual components, as well as the

Table 1. Average percentage composition of milk of various species

	Cow	Ewe	Goat
Protein	3·81	5·85	2·63
Fat	3·80	6·45	3·5
Lactose	0·75	4·47	4·15
Vitamins and minerals	0·75	0·83	0·79
Water	87·10	82·40	88·30

Biss, 1991.

enzymatic action of microbial constituents. The majority of cheeses are now made from cows' milk but that of ewe and goat is also widely used. *See* Milk, Dietary Importance

The blue cheese, Roquefort, is probably the most renowned of the ewes' milk cheeses, and it is said to have been produced for at least 2000 years. Greece is well known for its feta, which is a brined cheese also made from ewes' milk. There are many varieties, both hard and soft in most other countries where sheep are milked. *See* Sheep, Milk

A main characteristic of both sheep's and goats' milk is the very white colour owing to the lack of carotene; another is the very small size of the fat globules. While there a number of locally named goats' milk cheeses, the majority are commonly referred to under the single term 'chevres' and are eaten fresh.

Mozarella, best known of the Italian 'stretched curd' (pasta filata) cheeses, was traditionally made from buffaloes' milk, but a large proportion is now made from cows' milk. *See* Buffalo, Milk

The number of varieties of cheese are rapidly becoming too numerous to list. France has long boasted of having a cheese for every day of the year, but there are almost certainly double that number by now. That veritable 'bible' of world cheeses – *The Mitchell Beazley Pocket Guide to Cheese* (Carr, 1987) – lists 1200 in the latest edition and a visit to any gathering of Specialist Cheesemakers Associations demonstrates that more new and named varieties of cheese are continually being added to the lists.

There are basically three main types of cheese: hard, blue and soft.

The Hard Cheeses

Extra Hard

'Extra hard' is the term given to the low-fat, low-moisture, very hard grating cheeses, such as the parmesans – Parmegiano Reggiano and Grana Padana – Romano, Sbriz and Asiago. These cheeses are made in special copper vats or 'kettles' using thermophilic starters and very high scald temperatures. After forming, they are immersed in brine for several days before being left to mature for periods as long as several years.

Hard Pressed Cheeses

Hard pressed cheeses are the most popular in the UK. Cheddar, with 48% fat-in-dry-matter and 39% moisture, is the best known and, worldwide, is probably consumed in greatest quantities. The curd is 'texturized' after cutting and scalding. It is then milled and salted, placed in the traditional cylindrical moulds or, more commonly, in blocks for pressing to remove the final moisture. The cheeses are matured slowly in stores held at 15°C and 88% relative humidity, or when in film-wrapped blocks, at 4–6°C.

The cheeses are regularly inspected and graded during storage. The flavour of a mild Cheddar has developed sufficiently within 3–4 months, a medium cheese after 6 months and the mature cheese in 8–12 months. When a grader approaches a cheese to assess its quality, he or she removes a sample with a cheese iron, then looks at the colour and the appearance; after rolling it in the fingers to 'feel' the texture (body), smells it and, finally, tastes it. All these attributes combine to make a good cheese and each is specific to an individual cheese type.

Other UK cheeses, known as British territorials – Cheshire, Double Gloucester, Derby and Red Leicester, Wensleydale and Caerphilly – are also textured cheeses and are made by slight variations on the basic method; Cheshire, Lancashire and Caerphilly are moister cheeses with a crumbly texture, and ready to be marketed within about 6 weeks.

Hard, with Eyes

The eyes (gas pockets) are formed in firm, elastic-bodied cheeses by carbon dioxide produced by propionic acid bacteria (*Propionobacterium freudenreichii* subsp. *shermanii*) added to the starter cultures. There are two groups which come into this category: first, the Swiss-type cheeses, Emmental and Gruyère which are rubbed with salt after moulding; second, a miscellaneous group of cheeses (e.g. Tilsit) with smaller eyes and, frequently, smear-coated with *Brevibacterium linens* to ripen.

Semisoft

The term 'semisoft' is applied to the very popular continental cheeses, such as Edam and Gouda, which are eaten in large quantities in northern Europe. They are close-textured, mild, washed-rind cheeses in which the curd is lightly scalded so that it retains a higher percentage of lactose and moisture than in hard cheeses. In addition, some of the whey is replaced with water during the scalding stage and this dilutes the residual

Types of Cheese

lactose and restricts the production of acid. The cheeses are lightly salted by floating them in a brine bath for up to 10 days before final, short-time ripening.

Surface-ripened

Limburger, St Paulin and Munster are examples of semisoft, fresh curd cheeses which are ripened partly by proteolysis induced by the starter bacteria and the rennet, and partly by the characteristic reddish-brown surface growth of *Brevibacterium linens*, which develops within a few days of application.

Blue Cheeses

Internal-mould-ripened

The internal-mould-ripened cheeses include the blue-vein cheeses, e.g. Gorgonzola, Roquefort, Stilton; these are high-acid, semi-soft cheeses which are allowed to drain slowly rather than by pressing. The flavour develops in the cheese as a result of proteolytic and lipolytic changes brought about by the spread of the blue moulds. *Penicillium roquefortii* and *P. glaucum*, through the cheese after they have been pierced to allow the entry of air.

Soft Cheeses

Cheeses coming into the soft cheese category range from the fresh lactic cheeses, i.e. Petit Suisse, to the firmer types, Brie, Coulommier and Camembert.

Mould-ripened

Camembert and Lymeswold are examples of mould-ripened soft cheeses. The fresh cheese is shaped in a mould and the whey allowed to drain off. After demoulding, the cheeses are placed in stacks in a warm, humid room and sprayed with the white mould, *Penicillium albus* (*P. camemberti*). The cheese ripens, accompanied by development of the characteristic surface growth, within about 10 days. There are a number of varieties of surface-ripened cheeses, some of which develop as a result of microorganisms occurring naturally in the environment.

Lactic Cheese

The lactic types are the most simple of cheeses, made by draining the coagulum produced by lactic acid starter bacteria and eaten fresh.

Cottage Cheese

Cottage cheese is a soft curd cheese made from skim milk. The curd is diced and handled with extreme gentleness so that the cubes are left separate and cooked to retain a very high moisture content (80%). Flavouring and stabilizing agents can be added, as well as a cream dressing to separate the curd pieces.

Table 2. World factory production of cheese, including fresh, 1990

	Production ($\times 10^3$ t)
World total	14 555·8
EEC	4962·0
Other western European countries	507·6
Eastern Europe	3327·8
North America	3479·3
South America	417·2
Australasia	219·9
Rest of the world	1485·8

MMB England & Wales (1991) *EC Dairy Facts and Figures 1991*. Surrey: Milk Marketing Board of England and Wales.

Table 3. Per capita cheese consumption, 1989–1990

	Total (kg)	Fresh cheese (kg)
France	22·5	17·3
Finland	22·5	NA
Greece	22·1	0·1
FRG	18·6	8·2
Italy	18·1	4·7
Belgium	17·2	3·9
Israel	16·2	13·9
Sweden	15·5	0·9
Canada	15·3	1·2
The Netherlands	15·2	1·6
Denmark	14·7	1·1
USA	12·3	1·6
Austria	10·9	3·8
Australia	9·2	0·8
UK	8·6	1·0
Hungary	8·5	4·6
New Zealand	7·9	0·9
USSR	6·6	3·3
Ireland	5·5	NA
Spain	5·3	NA
Japan	1·2	0·1
India	0·2	NA

NA, not available.
Milk Marketing Board of England and Wales, International Dairy Federation, National Statistics.

Whey Cheese

A type of cheese popular in certain European countries is made from whey, usually obtained from the manufacture of hard cheese. Examples are the Italian ricotta or Norwegian Getost. The whey is neutralized and concentrated for several hours at high temperatures (85–90°C) to coagulate and precipitate the proteins together with residual fat. The curd obtained is drained and moulded to give a solid, but soft, cheese with a short shelf life. Some 5–10% of whole or skim milk can be added to increase the yield.

Processed Cheese

Processed cheese is a 're-cooked' cheese made from any variety of natural cheese, which is melted by heat and mixed with emulsifying agents – the sodium, potassium, calcium or ammonium salts of citric, phosphoric, polyphosphoric and tartaric acid. Processed cheese has a moisture content of not more than 48% under UK regulations. Cheese spread, with 20% fat and not less than 60% moisture, is another similar product.

The Marketplace

World production of cheese in 1990 was estimated at around 17 million tonnes. The bulk comes from the temperate regions where sophisticated dairy industries have grown up. Factory-made cheese – including fresh cheeses – added up to 14·5 million tonnes with the EEC countries accounting for 34% (see Table 2).

Most of the cheese produced is consumed by individual countries' home markets (see Table 3); only a small percentage is traded on the open market and now, of course, the volumes being produced in the Western countries are under pressure as a result of milk quotas and other devices introduced to reduce the overproduction of milk which has grown since World War II. World trade figures recorded by the Milk Marketing Board of England and Wales in its annual statistical review shows that less than 1 million tonnes (890 000 tonnes) enters the open market and, of this, the EEC offers 50%. In a similar context, the EEC provides almost 50% of the milk powder traded and just under 30% of the world's butter.

Bibliography

Androuet P (1981) *Un Fromage pour Chaque Jour*. Paris: Editions de Vergeures; published in collaboration with CIDIL, Paris.
Biss K (1991) Sheep and Goat Cheese. *Journal of the Society of Dairy Technology* 44(4): 104.
Carr S (ed.) (1987) *The Mitchell Beazley Pocket Guide to Cheese*. London: Mitchell Beazley Publishers.
Chapman HR and Sharpe ME (1981) Microbiology of cheese. In: Robinson RK (ed.) *Dairy Microbiology*, vol 2. Essex: Elsevier Science Publishers.
Corato R (1985) *Italian Cheeses – Pocket Guide*. Polenghi Lombardo SpA.
Rance P (1989) *The French Cheese Book*. London: Macmillan.
Scott R (1986) *Cheesemaking Practice* 2nd edn. Essex: Elsevier Science Publishers.

Pauline Russell
London, UK

Starter Cultures Employed in Cheesemaking

Starter cultures as we know them today are balanced combinations of lactic organisms. The original starters, however, were the result of a nonspecific natural souring of milk. The haphazard action of these natural clusters has been refined and developed to meet the demands of a modern dairy industry.

History of Cheese Starter Cultures

The progression from a natural souring to a form of starter probably occurred when the fermentation was slow or failed. It was observed that a more successful fermentation occurred if whey from the previous day's cheesemake was added to the fresh milk. This early form of culture transfer established the benefit of capitalizing on the proven ability of the previous day's culture and was also the precursor to the practice of daily transfer/propagation of cultures. The transferred culture was used to start the fermentation and hence cultures were called cheese starters.

In the early part of this century, scientists and commercial companies began to investigate these natural starters and examine the organisms they contained. As one would expect, in addition to the lactic acid bacteria it was found that there were a number of undesirable contaminants. Once purified, the cultures were maintained by continual subculturing under aseptic conditions in sterile media. From these original cultures the best were selected and made available to the cheesemakers in a liquid culture form as a pure lactic ferment.

These cultures, properly characterized, were freeze dried and have formed the basis of most modern cultures.

Starter Culture Organisms

The organisms isolated from the naturally derived starters are classified as lactic acid bacteria (LAB). There are a number of different organisms used in

Table 1. Distinguishing properties of the lactic acid bacteria found in starter cultures

Name	Shape	Growth temperature (°C)		% Lactic acid in milk	Isomer of lactate	Fermentation of			Citrate metabolism	NH₃ from Arg
		10	45			Lac	Glu	Gal		
L. lactis ssp. *lactis*	Coccus	+	−	0·8	L	+	+	+	−	+
L. lactis ssp. *cremoris*	Coccus	+	−	0·8	L	+	+	+	−	−
L. lactis ssp. *lactis* biovar. *diacetylactis*	Coccus	+	−	0·8	L	+	+	+	+	+/−
Leu. cremoris	Coccus	+	−	0·2	D	+	+	+	+	−
Str. salivarius ssp. *thermophilus*	Coccus	−	+	0·6	L	+	+	−	−	−
Lb. delbrueckii ssp. *bulgaricus*	Rod	−	+	1·8	D	+	+	−	−	+
Lb. helveticus	Rod	−	+	2·0	DL	+	+	+	−	−

Table 2. Mesophilic and thermophilic organisms used in cheesemaking

Mesophilic organisms
   (temperature range of growth 15–40°C)

Homofermentative:
Lactococcus lactis ssp. *lactis*
Lactococcus lactis ssp. *cremoris*

Heterofermentative:
Lactococcus lactis ssp. *lactis* biovar. *diacetylactis*
Leuconostoc cremoris

Thermophilic organisms
   (temperature range of growth 30–50°C)

Homofermentative:
Streptoccus salivarius ssp. *thermophilus*
Lactobacillus delbrueckii ssp. bulgaricus
Lactobacillus helveticus

cheesemaking and these can be divided into two basic groups – mesophilic (medium temperature with an optimum temperature of 30°C), isolated from dairies in Northern Europe, and thermophilic (high temperature with an optimum temperature of 45°C), isolated from the warmer Mediterranean countries (Table 2). A simple rule to find out the type of culture used in any of the old cheese varieties is to establish the country or area where the cheese originated. For example, the cultures used for UK cheese are mesophilic and those used for Italian varieties are thermophilic. Additional non-LAB cultures employed in secondary fermentation are *Propionibacterium shermanii*, *Penicillium camemberti*, *P. roqueforti* and *Brevibacterium linens* **See** Lactic Acid Bacteria

Composition of Starter Cultures

The original undefined cultures contain many strains of LAB, including strains from more than one genus. The individual strains each contributing in a slightly different way to the total culture and its overall characteristics. Organisms in the same group have similar properties but there will be variations, for example in their rate of acidification, production of aroma and carbon dioxide, proteolytic activity, production of antimicrobial compounds or phage type. Yet, despite these different characteristics, or perhaps in many instances because of them, they grow together in a mildly symbiotic relationship.

Mesophilic Mixed Multistrain

The survivors of the original starter cultures are described as mixed multistrain cultures (a typical culture will contain approximately 5% *L. lactis* ssp. *lactis*, 70% *L. lactis* ssp. *cremoris*, 10% *Leu. cremoris* and 15% *L. lactis* biovar. *diacetylactis*), undefined mixtures that have achieved a natural balance.

These cultures ferment milk to a final pH of 4·5, and exhibit general qualities of mildness, fullness of flavour and slow but steady acid production. These qualities are important for many cheese varieties and they are regularly used for the production of Cheshire, Camembert, Stilton, fromage frais, Edam and other varieties where small-hole formation or open texture is required.

Multistrain Cultures

The multistrain culture was the first stage in creating more defined cultures: strains of the same genus or specific properties were grouped together. This development was prompted by demands from Japan that the cheese supplied by New Zealand should not gas during shipment. These cultures are now commonly used for Cheddar and cottage cheese, where gas production or open texture can cause problems.

The multistrain cultures, although offering more specific characteristics, are susceptible to a virus (bacteriophage) which attacks and kills the culture. The problems associated with bacteriophage prompted research to improve the phage resistance of cultures.

Defined Strain Cultures

The development of defined cultures was pioneered in New Zealand and Australia. Cheese manufacturers had been asking for cultures with improved resistance to phage for use in Cheddar cheese production. The researchers initially screened strains for their resistance to phage but, additionally, they had to be good acid producers, with a clean flavour and good proteolytic activity. The final result of this research was the introduction of paired phage-resistant strains, used on a nonrotational basis with backup strains available should a phage develop to one or both of the strains.

Defined strain cultures are not restricted to two strains; they may contain more. It was established, however, that a balance between fast and slow strains is important to give good flavour characteristics. A predominance of fast strains can lead to harsh bitter flavours in Cheddar cheese. The balance of the culture is, therefore, important and must be designed to operate within the make parameters required.

The development of defined strains cultures was carried out to meet the demands of Cheddar production, but the principle is now applied to the specific need of other varieties. Strains selected for cottage cheese should have the ability to produce uniform acid throughout the vat and not be affected by natural antibodies in the milk. These antibodies will agglutinate some strains as part of a natural defence mechanism against foreign bodies. Strains with good proteolytic activity and sugar utilization are selected for mozzarella. Wherever specific properties are required, strains can be selected and combined to provide the characteristics required.

The Role of the Starter Culture in Cheesemaking

Cheese production converts a short shelf life product milk into a long shelf life product cheese. The starter contributes to many facets of the production and character of cheese:

(1) The primary role of a starter culture is the production of lactic acid from lactose. Starting from an initial milk pH of 6·6, the pH must be lowered to pH 4·7 in 4 h for cottage cheese, pH 5·25 in 4·5 h for Cheddar, pH 5·1 in 20 h for Gouda and pH 4·5 in 18 h for quarg. To achieve these results starter is added at, for example, 5% for cottage cheese and 0·2% for quarg.

Some cheese varieties can be made by direct acidification, such as cottage cheese and mozzarella for pizzas. However, the culture is responsible for more than just the acidification. The culture will control the development of nonstarter flora, inhibit pathogens, improve shelf life and, most importantly, contribute to flavour development.

(2) In addition to the acid produced by the LAB, the heterofermentative organisms produce volatile flavour compounds, such as diacetyl and carbon dioxide from citrate. The carbon dioxide produced assists in creating open texture in Cheshire and Stilton, and hole formation in other varieties, such as Edam, Havarti and Danbo.

(3) The final role of the starter organisms occurs during ripening. The starter organisms contribute a major source of both proteinase and peptidase enzymes, whose activity is of great importance in assisting to produce the flavour of mature cheese.

Lactococcus organisms have 95% of their proteinase activity associated with their cell wall, cleaving the milk protein into a range of peptides. The peptides are then further degraded by the intracellular peptidase enzymes.

Some of the peptides produced by the first-stage proteolysis can be detected as harsh and, possibly, bitter flavour notes. The peptidase enzymes will reduce the harsh or bitter flavour by further degrading the peptides to amino acids. However, the peptidase enzymes are prevented from acting on the bitter flavour peptides until death of the bacterial cell occurs and the enzymes are released into the cheese.

It is very important for the starter to provide a balanced proteolytic system if well rounded mature flavours are desired.

Role of Non-LAB Cultures

Included in the non-LAB group of cultures are cultures of bacteria, for example propionic acid bacteria and *Brevibacterium*, and moulds of the genus *Penicillium*.

Propionibacterium shermanii is used to produce large holes in Emmental. Propionic acid bacteria ferment lactic acid, producing propionic acid, acetic acid and carbon dioxide gas. The cheese is transferred after brining to a warm room at 21°C, after which the secondary fermentation commences, producing the large-hole formation and sweet flavour typical of Emmental.

Starter Cultures Employed in Cheesemaking

Brevibacterium linens is used as a surface-ripening culture and is identified by the characteristic red/orange colour as seen on Limburger but, additionally, is used to develop flavour in Esrom and Danbo.

Penicillium roqueforti has been isolated from Roquefort cheese and is used in Stilton and dana blue. All these cheeses must be pierced to allow oxygen to reach the mould spores within the cheese allowing the characteristic blue veining and flavour to develop.

Penicillium camemberti isolated from Camembert is used as a white surface ripening mould, extensively used on Brie and other varieties. These all have a large surface area to allow penetration of mould enzymes.

These microorganisms are all additional to the regular acidifying cultures, each contributing specific characteristics to the finished cheese.

Factors Affecting Culture Growth

When propagating cultures, certain criteria for growth need to be met. Milk, being the natural substrate for LAB, provides all the nutrients required. Lactose is the source of carbohydrate, casein provides the nitrogen and all the necessary minerals and vitamins are present in milk.

Cultures will continue to grow while nutrients are available, or until they are inhibited by the acid they produce. Too high a nutrient level may be inhibitory if the osmotic pressure is too high. Other factors which have an inhibitory or disturbing influence on culture growth include: antibiotic or sterilant residues in the media; high levels of lactic acid which will cause cells to lose activity and vitality; oxygen incorporated into the media which will retard growth and can lead to loss in activity; and variable temperatures during fermentation leading to culture imbalance or lack of activity. The nutritional and environmental conditions are easy to control. The most destructive agent to cell growth is, however, bacteriophage.

Bacteriophage or 'phage' is the term used to describe the virus-like material which can infect and destroy bacteria. They are tadpole-like in shape, having a head and tail (Fig. 1). If a phage is added to a susceptible culture in liquid suspension, the phage particles by lysing the bacterial cells will clear the liquid of the cells with simultaneous multiplication of phage particles. The various stages of phage attack on bacterial cells are well established.

(1) The tip of the tail of the phage particle attaches itself to the bacterial cell.
(2) The wall of the bacterial cell, at the point of attachment, is penetrated by a segment of the tail and DNA from the head of the virus is injected via the tail into the host cell.
(3) The viral DNA uses the bacterial cell replication enzymes for the construction of new phage particles.

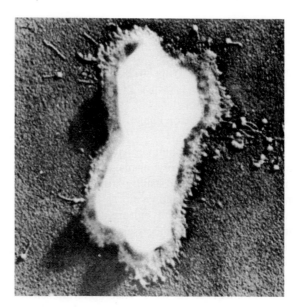

Fig. 1 Electron micrograph of bacteriophage active on *Lactococcus lactis* subsp. *lactis*.

(4) When phage synthesis is complete, the host cell ruptures, releasing many new phage particles.

The number of phage particles released when the host cell bursts is called the 'burst size', and the time lapse from attachment to burst is termed the 'latent period'. The burst size is between 50 and 200 and the latent period between 20 and 50 min.

Phage are relatively heat resistant, but are readily destroyed by hypochlorite and iodophor solutions. Cheese factories may become heavily infected with phage particles, which are readily airborne. Consequently, extreme precautions are necessary to avoid infection of starters at all stages of propagation and also of the milk for cheesemaking.

Quality Control

Only a limited assessment of the quality of liquid cultures can be made prior to use. Cultures can be stored for 24 h if cooled to 5°C, but this period allows only activity, vitality and phage results to be obtained. Viable cell numbers and bacterial contaminant results are not available until after the culture has been used.

The standard assessment of a bulk culture will be made on a 6 h activity test in reconstituted skim milk (RMS), a 6 h vitality test in pasteurized milk and a phage detection test also in pasteurized milk and incorporating the cheese temperature profile. There are various modifications of these tests, but the principle of the activity test is to assess the development in acidity over a set time at a set temperature and in a constant medium. The vitality test mimics a cheese make using pasteurized milk with rennet added; and acidity readings are taken from the whey. The phage detection test is an activity test using pasteurized milk. When control tubes are compared to ones with varying levels of filtered whey (living cells removed), the presence of phage related to the culture strains will be detected by a reduction in acidity compared to the control. Phage inhibits acid production by killing cells.

Standard plating techniques with selective media will detect contaminating organisms, and there is also a phage detection method using plating techniques. The presence of phage is shown up as clear zones where phage has inhibited the culture. These results are retrospective but very necessary for quality control purposes.

The only cultures which can be fully tested before use are the frozen, freeze-dried or concentrated cultures.

Developments so far have relied on strain selection, but future advances will employ genetic-engineering techniques.

A greater understanding of the genetic information contained in the bacterial cell will allow the introduction of specific segments of DNA which control specific characteristics. The use of natural genetic techniques and recombinant DNA technology will allow the construction of strains with improved characteristics, such as phage resistance, activity and flavour.

Bibliography

Daly C (1983) Starter culture developments in Ireland. *Irish Journal of Food Science and Technology* 7: 39–48

Davies FL and Law BA (eds) (1984) *Advances in the Microbiology and Biochemistry of Cheese and Fermented Milks*. Barking: Elsevier.

Lawrence RC, Thomas TD and Terzaghi BE (1976) Reviews of the progress of dairy science: cheese starters. *Journal of Dairy Research* 43: 141–193

Olson NF (1990) The impact of lactic acid bacteria on cheese flavour. *FEMS Microbiology Reviews* 87: 131–148

Sandine WE (1989) Use of bacteriophage-resistant mutants of lactococcal starters in cheesemaking. *Netherlands Milk Dairy Journal* 43: 211–219

Tamime AY (1990) In: Robinson RK (ed.) *Dairy Microbiology*, Vol. 2, pp 131–202. Barking: Elsevier.

C. R. Stilton
J.J. Saunders Ltd, Bath, UK

Chemistry of Curd Manufacture

Cheesemaking originated some 8000 years ago as a method of preserving milk. The process has developed to such a degree that, probably, 500–1000 varieties are now produced throughout the world with a total production in excess of 12 million tonnes per annum.

The single unifying characteristic of all cheeses is that they are produced by coagulation of the milk casein (the major fraction of the milk protein) to form a gel, which entraps the majority of the milk fat, unless skimmed milk is utilized. This is followed by a separation process in which the liquid whey is removed from the solid curds. Hence the casein, fat and colloidal salts of the milk are concentrated by a factor of 6–12 times into the curd, while most of the water, lactose, soluble salts and whey proteins are removed as whey. Table 1 shows the gross composition of typical samples of milk, a hard and a soft cheese and whey – note that such data are subject to wide variation. *See* Casein and Caseinates, Uses in the Food Industry; Whey and Whey Powders, Production and Uses

The great majority of cheeses are produced by enzymatic coagulation although some are coagulated by acid or a combination of acid and heat. This article describes the chemical processes involved in the formation and development of cheese curd. *See* Enzymes, Uses in Food Processing

Enzymatic Coagulation

The manufacture of rennet curd cheese usually involves acidification of the milk (typically to about pH 6·5 using starters which convert lactose to lactic acid), followed by enzymatic coagulation, cutting of the curd and drainage of the whey. The curd is then salted, moulded and allowed to ripen to the finished cheese. *See* Lactic Acid Bacteria; Starter Cultures

Enzymatic coagulation is a two-phase process. In the primary phase the casein micelles are destabilized as a result of proteolysis, while the secondary phase consists of aggregation of the destabilized micelles to form a gel.

Casein Micelles – The Basic Coagulation Unit

Casein accounts for approximately 80% of milk protein and consists of several molecular species of which the

Table 1. Typical composition of cows milk, hard and soft cheese varieties, and cheese whey

	Composition (%)				
	Water	Fat	Protein	Lactose	Ash
Milk	87	4	3·6	4·6	0·8
Cheddar cheese	37	33	25	1	4
Camembert	52	24	20	0·5	3·5
Whey	93·3	0·4	0·8	4·9	0·6

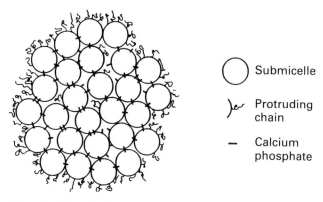

○ Submicelle

)⌁ Protruding chain

— Calcium phosphate

Fig. 1 Model of a casein micelle. Reproduced from Walstra P and Jenness R (1984) *Dairy Chemistry and Physics*. Chichester: Wiley.

principal ones are α_{s1}-, α_{s2}-, β- and κ-casein (in the approximate proportions 4:1:4:1). The soluble whey proteins, which account for the remaining 20% of milk protein, are not involved in the cheesemaking process (unless the milk is subjected to high-heat treatment which causes the whey protein to be denatured and complexed with the casein). The vast majority (95%) of the casein exists in association with calcium phosphate in colloidal structures called casein micelles which are 20–300 nm in diameter. The micelles are the basic unit involved in the transformation of milk to curd and cheese. Although the exact structure of micelles is not certain, it is generally accepted that they are composed of smaller particles of aggregated casein called submicelles and that the majority of the κ-casein exists on the outer surface. κ-Casein is amphipathic and the majority of the molecules are glycosylated to some extent. The amino terminal (N)-terminal two-thirds of the molecule is hydrophobic and is equivalent to the p-κ-casein fraction on renneting (see below). The remaining one-third from the carboxy (C) terminus is hydrophilic, anionic, contains a varying number of hydrophilic carbohydrate moieties and is equivalent to the soluble caseinomacropeptide (or glycomacropeptide) fraction on renneting. The N-terminal end is associated with the hydrophobic α- and β-caseins and colloidal calcium phosphate, and thus projects to some degree into the micelle. The remainder, probably most of the molecule, protrudes from the surface to give the micelle a 'hairy' appearance. The micelle may, therefore, have a structure similar to that shown in Fig. 1, with κ-casein positioned as schematically depicted in Fig. 2. Before rennet is added to milk, the micelles show no tendency to aggregate, perhaps for two reasons:

(1) The hydrophilic 'hairs' are anionic, giving the micelles an overall negative charge and a ζ potential between -10 and -20 mV. Electrostatic repulsion therefore provides a barrier to close approach between micelles.

(2) The 'hairy' outer layers of the micelles cannot interpenetrate and therefore aggregation is prevented by steric effects.

In essence, therefore, the hydrophilic region of κ-casein protects the micelles from aggregating and forming a coagulum.

Milk-clotting Enzymes and the Primary Phase of Coagulation

Rennet preparations from the stomachs of young ruminants are the traditional coagulants used in cheese manufacture. Calf rennet is the predominant coagulant although similar preparations can be made from kids or lambs. The major enzyme in rennet is chymosin.

Alternative clotting agents have been sought as there is a shortage of calf stomachs, and also to satisfy the market for vegetarian cheese. The proteinases may be used either as substitutes or to fortify traditional rennet preparations and include

- bovine, porcine and chicken pepsin;
- vegetable proteinases (traditionally used in Serra cheese in Portugal);
- chymosin produced by gene cloning in microorganisms (not yet widely available commercially);
- fungal proteinases (mainly from *Mucor miehei*, *M. pusillus* or *Endothia parasitica*). **See** Vegetarian Diets

Whether traditional rennet or a substitute is used, the major action is to hydrolyse the κ-casein at the Phe105–Met106 bond of the protein as shown schematically in Fig. 2. This bond is also very much more susceptible to acid hydrolysis than any other peptide bond in the molecule due to the primary structure and conformation of the surrounding amino acids. κ-Casein is therefore broken into the hydrophobic p-κ-casein, which remains attached to the micelle surface, and the hydrophilic caseinomacropeptide, which becomes detached from the micelle surface. In this way the majority of the protruding peptide 'hairs' are removed from the micelles, which is accompanied by a reduction in the ζ potential to between -5 and -7 mV. Thus, electrostatic and steric repulsion between micelles is greatly reduced and the micelles become destabilized. The hydrodynamic voluminosity of the micelles is also reduced.

The rate of κ-casein hydrolysis is affected by rennet concentration, Ca^{2+} concentration, ionic strength, temperature and pH. The optimum pH is in the range 5·0–5·5, although there is sufficient chymosin activity at the natural pH of milk (6·6–6·8) for clotting to occur. Many rennet curd cheeses are coagulated after acid development to a pH of about 6·4–6·6.

Chemistry and Microbiology of Cheesemaking

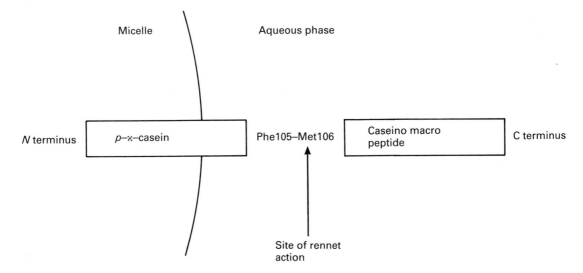

Fig. 2 Schematic diagram showing the possible orientation of κ-casein in the micelle, and the site of chymosin action.

Secondary Phase of Coagulation

Aggregation of the casein micelles can commence before the primary, enzymatic phase is complete. When approximately 85% of the κ-casein has been hydrolysed the micelles become destabilized to a critical level. The micelles then start to aggregate and the rate of aggregation increases until all the stabilizing caseinomacropeptide has been removed, after which the rate follows the Smoluchowski theory – i.e. the growth of molecular weight of the aggregate with time is linear. Initially the micelles form chain-like structures which link up to form a gel network which entraps the fat globules (if present). This process can be observed by electron microscopy. By the time that coagulation can be observed visually, the formation of a network is quite advanced.

The reasons for aggregation are not fully understood, but the process probably involves van der Waals attraction and hydrophobic interactions, as well as electrostatic interactions between amino acid residues of casein molecules in adjacent micelles. The presence of Ca^{2+} is critical to the mechanism, either due to the formation of cross-links between micelles, or to the neutralization of surface charges. In addition, colloidal calcium phosphate is essential for coagulation. Rennet coagulation time is, therefore, reduced by addition of Ca^{2+} and factors which affect the distribution of calcium in the milk (e.g. pH adjustments) will alter the aggregation rate.

The secondary phase is particularly temperature-sensitive. Coagulation does not take place below about 15°C even though κ-casein hydrolysis may be complete. Normally coagulation is carried out at about 31°C although the rate of aggregation is much higher at increased temperature.

Curd Development and Syneresis

Following coagulation the strength of the gel increases due to an increase in the number and strength of the attachments between micelles. Some authors suggest that cross-links are formed between micelles after they have come into contact. These involve the linking of phosphoryl groups of β-casein by Ca^{2+} bridges. Increasing the number of cross-links would result in an increase in gel strength. The strength of the gel relates to the yield and quality of cheese, and is determined by the composition and pretreatment of the milk plus the manufacturing methods.

After a period of gel development the curd is cut to permit syneresis (drainage of whey). Whey is actively expelled from the curd due to the force of the aggregation and resulting curd shrinkage. Control of syneresis is essential to the moisture content of the finished cheese. Many compositional factors such as pH, and Ca^{2+} and fat content, affect whey drainage. Increasing the fat level reduces syneresis by restricting casein aggregation and 'plugging' the channels in the curd through which the whey flows.

Coagulation by Acid or a Combination of Acid and Heat

Acid curd cheeses (e.g. quarg, cream, cottage) are usually consumed unripened and are prepared by acidification of milk to the isoelectric point (pI) using either starter organisms which produce lactic acid from lactose in the vat, or by addition of preformed acid or acidogen (e.g. glucono-δ-lactone). The four major caseins all have a pI at approximately pH 4·6 and are completely insoluble around this pH at normal curd-making temperatures (20–32°C.). If milk at 30°C is gradually acidified, gelation starts considerably before the pI – at approximately pH 5·1. As with enzymatic coagulation, this is at least partly due to a lowering of the ζ potential. Generally with colloidal proteins the ζ potential falls steadily with pH to become zero at the pI. The caseins are anomalous in this respect, having a mimimum ζ potential at pH 5·2, which more or less coincides with the onset of gelation. As the pH is further reduced, the ζ potential rises again before falling to zero at pH 4·6.

The destabilized (neutralized) casein again undergoes an aggregation process into chains and clusters of micelles, entrapping fat (if present) to form the curd, but there are differences from the formation of rennet curds. It is well established that acidification of milk results in solubilization of colloidal calcium phosphate so that at pH 5·1 almost all the calcium is removed from the micelles. In addition, some of the casein dissociates from the micelles (in the order $\beta > \kappa > \alpha_{s1}$) with a maximum solubility at approximately pH 5·4, the dissociation returning to zero at the pI. Hence the micelles are probably quite substantially disrupted before aggregation occurs, although much of the basic framework remains intact and they do not disintegrate completely.

Acid coagulation is temperature-dependent. The caseins remain soluble at the pI at $<6°C$, and the temperature of acidification will affect the texture of the resulting curd. Generally, acid curds are not as firm and do not drain as well as rennet curds.

Coagulation may also be brought about by acidification to pH 5·2–5·4 (using either lactic acid starters or added food grade acids such as lactic, acetic or citric acid) and heating to $>70°C$. Cheeses such as Ricotta, Chhana, Paneer and Queso Blanco can be prepared by this method. The milk protein system is extremely resistant to heat coagulation at its normal pH (e.g. milk may be heated to 140°C for 20 min before coagulation). This stability falls off markedly as the pH is reduced so that milk at pH 6·1 coagulates at 90°C and lower temperatures are required below this pH. The mechanism of heat gelation is not fully understood although it is not simple protein denaturation. Presumably, charge neutralization resulting from acidification accelerates the process. When temperatures $>80°C$ are used, as is usually the case for such cheeses, significant quantities of whey proteins are denatured and incorporated into the cheese.

Bibliography

Dalgleish DG (1987) The enzymatic coagulation of milk: In: Fox PF (ed.) *Cheese: Chemistry, Physics and Microbiology*, pp 63–96. London: Elsevier Applied Science.

Fox PF and Mulvihill DM (1990) Casein. In: Harris P (ed.) *Food Gels*, pp 121–173. London: Elsevier Applied Science.

Green ML and Grandison AS (1987) Secondary (non-enzymatic) phase of rennet coagulation and post-coagulation phenomena. In: Fox PF (ed.) *Cheese: Chemistry, Physics and Microbiology*, pp 63–96. London: Elsevier Applied Science.

Heertje I, Visser J and Smits P (1985) Structure formation in acid milk gels. *Food Microstructure* 4: 267–277.

Walstra P and van Vliet T (1986) The physical chemistry of curd making. *Netherlands Milk and Dairy Journal* 40: 241–259.

A. S. Grandison
University of Reading, Reading, UK

Chemistry and Microbiology of Maturation

Cheese Maturation (Ripening)

Most rennet-coagulated cheeses are ripened for at least 4 weeks before consumption. Cheese ripening involves several complex and dynamic biochemical processes which result in textural and flavour changes, unique for each variety. Notably, a 'green', rubbery, tough cheese with bland taste is converted into a 'mature', firm, elastic or soft-body cheese with a characteristic flavour.

The major biochemical changes which occur during ripening include lactose/lactate metabolism, proteolysis and lipolysis. These changes are brought about by the activities of residual rennet, enzymes from starter and nonstarter microorganisms, indigenous milk enzymes and exogenous enzymes added to the milk or cheese for specific functions. The composition of cheese (moisture, salt, pH) and ripening conditions (temperature, humidity) affect microbial growth enzyme activity and, consequently, the rate of ripening. *See* Enzymes, Uses in Food Processing

Rennets

'Rennet' was originally used to describe the milk-clotting enzyme preparation from the calf stomach, which contains the active digestive enzyme called chymosin (rennin). At present, the term 'rennet' is used broadly to describe all milk-clotting enzymes, including

(1) chymosin;
(2) bovine pepsin;
(3) porcine pepsin;
(4) chicken pepsin;
(5) *Mucor miehei* protease (MM);
(6) *Mucor pusillus* protease (MP);
(7) *Cryphonectria parasitica* (formerly *Endothia parasitica*) protease;

(8) fermentation-produced chymosin;
(9) blends of (1) and (2) or (3).

All the above enzymes, except porcine and chicken pepsins, are used for commercial cheesemaking. Rennet action during cheesemaking results in the conversion of milk into cheese.

A portion ($< 10\%$) of the rennet used in cheesemaking is retained in cheese. The amount of rennet retained depends on the pH of the milk at setting, the type and amount used and its ability to survive cooking temperatures used in cheesemaking. The retention of chymosin, bovine pepsin or porcine pepsin in cheese increases with decreasing pH of milk at which rennet is added (setting). However, the retention of proteases from *M. miehei*, *M. pusillus* and *C. parasitica* is independent of setting pH.

Starter and Nonstarter Microorganisms

'Starter' refers to a culture of lactic acid bacteria used for acid production, through the fermentation of lactose, during cheesemaking. Table 1 contains a list of starter and nonstarter microorganisms important in the ripening of major cheeses. *See* Lactic Acid Bacteria; Starter Cultures

Mesophilic starters (*Lactococcus lactis* subsp. *cremoris* (formerly *Streptococcus cremoris* or *Lc. lactis* subsp. *lactis* (formerly *S. lactis*)) are important in the ripening of Cheddar and Dutch-type (Gouda, Edam) cheeses. Thermophilic starters (*Streptococcus salivarius* subsp. *thermophilus* (formerly *S. thermophilus*) or *Lactobacillus delbruekii* subsp. *bulgaricus* (formerly *Lb. bulgaricus*)) are important in the ripening of Emmental-type (Swiss, Guyère) and Italian-type (Romano, Parmesan, Provolone) cheeses.

Other lactic acid bacteria (*Leuconostoc* spp., *Lc. lactis* subsp. *lactis* biovar. *diacetylactis* (formerly *S. diacetylactis*) or *Lb. helveticus*) play a role in the ripening of Dutch- and Emmental-type cheeses.

Microorganisms, other than lactic acid bacteria, significant to cheese ripening include *Propionibacterium shermanii* for Emmental-type cheese, moulds (*Penicillium roqueforti*, *P. glaucum*) for blue-veined varieties or *P. camemberti* for Camembert and Brie and *Brevibacterium linens* for Limburger.

Some cheese varieties contain nonstarter lactic acid bacteria (NSLAB), such as *Lactobacillus* spp. (*Lb. casei*, *Lb. plantarum*, *Lb. brevis*), *Pediococcus pentosaceus* and *Micrococcus* spp. Some of the biochemical processes which occur during cheese ripening are attributable to the activity of NSLAB.

Microbiological Changes

Starter bacteria multiply from 10^6–10^7 colony-forming units (cfu) ml^{-1} milk to $\sim 10^9$ cfu g^{-1} of fresh cheese.

There is a decline in starter population as ripening progresses. The rate of decline varies among cheeses and is dependent on the elimination of lactose (the primary source of energy), inhibition by salt and/or autolysis. Starter activity is inhibited when salt in the moisture (S/M) of cheese is $> 5\%$.

In Cheddar and Gouda cheeses, the starter population declines to $< 10^3$ cfu g^{-1} within the first few weeks while, in varieties like Provolone and Parmesan, cell densities remain high ($> 10^4$ cfu g^{-1}) even after 12 months of ripening.

In Emmental cheese, the maximum cell density of the lactic streptococci (10^9 cfu g^{-1} at the periphery and 10^8 cfu g^{-1} in the centre) is reached after about 3 h of pressing. The lactic and formic acids produced by the streptococci stimulate the growth of lactobacilli which reach cell densities of $\sim 10^9$ cfu g^{-1} after 10–20 h of pressing. The population of both lactic streptococci and lactobacilli declines after pressing and brining. The growth of propionibacteria is induced when the cheese is transferred to the warm room, which is usually at 20–25°C and 80–85% relative humidity (RH). Here, cell densities of propionibacteria reach 10^9 cfu g^{-1} in the centre, after 3 weeks.

In blue-veined cheeses, starter bacteria are inhibited by the high salt concentration (10% S/M). During the first few weeks of ripening (10°C, 96% RH), the cheese is pierced to admit air into the interior. This induces the growth of *P. roqueforti* to a maximum in ~ 90 days.

The growth of NSLAB in varieties like Cheddar begins after ~ 3 weeks of ripening. The cell densities of nonstarter lactobacilli may reach $\sim 10^7$ cfu g^{-1} in 10 weeks. Similar cell densities are reached by pediococci, while micrococci reach ~ 100 cfu g^{-1} during the same period.

Biochemical Changes

Lactose, Lactate and Citrate Metabolism

Lactose and to a lesser extent, citrate, are the primary carbon (energy) source for microorganisms in cheese. Both are catabolized to lactate (lactic acid) via a key intermediate, pyruvate, which serves as a precursor of various flavour and aroma compounds in cheese. *See* Lactose

The concentration of lactose in fresh cheese (1 day old) ranges from $< 0.1\%$ in Dutch- and Emmental-type cheese to about 1% in Cheddar. At S/M levels $< 5\%$, starter and NSLAB metabolize residual lactose to lactate, which may be produced in the L($+$) or D($-$) isomeric form, depending on the organism (Table 2). Lactic acid ($\sim 1.5\%$, in Cheddar) reduces the initial pH of cheese to < 5.3, and is a source of energy for some microorganisms, thereby serving as a precursor of flavour compounds.

Table 1. Microorganisms of importance in the ripening of cheese

Cheese category and Examples	Moisture content (% max.)	Starter	Other microorganisms
Very hard			
Parmesan	34	*Lb. delbruekii* subsp. *bulgaricus,*	Pediococci,
Romano	34	*S. salivarius* subsp. *thermophilus*	Micrococci,
			Propionibacterium sp.
Hard			
Cheddar	39	*Lc. lactis* subsp. *cremoris,*	*Lb. casei,*
		Lc. lactis subsp. *lactis*	*Lb. brevis,*
			Lb. plantarum
			Pediococci,
			Micrococci
Emmental	41	*S. salivarius* subsp. *thermophilus,*	
Gruyère	39	*Lb. delbruekii* subsp. *bulgaricus,*	
		Lb. helveticus, Lb. lactis,	
		Propionibacterium shermanii	
Gouda	45	*Lc. lactis* subsp. *cremoris,*	
Edam	45	*Lc. lactis* subsp. *lactis,*	
		Lc. lactis subsp. *lactis*	
		biovar. *diacetylactis, Leuconostoc* sp.	
Semisoft			
Limburger	52	*Lc. lactis* subsp. *cremoris,*	Yeasts, *Brevibacterium linens*
		Lc. lactis subsp. *lactis*	
Blue-vein mould			
Blue	46	*Lc. lactis* subsp. *lactis,*	*Penicillium roqueforti,*
Roquefort	45	*Lc. lactis,* subsp. *cremoris,*	Yeasts, micrococci
Gorgonzola	42	*Lc. lactis* subsp. *lactis*	
Stilton	42	biovar, *diacetylactis,*	
		Leuconostoc sp.	
Soft			
Brie	56	*Lc. lactis* subsp. *cremoris,*	*P. camemberti,*
Camembert	48	*Lc. lactis* subsp. *lactis*	*P. caseicolum,*
			P. candidum,
			Br. linens

L(+)-Lactate is metabolized by propionibacteria, in the pH range 5·0–5·3, to propionic acid, acetic acid and carbon dioxide (eqn [1]) in Emmental-type cheese. Some of the carbon dioxide produced accumulates in the cheese and forms holes, which are commonly called 'eyes'.

$$3\ CH_3CHOHCOOH \rightarrow 2\ CH_3CH_2COOH + CH_3COOH + CO_2 + H_2O \quad (1)$$
Lactic acid   Propionic acid   Acetic acid

In Cheddar cheese, NSLAB are capable of metabolizing lactose to produce ethanol and formic acid, both of which are undesirable in large quantities. The NSLAB may also oxidize lactate to acetate and carbon dioxide. Pediococci and lactobacilli convert L(+)-lactate to D(−)-lactate, resulting in a racemic mixture of both isomers after 6 months of ripening. D(−)-Lactate forms

an insoluble calcium salt which may crystallize in cheese and appear as undesirable white specks on cut surfaces. The injestion of high levels of D(−)-lactate by humans causes metabolic disturbances. *Lb. casei* and *Lb. plantarum* oxidize citrate to acetate and carbon dioxide, resulting in a gradual increase in acetic acid during Cheddar cheese ripening.

In Dutch-type cheeses, pyruvate, produced from citrate metabolism, is oxidized to diacetyl and carbon dioxide (eqn [2]) by *Lc. lactis* subsp. *lactis* biovar. *diacetylactis* and *Leuconostoc* spp.

$$2\ CH_3COCOOH + O_2 \rightarrow CH_3COCOCH_3 + 2\ CO_2 + H_2O \quad (2)$$
Pyruvic acid   Diacetyl

The metabolism of lactate and formation of alkaline nitrogen compounds (by proteolysis) result in an overall

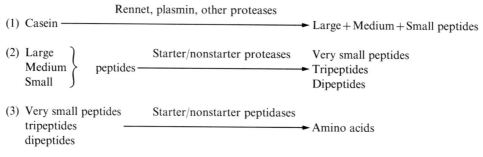

Scheme 1

increase in the pH of most varieties during ripening. After 6 months of ripening, the pH of Emmental-type cheese increases from ~5·3 to ~5·9 and those of Camembert and blue cheeses increase from ~4·8 to ~7. The pH of Cheddar cheese, however, increases only slightly (~0·2 pH unit) because the concentration of lactic acid remains high (1·2–1·9%), even after 12 months of ripening.

Proteolysis

Of the major milk proteins, α_{s1}-, α_{s2}- and β-casein predominate in cheese. Proteolysis involves the breakdown of these proteins and polypeptides therefrom by residual rennet, indigenous milk proteases and/or proteases/peptidases of starter and non-starter microorganisms. The effect of residual rennet on proteolysis is shown in Fig. 1. In general, the lowest level of proteolysis occurs in cheese made with porcine pepsin while the most extensive proteolysis occurs in cheese made with microbial rennets. *See* Casein and Caseinates, Uses in the Food Industry

Chymosin hydrolyses the Phe_{23}–Phe_{24} or Phe_{24}–Val_{25} bond of α_{s1}-casein to produce α_{s1}-I (α_{s1}-CN(f24/25–199)) peptide. The release of this peptide is probably the most important reaction responsible for the initial softening of cheese. Subsequent degradation of the α_{s1}-I peptide occurs during ripening.

Proteolysis of β-casein is less extensive than that of α_{s1}-casein in cheeses made with chymosin, bovine pepsin or porcine pepsin but more extensive breakdown of β-casein occurs in cheeses made with proteases from *Mucor miehei*, *M. pusillus* and *C. parasitica*.

Plasmin, an indigenous milk protease, hydrolyses all the caseins except κ-casein. Specifically, it hydrolyses β-casein to γ-caseins (β-CN(f29–209, 106–209 and 108–209)) and proteose peptone. The activity of plasmin is high in cheeses like Romano and Emmental which are manufactured using high cooking temperatures and is influenced by high pH.

Starter and nonstarter bacteria show very limited proteolysis towards whole caseins in cheese, although some strains of lactococci hydrolyse β-casein in solu-

Table 2. Isomers of lactic acid produced by lactic acid bacteria

Lactate isomer	Organism
L(+)	*Lc. lactis* subsp. *cremoris*
	Lc. lactis subsp. *lactis*
	Lc. lactis subsp. *lactis* biovar. *diacetylactis*
	S. salivarius subsp. *thermophilus*
D(−)	*Lb. delbruekii* subsp. *bulgaricus*
	Lb. lactis
	Leuconostac sp.
DL	*Lb. helveticus*
	Lb. plantarum
	Lb. brevis
	Lb. casei
	P. pentosaceus

tion. However, starter proteases and peptidases hydrolyse polypeptides, resulting from the action of rennet and/or indigenous milk proteases on caseins, to smaller peptides and amino acids essential for the development of flavour. The most common free amino acids in cheese include glutamic acid, methionine, asparagine, histidine, alanine, valine, phenylalanine, leucine and lysine. In Emmental-type cheese, proline is also present. *See* Amino Acids, Properties and Occurrence

Proteolytic enzymes from *Penicillium* and *Brevibacterium* spp. are major contributors to proteolysis in mould-ripened cheeses. Depending on the strain of *P. roqueforti* used, water-soluble nitrogen compounds in blue cheese may be as high as 50% of the total nitrogen content after 3 months of ripening.

A summary of the sequence of proteolytic events which take place during cheese ripening is shown in scheme 1.

Lipolysis

The action of lipase on triglycerides produces fatty acid(s), and mono- and diglycerides. Starter and nonstarter bacteria contain lipases which hydrolyse mono-

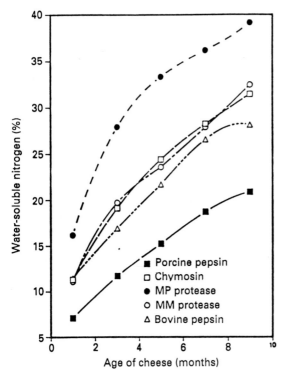

Fig. 1. Water-soluble nitrogen (% of total nitrogen) during ripening of Cheddar cheese made with identical milk-clotting activities of different enzymes.

and diglycerides, but have weak lipolytic activity towards unhydrolysed milk fat (triglycerides). Therefore, the concentration of free (C_4–C_{18}) fatty acids (FFA) in bacteria-ripened cheeses like Cheddar, Emmental-type and Dutch-type cheeses is low (0·1% in 3 month old Cheddar, increasing to <0·2% after 12 months of ripening). Cheddar cheese containing >0·2% FFA usually has a rancid flavour. *See* Fatty Acids, Properties; Triglycerides, Structures and Properties

The level of lipolysis during the ripening of blue-veined cheeses and some Italian varieties like Romano, Parmesan and Provolone is over three-fold greater than in Cheddar. Lipolysis in blue-veined cheeses is due to the activity of one (the acid enzyme) of the two (acid or neutral) types of lipases produced by *P. roqueforti*. Lipolysis in the Italian varieties is due to the activities of the exogenous esterases and/or lipases added during cheesemaking.

The sequential process of catabolism of fat during cheese ripening is as follows:

(1) liberation of FFA, and mono- and diglycerides from milk fat by lipase;

(2) oxidation of FFA to form β-keto acids (β oxidation);

(3) decarboxylation of β-keto acids to produce methyl ketones;

(4) reduction of methyl ketones to secondary alcohols.

The short-chain (C_4–C_{10}) fatty acids, methyl ketones (mostly 2-heptanone, followed by 2-nonanone and 2-pentanone) and secondary alcohols contribute to the characteristic flavour and aroma of cheese.

Other Chemical Changes

Small quantities of various organic compounds (e.g. aldehydes and esters, lactones, amines) present in cheese are products from the metabolism of free amino acids and fatty acids. For example, deamination of glycine and alanine produces methanol and ethanol, respectively; decarboxylation of tyrosine and histidine results in tyramine and histamine, respectively. The reduction of cystine/cysteine produces hydrogen sulphide, which reacts with methionine to form methanethiol. Methanethiol and hydrogen sulphide contribute to Cheddar cheese flavour.

Bibliography

Farkye NY and Fox PF (1990). Objective indices of cheese ripening. *Trends in Food Science and Technology* 1: 37–40.

Fox PF (ed.) (1991) *Cheese: Chemistry, Physics and Microbiology*, 2nd edn. London: Elsevier.

Fox PF, Lucey JA and Cogan TM (1990) Glycolysis and related reactions during cheese manufacture and ripening. *Critical Reviews in Food Science and Nutrition* 29: 237–253.

Robinson RK (ed.) (1990) *Dairy Microbiology*, 2nd edn, vol. 2. London: Elsevier.

Wong NP, Jenness R, Keeney M and Marth EH (eds) (1988) *Fundamentals of Dairy Chemistry*, New York: Van Nostrand Reinhold.

N. Y. Farkye
California Polytechnic State University, San Luis, USA

Manufacture of Extra-hard Cheeses

Classification, Definition, Examples

The extra-hard (or very hard) cheeses are a group of cheeses characterized by a long ripening time, and by production in large pieces having weights from 18 kg to more than 100 kg per whole cheese; they are produced principally in Mediterranean Europe with sheep's or cow's milk. The technology of production is thousands of years old, and the hard cheeses are characterized by having a low moisture content. *See* Sheep, Milk

Once they are ripe, their taste can be harsh and strong or delicate and fragrant, their structure is compact and friable, and they are used mainly for grating as a condiment. They play an important role in the Mediterranean diet.

The following cheeses are included in the group of extra-hard (or very hard) cheeses: grana, pecorino Romano, provolone piccante and caciocavallo, sapsagno and spalen.

Each grana (whole cheese) weighs 34–38 kg, and it is produced only in Northern Italy (Po Valley) using partially skimmed cow's milk. It is the best known cheese among those used for grating as a condiment and, in order to maintain all its fragrance, it should be grated just before use. The annual production is 190 000 tonnes, which means using more than 35% of the Italian whole-milk production.

The pecorino Romano cheese is one of the most ancient cheeses: a description of the cheesemaking process dating back to before Christ is available. It is produced in Sardinia and in the area around Rome, using only sheep's milk coagulated by means of rennet paste from lambs; whole cheeses range between 16 and 22 kg in weight, and its taste is typically strong.

The provolone piccante cheese and the caciocavallo cheese are typical stirred-curd cheeses, originating in, and very widespread in, the Mediterranean area. The large provolone piccante cheese is cylindrically shaped, and can weight up to 100 kg: it is produced with raw milk, rennet paste from kids and, once ripe, its taste is sharp, strong and very pleasant.

As far as the description of the manufacturing technology, both traditional and modern, of extra-hard cheeses is concerned, we are going to describe only that of the grana cheese, as it is the most well known.

Traditional Methods of Manufacture

The traditional method is not very different from methods used today, for it a feature of hard cheeses to apply technological rules which do not vary very much with the passing of time.

Up to about 100 years ago, grana cheese was very often manufactured in cheese factories designed following particular rules aimed at obtaining well-defined goals. Such a factory was a single, isolated building with an octagonal base, and walls free from windows. The height of the building was about 3 m, and the roof was supported by a wooden structure. Architecturally, such buildings are pleasant in appearance; a typical structure is shown in Fig. 1.

Inside, all the cheesemaking operations were carried out using direct-fire, milk heating and the typical structure allowed natural aeration.

According to tradition, raw milk obtained the evening before manufacture was poured into vats having a low height, but a large surface area, so as to facilitate

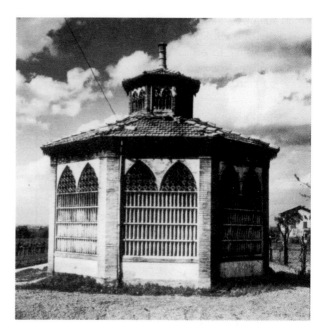

Fig. 1 Traditional dairy plant for grana cheese production.

separation of the cream; this process was necessary since grana cheese is produced with partially skimmed milk. The vats are either wood or tin-plated copper of sufficient volume to hold half of the milk necessary to produce a whole grana cheese, i.e. 250 litres. The creaming took place overnight and, in the morning, after the skimming operation, the milk was mixed with fresh milk, and cheese manufacture in a large copper vat could then start.

Up until the end of the 19th century, no starter cultures were added and, in order to reach the desired acidity, the polluting microflora collected during milking and in the cheesemaking operation was exploited; the vat was then left for a prolonged period which allowed a remarkable bacterial flora to develop. *See* Starter Cultures

Rennet of sucking calves was always used for coagulating the milk. After breaking the coagulum, very small curd granules, which had a very low moisture content, were obtained. The granules were smaller in dimension than rice grains, and the expulsion of whey was through the high 'cooking' temperature (53–54°C).

Originally the cheese vat had a capacity of 500 litres (so as to produce one whole cheese at a time), a truncated cone shape (inverted bell), was made of copper and had direct-fire heating.

Salting – using brine – was started 2 or 3 days after production, and continued for 25–28 days in separate brining rooms.

The ripening was carried out in stores at the prevailing temperature, i.e. under the influence of the seasons, temperatures varied from about 5 to 28°C. Ripening could last up to 24 months. During this long period, and especially in the first months, many manual operations were necessary in order to avoid the development of moulds on the cheese surfaces, and to obtain a smooth and even rind. Towards the end of the ripening period, the cheese was covered with a mixture of carbon black, umber and grape seed oil, so as to obtain a black colour and a characteristic shiny, bright appearance.

Modern Systems of Production

The current manufacturing technology of grana cheese shows, in comparison with the traditional one, some differences.

The current procedure uses raw milk, natural creaming and a high cooking temperature, but nowadays the technology also includes the addition of a starter culture, 'double cheesemaking', a rapid cheesemaking time, 'twins' production, controlled ripening as well as other changes which will be described later.

The whey starter culture was introduced at the end of the last century, and has a very complicated microbial composition. The prevailing bacteria are *Lactobacillus helveticus* together with *L. delbrueckii* subsp. *lactis* and subsp. *bulgaricus* and *L. fermentum*; thermophilic streptococci are generally absent. The culture is phage-resistant, has a high acidity capacity, a high thermophily, very good viability and is very easy to prepare. It is affected by the microbial characteristics of the milk and the environment where manufacture takes place, and it is the result of the action of several technological factors typical of each environment; due to its characteristics, it turns out to be an unrepeatable culture which cannot be replaced by the association of different strains in the laboratory. The activity of the natural whey culture is very important; primarily to produce an acid environment in the cheese (so inhibiting the gas-producing bacteria), to take part in the hydrolysis of proteins, as well as to take part in taste and fragrance formation. *See* Lactic Acid Bacteria; Whey and Whey Powders, Production and Uses

The 'double cheesemaking' process involves the transformation of milk from two milkings, and brings about the creaming of all the milk employed. From a practical point of view, this is a very important change, because by creaming at a temperature of 12–15°C, not only is the milk skimmed, but also many bacteria are carried out with the cream; an effect similar to that obtained through pasteurization.

This cold reduction in bacterial numbers leaves the cheesemaking properties of raw milk unchanged, a point of primary importance in grana cheese production.

This system is widespread in the whole production zone of grana Padano; the grana Parmigiano Reggiano cheesemakers keep to the traditional method of manufacture.

The 'rapid cheesemaking time' used today in grana cheese production refers to the time between the addition of rennet to the milk and the end of the curd cooking. At the end of the last century, the time was rather long – sometimes even 50–60 min – but today it is just 18–22 min.

The reasons for these changes include both the different conditions of milk production, and the introduction of thermophilic cultures of lactic acid bacteria. From a practical point of view, it allows better work organization, and more regular cheese quality standards.

The 'twins' production started with the replacement of the 500 litre vats with 1000 litre ones; the shape of the copper vat is unchanged, and is typical for this kind of cheese; the maximum capacity is 1000 litres of milk. As a consequence, two whole cheeses can be obtained each time, and these are called twins since they are the result of the division into two even parts of the curd obtained from 1000 litres of milk.

The number of grana cheese factories is still more than 1100 today, but a progressive transformation towards medium-to-large factories is taking place. As shown in Fig. 2, several copper vats may be found in one factory, but because the manufacture involves separate batches of milk of 1000 litres each there is neither real mechanization nor automation (not even cheese pressing is carried out mechanically). Nonetheless, the whole cheesemaking process in the vat is carried out in a short time, with a regular and precise sequence even in the case of large factories. Coagulum breaking, after a first phase which is still manual, and curd stirring up to complete cooking is carried out through simple mechanical means.

The long ripening stage is carried out in stores having controlled temperature, humidity and aeration: the temperature is 16–18°C, the humidity 85%, and the air change continuous without creating currents of air.

The ripening takes between 14 and 24 months (the grana Padano needs a shorter time in comparison with the Parmigiano Reggiano) and, during this period, the whole cheeses are often turned upside down: once a week in the first months, and then less frequently. The maintenance of the cheeses (turning upside down and brushing) is carried out mechanically by means of automatic systems.

The modern system for grana cheese production provides for milk cooling at 8°C for 12 h in sheds, then mixing with hot milk from the subsequent milking, thus allowing a single collection per day. If necessary, and in particular in areas where there is a high consumption of ensiled fodder, irregular fermentations can be avoided

Manufacture of Extra-hard Cheeses

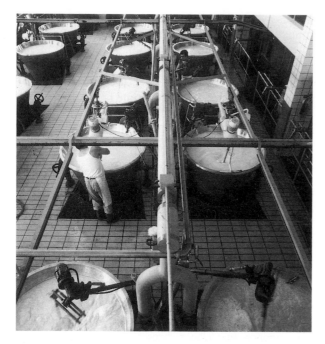

Fig. 2 Copper vats in a modern dairy plant for grana cheese production.

Table 1. Isomeric distribution of lactic acid with time in a grana cheese (values are in grams per litre)

0 h		2 h		4 h	
D(−)	0·90	D(−)	2·85	D(−)	3·99
L(+)	1·80	L(+)	4·47	L(+)	6·35
DL	2·7	DL	7·32	DL	10·34

22°Bé and temperature 16–17°C); the salting lasts 24–28 days.

(9) At the end of the salting and once the whole cheeses are dry, they are carried to the ripening store, kept at a temperature of 16–18°C and at a humidity of 85%.

Maturation and Storage

The grana cheese, after ripening, has the following average composition (%):

Protein	33·20	Moisture	32·00
Fat	27·50	Sodium chloride	1·60
Ash	4·80	Lactic acid	1·30

Due to the high content of protein in comparison to the low fat content, the grana cheese can be defined as a 'half-fat' cheese having a high protein content.

In the first hours of the life of a grana cheese, an intense fermentation process takes place, transforming the lactose into lactic acid. The pH value after 6 h is about 5·50 and after 16 hours 5·0, and the lactic acid is distributed as indicated in Table 1.

After 5 hours of fermentation, the lactose has dropped to about 1·6%, the accumulated galactose is slightly higher than 1% and the glucose reaches about 0·30%.

During the long ripening period, even the casein fractions undergo an intense hydrolytic reaction. β-Casein is rapidly hydrolysed in the first part of the ripening cycle, and its enzymatic degradation finishes within the first 12 months of ripening. However, α_{s1}-casein is degraded much more slowly. With reference to the total amount of hydrolysis products, about 30% is from β-casein, while those from α_{s1} casein form about 18%.

The release of amino acids increases progressively till about the 15th month of ripening and then becomes stable. When the cheese is ready to use, the amino acids form, on average, 22% of the total crude protein value and 7% of the cheese; as a consequence, grana cheese is one of the cheeses having a high content of free amino acids. In cheeses of first quality, serine increases progressively with the passing of ripening time and, at the end, it reaches about 1·5% of free amino acids; glutamine reaches 1% in the first 12 months and disappears once

through the partial elimination of bacteria by centrifugation. The main steps in Grana cheese production can be briefly described as follows:

(1) Milk is poured into 1000 litre vats having the dimension $4·50 \times 1·90 \times 0·25$ m for creaming, so that the milk reaches the copper, truncated coneshaped vats having a fat content ranging, depending on the region, from 2·00 to 2·30.

(2) After transfer of the partially skimmed milk to the 1000 litre copper vats, about 3% of natural whey culture is added as to reach an acidity (in lactic acid) in the mixture (milk + whey culture) of 0·19–0·20%; heating at 33°C follows, together with the addition of rennet (titre 1 : 100 000) – 2 g per 100 litres.

(3) Coagulation in 9–10 min and coagulum breaking in 3 min to obtain curd granules having the dimensions of rice grains.

(4) Heating (duration 7–8 min) to reach the cooking temperature of 54°C.

(5) Curd compaction at the bottom of the vat; the curd is then kept in the hot whey for about 45 min.

(6) Fresh paste (curd) extraction, splitting into two whole cheeses which are placed in the unfixed wood moulds; start of the pressing operation which is carried out not through mechanical means, but by loading each cheese with 20 kg weights.

(7) During the first 10 h, the cheeses are turned three to four times with cloth changes; after 15–20 h the cloths are removed and the wooden mould is replaced by a metal one.

(8) On the 3rd day the cheeses are brine salted (density

the ripening is finished and arginine, released during the ripening period, is degraded into ornithine. The presence of γ-aminobutyric acid indicates that anomalous fermentation processes have taken place. *See* Amino Acids, Properties and Occurrence

The hydrolysis of fat in grana cheese does not play an important role, in spite of the long ripening period. There is also a slight loss of vitamin A, a more remarkable loss of vitamin E, and a serious reduction of β-carotene from 640 to 100 μg per 100 g of cheese. *See* Carotenoids, Properties and Determination; Retinol, Properties and Determination; Tocopherols, Properties and Determination

The mineral component, composed of macro- and microelements, takes on a very precise character: calcium, phosphorus and magnesium are the elements present at higher levels: 1150 and 680 mg per 100 g as far as the first two are concerned, and 430 mg kg^{-1} for magnesium. The ratio of calcium–phosphorus is high (1·70) that is to say, much higher than that found in many other cheeses. *See* Calcium, Properties and Determination; Magnesium; Phosphorus, Properties and Determination

The average content of sodium is 650 mg per 100 g of grana cheese. Among the microelements, the content of zinc is very high. *See* Sodium, Properties and Determination; Zinc, Properties and Determination

The microbiological composition of grana cheese is characterized by two separate steps. The first concerns the very young cheese (first hours), and the second covers the first months, and even goes on till the end of ripening.

The lactic acid bacteria are very plentiful during the first period, and the flora is that of the starter, mainly composed of *L. helveticus*, reaching usually, after 12–14 h, 0.8–1×10^9 cells per gram of cheese and *L. fermentum* reaching maximum development in about 24–28 h with 120–140×10^6 cells per gram. In this first period, even *L. delbrueckii* subsp. *bulgaricus* and subsp. *lactis* are active. The development of this homo- and heterofermentative thermophilic, lactic acid flora plays a very important role in the commercial success of the final product, since it:

- ensures a rapid acidification of the fresh cheese;
- regulates the whey drainage;
- accumulates enzymes of the proteolytic system;
- causes the formation of small holes;
- produces volatile compounds;
- contributes to the formation of the cheese structure.

Figure 3 shows the formation of microcolonies of thermophilic lactic acid bacteria in grana cheese 12 h old.

In the second period, a nonstarter lactic acid flora develops consisting of coccoid lactic acid bacteria, e.g.

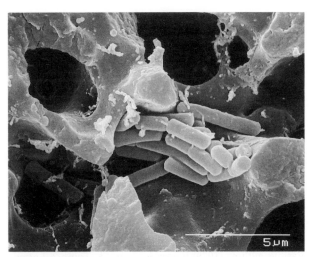

Fig. 3 Microcolony of rod-shaped lactic acid bacteria in a 24 h grana cheese.

Pediococcus acidilactici and rod-shaped bacteria, e.g. *L. casei* subsp. *casei*, subsp. *pseudoplantarum* and subsp. *rhamnosus*.

In the period of maximum development, that is, 25–40 days after production, this lactic acid flora reaches 60–80×10^6 cells per gram, but, for the remaining ripening period, the number decreases progressively. Pediococci are the most resistant forms, and are still present in the cheese at the time of consumption.

The metabolic activity of the mesophylic lactic acid bacteria contributes to the development of the ripening process, and its contribution to casein hydrolysis is very important.

Finally, there are the propionic bacteria, which are useful for the formation of the organoleptic characteristics of the cheese, so long as their development is limited to a few million cells per gram.

Specification and Standards

The grana cheese produced in the Po Valley can have the mark 'Parmigiano Reggiano' or 'Grana Padano', depending on the areas of production.

It is a half-fat hard cheese, cooked and slowly ripened, its colour is light straw-yellow, it has a compact, granulose and friable structure with flake-shaped radial fracture and a fragrant and delicate aroma. For its production, raw milk, half-skimmed through natural creaming, is used. To the milk is added a natural starter culture of thermophilic lactic acid bacteria developed in whey, and it is coagulated by means of rennet from suckling calves. The ripening lasts 18–24 months for Parmigiano Reggiano, and 13–15 months for grana Padano.

The ripe product, ready to eat, has:

- a cylindrical form with convex (lateral) sides, and the flat sides are also slightly convex;

- dimensions varying between 35 and 45 cm in diameter, and between 18 and 24 cm in height of the lateral side;
- a whole cheese weight between 32 and 34 kg;
- a hard, smooth, bright surface, having a natural uniform colour.

The grana cheese is principally used for grating as a condiment.

Bibliography

Various authors (1979) Il formaggio grana. Tomo 1. Latteria Didattica P. Marconi, Thiene (VI).

Various authors (1979) Il formaggio grana. Tomo 2. Latteria Didattica P, Marconi, Thiene (VI).

Various authors (1988) Atti giornata di studio "Ricerca triennale sulla composizione e su alcune peculiari caratteristiche del formaggio Parmigiano Reggiano". Reggio Emilia 28 marzo 1988. Consorzio del Formaggio Parmigiano Reggiano.

Bosi F, Bottazzi V, Vescovlo M, Scolari GL, Battistotti B and Dellaglio F (1990) Batteri lattici per la produzione di formaggio grana. I parte: caratterizzazione tecnologica di ceppi di lattobacilli termofili. *Scienza e tecnica Lattiero Casearia* 41: 105–136.

Bottazzi V (1979) *Microbiologia del Fermenti Lattici.* Modena: Aitel.

Fortina MG, Parini C, Manachini PG, Morelli L, Bottazzi V and Concari P (1990) Genotypic and phenotypic correlationships among some strains of *Lactobacillus helveticus*. *Biotechnology Letters* 12(10): 765–770.

Parisi O (1958) *Il Formaggio Grana*. Mucchi, Modena: Stem.

V. Bottazzi
Università Cattolica, Piacenza, Italy

Manufacture of Hard-pressed Cheeses

Definition of the Group

Cheese has been known to humans for thousands of years, but it was the development of large, hard-pressed cheeses such as Cantal and Gruyère, which made cheese transportable and established over a wider area. With the opening up of trade in the 16th and 17th centuries, transport and storage were of prime importance, and it was the resourceful Dutch who improved Edam cheese so that it was pressed more efficiently and had a well-protected rind. This early work was so effective that Edam remains one of the most popular and widely exported varieties. The most usual method of classification of cheese is by moisture content, which also acts as an indication of the keeping quality. The group defined as hard-pressed cheeses has a moisture content of 36–50%, thus excluding the extra hard (grating) cheeses such as Parmesan, Asagio and Sbrinz, but including some of the semihard types such as Caerphilly and Lancashire. Most countries have regulations determining the composition of cheeses, and the moisture and fat in dry matter (F in DM) in Table 1 are taken from the UK regulations.

Traditional Methods of Manufacture for Cheddar and Related Types

The method described is a general Cheddar method which covers most of the varieties in this group. Slight

Table 1. Hard and semihard cheese (moisture content 36–50%)

Cheese	Country of origin	Scalding temperature	Moisture max %	F in DM[a]	Semi-hard	Character
Cheddar	UK	Medium	39	48		Firm body, close texture, may be coloured
Derby	UK	Medium	42	48		Not so firm as Cheddar, close texture, uncoloured
Red Leicester	UK	Low	42	48		Firm body, flaky texture, highly coloured
Cantal	France	Medium	44	45		Firm body, more open texture, uncoloured
Double Gloucester	UK	Medium	44	48		Firm body, not so close textured as Cheddar, slight colour
Dunlop	UK	Medium	44	48		Smooth, close texture, uncoloured
Cheshire	UK	Low	44	48		Firm body, crumbly texture, may be coloured
Edam	Netherlands	Low	46	40	+	Pliant body, rubbery texture, uncoloured
Gouda	Netherlands	Low	45	48	+	Firm body, flexible texture, uncoloured
Wensleydale	UK	Low	46	48	+	Firm body, flaky texture, uncoloured
Caerphilly	UK	Low	46	48	+	Soft/firm body, close texture, uncoloured
Lancashire	UK	Low	48	48	+	Soft body, very crumbly texture, uncoloured

[a] F in DM, fat in dry matter.

alterations to the method can be used to produce varieties such as Cantal and double Gloucester. With cheeses, such as Cheshire, which differ from Cheddar in body, texture and maturation time, this is brought about by variations in the manufacture, i.e. increasing the starter inoculation rate together with a rapid make time, a lower scald temperature and a high moisture.

Treatment of the Milk

Cheese may be manufactured from raw or pasteurized milk. Most cheese produced in modern factories is made from pasteurized milk, resulting in a more uniform product.

Raw milk is standardized to a casein:fat ratio (0·68–0·72) or fat:SNF (solids not fat) ratio (0·33–0·46). The milk is then pasteurized at 72°C for 15 s and cooled to 30–32°C. *See* Milk, Processing of Liquid Milk

Addition of the Starter Culture

Starter is added either as a bulk starter usually at 1–2% (v/v), or as a DVS (direct vat starter) equivalent. The starters for Cheddar and related types are mesophilic homofermentative cultures of *Lactococcus lactis* subsp. *lactis* and *cremoris*. There is usually a ripening period of 30–60 min depending upon the type of starter added. DVS cultures require a longer ripening period. *See* Lactic Acid Bacteria; Starter Cultures

Addition of Annatto and Other Additives

Colour in the form of cheese annatto, and chemicals such as calcium chloride may be required by the recipe, and these are usually added during the ripening period. The colour of the cheese is an important characteristic and, to keep the colour constant, some cheesemakers follow the practice of adding varying amounts of annatto throughout the year to compensate for variations in the milk due to feeding and climatic conditions. Some varieties, such as red Leicester, have a definite requirement for colour stated in the recipe. Annatto for use in cheese is a colour extracted by sodium hydroxide from the seeds of the South American plant *Bixa orellana*. The pigment in annatto is the acid bixin which, in the alkaline form, becomes norbixin. *See* Colours, Properties and Determination of Natural Pigments

Successful coagulation of the milk depends upon the calcium balance and this may be disturbed, under certain circumstances, by the processing of the milk. The addition of calcium chloride, usually about 0·02%, will redress this.

Addition of Rennet

There are several types of rennet available to the cheesemaker:

(1) Standard rennet, which is derived from the stomachs of young milk-fed calves. The enzyme chymosin is extracted from the fourth stomach or vel by soaking for several days in a 10% sodium chloride solution.
(2) 50/50 rennet, which contains a proportion of bovine or porcine pepsin and pure calf chymosin.
(3) Microbial rennets, which are produced from moulds, such as *Mucor meihei* or *M. pusillus*, and bacteria such as *Endothia parasitica* and *Bacillus subtilis*. These rennets are suitable for the production of cheese for vegetarians.
(4) Plant rennets, which are not so widely used; however, in Portugal, the plant proteinase from a species of the genus *Cynara* is used for the production of Serra cheese.
(5) Genetically engineered chymosin is produced by cloning the allele(s) responsible for calf chymosin into host organisms such as *Kluyveromyces marxianus* var. *lactis*. This results in a chymosin identical to calf rennet.

Clotting times tend to be longer with pepsin rennets than with calf rennets. The development of so many coagulants has been brought about because of the increasing amounts of milk available for cheesemaking, and the decline in the slaughter of young calves. It is important for the cheesemaker to be aware of the characteristics of each of the rennets, and that care is taken when changing from one rennet to another. After pressing, approximately 6% of the enzyme is carried over into the curd where it is still active.

Rennet is usually diluted 5–6 times with cold potable water immediately before adding to the vat milk. This ensures an even distribution of the rennet in the milk when a stirring time of 3–5 min is allowed. A fact which may be overlooked in the use of rennet is its destruction by chlorine in the water used for dilution purposes, and it is a point of good management to avoid leaving rennet diluted for long periods. Coagulation occurs in 20–50 min, provided the temperature of the milk is maintained, and there is a degree of developed acidity.

Cutting the Curd

The purpose of cutting the curd is to expel moisture. The curd is cut into small cubes varying in size from 5 to 15 mm, depending upon the variety of the cheese. This gives an increased surface area from which the whey can be expelled. Many attempts have been made to automate this phase in the cheesemaking process, but the cheesemaker invariably judges the point of cutting by placing the hand or knife blade below the surface of the curd, and then gently lifting the finger or the blade until the coagulum breaks in a clean split with whey in the base. In small factories, the curd is cut with hand-held multibladed knives or wires whereas, in the larger factories, the knives or wires are mechanically operated.

Manufacture of Hard-pressed Cheeses

It is a point of good management that the blades of the knives be kept sharp, so that they cut the curd cleanly and do not damage it by tearing, thereby losing excessive amounts of fat into the whey. It is usual to cut the curd once lengthways and once across the vat with the vertical hand-held knives, and then once with the horizontal knife. The curd particles are then reduced to the required size with the vertical knife. The mechanical knives used in the larger vats operate at controlled speeds until the size of the curd particle is correct; they are then reversed for the stirring process.

Stirring and Scalding the Curd

Immediately after cutting the curd is stirred at a slow speed, and without heat, to allow it to 'heal', where the surface fat globules have been exposed and lost into the whey. Once the 'healing' process has occurred, the stirring speed may be increased. Heat is fed into the jacket of the vat in the form of steam or hot water, and the curds and whey are heated over a period of 30–60 min.

Scalding causes the curd to shrink and expel more whey, while the extra warmth speeds up the metabolism of the starter organisms trapped in the curd. Lactic acid is produced, the pH drops and the acidity assists in the expulsion of more whey.

Low-temperature scalds leave more moisture and lactose in the curd and produce a softer, more acid cheese which matures quickly, e.g. Wensleydale, Caerphilly and Lancashire.

High-temperature scalds produce a drier, firmer curd and a slower-maturing cheese, e.g. Cheddar.

The importance of a starter culture which produces acidity at a regular rate can now be seen – the faster the acid development, the greater the expulsion of moisture. The amount of lactose available in the curd for lactic acid production may be controlled by the scald temperature and reduction in pH but, in some washed curd varieties, the addition of hot water to the whey/curd mixture extracts the lactose by osmotic pressure into the diluted whey. This latter treatment results in a much more pliant or rubbery texture.

It is possible to apply heat to the curds and whey too quickly, thus cooking the outside of the curd particles, and locking in the moisture; this is known as 'case hardening'.

The maximum scald temperature is usually determined by the required moisture content of the cheese and heat tolerance of the starter bacteria. Mesophilic starter cultures will be inhibited at temperatures in excess of 40°C.

Pitching the Curd

It is the cheesemaker's decision whether or not the curds and whey are pitched, i.e. allowing the curd to settle and form a mass in the bottom of the vat. If the acidity development is rapid, it is normal to stir the curds until the whey is drawn. Where acid development is normal, the curds are pitched, when stirring ceases and the curd settles to the bottom of the vat to facilitate the removal of the whey.

Removal of the Whey

This is an important stage in the manufacture of all varieties of cheese. At this stage the acidity of the curd is greater than that of the whey, since the starter bacteria and casein are mainly enclosed in the former; the titratable acidity of the casein, contained in the curd, contributes to this. In cheese not textured in the vat or on coolers, and hence where little starter activity is required during the texturing (e.g. Edam and Gouda), the curd is removed from the whey into the moulds or hoops and pressed; the pH continues to fall until the cheeses are brined. In textured cheese curds (e.g. Cheddar) the whey is removed from the vat where the curds may then be textured, or the curds and whey are pumped onto drainage tables where the texturing takes place while the vats are being refilled. *See* Casein and Caseinates, Methods of Manufacture; Whey and Whey Powders, Production and Uses

During the cheddaring or texturing process, the starter bacteria continue to multiply as the pH falls. For Cheddar cheese the optimum pH is 5·20. Cheeses in the pH range 4·9–5·0 usually have a more crumbly texture. Cheddaring usually takes about 1 h, during which time the titratable acidity increases 0·05% every 10 min, and the curd changes from being fragile and crumbly to having a smooth texture which exhibits the characteristic 'chicken breast' texture (Fig. 1). This is caused by the increasing acidity which strips calcium from the relatively inert dicalcium paracaseinate to form monocalcium paracaseinate and free paracaseinate which gives the plastic properties to the resulting cheese.

With cheeses such as Cheshire, the curd is broken and kept separate while the acidity develops, so giving a more crumbly nature to the cheese.

Milling and Salting

Milling aerates and cools the curd, allows further drainage of whey and ensures uniform distribution of salt over the increased surface area. Most of the hard-pressed cheeses produced in the UK are dry salted, with the exception of Caerphilly, which is sometimes brined.

Dry salt levels are between 1·7 and 2·0%. Sufficient time must be allowed after salting to ensure adsorption onto the curd surfaces.

Manufacture of Hard-pressed Cheeses

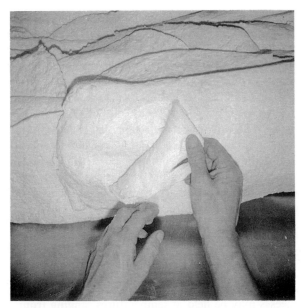

Fig. 1 The characteristic chicken breast texture of Cheddar cheese.

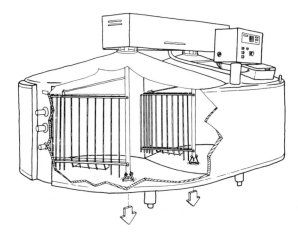

Fig. 2 A modern cheesemaking vat-type OCT. Reproduced by permission of APV Pasilac AS.

Pressing the Curd

The object of pressing is to form the loose curd particles into a compact mass and expel whey. In traditional methods of manufacture, the curd is filled into moulds or forms and pressed for 1–3 days. Pressure is applied gradually to avoid the entrapment of whey within the cheese. The temperature of the curd before pressing should be below 26°C or fat will be lost into the whey. In mechanised operations, the milled curd is pressed under vacuum and 18–20 kg blocks are cut from the pressed cheese. These blocks are then vacuum packed, coded, boxed, cooled and palletized into loads of approximately 1 tonne.

Recent Developments in Plant and Processing

Over the last 30 years, enormous strides have been made in the mechanization of cheesemaking. Unfortunately, these mechanized systems require large amounts of capital investment which is not always available.

Starting with milk treatment, the following systems exist and all are methods of reducing heat damage:

(1) Bactofugation or bacterial centrifugation. This has been in use for some years and removes bacteria from the milk in a high-speed centrifuge. This method is particularly effective in removing spore-forming bacteria; 80–90% of the bacteria from the original milk may be removed along with a small volume of milk, which is then sterilized and recombined with the cheese milk.
(2) Microfiltration, known as 'Bacto-catch'. This involves pumping milk through a ceramic filter with a pore size sufficient to allow the casein micelles and lactose molecules to pass but not large enough for the passage of bacteria or bacterial spores. The retentate, which contains a concentration of bacteria, spores and fat globules, is then subjected to UHT treatment before being fed back into the permeate. Dutch-type varieties are especially vulnerable to butyric acid fermentation, and nitrate has been used as a preventative measure for many years. This microfiltration system is particularly useful if nitrate addition to the cheese milk is not permitted.
(3) In-line standardization. These units are available for maintaining an exact fat:protein ratio. Standardization of protein by ultrafiltration is also possible. *See* Membrane Techniques, Principles of Ultra-filtration
(4) Sirocurd process for Cheddar cheese. In this system whole milk is first standardized and pasteurized, followed by fivefold concentration, which removes 80% of the milk volume as permeate. The retentate is then blended with a concentrated starter ($9 \times 10^7 \, g^{-1}$) and one-third of normal rennet usage; this is then held until a coagulum forms. The curd moves forward through a series of cylinders where cutting, scalding and syneresis take place. Eight per cent of the original volume is released in the syneresis stages; the manufacturing time is reduced by 1 h, and yield increases of 6–8% are claimed. This is a system which requires considerable capital investment. A careful study of yields and the quality of the cheese produced would be necesary to justify such expenditure.
(5) Curdmaking equipment. The traditional cheese vats used in curdmaking were open, with rounded ends and overhead cutting and stirring mechanisms. The capacity of the vats was 20000 litres. Modern cheese vats are enclosed tanks, either horizontal or vertical, with capacities of up to 26000 litres (Fig. 2). These vats are designed for renneting, cutting and scalding processes.

They have programmable controls and outlets for the drainage of 25 and 50% of the liquid volume, giving increased versatility.

(6) Texturing of the curd. For small-scale procuction, the curds and whey are delivered on to end-unloading curd tables which have an overhead, curd-manipulating apparatus. The curd is salted on the table, the end of the vat opened and the curd pushed into the mill, from where it is filled in weighed amounts into the moulds. This system allows quite a large amount of flexibility in the varieties of cheese made. For larger-scale systems, the curd may be delivered onto a system of conveyor belts where it is dry stirred or allowed to fuse. Milling and salting are in-line, and the system is designed for flexibility by varying the length of the conveyor belts and fitting stirrers for textured curds. This system is often used with a block former which fuses the curd under vacuum into 18–20 kg blocks. The curd is filled into a stainless steel tower under vacuum, and the blocks formed are consistent in weight, shape and size. The blocks are then vacuum sealed, coded and boxed, cooled and palletized into loads of approximately 1 tonne.

Cheese Ripening

This is a complex process which takes from 2 weeks to over 12 months. During this time, the tough flavourless curd changes, with the production of a flavour, aroma and texture characteristic of the variety. Changes also occur in the physical, chemical and organoleptic state of the cheese brought about by enzymes which are present in the curd from the starter bacteria, residual enzymes from rennet, somatic cells and the indigenous flora of the milk.

The chemical constituents involved in this process are protein, fat and carbohydrate.

Most of the lactose disappears within the first 10 days of manufacture, having been converted to lactic acid and small amounts of acetic and propionic acid, as well as carbon dioxide and diacetyl.

The proteins are water-insoluble, but are hydrolysed by enzyme action into more simple compounds, e.g. polypeptides–peptides and amino acids. These contribute to the flavour, and cause physical changes in the cheese, making it softer and creamier. *See* Flavour Compounds, Structures and Characteristics

Fat is not broken down to any great extent, but lipolytic enzymes produce glycerol and volatile fatty acids which contribute to the distinctive flavour of the cheese, and also influence the texture, making it smooth and velvety. It can be seen that the final flavour of the cheese is made up of a fine balance of a large number of compounds.

Accelerated ripening may be achieved within the UK legislation by two methods: (1) elevated ripening temperatures; (2) use of modified starter cultures.

By acceleration of ripening times, the producer reduces the cost of storage. The traditional ripening temperature for cheddar is 6–8 °C but, by increasing the temperature to 12–13°C, the ripening rate is increased by 50%. Today, there is a trend towards low-fat cheese, i.e. less than 17% fat. The problems connected with the production of low-fat cheese are bitter flavour and poor texture. The addition of a modified starter culture, which has been treated so that it no longer influences the production of acidity, but still possesses an enzyme system capable of degrading the bitter peptides, would seem to be the answer to these problems. This system works well at temperatures from 7 to 12°C.

Storage of Cheese

Maturation is influenced by temperature and humidity. Cheeses may be held at temperatures ranging from 5–12°C and at a relative humidity of 85–88%; this prevents excessive evaporation of moisture which can cause defects in the cheese rind. Traditional methods of treating the cheese after pressing include cloth bandages, paraffin wax or plastic coatings. Most modern factories now package hard cheese in vacuum-packed, barrier bags, which give excellent protection from mould spoilage and evaporation. Where this method of packaging is employed, the relative humidity need not be controlled.

Bibliography

Eck A (ed.) (1986) *Cheesemaking – Science and Technology*, 2nd edn. New York: Lavoisier Publications.

Flowerdew DW (Leatherhead Food Research Association) (1990) *A guide to the Food Regulations in the U.K.*, 4th edn., 1st supp. Leatherhead: The British Food Manufacturing Industries R.A.

Fox PF (ed.) (1987) *Cheese: Chemistry, Physics and Microbiology*. London: Elsevier.

Kosikowski FV (1982) *Cheese and Fermented Milk Foods*, 2nd edn. New York: Kosikowski.

Scott R (1986) *Cheese*, 2nd edn. London: Elsevier.

Valerie E Bines
Milk Marketing Board, Reading, UK

Cheeses with 'Eyes'

In the production of hard (and semihard) cheese, curd grains with relatively low water content are pressed into a loaf. Pressing is essential to form a coherent loaf of the dimensions specific to a variety of cheese, and a closed, firm rind. Several varieties desirably develop round to oval-shaped, shiny openings (eyes) in the cheese body during ripening; most representative are Swiss-type and Dutch-type varieties. The eyes result from carbon dioxide production by particular bacteria.

In Dutch-type cheeses, gas production results from the metabolic activity of lactic acid bacteria, deliberately added to the cheese milk to initiate lactic acid fermentation (starter culture). Besides homofermentative strains, the starter generally includes heterofermentative strains (see below) liberating carbon dioxide during the lactic acid fermentation; the main source for gas production, however, is the decomposition of citrate in milk by particular starter organisms. The degree of gas production favours the formation of relatively small eyes. Examples are Gouda and Edam cheese (The Netherlands) and Danbo (Denmark) *See* Lactic Acid Bacteria

In Swiss-type cheeses, lactic acid fermentation predominantly proceeds by homofermentative fermentation (see below), and eye formation results from gas production by propionic acid bacteria. These may originate from the raw milk used in cheesemaking, but are always added to the milk in the manufacture of cheese made from pasteurized milk (heat treatment of milk for 20 s at 72°C will kill these organisms). Examples of cheeses with large to very large eyes are Emmental (Switzerland), Jarlsbergost (Norway) and Maasdam-type cheese (The Netherlands). Some other varieties should show only modest propionic acid fermentation, and their ripening conditions are aimed to limit the degree of eye formation. Examples are Gruyère (Switzerland), Fontina (Italy) and Samso (Denmark). *See* Milk, Processing of Liquid Milk

Most varieties of hard cheese keep a dry rind during ripening. However, some are treated to develop a slimy surface of predominantly yeasts and coryneform bacteria producing specific flavour compounds, e.g. Gruyère and Appenzeller (Switzerland) and Tilsiter (Germany).

Openings in cheese do not always result from gas production; for example, inclusion of air bubbles in the curd may cause small holes in the cheese body. Finally, openings in cheese as eyes, cracks, etc., may result from undesirable growth of microorganisms producing gas (see *Microbial Defects with Gas Formation*, below)

Lactic Acid Fermentation

Fermentation of any cheese starts with the conversion of the milk sugar lactose by homo- or heterofermentative lactic acid bacteria. Homofermentative fermentation almost exclusively produces lactate, whereas heterofermentation leads to the production of lactate, acetate, ethanol and carbon dioxide. To control fermentation, a starter culture of lactic acid bacteria is added to the cheese milk.

This culture consists of strains of species of lactic acid bacteria with specific properties. Selection of starter organisms depends on the manufacturing conditions and the desired characteristics of the variety of cheese to be made. Starters for Swiss-type cheeses predominantly consist of homofermentative, thermophilic species (optimum growth temperature 38–45°C) – *Streptococcus thermophilus* and the lactobacilli, *Lactobacillus helveticus*, *L. lactis* and *L. delbrueckii* subsp. *bulgaricus* – which survive the high cooking temperature during manufacture (see *Cooking or Scalding*, below). Starters for Dutch-type varieties are composed of mesophilic bacteria (optimum growth temperature 20–30°C); they always contain homofermentative species, *Lactotoccus lactis* and/or *Lactococcus lactis* subsp. *cremoris* as the main lactic acid producers, and the heterofermentative *Leuconostoc mesenteroides* subsp. *cremoris* and/or the homofermentative *Lactococcus lactis* biovar. *diacetylactis* as citrate-fermenting organisms. *See* Starter Cultures

Lactic acid fermentation in cheese is generally completed within 24 h at maximum. The lower the pH as a result of this process, the more lactic acid is present in the undissociated form and acting as a preservative. The absence of lactose and a low pH hinder the development of undesirable microorganisms, which need a fermentable sugar or a higher pH for growth. Lactic acid bacteria grow best under microaerophilic conditions; during their growth in cheese they lower the redox potential (E_h), thus preventing any undesirable growth of aerobic microorganisms. These factors and the salting of cheese crucially contribute to its keepability.

Lactic acid greatly affects the taste of cheese and, by its effect on pH, the texture (see *Evolution of Eyes*, below) and the consistency of the product, e.g. elasticity or sliceability.

Propionic Acid Fermentation

Propionic acid fermentation mostly involves the species *Propionibacterium freudenreichii* var. *shermanii*. A small quantity of a culture of this organism may be added to the cheese milk, in addition to the lactic starter. Propionic acid bacteria prefer a low E_h for growth, which means anaerobic conditions. Their fermentation starts when the lactic acid fermentation has finished. To initiate fermentation, the cheese ripening temperature is raised to 18–25°C for a certain period of time (20–30 days). The propionic acid fermentation starts with the conversion of lactate and leads to production of propionate, acetate and carbon dioxide.

When sufficient eye formation has been achieved, the fermentation process is retarded by storing the cheese at a lower temperature. Propionic acid imparts a particular sweet taste to the cheese.

Cheeses with 'Eyes'

Evolution of Eyes

Normal eye formation in cheese is the result of gas – mostly carbon dioxide – production. Carbon dioxide easily dissolves in cheese moisture, so that in order to initiate eye formation a certain oversaturation of the moisture with the gas is necessary; small air bubbles in the cheese probably also serve as nuclei, facilitating that process. Various factors determine the development and size of gas holes in cheese: velocity and extent of carbon dioxide production within a particular time; water content of the cheese; rate of carbon dioxide diffusion in the cheese; size of the cheese (a larger surface to volume ratio favours the escape of more carbon dioxide into the environment); temperature of the cheese (at low temperatures, dissolution of carbon dioxide in cheese moisture is increased).

When the gas is produced too slowly, an oversaturated state does not develop and few or no holes are formed; when it is generated too rapidly the gas has insufficient time to diffuse and too many, too small holes may become visible. Large openings will also be produced by too high a rate of gas production. Cheese structure is of crucial importance to the shape of the holes: when it permits the cheese mass to 'flow', round eyes will be formed; otherwise, splits or cracks will result. Conditions most favourable for round-eye formation are a pH of 5·3 and a rather low salt content ($<2.5\%$).

Microbial Defects with Gas Formation

Some microbial defects are accompanied by excessive gas formation, negatively affecting the smell, taste and texture of the cheese. The most important defects of this type are as follows:

1. Butyric acid fermentation, caused by anaerobic clostridia, *Clostridium tyrobutyricum* in particular, which decompose lactate acid into butyric acid (awful smell), acetic acid, carbon dioxide and hydrogen gas. Hydrogen gas is almost insoluble in the moisture of cheese, and its production involves rapid formation of (large) eyes, splits or cracks, depending on the cheese consistency ('late gas blowing'). Silage, used as the cow's feed, is the main source of contamination of the raw milk. These bacteria are not destroyed by pasteurization of cheese milk, and because of their favourable chemical composition, especially pH, Dutch-type and, in particular, Swiss-type varieties are very vulnerable to this defect. The use of silage may therefore be prohibited in areas with Emmental cheese production. Other precautions to reduce the number of spores in milk and to limit the chance for butyric acid fermentation involve hygienic milking of cows, removal of the vast majority of spores from milk by centrifugal force (bactofuga-

tion), the use of some nitrate and egg-white lysozyme when these additions are legally accepted.

2. At the early stages of cheese production, coliform bacteria, e.g. *Enterobacter aerogenes*, may decompose lactose to a variety of substances, among them carbon dioxide and hydrogen ('early gas blowing'). This fermentation causes off-flavours and a bad texture in the cheese. The organisms are destroyed by pasteurization of cheese milk. Hygienic milking, particularly when cheese has to be made of raw milk, adequate pasteurization and strictly hygienic conditions during cheese manufacture help to prevent the defect. *See* Pasteurization, Principles

3. Even in cheese made from pasteurized milk, particular lactic acid bacteria (nonstarter organisms) may cause off-flavours and, through the excessive production of carbon dioxide, splits, cracks or too many or too large eyes (e.g. too large eyes in Dutch-type cheeses). Carbon dioxide production is most frequently caused by decarboxylation of amino acids. Hygienic conditions throughout the manufacturing process must be strictly maintained to prevent such defects.

Manufacture

Emmental is the most famous variety of Swiss-type cheese; its manufacture is therefore described in more detail. Some other hard-pressed cheeses with eyes will be discussed briefly.

Emmental is named after the valley of the river Emme in Switzerland. Originally, Emmental was manufactured by the Sennen, shepherds who watched their cattle during the summer on the Alps. There they made cheese from the milk. Early in the nineteenth century, production started in factories in the valleys. Nowadays, Emmental cheese is being manufactured outside Switzerland, e.g. in France and the FRG.

Traditional Manufacture of Round Wheel Emmental

The Milk

Raw, clarified cows' milk (pH 6·5) is standardized to about 3·0% fat.

Renneting

About 1000 l of milk are put into copper kettles. From this milk one cheese (weight up to 100 kg) is produced. The milk is warmed to 35°C, and a culture of lactic acid bacteria (0·15%) and of propionic acid bacteria (1 ppm) are added and mixed with the milk. The production of lactic acid is initiated. After 20 or 30 min, rennet, an extract from calf stomach, is added (15 ml per 100 l of milk) to the milk. The milk curdles.

Cutting and Harping

The curd is cut into cubes (about 3 mm³) with knives, called Swiss harps.

Cooking or Scalding

The curd–whey mixture is stirred for 40 min ('foreworking'). The curd particles shrink and expel whey ('syneresis'). The curd becomes firm and elastic. After foreworking the curd is cooked ('scalded') for 30 min at 50–53°C; this is achieved by injecting steam into the kettle jacket. During cooking, the curd is stirred continuously. The high temperature kills various nonthermoresistant bacteria (among them organisms that might otherwise cause cheese defects). The high temperature also crucially affects the degree of syneresis, determining the water content of the cheese. Curd particles lose more water and become more and more dry. The high temperature inactivates rennet enzymes, affecting proteolysis. Cooking is continued for 30–60 min ('postworking') until a desirable acidity of the curd–whey mixture (pH 6·3–6·4) has been obtained and curd particles show the correct physical properties. Stirring is stopped and the curd particles settle quickly on the bottom of the kettle.

Dipping

The high temperature of the curd favours deformation of the cheese during pressing. Consequently, the curd should be removed quickly from the kettle to the mould. For traditional Emmental the mould is a flexible wooden hoop and two wooden pressboards. The removal of the curd from the kettle ('dipping') involves a peculiar procedure. One side of a large, coarse cloth is fitted to a flexible steel rod. While keeping the rod with the fitted end of the cloth against the inner wall of the kettle, the cheesemaker moves the cloth under the curd, thereby holding the opposite, unfitted corners of the cloth to form a large bag. The rod is removed, the corners of the cloth are tied together and the curd is removed from the kettle by means of a chain and hydraulic lift. The curd mass (up to 100 kg) is permitted to drain briefly and transported into the round wooden hoop. The top area of the mass is covered with the cloth, provided with a wooden follower and pressed, applying pneumatic or hydraulic pressure.

Pressing

Pressing takes 12–20 h. At intervals (two or three times) the cheese is removed from the hoop, turned, re-clothed with a clean cloth and replaced under the press. Pressing results in a coherent loaf with the desired dimensions and a firm rind. Production of lactic acid is most substantial during pressing. After pressing, the pH of the cheese should be about 5·2. A lower pH would inhibit growth of the propionic acid bacteria during the 'warm room treatment'. The acid stimulates the loss of whey. The temperature in the pressing room is about 22°C.

Brining

After pressing, the cloth is removed and the cheese is marked for product identification. While still in the wooden hoop, the cheese is placed in saturated brine (23% sodium chloride) at 14°C. The top surface of the floating cheese is sprinkled with dry salt. The cheese is turned every day and salting of the top surface with dry salt repeated.

Cool Room Treatment

After brining, the cheese is stored for 2 weeks on a wooden shelf in a humid room at 14°C. It is turned every day and dry salt is sprinkled on the surface. During this period the cheese rind becomes firmer and salt is dispersing through the cheese mass.

Warm Room Treatment

After the 'cold storage', the cheese is stored for 5–8 weeks at 18–25°C. This treatment stimulates propionic acid fermentation with the production of carbon dioxide. Formation of eyes starts after 4 weeks. The colour of the rind changes from white to golden. To prevent the growth of moulds, the cheese is brushed every day with salty water, turned and sprinkled with salt. Too high a salt concentration in the cheese moisture inhibits the growth and fermentation of propionibacteria.

Maturation

When the cheese has attained the desirable shape with proper eye development, it is stored for 3–12 months in a cold room (7–14°C). Storage at this temperature retards the activity of the propionibacteria; eye development may continue at a much reduced rate. The cheese also acquires the characteristic sweet and nutty flavour, owing to the metabolic activity of the propionibacteria which produce propionate and acetate from lactate. Amino acids and short peptides, produced by the proteolysis of casein, are also responsible for the specific taste and flavour. *See* Casein and Caseinates, Uses in the Food Industry

Plasmin, the milk-indigenous proteinase, plays an important role in proteolysis, as do proteinases and peptidases of the thermophilic lactic acid bacteria (starter culture). Rennet enzymes, used to coagulate the milk, contribute negligibly to the decomposition of casein because the rennet is largely heat-inactivated during the manufacture of Emmental. The contribution

Cheeses with 'Eyes'

Table 1. Hard-pressed cheeses with eyes

Country of origin, and variety	Fermentation	Description of the eyes	Percentage fat in dry matter content	Form	Flavour
Switzerland					
Appenzeller	+	Round, regular, 0·5–1 cm	50	Low cylinder	Strong taste
Emmental	+0	Round, plentiful 1–3 cm	45–48	Cartwheel	Soft and nutty
Gruyère	+	Round, regular 0·5–1 cm	45–48	Cartwheel	Salty, fruity
Denmark					
Samso	+	Round, pea- to cherry-sized	30–45	Cartwheel	
Danbo	+	Round, few, pea-sized	10–45	Rectangular	Aromatic, strong taste
The Netherlands					
Edam	+	More or less round, pea-sized	40	Ball, waxy coating	Aromatic, strong taste
Gouda	+	More or less round, pinhead- to pea-sized.	48	Cartwheel	Creamy, mild
Maasdam	+0	Round, plentiful, 1–3 cm	45	Cartwheel	Sweet, soft
Italy					
Fontina	+	Holes	45	Low cylinder	Creamy, mild
Provolone	+	Few holes and splits	44	Varying	Aromatic sharp taste
FRG					
Tilsiter	+	Regular, round, 2–4 mm	30–50	Cartwheel	Aromatic, strong taste
Norway					
Jarlsbergost	+0	Round, pea- to cherry-sized	45	Cylinder	Mild, delicate, sweet

+, Lactic acid fermentation; 0, deliberate propionic acid fermentation.

of propionibacteria to proteolysis is significant. The presence of some copper in the cheese seems to control the action of the proteolytic enzymes and, by that, the development of taste and flavour. Decomposition of milk fat to fatty acids (lipolysis) also contributes to the taste. Milk indigenous lipase affects lipolysis in cheese made from raw milk; in cheese made from pasteurized milk, the enzyme is largely heat-inactivated. Proteolysis also affects the consistency of the cheese and, to a certain extent, its texture by producing some carbon dioxide from decarboxylation of amino acids, contributing to the enlargement of eyes. *See* Fatty Acids, Properties

Manufacture of Gruyère

Gruyère is another famous Swiss-type cheese, made from raw, unstandardized milk. Compared to Emmen-tal it differs significantly in flavour and dimensions: its body is more firm, and propionic acid fermentation is slight. Because of a lower temperature during the warm room treatment (14–18°C), Gruyère cheese shows only a few small eyes. Instead of the golden surface colour of Emmental, the rind of Gruyère is a red-brownish colour. This is caused by coryneform bacteria, e.g. *Brevibacterium linens*, which develop during ripening on the cheese surface, and cause the production of the characteristic taste, arising from sharp and distinct flavour compounds (e.g. ammonia). Growth of these bacteria is favoured by rubbing the cheese with a cloth moistened in brine containing the organisms during the early ripening period, every morning and evening but later only once a day. After about a month, the cheese acquires a grainy, red-brownish appearance. Gruyère is not only produced in Switzerland, but also in France.

Cheeses with 'Eyes'

Two subvarieties of French Gruyère are Beaufort and Comté.

Modern Production of Emmental

Modern cheese plants most frequently use stainless steel tanks instead of copper kettles; sometimes a little copper salt is then added to the cheese milk. Other methods have been introduced to mechanize and automate cheese production, e.g. apparatus for whey drainage, for vacuum moulding and for pressing more loafs at one time. Cheesecloth is no longer needed. The entire production, storage and maturation of the cheese is completely controlled. This means that the quality of the cheese is more constant and that the occurrence of defects is minimized.

Especially because of its large dimension, the traditional Emmental is not easy to pack and transport. Factories in the USA and FRG therefore produce Emmental as rindless blocks of cheese with various weights. Immediately after brining, the cheese is wrapped in plastic foil, vacuum-packed and ripened in the package. Such cheese does not have a firm rind. The package protects the cheese from drying out and from mould growth on its surface by hindering the diffusion of oxygen. The ripening time of rindless blocks of Emmental is 6–8 weeks.

Varieties

Several varieties of hard-pressed cheese develop round to oval-shaped eyes in different numbers owing to gas production caused mostly by lactic acid or propionic acid bacteria.

Taste and flavour of the cheese varieties depend, in the first place, on the type of fermentation that is initiated and on the time of maturation. On the other hand, taste and flavour are influenced by the treatment of the cheese surface during maturation.

Table 1 shows the names of the most famous hard-pressed cheese varieties. It also shows the characteristics of the cheese eye form and number, percentage fat in the dry mass, and the cheese form. An indication of the expected flavour and taste is given. Of course, there are more specific varieties in the different countries. The cheeses in Table 1, however, are the most famous of the hard-pressed cheese varieties with eye formation.

Bibliography

Catsberg CME and Kempen-van Dommelen GJM (1990) *Food Handbook*. Chichester: Horwood (Ellis).
Fox PF (1987) *Cheese: Chemistry, Physics and Microbiology*, vol. 2. Essex: Elsevier Science Publishers.
Kosikowski F (1977) *Cheese and Fermented Milk Foods*. Ann Arbor, Michigan: Edwards Brothers.
Reinbold GW (1972) *Swiss Cheese Varieties*. New York: Pfizer Inc.

C. M. E. Catsberg
Es Apeldoorn, The Netherlands
G. J. M. Kempen-van Dommelen
Hogeschool, Nijmegen, The Netherlands

Manufacture of 'Pasta Filata' Varieties

Cheeses of the pasta filata variety are made widely in central and eastern Europe from milk of the cow, horse, sheep and water buffalo. The term 'pasta filata' indicates that the curd has been pulled, kneaded or stretched. Curds produced from a typical enzyme and starter culture process are heated and then stretched and kneaded until a smooth plastic texture is formed. The stretched cheese is then ready to eat or stored until more flavour has developed, depending on the type of cheese being made. *See* Sheep, Milk; Buffalo, Milk

Probably the best known pasta filata cheeses are mozzarella and provolone. Other cheeses made by the pasta filata process are kaskavalsajt (Hungary), gilad (Israel), cascaval dalia and cascaval dobrogea (Romania), and kashkaval (Bulgaria). Italian varieties other than mozzarella and provolone include: provatura, scamorze (or scarmorze), caciocavallo, manteca, moliterno, foggiano and cartonese. These cheeses are different from each other in a variety of ways, including the type of milk, ageing or ripening, fat content, and addition of other flavourings, e.g. smoked or addition of peppers. Whatever the cheese variety, all are made via the same basic process, which will be discussed below.

Manufacturing

Since mozzarella cheese is the largest single pasta filata variety, its manufacture will be used as an example of the production of pasta filata cheeses. A flow diagram of the cheesemaking process can be seen in Fig. 1. The other previously mentioned varieties will vary in moisture and fat content, other ingredients (e.g. peppers, smoke flavouring) and type of milk (e.g. cow, sheep, goat, etc).

Milk

Originally, buffalo's milk was used in Italy, but today fresh cow's milk of high microbial quality is used for the production of mozzarella cheese. The milk is usually standardized to a specified butterfat level. The actual percentage of butterfat depends on the type of cheese being manufactured. For mozzarella, milk of 1·6–3·0% fat can be used, depending on whether a part-skim or whole-milk cheese is desired.

After standardization, the milk is pasteurized. In the past milk was not always pasteurized but most countries now require pasteurization due to possible foodborne pathogens in the milk. Pasteurization temperatures are 15 s at 74°C for a high-temperature short-time process and 30 min at 63°C for a batch process. *See* Pasteurization, Principles

Acid Development

Traditionally, mozzarella was made without addition of a starter culture; however, modern cheesemaking stand-ards make this impractical since the milk is usually pasteurized. In order to make a more consistent product, day after day, a starter is usually added to the milk. For mozzarella, the typical bacterial starter contains a mixture of *Streptococcus thermophilus* and *Lactobacillus delbrueckii* ssp. *bulgaricus*. Other bacterial strains that could be used are *Lactococcus lactis* ssp. *lactis*, *Enterococcus faecalis* (DK) and *L. lactis* spp. *cremoris*. All cultures are added to the milk in the range 0·5–1·5% by weight. *See* Lactic Acid Bacteria; Starter Cultures

The choice of starter culture also depends upon whether a more traditional or modern method of processing is done. In the traditional method, the curd is set, cut, drained and then iced until the pH of the curd is 5·1–5·3. This method usually takes 3 days. Today, in most modern cheese plants the curd is held at 30–32°C for 1–3 h until the pH reaches 5·1–5·3. When the pH is at this optimum level, the curd is at the ideal condition for mixing (stretching/kneading) and moulding.

Another method to produce mozzarella is to acidify the milk directly. Acetic, lactic, citric and hydrochloric acids have been used to acidify the milk and produce an acceptable cheese. The optimum curd pH (5·6) is higher than for curd produced using starter culture and less time is required to produce the cheese. Some companies may combine the use of starter and acid to increase production.

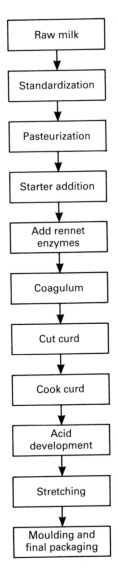

Fig. 1 Flow diagram of a typical process for pasta filata cheese.

Coagulation

After addition of the starter, the milk is allowed to ripen at the optimum growth temperature for the starter. Ripening time depends on the starter used but it is usually 30–50 min at 30–32°C. Ripening time may also be determined by a change in the milk acidity. Assuming the initial milk titratable acidity is 0·17%, the coagulant can be added when the titratable acidity is 0·19%.

Calf rennet or one of its microbial analogues is used to coagulate the milk. For mozzarella, enough rennet is added to coagulate the curd in 30 min at 30–34°C. This amounts to about 80 g of rennet per 500 kg of milk. Usually the rennet is diluted in water prior to addition to the milk. Once the rennet is added the milk is allowed to rest until optimum curd strength is obtained (usually 30 min).

Curd Cutting/Cooking

After the curd has reached its optimum strength it is cut into cubes using curd knives. The size of the cube will affect the moisture content of the cheese since smaller cubes produce an increased surface area and therefore greater moisture loss when the curd is cooked. Typically, the cutting is done with 1–2 cm knives. Once the

Manufacture of 'Pasta Filata' Varieties

curd is cut it is allowed to sit undisturbed for 15 min. Allowing the cut curd to rest helps prevent fat loss into the whey.

Whether the curd is cooked or not will depend on what final moisture content is desired. A high-moisture mozzarella is often not cooked at all but instead is held at the set temperature for 15–60 min with gentle stirring. Actual holding time may depend on acid development as well as cheese variety. Low-moisture mozzarella cheese (often called pizza cheese) is usually made of curds which have been cooked. The cooking is usually done by gradually raising the curd's temperature to the final cook temperature (40–45°C) in 35–60 min. Once the cook temperature has been obtained, the heated mixture of whey and curds is stirred for 10 min.

Draining Whey/Piling of Curds

When the cooking step is done, the whey is drained. For mozzarella, only half of the whey is usually drained and the curd may be stirred before being allowed to mat. Some cheesemaking methods call for draining the whey and then washing with warm water before allowing the curds to mat. After all the whey has been drained, the curd is cut into blocks and turned every 15–30 min until the optimum pH is attained. The curd blocks may be stacked one on top of the other like Cheddar curds are handled, depending on the type of cheese being made. In the traditional 3 day manufacturing method the mozzarella curds are cooled and refrigerated until the optimum pH for stretching is obtained. Once the proper curd pH (5·1–5·3) is reached the curd is ready to be milled and stretched.

Stretching

Before discussing the stretching procedure the chemistry of the cheese should be explained. The chemistry of the stretch is important because the production of a high-quality cheese does not depend on the skill of the person or the type of machine that stretches the cheese but rather on the chemical changes in the casein during the coagulation and acidification of the milk. Figure 2 shows a simple flow chart of what is happening to the casein during cheese manufacture. *See* Casein and Caseinates, Uses in the Food Industry

Rennet and starter culture are added to the milk. Casein in the form of calcium caseinate is hydrolysed by rennet to produce dicalcium paracaseinate which coagulates to form the curd. The starter culture produces lactic acid from lactose. Lactic acid lowers the pH causing some of the dicalcium paracaseinate to become monocalcium paracaseinate. It is the monocalcium paracaseinate that possesses the unique properties that

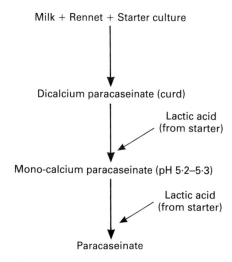

Fig. 2 Flow diagram of how casein changes to improve stretchability.

allow it to be stretched. Monocalcium paracaseinate is soluble in 5% sodium chloride and when heated to 54°C or higher the curd becomes smooth, pliable, stringy and retains the fat.

If too much acid is developed, the monocalcium paracaseinate is converted to paracasein. Paracasein is unable to retain the butterfat and will therefore affect the texture of the final product. Other ways to affect the stretchability adversely are homogenization of the cheese milk, some curd decolorization methods, and addition of emulsifying salts.

The actual process of stretching is fairly simple. The curd is milled into small cubes or strips and then covered with 72–82°C water. After a brief holding period the warmed curds are stretched using a revolving blender or wooden paddles. Alternatively, the milled curds are placed in a mechanical-mixer cooker which heats and stretches the curd simultaneously. Whichever method is used, the internal curd temperature should not exceed 57°C. The mixing/stretching continues until a smooth, long, white plastic mass is formed. Once the stretching is completed, the hot cheese may be moulded into balls or bricks of various sizes and then cooled. In the case of mozzarella, it is then brined in a 23% sodium chloride solution from 2 to 12 h depending on the size of the block of cheese. After brining, the mozzarella is ready for packaging and consumption. Brining will help in both flavour development as well as preserving the cheese.

Other Varieties

After brining begins, the manufacturing process changes depending on the variety being manufactured. One important difference between mozzarella and other types of cheese is the salt content. Mozzarella can

Manufacture of 'Pasta Filata' Varieties

contain 0·7–1·0% sodium chloride while Bulgarian kashkaval can contain up to 4% sodium chloride.

Milk source is another way the pasta filata cheeses vary from region to region. Kashkaval made in Bulgaria is made from a blend of cow, sheep or goat's milk, Balkan kashkaval is produced from sheep's milk, while a Yugoslav variety is produced only from cow's milk.

Provolone differs from mozzarella by its lower moisture content, and being aged for 2–12 months; some types of provolone are smoked. Smoking a cheese prior to ageing not only imparts the smoke flavour but it can also help reduce the moisture content. In addition to smoking, other flavours may be imparted by the addition of lipases (provolone), butter (manteca or manteche) and peppers (cartonese) to mention just a few.

Because of the heating of the curd, many shapes are possible. Provolone is an excellent example of this, ranging from small pear-shaped bells to the larger salami and giganta types. Kashkaval is usually flat and cylindrically shaped while mozzarella is typically spherical.

Cheeses which are ripened are usually ripened around 2–12 months. Ripening temperatures range from 4 to 16°C (provolone and kashkaval, respectively) in controlled-humidity ripening rooms. During the ripening stage, some water may be lost, lipids are hydrolysed, and proteins are cleaved by residual enzymes, thus contributing to each cheese's unique flavour.

Bibliography

Carić M (1987) Mediterranean cheese varieties: ripened cheese varieties: ripened cheese varieties native to the Balkan countries. In: Fox PF (ed.) *Cheese: Chemistry, Physics and Microbiology. Major Cheese Groups*, vol. 2, pp 257–276. London: Elsevier.

Fox PF (ed.) *Cheese: Chemistry, Physics and Microbiology. General Aspects*, vol. 1. London: Elsevier.

Fox PF and Guinee TP (1987) Italian Cheese. In: Fox PF (ed.) *Cheese: Chemistry, Physics and Microbiology. Major Cheese Groups*, vol. 2, pp 221–256. London: Elsevier.

Kosikowski F (1982) *Cheese and Fermented Milk Foods*, pp 179–212. Brooktondale, NY: FV Kosikowski.

Reinbold GW (1963) *Italian Cheese Varieties*, pp 14–23. New York: Charles Pfizer.

Scott R (1981) *Cheesemaking Practice*, pp 177, 269–272, 321. London: Applied Science.

Kevin L. Mackey
USDA, ARS, Eastern Regional Research Center, Philadelphia, USA

Soft and Special Varieties*

This article deals with a group of cheeses: cream cheese, cottage cheese and those cheeses manufactured from whey and/or by direct acidification, such as queso blanco.

Cream Cheese

Cream cheese is a soft unripened cheese containing 35% fat, 54% moisture and 7·5% protein (Table 1). It has a mild acid, creamy flavour. Neufchatel cheese is similar, with a lower fat content of 23%. Cream cheese is an important use of milk fat in many countries with annual production in 1989 of 172 000 tonnes in the USA and 11 900 tonnes in Canada.

Manufacture

Cream cheese can be manufactured by a variety of methods. All start with a fat-standardized cream (about 11%) which has been pasteurized at a temperature/time slightly above those of pasteurization, e.g. 68°C, 30 min. Excessive heat treatment inhibits whey drainage. This cream is then fermented at 22°C with a commercial lactic culture for 16 h, or at 30–32°C for 5 h; the mixture should attain a pH of 4·5–4·4. Some recommend the addition of a milk-coagulating enzyme, prior to incubation. Cream at pH 4·5–4·4 is a soft gel. *See* Pasteurization, Principles

Subsequently, in the traditional process, the coagulated cream is pumped or otherwise transferred to muslin bags. These bags are transferred to a cold room and allowed to drain overnight. A soft, fresh cheese results which is then packaged for consumption or for further processing.

Modern processes now all use a special centrifuge similar to that used for quarg. The coagulated cream is pumped to the centrifuge which separates it into whey and cream cheese; whey can also be separated by ultrafiltration. *See* Membrane Techniques, Principles of Ultra-filtration

Packaging is an important step for cream cheese. The traditional packaging is the 'cold-pack', which results in more flavour, a higher aroma and a body which is not sticky. However, the 'hot-pack' procedure is used commercially. A stabilizer, e.g. locust bean gum at 0·35%, and salt (1%) are added and the mixture is heated in a kettle or scraped-surface heat exchanger to 70°C, immediately homogenized at 136 atm (2000 psi), pumped to the filler and packaged hot. The 'hot-pack' cream cheese has excellent keeping quality (60 days or more). *See* Stabilizers, Types and Function

Use

Most cream cheese is sold as such and used by consumers as a spread or ingredient for cooked or

---

* The colour plate section for this article appears between p. 1146 and p. 1147.

Soft and Special Varieties

Table 1. Composition of cottage, creamed and Neufchatel cheeses

Component	Cream cheese	Neufchatel cheese	Creamed cottage cheese	Low-fat cottage cheese, −2%	Low-fat cottage cheese, −1%	Dry curd
Moisture	53·75	62·21	78·96	79·31	82·48	79·77
Fat	34·87	23·43	4·51	1·93	1·02	0·42
Protein	7·55	9·96	12·49	13·74	12·39	17·27
Carbohydrate	2·66	2·94	2·68	3·63	2·72	1·85

Source: USDA (1976) *Composition of Foods. Agriculture Handbook*, No. 8-1. Washington, DC: Agricultural Research Service.

uncooked dishes, such as cheesecake. Some is flavoured by manufacturers with condiments, such as pimento. An increasing amount is being used as a base or ingredient for spreads or chip dips flavoured with a wide range of fruits, spices, herbs and vegetables.

Cottage Cheese

Cottage cheese, as known in the 1990s, was first introduced in California and is now produced and consumed throughout North America and most countries with a developed dairy industry. It is sold almost exclusively as creamed cottage cheese with a mild, slightly acid flavour and aroma. It consists of small curd particles with a thick 'cream' between them of varying quantity and viscosity, depending on the brand; it is usually sufficiently thick that the mixture hangs together on a spoon. Other products, which are sometimes called cottage cheese, are a paste, like quarg, or are the uncreamed curd particles.

The size of the curd particles determines whether the creamed cottage cheese is termed 'large curd' or 'small curd'. The latter particles are about 4 mm and the former 8 mm in diameter, or larger.

Cottage cheese is a soft unripened cheese containing about 80% moisture. Creamed cottage cheese contains 4% fat and a low-fat cottage cheese, 2, 1 and, now, 0% fat (Table 1). Low-fat cottage cheeses usually contain more moisture than the full-fat creamed versions, with fat-free cheese replacing the fat.

Production of cottage cheese in Canada in 1989 was 30 000 tonnes, whilst in the USA in the same year 259 000 tonnes of creamed cottage cheese and 136 000 tonnes of low-fat cottage cheese were produced.

Manufacture of Curd

Pasteurized skim milk (72°C, 16 s) is fermented in large vats with a non-gas-producing lactic culture, at 22°C for 12–16 h (long set), at 32°C for 4 h (short set) or at some intermediate combination (intermediate set). The amount of culture varies from 0·5–1% (long set) to 5%

(short set). Rennet or a milk-clotting enzyme is added at a rate of 1 ml per 450 kg of skim milk.

It is important that the coagulum be cut at a constant pH of 4·6–4·8, the exact pH seeming to be a characteristic of the plant; a higher cutting pH gives a firmer cheese. It is also important that subsequent steps be kept as constant as possible. Cutting is done with wire knives: 1·2 cm spaces for large curd and 0·6 cm for small curd. Fifteen minutes after cutting, stirring and heating begin slowly, raising the temperature to 55°C over 90 min. After checking for firmness, the whey is drained. The curd is washed 2–3 times with water, the first at 15°C, the last at 4°C, each for a period of 15 min. After complete drainage of the wash water, the curd is ready for creaming.

Acidification can also be accomplished by acidulants without the use of lactic cultures. In commercial processes, phosphoric acid is added first to lower the pH partially. Then glucono-δ-lactone is added in an amount to decrease the pH to 4·7 or 4·6. This compound hydrolyses slowly in water to give gluconic acid and a normal coagulation of the milk. Subsequent steps are identical to those followed in the culture method. *See* Acids, Natural Acids and Acidulants

Creaming

The creaming mixture can and does vary depending on the characteristics desired. A low cream:curd ratio of 1:2 gives a drier-appearing product; a higher ratio (2:3 or 1:1) gives a more liquid, looser product. The mixture contains an amount of fat appropriate to the fat content of the final product, e.g., 12·0% fat for a fat content of 4·5% and a creaming ratio of 36:64.

To the creaming mixture is added salt (to give 0·8–1·0% salt in the creamed product), milk solids (skim-milk powder and whey solids) and a commercial blend of stabilizers or thickeners to thicken the cream.

Cream dressings can be further modified to increase the shelf life of the creamed cheese. Creamed cottage cheese is particularly susceptible to spoilage by psychrotrophs because of relatively greater exposure to contamination by spoilage microorganisms, and because of

Table 2. Some flavour ingredients added to creamed cottage cheese for sale in the UK

Onion and chives	Tandoori chicken
Pineapple	Tuna
Onion and cheddar	Ham and pineapple
Onion and peppers	Salmon and cucumber
Chives	Chicken and asparagus
Prawns	

the high water activity and low salt. Inhibitory cultures can be added, whose presence seems to inhibit pyschrotrophs. More stringent measures include fermentation of the cream dressing, or parts of it, with psychrotroph-inhibiting microorganisms.

In the creaming process, the cream dressing and curd are blended. The contact is usually for a minimum of 15–30 min because serum absorption from the dressing is a time-dependent process. The first mixture is relatively loose and some absorption is desirable to enable delivery of a uniform mixture of cream and curd to each package. The time allowed in the process determines to some extent the amount of stabilizers, the cream:curd ratio, etc. Then the creamed cheese is packaged.

The packaged cheese is cooled in the cold room to 4°C. The shelf life of the cheese can be 21–28 days in a well-controlled operation.

Equipment

The equipment can vary widely. In the simplest process, fermentation, cooking, curd washing, draining and creaming occurs in the same vat. The creamed curd is pumped to the filling machines.

In fully mechanized, high-production plants, the following can be used: washing towers to which either curd and whey or curd and the first wash water are pumped for further washing; continuous separators of curd from whey or wash water in which the mixture passes over a rotating perforated drum; creaming mixers into which dry curd falls and cream is added, blended and dispersed to the packaging machines. A continuous whey separator and washing apparatus is now used commercially and there will probably be further development in this area.

Use

Cottage cheese is used by consumers in salads and a little in cooking. Salad use has led to marketing cottage cheese with imaginative added ingredients in the UK (Table 2). Preparation and incorporation of some ingredients pose special technological and sanitary problems.

Cheese Produced by Direct Acidification and Thermal Processes

Several varieties of cheese are produced by direct acidification in combination with heating, while other cheeses, such as whey cheese, are produced by heating (evaporation) processes alone. These cheeses are often consumed fresh or used as ingredients in condiments in food preparation.

Latin American White Cheese

The term 'white cheese' is perhaps a misnomer, as most of the Latin American cheeses are manufactured from the milk of goats, sheep or buffaloes, which tends to make the cheese yellow when compared with cheeses manufactured from cows' milk. A variety of Latin American white cheeses are produced, but queso blanco and queso del pais are about the only varieties which are produced by direct acidification. Often these cultures are produced by using a rennet and a high degree of acid development. Cheeses, such as queso de prensas (El Salvador, Mexico, Venezuela) and queso estera (Columbia), are made from milk with the use of milk-clotting enzymes and starter. *See* Sheep, Milk; Buffalo, Milk

The manufacturing steps involved in the production of queso blanco, produced by direct acidification, consist of heating whole milk or partially skimmed milk (e.g. 3% milk fat) to 80–88°C and holding for up to 15 min to denature the whey proteins. A predetermined amount of food-grade acidulant is added to coagulate both the casein and denatured whey proteins from the hot cheese milk and yield a final cheese pH of 5·3–5·7. The acid is gently, but quickly mixed with the cheese milk with just sufficient stirring to ensure uniform distribution of the acidulant, otherwise curd structure is disrupted and yield is reduced. Usually 3 min stirring is sufficient for a 500 litre vat.

After about 15 min, the whey is drained from the vat and the curd is salted (up to 5% salt) to yield a fairly dry, soft and granular product. The curd is placed in forms at this point, or pressed to yield a more compact product with a lower moisture content. The production of queso blanco cheese continues to be done on a farm scale or in small factories.

The yield and composition of queso blanco varies considerably, but products with 15–17% milk fat, 51–58% moisture, 18–22% protein and 3·5–4·5% salt, are typical. Yields of 11–14·6% are common for this type of cheese and are higher than those for Cheddar due to both higher moisture and inclusion of the whey proteins.

Queso blanco is normally used as a fresh cheese. It has a creamy texture, acid flavour and is highly salted. It is often consumed with fruit or guava sauce in South American countries.

Paneer Cheese

Paneer cheese is also known as 'chana'. This cheese is produced primarily in India using buffalo's milk and a manufacturing procedure which is similar to that of the queso blanco. The composition differs slightly in that the product contains less moisture (53%) and more fat (25%) than the Latin American white cheese. Uses of paneer cheese include the preparation of sweetmeat and cooked vegetable dishes.

Ricotta Cheese

Ricotta is a high-moisture soft cheese which is prepared exclusively from whey (Italy) or from mixtures of whey and milk. Ricotta is often prepared from whole milk in North America, but this product is practically identical to queso blanco, except that fresh ricotta is not pressed.

Ricotta was first made in Italy from sweet whey obtained from the manufacture of other cheeses, such as Provolone; however, it is now made in many parts of Europe and North America by blending cow's milk and whey. It is sometimes called whey or albumin cheese, but has many other names including Ziger, Recuit, Sérac, Mejette, Ceracee, Broccio or Schottenziger.

Much of the world's ricotta production is still done in a batch system using open kettles, heated either directly or indirectly with steam. Ideally one should start with sweet whey which has no more than 0.2% titratable acidity, expressed as lactic acid (pH not less than 6.2). Often 10–25% milk is added to sweet whey to dilute the developed acidity in the whey component, improve curd cohesiveness, and thus yield.

The manufacture of ricotta by the traditional process consists of heating whey or mixtures of whey and milk from 82 to 93°C and then stirring in a food-grade acidulant as described for queso blanco. Only small amounts of acidulant are required. The pH should not drop below 5.9–6.1, otherwise the resulting cheese will lose sweetness. The denatured whey proteins rise to the surface, due to entrapped air. The curd is dipped off by means of a perforated ladle or a dipping cloth and may be hung to cool and drain. It can also be placed in perforated forms or spread on a curd table for whey drainage. At this point the curd is very soft, grainy and fragile and lacks cohesiveness. In some cases, the curd is pressed and marketed as dry ricotta.

Although ricotta cheese is relatively easy to prepare, the yield is generally quite low, e.g. 5–6% for Italian ricotta. This is a reflection of both low solids in the starting whey (6–7%) and recoveries of protein which average approximately 70–75%.

The composition of ricotta is quite variable and is highly dependent on the starting material. A blend of 5% milk with 95% whey will yield a curd with approxi-mately 68–73% moisture, 4–10% fat, 16% protein, and 4% lactose and minerals.

Ricotta production is a labour-intensive process and numerous attempts have been made to mechanize manufacture. Among the most notable inventions is an Italian process for continuous production. A blend of sweet whey and milk is continuously neutralized to pH 6.9–7.1 with sodium hydroxide followed by heating to 88–92°C and holding; in-line salt and acid injection are used. Sour whey or bulk lactic acid-producing starters can also be used as acidulants. The hot acidified whey (pH 5.9–6.1) is pumped into the bottom of a 'V'-shaped vat. The curd floats to the top of the vat where it is scraped off with a mechanized series of paddles onto a nylon mesh for whey drainage and cooling. The product is then collected in perforated containers to allow for additional expression of moisture, followed by packaging.

Ricotta is a soft, creamy product which has a mild, pleasant caramel flavour. This product is often consumed as such, but is also used extensively in Italian dishes, such as ravioli and lasagna. The product is also used as a base for chip dips, sour cream and cream cheese. Use as a replacement for Cheddar cheese in processed cheese food and spread has to be limited due to the poor melting properties of this product.

Cheese Prepared by Thermal Processes

Whey cheeses consist primarily of caramelized lactose as well as milk fat, minerals and protein present in the original whey. These products originated in the Scandinavian countries and are still produced primarily in Norway, Denmark and Sweden with limited production in North America. Cheese prepared from whey of bovine origin is called 'mysost', while cheese derived from goat's milk whey is termed 'gjetost'. Often buttermilk, cream or whole milk is added to the starting whey to give a softer cheese, referred to as 'primost'. Cheese manufactured solely from whole milk is called 'gomost'. *See* Whey and Whey Powders, Production and Uses

The traditional method of manufacture consists of heating sweet whey in an open kettle until a viscous mass is obtained. During the process, the albumins are denatured and skimmed off, but only to be added back towards the end of the evaporation process. At this point the cheesemaker has the option of adding cream or flavouring material. The product is constantly stirred while cooling to prevent the formation of large lactose crystals and then is packaged while still warm.

More recently, the process has been mechanized to increase efficiency and reduce labour costs by implementing double-effect evaporation. The whey or mixture of whey and cream is concentrated to 60% total solids and then finished in a round vacuum kettle to 80–

84% total solids. At the end of the process the product is heated at 95°C, under atmospheric pressure, to impart the desired colour, flavour intensity and plastic condition to the cheese. At the point the product is agitated, cooled and is filled directly into the final package or mechanically extruded by means of a butter printer and cut into the desired size prior to packaging.

The finished whey cheeses have usually a light tan colour with a smooth creamy body and a flavour of slightly sweetened, cream caramel. The product undergoes virtually no ripening due to the high osmolarity of the product. This cheese will keep for long periods of time providing it has been properly packaged to prevent surface growth of yeast and mould. Whey cheese contains approximately 35–40% lactose and about 30% fat, and serves as an excellent source of energy.

Bibliography

Emmons DB (1963) Recent research in the manufacture of cottage cheese. Parts 1 and 2. *Dairy Science Abstracts* 25: 129–137, 175–182.

Emmons DB and Tuckey SL (1967) *Cottage Cheese and other Cultured Milk Products.* New York: Chas. Pfizer.

Fox PF (1989) *Cheese: Chemistry, Physics and Microbiology.* vol. 2. New York: Elsevier.

Kosikowski FV (1982) *Cheese and Fermented Milk Foods.* Brooktondale, NY: Kosikowski and Associates.

Mair-Waldburg H (1974) *Handbuch der Käse. Käse der Welt von A–Z. Eine Enzyklopädie.* Kemptin (Allgäu): Volkswirtschafter Verbeg.

Robinson RK and Tamine AY (1991) *Feta and Related Cheeses.* London: Ellis Horwood.

USDA (1978) *Cheese Varieties and Descriptions.* Washington, DC: US Department of Agriculture.

D. B. Emmons and H. W. Modler
Centre for Food & Animal Research, Agriculture Canada, Ottawa, Canada

White Brined Varieties

Characteristic Properties

The production of brined (pickled) cheese varieties has long been limited to the Mediterranean and southeast European countries. Nowadays, the international recognition of brined cheeses and the dynamic growth in their demand have extended their production to other countries, including Denmark, Ireland, the UK, the USA, Australia and New Zealand.

Preservation in brine (pickle) is the main characteristic of this group of cheeses. The brine serves to preserve the cheese and prevent it drying out. Consequently, the composition and properties of these cheeses and those of the used brine are interrelated.

Brined cheeses are generally rindless, produced in the form of blocks of various shapes and sizes (cubes, bricks or segments), covered with salt brine or whey, and stored in wooden barrels, tins or laminated packages. Brined cheeses are marketed either fresh or after storage of up to one year.

Brined cheeses are characterized by their clean, acid, salty flavour. The high salt content of the cheese and brine allow for good keeping quality in hot climates without the need for cold storage.

Rapid developments in the technology of brined cheeses have been achieved during the last two decades; the application of ultrafiltration in the manufacture of feta cheese is one of the most outstanding.

Although all brined cheeses are subjected to the same practice of storage in pickle for extended periods, they differ significantly in their manufacturing technologies, composition and properties.

Classification

As shown in Table 1, brined cheeses include soft and semi-hard varieties, and nearly all of them are made by

Table 1. Classification of brined cheeses

Cheese	Country of origin	Milk used
Rennet-coagulated		
Soft cheeses		
Feta type (salting of curd)		
Feta	Greece	S, S plus G, C
UF-Feta	Denmark	C, R
Telemea	Romania	S, B, C
White pickled	Eastern Europe	S, C
Bli-Sir-O-Kriskana	Yugoslavia	S
Bajalo (Belo Salamureno Sirene)	Bulgaria	S, C
Brinza	USSR, Bulgaria	C
Chenakh	USSR	S
Akiavii	Syria, Turkey	S, G
Domiati (salting of milk)		
Domiati	Egypt	B, C R
UF-Domiati	Egypt	B, C, R
Dani	Egypt	S
Semihard cheeses		
Halloumi	Cyprus	S, G, C
Medaffara/Magdola	Sudan, Syria	S, B, C, R
Shenkalish	Syria	S
Acid-coagulated		
Mish	Egypt	Skim milk

S, sheep; G, goat; C, cow; B, buffalo; R, recombined milk.

rennet coagulation of milk. In general, brined cheeses can be made from different kinds of milk, but sheeps' milk is preferred for most of these varieties. *See* Sheep, Milk

Methods of Manufacture

Traditional Methods

Feta Cheese

Whole milk is heated to 65°C for 30 min (optional) and then cooled to 32–33°C; 1–3% starter (*Lactococcus lactis* plus *Lac. lactis* subsp. *cremoris*) is then added (optional); 20–30 ml of rennet (preferably lamb or kid rennet) per 100 l is used to coagulate the milk in 50–150 min; the curd is then cut into 2–3 cm cubes and left in the whey for 10–15 min, after which it is scooped into metal hoops 20 cm deep and left for 1 h; the hoops are transferred to a room (16–18°C), and the surface of the curd is lightly salted; the cheeses are turned upside down and left for 20 h; the curd is then cut into pieces (different sizes), placed in barrels in layers, and dry salted with 3% coarse salt over a period of 3 days; the barrels are topped up with 5% brine and left for 15 days, prior to being transferred to cold storage (4°C) until required. *See* Lactic Acid Bacteria; Starter Cultures

Telemea Cheese

Whole milk is heated to 60–68°C for 20–30 min; 0·5% starter (mesophilic bacteria plus *Lactobacillus casei*) is added at 28–31°C, followed by 25–30 ml of rennet per 100 l of milk and held at 30–34°C for 60 min; the curd is transferred into cheesecloth in layers; the resultant curd is cut crosswise with a long knife and pressed for 2 h; the cheese is cut into blocks and immersed in a salt bath (18–22% sodium chloride, NaCl) at 15–16°C overnight; the cheese is layered in tins, which are filled with acid (1·3–2% lactic acid), salted (4–5% NaCl) whey for one month, then stored at 5–10°C. *See* Whey and Whey Powders, Production and Uses

White Pickled Cheese

Whole milk is flash heated to 70°C, or to 68°C for 10 min (optional), and starter (sour milk or mesophilic bacteria, 0·5–1%) is added, followed by rennet (25–30 ml per 100 l of milk at 30–31°C) to complete coagulation in 60–70 min; the curd is ladled into a cheesecloth which is laid over a wooden frame, placed over a drainage table; the cheese is pressed by tightening the cloth and by the use of weights; the curd is cut into cubes (10 cm³) and immersed in saturated brine overnight; the cheese is packed into barrels, casks or tins which are filled with salted whey (8–12% NaCl).

Brinza

Milk is coagulated by rennet at 25–32°C for 40–90 min, after which the curd is transferred to the drainage table for cutting, turning and pressing (whey is removed in 2 h); the curd is cut into rectangular blocks (1 kg), and salted in brine at low temperature (10–12°C); the cheese is packed into wooden barrels or lacquered tins which are filled with brine or salted whey, then stored at 4°C or 12–20°C.

Bli-Sir-O-Kriskana

Starter (0·1%, *Lactococcus lactis* plus *Lactobacillus casei*) is added to the milk, followed by rennet (20–30 ml per 100 l at 30–32°C) in order to achieve coagulation in 70–90 min; the curd is cut horizontally and vertically, and left for 15–20 min; the curd is recut into smaller cubes and ladled into a cheesecloth; it is pressed for 1–4 h, then cut into cubes (10 cm³) for dry salting, or immersion in brine (20–25% NaCl) for 10–20 h at 12–15°C; the cheese is packed in parchment-lined casks or tins which are filled with brine (10–12% NaCl), and held at 12–15°C to ripen in one month; the cheese is stored at 10°C.

Bjalo (Belo Salamureno Sirene)

Milk is heated at 68°C for 10 min, then cooled to 31°C; 0·1–0·3% starter (*Lactococcus lactis* plus *Lactobacillus casei*) is added, followed by 20 ml of rennet per 100 l; coagulation time is 60–90 min; the curd is cut into cubes (2–3 cm³), which are ladled into a cheesecloth; the curd is then cut into strips, and the cloth tied over the curd; it is left to drain, then pressed for 4–5 h at 14–16°C; the curd is cut into pieces (12 × 12 cm), immersed in saturated brine or dry salt for 24 h, and packed into metal or plastic drums which are filled with brine (10–12% NaCl); the cheese is ripened for 2–4 weeks and stored at 4–8°C.

Domiati

Brine (5–15% NaCl) is added to the milk and stirred until dissolved; the salted milk is strained through cheesecloth, and heated to 60°C for 15 min (optional); after cooling to 37–42°C, rennet (30–40 ml per 100 l) is added to achieve coagulation in 2–3 h; the curd is scooped into wooden frames lined with cheesecloth, placed over a wooden board on a draining table, and allowed to drain for 3–4 h; the curd is broken and pressed to achieve complete drainage in 16–24 h; the cheese is cut into blocks and wrapped in cheesepaper; it is packed into 20 l tins filled with salted whey (from the same cheese) and stored at room temperature.

White Brined Varieties

Halloumi

Sufficient rennet is added to sheeps' milk to coagulate the milk at 34°C within 7–8 min; the curd is cut after 30 min into grains (1 cm³) and left for 10 min; after gently stirring for 10 min, then scalded at 60°C for 15 min; the curd is transferred to hoops, then pressed with weights (3 kg per kg of cheese) for 35 min; the pressed curd is cut into small blocks (10 × 10 × 3 cm) and transferred to deproteinated whey, then heated to 90–92°C for 30 min; the cheese is drained and sprinkled with dry salt and dried *Mentha viridis* leaves before conservation in brine.

Medaffara

Rennet is added to raw milk at 32–37°C for 40–60 min, and left to ripen (30–60 min); after curd cutting and partial removal of the whey, the cubes are left to ripen in the whey until they form a slim block about 2 m long; this ripened curd is then kneaded in hot water at 80°C for 10 min, after which black cumin spice (*Nigella sativa*) is added; the curd is shaped, while hot, to form a cord which is braided and then brined.

Equipment and Process Development

Industrial-scale production of brine cheeses is based on modification of the traditional methods. Normally, milk is pasteurized, starter is added, and the milk is coagulated with rennet in either open or closed cheese vats. The cheese curd is then transferred directly to a special table from which the whey is drained off through a perforated steel sheet at the bottom, or part of the whey is removed via a vibrating strainer before the curd is deposited on the table. After filling the table, it is covered with pressure plates and the curd is then pressed into one large cheese block, which is subsequently cut into retail sizes (0·25–1 kg). The cutting is performed with a special knife with preset cutting dimensions.

Most of the progress in the manufacture of brined cheeses has been achieved through the use of ultrafiltration (UF) techniques in the manufacture of feta and Domiati cheeses.

UF-Cast Feta Cheese

Two systems are in use for the production of UF-cast feta cheese:

1. Standardized pasteurized milk (12·5% total solids (TS), 3·5% fat) is ultrafiltered to give a retentate of 37–38% TS. The retentate is then pasteurized, homogenized and pumped from a balance tank by means of a finely controlled, positive pump to the filling, mixing and dosing aggregate. At the same time, precise amounts of

rennet, lipase, NaCl and acidulant (glucono-δ-lactone and blue phosphoric acid) are dosed into the concentrate before it reaches the filling head. The concentrate is aseptically filled into laminated 'tetrapacks' (250–500 g), or it can be packed into a special polymeric film and encased in a rectangular carton.

2. The UF-milk retentate (37–38% TS) is pasteurized, homogenized and directed into an intermediate tank. After cooling to 30°C, 3% mesophilic starter and lipase (4–8 g of lipase powder per 100 kg) are added. No time is allowed for acid development to take place. Before casting in tins (20 l), rennet is dosed in-line into the retentate. Filling takes place in three stages as each layer is coagulated separately. The tins are then forwarded to the portioning section, where the cheese is cut by a cutting machine equipped with three vertical knives. The cheese is salted with 4–5% salt, then dosed and spread automatically on top of the cheese; the tins are then closed.

UF-Structure Feta

Continuous coagulation of a retentate with 26% TS takes place in a coagulator, followed by automatic cutting of coagulum. The cheese grains are treated in permeate (from the UF process) where syneresis takes place. The cheese grains are filled into moulds, whey is drained off, and the finished cheese is cut into blocks, filled into tins and salted as described for cast feta.

UF-Domiati

Standardized pasteurized milk (12·5% TS, 3·5% fat) is concentrated by ultrafiltration to 35% TS. The retentate is homogenized, heated to 75°C for 1 min, and cooled to 34°C; 1% starter (mesophilic) and 5% NaCl are added, and the mixture is poured into trays (50 × 50 × 10 cm) and left to coagulate. The cheese is then cut into cubes (0·5 kg), and packed in 1 kg rigid plastic containers (consumer package) or in 20 l tins; the containers or tins are filled with 5% salted permeate and then closed.

Changes in the Composition of Brined Cheeses During Storage

Table 2 shows the average composition of some brined cheeses. General factors affecting the composition of other cheese varieties apply also to brined cheeses. These include type of milk, heat treatment received, and conditions and duration of storage. In addition, storage in brine plays a special and important role in determining the changes in composition of brined cheeses. This can be understood from the following:

- Brine provides a very high water activity for stored cheeses.

White Brined Varieties

Table 2. Average composition of some brined cheeses

Cheese	Moisture (%)	Fat/DM (%)	Total protein (%)	NaCl (%)	pH
Feta	48–54	48–52		4–5	4·3–4·6
Telemea	55	48–51		3–5	4·4–4·7
Bjalo	58–60	27–31	10–12	3–4	
Brinza	58	45–50		4–10	
Domiati (fresh)	60	40		8–10	6·6
Domiati (3 months)	54	45–50		6–8	3·7–4·2
Halloumi	35–48	38–5	24–30	2–5	5·3–6·1
Medaffara	53–54	17–22	21–24		5·1

- There is a continuous equilibrium in the distribution of soluble constituents between cheese and brine.
- There are ion exchange equilibria between Na^+Cl^- in the brine and the ions in the cheese.
- Brine partially solubilizes the protein matrix of cheese.
- Brine controls the cheese microflora; the surface microfloras are of limited or no significance.

In general, the changes occurring in brined cheeses can be described as follows.

Moisture Content

Depending on the initial moisture content, pH and concentration of brine, the moisture content of brined cheeses decreases on storage. This is obvious in Domiati cheese, where a 5–10% decrease in cheese moisture is normally observed during storage.

Nitrogenous Constituents

The different cheese proteins are subject to variable proteolysis: α-s-casein is extensively hydrolysed, while β- and p-κ-casein are less affected. An increase in the soluble constituents is normally observed during storage of brined cheeses. These compounds include peptides, amino acids and ammonia, but the formation of biogenic amines is very limited.

Milk Fat

The rennet used in brined cheeses traditionally contained pregastric lipases and, in developed technologies, lipase is added. Lipolysis is therefore one of the characteristics of brined cheeses. The mono- and diglyceride content of the cheese increases on storage with the formation of variable free fatty acids. However, the volatile fatty acids of brined cheeses contain a high percentage of acetic acid, originating from microbial fermentations. *See* Fatty Acids, Properties

Lactose

Fresh brined cheeses retain variable quantities of lactose, and those stored in salted whey have access to a continuous supply of lactose during storage. It is not surprising, therefore, to find measurable quantities of lactose in brined cheeses throughout the storage period. The presence of galactose in stored Domiati cheese has been reported.

Mineral Constituents

The calcium content of brined cheeses decreases as a result of acid development and ion exchange with NaCl in the brine; the phosphate content of cheese also decreases during storage. Changes in the Na^+ and Cl^- contents of cheese are dependent on (1) the concentration of the brine, (2) the initial NaCl content of cheese, and (3) any decrease in cheese moisture during storage. *See* Calcium, Properties and Determination; Phosphorus, Properties and Determination

Vitamins

Vitamin A is stable, but thiamin, riboflavin and nicotinic acid show variable decreases in cheese stored in tins. *See* Niacin, Properties and Determination; Retinol, Properties and Determination; Riboflavin, Properties and Determination; Thiamin, Properties and Determination

Volatile Flavour Compounds

Brined cheeses develop a mixture of short-chain fatty acids, mainly acetic acid and, to a lesser extent, C_{4-8} fatty acids. In feta cheese, several alcohols and carbonyl compounds increase in concentration on prolonged storage.

Microbiology

The microflora of Domiati cheese has received more attention than that of other brined cheeses. The total bacterial count generally reaches a maximum within a week of manufacture, and then declines rapidly. In

White Brined Varieties

Telemea cheese, the total bacterial count decreases rapidly within the first 2 months and slowly during prolonged storage. Streptococci are dominant in the early stages of pickling of Domiati cheese, and are then replaced with lactobacilli or lactobacilli and micrococci in the later stages of ripening, depending on the level of NaCl in cheese. Counts of nonlactic acid bacteria decrease steadily during storage. The total bacterial counts of UF-feta cheese, made either by direct acidification or with the use of cultures are generally lower than that of traditional cheeses.

The following bacterial species were found in good-quality Domiati cheese: *Enterococcus faecalis, Lactococcus lactis* subsp. *cremoris, Lactobacillus lactis, L. plantarum, L. casei* and *Leuconostoc mesenteroides* subsp. *cremoris*.

Several species of yeast have been isolated from Telemea and Domiati cheese, including *Torulopsis, Pichia, Cryptococcus, Hansenula, Saccharomyces,* and *Rhodotorula. See* Spoilage, Yeasts in Food Spoilage

The role of cheese microflora in the development of flavour and cheese ripening is not clear. However, several unconventional starters have been used to develop the desirable characteristic flavour in Domiati cheese, including *Enterococcus faecalis,* and *Pediococcus* sp.

The presence of *L. casei, L. plantarum* and *L. brevis* in large numbers is associated with the spoilage of UF-feta cheese, and can be controlled by the addition of nisin.

'Blowing' of tins is one of the reported defects in brined cheeses. Coliforms, including *Enterobacter aerogenes,* have been isolated from blown tins of Domiati cheese. The addition of more than 9% NaCl to cheese milk suppresses the growth of coliforms in Domiati cheese made from raw milk. Clostridia and micrococci are present in small numbers in UF-feta cheese (less than 10 per g), but they are of little significance. *See* Spoilage, Bacterial Spoilage

Nocardia-like organisms dominate the microflora of the surface-slime defect observed in Domiati cheese made from raw milk.

Structure

Electron microscopic examination of feta and Domiati cheese indicate that the internal structure of fresh cheese is composed of a framework of spherical casein aggregates, held together by bridges and enclosing fat. During storage in brine, the casein aggregates in Domiati cheese disintegrate into smaller spherical particles forming a loose structure. The casein particles in feta cheese coalesce as particles cling to one another, forming larger clumps than in Domiati cheese. The changes in the protein matrix during storage are generally responsible for the smooth body of ripened brined cheeses. These changes are likely to arise from (1) the partial loss of calcium from the cheese matrix into the brine, and (2) continuous proteolysis of α-s-casein, known for its important role in linking the cheese protein network.

Bibliography

Abd El-Salam MH, El-Shibiny S and Fahmi AH (1976) Domiati cheese. A review. *New Zealand Journal of Dairy Science and Technology* 11: 57–61.
Abou-Donia SA (1986) Egyptian Domiati soft white pickled cheese. *New Zealand Journal of Dairy Science and Technology* 21: 167–190.
Fox PF (ed.) (1987) *Cheese: Chemistry, Physics and Microbiology,* vol. 2. Essex: Elsevier Science Publishers.
Lloyd GT and Ramshaw EH (1979) The manufacture of Bulgarian-style Feta cheese. A review. *Australian Journal of Dairy Technology* 34: 180–183.
Scott S (1988) *Cheese Making in Practice* 2nd edn. Essex: Elsevier Science Publishers.

M. H. Abd El-Salam
National Research Station, Cairo, Egypt

Quarg and Fromage Frais

Acid fresh, unripened cheeses are produced throughout the world, but consumption is extremely variable even within individual countries. Besides Israel (*c.* 11 kg per head per annum), high consumption is observed in central Europe (Poland, 10 kg; FRG, 9 kg), Iceland (7 kg), Czechoslovakia and France (5 kg), and Hungary and Austria (4 kg) (for comparison: UK, 0·1 kg). About 30 to 40 different types of unripened cheeses are mainly made from cows' milk, but also from ewes' milk and especially from goats' milk, these latter products being rather popular in the Mediterranean countries. A common criterion for all cheeses of this class is the low pH value and a calcium content of 0·6–0·9% in the dry matter.

Historically, the lactic curd cheeses are mainly by-products of butter manufacture, i.e. they are produced from partly skimmed milk. Before 1888, the separation of cream occurred by gravitation. The milk was set at rest in a cool place in shallow pans, during which the cream and the skimmed milk became acid. After skimmed milk was clotted the coagulum was scrambled and drained of whey, either in cloths or in bags. Sometimes the curd was pressed or even washed to remove most of the whey. Handling of the lactic curd (quarg) was different in individual countries. In central Europe, for example, small cheeses were sometimes prepared from salted quarg, either mould-ripened (Korbkäse, Graukäse, Schabziger, etc.) or smear-ripened with yellow-reddish smear-forming, wild-type coryneformes (Harzer Käse, Mainzer Käse, Olmützer Quargel, etc.), or heated with a mild base (e.g. sodium hydrogen carbonate) and spiced to form cooked cheese. Originally, all these types of cheese had a variable content of fat, owing to the fact that creaming was more or less incomplete before the acid coagulation of the milk took place in the vats.

After introduction of the milk centrifuge in 1888, sweet skimmed milk became available, which could even be used for the production of lactic as well as rennet cheeses. However, in most countries, the consumption of lactic curd cheeses decreased constantly because of their very limited shelf life (less than 2 days), their often unclean flavour, bitterness due to proteolytic activity, and short consistency. In addition, the rather high fat content of the traditional products had made them much more tasty than the new products made from pure acid casein. Even in central Europe, where 'Quark' had a long tradition, the product remained a home-made one.

About the time of World War I, the taste of quarg was improved by adding about 2% buttermilk (which contains homofermentative lactic starters, and hetero-fermentative, aroma-producing lactic acid bacteria) as fermentation culture, e.g. starter to skimmed milk, and by combining the acid-induced formation of the curd with coagulation by renneting. This not only caused a change in the consistency (acid casein gels are hydrophilic, rennet-induced gels are hydrophobic with a tendency to syneresis, especially when heated (maximum 65°C)) but also permitted a certain heat-treatment of the curds which led to products with shelf lives of up to a week ('Dauerquark') at temperatures below 15°C. This development enabled the production and distribution of quarg outside of the home. At the same time, emigrants from Europe introduced into the northwest of the USA a variant of drained quark, namely 'cottage cheese', which became very popular, at least in North America.

Up to that time, fresh cheeses were prepared from unheated milk to avoid the precipitation of denatured whey proteins onto the casein, a change which induces a higher water-binding capacity in the protein, and gives a very soft, smooth consistency to the product. In the FRG in 1951 it was requested by law that milk used for unripened cheeses must be pasteurized (72–74°C for 20 s) in order to avoid health risks. This led to a further reduction of dry matter in quarg, and the new product, 'Speisequark', became very popular, particularly when enriched with cream. Up to that time, quarg had been mainly used for cooking and baking, but it then lost its cheese image and became a lactic acid dairy product for direct consumption, either sweet with fruit, or salty with herbs and spices.

The problem of limited shelf life was overcome by the development of special separators (up to $10\,000\,l\,h^{-1}$) for quarg in the 1950s. It became possible to produce Speisequark on a large scale with enclosed sanitary production lines, and avoiding recontamination during packaging. The shelf life of this product was extended to 22 days (12°C), even without adding preservatives. (In some countries, preservatives such as sorbic acid and hydrocolloids are used to prolong the shelf life of fresh cheeses.) Within a 10–15-year period, consumption of the new type of quarg increased in Germany about 10-fold, and production lines handling 200 000 kg of milk per day made the product a rather low-priced one. Consequently, new developments were necessary to overcome the resulting low profits of the dairies.

In the middle of the 1970s, a product ('Thermoquark') was developed which contained, besides the caseins, all of the whey proteins of milk. They were denatured by high-temperature heat treatment (82–92°C for 5–6 min) of the milk prior to fermentation, and special centrifuges were developed for the Thermoquark. Some manufacturers also started to add denatured whey protein concentrates – separated from heated whey either by the 'centri-whey' process or by ultrafiltration – to quarg. Since some dairies added up to 30% whey proteins to fresh cheeses, the International Dairy Federation and the German government limited the use of whey in fresh cheeses 'up to the natural whey protein content of the milk', i.e. 16–18% of the total milk protein. *See* Casein and Caseinates, Uses in the Food Industry; Membrane Techniques, Principles of Ultra-filtration; Whey and Whey Powders, Protein Concentrates and Fractions

Direct concentration of sweet milk up to 18% dry matter by ultrafiltration, fermentation and curd formation without whey drainage was extensively studied for the production of quarg, but without success, since calcium ions (Ca^{2+}), which are not removed from sweet milk by ultrafiltration, lead to the development of a bitter flavour in the product during storage. For this reason 'UF-Quark' is now produced by a method similar to thermoquark, mainly from high-temperature-treated milk and not from a milk concentrate; but the separation of the curd from the whey is achieved mechanically by concentrating the fermented milk by UF with stable membranes instead of a special separator. The benefit for the producer is that the dry matter of UF-quarg contains more lactose and ash in the dry matter compared to thermoquarg, that there is a saving in expensive protein. As a result of this development, the law in Germany was revised, and Speisequark must now contain at least 12% total protein; otherwise, the product must be named 'fresh cheese'.

The industrially produced fresh cheeses containing high amounts of whey proteins are heat treated at about 60°C before separating the whey by centrifugation or ultrafiltration, otherwise, it is impossible to obtain dry matter content of 18% and more. Lactic acid bacteria and their enzymes are inactivated at this temperature, as are the enzymes of the psychrotrophs. The shelf life of

Table 1. Mean composition of quarg from skimmed milk in the FRG within the last century

Product	Year	Dry matter (%)	Lactose (%)	Lactic acid (%)	Salts (%)	Protein (%)	Ratio of whey protein to casein	Milk content (kg) per kg of quarg
Traditional quarg	1871	32–35	2	1·5	1	27	0·02:1	10
Dauerquark	1910	23·3	3·5	0·9	0·9	18	0·04:1	6·7
Quark	1947	21	3·0	1·0	0·7	16·0	0·07:1	5·8
Speisequark	1951	17	3·0	0·8	0·7	12·5	0·04:1	4·8
Thermoquark	1977	17	3·2	1·0	0·8	12·0	0·19:1	3·9
UF-Quark	1985	17	3·7	1·3	1·3	10·7	0·20:1	3·4

Mean values from different sources.

unripened cheeses is nowadays not limited by bacterial contamination, but rather by a decline in sensory properties, e.g. from light-induced off-flavours. *See* Lactic Acid Bacteria; Pasteurization, Principles

A special group of products e.g. double cream cheeses, is made from quarg containing high levels of cream. Sometimes they are stabilized with hydrocolloids (not allowed in the FRG) and pasteurized by heating to 60–80°C for 2–5 min. Hot packaging guarantees a shelf life of at least 12 weeks. During the last few years, some rather unique products of this type, containing herbs and spices, have been produced with techniques and equipment used for the manufacture of processed cheese. Products with very high fat contents are made by adding emulsifiers (e.g. phosphates and citrates). Italy seems to be the leading country in the development of this type of product. *See* Emulsifiers, Phosphates as Meat Emulsion Stabilizers

Within the last 100 years, the character and composition of fresh cheeses have completely changed, at least where the quarg-type products are concerned. However, besides the newly developed varieties of product, the traditional products are still available, e.g. in shops for alternative food or in Italian speciality shops, so that the range of fresh cheeses available to modern day consumers has expanded greatly during the last decades. Table 1 demonstrates changes in the composition of quarg within the last century.

Production

Milk

The raw material for most fresh cheeses is (partly) skimmed milk, but some types are produced from (homogenized) full-fat milk or even from fat-enriched milk (up to 12%). In the case of Speisequark, it is usual to add the desired amounts of cream to the low-fat curd after separation of the whey. This is impossible in the case of highly structured products such as full-fat cottage cheese. Besides milk, considerable amounts of

buttermilk are used nowadays to produce fresh cheeses. Owing to the fact that most fresh cheeses have only a soft consistency, reconstituted milk from low-heat powder is also a rather good raw material; however, some $CaCl_2$ should be added. Some varieties of lactic cheese are prepared from milk–whey mixtures.

As already mentioned, heat treatment of the milk varies between zero and high heating, according to the individual products and the technology in use. However, it should be remembered that fresh cheeses do contain a low amount of their own flavour compounds and they are very sensitive to off-flavours from the milk used. Only raw milk of the best quality yields fresh cheeses with the typical and delicate flavour.

Acidification

Some (Mediterranean) fresh cheeses are prepared by direct acidification with lemon juice or vinegar, but nowadays commercially available lactic acid may be used, and even phosphoric acid has been mentioned as an acidulant. However, most fresh cheeses are produced by acidification of the milk with lactic acid bacteria, e.g. by fermentation. In the northern countries mesophilic starters are used and in the oriental areas with warm climates, thermophilic microorganisms, or even pure yoghurt cultures, are used.

Industrial production of fresh cheeses makes use of selected strains of *Lactococcus lactis*, and *Lact. lactis* subsp. *cremoris* to develop lactic acid, and sometimes *Lact. lactis* biovar. *diacetylactis* or *Leuconostoc mesenteroides* subsp. *cremoris* to form flavour compounds. To avoid proteolysis, which causes loss in yield and initiates off-flavours, *Lact. lactis* may be removed from some selected starters.

With thermophilic starters (optimum 43°C) it is more easy to limit acidification; *Lactobacillus acidophilus* is a typical species in use. For example, cultures with limited acidification not lower than pH 4·8–5·0 are produced by Biogarde® containing *Streptococcus thermophilus*, *Lactococcus lactis*, *Lact. lactis* biovar. *diacetylactis*, *Leuco-*

nostoc mesenteroides subsp. *cremoris*, *Lactobacillus acidophilus* and even *Bifidobacterium bifidum*. Labaneh and labneh, which are very popular in the Middle East, are acidified with thermophilic yoghurt starters. Industrially used starters should not produce gas (CO_2); this avoids problems in the production line, especially in the separators. *See* Starter Cultures

Normally, 0·5–1% starter is added to the milk at about 30°C. When pH 6·3 is reached (after about 1·5 h), rennet may be added (in this case, the milk is stirred well to distribute the enzyme), and in about 16 h the desired acidity of pH 4·5–4·55 is reached. During acid development, the milk should not be stirred. Clearly, acid development is strongly dependent on some important factors, which are part of the typical and individual technology for the different unripened cheeses.

Curd Formation and Treatment

Rennet, if any, is used in small amounts, e.g. 0·5–1·0 ml (1 : 10 000) per 100 l of milk for quarg.

Pure acid casein curds are rather sensitive to heat, a temperature around 43°C and a pH of 4·3 seems to be optimal for whey drainage. If the temperature is only a few degrees higher, the curd changes from dry to smeary. After cutting, traditionally prepared lactic curds are therefore normally filled into cheesecloths and drained at room temperature, and afterwards at low temperatures (4–5°C) for many hours.

In the case of renneted acid curds, heating up to 50–55°C for 1·5 h (cottage cheese) or even 60–64°C for 4–5 min (quarg) improves the syneresis of the coagulum. Owing to these effects, cottage cheese is prepared in a granular form; the curd is washed three times with water at decreasing temperatures (30°C, 16°C, 4°C) to remove lactose and to stabilize the pH value and shelf life.

Centrifugation of quarg curds is performed at about 40–44°C; ultra-filtration is performed over the same range of temperatures or even higher. Cooling of quarg takes place in special tubular coolers, and the product is transported through the line by positive pumps. At the end of the line, quarg mixer may be installed to enrich the product with cream, salt, fruits, stabilizers, etc. Fresh cheeses are normally packaged in plastic containers, glass jars, etc., preferably under aseptic conditions. Some types of fresh cheese with high contents of dry matter are sold as small, round or wedge-shaped bodies packaged in foil.

This is certainly true for the high-fat cream cheeses. They are produced from homogenized milk with 10% or more fat (with 9% fat the curd has the same specific weight as whey, so that centrifugal separation is impossible!). The acidified milk is heated to 80°C before separation. The total solids content of the hot drained curd is 44%, and after salting and cooling it becomes a viscous mass due to crystallization of fat.

Miscellaneous Products

Cottage cheese represents the most structured type of lactic cheese. 'Dry curd' quality (<0·5% fat) is produced from skimmed milk; cottage cheese (low-fat) contains 0·5–2% fat, and cottage cheese itself usually contains >4% fat. It is normally produced by treating the grains with a cream dressing. According to the size of the grains, it is distinguished as Californian-style, Popcorn-style and Country-style, as well as large- and small-curd style. Block-pressed cottage cheese is called Farmer's cheese.

Although cottage cheese is slightly salted (1% sodium chloride), the shelf life is often below 2 weeks, owing to the rather high pH values and sometimes poor bacteriological quality of the wash water. In the FRG, products with fats in the dry matter up to 20% are made, and manufacturing technologies involving ultrafiltration of the milk are also applied.

Quarg (Quark, Topfen, Koarg, Kwarg, Twarog, Tvorog, Taho, lactic cheese, fromage frais, etc.) is available with different levels of fat, up to 45% in the dry matter. With increasing fat content, the consistency changes from crumbly-dry to smooth, but this texture can be influenced by technology (e.g. dry-matter, casein and whey protein content). A foamed quarg is named Bresso. Whipped quarg with not more than 15% dry matter is fromage frais battu maigre. Baker's cheese is characterized by a high dry matter content (22–26%). Schichtkäse, like Cambridge and York, is prepared from layers of low-fat and high-fat lactic curd. Danish smoked quarg is named Rygeost.

Typical lactic curd, fresh cheeses with high fat in dry-matter contents are cream cheese (70% fat in dry-matter), Petit-Suisse (>70% fat in dry matter) and Demisee (40% fat in dry matter), Neufchatel (55% fat in dry matter), Doppelrahmfrischkäse (<85% fat in dry matter) and double cream cheese (>65% fat dry matter). Some of these products are stabilized with hydrocolloids, and the milk is homogenized. Products such as Philadelphia and Gervais, Boursin and Le Tartar (with herbs and spices) are internationally distributed.

A very-high-fat Italian fresh cheese is mascarpone (mascherpone). It is produced from full-fat cream, heated to 90°C, and acidified with citric acid. Whey drainage is performed at 8–10°C for 12–18 h. In the new Sordi process, cream (40–60% fat) is pasteurized, mixed with milk concentrate from ultrafiltration and acidified with citric acid in heated vats. After careful stirring, the product is packaged and stored for about 12 h in the cold to crystallize the fat. Mascarpone is very popular for sweet desserts.

Ricotta was prepared originally by the direct acidification of heated cheese whey from ewes' milk (ricotta di pecora). Many varieties of ricotta are now available, mainly from cows' milk (ricotta di vacca). The consistency varies between soft and dry (ricotta secca). Salted varieties (ricotta salata) as well as the smoked cheeses are used in the kitchen, whereas the unsalted product (ricotta tipo dolce), like the baked ricotta (ricotta salata al forno), are consumed directly as appetizers or desserts. Ricotta is named *requesón* in Spain and *requeijao* in Portugal.

Queso blanco (queso del pais, queso fresco) is also available in many varieties in the Spanish-speaking countries, but is now also manufactured in the USA. It is produced by a combined heat-acid process (82°C and pH 4·6–4·7). Citric acid is said to give the best results, but acetic acid is the most popular acidulant. This cheese can be fried without melting, and is used in the preparation of snack foods; with spices and tomato sauce or chili sauce it is consumed fresh. The organoleptic qualities can be improved using yoghurt starters instead of mesophilic starters. The moisture content is about 50–54%. *See* Acids, Natural Acids and Acidulants

Yoghurt starters are exclusively used in the production of labaneh and labneh. Labaneh is the pure acid curd from skimmed milk, and it can be stored for a long time in olive oil. Labneh is prepared from full-cream milk by acidification and by rennet coagulation. The dry matter content is approximately 40%. These products are the Middle East equivalents of quarg.

Last, but not least, the Swiss Zieger (named Seirass in Piemont, Cérat in Savoy) should be mentioned. Originally prepared by heating acidified whey, they are now also produced from mixtures of milk and whey, or even from skimmed milk. The cheese is white or somewhat yellow, spreadable, and crumbly-soft.

Bibliography

Drewes K (1952) *Die Herstellung und Beurteilung von Sauermilchquark.* Hildesheim: Mann-Verlag.

Eck A (ed.) (1987) *Cheesemaking* 2nd edn. New York: Lavoisier.

Fox PF (ed.) (1987) *Cheese: Chemistry, Physics and Microbiology*, vol. 1. Essex: Elsevier Science Publishers.

Klupsch HJ (1984) *Saure Milcherzeugnisse – Milchmischgetränke und Desserts.* Gelsenkirchen: Verlag Th. Mann.

Kosikowski FV (1977) *Cheese and Fermented Milk Foods*, 2nd edn. Ann Arbor: Edwards Bros.

Lehmann HR, Dolle E and Bücker H (1984) *Prozesslinien zur Herstellung von Frischkäse.* Oelde: Westfalia Separator.

Mair-Waldburg H (1974) *Handbuch der Käse.* Kempten: Volkswirtschaftlicher Verlag.

Robinson RK (ed.) (1986) *Modern Dairy Technology*, vol. 2. Essex: Elsevier Science Publishers.

Scott R (1986) *Cheesemaking Practice* 2nd edn. Essex: Elsevier Science Publishers.

Stieger W (1920) *Anleitung zur Quarkbereitung und zur Handkäsefabrikation* 3rd edn. Berlin: Paul Parey.

H. Klostermeyer
Technische Universität München, Freising-Weihenstephan, FRG

Processed Cheese*

Processed cheese, compared to natural cheese, is a new product with its origins in the beginning of the nineteenth century. Spoilage of natural cheese exported to distant places, especially those with hot climates, as the motive behind the trials adopted to improve the shelf life of cheese. Some of these trials succeeded in prolonging the keeping quality of soft or even semihard cheese by applying heat treatments, but the situation was not the same for hard cheeses, as a result of a shrinkage of the cheese protein by the heat, and separation of the water and fat phases. In 1912–1913, two Swiss workers, Walter Gerber and Fritz Settler, succeeded in solving these problems by heating hard cheese to which sodium citrate was added. This treatment was the real invention of processed cheese. Later, phosphate salts were introduced as emulsifying salts, and development of the processed cheese industry continued and different patents were granted. Kraft, in 1916, established the first commercial factory of processed cheese in the USA. Production and consumption of the processed cheese increased steadily and, today, large tonnages of natural cheeses are coverted to processed cheese. Production of processed cheese affects – directly or indirectly – dairy production in general in the following ways:

1. It encourages cheese production as a base for the manufacture of processed cheese.
2. It makes it possible to use second-grade cheese or cheese that has mechanical or surface defects.
3. At peak times of cheese production, young cheese could be precooked and stored until it is used for processed cheese. In this way it is possible to control the ripening and save the cost of fresh cheese storage for long periods in expensive stores.

Processed cheese products have many advantages over the natural cheese:

1. In most cases, processed cheese can be stored without refrigeration.
2. Processed cheese can be introduced in different shapes, flavours and physical properties, e.g. soft, firm, spreadable, in variable and attractive packages, and it has a relatively long shelf life.
3. It is free from pathogenic microorganisms.

---

* The colour plate section for this article appears between p. 1146 and p. 1147.

Nature and Type of Processed Cheese

Processed cheese is made by heating natural cheese from different types, ages and maturity in the presence of suitable emulsifying salts and with the help of mechanical agitation. In making processed cheese, the insoluble paracasein gel of the natural cheese, under the influences of heating and the action of emulsifiers and agitation, is changed to a paracasein sol – a homogeneous and flowing mass. This sol is changed again to a gel by the influences of cooling and polymerization forces. By understanding the role of different factors related to processed cheese manufacture, it is possible to control and select the characteristics of the end product – soft, firm, sliceable, spreadable, etc. *See* Agitation and Agitator Design

Processed cheeses can be grouped into three main products described below.

Pasteurized Processed Cheese

Pasteurized processed cheese is made of one or more lots of cheese of the same or different varieties. Water, salt, colouring and flavouring materials may be added. The moisture content of the processed cheese may exceed by not more than 1% the maximum permitted in the natural cheese from which it is made, while the fat content may not be less than that of the natural cheese; the processed cheese bears the name of the natural cheese from which it is made. The processing temperature varies from 80°C to 85°C and the pH of the end product ranges from 5·4 to 5·6. Good processed cheese has a smooth, compact and firm body, easily cut into slices.

Pasteurized Processed Cheese Foods

Processed cheese food resembles the above processed cheese but it contains more moisture and less fat. Optional ingredients may be added, including dried whey, dried skim milk, lactose, and organic acids. The moisture content should not exceed 44% and the fat content should be not less than 23%. The processing temperature is normally 85–90°C and the pH of the processed product is 5·6–5·8. Processed cheese food has a softer body and milder flavour than processed cheese. *See* Lactose; Whey and Whey Powders, Production and Uses

Pasteurized Processed Cheese Spread

The constituents of pasteurized processed cheese spread are similar to that used for making processed cheese food, but it contains more moisture in order to achieve a soft body and spreading properties. In many standards, the moisture content should not exceed 60% and the fat should not be less than 20%. This cheese is normally processed at high temperature (85–95°C) in the traditional cookers, and has a pH between 5·6 and 5·9. Binding agents may be added in amounts not exceeding 0·8% of the finished product to improve the water retention. Processed cheese spread is characterized by a mild flavour and a smooth, soft body that is easy to spread at room temperature.

Recently, a new version of processed cheese has been introduced under the name of 'imitation processed cheese': the natural cheese and the fat is replaced by caseinates, vegetable proteins such as soya bean protein, and a suitable vegetable oil. The processing conditions, i.e. emulsifiers, heating temperature and pH, are quite similar to that reported for processed cheese spread. *See* Casein and Caseinates, Uses in the Food Industry; Soya Beans, Processing for the Food Industry; Vegetable Oils, Applications

The limits of moisture and fat in processed cheese are quite flexible and may vary from country to country according to specific standards implemented in each country.

Raw Materials for Processing

The main materials used in the manufacturing of processed cheese include natural cheese, emulsifiers, water and other additives.

Cheese

Two main factors should be considered in selecting the cheese for processing – type and degree of maturity.

Type of Cheese

In general, all rennet cheeses, i.e. soft, semihard and hard cheese, can be used for making processed cheese, but it is common practice to use only hard and semihard cheeses, while soft cheese is used only for flavouring. The selected cheese should be checked for dry matter, fat, pH, protein content, age, and degree of maturity; in many countries, Cheddar cheese is preferred as a main base for processed cheeese. One type of natural cheese can be employed but it is more common to use more than one cheese with the aim of giving the desired body, texture and flavour to the final product. It is worth mentioning that good-quality natural cheese is essential for producing high-quality processed cheese. Second-grade cheese or cheese with mechanical defects can be used, but cheese with a putrid or rancid flavour must not be used, even in small quantities, as the fault will appear in the processed cheese.

Degree of Ripening

In general, hard cheeses may be grouped according to the degree of maturity:

- Fresh, green or young cheese, 1–2 weeks old.
- Medium ripened cheese, 2–4 months old.
- Ripened cheese, over 4 months old.

Natural cheeses of different degrees of maturity are selected for processing to obtain the required composition, physical properties and flavour in the processed cheese. Young cheese has a high level of intact casein as most of the cheese casein has not decomposed to soluble components; the ratio between insoluble casein nitrogen and the total nitrogen is called 'relative casein'. The higher the relative casein (90–95% in young cheese), the more stable the resultant processed cheese. Processing young cheese results in processed cheese of long structure, and the body tends to be smooth or firm according to the moisture content; it is difficult to use only young cheese in processing as it will result in a processed cheese of 'flat' flavour.

However, the long structure of young cheese can be altered by the action of various factors during processing. These factors are mainly related to the use of suitable emulsifying salts to attack the protein along with excessive agitation over quite a long period of time during the thermal process. Changing the long structure of young cheese to a short one of good spreadability is known as a creaming. During the creaming process, the large casein micelles, of low hydration in young cheese, are split into small casein micelles of increased surface area, hydration and, accordingly, good spreadability. Thus young cheese, with proper processing, is convenient as a main base for making processed cheese spreads containing high levels of fat-in-dry-matter (60–70%). The young cheese also contains the high level of intact casein necessary for stability; it is reported that stable processed cheese should have not less than 12% intact casein. As the ripening of fresh cheese progresses, its relative casein content decreases as a result of the breakdown of the protein; hence fully ripened cheese is normally added to the processed cheese blend (10–20%) only to give the desired flavour. It is too difficult to use fully ripened cheese as a main base for processing, as its intact casein is already degraded and is not able to give a stable emulsion.

Medium-ripened cheeses are normally blended with young cheese in different ratios for making processed cheese spread. If a high percentage of medium-ripe cheese is used in a processed cheese spread blend, there is no need for excessive processing to achieve the necessary creaming properties as the intact casein is, to some

Table 1. Suggested blends of natural cheeses for producing processed cheeses

Processed cheeses	Natural cheese (%)		
	Young	Medium-ripened	Fully ripened
Block	50–60	20–30	10–20
Food	30–40	50–60	10
Spread	50–60	30–40	10

extent, already decomposed. Different ratios of young, medium- and fully ripened cheese have been reported for the manufacture of processed cheese products. These ratios are not fixed figures, and may vary according to the type, characteristics and composition of the natural cheese; they may also vary in the presence of other dairy products, such as milk or whey powder. Some typical blends are presented in Table 1.

The storage of cheese for ripening is rather expensive; hence many attempts have been made to render young cheese, or even rennet curd, suitable for processing after a few days or weeks of manufacture. The addition of lipolytic and/or proteolytic enzymes was tried, as was cooking the curd in a lactic acid solution. Gouda et al. (1985) succeeded in using a hard cheese with a low pH (4·8–5·0), and the cheese was used a few days after manufacture as the main base for a good processed cheese spread. The main aim was to release calcium from the curd, and the process was employed on a commercial scale. *See* Enzymes, Uses in Food Processing

Emulsifiers

Natural cheese is basically an emulsion of oil-in-water, stabilized by the cheese protein. Heating and agitation, or changing the pH, will affect the protein which may lose all or part of its ability to effect stabilization; defective texture, water and fat separation will occur. In the presence of emulsifying salts, the separated water and fat reincorporate into the cheese mass, resulting in a homogeneous mixture. The action of emulsifying salts (melting salts) in processed cheese manufacture can be summarized as follows:

1. Removal of calcium from the protein system.
2. Breakdown and dispersion of the protein.
3. Hydration and swelling of the protein.
4. Control and stabilization of the emulsion system and the pH of the cheese.
5. Control of spoilage of the cheese.

See Emulsifiers, Phosphates as Meat Emulsion Stabilizers; Emulsifiers, Uses in Processed Foods

The major emulsifying salts which are used on a large scale are the sodium salts of citrates, monophosphates, diphosphates and polyphosphates. Sodium aluminium phosphate is also used. It is common practice to use a mixture of emulsifying salts rather than one salt to attain the general desired characteristics. The amount of emulsifiers used in processed cheese is normally 2–3% depending on type, maturity and amount of natural cheese in the blend.

Water

Water is very important for producing a stable emulsion. Emulsifying salts need water to dissolve and act properly on the casein. Water is added to the blend to give the required water content in the processed cheese. In calculating the amount of water, it should be borne in mind that heating by direct steam injection will add some condensed water to the blend. Water may be added at the start of processing, as in the case of block processed cheese, or in portions, as for processed cheese spread. The addition of only part of the water at the start of processing increases the concentration and action of the emulsifiers on the casein.

Additives

Optional ingredients may be added to the processed cheese blend for economic reasons, or to improve the shelf life and quality of processed cheese.

Dried Skim Milk and Dried Whey

Dried skim milk or whey can be used to replace part of the cheese solids in the blends for processed cheese food or spread. Skim-milk powder and whey powder promote the creaming process and improve spreadability, but the amount must not exceed 10% of the blend in order to avoid a sweet-salty taste – especially when young cheese is used – and to prevent browning and crystallization owing to excess lactose in the processed cheese.

Fats

Different fats may be added to the blend to increase the fat-in-dry matter content of the processed cheese. Heavy cream, butter or butteroil can be used as a source of fat. For processed cheese spread of defined total solids, increasing the fat content cause a decrease in the solids not fat (SNF) in the blend; hence young cheese of high intact casein should be used as the main base to give a stable emulsion; caseinates may also be used. The emulsifying salts used in processed cheese have no direct effect on the fat. *See* Fats, Uses in the Food Industry

Precooked Cheese

Precooked cheese may be used to improve the stability of the processed cheese. It is normally produced at peak times of cheese production when there is a volume of cheese above the capacity of the ripening rooms, or when the cheese is not fit for maturation. Pre-cooked cheese made from young cheese has a long structure and can be added to a processed cheese blend containing over-ripened cheese to improve its stability. Precooked cheese made from mature cheese has a short structure and can be used to promote the creaming property of a processed cheese spread. The amount of precooked cheese added to a blend varies according to the degree of maturity of the cheese in the blend and the type of processed cheese to be manufactured.

Flavouring Materials

Flavouring materials may be added to give a particular flavour to the processed cheese, or to improve the flavour, especially when young cheese is used. Among these materials, meat, ham, wines, fruit, spices and essences are of common use in processed cheese. Flavouring materials should be of good microbiological quality, and this can be attained by thermal treatment before addition to the blend. The physical properties of the processed cheese are not affected by the use of such additives. *See* Flavour Compounds, Structures and Characteristics

Binding Agents

Binding agents or stabilizers are sometimes added to processed cheese spread to absorb some of the water, and improve the stability of the cheese. The amount of stabilizers, if permitted, should not exceed 0·8% of the processed cheese. Gum arabic, locust bean gum, gelatin, pectin, carboxymethyl cellulose and agar are examples of such materials. *See* Stabilizers, Types and Function; Stabilizers, Applications

Preservatives

The addition of preservatives to processed cheese is prohibited in many countries. However, preservatives such as benzoic and sorbic acids are used to overcome the blowing of processed cheese. In addition, biological substances, such as Nisin, are used as inhibitory agents to prevent the growth of anaerobic spore-formers (clostridia), the main cause of blowing in processed cheese. Nisin is a polypeptide discovered in cultures of some varieties of *Lactococcus lactis*, and is commercially produced in powder form. Although Nisin is successfully used in many processed cheese factories, there is some doubt concerning its efficiency against some strains of clostridia. *See* Preservation of Food

Manufacturing of Processed Cheese

The steps involved in the manufacture of processed cheese can be summarized as follows.

Selection and Calculation of the Raw Materials

Two important factors must be considered in selecting the cheese for the blend: (1) the characteristics of the natural cheese, i.e. type, age, maturity, pH, fat, total solids and the physical properties; (2) the desired properties for the processed cheese, i.e. firmness, spreadability, etc.

The amount of cheese and other ingredients in the blend are calculated according to their fat and dry-matter contents, so that the product conforms to the legal standards of the specific type of processed cheese.

Cleaning

Hard and semihard cheeses selected for processing are subject to cleaning before use. Very hard rind, waxes or wrapping materials used to cover rindless cheeses, and surface defects must be removed manually or mechanically before processing.

Cutting, Mincing and Milling

The selected blocks of cheese are cut manually, or mechanically with special knives, into small slices suitable for the mincing machines. The slices are then minced or shredded through special mincing machines into fine granules, which are ground through roller mills to make them soft, smooth, and free from small, hard particles. Mincing and milling of the cheese enables the emulsifying salts to be in contact with the cheese, and eases the absorption of water and dispersion of the cheese protein.

Processing

Milled cheeses and other ingredients of the blend are placed in the processing kettle. Heating may be carried out directly by steam injection, indirectly, or by both methods to a temperature normally not less than 75°C to ensure a complete pasteurization of the processed cheese. Agitation during processing is important for a complete emulsification of the cheese blend. Processing kettles are operated either batch or continuously. They are available in various shapes and capacities. A normal kettle consists of two pans equipped with one movable cover which bears an agitator, steam injection nozzles, vacuum tubes and gauges for temperature and pressure. When processing is carried out in one of the pans, the other one is loaded with raw materials ready for processing.

The temperature and duration of processing is determined by the type of processed cheese, and by the condition of natural cheese in the blend. In general, a period of 2–4 min is required to reach the processing temperature, and the temperature is kept constant for a further 5–10 min. Block processed cheese is processed at 80–85°C for 8–15 min, and a processed cheese spread at 85–95°C for 8–15 min in a traditional kettle. The duration of processing is related to the speed of agitation. Stephan kettles are equipped with very fast agitators, so that a period of 4–5 min is enough for processed cheese spread. In some kettles, processing is carried under pressure at 130–140°C for a few seconds.

Homogenization

Homogenization is an optional operation used for processed cheese spreads, especially those that contain high fat contents, and is conducted directly after processing. It improves the consistency, stability and appearance of the processed cheese. Contamination during homogenization should be carefully avoided.

Packaging

The hot, flowing mass of processed cheese is transported manually in stainless steel buckets or by special pumps to the filling machines. Keeping the processed cheese quite hot in the filling machines eases the sealing of the packaging materials. Processed cheese is packed in thin aluminium foil coated with a special lacquer, in plastic membranes or in tins; it is packed in different shapes varying in weight from 3 g to 3 kg.

Storage

Directly after packing, the processed cheese is still quite warm (40–60°C), but it should be cooled down to room temperature in a time that varies according to the type of processed cheese. As a rule, processed cheese spread should be cooled quickly (30–60 min) to stop the creaming phenomenon; otherwise, overcreaming will cause fat and water separation and a defective texture. In cooling processed cheese spread, a space should be let between the boxes to ease the movement of the cool air. For block processed cheese, a long time (10–15 h) is needed to cool it down, but cooling that is too slow, especially in the presence of lactose, may result in browning or firming-up of the cheese, and may allow the growth of spore-forming microorganisms. After the cheese has been cooled down, it should be kept in a cold store (5–10°C). It is advisable to keep processed cheese above 0°C – to prevent the freezing of the product – and below 20°C; otherwise, surviving microorganisms, especially clostridia, may grow and cause defects. *See* Spoilage, Moulds in Food Spoilage

Defects in Processed Cheese

The two main defects of importance in processed cheese are microbiological defects and those of physiochemical origin.

Microbiological Defects

Microbiological defects are mainly related to the blowing of the processed cheese as a result of gas formation by anaerobic spore-formers (clostridia). Spongy texture and bad odour are indicators of a heavy contamination with clostridia.

In addition, mould growth may appear on the surface of poorly sealed packs of processed cheese. However, the use of raw materials of good microbiological quality, proper processing and the addition of permitted antimicrobial materials should minimize or eliminate these defects.

Defects of Physiochemical Origin

Too firm a block, results from one or more of the following:

- Low moisture content
- High casein content
- Use of the wrong emulsifiers
- Strong overcreaming
- Low pH.

Too soft a block may occur as a result of the following:

- High moisture content
- Unsuitable or insufficient emulsifiers
- Too high a pH
- Excessive processing
- Addition of milk or whey powder
- Use of too much mature cheese.

Inhomogeneous cheese could be the result of the following:

- Insufficient milling, especially of cheese with a hard rind
- Improper processing time, temperature or agitation
- Unsuitable or insufficient emulsifiers

- Use of raw materials of too low pH, particularly an acid-precipitated cheese or curd.

Gum-like spread could be caused by the following:

- Use of too much young cheese
- Insufficient processing to achieve proper creaming
- Absence of creamed, precooked cheese
- Addition of all the water at one time.

'Sticky spread' is the term used when the processed cheese adheres to the aluminium foil. This defect may be attributable to the following:

- Excess water content or all the water added at once
- The blend contains too much young cheese
- Proper creaming is not achieved
- No well-creamed, precooked cheese has been added
- The intact casein in the blend is insufficient.

The reasons for brittle spread are as follows:

- Overcreaming during processing
- Addition of too much overcreamed, precooked cheese
- Decrease of pH after processing or during storage.

Gas Formation

As result of a chemical reaction between the aluminium foil and the cheese, the resultant hydrogen can cause gas 'holes' on the cheese surface without odour formation. This defect can be attributed to the absence of, or use of, poor-quality, lacquering materials or to the use of an emulsifying salt which is too acidic or too alkaline.

Browning (Maillard Reaction)

Normal processed cheese colour is between white and pale yellow. Browning may occur directly after processing, or during storage, as a result of a reaction between amino compounds and reducing sugars. This defect may be caused by the following:

- Use of too high a processing temperature for a long time, especially in the presence of lactose
- Storage of the processed cheese at high temperature, particularly when the pH is high.

This defect is more common in processed cheese spread than in the block type. *See* Browning, Nonenzymatic

Crystallization

Crystallization is a defect which can be seen inside or on the surface of the cheese; a 'sandy' texture may result. The reasons for this defect may be as follows:

- Precipitation of calcium monophosphate, diphosphate, polyphosphate or citrate, particularly when excess emulsifier has been used

- Undissolved particles of emulsifier, owing to poor storage of the emulsifier or improper processing
- Use of precooked cheese with a sandy texture
- Precipitation of lactose crystals as a result of too much dried milk or whey in the blend
- Use of very mature cheese may result in white precipitates of some amino acids, such as tyrosine.

Water Separation

Water separation can take the form of small droplets inside the cheese, or wetting of the cheese surface. It is caused by the following factors:

- Too low a pH of the processed cheese
- Changes in the cheese structure (overcreaming)
- Unsuitable storage conditions, e.g. the cheese is subjected to mechanical pressure.

Fat Separation

Fat separation could be the result of the following factors:

- Use of too much mature cheese
- Insufficient or excess emulsifiers
- Too low a pH of the processed cheese
- Storage of the cheese for long time at high temperature.

Flavour Defects

Examples of the more common flavour defects are as follows:

- Sharp flavours, owing to use of too much mature cheese
- Flat flavour, owing to use of too much young cheese
- Salty taste, owing to use of salty cheese or excess emulsifiers
- Putrid taste, owing to use of putrid cheese or growth of clostridia
- Rancid taste, owing to use of rancid cheese and/or butter, or cheese ripened by moulds
- Chemical taste, owing to use of impure emulsifiers, addition of certain preservatives or stabilizers, or use of too salty cheese.

Bibliography

Fox PF (ed.) (1989) *Cheese Chemistry, Physics and Microbiology*, vol. 2. Essex: Elsevier Science Publishers.

Gouda A, El-Shabrawy E, El-Zayat A and El-Bagoury E (1985) Use of calcium caseinate in processed cheese spread making. *Egyptian Journal of Dairy Science* 13: 115–119.

Kosikowski FV (1978) *Cheese and Fermented Milk Foods*. Ann Arbor, Michigan: Edwards Brothers.

Meyer A (1973) *Processed Cheese Manufacture*. London: Food Trade Press.

Shimp LR (1985) Processed cheese principles. *Food Technology* 39(5): 63–70.

Thomas MA (1977) *The Processed Cheese Industry*. Bulletin D44. New South Wales: Department of Agriculture.

A. Gouda
Suez Canal University, Ismailia, Egypt

Dietary Importance

Cheese is the oldest way of preserving the nutrients in milk and is essentially a concentrated form of milk. Most cheese is made from cows' milk, but other milks including sheep's, goats' and buffalos' can also be used. The process used to make the cheese tends to determine the nutritional value. This article will review the nutritional value of different types of cheese, its role in the diet for different groups of the population and trends in cheese consumption around the world.

Hard Cheeses

Hard cheeses such as Cheddar and Cheshire retain most of the protein, fat, calcium and other minerals, and vitamins such as vitamin A, riboflavin (vitamin B_2) and vitamin B_{12}. Table 1 shows the nutrient composition of some hard cheeses. *See* individual nutrients

Hard cheese contains very little lactose as most is either lost with the whey during the cheesemaking process, or converted to lactic acid. The major protein in cheese is casein, which is a high-quality protein containing all the essential amino acids in roughly the proportions required by the body for health. Minerals in cheese, such as calcium and zinc, are particularly well absorbed and utilized (high bioavailability).

Low-fat hard cheeses are available in the UK. They typically contain about half the quantity of fat found in the traditional cheese and remain a valuable source of essential nutrients.

Soft Cheeses

Soft cheeses vary widely in nutritional composition, depending on whether they belong to the ripened or unripened varieties. Fresh, unripened cheeses, such as cottage cheese, are low in fat, relatively low in calcium, high in moisture and contain unfermented lactose. Very-low-fat versions are also available. On the other hand, a surface-mould-ripened cheese, such as Brie or Camembert, contains a high proportion of fat and protein and less water (Table 2). Mould-ripened soft cheeses have a slightly lower fat content than traditional hard cheeses. The addition of salt is an essential part of the cheese-making process. The salt is added to help preserve the cheese and to bring out the flavour.

Cheese from Unpasteurized Milk

Most of the cheese produced in the UK is made from pasteurized milk. However, there is a demand for cheese made with unpasteurized milk, as it is believed by some to have a superior flavour. Provided that the milk used has come from farms operating to the highest standards, so that the milk is free of pathogens, and that the creamery operates to the same high standards, the resulting cheese will not carry a health hazard.

Tyramine in Cheese

In common with foods such as red wine, hung game, soused herrings and yeast extracts, certain cheeses (e.g. mature Cheddar, Roquefort and Gruyère) contain an amino acid derivative known as tyramine.

In sensitive individuals, tyramine can provoke

Table 1. Nutritional composition (per 100 g) of some hard cheeses

	English Cheddar	Cheshire	Blue Stilton	Edam	Reduced-fat Cheddar
Energy					
(kcal)	412	379	411	229	261
(kJ)	1708	1571	1701	957	1091
Protein (g)	25·5	24·0	22·7	32·6	31·5
Carbohydrate (g)	0·1	0·1	0·1	Trace	Trace
Sugars (g)	0·1	0·1	0·1	Trace	Trace
Fat (g)	34·4	31·4	35·5	25·4	15·0
Saturates (g)	21·7	19·6	22·2	15·9	9·4
Monounsaturates (g)	9·4	9·1	10·3	7·4	4·4
Polyunsaturates (g)	1·4	0·9	1·0	0·7	0·4
Sodium (mg)	670	550	930	1020	670
Dietary fibre (g)	Nil	Nil	Nil	Nil	Nil
Vitamin A (μg)	336	387	386	200	182
Thiamin (mg)	0·03	0·03	0·03	0·03	0·03
Riboflavin (mg)	0·42	0·48	0·43	0·35	0·53
Nicotinic acid (mg)	0·09	0·11	0·49	0·07	0·09
Potential nicotinic acid from tryptophan (mg)	6·00	5·64	5·34	6·12	7·41
Vitamin B_6 (mg)	0·10	0·09	0·16	0·09	0·13
Folic acid (μg)	37	40	77	40	56
Vitamin B_{12} (μg)	1·2	0·9	1·0	2·1	1·3
Pantothenic acid (mg)	0·38	0·31	0·71	0·38	0·51
Biotin (μg)	3·1	4·0	3·6	1·8	3·8
Vitamin C (mg)	Trace	Trace	Trace	Trace	Trace
Vitamin D (μg)	0·26	0·24	0·27	0·19	0·11
Vitamin E (mg)	0·54	0·70	0·61	0·48	0·39
Vitamin K (μg)	N/A	N/A	N/A	N/A	N/A
Calcium (mg)	740	560	320	770	840
Chlorine (mg)	1010	830	1410	1570	1110
Copper (mg)	Trace	0·13	0·18	0·05	0·05
Iodine (μg)	46	(46)	(46)	N/A	N/A
Iron (mg)	0·2	0·3	0·3	0·4	0·2
Magnesium (mg)	26	19	20	39	39
Phosphorus (mg)	490	400	310	530	620
Potassium (mg)	79	87	130	97	110
Selenium (μg)	12	(11)	(11)	N/A	15
Zinc (mg)	2·3	3·3	2·5	2·2	2·8

N/A: no reliable figures available. ( ): estimate.
Source: Holland B, Unwin ID and Buss DH (1989) Milk Products and Eggs. The fourth supplement to McCance and Widdowson's *The Composition of Foods* 4th edn. Cambridge: Royal Society of Chemistry, and Ministry of Agriculture, Fisheries and Food.

Dietary Importance

Table 2. Nutrient composition (per 100 g) of soft cheese

	Soft, fresh				Surface-mould-ripened	
	Cottage cheese: plain	Fromage frais: plain	Fromage frais: plain, very low fat	Quark	Brie	Camembert
Energy						
(kcal)	98	113	58	74	319	297
(kJ)	413	469	247	313	1323	1232
Protein (g)	13·8	6·8	7·7	14·6	19·3	20·9
Carbohydrate (g)	2·0	5·4	6·5	3·8	Trace	Trace
Sugars (g)	2·0	5·4	6·5	3·8	Trace	Trace
Fat (g)	3·9	7·1	0·2	Trace	26·9	23·7
Saturates (g)	2·4	4·4	0·1	Trace	16·8	14·8
Monounsaturates (g)	1·1	2·1	0·1	Trace	7·8	6·9
Polyunsaturates (g)	0·1	0·2	Trace	Trace	0·8	0·7
Sodium (mg)	380	31	(33)	45	700	650
Dietary fibre (g)	Nil	Nil	Nil	Nil	Nil	Nil
Vitamin A (μg)	46	100	3	2	320	283
Thiamin (mg)	0·03	0·04	(0·03)	(0·04)	0·04	0·05
Riboflavin (mg)	0·26	0·40	(0·37)	0·30	0·43	0·52
Nicotinic acid (mg)	0·13	0·13	(0·14)	0·19	0·43	0·96
Potential nicotinic acid from tryptophan (mg)	3·24	1·59	1·81	3·43	4·53	4·91
Vitamin B_6 (mg)	0·08	0·10	(0·07)	0·08	0·15	0·22
Folic acid (μg)	27	15	(15)	45	58	102
Vitamin B_{12} (μg)	0·7	1·4	(1·4)	0·7	1·2	1·1
Pantothenic acid (mg)	0·40	N/A	N/A	0·44	0·35	0·36
Biotin (μg)	3·0	N/A	N/A	3·0	5·6	7·6
Vitamin C (mg)	Trace	Trace	Trace	1·0	Trace	Trace
Vitamin D (μg)	0·03	0·05	Trace	Trace	0·20	0·18
Vitamin E (mg)	0·08	0·02	Trace	Trace	0·84	0·65
Vitamin K (μg)	N/A	N/A	N/A	N/A	N/A	
Calcium (mg)	73	89	(87)	120	540	650
Chlorine (mg)	550	100	(89)	110	1060	1120
Copper (mg)	0·04	Trace	(0·01)	0·06	Trace	0·07
Iodine (μg)	N/A	N/A	N/A	4	N/A	N/A
Iron (mg)	0·1	0·1	(8)	Trace	0·8	0·2
Magnesium (mg)	9	8	(110)	11	27	2·1
Phosphorus (mg)	160	110	(8)	200	390	310
Potassium (mg)	89	110	(110)	140	100	100
Selenium (μg)	(4)	(2)	(2)	N/A	N/A	N/A
Zinc (mg)	0·6	0·3	(0·3)	0·9	2·2	2·7

N/A: no reliable figures available. ( ): estimate.
Source: Holland B, Unwin ID and Buss DH (1989) Milk Products and Eggs. The fourth supplement to McCance and Widdowson's *The Composition of Foods* 4th edn. Cambridge: Royal Society of Chemistry, and Ministry of Agriculture, Fisheries and Food.

migraine and skin rashes. This may occur, for example, in those taking drugs that block the enzyme monoamine oxidase, which metabolizes tyramine. *See* Migraine and Diet

Trends in Cheese Consumption

Table 3 shows consumption of cheese in different countries. Compared with most European countries,

cheese consumption in the UK is low. Consumption is particularly high in France and the Netherlands.

In the UK, cheese consumption has risen from 4·7 kg per person per year in 1966 to 8·1 kg per person per year in 1989, according to the *International Dairy Federation Annual Statistics* (Fig. 1). Data from the National Food Survey, conducted by the UK Ministry of Agriculture, Fisheries and Food, indicate that average household cheese consumption in 1989 was 114 g (4·07 oz) per

Dietary Importance

person per week. Cheese consumption is greater in higher income groups and smaller households. There are no strong regional differences.

Importance of Cheese for Different Groups

As a product of milk, cheese confers similar nutritional benefits. In particular it is a rich source of protein, calcium and vitamins A, B_2 (riboflavin) and B_{12}. It is also a useful source of highly bioavailable zinc. In addition, cheese is a very versatile food, which can be incorpor-

Table 3. Consumption of cheese (kg per person per year) in various countries

	Fresh, including cottage cheese	Other cheese, including processed cheese
Denmark	1·1	13·1
Sweden	0·9	14·6
France	7·0	15·3
Germany	8·0	10·1
Netherlands	1·5	13·3
Canada	1·2	14·1
Australia	0·8	8·4
UK	1·0	7·1
Japan	0·1	1·1

Source: IDF (1991) *Bulletin No 254* Brussels: International Dairy Foundation.

ated into many different dishes. It keeps well if properly stored in the refrigerator, wrapped in greaseproof paper and foil. Hard cheeses such as Cheddar freeze well and can be kept for up to 3 months. On thawing best results are achieved if the cheese is allowed to defrost gradually, preferably in the refrigerator.

Mild hard cheeses and fresh soft cheeses such as cottage cheese can be introduced into a child's diet from the age of 6 months. Cheese can be a useful snack food for children. It is one of the few foods which do not contribute to dental caries, and it may even have a protective effect against dental decay, perhaps by controlling the pH at the surface of the tooth. Some dentists recommend a small piece of cheese at the end of a meal for this reason. *See* Dental Disease, Role of Diet

Calcium requirements are particularly high during pregnancy, and cheese, an excellent source of calcium, is therefore a valuable food for pregnant women. However, as a precaution, pregnant women are advised to avoid mould-ripened soft cheese such as Brie and Camembert because of the increased chance of their containing *Listeria monocytogenes*, the bacterium which causes listeriosis. Most healthy people are unaffected by listeriosis, but pregnant women are at a greater risk. Fresh soft cheeses, e.g. cottage cheese and hard cheeses such as Cheddar, are considered safe in this respect. The pH of Cheddar and other such cheeses limits the growth of this bacterium, which prefers more alkaline conditions. *See* Listeria, Listeriosis

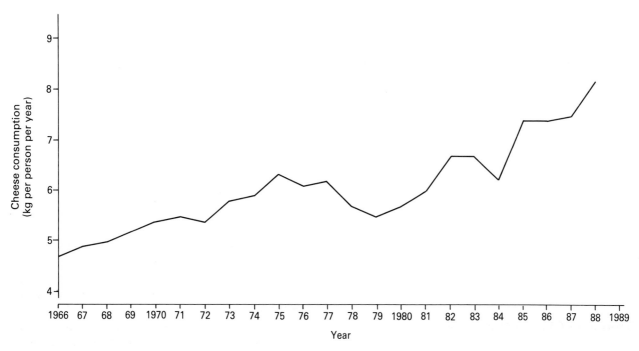

Fig. 1   Cheese consumption in the UK from 1966 to 1989 (IDF (1980) *Bulletin No 119*; (1989) *Bulletin No 241*; (1990) *Bulletin No 246*; (1991) *Bulletin No 254*. Brussels: International Dairy Foundation.)

For vegetarians who include dairy products in their diet, cheese can be an important source of protein, vitamin B_{12} and minerals. Vegans, who exclude all foods of animal origin, will require vitamin-B_{12}-fortified foods or supplements, since the vitamin is found only in dairy foods and other foods of animal origin, such as meat. *See* Vegan Diets; Vegetarian Diets

Hard cheeses, such as Cheddar, have a very low lactose content and can be a useful source of calcium and other essential nutrients for those people who are lactose intolerant. *See* Food Intolerance, Lactose Intolerances

Bibliography

Ministry of Agriculture, Fisheries and Food (1990) *Household Food Consumption and Expenditure, 1989*. London: Her Majesty's Stationery Office.

Renner E (1983) *Milk and Dairy Products in Human Nutrition*. Munich: Volkswirtschaftlicher Verlag.

Renner E (1989) *Micronutrients in Milk and Milk-Based Food Products*. London: Elsevier Applied Science.

Scott R (1981) *Cheesemaking Practice*. London: Applied Science Publishers.

Judy Buttriss
National Dairy Council, London, UK

CHEMICAL ANALYSIS

See Specific Analytical Techniques

CHERRIES

Cherry Taxonomy and Types

Commercially, the two most important cherry species are sweet cherry, *Prunus avium* L., and sour cherry, *Prunus cerasus* L., both tree fruits native to southeastern Europe and western Asia. They are closely related, graft compatible and will hybridize to form interspecific (Duke) cultivars. Sweet cherry (diploid, with a base chromosome number of 8, and a somatic number of 16) probably originated between the Black Sea and the Caspian Sea, but it spread into Europe in ancient times. Sour cherry (tetraploid, with a base chromosome number of 16, somatic chromosome number of 32) is native to the same areas as sweet cherry, and there is good evidence that crosses between *Prunus avium* and ground cherry, *P. fruticosa* Pall, gave rise to sour cherry. There are other cherry species, but most, e.g. Nanking cherry (*Prunus tomentosa*), have limited commercial value as fruits.

Sweet cherries can be divided into two major types based on fruit characteristics. Heart-type cherries are ovoid or heart-shaped with relatively soft flesh, often early ripening. Most of the commercially important cultivars, however, are of the Bigarreau type with firmer, crisp-fleshed fruit, ripening mid- to late season. Fruit flesh may be red or yellow, and the skin may be dark (red to nearly black) or light (yellow-red to yellow-white).

Many sweet cherry cultivars grown throughout the world originated in Europe, but a number of important ones were selected or bred in local cherry districts. European cultivars grown in the USA are Napoleon (Royal Ann), Black Tartarian, Eagle, Early Purple, Early Rivers, Elkhorn, Hedelfingen, Knight's Early Black, Lyon and Schmidt. The cultivars, Windsor, Van, Sam, Vista, Victor, Sue, Vega, Summit and Stella, were developed in Canada. Chinook and Rainier were developed in Washington. Bing, Lambert, Black Republican, Corum and Hoskins were selected and developed in Oregon. Chapman, Burbank, Bush Tartarian, and the new cultivars, Mona, Larian, Jubilee, Berryessa and Bada, originated in California. Recent introductions include Ulster and Hudson from New York, and Angela from Utah.

The most important sweet cherry cultivars in the western USA, where about 80% of the US crop is produced, are dark-fruited, crisp-fleshed cultivars – Bing (the leading cultivar in North America), Van and

Lambert – although others may be available because of their use as pollinizers. Firmness, colour, and soluble solids are all important market considerations, and growers in regions where summer rains are prevalent, e.g. eastern USA and eastern Europe, are at a disadvantage because the main cultivars are often the softer fleshed, rain-cracking resistant types, such as Emperor Francis, Hedelfingen, and Schmidt. Light-fleshed cultivars, Rainier, Napoleon (Royal Ann), Corum and Emperor Francis, are best for making into maraschino cherries (because pigment is undesirable), but some are grown for the fresh market. Napoleon is also used for canning. Bing is mainly a fresh market cultivar, and Lambert is used both for canning and fresh market. Black Republican and other very firm, dark cherries are good for freezing.

Sour cherry fruits are generally soft, juicy, and depressed-globose in shape, but colours may range from the Morello types, with red to dark red flesh and juice, to the Amarelle types, with nearly colourless juice and flesh.

Although there are several sour cherry cultivars grown in North America, ranging from the light red Early Richmond, the medium red-skinned Montmorency, to the late dark red English Morello, Montmorency is the standard. In western Europe, Schattenmorelle and Sternsbaer are common, but many others are grown in Russia, Yugoslavia, Romania and Hungary. Most, unlike sweet cherry, are more or less self-fertile and generally do not require pollinizers. Almost all of those grown in the USA and western Europe are harvested mechanically and sold for processing, primarily as a frozen or canned ingredient for use in manufactured food products such as pies, but in Europe and other areas for dried fruit products, juice, liqueur, and marmalade production, and for combination with yoghurt.

Production Areas

The USA, the Soviet Union and Germany are large producers of both sweet and sour cherries. In some areas of northern Europe, sour cherries are, after apples, the second most important fruit grown. Otherwise within Europe, sour cherry production is concentrated in eastern Europe, Yugoslavia, Hungary and Romania, while sweet cherry production is more common in western Europe, in Italy, Switzerland, France and Spain. In the USA sweet cherry production is mostly in the west, primarily in Washington, but also in Oregon and California. Most US sour cherry production occurs near the Great Lakes, primarily in Michigan, where 70–75% of the US crop is grown; added to New York, Wisconsin and Pennsylvania, this totals 90–95% of the US crop.

Maximum world production values for sweet and sour cherries are approximately 1 450 000 and 1 600 000 t, respectively. Wide annual supply fluctuations, especially regionally, in both sweet and sour cherries characterize production and create high risks in product availability and price change for producers, processors and marketers. Annual US sour cherry production has ranged, for example, from 63 600 to 141 000 t, but there has been a gradual downward trend in average production since the mid-1960s to about 125 000 t during recent years, with a farm value of about $50 000 000, but the processed value is at least three times that. Sweet cherry production, however, is increasing, especially as markets develop in Japan and the Far East of the Pacific Rim for fresh cherries grown in western USA and elsewhere. *See* Fruits of Temperate Climates, Commercial and Dietary Importance

Growth and Management

Flowering and Fruit Set

Sweet cherry flowers are in clusters of two to four, usually borne laterally on short spurs on 2-year-old twigs or near the base of longer 1-year-old shoots. Floral initiation takes place in July, after the crop is harvested, and only on buds where the subtending leaves open relatively early in summer. Flower buds are of the unmixed type and do not give rise to a lateral or bourse shoot. As a result, flowering spurs, unlike those on apples and pears, do not remain productive. Flowers generally have a single pistil, but in very hot summers may form two pistils that result in undesirable double fruits. With few exceptions, e.g. 'Stella' and its progeny, commercial sweet cherry cultivars are self-sterile (self-incompatible), and therefore require another cultivar for pollination. There are, however, intrasterile groups, where none of the group will cross-pollinate any other member of the group. Bing, Lambert and Napoleon are one such group.

Sour cherry flowers develop much like sweet cherry, with buds of two to four flowers on either spurs or lateral buds. Sour cherry cultivars range from compatible to self-incompatible. Montmorency, for example, is only partially compatible, but is always grown without a pollinator. Fruit set clearly limits yield of the fully incompatible cultivars, but overcropping may occur in other cultivars, with overflowering or excessive fruit set resulting in too few leaves or leaf buds to properly size the fruit.

In both sweet and sour cherries, flower development and fruit set may frequently be harmed by late frosts, although sour cherry is hardier and generally blooms later than sweet cherry. Wide annual supply fluctuations are consequently common in major growing areas for both species due to spring frosts or to low midwinter temperatures where lack of wood hardiness is a contributing factor. Sweet cherries are less hardy than apples, but some sour cherry cultivars may be as hardy as the apple cultivars, McIntosh or Northern Spy. In addition, the best quality sweet cherry cultivars tend to be more susceptible to rain cracking, and do best in regions with dry summer growing conditions. Fruits also develop good quality in regions often too cool for peaches or apricots. Climate also dictates that cherries be grown where winter chilling temperatures (about 1000 h for most sweet cherries, longer for sour cherry) are adequate to break rest; thus cherry culture is generally limited to cooler temperate regions.

Tree Size and Rootstocks

Tree size plays a central role in production of quality fruit. Dwarf trees have many advantages: light penetrates better, favouring photosynthesis, and the tree produces more and better fruit; spraying can be done more efficiently, usually with reduced use of chemicals; and dwarf trees are easier to harvest. Cherries are no exception, but dwarfing rootstocks have not been available for either sweet or sour cherry. The common rootstocks, 'Mazzard' and 'Mahaleb', only slightly affect tree size, if at all. 'Colt' is similar, and may be somewhat drought- and cold-susceptible. Recently, however, dwarfing rootstocks have been developed in several breeding programmes, and these are being tested. For example, of 17 cherry rootstocks developed in Giessen, Germany, most produce relatively large trees, but two give trees about 25% of the standard, and several developed in Belgium also seem promising.

Harvesting and Handling

Sweet cherries are almost all hand-harvested, particularly those intended for the fresh market. Avoiding pitting and bruising throughout harvest, sorting and packing are major problems in delivering high-quality fruit to the fresh market. Bruise susceptibility of some white- or yellow- fleshed cultivars may even require field packing to minimize loss. Mechanical harvesting of sour cherries for processing, however, has been a major technological development which substantially reduces grower costs. A grower and his family plus some high school students (a crew of six to eight) can mechanically harvest as much as 200–300 hand-pickers formerly did. The results include huge savings in direct labour costs, large reductions in housing costs, plus substantial savings in labour fringe costs. The US sour cherry industry became completely mechanically harvested during the 1970s, although there have since been additional improvements in equipment and techniques.

Some aspects of cherry processing have also substantially changed and this has led to greater efficiencies and product quality in the cherry industry. Almost all sour cherry processors have adopted electric-eye sorting equipment which substantially reduces in-plant sorting labour, and de-stemmer equipment efficiently removes the stems from mechanically harvested cherries. Although picking is still by hand, subsequent handling of sweet cherries for the fresh market has been improved dramatically very recently with the substitution of hydraulic flumes for conveyor belts to reduce bruising and pitting throughout sorting and packing.

Quality Factors

Colour and soluble solids (primarily hexose sugars and sorbitol) and fruit colour (depending on the type) are the best indicators of quality for both sweet and sour cherry, although fruit acid level may be important in sour cherry. Except for soluble carbohydrates and vitamins A and C, cherries are low in nutrients, but calcium, iron, magnesium, phosphorus and copper contents are high compared to apple, peach, grape and strawberry. High-quality cherries typically have at least 15% soluble solids, while sweet cherries should be nearer 20%. Standards for harvest and marketing may, however, often be lower. Optimum conditions also often vary with use. To facilitate brining (bleaching in sulphur dioxide solutions for maraschino cherries) fruit may be picked prematurely before colour and soluble solids are adequate for the fresh market. Stem fruit removal force is carefully monitored for sour cherries that will be mechanically harvested, and abscission may be brought on by treatment with ethephon, which releases ethylene, expediting abscission and fruit drop in response to mechanical shaking. *See* individual nutrients

Disorders, Diseases and Pests

Disorders

In processing brined sweet and sour cherries, the 'solution pocket' problem involves subepidermal splits in the flesh, which fill with brine solution and ruptured cell contents. Time of harvest, degree of turgidity at brining, temperature, or any procedures that reduce either the sugar or water content of the fruit, will tend to decrease the problem.

Rain cracking (swelling followed by rupture of the epidermis) of sweet cherries occurs mostly during the harvest period when the fruit is mature or nearly so and has been wet with rain for some time. Primary cause is absorption of water directly through the skin of the fruit and not through the root system. Cultivar cracking susceptibility has been tested extensively. In testing, Bing, one of the best quality cultivars, was worst, followed by Napoleon, Lambert, Emperor Francis, Giant, Schmidt, Yellow Spanish, and Montmorency, which did not crack. In another ranking, Bing invariably cracked very badly, and was followed by Lambert, Giant, Gil Peck, and Hedelfingen. In yet another test, Van, Merton Glory, Vega and Vista were very susceptible, while Emperor Francis, Schmidt and Sam were less, and Sue, Kristin, Ulster and Early Rivers were least susceptible. From the long-range viewpoint, breeding programmes under way may ultimately produce desirable crack-resistant cherries. It is not yet clear if cracking may be reduced by some chemical or hormonal treatments, e.g. calcium, aluminium, and lime sprays or auxin (NAA) and gibberellin (GA_3) applications, but in some parts of the world (e.g. Norway) covering trees with plastic film is widely used to avoid cracking, and the method is being tested elsewhere.

Pitting of sweet cherry is a condition in which areas near the surface of the fruit become sunken, forming dimples or pits. It may occur before or after harvest, and there are at least three different causes, the most common of which is bruising during handling; pitting may also result from feeding by sucking insects such as the soldier bug, and perhaps from physiological injuries, e.g. adverse low-temperature stress during post-harvest cooling or growing conditions.

Diseases

Bacterial canker, one of the most important sweet and sour cherry pathogens, is caused by two different pathogens, *Pseudomonas syringae* and *P. morsprunorum*, and is characterized by oozing of gum (gummosis) at infection sites. Disease development is most prevalent during the cool, wet periods of early spring.

Crown gall, caused by *Agrobacterium tumefaciens*, can affect sweet and cherry rootstocks and is characterized by galls forming usually near infection sites caused by wounds, sometimes man-made, e.g. cultivation injuries, or due to damage from subterranean chewing insects or rodents. Some rootstocks, however, are only moderately susceptible, and some hybrids may be tolerant.

Brown rot, caused by the fungi *Monilinia fructicola* or *M. laxa*, affects both sweet and sour cherries and reduces yield by infecting and decaying blossoms, twigs and fruit. Fruit decay after harvest is also a problem. The fungi persist in mummified fruits on the tree and the ground, and infection continues from these inocula the following spring. Growing regions with cooler and drier summers provide some relief.

Cherry leaf spot, *Blumeriella jaapii* (*Coccomyces hiemalis*), is the most serious disease affecting sour cherry and most ground cherries. Infection occurs in the spring on expanding leaves and continues throughout the season under favourable conditions, e.g. high humidity. Severely infected leaves become chlorotic and abscise, and if defoliation is severe, fruit may not ripen properly and tree vigour and hardiness are reduced. Powdery mildew (*Podosphaera ocyacanthae*) is similar.

Other fungal pathogens may sometimes be important, causing blights, crown or root rots, and replant (orchard re-establishment) problems. Cherry dieback is thought to be a complex of several disorders, one of which may be a mycoplasma. X-disease, leafhopper transmitted and often devastating, is also due to a mycoplasma.

Several viruses cause poor vegetative growth, reduce yields, and may even result in tree death, but others are symptomless. Among the most severe is *Prunus* necrotic ringspot virus which is pollen transmitted and present in all cherry growing areas of the world. Little Cherry (Prune Dwarf) disease is another pollen transmitted virus and very destructive. *Prunus* stem pitting disease is caused by the tomato ringspot virus and is spread by nematodes.

Pests

Bird damage can be very serious, and some areas may require protective netting to reduce predation. The cherry fruit fly passes the winter in the soil as a pupa; adult flies emerge in late spring, and females feed on surfaces of leaves and fruit and lay eggs in the nearly ripe fruit. On hatching, the larvae (maggots) feed on the fruit flesh. The larvae are easily killed by holding fruit near 0°C, but fumigation, often with methyl bromide, may be required to meet quarantine restrictions for shipping overseas. Other pests include black cherry aphid, plum curculio, European red mite, peach tree borer, and two-spotted mite.

Economic Problems and Future Developments

Although the sour cherry industry is facing a serious problem of excessive productive capacity and persistent oversupplies, this industry has adopted new technologies and practices in the last 10 years which substantially improve its cost efficiency and productivity. Much of the newly planted acreage uses efficient trickle irrigation and closely planted orchard systems that also involve hedging techniques. These recent new techniques, especially in combination, provide large increases in yields per hectare and hence substantial reductions in costs.

Considerable genetic diversity still exists in Eastern Europe and Russia, the centre of origin for both sour and sweet cherries. Although breeding programmes have been limited, exploiting that diversity should do much to overcome the growing, handling and processing problems that face growers using the industry standards – the sweet 'Bing' and the sour 'Montmorency'. Sweet cherry growers especially need dwarfing rootstocks and spur types for growth control, and all growers need disease and pest resistance, less self-sterility, and cultivars with a range of maturities so that there are longer seasons for fresh markets. Sweet cherry growers also need rain-cracking resistance and, for postharvest quality, resistance to bruising. Sour cherry growers need new cultivars for diversifying and strengthening marketing options (e.g. fresh and frozen juice products, dyes for cosmetics and the food processing industry) and dry stem scars and small freestone pits to facilitate handling and processing. A combination of new marketing strategies and products for sour cherries, and advances in breeding of both sweet and sour cherries, would clearly benefit the economic potential of the entire cherry industry.

Bibliography

Brown SK, Iezzoni AF and Fogle HW (1991) Cherries. In: Janick J and Moore J (eds) *Advances in Fruit Breeding*. In Review.

Iezzoni A, Schmidt H and Albertini A (1990) Cherries (*Prunus spp.*). In: J. N. Moore and J. R. Ballington, Jr. (eds) *Genetic Resources of Temperate Fruit and Nut Crops*, pp 110–173. Wageningen: International Society for Horticultural Science.

Perry R (1987) Cherry rootstocks. In: Rom RC and Carlson RF (eds) *Rootstocks for Fruit Crops*, pp 217–264 New York: Wiley Interscience.

Westwood MN (1978) *Temperate Zone Pomology*. San Francisco: WH Freeman.

Wayne Loescher
Michigan State University, East Lansing, USA

CHESTNUTS

Global Distribution

Castanea is a genus of about twelve species native to the north temperate regions, belonging to the family Fagaceae. The sweet chestnut (*Castanea sativa* Mill. Synonyms: *C. vulgaris* Lam., *C. vesca* Gaertn. and *C. castanea* Karst.) is native from southern Europe, north Africa and Asia Minor to China. It is cultivated in many parts of the Himalayas, especially in Punjab and the Khasia Hills. Naturalized in central, western and northern Europe, and introduced on Pacific Coast of the USA, it is commonly known as European, Spanish, Italian, Eurasian or sweet chestnut.

Description of Fruits

Fruits are in groups of one to three single-seeded nuts, often 2–3·5 cm in diameter. Shiny brown, with paler bases, they are thickly pubescent at the tip, bearing a short-stalked perigynium with its persistent styles. The seed has a large embryo but no endosperm. Nuts of the European chestnut are generally dark brown in colour and often lightly striped. The nuts contain an edible kernel, enclosed in a thin, tough and astringent skin (pellicle) and surrounded by a spinous, cup-like organ termed a cupule. The latter is a unique feature of the family. The kernel of European chestnut is often deeply grooved, with the fibrous pellicle folded into the grooves, making it difficult to separate this bitter covering from the kernel. There are several cultivars of chestnut, differing in the quality of kernels; the forms grown in India, for example, are inferior to those cultivated in Europe.

Cultivars

In the past, only two cultivars (CVS) were known – Aspleniifolia with narrow leaves, often linear and irregularly lobed, and Macrocarpa with large fruit – but, more recently, the following examples have been cultivated: Marron Combale, Marron Nousillard and Marron Quercy, which originated in France; all have very large, light- to dark-brown nuts and are very productive. Numbo and Paragon are the most frequently grown cvs in the USA; they have medium-large, roundish nuts of fair quality, and bear regularly. Ridgely, which originated in Dover, Delaware, has fair-sized nuts, of very good quality and flavour, with two to three nuts per bur; it is vigorous and productive. Rochester and Comfort are grown to a limited extent.

Commercial and Industrial Importance

Uses

Chestnuts are grown as ornamentals and for the edible nuts. Trees often bear nuts 2 or 3 years after planting.

Propagation is by budding or grafting on chestnut stocks. They are naturally tolerant of acid soils and present no special cultural difficulties on well-drained land. The chestnut blight may be injurious or fatal to susceptible species, and weevils may be troublesome.

The Fagaceae family is the source of some of the most important hardwood timbers of the world, the most notable being oak, beech and chestnut. The timber of the sweet chestnut is almost equal to oak in strength and durability, and the one is often substituted for the other. Coppiced chestnut is in great demand for fencing, which lasts for very many years even when not treated with creosote. The relatively hard, durable, fine-grained wood is easy to split but not easy to bend (density, 593–865 kg m^{-3}). It is used for general carpentry, railway ties, and the manufacture of cellulose. The bark and wood are used for tanning (see *Chemistry*, below). Wood and burs may be used for firewood or for the production of charcoal.

European chestnuts are grown for the kernels of the nuts, and are extensively eaten by humans and animals. The nuts are used as a vegetable, boiled, roasted, steamed, puréed, or in a dressing (stuffing) for poultry and meats. In some European mountainous regions, chestnuts replace wheat and potatoes in the form of chestnut flour, chestnut bread, and mashed chestnuts. Flour made of ground chestnuts is said to have provided a staple ration for the Roman legions. In Italy, chestnuts are prepared like a stew with gravy. Dried nuts are used for cooking purposes in the same way as the fresh nuts, or eaten like peanuts. They are also used in brandy, in confectionery, in desserts, as a coffee substitute, for thickening soups, and as a source of oil. The largest nuts, called marron, command the highest price and are used to make the famous French delicacy, *marrons glacés*. Culled chestnuts are safely used for fattening poultry and hogs, as well as for feeding cattle.

Yields

Yields average from 45 to 136 kg of nuts per tree. In 60–80-year-old stands in Russia, yields average 770 kg ha^{-1} and up to 1230 kg ha^{-1} in better stands. Italy reports *c.* 1100 kg ha^{-1} France *c.* 1500–2200 kg ha^{-1} and Spain *c.* 2800 kg ha^{-1}. In the best years, 5000 kg ha^{-1} are reported. Nuts are marketed to a limited degree, but are mostly locally cultivated and used.

Folk Medicine

The nuts, when crushed with vinegar and barley flour, have been said to be a folk remedy for indurations of the breasts. Reported to be astringent, sedative and tonic, European chestnut is a folk remedy for circulation problems, cough, extravasation, fever, haematochezia, hernia, hunger, hydrocoele, infections, inflammation, kidney ailments, myalgia, nausea, paroxysm, pertussia, rheumatism, sclerosis, scrofula, sores, stomach ailments and wounds. An aqueous infusion of leaves is used as a tonic, and is effective in paroxysmal coughs and irritable conditions of respiratory organs.

Chemistry

General

Castanea sativa leaves proved to contain two flavonoid aglycones (quercetin and myricetin) along with their glycosides. A study of *Castanea* species indicated that catechol tannins were more abundant in buds at the tip and base, while bud scales contained about 80% of the tannins of the whole bud. The leaves, bark and wood also contain tannins. It is only the wood (8–13% tannins), however, that is used in the tanning industry and for commercial preparation of the chestnut extract. Countries manufacturing the extract are France, Italy and the USA. Commercial liquid extracts contain 29–49% tannin, while solid extracts contain 56–76% tannin. *See* Tannins and Polyphenols

Nutritional Composition

The seed (100 g, dry wt.) is reported to contain 1·705–1·714 kJ (406–408 cal), 6·1–7·5 g protein, 2·8–3·2 g fat, 87·7–88·6 g total carbohydrate, 2·3–2·4 g fibre, 2·0–2·1 g ash, 30·3–56·8 mg calcium, 184–185 mg phosphorus, 3·4–3·6 mg iron, 12·6–32·3 mg sodium, 956–1705 mg potassium, 0·46 mg thiamin, 0·46 mg riboflavin, and 1·21–1·26 mg nicotinic acid. The USDA (US Department of Agriculture) reports a similar composition for roasted chestnuts. Thus roasted chestnuts (100 g dry wt.) are reported to contain 1·714 kJ (408 cal), 5·33 g protein, 3·66 g fat, 88·33 g total carbohydrate, 48·3 mg calcium, 178·3 mg phosphorus, 1·51 mg iron, 55 mg magnesium, 0·95 mg zinc, 0·85 mg copper, 3·33 mg sodium, 986 mg potassium, 0·4 mg thiamin, 0·3 mg riboflavin, 2·23 mg nicotinic acid, 40 μg vitamin A, 2 mg vitamin E, and 43·33 mg vitamin C. The chemical composition is similar to that of wheat; the starch is easily digested after cooking. Spanish chestnuts are reported to contain 2·87–3·03% ash, 9·61–10·96% total protein, 2·55–2·84% fibre, 73·75–77·70% total nitrogen-free extract, and 7·11–9·58% fat. Chestnuts from 19 natural stands in southern Yugoslavia showed a total fat content of 4–5%; oleic and linoleic acids predominated, followed by palmitic. *See* Wheat and individual nutrients

Handling and Storage

Harvesting

Traditionally, mature chestnuts have been gathered from the ground after they fall. Some cultivars stick, and shaking or jarring the limbs is useful. In other cultivars, burs open, and nuts fall to the ground. Burs which fall and do not open can be made to shed their nuts by pressure of the feet, or by striking with a small wooden mallet. Some harvesters use heavy leather gloves and twist nuts out of burs by hand. Unopened burs stored in a humid, cool 12–18°C location will continue to mature and open in a week. In gathering nuts, the collector usually has two pails or containers, one for first-grade, perfect nuts, the other for culls. Some sort of harvest mechanization is essential for the development of a chestnut orchard industry.

Storing

Fresh chestnuts contain 40–50% carbohydrate, mostly in the form of starch, about 5% oil, 5% protein and 40% moisture. They are highly perishable because they lose water rapidly at normal room temperature and humidity, causing the kernel to become hard and incapable of germinating. Numerous fungi and bacteria attack the nuts, causing decay and spoilage. High temperatures, as a result of remaining in the sun, causes rapid kernel deterioration. The nuts should be stored at 0–4°C under conditions of high humidity but no free moisture. *See* Storage Stability, Mechanisms of Degradation

Nuts should be picked up every morning and stored in sacks, if they are to be shipped at once. If they are to be kept for a while, they should be piled on the floor to sweat. The pile should be stirred twice a day for 2 days; then the nuts should be sacked. Nuts should always be stored in a manner so that air can circulate freely. A practical method for storing small quantities of nuts is to mix the freshly harvested nuts with dry peat moss in plastic bags, close the bags, and refrigerate. Properly stored, they will keep satisfactorily for 6 months and have even been kept for as long as 3 years.

Nuts to be eaten raw should be 'cured' for several days by allowing the kernel to dry to a spongy texture. The amount of free sugar and sweetness is maximized in this way.

Seed propagation

Chestnut seeds require a moist cold treatment of at least 1–2 months at 0–4°C to ensure good and uniform germination. Stored nuts should not be subjected to temperatures much below freezing (irreversible damage begins to occur around −4°C) or above 7°C.

Bibliography

Bailey LH and Bailey EZ (1976) *Hortus Third*. A Concise Dictionary of Plants Cultivated in the United States and Canada, pp 230–231. New York: Macmillan.

Duke JA (1989) *CRC Handbook of Nuts*, pp 90–92. Boca Raton, Florida: CRC Press.

Jaynes RA (ed.) (1979) *Nut Tree Culture in North America*, pp 111–127. Northern Nut Growers Association.

Nabiel A. M. Saleh
National Research Centre, Cairo, Egypt

CHICKEN

See Poultry

CHICORY BEVERAGES

Chichorium intybus L., the wild chicory, has been adapted to a 2 year vegetation cycle. The cultivation of chicory started in several European countries at the end of the 18th century and spread from there to other countries, e.g. the USA, India and South Africa. Only the root of the chicory plant is used for making various coffee beverages; the plant is shown in Fig. 1. This article describes the cultivation of chicory, the processing of the roots to roast and ground blends and to soluble beverage powders in which chicory is an ingredient. Furthermore, the composition of chicory and changes taking place during processing are discussed.

Cultivation, Drying and Roasting

In Central Europe, sowing is at the end of April or at the beginning of May. Three forms of seed are employed: ordinary naked seed, seed coated with dyes and fungicides, and seed pelleted with nutrients, fungicides and insecticides. Coated and pelleted seeds facilitate the control of the right sowing depth. Protection and the conditions for germination of the seed embryo are optimal in pelleted seed.

In order to produce chicory roots of a suitable size for industrial processing, a space of about 600 cm² per plant is recommended. The distance between the seed rows is usually 45 cm; pelleted seed are drilled within the row at a distance of 6 cm. After emergence and when the plants have reached the three- or four-leaf stage, they are thinned out to distances of about 14 cm in the row. The plant density should reach up to 160 000 plants per hectare in order to attain the right root size and a good field yield.

Chicory requires a vegetation period of about 160 days. In Europe, the chicory harvest is from the end of September to the middle of November. Machines are used which carry out the entire harvesting operation: cutting of leaves, lifting of the roots, their collection in containers and transfer to trailers. The yield of chicory roots varies from 30 to 45 tonnes ha⁻¹, depending on the climate, weather and soil conditions. The harvested chicory roots are delivered to the drying plant, where the quantity of roots is determined by weighing the trailer loaded and unloaded. The farmers are paid for the root weight reduced by the amount of soil present. The chicory roots are stored in long, extended heaps with heights of up to 3 m until processing.

Figure 2 illustrates the processing of fresh chicory roots to soluble powder. The drying of chicory is a seasonal operation which starts in central Europe at the beginning of October. The installation for washing the roots comprises several compartments; it operates on the counterflow principle and rinses the roots with clean water during discharge. The roots are cut into slices (6 × 22 mm cross-section and of varying length) and cubes (lengths of sides between 12 and 16 mm). Chunks are also produced, having a thickness of more than 16 mm.

Drying of chicory reduces the water content from about 75 to 12%. The most frequently used rotary drum driers are equipped with baffles inside and work continuously. Only those driers furnished with gas firing allow direct contact of the combustion gases with the cut material. The chicory moves in the slowly rotating drum in the same direction as the hot air is drawn through. The temperature of the hot air at the inlet reaches 400–500°C, at the outlet about 120°C. The dried chicory leaves the drum at a temperature of about 80°C. The necessary cooling and the final drying is accomplished on well-ventilated conveyor belts. The chicory fragments produced through breakage and abrasion are sifted off. Dried chicory with a water content of less than 12% is considered to be stable and can be kept in storage for several years.

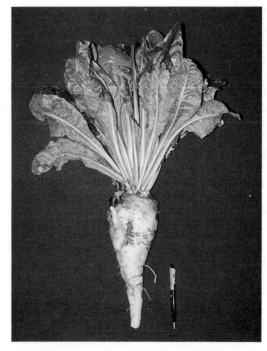

Fig. 1 Photograph of a harvested chicory plant.

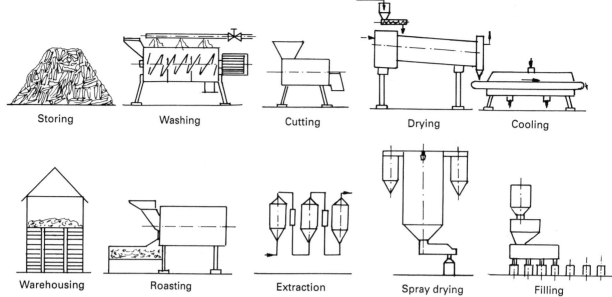

Fig. 2 Processing of fresh roots to soluble powder.

Roasting of chicory is conducted batchwise by employing drum roasters and long cycle times. Since smaller chicory pieces are roasted faster than larger ones, a narrow size distribution of the dried chicory should be used to obtain a homogeneous roast. The rotating drum is heated by a gas burner and charged with chicory. Vegetable oil in a quantity of about 1% of the chicory load is added to bind the dust and to prevent sticking of chicory to the roaster wall and baffles. The combustion gases are first directed around the drum and are then drawn through the drum. The moisture in the chicory is driven off and is removed by the combustion gases. In the later stages of roasting, the heat supply is reduced by steps and the heating gases are only drawn outside around the drum. The actual roasting takes place at temperatures of 170–180°C. After a roasting time of 60–80 min the chicory reaches the required colour and is discharged into the cooling screen. The total roast loss is in the range 15–25%. Roast and ground chicory is usually blended with coffee or cereals and marketed as coffee mixture or coffee substitute. *See* Coffee, Roast and Ground

Extraction and Spray Drying

Roasted chicory is more frequently extracted in blends with roasted coffee or roasted cereals than alone by itself. The common extraction with coffee or cereals is conducted in percolation batteries which consist of about six columns connected in series. Hot water is pumped into the column which contains the most spent roasted material, flows in an anticlockwise fashion through the plant and finally enters the column with

fresh roast material. The concentration of the draw-off extract depends on, among other things, the composition of the roast blend and varies from 15 to 30%. Each column with an exhausted blend is replaced by one with a new roast blend. The feed water temperatures may be up to 180°C with blends of coffee and chicory, or up to 140°C with blends of cereals and chicory. Heat exchangers placed between the columns lower the extract temperature in stages up to 90°C in the column with the fresh roast blend. The extraction yield and the draw-off concentration increase with higher temperature profiles. Since chicory contains a high proportion of soluble carbohydrate, it can be extracted efficiently at temperatures below 100°C. The extraction of roasted chicory by itself is performed in twin-screw conveyors or hydraulic piston presses. Pure chicory extracts are, for the most part, mixed with coffee or cereal extracts. The liquid extracts are sometimes concentrated before spray drying or mixed with glucose syrup in order to improve the drying properties of the extract. *See* Coffee, Instant

The spray drying of the liquid extracts with soluble solid contents of 30–45% is conducted in tall towers in which the extract is pumped under high pressure through nozzles and is dispersed into small droplets. In the upper part of the tower the water in the droplets evaporates in a flow of hot air, in the lower part the exhaust air is drawn off and the separated powder is collected in bins. The instant powders, which have a moisture content of about 3%, are filled into water vapour-tight containers such as jars with sealable lids.

Composition and Varieties

Based on dry matter the composition of two chicory varieties is given in Table 1. The water content of fresh

Table 1. Composition (grams per 100 g) of chicory varieties

| | Variety superior in | |
	Root quality	Field yield
Dry matter[a]	26·9	21·7
Extractable matter[b]	82·2	80·0
Composition[b]		
Inulin	64·1	57·8
Sucrose	5·3	7·8
Protein	4·5	5·5
Amino acids	1·1	1·5
Organic acids	2·6	3·2
Fibre	13·6	16·1
Minerals	4·0	5·0
Others	4·8	3·1

[a] Based on root weight.
[b] Based on dry weight.

Table 2. Yields (tonnes per hectare) of chicory varieties

| | Variety superior in | |
	Root quality	Field yield
Fresh roots	40·7	46·9
Dry matter[a]	10·9	10·2
Soluble acids[a]	9·0	8·1

[a] Calculated with the values of Table 1.

chicory roots is in the range 70–80% and is influenced by the variety, the soil and weather conditions. The solid matter of finely ground chicory roots is extractable in boiling water to an extent of 80%. Chicory is characteristic in that the main constituent of the roots is the polysaccharide inulin. This reserve carbohydrate with a molecular weight of approximately 6000 comprises up to 65% of the dry matter of the root. About 35 fructose molecules are linearly linked together with one glucose molecule at the end. The polymer chain of inulin is completed by a sucrose molecule and, therefore, it has no reducing power. In addition, chicory roots contain further carbohydrates, including usually contents of about 5% sucrose and 15% fibre substances. During extraction, the fibre remains insoluble in the residue. Nitrogenous compounds amount to about 6% and comprise protein and free amino acids. The content of organic acids is about 3%, of which tartaric acid and citric acid are about 30% each. Mineral substances show levels of about 5% in the root, the most important components being potassium, calcium, phosphate and sulphate. Furthermore, the roots contain lactucin and lactucopicrin in a total amount of about 0·4%. These sesquiterpene lactones are responsible for the bitter taste of fresh and dried chicory. Both lactones are completely decomposed during roasting. *See* Acids, Natural Acids and Acidulants; Amino Acids, Properties and Occurrence; Carbohydrates, Classification and Properties; Minerals, Dietary Importance; Protein, Chemistry

It is known from screening tests of chicory varieties that a negative correlation exists between the root quality and the field yield. Breeding of chicory aims at combining both attributes. A variety with a superior root quality has a higher content of inulin, and dry and soluble matter, and, conversely, a variety with a superior field yield has a high root weight, and a high content of protein and minerals. For these two opposing chicory varieties, yields of fresh roots and calculated yields of dry matter and soluble solids are given in Table 2. A cost calculation conducted for the processing of dried chicory from fresh roots results in a price differential of up to 20% for the use of roots from a quality variety. The total expenditure considerably diminishes for roots from a high-quality variety, since the required root quantity and the amount of water removed during drying is less.

Changes in Composition During Processing

Higher temperatures in the root heaps during longer storage periods induce the start of hydrolysis of the polysaccharide by the enzyme inulinase present in the roots. The generated sugars favour the loss of material as a result of respiration of the roots and by decay through microorganisms. Fresh roots should, therefore, not be stored for long periods at high temperatures in order to minimize inulin hydrolysis and other causes of losses. The ideal storage conditions are temperatures of about 5°C and air humidities of about 95%, which cannot normally be achieved in practice.

Very high temperature profiles during drying provoke puffing of the wet chicory pieces. Hollow spaces remain inside after drying which lower the firmness of the cubes or slices and increase the tendency to break more easily during transport. Chicory pieces with larger dimensions usually leave the drum drier still with moist centres. During storage, enzymatic hydrolysis of the inulin proceeds, at a rate dependent on the moisture content, and the sugar content increases. Dried chicory should normally show a bright colour, a low content of reducing sugar, a high content of extractable solids and inulin. Darker outer colours and burnt edges of dried chicory enhance water uptake during storage and make it more difficult to obtain a homogeneous roast. Higher sugar contents of dried chicory are sometimes accepted in view of the taste of the product, but they impair further processing due to the higher hygroscopicity.

Table 3. Characteristic values (grams per 100 g of dried matter) of dried and roasted chicory

		Roasted		
	Dried	Light	Medium	Dark
L-Colour value of powder	77·0	46·4	40·0	32·5
Extractable matter	83·1	82·8	82·2	78·3
pH value[a]	5·7	4·7	4·6	4·4
Acid degree[a,b]	12	27	31	40
Reducing sugars	1·9	8·4	14·1	12·1
Free fructose	0·5	2·4	4·6	3·4
Free glucose	0·1	1·0	2·2	1·9
Inulin and sucrose	67·1	52·6	39·1	24·8

[a] Measured in a 1% extract solution.
[b] Defined as milliequivalents of sodium hydroxide per 100 g of soluble solids.

Roasting of chicory results in the formation of specific colour, flavour and aroma compounds which are characteristic of the product. The constituents of chicory, such as inulin, sucrose, protein and free amino acids, partially or totally undergo various changes. Most alterations in the chemical composition are connected with two browning reactions, the Maillard reaction and the pyrolysis of the inulin. The Maillard reaction takes place between reducing sugars and amino groups of free amino acids and of the protein and leads to the melanoidins (brown polymeric materials) and to volatile aldehydes. They give chicory its typical flavour. The pyrolytic degradation of inulin yields high-molecular-weight caramel compounds and low-molecular-weight carbonyl compounds, such as aldehydes, ketones and organic acids. These compounds likewise contribute to the colour and the taste of roasted chicory. *See* Browning, Nonenzymatic

The analytical values in Table 3 illustrate the changes in the carbohydrate composition and the free acidity during roasting of chicory. The decomposition of inulin and the formation of free acids steadily proceed with increasingly darker roasting. The contents of reducing sugars, of fructose and of glucose first increase during roasting, reach a maximum and decrease again. The content of reducing sugars in, for example, cubes or slices reaches a maximum value of 15%. Light and medium roasted chicory are extractable in boiling water to about 80%, whereas the extractable content of dark roasted chicory falls to below this value. Insoluble matter is formed by the strongly exothermic pyrolysis of inulin and lowers the amount of extractable material, especially of dark roasted chicory. The heat inside the chicory pieces generated by this reaction accelerates the roasting and leads to charring of the cores.

During extraction, free acids already present in roasted chicory induce the hydrolysis of inulin to monosaccharides. Fructose, itself thermally unstable, is subjected to further decomposition, the extent of which depends strongly on the extraction conditions. Shorter extraction times and lower water temperatures are considered favourable to minimize the amount of free fructose and free acids in the chicory extracts. The analytical values stated in Table 4 show that temperatures below 100°C should be applied for the extraction of chicory.

Fructose has a steeper sorption isotherm than inulin and is very hygroscopic. As a result, light roasted chicory with more inulin and less fructose is preferably used for the production of instant powders. Chicory extracts have a higher hygroscopicity and an increased stickiness in contrast to coffee or cereal extracts. Spray drying of extracts containing chicory soluble solids is more difficult and requires certain precautions. For example, the output capacity of the spray drier is reduced by extracts produced from roasted coffee–chicory or cereal–chicory blends and, in particular, by pure chicory extracts. *See* Fructose

Taste and Physiological Effects

Infusions of light roasted chicory have a sweetish and mild flavour. In combination with coffee or cereals the chicory imparts to the beverage a smooth and round taste. With darker roasting of the chicory, the sweet taste diminishes and the strength, acidity and bitterness of the brew increase.

Information concerning the physiological effects of roasted chicory is exceedingly scarce. A lot of practical advice compiled over the years, regarding natural medicine, is found in ancient literature. According to this knowledge, infusions of roasted chicory are beneficial and contribute to the well-being of the body. Chicory brews are supposed to be mild diuretics and are said to have sedative effects. It has been known for a long time that chicory promotes digestion by stimulating the secretion of the gastrointestinal glands and, especially, that it increases bile production. Modern scientific studies confirm the conclusions previously cited. The tests performed with animals and humans substantiate the fact that chicory is perfectly safe and has no adverse effects. Some physiological effects were thought to be related to the sesquiterpene lactones contained in fresh or dried chicory. These lactones are decomposed during roasting and do not play a part in roasted chicory. Some investigations point out that the digestion of milk is facilitated by the addition of chicory. The finer milk particles formed in the stomach are more easily digested. Soluble chicory powders can contain up to 60% inulin or oligomeric compounds derived from it. These fructose oligomers are not metabolized either by the gastric acidity or enzymes and behave as soluble

Table 4. Increase of free acids and free sugars during storage of a liquid chicory extract (23% dry matter, 61% inulin and sucrose) for 1 h at different temperatures

	Original	Treated at				
		60°C	80°C	100°C	120°C	140°C
pH value of extract	4·7	4·7	4·6	4·5	4·1	3·6
Acid degree[a]	21	22	23	26	34	68
Free fructose[b]	2·7	3·0	3·7	8·2	54·3	44·7
Free glucose[b]	1·2	1·2	1·4	1·7	5·3	8·8

[a] Defined as milliequivalents of sodium hydroxide per 100 g of soluble solids.
[b] Grams per 100 g of dry matter.

fibre. Inulin is only slightly fermented in the colon by bacteria. The mild laxative effect of inulin could explain the role of chicory as an intestinal regulator. Partially hydrolysed chicory extracts have a high fructose content; these extracts could be used in diabetes therapy. *See* Coffee, Physiological Effects

Use as an Adulterant and Analysis

Roast and ground coffees or instant coffee powders may be adulterated by mixing chicory with coffee after roasting, before extraction or even after drying. Microscopic, physical and chemical methods are applied to detect and to analyse the adulteration of roasted or soluble coffee with chicory. Cell structures from chicory can be identified by the examination of suspicious samples of roasted coffee under the microscope. The extractability of roasted coffee and roasted chicory differ enormously: finely ground coffee is extractable in boiling water to about 30%, chicory to about 80%. From the increase in coffee extractability the portion of chicory in roast and ground coffee can be estimated.

Several methods depend on the analysis of specific constituents only present in coffee or chicory. The determination of the content of total fructose appears most suitable, since the content of fructose in chicory is relatively high compared to the content of caffeine and chlorogenic acids in coffee. Although all these methods detect adulteration of coffee, it is difficult to specify the blend quantitatively. *See* Adulteration of Foods, History and Occurrence

Bibliography

Beitter H and Schröder C-H (1970) *Handbuch der Lebensmittelchemie*, vol. VI, pp 96–138. Berlin: Springer-Verlag.
Clarke RJ and Macrae R (1987) *Related Beverages, Coffee*, vol. 5: London: Elsevier.
Maier HG (1981). *Kaffee*, pp 146–194. Berlin: Parey.

Karl Löhmar
Dereco, Ludwigsburg, FRG

CHILDREN

Contents

Nutritional Requirements

Assessment of Nutritional Status

The most commonly used index of normal nutrition is growth. In healthy infants, bodyweight and height should be monitored at monthly or bimonthly intervals during the first year of life, and less frequently thereafter, and compared to standard growth charts. Development of typical clinical signs of nutritional deficiencies, such as skin and hair decoloration, mucosal lesions, etc., is extremely rare in developed societies, but may appear secondary to diseases which impair nutrient intake, absorption or utilization. *See* Nutritional Status, Anthropometry and Clinical Examination

Nutrition from 1 to 5 Years of Age

The first 5 years of life are among the periods of more rapid growth. Major changes also occur in the relative size of body regions and in the proportions of water, fat and lean mass tissues. Over these years, nutrition must accommodate a changing pattern of energy, protein and micronutrient needs. *See* Infant Foods, Weaning Foods; Infants, Weaning

The growth pattern after the first year of life shows periods of both rapid and slow gain in stature and weight. Children tend to grow 12 cm during the second year, 9 cm on the third, and 7 cm or less thereafter. *See* Growth and Development

After the first year, healthy children should be able to eat virtually the same as the adult members of the family. Indeed, it is at this stage that family dietary practices have the most significant impact on the child's preferences and food intake patterns. It is thus important for parents to be aware of their role in educating and forging sound dietary habits in their children.

The feeding behaviour of children at this age is much more variable than previously. Children have a much wider repertoire of eating behaviours, and should be allowed, within reason, to practise them. As a rule, a healthy child should be allowed to eat as much or as little as he or she wishes. Forced feeding or threats around food do not lead to good nutrition, but rather to sometimes long-term confrontation, to the detriment of actual food intake. Furthermore, there is evidence that healthy children have a quite accurate mechanism of maintaining energy balance by compensating for deficient or excessive food intake over periods of days or even weeks. *See* Infants, Feeding Problems

Nutrition over 5 Years of Age

The growth pattern between 5 and 10 years of age is usually more stable than during earlier years, averaging about 5 cm per year. Weight gain is around 2 kg per year at 5–6 years of age, and increases rapidly as puberty approaches, reaching as much as 4 kg per year by age 10. Physical activity also increases markedly during school years, as children become more involved in sports and outdoor activities in general.

Recommended Nutrient Intakes

The nutritional recommendations for older children do not differentiate by sex until 10 years of age. At that

Table 1. Recommended energy and protein intake in children aged 1 to 10 years[a]

Age (years)	Energy (kcal per kg per day)	Protein (g per kg per day)
1–2	105	1·20
2–3	100	1·15
3–5	95	1·10
5–7		1·0
Boys	90	
Girls	85	
7–10		1·0
Boys	78	
Girls	67	

[a]WHO (1985).

Table 2. Essential amino acid requirements during childhood[a]

Amino acid (mg per g of crude protein)	Preschool child (2–5 years)	Schoolchild (5–10 years)	Adult
Histidine	19[b]	19[b]	16
Isoleucine	28	28	13
Leucine	66	44	19
Lysine	58	44	16
Methionine and cystine	25	22	17
Phenylalanine and tyrosine	63	22	19
Threonine	34	28	9
Tryptophan	11	9[b]	5
Valine	35	25	13

[a]WHO (1985).
[b]Values interpolated from requirement versus age curves.

time, clear changes in body composition and activity patterns take place, which are to be reflected in nutrient requirements.

Protein and energy requirements

The WHO (World Health Organization) guidelines recommend that the caloric requirements be calculated from measurements of actual energy expenditure. However, the information available is insufficient to apply this criteria for children aged 5 to 10 years. Thus estimates of energy needs are based on dietary intake data. These data were compiled by the WHO (Tables 1 and 2), based on usual intake of healthy children in developed countries, and thus reflect dietary practices and lifestyles typical of these societies. In developing

Table 3. Recommended daily intakes of vitamins and minerals for children aged 1–10 years[a]

	Age of child (years)		
	1–3	4–6	7–10
Weight (kg)	13	20	28
Height (cm)	90	112	132
Vitamins			
A (μg RE)	400	500	700
D (μg)	10	10	10
E (mg α-TE)	6	7	7
K (μg)	15	20	30
C (mg)	40	45	45
B_6 (mg)	1·0	1·1	1·4
Folate (μg)	50	75	100
B_{12} (μg)	0·7	1·0	1·4
Minerals			
Iron (mg)	10	10	10
Calcium (mg)	800	800	800
Phosphorus (mg)	800	800	800
Zinc (mg)	10	10	10
Iodine (μg)	70	90	120
Selenium (μg)	20	20	30

[a]US National Research Council (1989).
RE: retinol equivalents. α-TE: α-tocopherol equivalents.

countries, and perhaps in lower socioeconomic groups of developed societies, children may have additional caloric requirements due to extra physical activity, for instance to walk to school, or to work in the field. These differences have not been quantified, but the WHO recommendations for caloric intake include an extra 5% allocation to 'allow for desirable physical activity'. *See* Energy, Energy Expenditure and Energy Balance;

There are also little data on nitrogen balance in school children, and therefore recommended levels of protein intake are based on estimates of protein absorption, nitrogen retention for growth, and obligatory nitrogen losses. *See* Protein, Requirements

Vitamins and minerals

Overall, the recommended levels of micronutrients for older children vary little from those for preschool children (Table 3). Vitamin A is calculated, after 2 years of age, by extrapolation from adult levels relative to bodyweight, yielding slightly higher values for schoolchildren: 700 versus 500 μg of retinol equivalents. Minor adjustments on recommended intakes of vitamin E, C, folate and B_6 also occur, as well as for iodine and selenium. Major adjustments in recommended intakes will take place with the onset of adolescence. *See* Dietary Reference Values

Food Additives

Over the years, several investigators have proposed that certain food additives could have a major behavioural impact on young children. But in spite of many years of research and controversy, there is no compelling evidence supporting those claims. Nevertheless, there are documented intolerances to some additives such as sodium glutamate and sulphites in adults, which can also occur in children.

Dental Development

Dental development is another important milestone during school age. Dental caries can appear early, and some surveys found that over 50% of children aged 3–4 years of age had dental caries. Major nutrients related to dental development are fluoride, and vitamin D, calcium and phosphorus (enamel formation), vitamins A and C, zinc and folate (gum integrity). Adequate intake of these nutrients is usually not a problem in developed societies. Of more practical importance are, perhaps, a number of dietary habits which may favour dental caries: excessive use of sugar and other fermentable carbohydrates, the nursing bottle syndrome (the baby is allowed to fall asleep while sucking a sweetened beverage, or even human milk), and poor dental hygiene. *See* Dental Disease, Aetiology of Dental Caries; Sucrose, Dietary Sucrose and Disease

A Prudent Diet for Children

There is growing awareness of the importance of diet in the development of chronic diseases, e.g. obesity and coronary heart disease. A number of changes in the current dietary practices of developed societies have been proposed, although the long-term impact of these changes is still unclear. There is also the question of how early in life a 'prudent' diet should be adopted. Special issues of nutrition in childhood, such as nutrient density, protein digestibility, and micronutrient requirements, need to be recognized. For example, there must be awareness of the potential negative impact that high-fibre or all-vegetable diets may have on protein digestibility, mineral bioavailability and energy density. *See* Dietary Fibre, Effects of Fibre on Absorption

Bibliography

Caballero B (1985) Food additives in the pediatric diet. *Clin. Nutr.* 4: 200–206.
Committee on Nutrition, Massachusetts Medical Society (1989) Fast food fare. *New England Journal of Medicine* 321: 752–756.

National Research Council, US National Academy of Sciences (1989) *Recommended Dietary Allowances* 10th edn. Washington DC: National Academy Press.

National Research Council, US National Academy of Sciences (1990) *Diet and Health*. Washington DC: National Academy Press.

WHO (1985) Energy and Protein Requirements. FAO/WHO/UNU Expert Consultation. *WHO Technical Report Series* 724.

Benjamin Caballero
The Johns Hopkins University, Baltimore, USA

Nutritional Problems

Rickets

Deficiency of vitamin D in the growing child leads to rickets (see Fig. 1), a metabolic disorder common in English and American polluted cities during the Industrial Revolution. The cause was secondary to poor nutrition, arising from both financial and educational poverty as well as the result of a hazy, smoggy atmosphere with little exposure to sunshine, or ultraviolet (UV) radiation. Adequate sunshine is not the entire explanation because rickets was common in the 1940s in Southern California and today in India. Furthermore, from October to March no UV light reaches the earth's surface in the UK and consequently vitamin D is not formed in the skin during that period. The incidence of rickets declined after the 1927 discovery that UV irradiation of ergosterol, a vitamin D plant derivative, increased its antirachitic effect.

Skin synthesis is the major source of vitamin D, and tanning prevents further formation. Black infants have lower circulating vitamin D levels than white children. This is because white skin allows vitamin-D-inducing wavelengths to pass through but black skin filters UV radiation under wavelengths of 436 nm. With the development of vitamin-D-fortified milks and milk products rickets has decreased in incidence. However, in some countries, cows' milk is not routinely fortified. Human milk contains almost 20 times more of this vitamin than unmodified whole cows' milk, yet in the USA a revival in breast-feeding has been linked to an increase in cases of nutritional rickets. *See* Cholecalciferol, Physiology

Rickets was described in Asian immigrants in Glasgow, Scotland in 1956. An estimate of the 1977 incidence of clinically overt rickets among UK Asians aged 0–16 years was 4 cases per 1000 in London and 10 per 1000 in the Midlands and the north of England. Rickets seemed to increase in the UK from 1960 to 1973 and then decrease. Pregnant Asian women with osteomalacia risk having infants with neonatal convulsions as a result of hypocalcaemia. Typically, rickets is seen in breast-fed premature infants and is especially prevalent in those born to Asian mothers in the UK. Rickets has also been described in the fetus. Adolescent Asian rickets, characteristically in children 8–14 years old may present with gross genu valgum (knock kee) and aching joints. Other clinical features include leg bowing, poor linear growth, delayed dental eruption, and impaired closure of the skull's fontanelle. Other skeletal deformities may develop.

Causes

The causes of rickets in children are as follows:

1. Inadequate exposure to sunlight.
2. Inadequate vitamin D intake.
3. Malabsorption of vitamin D, e.g. coeliac disease, short bowel syndrome, bacterial overgrowth in the bowel, deficiency of bile salts, cystic fibrosis, etc.
4. Increased enzyme activity: anticonvulsants (phenobarbitone and/or phenytoin) will increase metabolic degradation of $25(OH)D_3$ by stimulating hepatic microsomal enzymes.
5. Decreased enzyme activity: vitamin-D-dependent rickets (pseudovitamin D deficiency; deficiency of the renal enzyme, 25-hydroxyvitamin D 1α-hydroxylase).
6. Acquired deficiency of 1α-hydroxylase, e.g. chronic renal failure.
7. Failure of 25-hydroxylation, e.g. chronic liver failure.
8. Fanconi's syndrome – phosphaturia: the principal component of the disorder results in hypophosphataemic rickets.

Diagnosis

Diagnosis is radiological. In active rickets there is 'cupping' and 'fraying' of the distal ends of the forearm bones, and parts of the skull are demineralized.

Biochemical Findings

The following biochemical findings are characteristic of rickets:

1. Increased plasma alkaline phosphatase (of bone origin).
2. Phosphate reduced or normal.
3. Calcium reduced or normal.
4. Serum parathyroid hormone normal or increased.
5. Generalized amino-aciduria.

Reactive secondary hyperparathyroidism can complicate interpretation of biochemical diagnostic data.

Treatment

Adequate amounts of dietary calcium and phosphate should be ensured with vitamin D therapy.

Obesity

It is a tragic irony that the commonest nutritional problem in affluent countries is obesity, in sharp contrast to the undernutrition in less privileged societies. Obesity is the presence of excessive body fat and the visual identification of severe obesity is readily made. Weight in itself is an unsatisfactory way to assess fatness and particularly so in younger children where there is a poor relationship between weight and fat. *See* Obesity, Aetiology and Assessment

In adults one indicator of obesity is Quetelet's index which determines the body mass, or (weight)/(height)^2, but in children it is less useful because of a variation with age. However, this parameter can be related to a theoretical child with height and weight upon the 50th centile, and the measure then gives a percentage value: 90% indicates underweight, 90–110% normal weight, 110–120% overweight, and >120% obese.

Clinical examination needs to include an assessment of pubertal development and anthropometry which must be carefully evaluated. In addition, the observer ought to be aware of particular disorders associated with obesity, e.g. Down's syndrome, Prader–Willi syndrome, Klinefelter's syndrome and the Laurence–Moon–Biedl syndrome, as well as some endocrine diseases (hypothyroidism, Cushing's syndrome. *See* Down's Syndrome – Nutritional Aspects; Prader-Willi Syndrome – Nutritional Management

Body fatness can be assessed with a skin fold calliper, a tape measure, a stadiometer and weighing apparatus. Centile charts for triceps skin fold thickness, in boys and girls, are available. Values exceeding the 97th centile are indicative of obesity. *See* Obesity, Fat Distribution

Prevalence

As many as one third of the population of some industrialized nations are obese; in North America obesity affects 25% of children and adults, yet in other communities, such as Finland, it affects only 3%.

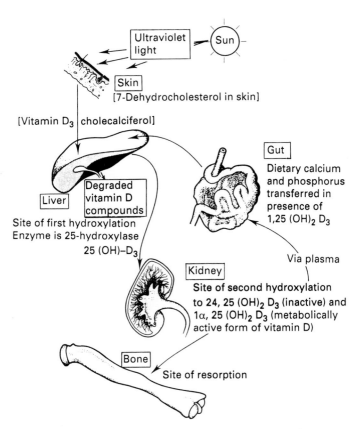

Fig. 1   Vitamin D is derived from the diet and from the effect of UV light on the skin. It is hydroxylated in the liver (25(OH)D$_3$) and undergoes a second hydroxylation in the kidney to the biologically active form, 1,25-dihydroxycholecalciferol (1α,25(OH)$_2$D$_3$), which acts on the gut and bone to increase gut absorption. 24,25(OH)$_2$D$_3$ is 24,25-dihydroxycholecalciferol. (Courtesy of Professor P Byrne.)

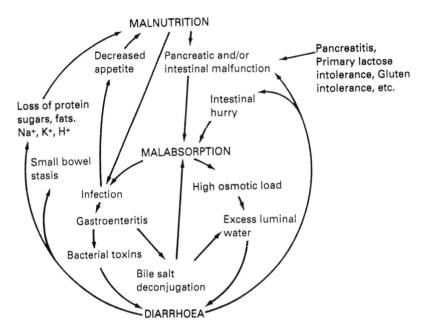

Fig. 2 The vicious cycle of diarrhoea and malnutrition. (Courtesy of WF Balistreri.)

Aetiology

It is uncommon for a child to be obese because of an underlying pathological condition (e.g. Prader–Willi syndrome or the Laurence–Moon–Biedl syndrome). Obesity develops only if there is a positive energy balance; this is contrary to some views – there are opinions which imply that not all obese children eat excessively. Overweight children are less active than their leaner counterparts and this pattern of reduced physical activity is of importance.

Many factors are involved in the aetiology of fatness, including behavioural problems, feeding patterns within the family, nature of newborn feeding, attitude of parents and siblings to obesity and physical activity.

Management

Specialized obesity clinics have many advantages, particularly if located at school. Serial measures of height, weight and skin fold thickness need to be recorded. Whatever the cause of obesity, management must include a reduction in intake of energy. Regular exercise also aids weight loss. Behavioural therapy has been shown to have a role. Anorectic drugs are only a transient aid because the original obesity will reappear after a time. *See* Obesity, Treatment

A multidisciplinary support group made up of parents, peers, nutritionist, paediatrician and a therapist or clinical psychologist has in theory much to offer. Food fads or 'crash diets' are potentially dangerous and must be avoided in childhood, if not in adulthood too.

Parents of children under 5 need advice to avoid offering a high intake of fat and sugar. Instances of moderate obesity can be managed by allowing the children to grow into their present weight.

As 450 g of excess bodyweight represents 14·7 MJ, a daily reduction of 2 MJ is needed to lose 450 g of weight a week.

Greater affluence will inevitably mean that an ever increasing number of youth will be obese, with all the associated phenomena. Determined educational and nutritional efforts must be adopted to avoid this scourge of life in privileged communities.

Protein–Energy Malnutrition (PEM)

Formerly known as protein–calorie malnutrition, PEM, is a major global problem and one which arouses much controversy even in terms of its classification. Although PEM is rare in adults it is responsible for a high mortality and indeed morbidity amongst children in developing countries. At one end of the spectrum PEM includes marasmus, and at the other the distinct syndrome of kwashiorkor, with intermediate deficiencies between both polarities (see Fig. 2). *See* Protein, Deficiency

Within this band there are deficiencies of specific dietary constituents, particularly folate and vitamin A. Many children with severe PEM have infestations due to *Giardia lamblia*, *Strongyloides stercoralis* or *Ascaris lumbricoides*. Tuberculosis, bronchopneumonia and measles are significant secondary complications.

Anorexia plays a dominant role in PEM, as does the presence of small bowel mucosal atrophy. These pheno-

Table 1. Comparison of marasmus and kwashiorkor

	Marasmus	Kwashiorkor
Weight	↓↓↓	↓↓
Oedema	− − −	+ + +
Depigmentation	− − −	↑↑↑
Hair changes	±	+ +
Vitamin levels	↓↓↓	↓↓
Small intestine – villous atrophy	+ +	+ + +
Lactase, sucrase, maltase	↓↓	↓↓↓
Pancreatic enzymes	↓	↓
Fatty liver	+	+

Modified from Gryboski J and Walker WA (1983) *Gastrointestinal Problems in the Infant* 2nd edn. Philadelphia: WB Saunders.
↓, slightly reduced; ↓↓, moderately reduced; ↓↓↓, markedly reduced.

mena may be accompanied by the presence of both a protein-losing enteropathy and iron deficiency. *See* Anorexia Nervosa

These disorders can be grouped together. Some workers regard marasmus as successful adaptation to nutritional stress, and kwashiorkor as the failure of such an attempt. A comparison of kwashiorkor and marasmus is given in Table 1. *See* Kwashiorkor; Marasmus

Malnutrition and its associated infections causes the death of many millions. However, the mortality can be as low as 5% where the children are taken to specialized resuscitation centres.

Protein–energy malnutrition is not limited to non-industrialized countries. Fad and strict vegetarian diets as well as medically unsupervised elimination regimes all have the potential for causing PEM. *See* Vegetarian Diets

Lack of nutritional knowledge and financial resources within a household, the community or society at large are responsible for the appalling childhood mortality and morbidity seen in PEM. Malnutrition ought to be regarded as the consequence of adverse social and economic conditions rather than a primary medical problem. Simple measures, such as the encouragement of breast-feeding, personal hygiene, improved sanitation and the establishment of adequate and safe drinking water, would do much to prevent the many potentially hazardous enteric infections seen in malnourished infants and children.

Food Fads

Food fads are not only potentially dangerous for adults but also particularly hazardous in childhood. Apart from human milk for babies and young infants there is no other single food which supplies all nutritional needs, yet food faddism seems increasingly attractive to many seeking 'healthy foods' and a diet free of all alleged

contaminants. *See* Food Fads and Fallacies; Health Foods, Definition and Dietary Importance

As food technology becomes more sophisticated and food processing is seen as an adulteration of our food, some will turn and seek alternatives via the use of 'natural, organic and health foods' – all loose terms. There is an organic food myth and we do not even have an acceptable definition of 'organic foods' – a term introduced by the late JI Rodale. Consumers presume such food is grown in soil free of artificial fertilizer, is pesticide-free and does not contain additives, preservatives, hormones or antibiotics, etc. There is no evidence to support the contention that 'organic foods' are healthier for the consumer. Man-made vitamins are as effective as 'natural vitamins'. Food grown in rich soil is not nutritionally dissimilar to that found in poor soil. Unfortunately, disinformation by the health food movement has facilitated the public acceptance of food mythology as a reality. Nutrition is a subject that is ill-understood by many. *See* Organic Foods

Tragically, children have died from malnutrition when fed weird and unconventional diets. Growth failure and anaemia were found in a small group of infants fed a formula of barley water, corn syrup and whole milk.

Faddism can result in many diverse and potentially dangerous outcomes. There are those who expect their children to survive solely on fruit ('fruitarians'); others are committed to a diet of raw foods. The discovery of fire 40 000 years ago by primitive humans brought an end to reliance on diets comprised solely of raw food. Some uncooked foods are toxic and unsafe, e.g. meat might become contaminated by bacteria, and raw foods may contain substances that interfere with vitamin B_1 (antihistaminases). Raw red kidney beans possess natural toxins (haemagglutinins). The Zen-macrobiotic diet has been associated with deaths. The ever increasing restrictive nature of this diet is such that ultimately only cereals are used, with disastrous consequences. *See* Macrobiotic Diets

Embroiled in this widening saga of unconventional diets is the use of vitamin supplements in megadoses. It is now increasingly evident that such therapy is metabolically hazardous, particularly for children. *See* Health Foods, Dietary Supplements

Food Intolerance and Aversion

There are few subjects that are so enigmatic, confusing and clouded with anecdotal clutter as that of food adversion (intolerance) and aversion (psychological intolerance or avoidance). It has been suggested that the term 'allergy' be applied only to those with immediate allergic responses to food and with the presence of specific immunoglobulin E (IgE) antibodies. Mast cells, basophils, eosinophils, macrophages and platelets can all be activated by IgE antibodies, causing the release of preformed or instant mediators. *See* Food Intolerance, Types; Food Intolerance, Food Allergies; Food Intolerance, Lactose Intolerances

Food Intolerance

Clinical manifestations of food intolerance may include diarrhoea, abdominal pain, failure to thrive, urticaria, eczema, migraine, behavioural disturbance, and inflammatory bowel disease.

Food intolerance is an adverse and reproducible reaction which can be caused by the following:

1. *Allergic reaction(s)*, which implies an unpleasant and immediate response to food(s); the mechanisms may be via IgE antibody formation, a T-cell-mediated reaction, or the systemic formation of antigen–antibody complexes.
2. *Pharmacological factors*, e.g. tyramine; there is a high concentration of tyramine in fermented cheese and this can elevate the blood pressure and produce symptoms. Caffeine in coffee and tea, in the hypersensitive, can cause symptoms such as anxiety and tachycardia.
3. *Toxic effect*, e.g. mycotoxins from storage of foods contaminated with moulds.
4. *Enzyme deficiency*, e.g. lactose intolerance caused by alactasia: it has been suggested that a deficiency of the enzyme, phenolsulphotransferase, may have a role in food-induced migraine.
5. *Food fermentation*: bacteria in the colon, particularly *Proteus morganii*, can produce decarboxylase, an enzyme that will convert dietary histidine to histamine. However, as histamine does not cause an immunological reaction its effect is pseudoallergic.
6. *Other intolerances*: *Tartrazine* is a common colouring substance contained in many foods, soft drinks and pharmaceutical products; its mechanism of action may be meditated by IgD antibodies; benzoates or sulphur dioxide preservatives and butylated hydroxyanisole or butylated hydroxytoluene antioxidants may have similar effects; manifestations of symptoms caused by food additives include urticaria, asthma, migraine, and rhinitis.

Acetylsalicylic acid (ASA), present in vegetables and fruits, can cause a range of symptoms in sensitive patients, including asthma, urticaria and rhinitis; synthetic salicylates are found as flavouring products.

Food Aversion

Food aversion, in contrast to adversion, is the result of either psychological intolerance or food avoidance. For a comprehensive and balanced account of this topic see Royal College of Physicians/British Nutrition Foundation (1984).

Pathogenesis

The permeability of the gastrointestinal tract mucosa to food allergens is believed to be a major factor in the pathogenesis of antigenic food reactions. It is known that intestinal permeability is increased following an acute gastroenteritis. Temporary changes in the gut have been demonstrated after rotavirus enteritis by studying the differential permeation of the sugars, lactose, lactulose and rhamnose. Studies using the inert probe, polythylene glycol, have shown increased intestinal permeability in allergic children which has been impeded by disodium cromoglycate. Moreover, using a radioimmunological method for measuring serum concentration of human α-lactalbumin, preterm infants have an increased absorption of macromolecules compared with that seen at term. Excessive uptake of such antigens might be associated with subsequent allergy in childhood, or even adulthood.

The integrity of the bowel mucosa is maintained in part by secretory IgA and the glycocalyx (a glycoprotein secretion coating the bowel enterocytes) as well as the mucosa-associated lymph tissues (MALTs). It has been suggested that following food challenge there is the deposition of immune complexes in different target organs and sites which can result in migraine, arthralgia or eczema.

Treatment

Treatment is often unsatisfactory because of difficulties in identifying and then removing the offending allergen(s). Disodium cromoglycate has been of some help and the next generation of so-called mast cell membrane stabilizers or food hyposensitization techniques might be more effective than those presently used. *See* Food Intolerance, Elimination Diets

Almost every food consumed by humans has been cited as an allergen in the literature. Many food dyes that have a low molecular weight and are not allergens in themselves act as haptens and become allergenic if linked to a large protein molecule.

Food Additives, Salicylates and Hyperactivity

Paediatricians and nutritionists seem to polarize themselves into either protagonists or vehement opponents of Dr Feingold's theory, which postulates that hyperkinesis can be managed in 30–50% of children by eliminating artificial food colouring matter, preservatives and other additives from the diet, and by eliminating fruits and vegetables containing natural salicylates. The major symptoms of this psychological disorder are over-activity, distractibility, restlessness, impulsive behaviour, and a short attention span, identifying this syndrome as a conduct disorder. British practice confines the diagnosis to those with epilepsy, mental subnormality or a recognizable neurological disease.

Hyperkinesis is probably not a single entity and the aetiology is multifactorial. Unfortunately, it is now accepted that as many as 50% of all children with this disorder show some of its features in adulthood.

Bibliography

Bender AE (1985) *Health or Hoax?* Goring-on-Thames: Elvendon Press.

Bentley D and Lawson M (1988) *Clinical Nutrition in Paediatric Disorders.* London: Baillière Tindall.

Brostoff J and Challacombe SJ (1987) *Food Allergy and Intolerance.* London: Ballière Tindall.

Dobbing J (1987) *Food Intolerance.* London: Ballière Tindall.

Hoorweg J and Niemeijer R (1989) *Intervention in Child Nutrition.* London: Kegan Paul International.

Jukes TH (1974) The organic food myth. *Journal of the American Medical Association* 230 (No. 2): 276–277.

Lawson DEM (1981) Dietary vitamin D: is it necessary? *Journal of Human Nutrition* 35: 61–63.

Mankin HJ (1990) Rickets, osteomalacia and renal osteodystrophy. *Orthopedic Clinics of North America* 21 (No. 1): 81–96.

Poskitt EM (1987) Management of obesity. *Archives of Disease in Childhood* 62: 305–310.

Reinhardt D and Schmidt E (1988) *Food Allergy. Nestlé Nutrition Workshop Series*, vol. 17. New York: Vevey/Raven Press.

Rosenbaum M and Leibel RL (1988) Obesity. Pathophysiology of childhood obesity. *Advances in Pediatrics* 35: 73–110.

Royal College of Physicians/British Nutrition Foundation (1984) Food intolerance and food aversion. A joint report of the Royal College of Physicians and the British Nutrition Foundation. *Journal of the Royal College of Physicians London* 18 (No. 2): 4.

Walker AF (ed.) (1990) *Applied Human Nutrition for Food Scientists and Home Economists.* Chichester: Horwood (Ellis).

Walker-Smith JA and McNeish AS (1986) *Diarrhoea and Malnutrition in Childhood.* Oxford: Butterworth Heinemann.

Wharton BA (1987) *Nutrition and Feeding of Preterm Infants.* Oxford: Blackwell Scientific Publications.

Donald Bentley
Ealing Hospital, Southall, UK

CHILLED STORAGE

Contents

Principles

Basic Theory

The complete chill chain for a food will contain many of the following unit operations: prechilling preparation, primary or secondary chilling, storage, transportation and display. Storage, transport and display are temperature maintenance operations. Chilling results in a substantial decrease in the mean temperature of the product, whilst during the preparatory treatment there can be a range of temperature responses from a large gain to a small decrease in the temperature of the foodstuff.

The initial and final temperatures, and the maximum and minimum desirable rates of temperature reduction during chilling depend on the food being processed. In all cases the final product temperature must be above the initial freezing point of the food, but in a number of products biological factors dictate higher storage temperatures.

The principal factors which control the rate of heat and mass transfer during cooling are independent of the foodstuff. Heat can be lost from the surface of a body by four basic mechanisms: radiation, conduction, convection or evaporative cooling. *See* Heat Transfer Methods

To determine the rate of heat transfer (Q_r) by radiation from food the following approximation may be applied:

$$Q_r = \varepsilon A \sigma (T_s^4 - T_e^4), \qquad (1)$$

where ε is the emissivity and A is the surface area of the food, σ the Stefan–Boltzman constant and T_s and T_e the temperature of the surface and the enclosure, respectively. To achieve substantial rates of heat loss by radiation, large temperature differences between the product and the enclosure are required. Such differences are not normally present during food-cooling operations, except in the initial chilling of bakery products.

The rate of one-dimensional heat transfer (Q_{cd}) by conduction is given by

$$Q_{cd} = kA \frac{\partial T}{\partial x}, \qquad (2)$$

where k is the thermal conductivity of the medium through which the heat is passing and $\partial T / \partial x$ the temperature gradient.

Physical contact between the product and a cooler surface is required to extract heat by conduction. The irregular shape of most foodstuffs precludes this mechanism in many applications. However, the rate at which heat can be conducted away from the surface is not the sole criterion that governs the time taken to cool a product. Heat must also be conducted from within the product to its surface before it can be removed. Most foodstuffs are poor conductors of heat and this imposes a severe limitation on attainable chilling times for either large individual items or small items cooled in bulk.

The rate of mass transfer (M) from the surface of an unwrapped food is described by the equation

$$M = mA(P_s a_w - P_m), \qquad (3)$$

where m is the mass transfer coefficient, A is the area, P_s is the saturated vapour pressure at the surface, a_w is the water activity and P_m is the vapour pressure above the food surface. The heat loss due to evaporation (Q_e) can be obtained by multiplying M by the appropriate latent heat. The heat lost in the evaporation of water from the surface of the product is a minor component of the total heat loss for most foodstuffs. However, in a number of specific cases it can be the primary cooling agent.

Most food chilling systems rely on convection as the principal means of heat removal. The rate of one-dimensional heat transfer (Q_c) by convection is given by

$$Q_c = h_c A (T_s - T_a), \qquad (4)$$

where h_c is the convection or film heat transfer coefficient and T_a the temperature of the cooling medium. The most common media are air or water, although salt solutions, sugar brines and other refrigerants have been used. Each combination of product and cooling system can be characterized by a specific surface heat transfer coefficient. The value of the coefficient depends on the shape and surface roughness of the foodstuff and to a much greater degree on the thermophysical properties and velocity of the medium.

Chilling Methods for Solid Foodstuffs

Moving Air

This is the most widely used method as it is economical, hygienic and relatively noncorrosive to equipment. Systems range from the basic in which a fan blows the cooled air around an insulated room, to conveyor blast chilling tunnels or spirals. Low rates of heat transfer are attained in air-cooling systems, but this is not important if conduction within the product is the rate-controlling factor. A major disadvantage is excessive dehydration from the surface of any unwrapped product, whilst the need to avoid surface freezing limits the lowest air temperature that can be used. In practice, air distribution is a major, often overlooked, problem.

A batch system where warm food is placed in refrigerated rooms is the most common method of chilling. Individual items such as carcasses, tuna or bunches of bananas are hung from rails, smaller products are placed on racks or pallets, and bulk fruits and vegetables are placed in large bins.

Conveying products overcomes problems of uneven air distribution since each item is subjected to the same velocity/time profile. In the simplest continuous systems, the food is suspended from an overhead conveyor and moved through a refrigerated room. This process is often used in air chilling of poultry or in prechilling of pork carcasses. Some small cooked products are continuously chilled on racks of trays which are pulled or pushed through a chilling tunnel using a simple mechanical system. In more sophisticated plants the racks are conveyed through a chilling tunnel in which the refrigeration capacity and air conditions can be varied throughout the length of the tunnel.

In larger operations it is more satisfactory to convey the cooked products through a linear tunnel or spiral chiller. Linear tunnels are far simpler constructions than spirals but require more space.

Hydrocooling/Immersion Cooling

Hydrocooling is probably the least expensive method of achieving rapid cooling in small products. The product is immersed in, or sprayed with, cool water, either at ambient temperature or near $0°C$. Practical systems vary from simple unstirred tanks to plants where the product is conveyed through agitated tanks or under banks of sprays. Such systems are typically used for celery, asparagus, peas, sweet corn, carrots, peaches, etc.

Immersion chilling is also used for larger products. Most poultry to be frozen is initially cooled by immersion in chilled water or an ice/water mixture. The procedure is very fast and the birds gain weight during the process. The maximum weight gain is controlled by legislation.

An alternative system to air or immersion is spray chilling. Practical spray chilling systems use a combination of air and sprays for the initial part of the chilling period and then air only for the rest of the chilling cycle. The sprays of cold water at 2–3°C are not applied continuously but in short bursts. The main advantage claimed for these systems is reduced weight loss.

Plate Cooling

With thinner materials a plate cooling system has the potential to halve the cooling time required in an air blast system. Continuous horizontal and rotary plate freezing systems have been produced commercially and could be modified to operate at higher temperatures. Such systems tend to be expensive, especially if automatic loading and unloading is required, but have low running costs. Designs have been produced for continuous-belt coolers.

Ice or Ice/Water Chilling

Chilling with crushed ice or an ice/water mixture is simple, effective and commonly used for fish cooling. Individual fish are packed in boxes between layers of crushed ice, which extract heat from the fish and consequently melt. The temperature of the 'coolant' remains at a constant 0°C until all the ice has turned into water. The process is labour intensive, although automatic filling systems have been developed. Cabbage and root crops are also cooled with crushed ice. *See* Fish, Sources

Vacuum Cooling

Solid products having a large surface area:volume ratio and an ability to release internal water are amenable to vacuum cooling. The products are placed in a vacuum chamber and the resultant evaporative cooling removes heat from the food. In general terms, a 5°C reduction in product temperature is achieved for every 1% of water that is evaporated. Prewetting is commonly applied to facilitate cooling without loss of weight.

Vacuum cooling is rapid and economical to operate because of low labour costs, but the capital cost of the large vacuum vessels is high. Large amounts of lettuce, celery, cauliflower, green peas and sweet corn are vacuum cooled.

Cryogenic Cooling

Avoiding surface freezing of the product is the main problem in using liquid nitrogen or solid carbon dioxide for chilling. Continuous chilling systems using liquid nitrogen either immerse the product in the liquid, spray the nitrogen onto the surface or vaporize the nitrogen in a forced draught and pass it over the surface of the foodstuff.

Direct spraying of liquid nitrogen on to a food product, whilst it is conveyed through an insulated tunnel, is the most common method. Surface freezing is still a problem, but an extra refrigeration effect is obtained by precooling the food with the cold gas produced by the vaporization.

Chilling Methods for Liquid Foodstuffs

The majority of liquid foodstuffs require cooling after a heat processing operation, such as cooking, pasteurization or sterilization. Milk is cooled at the point of collection to maintain its quality, unpasteurized fruit juices are cooled immediately after production, whilst fermented beverages are often cooled during primary and secondary fermentation, and before storage. *See* Fermented Milks, Products from Northern Europe; Milk, Processing of Liquid Milk; Pasteurization, Principles

In simple or small-scale processes, containers of hot liquids are allowed to cool in ambient air or are placed inside chill rooms. Other cooling systems for liquid foods rely on direct expansion refrigeration, the use of a secondary refrigerant which is passed through or around the foodstuff, vacuum cooling or a combination of liquid and vacuum.

Batch coolers for liquid foods range in capacity from 100 to 10 000 litres with the foodstuff contained in a stainless steel vessel. The cooling medium may circulate through the jacket of the vessel, through a coil immersed in the liquid, or both. Most vessels are provided with agitators to improve convective heat transfer and stop temperature stratification. One common method used to decrease cooling times in a closed vessel is to apply a vacuum to produce evaporative cooling.

Continuous cooling used to be achieved in falling film or surface coolers in which the hot liquid was pumped over the top of a horizontal bank of refrigerated coils and flowed down over the cooled surfaces. These systems have now been replaced by totally enclosed coolers. Double-pipe coolers have also been employed in specialized applications, but have a limited heat-transfer surface. Multiplate coolers are extensively used for liquid foods. They have the highest available heat transfer surface, lowest material requirements, maximum efficiency, are very flexible in operation and are easy to clean. In certain applications, such as beer and wine cooling, multitube coolers that have a much higher resistance to pressure and can use primary refrigerants have advantages over multiplate coolers.

Principles

Scraped-surface heat exchangers can have advantages in the cooling of very viscous liquid foods and where surface fouling is a potential problem.

Chilled Storage

Theoretically, there are clear differences between the environmental conditions required for chilling, which is a heat removal/temperature reduction process, and storage where the aim is to maintain temperature. However, in many air-based systems chilling and storage take place in the same chamber and, even where two separate facilities are used, in many cases not all the required heat is removed in the chilling phase. With some fruits and vegetables, the rate of respiration during storage is sufficient to require heat removal if product quality is to be maintained. *See* Storage Stability, Mechanisms of Degradation; Storage Stability, Parameters Affecting Storage Stability

Bulk Storage Rooms

Most unwrapped meat and poultry and all types of unwrapped foods are stored in large, air-circulated rooms. To minimize weight loss, air movement around the unwrapped product should be the minimum required to maintain a constant temperature. With wrapped products, low air velocities are also desirable to minimize energy consumption. However, many storage rooms are designed and constructed with little regard to air distribution and localized velocities over products. Horizontal-throw refrigeration coils are often mounted in the free space above the racks or rails of product, and no attempt is made to distribute the air around the products. Using air socks, it is claimed that an even air distribution can be maintained with localized velocities not exceeding 0.2 m s^{-1}.

Controlled-Atmosphere Storage Rooms

Controlled-atmosphere storage rooms were developed for specialized fruit stores, especially those for apples. Interest is growing in the application of this technique to other commodities including meat and fish. In addition to the normal temperature control plant, these stores also include special gas-tight seals to maintain an atmosphere which is normally lower in oxygen and higher in nitrogen and carbon dioxide than air. Additional plant is required to control the carbon dioxide concentration, generate nitrogen and consume oxygen. *See* Controlled Atmosphere Storage, Applications for Bulk Storage of Foodstuffs

There is growing interest in the use of controlled atmosphere retail packs to extend the chilled storage and display life of meat and meat products. Since the packs insulate the products, efficient precooling before packaging is important.

Transportation

Developments in temperature-controlled transportation systems for products have been one of the main factors leading to the rapid expansion of the chilled-food market. The sea transportation of chilled meat from Australasia to European and other distant markets, and road transportation of chilled products throughout Europe and the Middle East is now common practice. Air freighting is used for high-value perishable products, such as strawberries, asparagus and live lobsters.

Overland Transport

Overland transportation systems range from 12 m refrigerated containers for long-distance road or rail movement of bulk chilled product to small uninsulated vans supplying food to local retail outlets. The majority of current road transport vehicles for chilled foods are refrigerated using either mechanical, eutectic plates or liquid nitrogen cooling systems. Irrespective of the type of refrigeration equipment used the product will not be maintained at its desired temperature during transportation unless it is surrounded by air or surfaces at or below that temperature. This is usually achieved by a system that circulates moving air, either forced or by gravity, around the load. Inadequate air distribution is probably the principal cause of product deterioration and loss of shelf life during transport. Conventional forced air units usually discharge air over the stacked or suspended products either directly from the evaporator or through ducts towards the rear cargo doors. Because air takes the path of least resistance, it circulates through the channels which have the largest cross-sectional area. These tend to be around rather than through the product. If products have been cooled to the correct temperature before loading and do not generate heat then they only have to be isolated from external heat ingress. Many trucks are now being constructed with an inner skin that forms a return air duct along the side walls and floor, with the refrigerated air being supplied via a ceiling duct.

Sea Transport

Recent developments in temperature control, packaging and controlled atmospheres have increased substantially the range of foods that can be transported around the world in a chilled condition. Control of the oxygen and carbon dioxide levels in shipboard containers have allowed fruits and vegetables, such as apples, pears, avocado pears, melons, mangoes, nectarines, blueberries and asparagus, to be shipped from Australia and New Zealand to markets in the USA, Europe, Middle East and Japan.

International Standards Organization (ISO) containers for food transport are 6 or 12 m long, hold up to 26 tonnes of product and can be 'insulated' or 'refrigerated'. The refrigerated containers incorporate insulation and have refrigeraton units built into their structure. Insulated containers involve either plug-type refrigeration units or may be connected directly to an air-handling system in a ship's hold or at the docks. Close temperature control is most easily achieved in containers that are placed in insulated holds and connected to the ship's refrigeration system.

Air Transport

Although air-freighting of foods offers a rapid method of serving distant markets, there are many problems because the product is unprotected by refrigeration for much of its journey. Up to 80% of the total journey time is spent on the tarmac for transport to and from the airport. Perishable cargo is usually carried in standard containers, sometimes with an insulating lining and/or dry ice, but is often unprotected on aircraft pallets.

Retail Display

The retail display of chilled foods was the weakest link in the cold chain. However, in the UK, the Food Hygiene (Amendment) Regulations 1990 now require food retailers to maintain the temperature of certain chilled foods below 8°C during storage, transport and display. For some foods this temperature will be reduced to 5°C in 1993.

The required retail display life and consequent environmental conditions for wrapped chilled products differ from those for unwrapped products. The desired display life for wrapped meat, fish, vegetables and processed foods ranges from a few days to many weeks and is primarily limited by microbiological considerations. Retailers of unwrapped fish, meat and delicatessen products normally require a display life of one working day.

Display cabinets for delicatessen products are available with gravity or forced convection coils, and the glass fronts may be nearly vertical or angled up to 20°. In the gravity cabinet, cooled air from the raised rear mounted evaporator coil descends into the display well by natural convection and the warm air rises back to the evaporator. In the forced-circulation cabinets, air is drawn through an evaporator coil by a fan and then ducted into the rear of the display, returning to the coil after passing directly over the products, or forming an air curtain, via a slot in the front of the cabinet and a duct under the display shelf.

Although the same cabinets can be used for wrapped foods, most are sold from multideck cabinets with single or twin air curtain systems. It is important that the front edges of the cabinet shelves do not project through the air curtain since the refrigerated air will then be diverted out of the cabinet. On the other hand, if narrow shelves are used the curtain may collapse and ambient air can be drawn into the display well. External factors such as the store ambient temperature, the siting of the cabinet and poor pretreatment and placement of products substantially affect cabinet performance.

Bibliography

Anonymous (1974) *ASHRAE Handbook and Product Directory. Applications.* New York: American Society of Heating, Refrigeration and Air Conditioning Engineers.

Anonymous (1979) *Recommendations for Chilled Storage of Perishable Produce.* Paris: International Institute of Refrigeration.

Gormley TR (1990) *Chilled Foods – The State of the Art.* Barking: Elsevier.

Jowitt R, Escher F, Hallstrom B, Meffert HFTh, Speiss WEL and Vos G (1983) *Physical Properties of Foods.* Barking: Applied Science.

Perry RH and Chilton CH (1973) *Chemical Engineers' Handbook*, 5th edn. Tokyo: McGraw-Hill.

Stephen James
University of Bristol, Bristol, UK

Attainment of Chilled Conditions

The purpose of the chill chain is first to reduce the temperature of a food to below a set temperature and henceforth maintain it at or below that temperature. Since the growth of both pathogenic and food spoilage organisms is very temperature dependent, the rapid attainment and maintenance of low temperatures is important to food safety and shelf life. In this article the cooling rates and temperatures that can be attained and maintained are discussed together with the limiting physical factors.

The speed at which a food can be cooled can either be limited by the rate of heat removal from its surface or internal conduction. Heat removal from the surface is a direct function of the surface heat transfer coefficient (h). Typical values of h range from 5 W m^{-2}°C^{-1} for slow-moving air to 500 W m^{-2}°C^{-1} for agitated water. Table 1 shows that, at low values of h, a 10-fold increase (5–50 W m^{-2}°C^{-1}) makes a substantial (3·2- to 4·2-fold) reduction in cooling time (Table 1). A further 10-fold increase from 50 to 500 W m^{-2}°C^{-1} decreases the cooling time threefold for a 2 cm thick slab, but only results in a 60% reduction at a thickness of 8 cm. This indicates that, in the thicker material, internal heat conduction is becoming rate controlling.

Primary Chilling

Primary chilling after harvest or slaughter is usually applied to large individual items or small items cooled in bulk. Air cooling is often used in primary chilling because internal conduction controls the rate the products can be cooled. Data from the cooling of beef sides (Fig. 1) illustrate the relative influence of air temperature and air velocity. The data in Fig. 1 are presented as a plot of the logarithm of temperature against time and, provided air temperatures are chosen to avoid substantial surface freezing, it is quite feasible to determine the cooling time for any other air temperature. The fractional unaccomplished temperature on the y axis can be replaced by the meat temperature calculated from $y = (t - t_f)/(t_i - t_f)$, where t is the meat temperature, t_i is the initial meat temperature and t_f is the air temperature.

Cooling in air at a constant 4°C (compared with 0°C) will, at 3 m s^{-1}, increase the time to reach 7°C in the deep leg of a 100 kg side from 20·3 to 27·7 h (36% increase) and, at 0·5 m s^{-1}, that of a 220 kg side from 45·9 to 68·3 h (49% increase).

Secondary Chilling

Cooking rarely eliminates all food poisoning organisms, and a number survive as spores which will germinate and grow if cooling rates are slow. Rapid reduction in surface temperature retards microbial growth and consequently extends shelf life. This is especially important when chilling cooked products that will eventually be consumed cold or in a warm reheated state. Rapid rates of cooling are required without surface freezing. The problem is complicated in two-compartment ready meal consumer packs which typically contain rice or pasta in one compartment, and a meat or fish-based product in the second, because the thermal properties of the two items are often very different, and may be filled to different depths. Air at -10°C and 5 m s^{-1} produces a cooling time of 34 min, but substantial quantities of the product are frozen. At an air velocity of 0·5 m s^{-1} the cooling time is doubled but only a small area of the rice is frozen. With higher air temperatures the extent of freezing is reduced. A cooling time of approximately 0·75 h is achieved at -5°C and 5 m s^{-1} with acceptable freezing.

The importance of achieving a minimum required air velocity around small products is clearly demonstrated by data obtained from cooling pork pies (Fig. 2). To guarantee that all the crust remained above -2°C on the unwrapped 400 g (70 mm high, 95 mm diameter) pies, an air temperature of $-1·5 \pm 0·5$°C was used. At this temperature a small increase in air velocity from 0·5 to 1·0 m s^{-1} reduced the cooling time by 85 min (almost 30%). Even at very high velocities ($> 6·0$ m s^{-1}) appreciable reductions in cooling time were still being achieved.

Rapid rates of temperature reduction can be achieved in trays of cooked product, such as mince, baby foods and poultry portions, when cooled under vacuum. Cooked turkey carcasses (10 kg) can be cooled from 80 to 10°C in less than 1 h, but the rate of pressure reduction must be carefully controlled if textural quality is to be maintained.

Storage, Transport and Display

In general, after initial chilling, as a chilled product moves along the chill chain it becomes increasingly difficult to control and maintain its temperature. Temperatures of bulk packs of chilled product in large storerooms are far less sensitive to small heat inputs than single consumer packs in transport or open display cases. If primary and secondary cooling operations are efficiently carried out, then the food will be reduced below its required temperature before it is placed in store. In this situation, the store's refrigeration system is only required to extract extraneous heat that enters through walls, door openings, etc.

Even when temperature-controlled dispatch bays are used, there is a slight heat pick up during loading. In bulk transportation the resulting temperature rise is small and the vehicle's refrigeration system rapidly returns the product to the required temperature. Larger problems exist in local multidrop distribution to individual stores. There is a large heat input every time the

Table 1. Predicted cooling time (h) from 40°C to 2°C at the centre of meat slabs in systems operating at -1°C

| Cooling method | h (W m^{-2}°C^{-1}) | Meat thickness (cm) | | |
		2·0	4·0	8·0
Air (still)	5	5·0	11·0	24·0
Air (5 m s^{-1})	50	1·2	2·8	7·4
Plate	360	0·7	1·8	5·5
Immersion	500	0·4	1·2	4·4

Attainment of Chilled Conditions

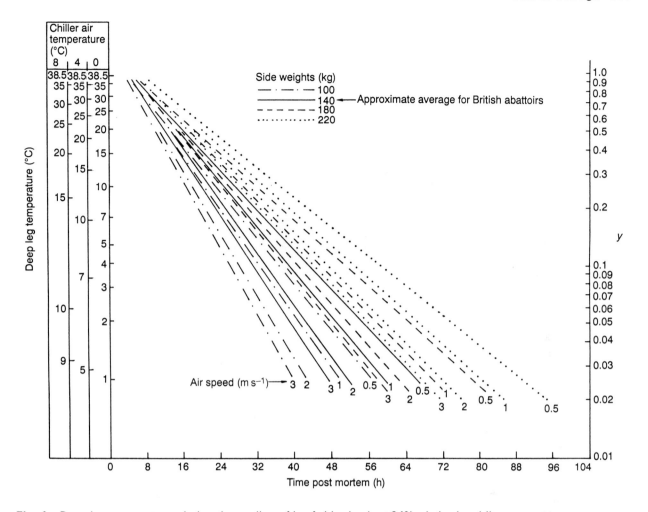

Fig. 1 Deep leg temperatures during the cooling of beef sides in air at 94% relative humidity.

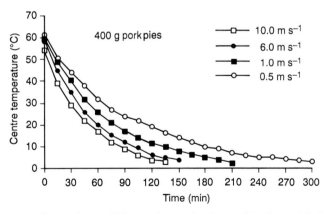

Fig. 2 Temperature at slowest cooling point in 400 g pork pies in air at $-1.5°C$ and 10, 6, 1 and 0.5 m s^{-1}.

doors are opened and product is unloaded, small packs rapidly rise in temperature and the vehicle often lacks the refrigeration capacity or time to recool the food.

Surveys carried out in the UK, Denmark and Sweden (Fig. 3) have revealed a very wide range of temperatures within foods on retail display. Before 1 April 1991, when the new Food Hygiene (Amendment) Regulations 1990

were implemented, there were no regulations in the UK to cover the temperature of chilled foods during distribution or retail display. The regulations, which are to be fully implemented over a 2 year period, divide the majority of chilled foods into two groups: one group, consisting of the most *Listeria*-sensitive foods, must have a maximum temperature during storage, transport

Attainment of Chilled Conditions

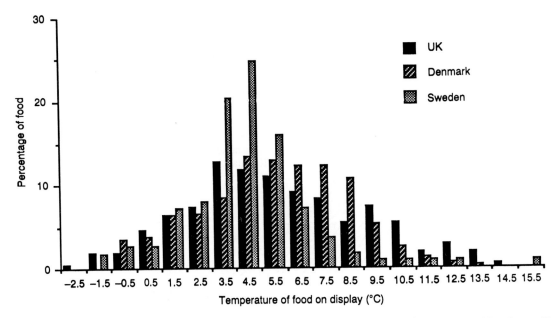

Fig. 3 Temperature of chilled foods in retail display cabinets in Denmark[a], Sweden[b] and United Kingdom[c]. (Data from [a]Bogh-Sorensen L, [b]Olsson P and [c]Rose S.)

Table 2. Maximum temperature measured, and increase in bacterial numbers (generations) during 1 h in car followed by 5 h in a domestic refrigerator

Product	Conditions	Maximum temperature (°C)	*Pseudomonas*	*Clostridium*
Paté	Ambient car	25	1·5	0·4
	Cool box car	13	<0·4	0
Raw Chicken	Ambient car	24	1·6	0·2
	Cool box car	4	0	0
Cooked Chicken	Ambient car	28	1·8	0·7
	Cool box car	12	0	0
Prawns	Ambient car	37	1·3	1·6
	Cool box car	14	0	0
Brie cheese	Ambient car	28	2·2	0·8
	Cool box car	12	0	<0·1

and display of 5°C, whilst foods considered less sensitive must be maintained below 8°C. Consistent monitoring of this new legislation should substantially improve the bacterial quality of chilled food when it is purchased by the consumer.

Domestic

Although legislation, such as that introduced in the UK, should ensure that food producers and retailers maintain acceptable product temperatures during the distribution chain, they lose control when the product leaves the retail store. After a chilled product is removed from a display cabinet it spends a period outside a refrigerated

environment whilst it is carried around the store and then transported home.

Investigations have compared unprotected transportation in a car boot with that in an insulated box. Initial product temperatures measured when the food reached the car ranged from 4 to over 20°C. Some product temperatures on samples placed in the boot rose to approaching 40°C (Table 2) during the 1 h car journey, whilst most of the samples placed in the insulated box cooled during the car journey except for a few at the top of the box which remained at their initial temperature. Small products, i.e. prawns, showed the highest temperature changes during transport. Thicker products like cooked chicken were less influenced. After being placed in the domestic refrigerator, it was approximately 5 h before the temperature was reduced below 7°C.

Attainment of Chilled Conditions

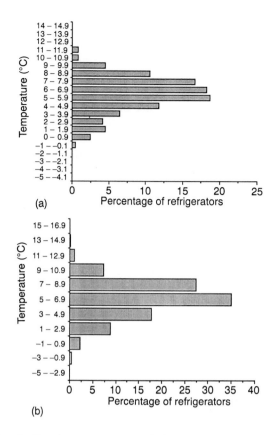

(a)

(b)

Fig. 4 Food temperatures and air temperatures measured in domestic refrigerators in 252 households in UK. (a) Percentage of food with temperature in stated range and (b) percentage of refrigerators with overall average temperatures within stated range.

Predictions made using a mathematical model that calculates bacterial growth from temperature/time relationships indicated that increases of up to 1·8 generations in bacterial numbers (Table 2) can occur during this transport and domestic cooling phase. The model assumes that bacteria require a time to acclimatize to a change in temperature (the lag phase) and that no acclimatization had occurred during display. If this rather optimistic assumption was not made, then up to 4·2 doublings of *Pseudomonas* spp. and growth of both *Salmonella* and *Listeria* spp. were predicted. Very small increases in bacterial numbers (< 0·4 generations, Table 2) were predicted when the insulated box was used, due to the lower product temperatures.

Chilled foods spend a period of between a few minutes and many days stored in domestic refrigerators. The average food temperature measured in a survey of refrigerators in 252 UK households was approximately 6°C (Fig. 4(a)). However, in over 15% of the refrigerators the average food temperature was above 8°C. In a typical UK refrigerator a chilled food would spend over 35% of its time in an air temperature above 7°C (Fig. 4(b)).

Bibliography

Anonymous (1972) *Meat Chilling – Why and How? MRI Symposium*, No 2. Bristol: Langford.

Anonymous (1986) *Proceedings of the International Institute of Refrigeration: Recent Advances and Developments in the Refrigeration of Meat by Chilling*, Bristol.

Evans JA, Stanton JI, Russell SL and James SJ (1991) *Consumer Handling of Chilled Foods: A Survey of Time and Temperature Conditions*. London: Ministry of Agriculture, Fisheries and Food.

Ramila A, Valin C and Taylor AA (1988) *Accelerated Processing of Meat*. London: Elsevier.

Stephen James
University of Bristol, Bristol, UK

Chemical and Physical Considerations

Quality and economic considerations are often the most important factors that govern the choice of a chilling system and the subsequent chilled chain for a particular foodstuff. Since the microbiological aspects are covered elsewhere, quality considerations in this article relate to organoleptic and nutritional changes. Chemical and biochemical changes within foods cause modifications in the appearance, taste or texture that can limit its high-quality shelf life. These changes are not always detrimental to the eating quality of the food. For example, biochemical changes, referred to as 'conditioning' or 'ageing', that occur in meat after slaughter lead to improvements in both its texture and taste.

In general with meat and fish-based foods, the longest high-quality shelf life is achieved by rapidly reducing the temperature of the food and then maintaining it at a temperature very close to its initial freezing point. However, this is not true of all foods. For example, tropical fruits such as bananas suffer discoloration at temperatures below 12°C, whilst salad vegetables such as cucumbers lose their textural properties at temperatures below 6°C. Different cultivars of tomato suffer damage called 'water soaking' and softening at temperatures below 7 or 10°C, pitting and russeting occur in beans below 7°C, and brown core in apples below 2°C.

Primary and Secondary Chilling

Quality Considerations

In the majority of foods, fast cooling is beneficial, but there are instances where excessively rapid chilling rates cause quality problems in particular foods. For example, a serious defect known as 'woolly texture' can be produced in rapidly cooled peaches. Biochemical constraints lead to toughening if the lean tissue of beef or lamb is reduced to 10°C or below within 10 h of slaughter. Due to differences in the biochemistry of pork muscle, the same temperature has to be achieved within 3 h to cause toughening. *See* Meat, Preservation

Different foodstuffs exhibit particular quality advantages as a result of rapid chilling. In meat the pH starts to fall immediately after slaughter and protein denaturation begins. The result of this denaturation is a pink proteinaceous fluid, commonly called 'drip', often seen in prepackaged joints. The rate of denaturation is directly related to temperature and it therefore follows that the faster the chilling rate the less the drip. With both pork and beef the use of rapid rates of chilling can halve the amount of drip loss. Fish passing through rigor mortis above 17°C are to a great extent unusable because the fillets shrink and become tough. A relatively short delay of an hour of two before chilling can demonstrably reduce shelf life. In a different commodity area, freshly harvested sweet corn loses 5, 20 or 60% of its sugar content after 24 h in air at 0, 10 and 30°C respectively. Prompt cooling is clearly required if this vegetable is to retain its desirable sweetness. Similarly, the ripening of fruit can be controlled by rapid cooling, the rate of ripening declining as temperature is reduced and ceasing below about 4°C. **See** Fish, Processing; Ripening of Fruit

Rapid cooling is often desirable with cooked products to maintain quality by eliminating the overcooking that occurs during slow cooling. For vitamin retention, the time taken to reduce the centre temperature from 80°C to 15°C is a critical factor. The vitamin C content in meals is reduced by 1–12% if cooling is carried out in 0·5 h, by 2–17% if the time is increased to 2 h, and by 10–38% when cooling takes 5 h. *See* Ascorbic Acid, Properties and Determination

Economic Considerations

It is clear from restrictions already detailed that attempts to increase chilling rates are complicated by many factors, but there are a number of clear advantages in production economics if faster cooling can be achieved. Most foods are of high value and any increase in the rate of product throughput will improve cash flow and utilize expensive plant more efficiently. For example, in a high-throughput baking line (> 1000 items per hour) the 7% increase in throughput, which would be achieved by raising the air velocity from 6 to 10 m s^{-1} and consequently reducing the cooling time of 400 g pies by 10 min, could justify the higher capital and running costs of larger fans. The power required by the fans to move the air within a chill room increases with the cube of the velocity. A fourfold increase in air velocity from 0·5 to 2 m s^{-1} results in a 4·4 h (18%) reduction in chilling time for a 140 kg beef side, but requires a 654-fold increase in fan power. Increasing air velocity to 3 m s^{-1} only achieves an extra 6% reduction in chilling time. In most practical situations, where large items (e.g. meat carcasses, tuna, bins of vegetables) are being cooled it is doubtful whether an air velocity greater than 1 m s^{-1} can be justified.

Efficient chilling produces a reduction in weight loss which results in a higher yield of saleable material. Most foods have a high water content and the rate of evaporation depends on the vapour pressure at the surface. Vapour pressure increases with temperature and thus any reduction in the surface temperature will reduce the rate of evaporation. The effect of air temperature and velocity on evaporative weight loss during chilling is dependent upon the end point of the chilling process (Fig. 1(a) and (b)). When chilling for a set time, weight loss increases as temperature decreases and velocity increases. The opposite effect is found when chilling to a set temperature.

Alternative chilling treatments can produce large increases in throughput and reductions in weight loss over conventional treatments (Table 1). The cash savings that result from the reduced weight losses can substantially increase the overall profits of many slaughtering operations (Table 1).

Commercial Storage, Retail Display and Domestic Storage

Packaged Food

Most packaging systems substantially reduce evaporative weight loss from the surface of the product, and many retard the rate of chemical degradation. The use of modified atmospheres or opaque packaging can limit colour changes during the chilled storage of meat, fish and fruits.

Losses in vitamin content tend to be reduced at lower storage and display temperatures. Vitamin C losses from lettuce average 4·8, 5·6 and 6·6% per day at temperatures of 1, 5 and 10°C, respectively. Larger effects of temperature are found in French beans with equivalent losses of 1·9, 3·0 and 5·1% per day. No losses were reported in carrots at the three temperatures.

Oranges and pineapples are examples of foods that have an optimum temperature for vitamin C retention. In oranges, a 10% loss per month at 10°C increases to 12% at 5°C and 26% at 0°C. Raising the storage temperature above 10°C also increases the rate of loss to 13% at 15°C and 22% at 30°C. A similar optimum at 10°C is found in pineapples.

Vitamin B$_6$ retention is also a function of both storage temperature and species. Loss from lettuce and French

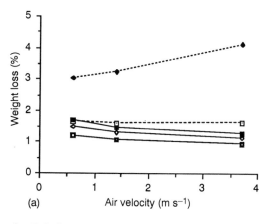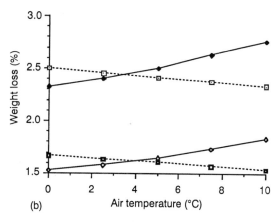

Fig. 1 Relationship between weight loss and (a) air velocity for lamb carcasses (– – –□– – –, 4 h; - - - -◆- - - -, 22 h, ——□—— 13°C, ——◇—— 7°C, ——■—— 4°C); and (b) air temperature for beef sides when chilling for either a set time or to a final temperature (- - - -□- - - -, thin 18 h; ———◆———, thin 10°C; - - - -□- - - -, fat 18 h; ———◇———, fat 10°C).

beans increases twofold and threefold, respectively as the temperature is increased from 1 to 10°C. No change was reported in parsley or carrots. *See* Vitamin B₆, Properties and Determination

Unwrapped Food

Changes in appearance are normally the criteria which limit storage and display of unwrapped foods, commercial buyers or domestic consumers selecting fresh or newly loaded product in preference to that displayed or stored for some time. Deterioration in appearance has been related to degree of dehydration in red meat

(Table 2), and similar changes are likely to occur in other foods. Apart from any relationship to appearance, weight loss is of considerable importance in its own right. The direct cost of evaporative loss from unwrapped foods in chilled display cabinets in the UK is in excess of £5 million per annum.

In the equation which governs weight loss, the mass transfer coefficient m is a function of air velocity with typical values ranging from approximately 2×10^{-8} kg m^{-2} s^{-1} Pa^{-1} at 0·25 m s^{-1} to 14×10^{8} kg m^{-2} s^{-1} Pa^{-1} at 1·5 m s^{-1}. The vapour pressure difference $(P_s a_w - P_m)$ is a function of surface temperature and dryness, and the temperature and relative humidity of the air.

Table 1. The weight loss (percentage saving over conventionally chilled controls), cooling time to 10°C for each treatment, drip loss from loin chops (total work done at 24 h post mortem) and annual saving for each treatment compared with the conventional chill used as a control for an abattoir slaughtering an average of 1000 pigs per week (74 kg dead weight at £0·90 per kg)

Chilling treatment	Weight loss at 24 h (%)	Cooling time to 10°C		Drip (%)	Texture work (J)	Saving (£)
		Deep leg (h)	Surface leg (h)			
Ultrarapid						
Side	1·13 (0·85)	>7·0	5·0[a]	2·3	0·18	28 300
Whole carcass	1·10 (1·01)	>8·0	4·0[a]	0·9	0·21	33 600
Ultrarapid two stage	2·00 (0·29)	7·0	—	0·2	0·23	9600
Immersion	0·32 (2·08)	5·4	3·6	1·5	0·30	69 200
High humidity	1·96 (0·21)	12·9	8·7	0·8	0·20	7000
Delay + high humidity	1·93 (0·24)	14·8	9·1	1·0	0·20	8000
Delay + spray	0·95 (1·22)	14·1	9·2	1·0	0·20	40 600
Rapid + high humidity	1·53 (0·64)	11·6	1·3	0·9	0·21	21 300
Rapid + conventional	1·67 (0·50)	11·5	1·6	1·0	0·24	16 600

[a] Measured at intersection of lean and fat.
[b] Work done in shearing cooked samples.

Table 2. The relationship between evaporative weight loss and the appearance of sliced beef topside after 6 h of display

Evaporative loss (g cm^{-2})	Change in appearance
$\leqslant 0.01$	Red, attractive and still wet; may lose some brightness
0.015–0.025	Surface becoming drier, still attractive but darker
0.025–0.035	Distinct obvious darkening; becoming dry and leathery
0.05	Dry, blackening
0.05–0.10	Black

In storage rooms at temperatures in the range 0–2°C, 76–90% relative humidity, the average weight loss from cauliflower, French beans and green peas is between 0·1 and 0·4% per day. Under conditions typical of domestic refrigeration, 4–8°C and 70–90% relative humidity, weight losses from the same products range from 0·3 to 3·0% per day. In a nonrefrigerated ambient store, 16–24°C and 50–70% relative humidity, losses are even higher in the range between 1·0 and 4·0% per day.

The relative effect of air temperature, velocity and humidity on weight loss in retail display are demonstrated in Fig. 2. Changes in relative humidity have a substantial effect with a reduction from 95 to 40% increasing weight loss over a 6 h display period by a factor of between 14 and 18. The effect of air velocity on weight loss is compounded by that of relative humidity. Raising the air velocity from 0·1 to 0·5 m s^{-1} has little effect on weight loss at 95% relative humidity, but increases the loss by a factor of between 2 and 2·4 at 60% relative humidity. A temperature change from 2 to 6°C has a far smaller effect on weight loss than changes in either relative humidity or velocity.

In further work, a model developed to predict the rate of weight loss from unwrapped meat under the range of environmental conditions found in chilled retail displays showed that it was governed by the mean of the conditions. Fluctuations in temperature or relative humidity had little effect on weight loss, and any apparent effect is caused by changes in the mean conditions.

There is a conflict between the need to make the display attractive and convenient to increase sales appeal and the optimum display conditions for the product. High lighting levels increase the heat load and the air temperature in the cabinet rises. This rise increases the temperature difference across the evaporator coil and the air entering the cabinet is dehumidified. Consequently the rate of evaporative weight loss from foods on display is increased.

Bibliography

Anonymous (1974) *ASHRAE Handbook and Product Directory. Applications.* New York: American Society of Heating, Refrigeration and Conditioning Engineers.

FR and PERC (1992) *Publications on the Refrigeration and Thermal Processing of Food.* Bristol: University of Bristol.

Gormley TR (1990) *Chilled Foods – The State of the Art.* Barking: Elsevier.

International Institute of Refrigeration (1979) *Recommendations for Chilled Storage of Perishable Produce.* Paris: International Institute of Refrigeration.

International Institute of Refrigeration (1985) *Technology Advances in Refrigerated Storage and Transport.* Orlando: International Institute of Refrigeration. Commissions D1, D2 and D3.

International Institute of Refrigeration (1986) *Recent Advances and Developments in the Refrigeration of Meat by Chilling.* Bristol: International Institute of Refrigeration. Commission C2.

International Institute of Refrigeration (1990) *Progress in the Science and Technology of Refrigeration in Food Engineering.* Dresden: International Institute of Refrigeration. Commissions B2, C2, D1, D2/3.

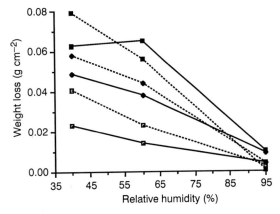

Fig. 2 Weight loss from samples of beef steak under simulated display conditions: ——□——, 2°C, 0·1 m s^{-1}; ——◆——, 2°C, 0·3 m s^{-1}; ——■——, 2°C, 0·5 m s^{-1}; ----□---, 6°C, 0·1 m s^{-1}; ----◆----, 6°C, 0·3 m s^{-1}; ----■----, 6°C, 0·5 m s^{-1}.

Chemical and Physical Considerations

Zeuthen P, Cheftel JC, Eriksson C, Gormley TR, Lonko P and Panlus K (1990) *Chilled Foods: The Revolution in Freshness.* Barking: Elsevier.

Stephen James
University of Bristol, Bristol, UK

Microbiological Considerations

Most biological reactions depend to some extent on temperature; in general, the lower the temperature the lower the rate of the reaction. Microbial growth is no exception to this and, as the temperature is reduced, the rates of activity and growth are generally slower. This phenomenon has been exploited over the years to control the microbiological spoilage of foods and thus to prolong shelf life. Today, therefore, refrigeration is widely used to extend the time for which food can be kept prior to consumption.

The temperature at which refrigerators should operate depends to some extent on the type of food stored in them. The UK Food Hygiene Regulations (1990) define storage temperatures which vary from 'below 5°C' for smoked or cured products, sandwiches, cut cheeses, cooked food containing meat, fish, eggs, cereals or vegetables, to 'below 8°C' for 'other relevant food'. Domestic refrigerators should normally be operated at 4°C or less, and the microbiology of chilled or refrigerated foods after purchase by the consumer should perhaps be considered for those organisms which can grow at 4°C or below. Nevertheless, the performance of such refrigeration systems is rarely measured by thermometer, and the temperatures that prevail in refrigerators or cold rooms, considered to provide adequate chilled storage for foods, can vary considerably. In this discussion, therefore, the microbiology of organisms whose activity is significant below 10°C will be discussed.

Chilled Storage of Foods

Not all microorganisms have the ability to grow at refrigeration temperatures. Many of the Gram-positive spoilage organisms (e.g. most lactic acid bacteria), most coliforms and the majority of pathogens do not grow significantly in chill conditions. However, there is an increasing list of pathogens and spoilage organisms which are now considered to multiply under chilled conditions.

Psychrotrophic microorganisms can be defined as those showing significant growth below 10°C, although many of these are also capable of growth at considerably higher (mesophilic) temperatures. Relatively few true psychrophiles (i.e. organisms that can only grow at low temperatures) are currently of interest to the food microbiologist, and, therefore, psychrotrophs are the organisms of major concern in any study of the refrigerated storage of food. These microorganisms are important both from the point of view of their spoilage potential and because of their public health significance.

Psychrotrophic Spoilage

The most common psychrotrophic spoilage organisms in low-acid, high-moisture foods, such as milk or raw meat, are the Gram-negative rods such as *Pseudomonas* spp. and the *Acinetobacter/Moraxella* group. These are widespread in nature and grow rapidly at refrigeration temperatures, having an average generation time at 7°C of about 7 h. As a general rule, therefore, they may be considered to show a daily 10-fold increase in numbers per day at this temperature. In contrast to the saccharolytic (acid-producing) spoilage caused by many mesophilic organisms, these Gram-negative rods tend to produce proteolysis and lipolysis. Thus, psychrotrophic spoilage is characterized by bitter or lipolytic taints due to the break down of proteins to give bitter peptides or the break down of lipids to give rancid off-flavours instead of the rather 'sour' or 'cheesy' off-flavours usually found as a result of spoilage at higher temperatures. These taints appear only when there are relatively high levels of spoilage organisms, the spoilage becoming detectable when contamination has reached a level of 10^7 to 10^8 organisms per gram of foodstuff. This appears to apply to a wide range of foods, from dairy products such as pasteurized milk, to raw chicken and beef.

Gram-negative psychrotrophs (especially in the genus *Pseudomonas*) grow so rapidly in low-acid, high-moisture foods at refrigeration temperatures that at the end of shelf life they will be the predominant microorganisms, irrespective of their proportion in the original foodstuff. Several of these organisms are also able to grow at warm temperatures and, consequently, they appear in the mesophilic colony count (which is undertaken at 30°C). Thus, after a few days of refrigerated storage, the psychrotrophic colony count and the mesophilic colony count become similar, since the two tests are able to detect the same group of organisms (Fig. 1).

Another group of spoilage organisms of major significance are the psychrotrophic members of the genus *Bacillus*. These are metabolically less active than the Gram-negative psychrotrophs, having a lag phase of 2–7 days, when they grow at about one-third of the speed. They compete poorly, therefore, but can be a cause of spoilage if Gram-negative psychrotrophs are absent. Psychrotrophic clostridia (obligately anaerobic spore-formers) are also found in foods, although less

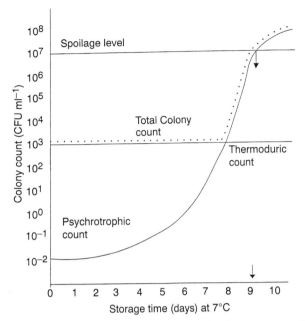

Fig. 1 Relationship between the total colony count and the psychrotrophic count observed in a food stored at 7°C.

often than *Bacillus* spp. There is only one major pathogenic species within the psychrotrophic clostridia (*Clostridium botulinum* type E) which has been reported to grow at 3·3°C.

Psychrotrophic bacteria are usually inhibited at low pH values (as in delicatessen salads, fruit juices, pickles or yoghurt), or when the water activity (a_w) is lowered by drying, or by the addition of salt or sugar (as in hard cheeses, bacon or jam). In many foods, combinations of these parameters are used to delay the multiplication of spoilage bacteria, and dried or acid foods are thus less perishable than low-acid, high-moisture products, yeasts and moulds being the major spoilage organisms.

In yoghurt (pH about 4·0–4·2), yeasts often gain access via the addition of fruit. During storage (especially if a low temperature is not maintained), they ferment the fruit sugars or the added sucrose and produce carbon dioxide gas which can result in exploding containers. Moulds can grow under similar conditions to yeasts but, unlike fermentative yeasts, they require some molecular oxygen for growth. Moulds tend, therefore, to be found as spoilage organisms on the surfaces of foods, such as Saran-wrapped hard cheese or non-vacuum-sealed jam. Vacuum-packed products rarely support a vigorous growth of moulds unless the integrity of the pack has been breached.

The Growth of Pathogens in Chilled Foods

Traditionally, the refrigerated storage of foods has been considered not only as a means of delaying spoilage, but also of reducing the risk of food poisoning. It was thought that pathogens do not grow at low temperatures, but this is now known to be untrue. There is an ever-expanding list of psychrotrophs that have been linked with disease. For many years, the only psychrotrophic organism of food poisoning significance was thought to be nonproteolytic *C. botulinum*, notably type E. Over the last 20 years, however, organisms such as *Aeromonas hydrophilia*, *Bacillus cereus*, *Escherichia coli*, *Listeria monocytogenes* and *Yersinia enterocolitica* have all been shown to grow at refrigeration temperatures, and to have been implicated in outbreaks of disease. The most widely publicised of these 'emerging pathogens' is *L. monocytogenes*, but the evidence that this or any of these species poses a significant threat to the consumer is scant. Nevertheless, because of the increasingly sophisticated techniques for investigating outbreaks of disease and for establishing the causative agents, the presence of these organisms in foods is now being questioned more closely.

The temperature ranges over which the growth of pathogens is currently considered to occur are listed in Table 1. Many of the organisms listed in the table fail to compete well with Gram-negative psychrotrophs at low temperatures and, for most properly refrigerated foods, they are of little consequence unless the spoilage competitors are eliminated. Microbial competition thus plays an important part in the safety of chilled foods. At the end of shelf life, for example, the level of psychrotrophic *B. cereus* in pasteurized milk or bakery products such as custard tarts depends on the competitive microflora. The growth rate for these strains of *B. cereus* at 7°C is about one-third that of *Pseudomonas* spp. Thus, in the presence of Gram-negative bacteria spoilage occurs in about 7 days, well before the pathogen is likely to have increased significantly in numbers. The risk of *B. cereus* food poisoning is, therefore, minimized. In the absence of Gram-negative bacteria, the shelf life of pasteurized milk at 7°C is about 3 weeks. This might be desirable to the consumer, but the predominant spoilage organism after that time might be *B. cereus*, and this would increase the risk of food poisoning. Attempts to extend the shelf life of chilled foods by eliminating Gram-negative contamination may, therefore, actually expose the consumer to unexpected risks.

A similar situation exists with *L. monocytogenes*. This organism has received much attention in recent years, despite the fact that only three cases of food poisoning have ever been recognized by the UK Department of Health in England and Wales. This is compared with approximately 35 000 cases per year of salmonellosis and a similar number of cases due to *Campylobacter* spp. It is unlikely that *L. monocytogenes* is a hazard in short shelf life products such as pasteurized milk, again due to the presence of Gram-negative bacteria. However, in soft cheeses the pseudomonads are inhibited by the

Table 1. Temperature range (°C) of growth of food poisoning bacteria

Organism	Vegetative cell	Germination and outgrowth of spore	Toxin production	
			Range	Optimum
Aeromonas hydrophila	1–42	—	—	—
Bacillus cereus	4–48	4–59	15–?	—
Campylobacter spp.	25–45	—	—	—
Clostridium botulinum				
Proteolytic	12·5–50	15–42	12·5–?	29
Nonproteolytic	3·3–45	5–37	3·3–?	26
Clostridium perfringens	5–50	—	—	37
Escherichia coli	4–45	—	—	—
Listeria monocytogenes	0–45	—	—	—
Salmonella spp.	4–45	—	—	—
Staphyloccocus aureus	6·7–45	—	15–40	37
Vibrio cholerae	10–40	—	—	—
Vibrio parahaemolyticus	5–44	—	—	—
Yersinia enterocolitica	4–42	—	—	—

Data from Gibson DM (1989) Pathogenic bacteria in chilled foods. *In*: Zeuthen P, Cheftel JC, Eriksson C, Gormley TR, Linko P and Paulus K (eds) *Chilled Foods: The Revolution in Freshness, Processing and Quality of Foods*, vol. 3, p 3·53–3·67. London: Elsevier.

slightly raised salt level which gives these products a correspondingly longer shelf life. *L. monocytogenes* is quite capable of withstanding moderately high salt levels, and thus might be allowed unrestricted growth in the absence of competition. The solution to this problem can only be to minimize the presence of *L. monocytogenes* in production premises (and hence in the food), and to limit its potential for growth, if contamination has occurred, by effective temperature control and limiting the shelf life. The former may not only be impractical and expensive, it may also be impossible. Thus, if such products are to continue to exist on our supermarket shelves, low temperatures must be maintained so that high levels of *L. monocytogenes* cannot develop in the product before consumption.

Staphylococcus aureus is not a psychrotrophic pathogen, but it is important to ensure that it is not present in chilled foods, and especially that it has not grown in the ingredients prior to preparation. The organism produces an emetic enterotoxin which is responsible for the disease. Whilst the organism itself is killed by pasteurization, the toxin is exceptionally heat resistant, and may remain in food long after the organism has died. In poorly prepared chilled foods, therefore, staphylococcal food poisoning may result if ingredients in which the organism can grow have been mishandled and kept too warm, even though the final product may have been stored under appropriate chilled conditions until consumption.

Heat Resistance and Postprocess Contamination

Food spoilage depends on many factors, notably the initial flora of the final product and the relative growth rates of the various species present. Because many foods are heat processed, the heat resistance of the species in the initial flora is a major factor in determining the final microflora.

All Gram-negative organisms are heat sensitive and are destroyed at temperatures well below boiling point. Indeed, none have been reported to survive the pasteurization process of 72°C for 15 s which is applied to milk to render it free from pathogens, and any foodstuff which has been given such a heat treatment may be expected to be free from Gram-negative organisms. Most foods, however, are not handled aseptically after heat treatment, and these organisms can regain access as post-process contaminants (PPCs) if strict hygiene is not observed. If the heat-treated product is kept free from PPCs during subsequent chilled storage, only heat-resistant psychrotrophs from the initial microflora (i.e. psychrotrophic spore-formers, *Bacillus* spp. and *Clostridium* spp.) will be able to grow and cause spoilage. Similarly, most pathogens are destroyed by pasteurization and should thus be absent from properly cooked foods. Those food-borne pathogens which may be present in the raw food and survive pasteurization (*B. cereus*, *C. botulinum* and *C. perfringens*) all produce spores, and these may subsequently germinate into vegetative cells if not inhibited either by the product composition (as in cured meats) or the storage temperature (as in pasteurized milk). However, spore germination is often slow or nonexistent at low temperatures (and indeed *C. perfringens* spores may even die during cold storage), and the growth rates of the resulting vegetative cells, even at 10°C, is also low. Thus, these species generally do not appear to be a major concern for properly refrigerated foods.

Because the growth rates of psychrotrophic sporeformers at refrigeration temperatures are much lower than those of the Gram-negative bacteria, pasteurized products which have been packaged to avoid PPCs and subsequently kept under refrigeration may have a considerably extended shelf life (possibly as much as 3–4 times longer than in the presence of Gram-negative PPCs). Storage temperature and the presence of PPCs both affect the spoilage microflora and shelf life in low-acid, high-moisture foods. One or two cells of a Gram-negative psychrotroph per 100 ml of pasteurized milk stored below 11°C can cause proteolytic spoilage and seriously curtail the shelf life. In the absence of PPCs, storage above 11°C permits the growth of thermoduric (Gram-positive), mesophilic microorganisms present in the initial microflora to cause saccharolytic spoilage. Shelf life is the not related to PPCs, but depends on the initial thermoduric microflora.

Postprocess contamination is also especially important in composite foods, such as pizza, which are assembled from a variety of ingredients. Yeasts and moulds found on hard cheese, for example, may be of no consequence in the block of cheese itself, but when cheese is used in the topping for a pizza with a higher a_w, these organisms may become the major spoilage microflora. Apparently minor recipe changes can thus seriously affect the shelf life of a composite food.

On the other hand, reducing the level of contamination is not necessarily the most effective means of extending shelf life. Shelf life depends to a great extent on two factors: the microflora of the food and the temperature at which the food is stored. Reducing either of these factors will extend the shelf life. However, reducing the level of contamination by half would only extend the time taken for spoilage to occur by one generation time. For a psychrotrophic pseudomonad at 7°C, this would be about 7 h. Control of storage temperature is much more effective.

Reducing the storage temperature from 7 to 4°C would halve the growth rate and, therefore, extend shelf life, e.g. from 7 to 14 days. Thus, for extension of shelf life, it is more effective to control temperature than to make minor improvements in production hygiene.

Storage Under Modified Atmospheres

The Gram-negative psychrotrophic bacteria (notably *Pseudomonas* spp.) are mostly highly aerobic and fail to grow in the absence of oxygen. Carbon dioxide has a bacteriostatic effect on them even in the presence of oxygen. Therefore, the microbiological shelf life of many foods can be extended by packaging under vacuum or in an atmosphere containing mixtures of gases. This is particularly important for foods, such as raw meat, which are naturally contaminated with Gram-negative bacteria.

Under modified atmospheres, the main cause of spoilage tends to be the slower-growing psychrotrophic lactobacilli. Vacuum packaging may also encourage the growth of clostridia, especially if low temperatures are not fully maintained. Although many clostridia are merely spoilage organisms, the genus does include *C. botulinum*, which causes the often (and rapidly) fatal disease botulism. Any process which might encourage the growth of this pathogen must be investigated thoroughly.

Reheating of Chilled Foods

Post-process contamination may occur in both the factory and the home. Thus, despite our best efforts at hygienic food production, it is essential that foods are cooled rapidly after heat processing, stored at a low temperature, reheated rapidly to a temperature above the range of growth and held at a high tempertaure before serving. This is especially important in commercial cook–chill operations where foods are reheated and may be held hot for several hours before consumption.

Table 1 shows that pathogenic species may be metabolically active over the temperature range 0–59°C. Generally, foods are not stored at 0°C but should be stored as close to this temperature as is practically possible. At the other end of the range, foods must be held above 59°C to ensure their safety, and indeed the UK Food Hygiene Regulations require that reheated foods are held above 63°C.

It is essential that the food passes through the 'danger zone' as rapidly as possible. Equally, it is important that foods are reheated only once. In the past it has been assumed that some pathogens, such as *Salmonella* and *Listeria*, spp. have a minimum infectious dose so that the ingestion of relatively large numbers of cells was necessary to cause food poisoning. Recent evidence, however, suggests that illness can be caused by the consumption of only a few cells. With susceptible individuals, therefore, it cannot always be assumed that there is a safe level of pathogens in foods.

Each time food is heated or cooled some microbial growth (either of pathogens or of spoilage organisms) is inevitable. Thus, repeated heating and cooling will result in microbial growth and, in the case of pathogens, the organisms may eventually achieve levels in excess of the infectious dose. Furthermore, if foods are repeatedly heated and handled nonaseptically to remove a serving on each occasion, the potential for contamination (e.g. via utensils) is greatly increased. Finally, the danger of food poisoning is further increased, because repeated heating and cooling may destroy the spoilage organisms, allowing pathogens to grow unrestrictedly in the absence of competitors.

Particular care is needed to ensure adequate reheating of food when using microwaves. Although microwave ovens are capable of heating food rapidly, the heating effect within the food may be nonhomogeneous, some parts of the food being raised to near boiling point whilst other parts may barely rise above blood heat. Pathogenic microorganisms, if present, may therefore survive in the cooler parts. This is not likely to be of any major consequence if the food is consumed immediately, as high numbers of pathogens are not likely to be present. However, if the food is not consumed within a few hours, or if it is allowed to cool and is then reheated on another occasion, the surviving pathogens will recolonize the cooked food and may grow to high levels, increasing the risk of food poisoning. Microbial competition is generally not used as a means of preventing the multiplication of pathogens, other than in fermented products such as cheese, yoghurt or fermented meats or vegetables. However, the importance of a competitive spoilage microflora must not be underestimated. Although spoilage organisms may limit the shelf life of the product, their presence does result in sensory spoilage so that the food is discarded before pathogens have been able to grow significantly.

Food poisoning depends on the number of organisms ingested and the susceptibility of the individual – both of which are highly variable factors. In general, however, high numbers of organisms are more likely to result in disease than low numbers. Maintaining food at a low temperature will restrict, if not prevent, the growth of pathogenic microorganisms and thus minimize, but not necessarily eliminate, the risk of food poisoning.

In conclusion, it is neither possible nor desirable that we should live in a sterile environment or eat only foods from which microorganisms have been eradicated. What is important is to minimize the contamination of foods and to limit microbial growth by hygienic production and appropriate storage conditions. In today's technological world, we rely more and more on refrigeration to extend the shelf life and maintain the safety of our food. Unless we also ensure that foods are stored at the correct temperature we are likely to be faced not only with an increase in food poisoning but also unnecessary spoilage at immense cost to the community.

Bibliography

Cousin MA (1982) Presence and activity of psychrotrophic microorganisms in milk and dairy products: a review. *Journal of Food Protection* 45(2): 172–207.

Prentice GA and Neaves P (1988) *Listeria monocytogenes* in food: its significance and methods for its detection. *Bulletin of the International Dairy Federation* 223.

Russel AD and Fuller R (eds) (1979) Cold tolerant microbes in spoilage and the environment. *Society for Applied Bacteriology Technical Series* 13.

Silliker JH, Elliott RP, Baird-Parker AC, Bryan FL, Christian JHB, Clark DS, Olson Jr JC and Roberts TA (eds) (1980) *Microbial Ecology of Foods*, vols I and II. London: International Commission for Microbiological Specifications for Foods/Academic Press, London.

G. A. Prentice
Grampian Food Technology Centre, Aberdeen, UK
P. Neaves
Milk Marketing Board of England and Wales, Thames Ditton, UK

Use of Modified Atmosphere Packaging

Definition of Terms

The preservative effect of chilling can be greatly enhanced when it is combined with control or modification of the gas atmosphere surrounding the food. The normal composition of air by volume is 78% nitrogen (N_2), 21% oxygen (O_2), 0.9% argon (Ar), 0.3% carbon dioxide (CO_2), and traces of nine other gases in very low concentrations. In general, the atmosphere is changed by increasing or decreasing the concentration of O_2, and/or by increasing the concentration of CO_2.

Two terms are in general use concerning procedures that involve changes in the gas atmosphere around perishable produce held in bulk storage. In *controlled-atmosphere storage* (CAS), the gas composition inside a food storage room is carefully monitored, and through the use of adsorbers which remove CO_2, and air vents to increase the O_2 concentration, the atmosphere can be actively controlled to within quite close tolerances. In contrast, *modified-atmosphere storage* (MAS) involves holding the food in an airtight storage room and allowing the respiratory activity of the fresh produce and the growth of microorganisms to change the composition of the atmosphere. Oxygen concentrations as low as 0%, and CO_2 concentrations of 20% or higher can be produced.

In contrast to bulk storage, several terms are used to describe changes in the gas atmosphere inside individual packages of food. *Controlled-atmosphere packaging* (CAP) is, strictly speaking, the enclosure of food in a gas-impermeable package, inside which the gaseous environment with respect to CO_2, O_2, N_2, water vapour and trace gases has been changed and is selectively controlled. Using this definition, there are no CAP systems in commercial use.

Modified-atmosphere packaging (MAP) is the enclosure of food in a package, inside which the atmosphere is modified with respect to CO_2, O_2, N_2, water vapour and trace gases. This modification is generally achieved using one of two processes: by removing air and replacing it with a controlled mixture of gases, a procedure generally referred to as *gas flush packaging*; or by placing the food in a gas impermeable package and removing the air, a procedure known as *vacuum packaging*. In vacuum packaging, elevated CO_2 levels of 10–20% can be produced by microorganisms, as they consume residual O_2, or by respiring produce.

Principal Factors in MAP

The principal factors in a successful MAP operation are as follows: the choice of gas or gas mixture and its effect on the product; the use of a suitable packaging material; and the packaging machine. Overriding all of these is close control of temperature throughout the packaging, distribution and retailing of the MAP products, and this factor is discussed further in the following article.

Choice of Gas

The choice of gas, or gas mixture, used to replace air depends largely on the nature of the food and its principal mode(s) of deterioration. Microbial growth and oxidation are commonly the two major deteriorative modes; thus the concentration of oxygen is frequently reduced and, in some cases, completely removed. Carbon dioxide inhibits the growth of a wide range of microorganisms. In aerobic systems, atmospheres containing 20–30% CO_2 are used (greater concentrations have little additional inhibitory effect on spoilage floras), and in anaerobic systems, atmospheres of 100% CO_2 may be used. *See* Spoilage, Bacterial Spoilage

Carbon dioxide is highly soluble in water and oils and will therefore be absorbed by the food until equilibrium is attained. For example, at $0°C$ and a partial pressure of 101 kPa of CO_2, the solubility of CO_2 is $3·4$ g kg^{-1} of water. In water, more than 99% of the carbon dioxide exists as the dissolved gas, with less than 1% as carbonic acid (H_2CO_3) which partly dissociates to give H^+, HCO_3^-, and CO_3^{2-}. The absorption of CO_2 by moisture in a sealed package creates a partial differential in pressure between the inside and outside of the package, resulting in a partial or complete collapsing of the package around the food, depending on the relative proportions of product and gas.

Nitrogen is used to purge air from a package to achieve a sufficiently low level of O_2 to prevent aerobic microbial spoilage. It also frequently functions as a filler gas in MAP to reduce the concentration of other gases in the package and to keep the package from collapsing as CO_2 dissolves into the product.

Since containers for gas packaging are comparatively good gas barriers, the internal atmosphere will be modified by the food during storage. The relative volumes of gas and food are therefore important in determining the progress of the changes in concentration of gases during storage, and cognizance must also be taken of the high solubility of CO_2 compared to the relatively low solubility of O_2 and N_2 in foods.

Choice of Packaging Material

The choice of packaging material is an important factor in any MAP operation. A low water vapour transmission rate, together with a high gas barrier must generally be achieved. Virtually all MA packages are based on thermoplastic polymers. A point that should be remembered is that all packages made purely from such materials allow some gas transmission, even at chill temperatures. Thus, over the relatively long storage times for which many MAP foods are held, there will be transport of gases through the package walls. The comparative dearth of gas permeability data for thermoplastic polymers at chill temperatures and high relative humidities makes prediction of the extent of such gas transport tenuous.

The packaging material also needs to have the mechanical strength to withstand machine handling and subsequent storage, distribution and retailing. Materials in use are laminations or coextrusions of polyethylene with polyester or nylon, with or without the addition of a 'high' barrier layer of vinylidene chloride–vinyl chloride copolymer or ethylene–vinyl alcohol copolymer, depending on the barrier required.

Choice of Packaging Machinery

Packaging machinery requirements are obviously related to methods of packaging, of which there are principally two: thermoforming and pillow packaging. The thermoforming method involves the use of a rigid or semirigid base material which is thermoformed into a tray. After loading of the product, the tray passes into a chamber in which the air is evacuated and the desired gas or gases introduced. Simultaneously, a top lidding material is drawn over the tray and sealed to the lip edge. This system has the advantage of being able to evacuate air from the package before flushing with gas so that, in

Use of Modified Atmosphere Packaging

the case of cellular products, a low residual O_2 level in the package can be achieved.

The pillow wrap or horizontal form-fill-seal machine employs a single reel of flexible packaging material which is formed into a tube and the two edges are heat sealed. The product is passed into this tube which is vented of air with a flushing gas prior to sealing.

Applications of MAP

MAP has found application in three major groups of foods: flesh foods, horticultural products and cereal-based products. Each of these will be discussed in turn.

Flesh Foods

Fresh Meat

The use of increased concentrations of CO_2 to extend the shelf life of chilled meat is hardly a new technique, having been devised by Moran and co-workers at the Low Temperature Research Station in Cambridge, England, in the early 1930s. However, it only became a commercial reality for retail packaging during the 1970s. The systems used for MAP of fresh meat can be classified into three categories: high-oxygen, low-oxygen and high-carbon-dioxide.

High-oxygen MAP

High-oxygen MAP systems, which have atmospheres of about 30% CO_2 and up to 70% O_2, are used both to extend the colour stability and to delay microbial spoilage of display-packaged meat. The commercial objective is usually to obtain a product life sufficient to permit meat cutting and retail pack preparation at a central facility. Although the colour stability and the time to spoilage are approximately doubled by high-O_2 MAP, this extension in shelf life is not wholly adequate for many commercial purposes; its suitability for display packaging will depend largely on commercial circumstances.

Low-oxygen MAP

Carbon dioxide gas flush In these packages, the air is largely displaced by CO_2, either by itself or mixed with N_2. In general, the shelf life extension is similar to that achieved with vacuum packaging, higher concentrations of CO_2 leading to a longer shelf life.

Nitrogen gas flush Although the formation of metmyoglobin on the surface is reduced when the package is flushed with N_2, the N_2 also dilutes the CO_2 produced by tissue respiration, prolonging the time required for the concentration to accumulate to levels sufficient to inhibit growth of spoilage bacteria.

Despite there being little commercial use of N_2 flushing with fresh meat, several studies have confirmed that 100% N_2 is as effective as vacuum for storing fresh meat joints, the only advantage being reduced exudate, caused by less mechanical pressure on the meat compared to when it was vacuum packaged.

High-carbon-dioxide MAP

The solubility of CO_2 in muscle tissue of pH 5·5 at 0°C is approximately 960 ml kg^{-1} of tissue at standard temperature and pressure (STP). As the temperature increases, the solubility decreases by 19 ml kg^{-1} for each 1°C rise. As tissue pH increases, the solubility decreases by 360 ml kg^{-1} for each pH unit. If CO_2 alone is added, the pack will collapse around the meat as gas is absorbed, unless CO_2 is added in excess of the quantity required to saturate the meat at atmospheric pressure. When mixtures of gases are used, the less soluble N_2 and unrespired components of the gas mixture maintain a volume of gas at atmospheric pressure around the meat that is less than the volume added initially.

Until recently, concern has been expressed about the discoloration of the surface of meat stored in high concentrations of CO_2. It is unlikely, however, that CO_2 is the cause of such discoloration, traces of O_2 remaining in the package after evacuation being a more likely reason. Vacuum packing lamb in gas-permeable bags before packaging them in a 'master' foil-laminate bag with CO_2 has resulted in storage lives of up to 16 weeks at −1°C.

Poultry

Although most poultry meat used to be sold in the form of whole, oven-ready carcasses, there is now an increasing demand for cut-up portions and a variety of other further processed products, both raw and cooked.

Atmospheres enriched with CO_2 have been advocated for extending the shelf life of poultry products. For chicken meat, 20% CO_2 can be as effective as 80% over one week's storage at 2°C, but higher levels are needed for longer shelf life. Storage lives of up to 35 days have been obtained under certain closely controlled conditions.

A wide range of manufactured poultry products has been developed, including rolls, roasts, burgers and sausages. However, in most cases very little information is available on either keeping quality or the influence on shelf life of particular gas mixtures and packaging materials.

Use of Modified Atmosphere Packaging

Fish

Commercial use of MAP to extend the shelf life of fishery products has been limited by the potential of *Clostridium botulinum* growth and toxin production in refrigerated, MAP fish, without any sensory evidence of spoilage. Despite these concerns, fillets of fresh fish in MAPs stored continuously at temperatures below $3°C$ have appeared in European supermarkets. No cases of botulism have been associated with the consumption of such products thus far. *See Clostridium*, Occurrence of *Clostridium botulinum*; Fish, Spoilage

Effective gas compositions vary according to fish species, with low O_2 concentrations being used with fatty fish which are susceptible to oxidative rancidity. In general, gas mixtures for nonfatty fish would be 30% O_2, 40% CO_2 and 30% N_2, and for smoked and fatty fish 40% CO_2 and 60% N_2.

Problems caused by a CO_2 level that is too high include pack collapse, increased drip, CO_2 taint which gives an acid flavour to certain species of fish, and clouding of the eyes.

Although some claims have been made of a shelf life of up to 3–4 weeks for the refrigerated storage of MAP fish, this is generally considered to be unrealistic. General target shelf lives of these products are in the range of 10–14 days, but may reach 18–20 days if the temperature is very tightly controlled.

Horticultural Products

Fresh Fruit and Vegetables

In contrast to the flesh foods discussed above, fruit and vegetables are still living tissues when they are held in MAP. The techniques for increasing the shelf life of apples by holding them in atmospheres containing very low O_2 and high CO_2 were first devised by Kidd and West at the Low Temperature Research Station in Cambridge, England, in the 1920s. In 1932 they reported on its use with tomatoes. Polymeric films have been used for packaging of horticultural products since the 1940s. Early work in the area stressed the primary role of packaging to reduce transpiration, with many studies encouraging film perforation to avoid the development of injurious atmospheres in packages.

Today, interest centres on the development of non-perforated polymeric films which have the desired permeability characteristics so that MAs appropriate for the particular commodity and its storage temperature can be developed and maintained. In addition, the film must have the ability to cope with fluctuating storage conditions (e.g. temperature, humidity and light) without injurious atmospheres developing.

Despite almost 50 years of research and hundreds of publications reporting the many experiments that have been conducted in this area, there is surprisingly little commercialization of MAP for horticultural produce.

Two methods of creating MA conditions within packages of fruit and vegetables are used: passive MA and active MA.

Passive MA

An atmosphere high in CO_2 and low in O_2 passively evolves within a sealed package over time as a result of the respiration of the commodity. Ideally, the gas permeabilities of the packaging film are such that sufficient O_2 can enter the package to avoid the occurrence of anoxic conditions and anaerobic respiration; at the same time, excess CO_2 can diffuse from the package to avoid injuriously high levels. Given the simplicity of this approach and the many interrelated variables that affect respiration rate, it would indeed be surprising if appropriate passive MA systems could be developed for all horticultural commodities.

Active MA

The air inside the package is removed, by pulling a vacuum, and then replaced with a specific gas mixture, thus creating the desired MA immediately after packaging (compare this to the passive approach, which may require a week or longer before achieving the same gas composition).

In addition, several types of adsorbers are available which can be used inside the package to delay the climacteric rise in respiration for some fruits by adsorbing ethylene (C_2H_4); to prevent the build-up of CO_2 to injurious levels by adsorbing CO_2, and to lower the concentration of O_2 through the use of O_2 adsorbers. Obviously, the use of gas adsorbers adds considerably to the cost, so that their use is limited to those commodities for which it is cost-effective. Recently, films which have the ability to adsorb gases (in particular, C_2H_4) have been developed and their use is likely to become widespread.

Few polymeric films have gas permeabilities that make them suitable to use for MAP. Those most likely to be suitable include low-density polyethylene, plasticized poly(vinyl chloride), polystyrene and ethylene-vinyl acetate copolymer.

Cereal-based Foods

Fresh Pasta

The production of pasta involves kneading of the dough, followed by extrusion or lamination and then drawing. In the case of special pasta, this latter stage is accompanied by filling, using a cooked meat or vegetable–cheese mixture, thus resulting in a wide variety of microbiological flora.

Fresh pasta products are not usually subjected to pasteurization but are refrigerated for retail distribution. The microbiological quality of fresh pasta will thus depend on the quality of the raw materials, the cleanliness and hygiene of the processing environment and equipment, and the handling of the product during production and packaging. In addition, the temperature of the product during storage, distribution and retailing is crucial with respect to microbiological quality. *See* Pasta and Macaroni, Methods of Manufacture

The use of MAP has become widespread for fresh pasta products. Typical gas compositions used are 100% N_2 or 70–80% CO_2 and 20–30% N_2, the pasta having a recommended shelf life of around 4 weeks when stored at 4°C.

The actual packaging materials used for fresh pasta products depend on whether or not the product is pasteurized (in which case the package must be able to withstand the pasteurization process without deforming) and whether or not the product is to be heated in its package in a microwave by the consumer (in which case the package must be able to withstand domestic microwave temperatures). For products that are not pasteurized, nor intended to be heated in their package, a rigid tray of poly(vinyl chloride)–polyethylene, onto which is sealed a polyamide–polyethylene film, is common. However, if microwave heating is used, the rigid tray is usually made from crystalline polyethylene terephthalate, and the film may be based on vinylidene chloride-vinyl chloride copolymer-coated polypropylene or polyethylene terephthalate.

Refrigerated Dough Products

Refrigerated leavened batters and doughs for biscuits, nut breads and the like have been commercially packaged in tubes made of double-wound vinylidene chloride–vinyl chloride copolymer clipped at both ends. The clips are applied to a continuous tube full of the batter, the diffusion of O_2 and CO_2 into and out of the package being hindered not only by the tightly bunched film at the ends of the tube, but also by the dried batter filling the interstices.

For biscuit and roll doughs, the usual container is the composite spiral-wound can, the cylindrical body of which is composed mainly of aluminium foil laminated to kraft paper. The lid is of tin plate and is made to fit tightly into the end of the can. The cans are not completely filled at the time of sealing but, as the leavening system continues to produce CO_2, the dough expands so that it ultimately fills the can completely and

exerts a pressure of 30·3–131·3 kPa. The sealed cans can be warmed for a few hours to accelerate the gassing reaction.

Normal shelf life is considered to be about 13 weeks and depends on the season, type of product and efficiency of the distribution system. Spoilage is indicated when the can bursts as a result of increased internal pressure (the result of metabolic activities of yeasts and bacteria) or of weakening of the can's structure as liquid leaks from the interior of the can into the fibre body. *See* Spoilage, Yeasts in Food Spoilage

Bibliography

Brody AL (ed.) (1989) *Controlled/Modified Atmosphere/Vacuum Packaging of Foods.* Trumball, Connecticut: Food and Nutrition Press.

Gill CO (1990) Controlled atmosphere packaging of chilled meat. *Food Control* 2: 74–78.

Inns R (1987) Modified atmosphere packaging. In: Paine FA (ed.) *Modern Processing, Packaging and Distribution Systems for Food,* chapter 3. Glasgow: Blackie and Son.

Matz SA (1989) *Bakery Technology: Packaging, Nutrition, Product Development, Quality Assurance.* Essex: Elsevier Science Publishers.

Robertson GL (1992) *Food Packaging: Principles and Practice.* New York: Marcel Dekker.

G. L. Robertson
Department of Consumer Technology, Massey University, New Zealand

Effect of Modified Atmosphere Packaging on Food Quality

Quality is taken to include microbial quality, chemical quality and sensory quality, and all these combine to produce a product which is appealing, safe and nutritious to consume until the end of its intended shelf life.

The shelf life and quality of any MAP (modified-atmosphere packaging) food is influenced by a number of factors. These include the nature of the food, the gaseous environment inside the package, the nature of the package, the storage temperature, and the packaging process and machinery.

Gaseous Environment

The presence of carbon dioxide (CO_2) is important because of its biostatic activity against many spoilage organisms which grow at chill temperatures. In general, the inhibitory effects of CO_2 increase with decreasing temperature, primarily because of the increased solubility of CO_2 at lower temperatures; dissolution of CO_2

in water lowers the pH and consequently slows reaction rates. The overall effect of CO_2 is to increase both the lag phase and the generation time of spoilage microorganisms; however, the specific mechanism for the bacteriostatic effect is not known.

While CO_2 inhibits some types of microorganisms, it has no effect on others. Furthermore, to be an effective biostat, it must dissolve into the aqueous portion of the product. Although the growth of anaerobic pathogens will be inhibited by the presence of oxygen (O_2), the shelf life of the food will not necessarily be extended. *See* Spoilage, Bacterial Spoilage

Temperature

Temperature is the single most important factor which influences the quality of MAP foods. The rates of deteriorative reactions in foods, whether they be enzymic, chemical or biochemical, as well as the rates of microbial growth, depend very much on the temperature, and the desired shelf life of MAP foods will only be achieved if the temperature is kept closely controlled during storage. *See* Spoilage, Chemical and Enzymatic Spoilage

One of the major concerns with MAP foods is temperature abuse, i.e. holding the food at temperatures above chill temperatures, such that the growth of pathogens is accelerated. In addition, because the biostatic effects of CO_2 are temperature-dependent, a rise in temperature during storage could permit the growth of microorganisms which had been inhibited by CO_2 at lower temperatures. If O_2 were present in the package, growth of aerobic spoilage organisms during periods when the food was at nonrefrigerated temperatures would alert consumers to temperature abuse via the appearance of undesirable odours, colours or slime. However, the absence of O_2 will favour the growth of anaerobic microorganisms (including *Clostridium botulinum*) over aerobic spoilage organisms. It should be noted that both aerobic and anaerobic pathogens can grow at temperatures as low as 4°C and produce toxin without any sensory manifestation of food deterioration. *See* Clostridium, Occurrence of *Clostridium botulinum*

Food Safety

Although much information exists in the general area of MAP technology, research on the microbiological safety of these foods is still lacking. The great vulnerability of MAP foods from a safety standpoint is that with many modified atmospheres containing moderate to high levels of CO_2, the aerobic spoilage organisms which usually warn consumers of spoilage are inhibited, while the growth of pathogens may be allowed or even stimulated.

In the past, the major concerns have been the anaerobic pathogens, especially the psychrotrophic, nonproteolytic clostridia. However, because of the emergence of psychrotrophic pathogens such as *Listeria monocytogenes*, *Aeromonas hydrophilia* and *Yersinia enterocolitica*, new safety issues have been raised. This stems mainly from the fact that the extended shelf life of many MAP products may allow extra time for these pathogens to reach dangerously high levels in foods. *See* Aeromonas; *Listeria*, Properties and Occurrence; *Yersinia enterocolitica*, Properties and Occurrence

To minimize problems with pathogens inside MAP foods, the foods should be of the highest microbiological quality at the time of packaging; they should be processed and packaged under high standards of hygiene and sanitation; their temperature should be reduced as rapidly as possible, and the temperature during distribution should be rigidly maintained as low as required to avoid anaerobic pathogen growth. If the above requirements are compromised in any way, serious public health hazards could result from ingestion of the MAP food.

Quality of Specific MAP Foods

Flesh Foods

Fresh Meat

Appearance is probably the most important attribute by which consumers judge the quality of meat. In particular, colour is regarded by the consumer, rightly or wrongly, as an indication of freshness and good quality. In fact, there is little correlation between the colour of raw meat and eating quality, but the mistaken belief that there is remains, and maintaining optimum colour during retailing has become one of the prime objectives of meat packaging.

Myoglobin is the principal pigment of fresh meat and the form that it takes is of prime importance in determining the colour of the meat. The colour of fresh meat depends chiefly on the relative amounts of the three pigment derivatives of myoglobin present at the surface: reduced myoglobin, oxymyoglobin and metmyoglobin. Reduced myoglobin is purple in colour and predominates in the absence of oxygen. The bright red colour of oxymyoglobin results when reduced myoglobin is oxygenated or exposed to oxygen; this is commonly known as 'bloom'. Metmyoglobin is brown in colour and exists when the oxygen concentration is between 0·5% and 1%, or when meat is exposed to air for long periods of time. *See* Meat, Structure

The O_2 level during storage determines the effectiveness of colour retention. Many workers have concluded that mixtures of 75–80% O_2 with 25–15% CO_2 are the most effective, but there have been reports of off-odours

Effect of Modified Atmosphere Packaging on Food Quality

and rancidity in meats stored in high O_2 concentrations. Both the colour stability and time to spoilage are approximately doubled by high-O_2 MAP. However, because O_2 is respired and CO_2 is highly soluble in meat, the package atmosphere tends to alter as storage proceeds, and high-O_2 MAP is thus not suitable for prolonged storage of red meat.

In low-O_2 MAP systems when air has been largely displaced by CO_2, red meats rapidly discolour because of the low oxygen concentrations. Consequently, a low-O_2 MAP system is generally considered unsuitable for use in retail packs of red meats.

As an inert gas, nitrogen is convenient for gas packaging; it is generally considered a neutral filler as it influences neither the colour of the meat nor its microbiological quality. If the air in the package is removed prior to the addition of nitrogen, the effect on meat is similar to that of vacuum packaging, except that residual oxygen is diluted and metmyoglobin formation on the surface should be less pronounced than with a vacuum.

While colour may be the most visible quality feature, the main cause of deterioration is the growth of microorganisms on the meat surface. If allowed to develop freely, they may cause undesirable odours and flavours, and eventually make the meat unsaleable. The bacteria that develop on fresh meat stored in air are mainly pseudomonads, which grow rapidly and are responsible for the putrefactive spoilage which normally ends shelf life. They do not grow in the absence of O_2 and are also inhibited by concentrations of CO_2 in excess of 20%. Lactic acid bacteria grow readily in the absence of O_2 and in the presence of CO_2. *See* Lactic Acid Bacteria; Meat, Preservation

In high-O_2 MAP, growth of aerobic organisms is inhibited, but not suppressed, by moderate concentrations of CO_2. In low-O_2 MAP, the inhibitory effect of CO_2 on the aerobic flora is augmented, to various degrees, by limited availability of O_2, and the CO_2 concentration may be sufficiently high to slow the growth of species tolerant to anaerobic conditions. In high-CO_2 MAP, O_2 deprivation prevents growth of aerobic species, while high concentrations of CO_2 inhibit growth of the species tolerant of anaerobic conditions.

Successful packaging must therefore maintain the attractive appearance of the meat and delay microbiological spoilage. The composition of the gas atmosphere in MAP determines both the colour of the meat and the nature of the microbiological spoilage which develops on its surface.

Poultry

Raw poultry meat is a perishable commodity of relative high pH (5·7–6·7) which readily supports the growth of microorganisms when stored under chill or ambient conditions. The organisms most often associated with foodborne disease in poultry and poultry products include (in order of importance) *Salmonella* spp., *Staphylococcus aureus*, *Clostridium perfringens*, and then *Bacillus cereus* and *Campylobacter jejuni*. With respect to the safety of MAP chicken, the possible problem organisms would be *Campylobacter jejuni*, which may be able to survive better in a MAP product, and *Listeria monocytogenes* and *Aeromonas hydrophilia*, which may, because of the extended storage lives of the MAP products, have an additional time to grow to potentially high numbers. Although *Clostridium perfringens* may be able to survive better in some MAP than in air, it would not be able to grow at the chill temperatures commonly used for MAP products. Most studies on the extension of shelf life using CO_2 in MAPs have concentrated on the suppression of spoilage organisms rather than the survival and growth of pathogens. *See Bacillus*, Occurrence; Campylobacter, Properties and Occurrence; *Clostridium*, Occurrence of *Clostridium perfringens*; Poultry, Chicken; Poultry, Ducks and Geese; Poultry, Turkey; *Staphylococcus*, Properties and Occurrence

Fish

Spoilage of fish results from changes brought about by chemical reactions such as oxidation, reactions due to the fish's own enzymes, and the metabolic activities of microorganisms. Although the chemical composition and microbial flora of fish vary considerably between species, different fishing grounds and season, spoilage of salt- and freshwater fish appears to occur in essentially the same manner. *See* Fish, Spoilage

However, there are significant differences in the application of MAP to meats, including poultry, and to fish. It is generally accepted that the internal flesh of healthy, live fish is sterile; microorganisms that exist on fresh fish are generally found in the gills, the outer slime, and the intestines. The post mortem changes leading to spoilage depend principally on the chemical composition of the fish, its microbial flora and subsequent handling, processing and storage.

Immediately post mortem, a whole series of tissue enzyme reactions begin the process of autolysis (basically, self-digestion of the fish muscle) which leads eventually to spoilage. The autolytic enzyme reactions predominate for 4–6 days at 0°C, after which the products of bacterial activity become increasingly evident with the appearance of undesirable odours and flavours. The rates of the autolytic changes are determined by many factors, the most important being temperature, pH, availability of O_2 and the physiological condition of the fish before death.

As spoilage proceeds, there is a gradual invasion of the flesh by bacteria from the outer surfaces. Breakdown

Effect of Modified Atmosphere Packaging on Food Quality

of the muscle structure only occurs after spoilage has proceeded well beyond the point of rejection. The development of objectionable slimes, odours and flavours results mainly from bacterial activity.

The third type of spoilage is chemical spoilage, primarily oxidation of the fat compounds leading to the development of rancid flavours. Because fish has a much higher content of polyunsaturated fat than meat, it is more prone to the development of oxidative or rancid flavours.

The effects of MAP on fish are similar to those described above for meat and poultry. The normal spoilage bacteria which cause off-odours and flavours are inhibited, and microorganisms not usually involved in aerobic spoilage eventually predominate. These are microorganisms such as streptococci and lactobacilli, which are less affected by the elevated CO_2 atmosphere and which grow more slowly than the normal aerobic spoilage bacteria. Because the microorganisms that predominate under MAP also cause less noticeable and less offensive organoleptic changes, the net result is a significant extension of shelf life under MAP at refrigeration temperatures.

It must be stressed that MAP alone is not capable of providing the safety required for extended storage of fish with respect to outgrowth and toxin production by *C. botulinum* type E in the absence of a fail-safe mechanism by which storage temperature could be maintained at 0°C. In order to effectively utilize the extended shelf life aspect of MAP, some intervention is needed to assure the delay of toxin production should even mild temperature abuse occur.

High temperature abuse (21–27°C) for periods of 12–24 h is a major concern since MAP fish generally do not become overtly spoiled under these conditions, yet may be toxic, whereas fish held at the same temperatures under similar aerobic conditions begin to become putrid before toxin production occurs. If MAP fish are held at very high refrigeration temperatures (greater than 10°C), no strong spoilage signals develop in advance of *C. botulinum* toxin production.

Fruit and Vegetables

Fruit and vegetables are living tissues and therefore respire during storage. Respiration involves the oxidation of energy-rich organic substrates, normally present in cells, such as starch, sugars and organic acids, to simpler molecules (CO_2 and H_2O) with the concurrent production of energy and other molecules which can be used by the cell for synthetic reactions. When the process takes place in the presence of molecular oxygen, respiration is said to be aerobic. If hexose sugar is used as the substrate, the overall equation can be written as follows:

$$C_6H_{12}O_6 + 6O_2 \rightleftharpoons 6CO_2 + 6H_2O + energy \qquad (1)$$

Temperature is the most important environmental factor in the post-harvest life of horticultural products because of its dramatic effect on the rates of biological reactions, including respiration.

A simple consideration of equation (1) suggests that if the CO_2 in the atmosphere were augmented (or the O_2 decreased), the respiration rate and the storage life would be extended. Reduction of the O_2 concentration to less than 10% provides a tool for controlling the respiration rate and slowing down senescence, although an adequate O_2 concentration must be available to maintain aerobic respiration.

The respiration rate of a commodity inside a polymeric film package depends on the kind of commodity, its stage of maturity and physical condition, the concentrations of O_2, CO_2 and ethylene (C_2H_4) inside the package, the quantity of product within the package, the temperature and, possibly, the intensity of light. Suffice it to say that the interplay of these factors leads to a complex situation about which it is difficult to make quantitative predictions.

It is impossible to make any specific predictions about the magnitude of the effect of a change in temperature on MAP since a number of key, interrelated factors are involved. Any change in temperature will affect the respiration rate; it will also affect gas diffusion between the cell sap and the intercellular spaces, the solubility of gases in liquids decreasing with increasing temperature. In addition, any change in temperature will affect the permeability of the plastic film surrounding the fruit or vegetable.

Cereal-based Products

Fresh Pasta

Fresh pasta is a low-acid product (pH > 4·6). Some manufacturers pasteurize the pasta after packaging, using hot air and/or microwaves. These pasteurized fresh pasta products fall into the category of REPFEDs, i.e. refrigerated, processed foods with extended durability. If the pasteurization process is carried out adequately, all vegetative bacteria and moulds present are killed. However, spores of many bacteria (including *C. botulinum*) can survive the heating process. If these foods are stored at temperatures between 3·3°C and 10°C, there may be risk of botulism if spores of group II (nonproteolytic strains) survive the heating process during preparation. *See* Pasta and Macaroni, Methods of Manufacture

Effect of Modified Atmosphere Packaging on Food Quality

Heating before consumption may not always be sufficient to ensure complete inactivation of botulism toxin. In order to ensure that the risk of botulism from these foods is adequately controlled, REPFEDS must be stored at a temperature lower than 3·3°C. If this temperature cannot be guaranteed, the storage time has to be limited. In temperature-abused products it has been shown that the a_w of fresh pasta is a principal factor in preventing botulinal toxin production by proteolytic *C. botulinum*; while most flat noodles are below the a_w limit for botulinal toxin production, most filled pasta has a_w values which permit toxin production if temperature abuse occurs.

Refrigerated Dough

The three preservation principles relied upon in refrigerated doughs are (1) an anaerobic atmosphere resulting from the generation of CO_2 by a leavening system, (2) relatively low water activities in the aqueous phase of the dough or batter, and (3) low temperatures (0–5°C) at which the products are stored and distributed. These conditions are generally met without any great difficulty and no serious quality problems have been reported with this class of MAP product. *See* Water Activity, Effect on Food Stability

Bibliography

Brody AL (ed.) (1989) *Controlled/Modified Atmosphere/Vacuum Packaging of Foods*. Trumball, Connecticut: Food and Nutrition Press.

Farber JM (1991) Microbiological aspects of modified-atmosphere packaging technology – a review. *Journal of Food Protection* 54: 58–70.

Gill CO (1990) Controlled atmosphere packaging of chilled meat. *Food Control* 2: 74–78.

Robertson GL (1992) *Food Packaging: Principles and Practice*. New York: Marcel Dekker.

G. L. Robertson
Department of Consumer Technology, Massey University, New Zealand

Packaging Under Vacuum

The Role of Oxygen in Food Spoilage

The presence of oxygen is one of the major factors of spoilage of foods and causes:

(1) oxidation reactions, damaging vitamins, fatty substances, pigments, flavouring substances which are often catalysed by enzymes;

(2) growth and activity of aerobic microorganisms (aerobic bacteria, yeasts, moulds). *See* Oxidation of Food Components

It is therefore essential, in order to prolong the freshness of foodstuffs, to eliminate the presence of oxygen in contact with the foodstuff itself and to prevent further access of oxygen during storage. Vacuum packaging is one of the simplest and most widely used systems to achieve this objective. This type of packaging has encountered an increasing success starting from the late 1950s, in parallel with the development of the technology of plastics owing also to the changes in the distribution chain of perishable foods requiring increased hygiene and storage life.

This article outlines the principles of vacuum-packaging technology, the features of the packages utilized and describes the main fields of application of vacuum packaging to chilled foods.

Vacuum Packaging: A Definition

'Vacuum packaging' is a term improperly but commonly used to define a packaging system which implies the reduction of the partial pressure of atmospheric gases (oxygen being 20% of them) inside a package. A vacuum inside a package can be obtained mainly through two systems:

- steam flushing of the headspace;
- sucking of air from the package headspace by means of equipment (vacuum chamber, nozzle) based on a vacuum pump.

The former system is mainly utilized in hot packaging of shelf-stable products which are generally packaged in rigid containers. The elimination of air is achieved by means of a steam flush which replaces atmospheric gases inside the package; steam condensation in the package headspace after chilling reduces the inner gaseous pressure. The latter system is the one commonly utilized for packaging of perishable foodstuffs which have to be stored in chilled conditions. In this case, packaging equipment based on a vacuum pump is generally utilized in combination with flexible packages which, after evacuation, are closed hermetically (by means of a seal or sometimes a tight clip) and collapse on the packaged product once the package is exposed to atmospheric pressure. Depending on the type of equipment employed, a residual pressure of atmospheric gases as low as 500 Pa can be obtained in the package.

Figure 1 illustrates the main systems utilized for evacuating flexible packages:

(1) nozzle (Fig. 1(a));
(2) single vacuum chamber (Fig. 1(b));
(3) divided vacuum chamber (Fig. 1(c)).

Packaging Materials Utilized for Vacuum Packaging

Plastics are the main raw material utilized for manufacturing the flexible materials employed in vacuum packaging of chilled foods. These materials must have the following properties:

- flexibility;
- mechanical resistance to various forms of abuse (abrasion, puncture, flex cracking);
- gas barrier properties adequate to the application requirements (generally expressed as gas permeation rates);
- thermosealability or clippability;
- good optics (haze and gloss);
- printability;
- suitable dimensional behaviour (dimensional stability to heat, formability after heating, shrinkability after heating).

To combine and balance to the required level the above properties it is often necessary to mix different types of individual materials. Different resins can be mixed together (resin blends), resin additives (such as plasticizers, pigments, stabilizers, slip agents, etc.) can be used and, more commonly, a multilayer material is produced, each layer being composed of a distinct individual material which imparts its properties to the overall structure.

Individual components most commonly used in manufacturing flexible materials utilized for vacuum packaging are listed below, together with their abbreviations and main properties:

- polyethylene (PE)—sealability, formability, moisture barrier, low cost;
- polypropylene (PP)—moisture barrier, thermal resistance, dimensional stability;
- ethylene–vinylacetate copolymer (EVA)—easy sealability, thermal shrink properties;
- ionomers—mechanical strength, easy sealability, grease resistance, formability;
- polyamides (PA)—mechanical strength, gas barrier, formability;
- polyesters (PET)—mechanical resistance, heat resistance, gas barrier;
- ethylene–vinylalcohol copolymer (EVOH)—gas barrier, easy processability in coextrusion;
- polyvinylidenechloride (PVDC)—gas barrier, grease barrier.

PE, PP, EVA and ionomers are classified in the wide family of resins called polyolefins. Aluminium foils and vacuum-metallized plastic films are also utilized because of the excellent gas barrier properties of aluminium.

Multilayer materials are manufactured using various techniques:

(1) coextrusion—the molten resins are combined in the final structure by extruding them through a round or flat extrusion die which keeps them separate in discrete layers;
(2) lamination—previously extruded plastic films and, sometimes, aluminium foil, are joined together by means of glues (glue lamination) or with resins which have adhesive properties (extrusion lamination);
(3) coating—pre-extruded films are coated with a layer of molten or dissolved resin (a latex).

Package Configurations Used for Vacuum Packaging of Chilled Foods

These can be classified into four main categories: shrink bags such as Cryovac*, pouches, thermoformed packages, and skin packages such as Darfresh*.

Shrink Bags

Shrink bags are available in the form of premade bags which can be prepared in different packages (e.g. taped bags) to allow their utilization on automatic equipment. The main feature of these bags is their capability to shrink when exposed for a short time to heat (for instance a few seconds at 90°C). This behaviour is the consequence of treatment imparted to the packaging material during its production (oriented polymeric chains which retain a built-in tension, making them able to shrink when relaxed by heating).

Shrinking increases the packaging material thickness (which varies between 40 and 120 μm), improving mechanical resistance and gas barrier properties, determines a tighter package around the product, limiting dripping out of juices in moist products such as meat, and improves the appearance by eliminating excess of packaging material around the product. Shrink bags at the onset of their introduction on the market in the 1950s were monolayer PVDC materials, but subsequent technological evolution gave rise to complex coextruded multilayer structures having polyolefins as the main components and gas barrier layers made of PVDC or EVOH.

Some materials are electronically cross-linked to improve mechanical properties.

Shrink bags are used for vacuum packaging of industrial units of fresh meat, processed meat and cheese, and for consumer units of processed meat and cheese.

Cryovac* and Darfresh* are registered trademarks of W. R. GRACE.

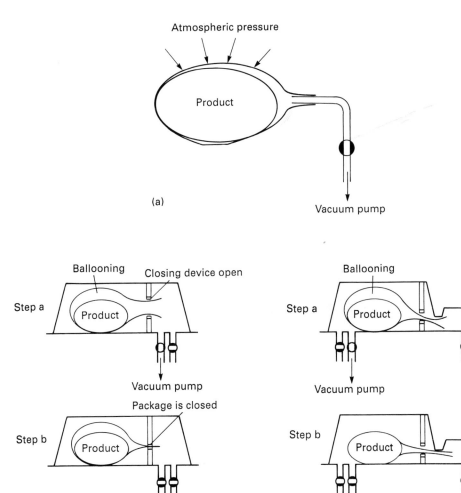

Fig. 1 The main systems utilized for obtaining vacuum packages. (a) The nozzle system. Air is extracted from the package (a bag or a pouch) through a nozzle and then the package is closed. This is the simplest way of extracting the air, however, it does not allow high levels of vacuum in the package. (b) This is the most common system utilized for evacuating bags, pouches and thermoformed packages. (c) Divided vacuum chamber. This allows better evacuation of the package headspace by using two separate chambers where a vacuum is applied sequentially.

Pouches

Pouches can be utilized in two forms:

- premade plastic envelopes of different sizes which are loaded with the product, then evacuated and sealed in vacuum chambers;
- in-line prepared pouches from machines using rollstock material (horizontal form fill seal and vertical form fill seal machines).

The above machines, starting from a flat web, produce a film tubing which can be either horizontal or vertical (hence the different definitions) which is filled with the product, sealed transversely and cut into final packages.

The machines can be equipped with a vacuum chamber to evacuate the pouch before final sealing. Form fill seal machines are widely employed in food packaging; however, their utilization for vacuum packaging of perishable foods is rather limited as thermoforming is preferred whenever a high packaging output and automation of packaging operation is required.

Premade pouches are commonly utilized for vacuum packaging of industrial units of fresh red meat such as whole primal cuts, processed meat (ham, bacon, salami, bologna) and cheese. Typical structures of materials for pouches, obtained by means of glue or extrusion lamination, are based on bioriented PA6 or PET (biorientation plus heat setting enhances dimensional stability and mechanical resistance) which can be coated with PVDC to increase gas barrier properties and are laminated to suitable sealing layers (PE, EVA or PP and ionomers when heat resistance for pasteurization or cooking in the package is requested). For long storage life applications (pasteurized cooked ham or sausages) where maximum gas barrier properties are needed, aluminium foil is also used.

The total thickness of the above materials varies between 70 and 250 μm, the higher thicknesses being employed for heavy and hard products.

Thermoformed Packages

These are obtained on continuous thermoforming machines which use rollstock materials. Two rolls are used, one for the bottom web which is unwound, heated by a warm plate and formed into cavities where the product to be packaged is subsequently loaded, and a second one, the top web, which is sealed onto the bottom web inside a vacuum chamber from which the air has been removed. Thermoforming is widely applied to packaging of perishable foodstuffs because of the flexibility of the process, the packaging speed and the ease of automation.

A wide variety of packaging materials is utilized. Bottom webs are generally based on PA laminated or coextruded with all types of polyolefins. PVDC or EVOH are used when high gas barrier properties are needed. Some bottom webs are also heat shrinkable after thermoforming.

Top webs are generally laminated structures similar to the ones used for pouches, the thickness of which seldom exceeds 100 μm. Metallized materials are often used in the top web formulation.

Thermoforming is utilized for packaging many kinds of perishable products, both consumer and industrial units, including whole ham and fresh meat primal cuts, with the exception of the biggest units of cheese and processed meat.

Skin Packages

Skin packaging represents an evolution of thermoforming where the top web is softened by means of heat and subsequently formed onto the packaged product.

The bottom web can be either flexible or rigid and can be preformed into a tray or a product-sized cavity into which the product to be packaged is loaded.

In skin packaging the top film conforms tightly to the product shape with advantages in terms of appearance, limited product crushing due to vacuum, and the possibility of contour sealing around the product, limiting the exudation of liquids from the product. Because of its appealing appearance and the high cost of the packaging materials, skin packaging utilization is limited to consumer or family units of meat (both fresh and processed), fish, prepared meals and cheese.

Top webs are usually based on ionomeric resins or on coextruded structures of polyolefins. PVDC or EVOH provides the necessary gas barrier.

Bottom webs are generally either laminated or co-extruded structures similar to the ones used for thermoforming.

When a rigid tray is required polyvinylchloride (PVC), polystyrene (PS) or PET is employed.

Influence of Vacuum Packaging on the Storage Behaviour of Chilled Foods

Fresh Meats and Poultry

Meats contain an abundance of nutrients necessary for the growth of microorganisms; they are particularly rich in soluble organic substances such as carbohydrates, amino acids and nucleotides. Therefore, spoilage of fresh meat and poultry during chilled storage is mainly due to the growth of aerobic psychrophyllic bacteria belonging to the Pseudomonadaceae family and to the *Moraxella–Acinetobacter* group. Growth of these bacteria results in development of off-odours (due to hydrogen sulphide, ammonia, amines and indole) and bacterial slimes which contribute to meat discoloration. *See* Spoilage; Bacterial Spoilage

Vacuum packaging in oxygen-impermeable materials limits oxygen supply to the typical aerobic spoilage microflora, providing conditions suitable only for the slower-growing lactic acid bacteria, which in chilled conditions require several weeks to produce off-odours. *See* Lactic Acid Bacteria

In addition, vacuum packaging has an impact on meat colour, which is mainly due to the presence in the muscle tissue of myoglobin, a conjugated protein where the protein moiety (globin) is bonded to a haem group.

The iron atom of the haematin nucleus can form complexes with different ligands and can be either in the ferrous (Fe^{2+}) or ferric (Fe^{3+}) oxidation state. The globin can be either in the native or denatured state.

Among the different complexes of haem, globin and ligands, three are important in fresh meat.

- oxymyoglobin, with oxygen as the ligand and iron in the ferrous state, characterized by a bright red colour;
- myoglobin, with water as the ligand and iron in the ferrous state, characterized by a purplish red colour;
- metmyoglobin, with water as the ligand and iron in the ferric state, characterized by a brown colour.

Oxymyoglobin is the pigment normally present on the surface of meat exposed to air, and gives the meat its bright and attractive colour.

During storage, as a consequence of the growth of aerobic bacteria which reduce the availability of oxygen on the meat surface, and of the reduction in the capability of the meat to reduce its own metmyoglobin level, metmyoglobin tends to predominate, imparting its brown colour to the meat surface, which contributes to consumer rejection of the product.

In vacuum-packaged meat, as a consequence of preventing oxygen access to the meat surface, the pigment is of the myoglobin colour and the meat appears darker than a sample exposed to air or packaged in modified atmospheres. Displaying of vacuum-packaged consumer units of fresh meat can create problems of consumer acceptance because of the purplish colour of the meat surface. In this case, proper consumer warning has to be given to explain the origin of the colour and the advantages of vacuum packaging in terms of prolonged storage life. *See* Controlled Atmosphere Storage, Applications for Bulk Storage of Foodstuffs

The storage life at 0–2°C of fresh primal meat vacuum packaged in bags or pouches is 4–8 weeks, allowing full ageing of meat types such as beef which require maturation. Consumer units in the form of meat slices have a storage life of 2–3 weeks.

Processed Meats

It is useful to classify the many existing types of processed meats into two main categories of products:

- products having high-activity water, the production processes of which often imply cooking (frankfurters, patties, bologna, fresh sausages, cooked ham, luncheon meats);
- cured products with low-activity water (raw ham, salami, bacon).

The spoilage of the former category of products can be due to surface drying, fat oxidation, discoloration or to microbiological factors (sliminess, souring, greening). The latter category of products is less susceptible to spoilage caused by bacteria. Rancidity, discoloration and mould growth are the most common limiting factors for storage life. *See* Meat, Structure; Spoilage, Moulds in Food Spoilage

All the above products can benefit from vacuum packaging, which avoids surface drying, mould growth and greatly slows down the oxidation of fat and pigments. Pasteurizable packages are also commonly used for microbial stabilization of some products (cooked ham, patties and frankfurters). Furthermore, cook-in-the-package technology has been developed for production of cooked ham, allowing optimization of the production process, hygienic quality and yield.

The chilled storage life of vacuum-packaged processed meats is very variable, depending primarily upon product composition and packaging material characteristics and can vary from a couple of weeks (certain types of fresh sausages) to several months (cured products and pasteurized or cook-in-the-package products).

Cheese

Vacuum packaging is mainly applied to hard and semihard types of cheese, both for industrial and consumer units, and its effect in storage life extension is due mainly to:

- elimination of surface drying;
- slowing down of fungal growth;
- limitation of oxidation of fatty substances.

An interesting application of vacuum packaging is the curing in the package technology which is utilized for certain types of cheeses (Emmenthal, Gouda, Edam). The cheese is vacuum packaged at an early curing stage and cured inside the package. This technique improves yield (limiting rind formation and water loss) and allows a certain product standardization. Curing in the package is particularly demanding in terms of gas transmission properties of the packaging material; a good compromise is necessary between a sufficiently high carbon dioxide permeability to allow the escape of gas formed inside the cheese during curing and a sufficiently low oxygen transmission rate to avoid mould growth. The gas transmission rate requirements can vary from cheese type to cheese type and also depend upon production conditions, which are often variable among different dairies. *See* Cheeses, Cheeses with 'Eyes'

Fish

Wet fish is probably the most perishable type of foodstuff because of the high content of soluble substances in the flesh, many of which contain nitrogen, and triglycerides characterized by polyunsaturated fatty acids (in fatty types of fish such as clupeids, salmonids and scombroids). In addition, fish flesh is characterized by a high level of enzymatic activity which plays a major role in the early stages of spoilage. *See* Fish, Spoilage

Vacuum packaging retards the growth of aerobic spoilage bacteria and limits the oxidation of fat. However, vacuum-packaged fish is very perishable and has to be carefully stored at temperatures below 2°C, the normal storage life being 5–7 days. Prepackaged consumer units of wet fish, utilizing skin packages, have been recently introduced at a commercial level due to the need for a distribution system capable of handling in a relatively easy way a product characterized by bad smells, dripping out, and hygienic and preparation problems at the consumer level. For processed fish (smoked, salted, pickled), vacuum packaging is commonly utilized because it limits the spoilage factors of this kind of product (mainly fat oxidation and mould growth). The storage life of vacuum-packaged processed fish depends upon the water activity level, ranging between 2–3 weeks for slightly salted fish and a few months for highly salted ones.

Prepared Foods

Vacuum packaging is also utilized for a wide range of prepared foods (delicatessen products, cooked meats and poultry, prepared meals, salads).

The spoilage mechanism and perishability of these products is related to their chemical composition (pH, additives) and heat treatment (pasteurization), and therefore their storage life is very variable, ranging from 2 weeks to several months.

An interesting application of vacuum packaging to prepared foods is the cook-in-the-package technique, which implies packaging under vacuum of raw or partially cooked foods which are cooked inside the package, pasteurized (when required), chilled and stored and reheated and unpackaged at the time of consumption. This technology allows the rationalization of meal preparation in central units (e.g. in institutional kitchens and restaurant chains) because of the storage life of the prepared meal (1 week or more) and it has been also introduced to food-processing plants to prepare meals to be distributed chilled at the retail level.

Bibliography

Benning CJ (1983) *Plastics Films for Packaging*. Lancaster, PA: Technomics.

Jay JJ (1978) *Modern Food Microbiology*, 2nd edn. New York: Van Nostrand.

Mathlouthy M (1986) *Food Packaging and Preservation: Theory and Practice*. London: Elsevier.

Rizvi SSH (1981) Requirements for foods packaged in polymeric films. *Critical Review in Food Science and Nutrition* 14: 111–134.

Rizvi SSH (1984) *Flexible Material Properties that Influence Shelf-life*. Proceedings of the Meat Industry Research Conference, American Meat Science Association, New Orleans.

Sacharow S and Griffin Jr RC (1970) *Food Packaging*. Westport, CT: AVI Publishing.

M. Rossi
Cryovac, Passirana di Rho, Italy

CHLOROPHYLL

Chlorophylls are the green pigments which take part in photosynthesis, the most important biological process occurring in photosynthetic biomembranes. Because of their widespread occurrence in a variety of vegetables, fruits, legumes and other plant products, chlorophylls play a vital role in the acceptability of food commodities. For instance, a radical shift in the colour of food, even though accompanied by no change in flavour of texture, can make the food completely unacceptable to consumers. This article covers topics concerning the occurrence of chlorophylls, their physicochemical properties, their stability and use as colourants and analysis

in food products. *See* Colours, Properties and Determination of Natural Pigments

Occurrence in Foods

Chlorophylls occur in the membranes of chloroplasts, the organelles that hold chlorophylls close to the cell wall, and carry out photosynthesis in plant cells. In the biosphere at least nine types can be identified; but only two types, chlorophylls a and b, are of interest from the viewpoints of food science and technology. The other types such as chlorophylls c, d and e, bacteriochlorophylls a and b and chlorobium chlorophylls occur only in microorganism and algal biomass.

Leafy vegetables, green peppers, cucumbers and unripe fruits are the main sources of chlorophylls in edible foods. Fresh green vegetables and fruits generally contain chlorophylls a and b, together with small amounts of their derivatives. The ratio of chlorophylls a and b ranges from 2·8:1 to 4·6:1 in vegetables of a dark green colour (spinach, brussels sprouts, broccoli, kale, cucumbers, green peppers, etc.) and from 1·5:1 to 2·5:1 in light green-coloured vegetables and fruits (green tomatoes, green peas, snap beans, turnip greens, okra, unripe apples, kiwifruit, etc.). These ratios can be significantly modified by growth conditions and environmental factors.

In food preservation, raw materials are often subjected to a moist heat treatment called blanching. This process induces formation of the C10 epimers of chlorophylls a and b. The concentration of these isomers is proportional to the severity of heating during blanching. Thus, chlorophylls a, a, b and b are found abundantly in blanched vegetables and fruits. *See* Heat Treatment, Chemical and Microbiological Changes

In the case of prolonged heat treatments, as in canning, almost all chlorophylls are converted to magnesium- and phytol-free derivatives (Table 1). Characteristic formation of a dull green or brown colour is evident in canning. It is also obvious from several investigations that chlorophylls a and b are absent in canned foods unless stabilizing agents are used and/or pH adjustment of canning water to neutral or slightly alkaline is made before canning. Magnesium-free derivatives, particularly pheophytins, are predominant pigments in pickled vegetables and fruits. The change from green to dull brown is an important index of the complete ripeness of the pickled products. Due to the increased activity of chlorophyllases, phytol-free chlorophyll derivatives become easy to detect in some types of pickles, which may contain around 25% of chlorophyllides and pheophorbides in the total pigments. *See* Canning, Quality Changes During Canning

Depending upon the conditions of dehydration processes, dried products vary in the content and composition of their chlorophylls. Under typical conditions of drying, chlorophylls a and b make up the highest proportion of the pigments in dried products such as celery, spinach, mint, maluhiya, green peas, etc. On the other hand, pheophytin and pheophorbides are predominantly present in vegetables dried by either severe heating or natural sun drying without a predrying blanching step.

Physicochemical Properties

Chemical Properties

Chemically, chlorophylls are complex organic molecules composed of four pyrrole rings. The central magnesium atom is bonded covalently to two nitrogen atoms. Additionally, two more coordinate bonds are formed when the other nitrogen atoms share two electrons with the magnesium (see Fig. 1). The chemical nature of pyrrole rings enables chlorophyll to associate readily with lipophilic components such as phospholipids as well as membrane proteins. Association of chlorophyll with neutral lipids and carotenoid pigments

Table 1. Concentration (mg per g of dry weight[a]) of chlorophylls a and b, pheophytins a and b; and pyropheophytins a and b in fresh, bleached and heated spinach processed at 121°C for various times

	Chlorophyll		Pheophytin		Pyropheophytin		
	a	b	a	b	a	b	pH[b]
Fresh	6·98	2·49					
Blanched	6·78	2·47					7·06
Processed (min)[c]							
2	5·72	2·46	1·36	0·13			6·90
4	4·59	2·21	2·20	0·29	0·12		6·77
7	2·81	1·75	3·12	0·57	0·35		6·60
15	0·59	0·89	3·32	0·78	1·09	0·27	6·32
30		0·24	2·45	0·66	1·74	0·57	6·00
60			1·01	0·32	3·62	1·24	5·65

From Schwartz SJ and von Elbe JH (1983) *Journal of Food Science* 48: 1303, with permission.
[a] Estimated error ±2%; each value represents the average of three determinations
[b] The pH was measured after processing but before pigment extraction.
[c] The process times listed were measured from the time the internal product temperature reached the retort processing temperature.

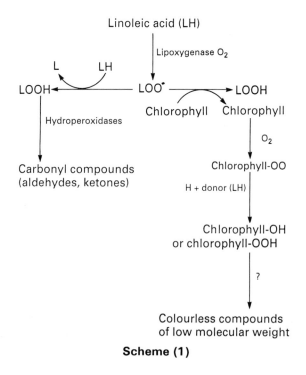

Compounds	Mg	R_1	R_2	R_3
Chlorophyll a	+	CH_3	Phytol	CO_2CH_3
Chlorophyll b	+	CHO	Phytol	CO_2CH_3
Chlorophyllide a	+	CH_3	H	CO_2CH_3
Chlorophyllide b	+	CHO	H	CO_2CH_3
Pheophytin a	−	CH_3	Phytol	CO_2CH_3
Pheophytin b	−	CHO	Phytol	CO_2CH_3
Pyropheophytin a	−	CH_3	Phytol	H
Pyropheophytin b	−	CHO	Phytol	H
Pheophorbide a	−	CH_3	H	CO_2CH_3
Pheophorbide b	−	CHO	H	CO_2CH_3

Fig. 1 Chemical structure of chlorophylls and their derivatives.

roxylated chlorophyllides which are extremely soluble in water and water-miscible solvents.

Chlorophyllase (EC 3.1.1.14) is the enzyme which hydrolyses chlorophyll to chlorophyllide and phytol. This enzyme occurs widely in plant tissues accompanying chlorophyll. It is of note that this enzyme also functions in the synthesis of chlorophyll itself by catalysing esterification of the phytol group to chlorophyllide in the final stage of biosynthesis. Chlorophyllase-catalysed hydrolysis is activated during handling and processing of foods by different mechanisms, including denaturation of chloroplastin (such as in prolonged heat treatment and brining) as well as the availability of some essential cofactors such as Ca^{2+} ions and activating phenolics. On the other hand, retardation of enzymatic hydrolysis of chlorophyll is a likely consequence of the presence of inhibitors and the reduction of water content of raw materials to a low level. *See* Coenzymes

Oxidation of chlorophyll by molecular oxygen is catalysed by metallic ions and/or biological oxidants such as oxidizing enzymes. As the loss of chlorophyll colour often accompanies this type of reaction, it is commonly known as chlorophyll bleaching. As an intermediary of bleaching, hydroxylated and allomeric chlorophyll products are implicated in raw materials of edible foods. These compounds are very unstable and are swiftly converted to colourless degradation products. Of the biological oxidants, lipoxygenases (linoleate:oxygen oxidoreductase), hydroperoxide-decomposing enzymes and peroxidases are of special importance. Lipoxygenases co-oxidize chlorophyll pigments throughout their action on fatty acids possessing

is facilitated by phytol, the C_{20} monounsaturated alcohol, which is esterified by a propionic acid residue at position 7. *See* Carotenoids, Properties and Determination; Phospholipids, Properties and Occurrence

The phytol side-chain is therefore responsible for the hydrophobicity of chlorophylls and their derivatives. Once the phytol is released, through hydrolysis, the solubility of chlorophyll in water and other polar organic solvents increases markedly. The formation of more polar derivatives, namely phytol-free chlorophyllides, arises from hydrolysis, and is catalysed by acids, alkalis or chlorophyllases. In acid-catalysed hydrolysis, another reaction, release of magnesium, is also initiated to produce pheophorbides. Conversely, hydrolysis by alkalis raises the stability of the magnesium atom in the chlorophyll molecules, resulting in bright green-coloured chlorophyllides. It is rather interesting, however, that hydroxylation at some positions on the molecule is initiated, through alkaline hydrolysis in particular, when the process involves heating. Products likely to result from this reaction may include mono- or polyhyd-

Linoleic acid (LH)

Lipoxygenase O_2

L LH

$LOOH \leftarrow LOO^{\bullet} \rightarrow LOOH$

Chlorophyll   Chlorophyll

Hydroperoxidases

O_2

Carbonyl compounds (aldehydes, ketones)

Chlorophyll-OO

H + donor (LH)

Chlorophyll-OH or chlorophyll-OOH

?

Colourless compounds of low molecular weight

Scheme (1)

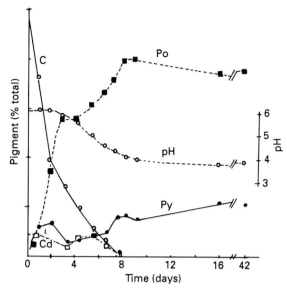

Fig. 2 Changes in chlorophylls (C), chlorophyllides (Cd), pheophytins (Py) and pheophorbides (Po) in brined cucumbers (White RC, Jones ID and Gibbs E (1963) *Journal of Food Science* 28: 431, with permission).

a *cis,cis*-1,4-pentadiene system such as linoleic, linolenic and arachidonic acids. A generally cited mechanism of lipoxygenase-catalysed chlorophyll bleaching, is shown in scheme [1].

Although convincing evidence is available on the role of lipid hydroperoxidases in promoting the oxidative destruction of chlorophylls, the mechanism with which they interfere is still obscure. As for peroxidase-dependent bleaching, some phenolics are essential for this type of degradation. The short-lived radicals generated during peroxidase–hydrogen peroxide reaction are likely to be involved in the biochemical pathway. For complete inactivation of the above-mentioned enzymes an excessive period of blanching is needed. This, however, initiates thermal degradation of chlorophyll, causing a remarkable loss in green colour. The optimal blanching time, therefore, should not exceed 1 min for the maximum retention of chlorophylls.

Substitution of the Mg^{2+} ion by two protons occurs most readily in acidic conditions, producing mainly pheophytins. Being acid catalysed, pheophytin formation (pheophytinization) is more frequent during the course of pickling and vigorous heating (see Fig. 2). It is of interest to note that the acidity of plant cell vacuoles makes it difficult to avoid pheophytinization. In addition, there are specific membrane-bound enzymes responsible for the release of the Mg^{2+} ion from the chlorophyll molecule. This enzyme is activated upon the disintegration of plant tissues.

On exposure to a mild heat treatment, chlorophyll undergoes an epimerization reaction at C10. As a consequence of this stereoisomerization the so-called a′

and b′ derivatives are formed. Moreover, prolonged heating can induce decarbomethoxylation at the same position, giving rise to pyroderivatives which are found in canned vegetables and refined oils in appreciable amounts.

Spectral Characteristics

Chlorophylls absorb light energy in the red and blue regions of the spectrum. This property is attributable to the occurrence of electronic transitions, for instance in the porphyrin structure, which create absorption bands typical for chlorophylls. The difference in primary structure between chlorophylls a and b makes it possible to distinguish them according to the shape and position of their absorption bands. Both are characterized by four main bands between 500 and 700 nm in the visible region and one or two large bands around 400 nm in the near-violet region (see Fig. 3). Once the porphyrin structure is broken, absorption in the violet or near-violet region becomes difficult to detect. In addition, substitution of the Mg^{2+} ion by protons or metallic ions causes the major absorption maxima to shift to shorter wavelengths in the near-violet region and to longer wavelengths in the red region of the spectrum, while no substantial change is noticed in the spectral characteristics as a result of the release of the phytol group. Factors likely to affect the absorption maxima of chlorophylls and their derivatives include solvent polarity, freshness of chlorophyll preparations and the atmospheric conditions under which chlorophyll extracts are stored before measurement. On this account, determination of the specific absorption coefficient (SAC) should be carried out in freshly prepared extracts using pure solvents.

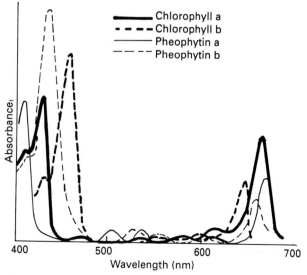

Fig. 3 Absorption spectra of chlorophylls and pheophytins.

Chlorophyll absorbs light of high energy, resulting in excitation and subsequent fluorescence. Exploiting this property, very sensitive detection of chlorophyll compounds can be achieved by fluorescence. The shape and positions of fluorescence spectra of chlorophylls a and b are similar to those observed in ultraviolet and visible spectra. However, because magnesium- and phytol-free derivatives have the same spectral characteristics as the original chlorophylls, application of fluorometry for differentiation is not possible.

Due to the characteristic motion of various functional groups present in chlorophyll (methyl, carbonyl, amide, etc.), vibrational transitions and, hence, characteristic and useful infrared spectra are generated on absorption of infrafred radiation. The modes of vibration of each group are very sensitive to changes in chemical composition, conformation and environment, and chemical groups not accessible to ultraviolet–visible spectroscopy can be studied. *See* Spectroscopy, Infrared and Raman

Chlorophyll can also be studied by nuclear magnetic resonance, mass spectroscopy and circular dichroism to assist structural elucidation. *See* Mass Spectrometry, Principles and Instrumentation; Spectroscopy, Nuclear Magnetic Resonance

Stability in Processed Foods

In general, chlorophylls are relatively unstable especially when exposed to unfavourable conditions, which are likely to occur during food processing. There is no denying the fact that processing can rupture cells and changes the permeability of the plastid membrane, leading to the release of chlorophylls into the cell. When chlorophylls come in contact with acids present in protoplasm or vacuoles, pheophytinization reactions take place. It is difficult to retain chlorophyll in processed foods, but chlorophyll stability can be raised during processing and storage of processed foods by careful control of conditions.

Adjustment of pH to neutral or slightly alkaline conditions retards pheophytinization reactions. This explains why sodium bicarbonate or buffering materials are added to green vegetables before processing. However, this procedure is not recommended for processing all varieties of vegetables because, at a high pH value, as a result of cellulose hydrolysis, a rapid decay of vegetable structure occurs. To obtain products having the desired pleasant colour and firm texture, calcium and magnesium salts are added together with buffering materials. These salts, due to their reaction with pectic substances, give rise to a firm texture.

Chlorophyll stability can also be raised chemically by addition of some metal ions such as copper and zinc. These ions complex with chlorophylls to form stable green-coloured compounds. Such complexing reactions do not commence until at least 25 mg kg^{-1} of the mineral are present with the ratio of metal to chlorophyll being approximately 1:1. In processed foods this phenomenon is known as regreening or green colour reversion.

It is quite possible to modify processing methods so as to reduce thermal degradation of chlorophylls. In comparison with conventional heat processing, the application of a high-temperature short-time (HTST) method does little damage to chlorophylls. The combination of pH adjustment and an HTST method offers the possibility of retaining the maximum green colour of processed foods. This improvement, however, is not easily achieved for the simple reason that pH stability requires large amounts of food additives that make the products almost unacceptable to consumers.

The rate of chemical alteration of chlorophyll at freeze storage is, of course, lower than at refrigeration or ambient temperatures. This is also due to the lower water activity in frozen foods. However, degradation of chlorophyll in some vegetables occurs even at $-18°C$. Factors likely to have a significant effect on chlorophyll stability during freeze storage include pH, temperature, water activity, storage time and physical state of frozen foods. *See* Freezing, Structural and Flavour Changes

Chlorophylls as Food Colorants

Unlike other plant pigments, such as carotenoids and flavonoids, chlorophylls are not commonly used as food colorants. At the beginning of this century, copper compounds and then organic dyes such as tartrazine and Green S were occasionally used to dye canned vegetables, in particular, canned peas. Synthetic dyestuffs are now less widely used as food additives and, along with other natural colours, attempts have been made to use chlorophyll to colour foods. Chlorophyll is difficult to use for this purpose, because of its low stability and water solubility. Nowadays, phytol-free sodium chlorophyllin, in which the Mg^{2+} ion is replaced by Cu^{2+}, is safely used. Its special features are its bright bluish-green colour, moderate solubility, resistance to heat treatment and, more importantly, its nontoxic nature. To both producers and consumers these features are welcome and appealing. Mono- or polyhydroxylated chlorophyllides produced by oxidation, as well as zinc or copper complexes of pheophorbides are other pigments applicable for the safe coloration of foods provided that the amount of metal the latter compounds contain is small so as not to represent a toxicity hazard. *See* Coronary Heart Disease, Antioxidant Status

Analysis of Food Chlorophylls

Since they have prenyl structure, chlorophylls are water-insoluble and, therefore, their isolation and extraction from plant tissues have to be carried out by means of organic solvents. Efficiency of extraction can be raised by disintegrating the samples in the presence of a suitable organic solvent to avoid oxidative degradation. Apart from aliphatic and aromatic hydrocarbons, various solvents or solvent mixtures can be used to extract chlorophylls. The complete extraction of such pigments is dependent upon the polarity of the solvent system employed. In general, an initial step with pure acetone may be essential for the full recovery of chlorophylls. Addition of water to the solvent increases its extractability. The percentage of water, however, should not exceed 20%; above this level the less polar chlorophyll a and magnesium-free pheophytins are only partially recovered. Combinations of the less polar solvents (carbon, tetrachloride, hexane, ethers, chloroform, etc.) and more polar ones (methanol, ethanol, ethyl, acetate, etc.), at an approximate ratio of 2:1, are better choices for the complete extraction of chlorophylls and their derivatives from water-containing, dry and lyophilized products. Some procedures recommend the use of alcohols at the disintegration step for removing water from the samples. Following filtration, the pigments in the alcohol fraction should be transferred to the water-free epiphase by gentle shaking with a sufficient volume of the less polar solvent.

To avoid chemical alterations during conventional extraction, some modifications seem to be necessary. They may include the use of calcium carbonate, magnesium carbonate, sodium carbonate, ammonium hydroxide, dimethylaniline or dimethylformamide to slow down pheophytinization reactions. Although heating promotes isomerization of chlorophylls, rapid boiling followed by immediate cooling of the samples may be applied before grinding to retard completely enzymatic oxidation and hydrolysis.

Spectrophotometric Analysis

Spectrophotometry is a fundamental means of chlorophyll analysis. An an important step in this analysis, the SAC is estimated for each chlorophyll compound at the maximum wavelength of light absorption in a freshly prepared solution. This coefficient, which is further affected by the polarity of the solvent system, is indispensible for the derivation of accurate equations for the quantification of the total and individual chlorophylls. Table 2 shows some of the derived equations

Table 2. Equations for the determination of the concentration of chlorophyll a (C a), chlorophyll b (C b), total chlorophylls (C a+b), pheophytin a (Ph a), pheophytin b (Ph b) and total pheophytins (Ph a+b) in leaf pigment extracts for solvents of different polarities. A is absorbance

Chlorophylls	Pheophytins
Diethyl ether (pure solvent)	
$C\,a = 10.05\,A_{660.6} - 0.97\,A_{642.2}$	$Ph\,a = 17.87\,A_{666.6} - 3.58\,A_{654.2}$
$C\,b = 16.36\,A_{642.2} - 2.43\,A_{660.6}$	$Ph\,b = 24.62\,A_{654.2} - 8.46\,A_{666.6}$
$C\,a+b = 7.62\,A_{660.6} - 15.39\,A_{642.2}$	$Ph\,a+b = 9.41\,A_{666.6} + 21.03\,A_{654.2}$
Ethanol, 95% (v/v)	
$C\,a = 13.36\,A_{664.2} - 5.19\,A_{648.6}$	$Ph\,a = 42.41\,A_{662.2} - 23.28\,A_{654}$
$C\,b = 27.43\,A_{648.6} - 8.12\,A_{664.2}$	$Ph\,b = 55.67\,A_{654} - 45.53\,A_{662.2}$
$C\,a+b = 5.24\,A_{664.2} + 22.24\,A_{648.2}$	$Ph\,a+b = 32.39\,A_{654} + 3.12\,A_{662.2}$
Acetone (pure solvent)	
$C\,a = 11.24\,A_{661.6} - 2.04\,A_{644.8}$	$Ph\,a = 516.7\,A_{653.4} - 501.2\,A_{652.6}$
$C\,b = 20.13\,A_{644.8} - 4.19\,A_{661.6}$	$Ph\,b = 732.5\,A_{625.6} - 725.1\,A_{653.4}$
$C\,a+b = 7.05\,A_{661.6} + 18.09\,A_{644.8}$	$Ph\,a+b = 321.3\,A_{652.6} + 208.4\,A_{653.4}$
Methanol (pure solvent)	
$C\,a = 16.72\,A_{665.2} - 9.16\,A_{652.4}$	$Ph\,a = 43.77\,A_{654.2} - 33.4\,A_{647.6}$
$C\,b = 34.09\,A_{652.4} - 15.28\,A_{665.2}$	$Ph\,b = 50.71\,A_{647.6} - 36.32\,A_{654.2}$
$C\,a+b = 1.44\,A_{665.2} + 24.93\,A_{652.4}$	$Ph\,a+b = 7.45\,A_{654.2} + 17.31\,A_{647.6}$

Data from Lichtenthaler HK (1987). Chlorophylls and carotenoids: pigments of photosynthetic biomembranes. *Methods in Enzymology* 148: 350–382.

involving estimated SAC values of chlorophylls and their derivatives. By applying these equations it is possible to determine accurately the concentration of chlorophylls as well as the ratio of a to b forms even when naturally occurring carotenoid pigments are present in the extracts. Recent developments in spectrophotometers, which exhibit automatic baseline correction and programmable peak picking and scanning, allow better selection of wavelengths and redetermination of the SAC. The redetermined SAC values for any pigment in one solvent can be compared directly with those in another solvent. The same holds true for the determination of the ratios of a to b forms of chlorophylls and phyeophytins.

Fluorescence spectroscopy is also applied to chlorophyll analysis. Due to the high sensitivity of fluorescence detectors, small quantities (picomoles) of chlorophyll can be estimated. The accuracy of fluorometric analysis increases considerably when appropriate equations are available and convenient solvents are employed. Nuclear magnetic resonance, infrared, mass spectrometry and circular dichroism spectra are suitable for identification and structural elucidation, but unsuitable for quantification of chlorophylls.

Chromatographic Analysis

Even though spectrophotometric methods are accurate, they are not suitable for simultaneous determination of chlorophylls and their derivatives, which exist as mixtures in biological samples. Separation and determination of the individual components of such a mixture are achieved through chromatography.

Column chromatographic methods with a nonreactive adsorbent is suitable for the isolation of large quantities of chlorophylls a and b, but it is not possible to separate and analyse the structurally similar compounds. This technique is rather slow, but column chromatography with chemically modified adsorbents such as diethylaminoethanol (DEAE)–cellulose, DEAE–Sepharose, CL-6B, Sephadex LH-20, etc., can be used to fractionate and prepare chlorophylls a and b and to eliminate other pigments in a much shorter time.

Thin-layer chromatography (TLC) is widely used in chlorophyll analysis, as a very cost-effective technique. However, inorganic adsorbents (silica gel and kieselguhr) used in the TLC separation of chlorophylls may cause chemical alterations of the compounds. Artefact formation during TLC analysis may be minimized by:

(1) using thin organic layers of sucrose, glucose, cellulose and, more recently, reversed-phase high-performance materials;
(2) modifying the resolution of chlorophyll compounds on cellulose by adding pyridine to light petroleum ether or n-heptane.

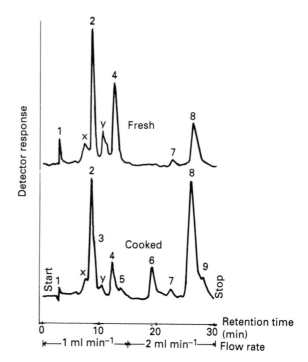

Fig. 4   Separation of chlorophyll-type pigments of fresh and cooked green peas on chromsil C_{18} columns eluted with acetonitrile methanolethyl acetate (53:40:7, v/v/v). Detection at 650 nm: (1) chlorophyllid b, (2) chlorophyll b, (3) chlorophyll b', (4) chlorophyll a, (5) chlorophyll a', (6) pheophytin b, (7) unidentified, (8) pheophytin a, (9) pyropheophytin a, (x) and (y) oxidation products of chlorophylls b and a, respectively.

Full separation of derivatives with similar structures, however, requires a two-dimensional TLC procedure with separate developing systems. Recently, the advent of reversed-phase high-performance TLC (HPTLC) has opened up new possibilities for the separation of chlorophylls. As a choice of developing systems, protic solvents (water-containing alcohols) are better than aprotic ones (consisting of acetone and acetonitrile) for the separation of chlorophyll components by HPTLC. *See* Chromatography, Principles; Chromatography, Thin-layer Chromatography; Chromatography, High-performance Liquid Chromatography

The advantages of high-performance liquid chromatography (HPLC), such as speed, high resolution, relatively short analysis time and sensitivity, make it superior to other techniques for the determination of chlorophylls and their derivatives. Complete analysis of chlorophyll compounds by this technique is not an easy task, due to differences in polarity of these compounds and the interaction of carotenoids which occur alongside chlorophylls in the membrane of chloroplasts. Recently developed variable-wavelength detectors with rapid scanning units assist in diminishing the above difficulty. Diode array detectors indicate the peak purity of the separated components and provide three-dimensional or contour maps for the whole separation, i.e. absorbance versus wavelength versus time. They also assist in choosing the most suitable wavelength at which no interference occurs with the other pigments.

Both adsorption and partition chromatography can be used in HPLC for chlorophyll analysis. Unlike normal-phase materials, hydrophobic reversed phases are extensively used with both isocratic and gradient elution, as their columns can be equilibrated rapidly and do not initiate artefact formation. With respect to the most suitable mobile phases for HPLC of chlorophylls, various mixtures of organic solvents may be used. In the case of normal-phase columns, nonaqueous mixtures of acetone/hexane, alcohol/hexane, isooctane/ethanol, heptane/diethyl ether/acetone, etc., are commonly used to separate chlorophylls b, b′, a, a′ and pheophytins under gradient elution conditions. With reversed-phase columns, elution of different components may be further modified by using ion supression, ion pairing and buffered or high ionic strength mobile phases. In gradient elution, it is necessary to start with a mobile phase consisting of water and alcohols to ensure separation of the more polar derivatives. The final gradient would be run with decreasing polarity to elute chlorophylls a and b and pheophytins. Application of such a complex gradient elution, however, implies a loss of time and labour and, in addition, is uneconomic. Achieving a fast and effective one-step HPLC procedure under isocratic elution conditions has been the aim of several investigations. The following are the major findings of research in this direction:

(1) resolution of chlorophyll compounds from reversed-phase columns can be improved by using a nonaqueous mobile phase of moderate polarity with an elution system of increasing flow rate (see Fig. 4);

(2) addition of salts or buffering materials (1–2%) to aqueous mobile phases improves resolution of chlorophyll pigments and protects them from pheophytinization reactions induced by acidity of both stationary and mobile phases used;

(3) use of fluorometric detectors having high sensitivity allows estimation of chlorophylls even when they exist at very low concentrations. These detectors make the analysis of samples of small size possible.

Bibliography

Czygan FC (1980) *Pigments in Plants*. New York: Gustav Fischer.

Daood HG, Czintokai B, Hoschke A and Biacs P (1989) HPLC of chlorophylls and carotenoids from vegetables. *Journal of Chromatography* 472: 296–302.

Goodwin TW (1976) *Chemistry and Biochemistry of Plant Pigments*, 2nd edn. New York: Academic Press.

Gross J (1987) *Pigments in Fruits*. London: Academic Press.

Macrae R (1988) *HPLC in Food Analysis*, 2nd edn. London: Academic Press.

Schwartz SJ and Vorenzo TV (1990) Chlorophyll in foods. *Critical Reviews in Food Science and Nutrition* 29: 1.

Vernon LP and Seeley GR (1966) *The Chlorophylls*. New York: Academic Press.

H. G. Daood
Central Food Research Institute, Budapest, Hungary

CHOCOLATE

See Cocoa

CHOLECALCIFEROL

Contents

Properties and Determination
Physiology

Properties and Determination

Physical Properties

Cholecalciferol (9,10-seco(5Z,7E)-5,7,10(19)-cholesta-trien-3β-ol), commonly referred to as vitamin D_3, exists in the pure form as white crystalline needles. Referred to as a 'fat soluble' vitamin, it is insoluble in water but is readily soluble in most organic solvents, notably hydrocarbons, chlorinated hydrocarbons and alcohols. A closely related substance, ergocalciferol (9,10-seco(5Z,7E)-5,7,10(19),22-ergostatetraene-3β-ol), will also be occasionally referred to in the text. Described more simply as vitamin D_2, it is physically, chemically and nutritionally similar to cholecalciferol. The term 'vitamin D' usually implies collectively both cholecalciferol and ergocalciferol together with any other active isomers and metabolites. Relevant physical properties are listed in Table 1.

Chemical Properties

Cholecalciferol is described in terms of steroid nomenclature and numbering (Fig. 1). The '9,10-seco' prefix is added to denote the bond cleavage and the opening of the typical steroidal ring structure, an essential feature necessary to impart antirachitic activity. This cleavage is generally induced by ultraviolet (UV) irradiation of the precursor compound, 7-dehydrocholesterol (provitamin D_3), and occurs in the skin during exposure to sunlight. The previtamin D_3 so formed subsequently undergoes temperature-dependent equilibration to vitamin D_3. This process, along with the requirement for further hydroxylation challenges its original classification as a vitamin; it is currently more accurately regarded as a prohormone.

Any homologue which possesses antirachitic activity is referred to as a D vitamin and each of the several compounds sharing this property elicits a unique and selective biological response (Fig. 1). Common structural features of these substances are the β stereochemistry of the 3-hydroxy substituent and the cis conformation of the double bond at C5. While the 3-hydroxy substituent does not have an overwhelming influence on biological activity, other structural features such as the A ring configuration and side-chain length appear to be more critical. Thus, while alterations to the side-chain result in diverse activity, only vitamins D_2 and D_3 are of prominence therapeutically and commercially. They are usually obtained either by extraction from natural oils or via chemical synthesis.

It is widespread practice to express vitamin D concentration in food in international units (iu), rather than on a weight basis (1 iu is equivalent to 0.025 μg of either calciferol, although this equivalence in humans is occasionally challenged). This can be a useful concept because it reflects the nutritional status where several components of different biopotency coexist within a product. Nevertheless, there is some move back to mass units, particularly in supplemented foods where the contribution of cholecalciferol is dominant.

The stability characteristics of cholecalciferol have received considerable attention because they play a major part in the shelf life of marketable products. Under conditions of low thermal, photochemical and oxidative stresses, cholecalciferol is stable for several years. However, when added to foods and exposed to

Table 1. Physical properties of the calciferols

	Cholecalciferol	Ergocalciferol
Molecular weight	384·62	396·63
Empirical formula	$C_{27}H_{44}O$	$C_{28}H_{44}O$
Melting point (°C)	84–85	115–118
λ_{max} (nm)	264·5	264·5
Extinction coefficient, $E_{1\,cm}^{1\%}$ in hexane	485	459
Optical rotation in chloroform	$+52°$	$+52°$

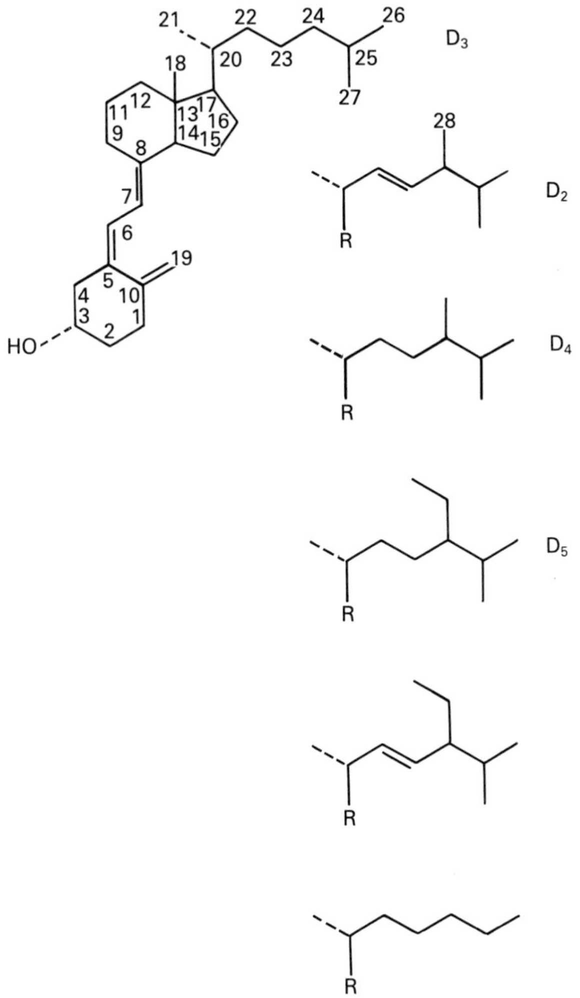

Fig. 1 The chemical structure of cholecalciferol (vitamin D₃) indicating the carbon numbering system of the molecule. Related calciferols with different side-chain configurations are also given, including ergocalciferol (vitamin D₂).

the side-chain of ergocalciferol imparts additional lability to the molecule.

Losses during storage are also known to occur in foods, and vary considerably between food types and conditions of storage. Thus, low temperatures and absence of light will minimize losses in manufactured foods, as will vacuum packaging or nitrogen flushing. Foods containing natural, or added fat-soluble antioxidants such as vitamin E and carotenoids will, in general, exhibit superior cholecalciferol conservation. *See* Antioxidants, Natural Antioxidants; Antioxidants, Synthetic Antioxidants

Occurrence and Forms in Foods

Most natural foods are limited in their content of active vitamin D components. 7-Dehydrocholesterol (provitamin D₃) and ergosterol (provitamin D₂) are widely distributed within the animal and plant kingdoms and supply a potentially good dietary source of vitamin D for humans, the extent being dependent upon the individual's pattern of exposure to sunlight. In particular, provitamins are abundant in fish, eggs, yeast, liver, milk and some vegetables such as mushrooms and cabbage.

Vitamin D itself is generally present at low levels in unfortified foods derived from animal sources. Marine fish and fish liver oils possess significant amounts, while meat, milk and eggs contain lesser quantities. Plants and vegetable oils contain negligible levels (<2% RDA). Table 2 provides a list of the richest food sources of vitamin D and their approximate concentrations.

In addition, previtamin D isomers invariably coexist with cholecalciferol and ergocalciferol. Previtamin concentrations are proportional to the calciferols and are influenced by thermal conditions during food processing and storage. Higher temperatures increase the previtamin:vitamin ratio. Although the previtamins are biologically active precursors, they are not always accounted for in nutritional tables due to analytical difficulties in their determination.

Some foods also contain small but significant quantities of hydroxylated metabolites. These compounds are highly bioactive and are found in edible tissues (meat, liver) and fluids (milk) as a result of their biosynthesis wtihin the live animal. The most predominant and biologically important compounds are 25-hydroxy-vitamin D and 1,25-dihydroxyvitamin D, while other trihydroxy metabolites may also be present.

Use in Food Fortification

The supplementation of food products with vitamin D is a contentious issue because of the toxicological conse-

industrial processes, degradation is commonplace. Light (UV) causes significant losses through the production of inactive substances such as toxisterol, suprasterol, lumisterol and tachysterol, in a process which is accelerated by heating (Fig. 2). Cooking temperatures above 100°C, even in the absence of light and air, will cause isomerization through ring closure to the pyrocholecalciferols. Cholecalciferol is also sensitive to low pH and, if subjected to an acidic environment, will irreversibly rearrange to the inactive isotachysterol via the 5,6-*trans* isomer. These reactions (illustrated in Fig. 3) are complex and will occur to an extent determined by the overall environment to which cholecalciferol is exposed. The reactions largely involve alterations to ring structure and so affect ergocalciferol and other D vitamins in a similar manner. It is generally acknowledged that ergocalciferol is less stable than cholecalciferol. This may imply that the double bond in

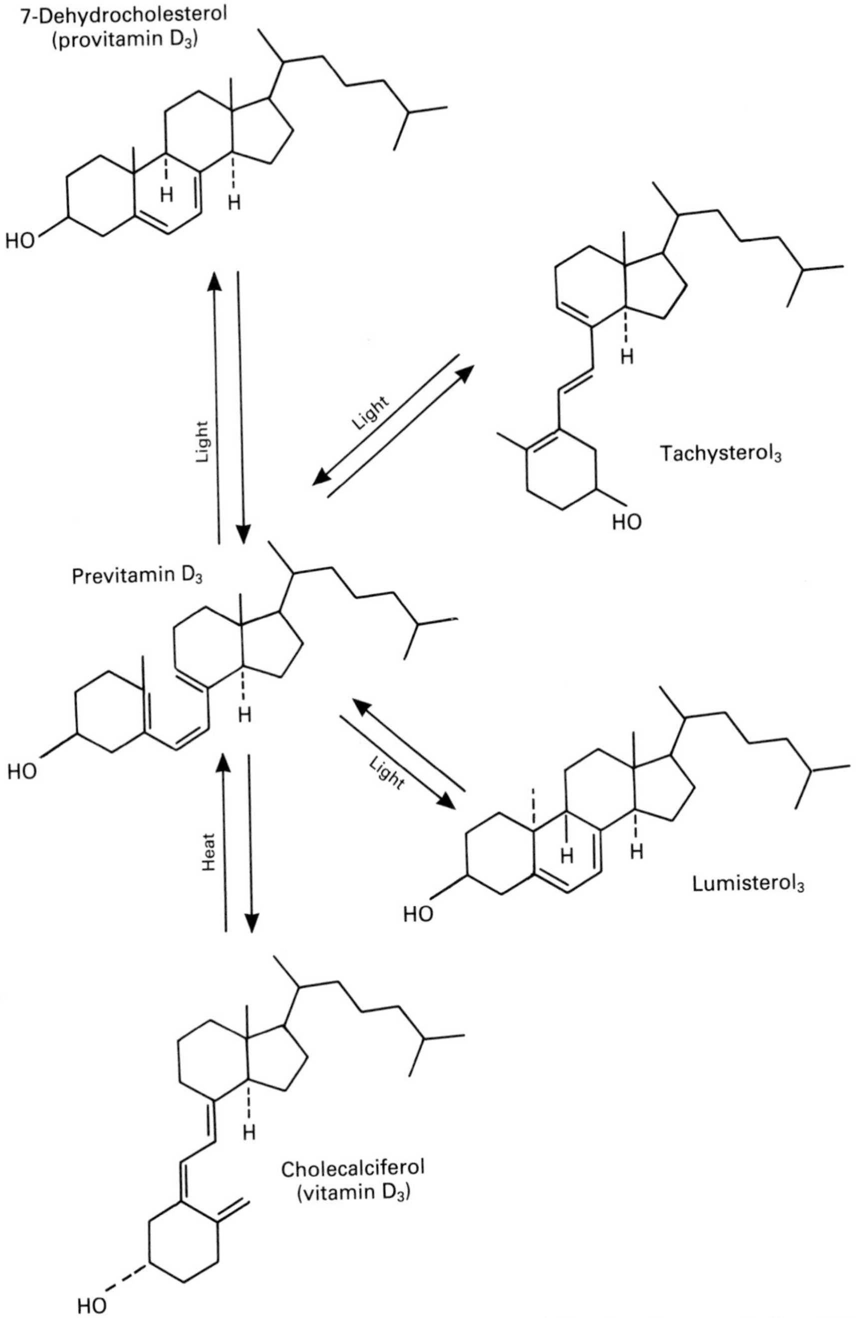

Fig. 2 The major photochemical reactions of cholecalciferol. Ergocalciferol undergoes similar reactions. Overirradiation products are not shown.

quences of overdose. While adequate exposure to sunlight will generally negate the need for this practice, modern Western life-styles (including the recent trend to reduce the intake of dietary fat), and climatic variables, justify its continuation. *See* Food Fortification

As many diets will not supply the 10 μg (400 IU) of vitamin D required per day, some additional source is generally recommended by nutritionists. The balance of vitamin can be obtained from specially prepared natural sources (concentrated fish oils) or from consumption of artifically fortified food products. In this way, the onset

of diet-induced bone disease is minimized, particularly in infants, the sick and the elderly. Legislation in many countries governs fortification strategies.

Cholecalciferol is the most common D vitamin additive, ergocalciferol being less frequently used for human nutrition. Difficulties potentially arise in delivery of the vitamin to the consumer as a consequence of its intrinsic hydrophobic and labile nature. Common vehicles are margarine, milk and milk powders, while a number of cereal products and various dietetic formulations contain vitamin D as part of their primary purpose.

Properties and Determination

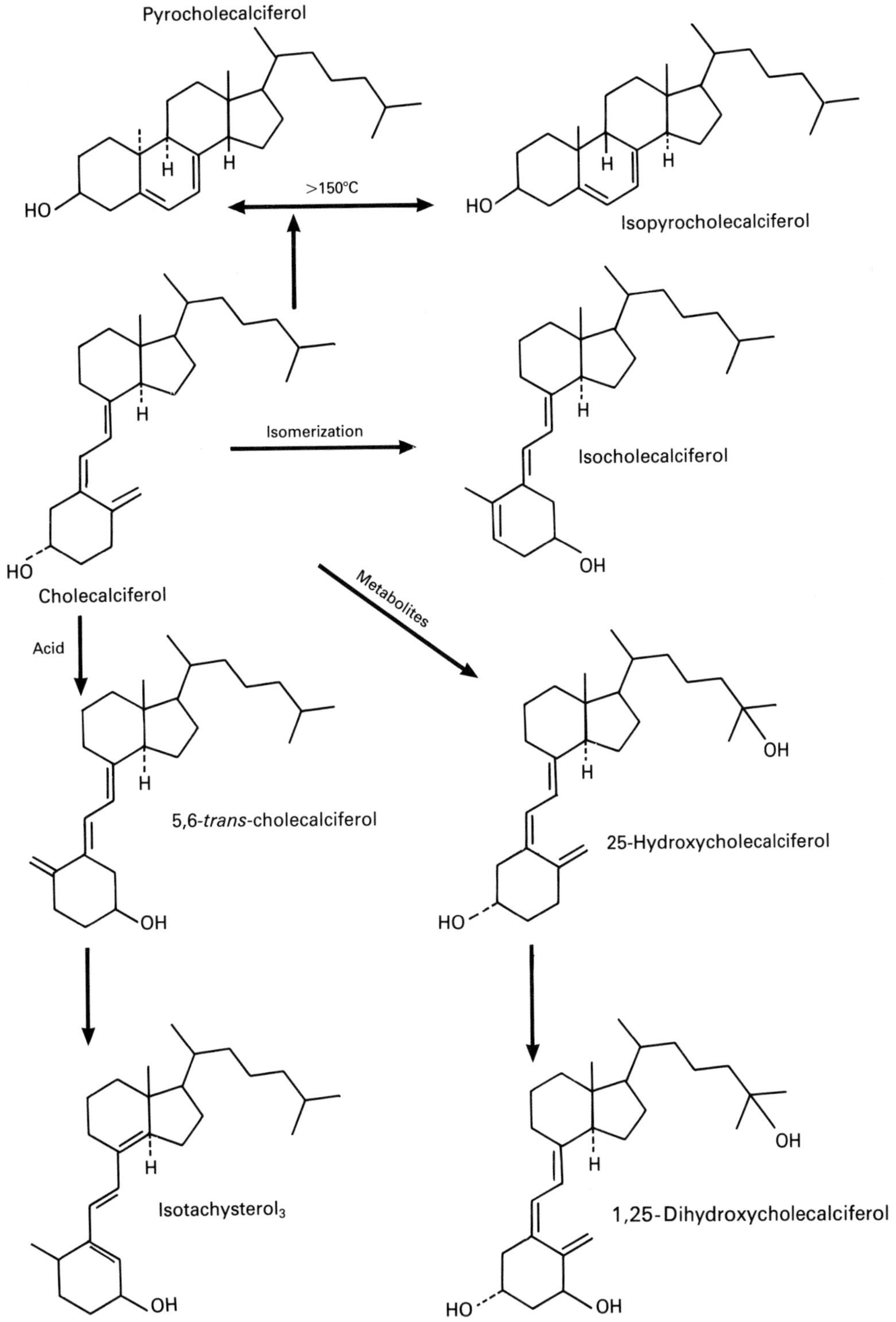

Fig. 3 The major degradation reactions of cholecalciferol as relevant to foods.

Cholecalciferol can be easily incorporated into fat- and oil-based foods by simple dissolution. It is common to add both vitamin D and vitamin A (retinol) to these foods. A protective phenolic antioxidant (e.g. 3-tert-butyl-4-hydroxyanisole (BHA), tert-butylhydroquinone (TBHQ), tocopherol) is usually incorporated at the same time. For powdered foods, cholecalciferol is added in an encapsulated 'beadlet' form, protected by a gelatine or acacia barrier and incorporating stabilizers and carrier. If the blending of the vitamin and food is performed by dry mixing, then cholecalciferol is maintained in its protected environment, ensuring enhanced shelf life. However, attaining uniform dispersion remains a problem and particle sizes must be carefully

Table 2. Typical vitamin D content of various foods

	Vitamin D content of edible portion (μg per 100 g)[a]
Natural food products	
Fish liver oils	150–3800
Fish	2–30
Egg yolk	5–8
Mammalian liver	0·5–4
Mushrooms	1–3
Butter	1·5–2
Meat	0·2–2
Cheese	0·1–1
Liquid whole milk (raw)	0·05–0·15
Green vegetables (typical)	0·005 (approx.)
Supplemented food products	
Dietary formulae (milk and soya based)	3–14
Whole milk powders	6–12
Margarine	8–10
Infant formulae	5–9
Liquid milk	0·75–1·25

[a] To convert to iu per 100 g, multiply by 40.

controlled to avoid redistribution during packaging, transport and storage. Alternatively, these difficulties can be overcome using 'wet-blending' procedures, but the vitamin is inevitably released from within its stabilized form into direct contact with the bulk food. Consequently, the receiving environment must be designed to minimize the potentially rapid degradation of the cholecalciferol supplement. *See* Retinol, Physiology

Analytical Considerations

While it is clinically important to measure the hydroxylated metabolites, food scientists have been largely concerned with vitamin D itself, at both endogenous and supplemental levels.

The quantification of the parent secosteroid in foods is complicated by several factors, including low concentration, overwhelming excesses of other lipophilic components, limiting spectral properties (nonselective λ_{max}, low absorptivity), absence of native fluorescence, thermal instability and the requirement to differentiate cholecalciferol from ergocalciferol.

Historically, curative and prophylactic bioassay techniques, based on the antirachitic quality of vitamin-D-containing food, have been used extensively and have the advantage of estimating the true (species specific) physiological response. Although sensitive, disadvantages of time, cost and poor precision moderate against the use of bioassays in routine food analysis.

Competitive protein-binding radioassay techniques, utilizing a vitamin D receptor, have been exploited more recently, especially in clinical assays. Such biochemical recognition methods offer advantages in sensitivity and specificity, but extensive sample purification is mandatory in order to avoid end-point interference from food artefacts. Lack of binding discrimination between vitamins D_2 and D_3 as well as the need for radioactive tracers and lengthy incubation periods remain problematic within the food industry. *See* Immunoassays, Radioimmunoassay and Enzyme Immunoassay

Physicochemical determination by UV spectrophotometry or colorimetry without prior separation, is clearly impracticable except for highly simplified food matrices, since the spectral properties of the parent or derivative calciferol species are insufficiently characteristic. Even high potency pharmaceutical preparations still require scrupulous clean-up procedures in order to minimize spectral interference.

The development of instrumental chromatographic techniques has revolutionized the task of vitamin D estimation in both food and clinical samples. Although novel detection methods exploiting fluorescence derivatization or electrochemical techniques are presently under investigation, contemporary UV approaches still require the inclusion of rigorous purification procedures, since this detection mode remains inherently nonspecific.

Isolation, Extraction and Clean-up

Vitamin D is vulnerable to oxygen, light, low pH and is also subject to reversible isomerization when heated. Therefore adequate precautions are essential throughout any analytical procedure to avoid loss of the target analytes.

All chemical extraction techniques exploit the inherent lipophilic property of this vitamin and a vitamin-rich fraction is separated from other food components either by saponification or by total lipid extraction.

Saponification

Alkaline hydrolysis is a convenient way to eliminate the bulk of neutral lipids and is particularly favoured in high-fat foods and those of an intractable nature. This popular technique is also advantageous for products containing encapsulated supplements and when relatively large sample quantities are needed for reasons of assay sensitivity or analyte heterogeneity.

While some authors report the use of high-temperature saponification, strategies such as direct measurement or use of conversion factors are then needed to account for the consequent elevated levels of previtamin D. These concerns can significantly complicate the assay and may be avoided through the use of overnight hydrolysis at ambient temperature, which additionally offers operational simplicity. It is considered mandatory during extraction to include a protective antioxidant and to purge with inert gas. Vitamin D, along with the other fat-soluble vitamins, sterols, carotenoids and hydrocarbons, remain in the nonsaponifiable fraction. Enzymatic hydrolysis with lipase has been suggested as an alternative to saponification, thereby minimizing possible degradation and facilitating concurrent recovery of the alkali-unstable vitamin K, if required.

The nonsaponifiable fraction containing the calciferol is rapidly and conveniently partitioned into a solvent mixture of hexane and diethylether with good recovery, although other solvent systems have also been cited in the literature. Following washing to remove hydrophilic remnants and excess alkali, the organic phase is dried and evaporated to recover an enriched crude extract. This will generally require further clean-up prior to quantification, dependent on the vitamin D concentration and level of coextractives.

Total Lipid Extraction

The risks of thermal equilibration with previtamin D and potential degradation of vitamin D have been avoided through an initial lipid extraction. A variety of solvent systems have been recommended depending upon sample type and fat content. A consequence of employing such a technique for foods is the need to isolate the vitamin components from high-molecular-weight fractions (triglycerides, phospholipids) by gel-permeation and/or adsorption chromatography. Various protocols have been advocated which, while successful, contribute complexities to the assays which are difficult for most quality control laboratories to manage.

This extraction route has been commonly applied to low-fat clinical specimens (such as plasma), and fat reduced fortified foods (e.g. skim milk). It is also useful when vitamin D and its metabolites are to be estimated concurrently. The literature consensus seems to support the view that saponification is more appropriate when complex and poorly characterized foods are to be assayed.

The concentrations of cholecalciferol are generally low, even after isolation of the crude extracts. Further clean-up to remove substantial quantities of sterols and other unsaponifiable material is usually incorporated prior to analysis. Such strategies may be as simple as cholesterol precipitation or as complex as multistage semipreparative chromatography, depending on both sample type and the sophistication of subsequent analytical techniques. Often at this stage, analysts may expediently utilize the convenience of prepacked solid phase extraction cartridges. Usually, the adsorption mode with activated silica is selected, producing an extract of higher vitamin D content and fewer potential interferences. These disposable cartridges are now widely replacing the earlier techniques of open-column or thin-layer chromatography (although the latter is still occasionally used for clean-up or qualitative 'spot testing').

Chromatography

Quantification of enriched vitamin extracts is achievable by applying gas–liquid chromatography (GLC) techniques although the thermal instability of vitamin D at operating temperatures results in formation of pyro and isopyro peaks of both parent or derivative forms. This problem has been successfully avoided by prior conversion to the thermostable isotachysterol isomers. Modern GLC now benefits from the use of capillary columns and ultrasensitive mass-selective spectrometric detectors, but the extensive manipulative procedures still make GLC less attractive than other technologies for routine food analysis. *See* Chromatography, Gas Chromatography

High-performance liquid chromatography (HPLC) has led to continuing improvements in the assay of vitamin D (and its metabolites) in foods and has now superseded GLC. While additional clean-up is not always unavoidable, derivatization procedures are unnecessary in the majority of schemes. Furthermore, the ambient and nondestructive features inherent in

HPLC are more compatible with the lability properties of this, and other, vitamins. *See* Chromatography, High-performance Liquid Chromatography

In the absence of useful native fluorescence or stable electrochemical viewing modes and the current infancy of commercial on-line liquid chromatography–mass spectroscopy (LCMS) interfaces, the use of UV spectrophotometric detection is universal.

The modest spectral properties of vitamin D often require a semipreparative HPLC fractionation step before an analytical HPLC stage can be undertaken. Spectral selectivity is further gained by the judicious use of either wavelength ratioing or full spectrum (e.g. diode array) detection. Alternative choices to attain additional specificity and selectivity include the use of off-line competitive protein binding assay or the precolumn conversion of cholecalciferol to its bathochromically shifted isotachysterol.

In view of the differing selectivities of normal-phase and reversed-phase HPLC, many researchers have concluded that the assay benefits by combining the two modes. This multidimensional technique exploits the fact that cholecalciferol and ergocalciferol are unresolved on silica columns yet are completely separated using C18 reversed-phase columns. There are a number of reported methods which employ reversed-phase chromatography during clean-up, either low pressure or HPLC, followed by normal-phase quantitation. This regimen is generally of use where both calciferols are known to coexist in the sample or where the sample is not well defined in terms of its vitamin D content.

Silica chromatography can be used during the preparative step and the two vitamins collected in a single fraction before application to a reversed-phase column. This allows one vitamin to be used as an internal standard for the other, greatly decreasing the cumulative assay errors introduced by isomerization and manipulative losses. The method can be used where only one vitamin is present as is usually encountered in the food industry. Chromatograms of a fish oil taken through this analytical procedure are shown in Fig. 4. The endogenous vitamin is cholecalciferol, allowing internal standardization with ergocalciferol. Solvent incompatibility between normal and reversed-phase modes unfortunately restricts the opportunity to automate this multidimensional procedure through the use of on-line column switching procedures.

The elution positions of previtamin D_3 and provitamin D_3 are shown in Fig. 4(a). They are well separated from vitamin D_3, thus allowing potential differentiation of the species. Other calciferols shown in Figs. 2 and 3 can be similarly resolved. On silica columns, using hydrocarbon/alcohol mobile phases, the major isomers elute in the sequence previtamin $D_3 <$ *trans*-vitamin $D_3 <$ lumisterol$_3 <$ isotachysterol$_3 <$ vitamin $D_3 <$ tachysterol$_3 <$ provitamin $D_3 <$ hydroxymetabolites. The pyrocalci-

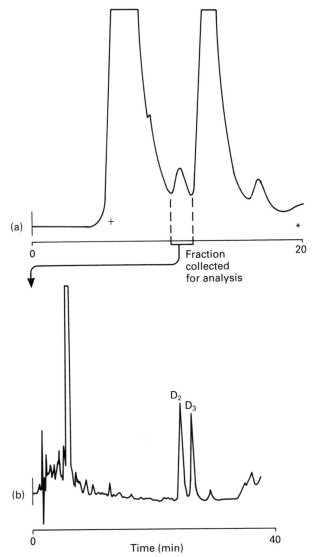

Fig. 4 HPLC chromatograms showing the analysis of cholecalciferol in halibut liver oil. An internal standard of ergocalciferol (D_2) was used throughout the analysis. (a) The semipreparative clean-up stage. A Brownlee (25 cm × 10 mm) silica column was used with a mobile phase of 1% 2-propanol in hexane, flowing at 3 ml min^{-1}. Detection was by UV at 280 nm (0.04 aufs). The unsaponifiable fraction from 2.5 g of fish oil was dissolved in 1 ml of mobile phase and injected. The fraction collected and evaporated for quantitative analysis is shown. The elution positions of previtamin D_3 (+) and provitamin D_3 (*) are shown. (b) A reversed phase C18 Column (Waters 5 μm Radial-PAK) was used for analyte quantification. A mobile phase of methanol/water/tetrahydrofuran (90:8:2 v/v/v) at a flow rate of 2 ml min^{-1} was used. The injection volume was 100 μl, representing the cholecalciferol (D_3) content of 0.25 g of oil. Detection was at 280 nm (0.005 aufs).

ferols elute close to lumisterol$_3$. The most likely interfering isomer is tachysterol$_3$ which elutes close to vitamin D_3 in both normal and reversed-phase analyses. Interestingly, the retention sequence of previtamin D_3, vitamin D_3 and provitamin D_3 is the same, regardless of which separation mode is used.

Bibliography

Ball GFM (1988) *Fat-Soluble Vitamin Assays in Food Analysis. A Comprehensive Review*. London: Elsevier.

Belitz H-D and Grosch W (1987) *Food Chemistry*, pp 305–319. Berlin: Springer-Verlag.

Collins ED and Norman AW (1991) Vitamin D. In: Machlin LJ (ed.) *Handbook of Vitamins*, pp 59–98. New York: Marcel Dekker.

Friedrich W (1988) Vitamin D. In: *Vitamins*. pp. 143–216. Berlin: de Gruyter.

Indyk H and Woollard DC (1984) The determination of vitamin D by high performance liquid chromatography. *New Zealand Journal of Dairy Science and Technology* 19: 1–6.

Jones G, Seamark DA, Trafford DJH and Makin HLJ (1985) Vitamin D: cholecalciferol, ergocalciferol and hydroxylated metabolites. In: De Leenheer AP, Lambert WE and De Ruyter MGM (eds) *Modern Chromatographic Analysis of the Vitamins*, pp 73–128 New York: Marcel Dekker.

Lawson DEM (1985) Vitamin D. In: Diplock AT (ed.) *Fat-Soluble Vitamins. Their Biochemistry and Applications*. London: Heinemann.

Macrae R (1988) *HPLC in Food Analysis*, 2nd edn. London: Academic Press.

Parrish DB (1979) Determination of vitamin D in foods. *CRC Critical Reviews in Food Science and Nutrition* 12: 29–57

Sherman HC and Smith SL (1931) Vitamin D. In: *The Vitamins*, 2nd edn. pp. 293–335. *American Chemical Society Monograph Series*. New York: Chemical Catalog Company.

Strohecker R and Henning HM (1965) Vitamin D. *Vitamin Assay, Tested Methods*, pp 254–282. Verlag Chemie.

Wagner AF and Folkers K (1975) *Vitamins and Co-enzymes*, pp 330–362. New York: Krieger.

D.C. Woollard
Ministry of Agriculture and Fisheries, Auckland, New Zealand
H.E. Indyk
Anchor Products, Waitoa, New Zealand

Physiology

Vitamin D generates a wide spectrum of biological responses in various target tissues by mechanisms similar to classical steroid hormones. The most potent biologically active metabolite of vitamin D is $1\alpha,25$-dihydroxyvitamin D_3 $[1,25(OH)_2D_3]$ which is synthesized from its precursor or prohormone form, vitamin D_3. Research in the last several years has unequivocally established the true identity of $1,25(OH)_2D_3$ as a bona fide steroid hormone rather than a vitamin. The pleiotropic effects of vitamin D are primarily mediated by the hormonal form of vitamin D, i.e. $1,25(OH)_2D_3$, both in classical tissues such as intestine, bone and kidney, and in a host of nonclassical tissues such as pancreas, muscle, skin, immune and haemopoietic system. *See* Hormones, Steroid Hormones

Physiologically, $1,25(OH)_2D_3$ not only serves to modulate mineral homeostasis but it also plays a role in the processes of osteogenesis, modulation of immune response, pancreas and muscle function, differentiation and growth of skin epidermal cells, and in haemopoietic tissue. The mechanism of genomic action of $1,25(OH)_2D_3$ parallels that of other classical steroid hormones in that it binds specifically with high-affinity nuclear receptors. The steroid–receptor complex then interacts with specific *cis*-acting regulatory DNA sequences to effect the induction or repression of hormone-sensitive genes. The receptor for $1,25(OH)_2D_3$ that mediates its hormonal effects shares strong structural resemblance with other classical steroid hormone receptors, such as those for glucocorticoid, oestrogen, progesterone, retinoic acid and thyroid hormones. An overview of the vitamin D endocrine pathway, covering aspects related to vitamin D metabolism, regulation and function, will be summarized in this article.

History

Historically, the discovery of vitamin D has been closely linked to rickets, which is a disorder of the bone. Experiments demonstrating the ability of heated, aerated cod liver oil to cure rickets led to the identity of a new vitamin, termed vitamin D by EV McCollum. The manifestation of rickets as a result of a dietary deficiency of vitamin D was subsequently established from the nutritional studies carried out by Sir Edward Mellanby.

Metabolism of Vitamin D_3

In order to execute its biological functions, vitamin D must undergo metabolic transformations involving hydroxylation at the C1 and C25 positions.

Skin Synthesis

Upon exposure to sunlight, the epidermal cutaneous reservoir of provitamin D_3 (7-dehydrocholesterol) is photolysed to previtamin D_3, which undergoes isomerization via a nonphotochemical rearrangement to yield vitamin D_3 at a rate dictated by the temperature of the skin. During prolonged exposure to sunlight, previtamin D_3 is photoisomerized into two biologically inert sterols, lumisterol and tachysterol, thereby preventing the excessive accumulation of previtamin D_3.

Absorption

Bile salts in the intestine have been implicated in the absorption of vitamin D that is obtained through the diet. In the rat and human, the absorption of vitamin D by intestinal epithelial cells occurs through the lacteal system into the chylomicrons and, consequently, into the bloodstream.

Transport

A specific plasma transport protein, known as the vitamin-D-binding protein (DBP), mediates the transport of vitamin D_3, derived either from photobiosynthesis in the skin or from dietary sources through the blood compartment. Vitamin-D-binding protein is an α-globulin protein with a molecular weight of 58 000 Da in humans.

Storage

The major storage depots of vitamin D and $25(OH)D_3$ in humans are the adipose and muscle tissue. The blood compartment, however, contains the highest concentrations of vitamin D compared to other tissues.

Hepatic Metabolism of Vitamin D_3

The vitamin D that is delivered to liver by DBP is metabolically activated by an obligatory hydroxylation at the C25 position to yield $25(OH)D_3$, which represents the major circulating form of vitamin D. This enzyme reaction is mediated by a mixed-function oxygenase(s), known as the vitamin-D_3-hydroxylase, present in liver microsomes and mitochondria.

Renal Metabolism of $25(OH)D_3$

In the kidney, which serves as an endocrine gland for vitamin D, $25(OH)D_3$ is converted by key hydroxylations at the C1 or C24 positions to form $1,25(OH)_2D_3$, or $24,25(OH)_2D_3$, respectively. The hydroxylation at the C1 position is catalysed by the 25-hydroxyvitamin-D_3-1α-hydroxylase (1-hydroxylase) which is located in the mitochondria of the proximal tubules in the kidney. The enzyme is a mixed-function oxidase, comprised of three proteins – renal ferredoxin reductase, renal ferredoxin and cytochrome P-450 – which are all integral components of the mitochondrial membrane; the former two components serve to transfer electrons from the reduced form of nicotinamide adenine dinucleotide phosphate (NADPH) to the cytochrome P-450. Cytochrome P-450 provides the substrate binding site and catalytic site which reduces one molecule of oxygen to yield water and one hydroxyl function, which is transferred to the substrate $25(OH)D_3$ at the stereospecific site.

The 24-R hydroxylase is also a mixed-function oxygenase and is responsible for the 24-hydroxylation of $25(OH)D_3$ in the kidney. Apart from these 3 major metabolites, 33 other metabolites of vitamin D_3 have been isolated and chemically characterized.

Regulation of Vitamin D Metabolism

Regulation of $1,25(OH)_2D_3$ Formation

The renal biosynthesis of $1,25(OH)_2D_3$ appears to be the key determinant of the regulation of vitamin D_3 metabolism. Regulation of 1α-hydroxylase activity and the consequent production of $1,25(OH)_2D_3$ are dependent on three important factors: (1) plasma $1,25(OH)_2D_3$ levels; (2) parathyroid hormone (PTH); and (3) the serum concentration of calcium and phosphorus.

The key modulator of $25(OH)D_3$-1-hydroxylase activity is the $1,25(OH)_2D_3$ status of the animal itself. When circulating levels of $1,25(OH)_2D_3$ are low, synthesis of $1,25(OH)_2D_3$ is maximum while production of $24,25(OH)_2D_3$ becomes negligible. However, when circulating levels of $1,25(OH)_2D_3$ are high, or with the exogenous addition of $1,25(OH)_2D_3$, the situation is reversed.

Two other major regulators of $25(OH)D_3$-α-hydroxylase are serum calcium ions (Ca^{2+}) and PTH. Under conditions of hypocalcaemia in intact animals, $25(OH)D_3$-1-hydroxylase enzyme activity is markedly elevated, and $25(OH)D_3$-24-hydroxylase is suppressed. This scenario is reversed with hypercalcaemia. The hypocalcaemic stimulation of $1,25(OH)_2D_3$ production is mediated by PTH. Under low serum calcium conditions, parathyroid glands, acting as ionized Ca^{2+} sensors, secrete more PTH. The increased PTH thus released stimulates the $25(OH)D_3$-1-hydroxylase and decreases the activity of $1,25(OH)_2D_3$-24-hydroxylase. In addition, $1,25(OH)_2D_3$ and $24,25(OH)_2D_3$ operate in a feedback loop to modulate and/or reduce the secretion of PTH. *See* Calcium, Physiology

Catabolism and Excretion

The catabolism of $1,25(OH)_2D_3$ to more polar seco-steroids involves a variety of chemical reactions that include oxidative cleavage of the side-chain.

Studies in humans have shown that glucuronide conjugates of $1,25(OH)_2D_3$ are eliminated in the faeces upon administration of radiolabelled $1,25(OH)_2D_3$.

Analogues of $1,25(OH)_2D_3$

Several analogues of vitamin D_3 that are endowed with selective biological activity have been designed based on knowledge of vitamin D chemistry.

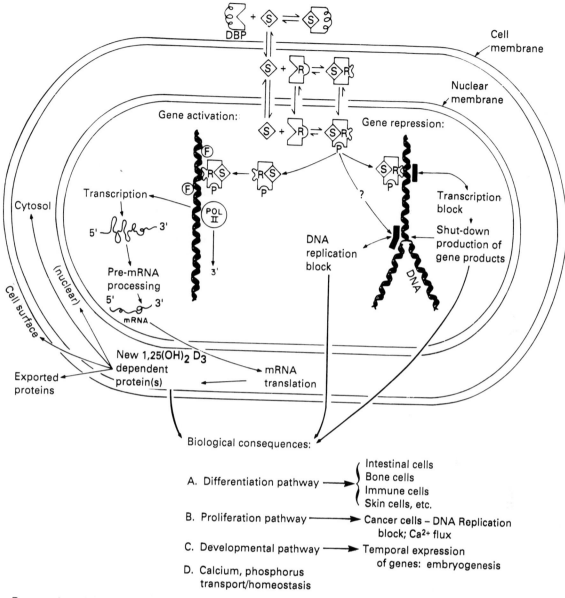

Fig. 1 Proposed model for the mechanism of action of the steroid hormone, $1,25(OH)_2D_3$. DBP, serum vitamin-D-binding protein; S, $1,25(OH)_2D_3$ steroid; R, receptor; P, phosphorylation; F, transcription factor; DNA, deoxyribonucleic acid; mRNA, messenger ribonucleic acid; POL II, DNA-directed RNA polymerase II.

Fluoro analogues, such as $24R\text{-}F\text{-}1,25(OH)_2D_3$, 24,24-difluoro-25-hydroxyvitamin D_3 and 24,24-difluoro-1,25-dihydroxyvitamin D_3, have been shown to possess biological activity. Other known analogues of vitamin D which show therapeutic potential are 1α-hydroxyvitamin D_3, dihydrotachysterol₃; 3-deoxy-1α-hydroxyvitamin D_3 and 3-deoxy-1,25-dihydroxyvitamin D_3.

Hormonal Action of 1,25-Dihydroxyvitamin D₃

Vitamin D serves essentially to regulate the calcium and phosphorus homeostasis in all vertebrates. The steroidal actions of $1,25(OH)_2D_3$ are mediated by intracellular high-affinity receptors present in the nucleus of target cells. Binding of the hormone $1,25(OH)_2D_3$ to its receptor results in the activation of the receptor; the hormone–receptor complex then interacts with specific *cis*-acting deoxyribonucleic acid (DNA) sequence elements, known as hormone response elements (HREs). This interaction culminates in either induction or repression of specific target genes. A schematic depiction of the hormonal actions of $1,25(OH)_2D_3$ is shown in Fig. 1.

A wide array of genes have been shown to be either upregulated or downregulated by $1,25(OH)_2D_3$ (see Table 1). The most extensively studied $1,25(OH)_2D_3$-sensitive gene at the molecular level is the bone-specific

Table 1. Classification of genes regulated by $1,25(OH)_2D_3$

Biochemical category	Gene or gene products	Regulation (↑, up; ↓, down)
Mineral homeostasis	Calbindin-D_{28K}	↑
	Calbindin-D_{9K}	↑
	Carbonic anhydrase	↑
	Alkaline phosphatase	↑
	Metallothionein	↑
Bone	Osteocalcin	↑
Extracellular matrix	Matrix-*gla*-protein	↑
	Collagen type I	↓
	Fibronectin	↑
	Osteonectin	↑
Cell surface differentiation antigens	6_3D_3	↑
	Mac-1	↑
	I a(Class II MHA)	↑
	F_c receptors	↑
	C_3 receptor	↑
Immunoglobulin production	IgG, IgM	↓
Oncogenes	c-*myc*	↓
	c-*myb*	↓
	c-*fos*	↑
	c-*fms*	↑
	c-KI-*ras*	↑
Chromosomal protein	Histone H4	↓
Growth factors	Interleukin-1	↑
	Interleukins 2 and 3	↓
	γ-Interferon	↓
	EGF-receptors	↑
	Transforming growth factor	↑
	Tumour necrosis factor-α	↑
Phosphorylation	Protein kinase C	↑
Peptide hormones	Preproparathyroid hormone	↓
	Prolactin	↑
	Thyrotropin-stimulating hormone	↑
	Calcitonin	↓
Polyamine biosynthesis	Ornithine decarboxylase	↑
	Spermidine *n*-acetyl transferase	↑
Mitochondrial genes	ATP synthetase	↑
	Cytochrome oxidase I, III	↑
Melanin synthesis	Tyrosinase	↑
Lipid metabolism	Diacylglycerol acyl transferase	↑
Cholinergic activity	Choline acetyl transferase	↑
Cyclic nucleotides	Adenylate cyclase	↓
Vitamin D_3 metabolism	$25(OH)D_3$-1-α-hydroxylase	↓
	$25(OH)D_3$-24-hydroxylase	↑

Abstracted from Minghetti and Norman (1988).

osteocalcin gene which is transcriptionally upregulated by $1,25(OH)_2D_3$. The vitamin D response element (VDRE) in the promoter of the osteocalcin gene has been defined only recently, and the sequence of this response element bears a striking similarity to those of the thyroid hormone and oestrogen response elements.

The recent cloning and sequencing of the avian, rat and human vitamin D_3 receptor complementary DNAs (cDNAs) indicate great sequence homology between vitamin D receptors and other steroid or thyroid hormone receptors. The receptor is a labile, soluble protein, sedimenting in high salt–sucrose gradients at $3 \cdot 1–3 \cdot 7 s$ (52 000–60 000 Da). It binds the ligand $1,25(OH)_2D_3$ with high affinity (K_D, $1–50 \times 10^{-11}$ M).

The distribution of $1,25(OH)_2D_3$ receptor in different tissues has been determined (Minghetti and Norman, 1988) using monoclonal antibodies against rat and human receptors:

1. Normal tissues: bone (osteoblasts); cardiac muscle; cartilage (chondrocyte); circulating lymphocytes (activated); circulating monocytes; colon; intestine; kidney (proximal and distal tubules); mammary tissue; ovary; pancreas (β cell); parathyroid gland; parotid gland; pituitary gland; placenta; skeletal muscle; skin (epidermal cells and fibroblasts); testes; thymus; thyroid (c-cells); uterus.
2. Malignant tissues or cell lines: breast carcinoma; cervical carcinoma; colon carcinoma; fibrosarcoma; medullary thyroid carcinoma; melanoma; myeloid or lymphocytic leukaemia; osteosarcoma; pancreatic adenocarcinoma; transitional cell bladder carcinoma.

Structurally, the $1,25(OH)_2D_3$ receptor is comprised of distinct functional domains that are organized into the ligand-binding domain oriented near the *C*-terminus of the receptor, a DNA-binding region towards the *N*-terminus, and a hinge region in between these two domains. The hinge region bears antigenic determinants as well as putative transactivating sequences that are known to augment transcriptional activation. Characteristically, the DNA binding region bears positionally conserved cysteine residues which are configured into two DNA binding 'finger' motifs, probably by coordinating with zinc ions (Zn^{2+}) – a feature typical in other steroid hormone receptors such as those for glucocorticoids, thyroid hormone, oestrogen, progesterone, retinoic acid, etc. The *N*-terminus of the receptor contains hypervariable amino acids and transactivating sequences.

One of the major molecular markers of the receptor-mediated interaction of $1,25(OH)_2D_3$ is the induction of a calcium binding protein named calbindin-D (Norman *et al.*, 1982). The protein exists as a 28 000 Da (calbindin-D_{28K}) species in the mammalian kidney and brain, and in the avian system, while in the mammalian intestine and placenta a smaller form is expressed (calbindin-D_{9K}).

Functions of Vitamin D

Classical Target Tissues

In the classical target tissues, such as intestine, bone and kidney, $1,25(OH)_2D_3$ – largely in conjunction with

PTH – serves to regulate mineral homeostasis such that serum calcium and phosphorus levels are maintained within a physiological range that can support normal mineralization of bone.

At the intestine, $1,25(OH)_2D_3$ primarily stimulates the active transport of Ca^{2+} and inorganic phosphate P_i via mechanisms that involve calbindin D. Available evidence suggests that calbindin D may be involved in protecting the cell (as a buffer) against large fluxes of Ca^{2+} which result from active transport induced by $1,25(OH)_2D_3$.

In addition to the genomic effects of $1,25(OH)_2D_3$, recent studies have shown that $1,25(OH)_2D_3$ can stimulate the rapid (2–4 min) transport of calcium, termed transcaltachia, via a receptor-mediated process, albeit one independent of gene activation.

In the kidney, $1,25(OH)_2D_3$ functions in concert with PTH to enhance renal Ca^{2+} reabsorption, besides regulating its own biosynthesis by feedback inhibition of renal 1-hydroxylase.

$1\alpha,25$-Dihydroxyvitamin D_3 plays an important role in bone growth, development and differentiation, and supports bone mineralization indirectly by supplying the minerals calcium and phosphorus via their enhanced intestinal absorption. In addition, $24,25(OH)_2D_3$ has been shown to promote the bone mineralization process.

Nonclassical Target Tissues

The $1,25(OH)_2D_3$ hormone promotes differentiation of cells in the haemopoietic system. Such effects of $1,25(OH)_2D_3$ offer a therapeutic prospect for leukaemia.

In the immune system $1,25(OH)_2D_3$ acts as an immuno-modulator, regulating the functional performance of cells involved in the immune response. *See* Immunity and Nutrition

Insulin production by the endocrine pancreas is influenced by vitamin D status in that the blunted secretion of insulin and impaired glucose tolerance seen in vitamin-D-deficient conditions are corrected by treatment with vitamin D_3 and/or $1,25(OH)_2D_3$. $1,25(OH)_2D_3$. *See* Glucose, Glucose Tolerance and the Glycaemic Index

Myopathy and abnormalities in muscle contraction seen in patients afflicted with metabolic bone disease are amenable to correction with vitamin D therapy. *See* Bone

$1\alpha,25$-Dihydroxyvitamin D_3 induces differentiation of keratinocytes in skin and exerts antiproliferative effects on these epithelial cells. Such an effect of $1,25(OH)_2D_3$ in the skin has prompted the use of $1,25(OH)_2D_3$ analogues for treatment of psoriasis, which is hyperproliferative disease of the skin.

Nutritional Requirements for Vitamin D

Adequate exposure to sunlight on a regular basis is a chief determinant of the vitamin D nutritional status in humans. The vitamin D requirements may also be influenced by the dietary composition of Ca^{2+} and P_i, age, sex and skin pigmentation.

By definition of the League of Nations in 1933, one international unit (iu) of vitamin D_3 is stated to be 25 ng. The current allowance of vitamin D_3 recommended by the US National Research Council is 400 iu per day. Since clinical rickets is manifested predominantly in a growing child, the recommendations of the committee of the Food and Agriculture Organization (FAO) and World Health Organization (WHO) are 400 iu per day for children up to the age of 6; thereafter a daily allowance of 100 iu per day has been recommended.

Disease States Related to Vitamin D

In humans, diseases related to vitamin D can arise because of (1) altered availability of vitamin D, (2) altered hepatic conversion of vitamin D_3, (3) impaired renal metabolism of $25(OH)D_3$, or (4) variation in end-organ responsiveness to $1,25(OH)_2D_3$.

Renal Disorders

Chronic renal failure, also known as renal osteodystrophy, is characterized by impaired renal production of $1,25(OH)_2D_3$ and intestinal malabsorption of calcium which can often lead to derangements in skeletal metabolism and hyperparathyroidism. These symptoms are alleviated by $1,25(OH)_2D_3$ administration. In 1977, in the USA, the Food and Drug Administration (FDA) approved the prescription use of $1,25(OH)_2D_3$ for renal osteodystrophy.

Vitamin-D-resistant Rickets

Also known as familial X-linked hypophosphataemic rickets, vitamin-D-resistant rickets is characterized by a primary phosphate leak in the kidney, skeletal deformities and hypophosphatemia. A combination of oral phosphate and $1,25(OH)_2D_3$ is effective in treating these patients.

Vitamin-D-dependent Rickets

Vitamin-D-dependent rickets is also referred to as hereditary hypocalcaemic vitamin-D-resistant rickets, and is classified into type I and type II disease states.

Type I rickets is believed to arise as a result of an inborn error in the renal 1-hydroxylase enzyme. The clinical features include hypocalcaemia, hyphosphataemia, and several rachitic lesions. These symptoms can be treated with pharmacological doses of vitamin D_3 or low doses of $1,25(OH)_2D_3$.

Point mutations in the receptor gene have been shown to be responsible for the defective receptors seen in children with *type II rickets*. The clinical manifestations are defective bone mineralization, decreased intestinal calcium absorption, hypocalcaemia, and increased serum $1,25(OH)_2D_3$ levels. To date, a point mutation in a steroid receptor gene resulting in the loss of functional activity has been demonstrated only for the vitamin D receptor and is therefore unique in this respect.

Diseases of Parathyroid

Hypoparathyroidism

Hypoparathyroidism exhibits hypocalcaemia as a major clinical consequence and is corrected with large doses of vitamin D or physiological doses of $1,25(OH)_2D_3$.

Hyperparathyroidism

Increased $1,25(OH)_2D_3$ levels, enhanced intestinal absorption of calcium (contributing to hypercalciuria), and nephrolithiasis are typical of this disorder.

Pseudohypoparathyroidism

Pseudohypoparathyroidism results from a state of resistance to PTH. The biochemical abnormalities are hypocalcaemia, hyperphospataemia, elevated serum PTH, and decreased serum $1,25(OH)_2D_3$ levels.

Disorder of Bone

Clinically, a deficiency in vitamin D manifests as rickets in children and osteomalacia in adults. Hypocalcaemia, hypophosphataemia, increased alkaline phosphatase, and decreased $25(OH)D_3$ levels are some of the salient biochemical abnormalities, all of which can be ameliorated by vitamin D administration.

Conclusion

Vitamin D exhibits a wide range of biological actions in both classical and nonclassical target tissues via pathways analogous to classical steroid hormones. Classically, vitamin D has been known to act as a calciotropic hormone which works to effect mineral homeostasis in higher animals. In this respect the daughter metabolite of vitamin D_3, $1,25(OH)_2D_3$, mediates the effective absorption of calcium in the intestine which is the principal site of $1,25(OH)_2D_3$ action. Many diverse pleiotropic effects mediated by $1,25(OH)_2D_3$ have been identified in recent years and studied extensively. These include the involvement of $1,25(OH)_2D_3$ in a variety of cellular processes involving endocrine, immune and cell differentiation functions. The recent discovery of the VDRE in the promoter region of a $1,25(OH)_2D_3$-sensitive gene – osteocalcin – establishes unequivocally the steroidal mode of vitamin D action.

Bibliography

Cooke NE and Haddad JG (1989) Vitamin D binding protein (Gc-globulin). *Endocrine Reviews* 10: 294–307.

Haussler MR, Mangelsdorf DJ, Komm BS *et al.* (1989) Molecular biology of the vitamin D hormone. *Recent Progress in Hormone Research* 44: 263–305.

Henry HL and Norman AW (1984) Vitamin D: metabolism and biological actions. *Annual Review of Nutrition* 4: 493–520.

Minghetti PP and Norman AW (1988) $1,25(OH)_2D_3$-Vitamin D_3 receptors: gene regulation and genetic circuitry. *The FASEB Journal* 2: 3043–3053.

Nemere I and Norman AW (1991) Transport of calcium. In: Field M and Frizzell RA (eds) *Handbook of Physiology*, sect. 13, pp 337–360. Bethesda: American Physiological Society.

Norman AW, Roth J and Orci L (1982) The vitamin D endocrine system: steroid metabolism, hormone receptors and biological response (calcium binding proteins). *Endocrine Reviews* 3: 331–366.

Anita C. Maiyar and Anthony W. Norman
University of California, Riverside, USA

CHOLESTEROL

Contents

Properties and Determination

Cholesterol is a well-known and commonly determined lipid component and an important intermediate in the synthesis of steroid hormones. It is a sterol ($C_{27}H_{45}OH$) that occurs notably in animal fats and oils, bile, gallstones, nerve tissues, blood, brain, plasma and egg yolk. Cholesterol is the most common animal sterol and is also found in trace amounts in vegetable fats and oils, seaweeds and green leaves. Cholesterol was first found in gallstones and derives its name from the Greek *kholé* (bile) and *stereos* (solid). The determination of cholesterol in serum and foods is of significance because of the implication of cholesterol in the aetiology of arteriosclerosis and coronary heart disease. *See* Atherosclerosis; Coronary Heart Disease, Intervention Studies

Structure

A systematic study of the chemistry of cholesterol began at the end of the 19th century. The classic work of Wieland, Vindaus, Diels, Rosenheim and King led to the formulation of the structure of cholesterol in 1932. The fundamental carbon skeleton of the cholesterol molecule is the cyclopentanoperhydrophenanthrene ring. The structure of cholesterol is shown in Fig. 1. The hydroxyl group on C3 is connected by a 'solid' bond (β orientation) and the hydrogen by a 'dashed' bond (α orientation), depicting the naturally occurring β-cholesterol. Atoms connected by solid bonds (β orientation) are regarded as projecting in front of the plane of the steroid ring, and those connected by dashed bonds (α orientation) as lying behind the plane. The molecular weight of cholesterol is 384·64. Cholesterol consists of 83·87% carbon, 11·99% hydrogen and 4·145% oxygen by weight. The formal chemical name of the molecule is cholest-5-en-3β-ol. Because the cholesterol nucleus contains eight centres of asymmetry, approximately 240 isomers of the molecule are possible. However, only two carbon centres (C3 and C5) appear to be involved in naturally occurring cholesterol isomers. In some of the earlier scientific literature, cholesterol is referred to as 'cholesterin'.

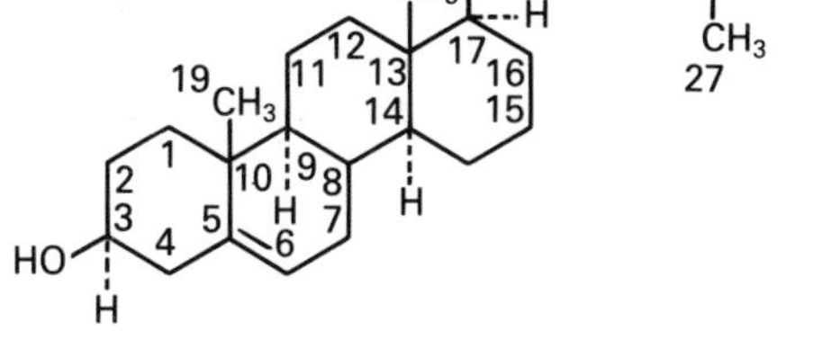

Chemical Characteristics

Cholesterol is a glistening, white, soapy, crystalline substance that is practically insoluble in water (about 0·2 mg per 100 ml). It is slightly soluble in alcohol (1·29% w/w at 20°C) and more soluble in hot alcohol (100 g of saturated 96% alcoholic solution contains 28 g of cholesterol at 80°C). One gram of the compound dissolves in 2·8 ml of ether, 4·5 ml of chloroform or 1·5 ml of pyridine. Cholesterol is also soluble in benzene, hexane, petroleum ether, oils, fats and aqueous solutions of bile salts. It crystallizes easily from absolute alcohol, acetic acid, ether and similar solvents as colourless rhombic plates with one or more characteristic notches in the corners. Because cholesterol has an unsaturated bond, it will accept up to two halogen atoms. Cholesterol is not saponifiable.

Cholesterol gives a number of colour reactions that are useful to test for the molecule both qualitatively and quantitatively. The Salkowski reaction produces a series of colours when a chloroform solution of cholesterol is stratified over concentrated sulphuric acid. The acid assumes a yellowish colour with a green fluorescence, whereas the chloroform layer first becomes bluish red, and then gradually changes to a violet-red. If the chloroform layer is decanted into a porcelain evaporating dish, it changes from violet-red to violet, to green, and then to yellow. Another test, the Liebermann–Burchard reaction, which consists of adding acetic anhydride and concentrated sulphuric acid (under conditions as nearly anhydrous as possible) to a chloroform solution of cholesterol, results in an initial blue to violet

Fig. 1 Structure of β-cholesterol showing carbon atom numbering.

colour that changes to emerald green. Under carefully controlled conditions, the intensity of the green colour produced is proportional to the amount of cholesterol present.

Free cholesterol unites with digitonin, a glycosidic saponin, to form cholesterol digitonide; cholesterol esters do not form such compounds. Cholesterol digitonide is insoluble in petroleum ether; cholesterol esters are freely soluble in petroleum ether. This difference in solubilities is useful to test both qualitatively and quantitatively for free versus esterified cholesterol.

Fieser showed that the melting point of cholesterol, which had been purified by recrystallization from acetic acid, was 149·5–150·0°C. Radin and Gramza indicated that the acceptable melting point of recrystallized cholesterol was 149·3–151·3°C. The *Merck Index* indicates that the melting point of anhydrous cholesterol is 148·5°C and the boiling point is 233°C at 0·5 mmHg and 360°C at 1 atm (760 mmHg). At 360°C some decomposition occurs.

Primary Cholesterol Standard

The requirements for primary standards become progressively more stringent as methods are developed that are more sensitive and more compound-specific; such is the case for cholesterol. Primary standards are chemical substances that, by virtue of their purity, can be weighed directly for the preparation of solutions with known concentrations. Primary cholesterol standards are expected to be at least 99% pure. Cholesterol stored at room temperature, unprotected by a nitrogen cover, will undergo autoxidation over an extended period. In addition, ultraviolet light will produce structural changes in cholesterol unless amber glass containers are used. Consequently, various amounts of cholesterol oxidation products may be present in what was initially pure cholesterol. Among the cholesterol oxides that have been identified in stored cholesterol are 7-ketocholesterol, 20-hydroxycholesterol, and 24-, 25- and 26-hydroxycholesterol. Therefore, primary standards that have been stored must be checked and may need to undergo repurification before use. Crystalline standards should be stored in small amounts over a desiccant such as silica gel at −20°C in the dark.

Cholesterol may be recrystallized from ethanol or acetic acid, or as the dibromide. A cholesterol preparation may be added to absolute ethanol, which is gently heated until the cholesterol dissolves and is then cooled to room temperature. The precipitated cholesterol is collected on a filter, washed with a small volume of diethyl ether, dried overnight in air, and dried in an oven at 90°C for 2 h. Cholesterol is recrystallized from boiling glacial acetic acid solution, which is then cooled to room temperature in an ice bath. The crystals are collected on a filter, washed with acetic acid and methanol, and dried as described above.

The recrystallization of cholesterol by the dibromide method (Schoenheimer) is a more arduous task than the recrystallization from either ethanol or acetic acid, but it produces a superior product. A bromine solution is added to the cholesterol solution. A white paste is produced that is then transferred to a filter and washed with acetic acid until the filtrate is colourless. Zinc dust is then added to a suspension of the white material in diethyl ether and glacial acetic acid (750:10 v/v); the reaction produces evolution of hydrogen. The resultant white precipitate of zinc salts is dissolved in water, and the ether solution is decanted. The water contains any excess solid zinc. The ether solution is washed in a separatory funnel with acid solution and neutralized with sodium hydroxide solution. Methanol is added to the ether solution, and most of the ether is evaporated on a steam bath as the purified cholesterol begins to crystallize. The crystallization proceeds more rapidly as room temperature is approached. The product is collected on a filter and dried as described above.

The cholesterol purified by the above methods may be characterized by the colour reactions discussed above (Salkowski and Liebermann–Burchard). Other colour tests, such as the formaldehyde–sulphuric acid test, may be used. In this test, formaldehyde–sulphuric acid solution is added to a solution of cholesterol dissolved in chloroform. The solution, which turns cherry red, is poured into another tube, and two to three drops of acetic anhydride are added. A blue colour develops. These colour tests have been adapted to form the basis of spectrophotometric measurements. The results of the purified products are determined by reference to a standard of known purity.

Purity of cholesterol standards may be assessed by using melting point and boiling point determinations, microscopic comparison of the crystals with a pure reference material, and infrared and ultraviolet–visible spectra. The spectrum of the cholesterol standard is compared with that of a pure crystalline reference material.

Classic colorimetric tests, microscopic examinations and melting point determinations have been supplemented with more modern techniques, such as mass spectrometry, nuclear magnetic resonance spectrometry, gas chromatography (GC) and high-performance liquid chromatography (HPLC) for determining the purity of prepared crystalline cholesterol. No one test in itself is sufficient to determine purity. Confirmation of results requires a minimum of two tests, which should preferably be chemically or physically unrelated. *See* Chromatography, High-performance Liquid Chromatography; Chromatography, Gas Chromatography; Mass Spectrometry, Principles and Instrumentation; Spectroscopy, Nuclear Magnetic Resonance

A serum reference material for determining serum cholesterol is normally used for both manual and automated methods. A serum reference material may be prepared by filtering pooled human serum through clarifying and 'sterilizing' filters. Stable serum preparations of cholesterol, with concentrations ranging from 100 to 400 mg dl^{-1}, may be made by adding an alcohol-precipitated cholesterol-rich protein from human serum to bovine, horse or human serum. Aliquots of the preparation should be stored in sealed vials or ampoules at a temperature of $-20°C$ or below. The stability of these preparations is similar to that of human serum. These sterile preparations may be shipped at room temperature for periods of up to 5 days. The concentrations of some commercial reference sera may vary considerably if the Abell–Kendall method is used as the reference assay. The Abell–Kendall procedure includes an initial step in which the serum is treated with alcoholic potassium hydroxide to liberate the cholesterol from the lipoprotein complexes and to saponify the cholesterol esters. The total cholesterol is extracted into a measured volume of petroleum ether. The cholesterol in an aliquot of the petroleum ether extract is measured by means of the Liebermann–Burchard colour reaction. All commercial reference sera should be checked against serum reference materials and standardized by the reference cholesterol method (Abell–Kendall method).

Colorimetry-based Analytical Methods

Routine lipid testing in clinical settings generally includes serum determination of triglycerides and cholesterol, and a more recent trend has been to include lipoprotein–cholesterol determination. The literature contains more than 200 methods or modifications for measuring serum cholesterol. This number is perhaps an indication of the difficulties of developing a reliable assay. Free cholesterol and cholesteryl esters may be determined separately, but it is common practice to determine the two together as 'total cholesterol'. *See* Spectroscopy, Visible Spectroscopy and Colorimetry

The Liebermann–Burchard reagent has had a central role in much of the methodological development of cholesterol measurement systems. Since Grigant introduced a procedure for the quantitative estimation of cholesterol in 1910 by using the Liebermann–Burchard reagent (developed between 1885 and 1890), numerous modifications of the method have appeared in the literature. Most of the deviations from earlier methods consist of changes in extraction and colour development.

The reaction of cholesterol with sulphuric acid in acetic anhydride (Liebermann–Burchard) to form a coloured product has provided the basis for many subsequent methods. These methods may be catego-rized into three groups: (1) direct, in which the serum is added directly to the colour reagent; (2) extraction, in which cholesterol is extracted into an organic solvent before it is added to the colour reagent; and (3) hydrolysis, in which the esterified cholesterol is hydrolysed before solvent extraction and colour development. Many methods utilize acetic anhydride, acetic acid, or ferric chloride to develop colour. Specificity is enhanced by prior extraction techniques. Values for cholesterol are usually higher by direct and automated methods than by manual, extraction or hydrolysis methods. The colour development of these various procedures obeys the Lambert–Beer law, which states that the absorbance is directly proportional to the concentration.

The direct methods are simple and convenient, but are subject to interference from compounds normally present in serum, such as bilirubin and proteins. Much of this interference is eliminated by extracting the cholesterol with a solvent before the colour development reaction is initiated. Esterified cholesterol in serum should be hydrolysed before a total cholesterol determination is made because more colour is produced by esterified cholesterol than by free cholesterol. Failure to hydrolyse results in an overestimation of total cholesterol. Standard solutions of cholesterol must be reacted with the colour reagent to determine when the colour has developed its maximum intensity. Colour reagents should be added to test solutions and standard solutions at fixed intervals, for example, every 30 or 60 s. When the colour intensity of the standard solutions has reached its maximum, the colour intensities of the test solutions should be read according to the preparation schedule, for example, every 30 or 60 s. The time required for the colour to develop its maximum intensity is influenced by the ambient temperature and the composition of the individual batches of prepared reagents.

The American Association of Clinical Chemistry has suggested three methods for small laboratories that need a manual procedure for estimating total serum cholesterol. These procedures are an enzymatic method, the iron–uranyl acetate method (Parekh–Jung) and the Liebermann–Burchard reagent method. The modified Liebermann–Burchard reagent method, in both manual and automated forms, is widely used by small clinical laboratories. This discussion focuses on the manual manipulation of the method for clarity of the chemistry. The Liebermann–Burchard colour reaction was discussed above with regard to primary standards. In the modified method, the cholesterol is extracted from serum test samples into 2-propanol to eliminate interfering substances. A measured aliquot of the extract is evaporated before the Liebermann–Burchard colour reagent is added. If the reagents are added directly to the extract, it is difficult to control the rate of colour reaction under manual conditions. The heat produced from the exothermic reaction of 2-propanol with sulphuric acid cannot be controlled sufficiently to allow reproducible measurements. However, under stringent automated conditions this problem can be circumvented. After a timed incubation and colour-development period, the absorbance is measured at 630 nm. In this method, reference serum and serum test samples are treated in the same manner. According to the American Association for Clinical Chemistry, recoveries of cholesterol added to serum were 98–101% over a linear range of cholesterol concentrations of 0·8–4·0 g l⁻¹. This method may be used to determine cholesterol in food and tissue extracts that have been cleaned in a separating funnel before being dried and redissolved in 2-propanol. Crystalline cholesterol is used as the primary standard for these test samples.

An estimation of the relationship of unesterified cholesterol to cholesterol ester can be made with another modification of the Liebermann–Burchard method. Unesterified cholesterol in serum is precipitated as the digitonide from ethanol–ether solution. The solvent is evaporated and the esters are extracted from the residue by adding petroleum ether, bringing the solution to a boil, cooling and centrifuging, and collecting the supernatant. The supernatant is processed as in a total cholesterol determination. The resultant value is a measure of the esterified cholesterol in the serum test sample.

The Parekh–Jung manual method is used in many clinical laboratories. This method is based on the precipitation of proteins and associated substances with ferric acetate–uranyl acetate reagent. The mixture is centrifuged and the resultant supernatant is treated with sulphuric acid–ferrous sulphate colour reagent. After a 20 min incubation and colour-development period, the absorbance is measured at 560 nm.

The enzymatic method for the determination of total serum cholesterol is frequently used both manually and in an automated setting. The enzyme method is of limited value when either aqueous or pure alcohol standards are used. The method may be calibrated accurately with a homogeneous and stable serum pool. The method provides a direct measure of serum cholesterol. The enzymatic analytical determination is calibrated by using serum labelled with a target value assigned by an accepted reference method (e.g. the Abell–Kendall method). *See* Enzymes, Use in Analysis

Although cholesterol in serum is primarily free, cholesterol associated with lipoproteins is esterified. Cholesteryl esters are freed from the lipoproteins and enzymatically hydrolysed by cholesterol-ester hydrolase to free cholesterol and fatty acids. The free cholesterol is then oxidized by cholesterol oxidase to cholest-4-en-3-one and hydrogen peroxidase. The peroxide, in the presence of peroxidase, oxidatively couples with phenol and 4-aminoantipyrine to produce a quinoneimine dye.

The absorbance values at 560 nm are proportional to the concentration of total cholesterol in the serum test sample. The absorbance obeys the Lambert–Beer law over a wide concentration of up to about 5·5 g of cholesterol per litre. An estimate of the relationship of unesterified cholesterol to cholesterol ester is made by subtracting the free cholesterol value (the enzyme cholesterol esterase is withheld from the working test reagent) from the total cholesterol value. The enzymatic method has also been successfully used to determine the cholesterol content of foods. For this purpose, the cholesterol is extracted with a chloroform–methanol solvent, and crystalline cholesterol is used for calibration. A survey of the literature indicates that the coefficient of variation for this method is about 1–3%.

The Abell–Kendall method is generally accepted by clinical chemists as the total cholesterol reference method. The results obtained by other methods are nearly always compared with those obtained by the Abell–Kendall method. The method, however, does not lend itself well to analysis of large numbers of test samples. A saponification step generally precludes the development of an automated version of the method. The serum or plasma is saponified with alcoholic potassium hydroxide. The free cholesterol (from both unesterified and esterified cholesterol) is extracted into petroleum ether and dried; the cholesterol is determined photometrically by a modified Liebermann–Burchard reagent (acetic anhydride–sulphuric acid–acetic acid) at 620 nm. The results of this method are in good agreement with those obtained by the Schoenheimer–Sperry method.

No discussion of colorimetric cholesterol methodology is complete without a brief discussion of the separate determination of blood cholesterol and cholesterol esters that was originally developed by Bloor and Knudson in 1916. Practically all methods for separating free and esterified cholesterol emulate their work. Bloor and Knudson adapted the Windaus cholesterol digitonin precipitation method to separate cholesterol from its esters in small amounts of blood. The method consists of the determination of total cholesterol in an aliquot of an alcohol–ether extract of blood and the determination of cholesterol esters in another aliquot after precipitation of the free cholesterol by digitonin. The difference between the two values represents free cholesterol. The colour reagent and colour development were previously used by Liebermann–Burchard.

Gas Chromatographic (GC) Analysis

GC is used to measure cholesterol as free cholesterol, as the trimethylsilyl ether derivative, or as cholesteryl butyrate. Although colorimetric methods have been used in the past to measure the cholesterol content of foods, body fluids, and tissues, they have been, for the most part, cumbersome and not compound-specific in many applications. Agricultural chemists, biochemists, nutritionists, and food scientists began to explore the use of GC for measuring sterols in the mid-1970s. Although blood cholesterol determinations by GC can be fairly easy to accomplish, GC is not widely used as a routine clinical technique for determining cholesterol. The most probable reasons for this are the difficulties of automating the preparative stages and the fact that adequate colorimetric assays currently exist. Most chromatographic determinations of cholesterol are found in the research environment, in food and nutrition analytical laboratories, and in government regulatory laboratories.

All GC methods use a column stationary phase that is classified as nonpolar, typically methyl silicone (SE-30). In one method, the test sample is saponified, and the unsaponifiable materials are analysed by GC. This method performs well for most products, but not for those that contain measurable amounts of α-tocopherol in addition to cholesterol. The retention times of α-tocopherol and cholesterol are nearly identical and, therefore, an analysis for either compound is not feasible in the presence of the other. The α-tocopherol may be present naturally, or may be added as a nutritional supplement or antioxidant. *See* Tocopherols, Properties and Determination

Another approach is to saponify the test sample, extract the unsaponifiables, and derivatize the unsaponifiable compounds before GC analysis. The official method of the Association of Official Analytical Chemists (AOAC) uses this approach to form trimethylsilyl ethers (Punwar method). Another well-established method uses the classic butyric anhydride–pyridine reaction to attach a C_4 ester at position 3 on the A ring of the sterol to form cholesteryl butyrate. During GC analyses, both derivatives function equally with respect to response, reproducibility, and reliability. The trimethylsilyl ethers create problems over an extended series of analyses. Detector sensitivity drops drastically, and the detector must be disassembled, thoroughly cleaned, and reinstalled to restore sensitivity. The butyrate derivatives burn cleanly in the hydrogen flame ionization detector and do not degrade detector sensitivity. The procedure for preparing the trimethylsilyl derivative is somewhat less tedious than that for preparing the buyrates.

The GC official method of the AOAC determines cholesterol as the trimethylsilyl ether on a $2 \cdot 4$ m $\times$ 3 mm internal diameter silanized glass column packed with 0·5% Apiezon L on 80–100 mesh Gas-Chrom Q (Alltech Associates/Applied Science, Deerfield, Illinois). An alternative column may be used that consists of a 1·8 m $\times$ 4 mm internal diameter glass column packed with 1% SE-30 on 100–120 mesh Gas-Chrom Q (Alltech Associates/Applied Science, Deerfield, Illinois). In this method, one column is maintained at 230°C and the carrier gas flow is adjusted to elute the trimethylsilyl ether of cholesterol in 9–11 min. An internal standard of 5α-cholestane is used and test samples containing 0·5–1 g of fat are extracted with chloroform–methanol–water (50:100:40 v/v/v).

A GC method based on steryl butyrates has been incorporated into a total-lipid analytical system (Sheppard–Hubbard system) for determining total lipids, fatty acid composition, and cholesterol in foods from extraction of a single test portion. The system is widely used in university, food quality control, commercial and regulatory laboratories to determine the lipid components required for fatty acid and cholesterol labelling. The system has also been used to identify adulterated foods. This analytical system uses an aliquot of the fatty acid methyl ester preparation to prepare cholesteryl butyrate and other sterols. The fatty acid methyl esters are not affected by the reaction that forms the butyrate derivatives of the sterols. On the SE-30 column, the fatty acid methyl esters elute near the solvent front and before the appearance of the butyrates of the tocopherols and the sterols. In this system, external calibration is used. However, internal standards can be used if the internal standard peak is situated very close to the peak being measured and if there are no interfering peaks from compounds such as squalane, squalene or cholestane in the test sample. Generally, in this system there are too many peaks from the matrix to have a clear retention time available for internal standards.

The relative retention times for some sterols are 1·0 for cholesteryl butyrate, 1·15 for brassicasteryl butyrate, 1·3 for campesteryl butyrate, 1·4 for stigmasteryl butyrate and 1·6 for sitosteryl butyrate. Free cholesterol and other sterols can be easily separated with a 15 m $\times$ 0·242 mm, SE-54, wall-coated, fused-silica capillary column operated at 250°C with a helium flow rate of 0·74 ml min^{-1}. The sequence of compound appearance the same as that for SE-30 packed columns.

High-performance Liquid Chromatography (HPLC)

HPLC is increasingly being used to determine cholesterol and other sterols in foods and tissue extracts. However, like GC, HPLC is not generally used in routine clinical analyses performed with automated clinical multiple analysis systems based on colorimetric or fluorometric assays. Sterols that can be separated by GC usually cannot be separated by an HPLC system. One HPLC system in widespread use determines the benzoate ester of cholesterol on a $300 \times 3 \cdot 9$ mm internal diameter μBondapak C_{18} column with a 100% methanol mobile phase and a variable wavelength ultraviolet detector set at 230 nm. GC and HPLC determinations of cholesterol in a variety of foods show that the two techniques yield statistically identical results. Amounts as low as 10 ng of cholesterol benzoate can be determined using HPLC.

Bibliography

Brumley WC, Sheppard AJ, Rudolf TS, Shen C-SJ, Yasaei P and Sphon JA (1985) Mass spectrometry and identification of sterols in vegetable oils as butyryl esters and relative quantitation by gas chromatography with flame ionization detection. *Journal of the Association of Official Analytical Chemists* 68: 701–709.

Christie WW (1987) *High-Performance Liquid Chromatography and Lipids: A Practical Guide*, 1st edn. New York: Pergamon Press.

Faulkner WR and Meites S (eds) (1982) *Selected Methods for the Small Clinical Chemistry Laboratory*, vol. 9, pp 157–183. Washington, DC: American Association of Clinical Chemistry.

Fieser LF and Fieser M (1949) *Natural Products Related to Phenanthrene*, 3rd edn, chapt. III. New York: Reinhold.

Macrae R (1988) *HPLC in Food Analysis*, 2nd edn. London: Academic Press.

Sheppard AJ, Newkirk DR, Hubbard WD and Osgood T (1977) Gas–liquid chromatographic determination of cholesterol and other sterols in foods. *Journal of the Association of Official Analytical Chemists* 60: 1302–1306.

Windaus A (1932) Uber die Konstitution des Cholesterins und der Gallensauren. *Zeitschrift für Physiologische Chemie* 213: 147–187.

Yasaei P, Sheppard AJ, Brumley WC, Mazzola EP and Aldridge MH (1989) Structural proof of cholesterol isolated from plants. II. Identification and verification by ^{13}C nuclear magnetic resonance spectroscopy and mass spectrometry. *Journal of Micronutrient Analysis* 5: 259–267.

Yasaei P, Sheppard AJ, Rudolf TS, Shen C-SJ and Aldridge MH (1989) Structural proof of cholesterol isolated from plants. I. Isolation and preliminary identification by chromatography and infrared spectroscopy. *Journal of Micronutrient Analysis* 5: 245–238.

Alan J. Sheppard, Jean A. T. Pennington and Roger G. O'Dell
Food and Drug Administration, Washington, DC, USA

Absorption, Function and Metabolism

Cholesterol is one of the most ubiquitous compounds in the body, being a vital structural component of every cell. In humans, cholesterol represents about 0·2% of bodyweight. Table 1 details the distribution of cholesterol in the body of a 'normal' 70 kg man.

The cholesterol present in the intestine is derived principally from three sources – the diet which contributes 300–400 mg in the average subject, the bile which contributes 750–1250 mg daily, and the intestinal wall whose contribution is small. Biliary cholesterol is derived from hepatic synthesis which amounts to about 9–13 mg per kilogram of bodyweight per day. In general, the amount of cholesterol absorbed ranges from 30 to 60%.

Absorption

Dietary fat, including cholesterol, enters the small intestine from the stomach as a coarse emulsion. In the duodenum this coarse emulsion is acted upon by pancreatic juice and bile. The former contains two enzymes, each of which has a different specificity. One, pancreatic lipase, acts on the triglyceride component of the digesta to split off the fatty acids at the 1- and 3-positions to yield a 2-monoglyceride. The other is phospholipase A, which removes the fatty acid in the 2-position of phospholipids to give lysolecithin, which is a strong detergent. Bile contains bile salts (amides of bile acids) which are powerful emulsifiers; they are amphiphiles, meaning they are soluble in both water and lipids. In water under proper conditions amphiphiles spontaneously form small, highly charged aggregates called 'micelles'. These aggregates solubilize the polar lipids, monoglyceride and phospholipids to produce mixed micelles. Mixed micelles have the capacity to incorporate appreciable quantities of insoluble lipids such as fatty acids or free cholesterol. The principal pathway for absorption of fats is by way of micellar solutions. A human lipid micelle containing 1 mol of bile acid will also contain 1·40 mol of fatty acid, 0·15 mol of lysolecithin and 0·06 mol of cholesterol. The means by which the micelle enters the intestinal mucosal cell is still not completely elucidated. However, the cholesterol which reaches the mucosa mixes with that already present, most of it ($\geqslant 80\%$) if re-esterified (most commonly with oleic acid) and is released into the lymph. *See* Bile; Carcinogens, Carcinogenic Substances in Food

The steps involved in cholesterol absorption can be summarized as:

(1) Dietary cholesterol, free and esterified, enters the duodenum as a coarse emulsion. Most dietary cholesterol is in the unesterified form, but some sources, such as liver, may contain appreciable quantities of cholesteryl ester.

(2) The dietary cholesterol is mixed with endogenous cholesterol and the esterified cholesterol is hydrolysed.

(3) A micelle of free cholesterol, bile acid or bile salt, lysolecithin and monoglyceride is formed.

(4) Micellar cholesterol enters the cell where it mixes with endogenous cholesterol.

Table 1. Distribution of cholesterol in a typical 70 kg human

Tissue	Weight (kg)	Cholesterol content		
		Weight (g)	Wet weight (%)	Total (%)
Brain, nervous system	1·6	32·0	2·00	22·9
Connective tissue, adipose tissue, fluids	12·1	30·2	0·25	21·6
Muscle	30·0	30·0	0·10	21·5
Skin	4·2	12·6	0·30	9·0
Blood	5·4	11·3	0·21	8·1
Bone marrow	3·0	7·5	0·25	5·4
Liver	1·7	5·1	0·30	3·7
Heart, lungs, spleen, kidneys, blood vessels	2·0	5·0	0·25	3·6
Alimentary tract	2·5	3·8	0·15	2·7
Adrenals	0·012	1·2	10·00	0·9
Skeleton	7·0	0·7	0·01	0·5
Glands (other than adrenal)	0·10	0·2	0·20	0·1
Total	69·6	139·6	—	100·0

(5) Cholesterol present in the mucosal cells is esterified and released into the lymph.

Transport

Cholesterol and other lipids are transported in the plasma as part of a continuum of lipid–protein complexes whose hydrated density is less than $1·210 \text{ g ml}^{-1}$. Other plasma proteins, which have minimal transport functions, exhibit a hydrated density of about $1·33 \text{ g ml}^{-1}$. These particles, called lipoproteins, may be separated and classified by electrophoresis, or by their rates of flotation in the ultracentrifuge. The lipoproteins may also be separated by column chromatography techniques. Electrophoresis was a very popular technique for lipoprotein separation and identification but is not used widely anymore. However, some of the terminology associated with electrophoresis is still in vogue. In most laboratories rapid precipitation of high-density lipoprotein (HDL) is accomplished using heparin or dextran sulphate or phosphotungstic acid. *See* Lipoproteins

The chylomicrons which are released into the lymph primarily contain triglycerides with a small amount of cholesterol, phospholipid and protein. As the lipoproteins increase in density their composition alters with a loss of triglyceride and concomitant increase in cholesterol and protein. Although the lipoproteins are described serially in this fashion (Table 2–4) their appearance is not due to a direct cascade effect. The lipoproteins are not all derived from the same source and their interactions are described below.

The chylomicrons emerge from the gut with their core of mostly triglycerides, carrying apoproteins B (apo B) and C (apo C) in their membrane. They acquire more apo C from HDL, lose some of their triglycerides, and become very low-density lipoprotein (VLDL) particles. Lipoprotein lipase removes more of the triglyceride from VLDL to form intermediate-density lipoprotein (IDL). During the formation of IDL much of the apo C is released and apo E is taken up from HDL. IDL is catabolized in the liver or converted to LDL with loss of apoproteins C and E. HDL is secreted as a discoidal molecule rich in apo A and apo E. Nascent HDL is converted to a circulating form of HDL by the action of the lecithin–cholesterol acyltransferase (LCAT) enzyme

Table 2. Physical characteristics of normal human plasma lipoproteins

Lipoprotein class[a]	Density (g ml^{-1})	Molecular weight (dalton $\times 10^{-6}$)	Diameter (Å)	Electrophoretic mobility
Chylomicron	<0·95	10^3–30^4	10^3–10^4	Origin
VLDL	0·95–1·006	5	250–750	Pre-β
IDL	1·006–1·019	4·5	250	Pre-β_1
LDL	1·019–1·063	2	200–250	β
HDL$_2$	1·063–1·120	0·39	70–120	α_1
HDL$_3$	1·120–1·210	0·19	50–100	α_1

[a] VLDL, very low-densitylipoprotein; IDL, intermediate-density lipoprotein; LDL, low-density lipoprotein; HDL, high-density lipoprotein.

Table 3.   Chemical composition (%) of normal human plasma lipoproteins

	Chylomicron	VLDL	IDL	LDL	HDL$_2$	HDL$_3$
Triglyceride	85	55	30	10	5	4
Phospholipid	10	15	22	20	30	23
Free cholesterol	1–3	5–10	8	7–10	5	3–4
Esterified cholesterol	3–5	10–15	22	35–40	16	12
Protein	2	10	15	20	40	50–55
Major apoproteins[a]	B	B	B	B	AI	AI
	CI	CI	CII		AII	AII
	CII	CII	CIII		E	
	CIII	CII	E			
	E	E				

[a] 5% or more of total apoprotein content.

to yield plasma HDL with its core of cholesteryl ester and carries apoproteins A, C and E. HDL particles act as reservoirs for the apo C and apo E which are recycled in the course of metabolism of the triglyceride-rich lipoprotein species. HDL, LDL and IDL are all catabolized by the liver or by peripheral tissue. LCAT is an enzyme which esterifies free cholesterol with the fatty acid in the 2-position of lecithin (Fig. 1).

Most of the cholesterol in plasma is carried in LDL and the concentration of LDL (or cholesterol) in plasma has been correlated positively with risk of coronary heart disease (CHD). The clarification of the pathway by which LDL is taken up by cells (receptor pathway) and how that regulates the synthesis of cholesterol in those cells earned the Nobel Prize for Brown and Goldstein several years ago. The receptor pathway accounts for about half of overall LDL catabolism.

Briefly, in the receptor pathway LDL is bound to specific receptors located on the cell membrane which recognize apo B. The LDL particle is internalized and degraded in the lysosomes with the release of cholesterol. The cholesterol released in this process regulates the production of new receptors and also suppresses the synthesis of the rate-limiting enzyme for cholesterol

Table 4.   The major apolipoproteins

Designation	Lipoprotein	Molecular weight
AI	HDL, CM	28 000[a,b,c]
AII	HDL, CM	16 000[a]
AIV	HDL, CM, VLDL	46 000[d]
B100	LDL, VLDL	550 000[a,e,f]
B48	CM	250 000[a,g]
CI	HDL, CM	6000[h]
CII	HDL, CM, VLDL	7000[i]
CIII	HDL, CM, VLDL	7000[j]
E	CM, VLDL, HDL	34 000[k]

[a] Structural component.
[b] Activator of lecithin–cholesterol acyltransferase (LCAT).
[c] Involved in reverse cholesterol transport.
[d] Unknown at present.
[e] Involved in synthesis and secretion of VLDL.
[f] Binds to LDL receptor.
[g] Activates LCAT.
[h] Activates lipoprotein lipase (LPL).
[i] Affects LPL activity.
[j] Binds to hepatic lipoprotein receptors.
[k] Receptor ligands.

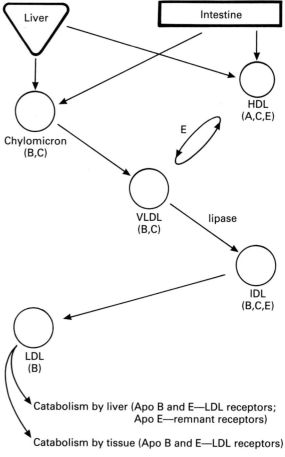

Fig. 1   Outline of lipoprotein metabolism (letters in parentheses refer to apolipoproteins).

Absorption, Function and Metabolism

synthesis, 3β-hydroxy-3-methylglutaryl-CoA reductase (HMG-CoA reductase). Genetic conditions or other factors (dietary, physical or pharmacological) which affect the receptor pathway will lead to elevated plasma cholesterol levels. In the popular press, LDL cholesterol is called the 'bad' cholesterol, which differentiates it from HDL cholesterol or the 'good' cholesterol.

The level of cholesterol in the plasma is one of the major risk factors for CHD. Among the other major risk factors are cigarette smoking, and high blood pressure, and some would add diabetes and obesity. Many other risk factors have been identified. Plasma triglyceride levels were considered to represent a risk of CHD about 40 years ago, then were relegated to an unimportant niche in the risk hierarchy but have been making a come-back in the past few years. *See* Atherosclerosis; Coronary Heart Disease, Intervention Studies; Hyperlipidaemia

It should be borne in mind that a risk factor is statistical in nature and represents a statistical diagnosis. In the absence of anything more accurate the risk factors represent the best indicator of CHD and normalizing levels of plasma lipids and hypertension as well as cessation of cigarette smoking demand our attention. *See* Hypertension, Physiology

It is important to call attention to fluctuations in plasma cholesterol. After earlier doubts it is now agreed that such fluctuations do indeed occur, but their origin remains unknown. Elevation in cholesterol levels can occur during periods of stress and there are a number of examples of seasonal variations. Very generally, levels are elevated in winter months and reduced in summer, but such changes do not occur in all subjects nor do they occur to the same extent in all subjects. Suffice it to say that many clinicians now feel that several determinations of plasma cholesterol levels may be needed before making any diagnosis.

Biosynthesis

The biological analysis of cholesterol is an area of research that captured the imagination of scientists for years. Early this century the observation that mice fed only on bread continued to grow and that their total body cholesterol continued to increase provided the first evidence that the mammalian organism can synthesize this complex molecule. However, it was the advent of stable and radioactive isotopes of carbon and hydrogen that provided the evidence that all 27 carbon atoms of the cholesterol molecule could be derived from the two carbon atoms of acetic acid. Block and his colleagues fed acetate labelled in the carboxyl group with ^{13}C and in the methyl group with ^{14}C to rats and showed that 15 of the 27 carbon atoms of cholesterol were derived from the acetate methyl group and the other 12 came from the

carboxyl group. The methyl/carboxyl ratio in the nucleus was 10·9 and in the side-chain it was 5/3. Still, since 27 is not divisible by 2 it was evident that carbon atoms were added or lost in the course of the synthetic process. It is beyond the scope of this article to follow the research and thinking that went into the solution of this problem. The pathway as we now know it is outlined below.

Two molecules of acetate (CH_3COO^-) combine to form acetoacetate ($CH_3COCH_2COO^-$). Condensation with another acetate molecule gives 3β-hydroxy-3-methylglutarate (**1**). The intermediates all react as

(1)

derivatives of coenzyme A, so that at this stage we have 3β-hydroxy-3-methylglutaryl-CoA or HMG-CoA. One carboxyl group of HMG CoA is reduced to give mevalonic acid (**2**). This step, the reduction of HMG to

(2)

mevalonate by an enzyme called HMG-CoA reductase, is the rate-determining step in the biological synthesis of cholesterol.

Mevalonate is phosphorylated at the hydroxyl position and then decarboxylated to yield the terpenoid compound 3-isopentenylpyrophosphate (**3**). As a historical

(3)

note, before the structure of cholesterol was known accurately, the Nobel Laureate Leopold Ruzicka, a Yugoslavian-born Swiss chemist, formulated the isoprene rule which predicted that most complex organic natural products would be synthesized by a mechanism involving condensation of isoprenoid units. Cholesterol is no exception.

Isopentenyl pyrophosphate (**4**) can isomerize to give γ,γ-dimethallyl pyrophosphate (**5**) and one molecule of each form condenses to give a C_{10} terpenoid, geranyl pyrophosphate (**6**) (eqn [1]; PP denotes the pyrophosphate group).

Absorption, Function and Metabolism

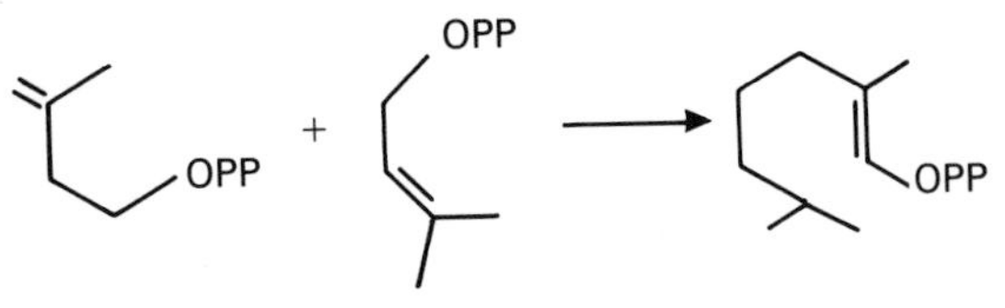

(1)

(4)   (5)   (6)

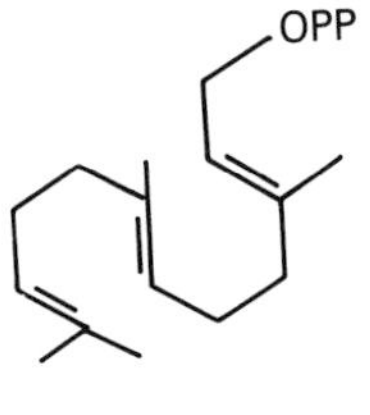

(7)

Geranyl pyrophosphate condenses with one molecule of isopentenyl pyrophosphate to yield a C_{15} terpenoid, namely farnesyl pyrophosphate (7). Two molecules of farnesyl pyrophosphate condense to give squalene (8), a $C_{30}H_{50}$ hydrocarbon. Thus a succession of six C_5 units have condensed to provide a C_{30} hydrocarbon, squalene.

Squalene is a straight-chain hydrocarbon but it can be drawn in such a fashion as to show that with three appropriate ring closures it can give a C_{30} molecule with a steroid nucleus. Indeed, under the influence of the enzyme squalene oxidocyclase and in the presence of oxygen squalene cyclizes to lanosterol (9), the sterol present in sheep fat (eqn [2]). During a series of oxidations, hydrogenations and double-bond shifts lanosterol loses three methyl groups, the double bond at the 8,9-position shifts to the 5,6-position, the double bond in the side-chain is reduced and the result is cholesterol.

The major site of cholesterol synthesis is the liver but it can be synthesized by virtually every other mammalian tissue with the possible exception of the aorta. The next major site of cholesterol synthesis after the liver is the intestine. Most of the cholesterol synthesized by the rat is made in the liver but in other species the contribution of extrahepatic tissue may be substantial. Dietschy and Wilson summarized the level of sterol synthesis by a number of tissues of the rat and monkey (Table 5).

Synthesis of cholesterol is under feedback control.

Thus, liver synthesis of cholesterol virtually ceases in rats or dogs fed cholesterol. In man synthesis has been seen to decline by 40–60%. Cholesterol synthesis is also under hormonal control. Insulin enhances synthesis whereas glucagon or glucocorticoids inhibit it. Thyroid hormone increases cholesterogenesis while thyroidectomy (chemical or surgical) inhibits it. Hypophysectomy abolishes hepatic cholesterol synthesis in rats. Feedback control of cholesterogenesis is lost in tumour tissue. *See* Hormones, Thyroid Hormones

A number of pharmacological agents have been shown to influence cholesterol synthesis. The step at which synthesis is inhibited is unique for each compound. Today a series of compounds which inhibit HMG-CoA reductase activity is being used to treat hypercholesterolaemia.

Metabolism

Cholesterol serves many functions in the organism. In the brain and nervous tissue it appears to act as an insulator; it is a lubricant in the skin and it is a precursor of a number of biologically important compounds such as corticosteroids, gonadal hormones and vitamin D. *See* Cholecalciferol, Physiology; Hormones, Steroid Hormones

The principal products of cholesterol catabolism are the bile acids. The degradation of cholesterol to give the primary bile acids, cholic and deoxycholic acids, occurs in the liver. Conversion of cholesterol to bile acids entails stereospecific hydrogenation of the 5,6-double bonds; epimerization of the 3β-hydroxyl group; introduction of additional α-hydroxyl groups at C7 (to give chenodeoxycholic acid) and at C7 and C12 (to give cholic acid); and scission of the side chain between C24 and C25 to yield a C24 carboxylic acid (eqn [3]). The intestinal microflora dehydroxylate the primary bile acids at C7 to yield the secondary bile acids – deoxycholic (from cholic) and lithocholic (from chenodeoxycholic).

The nuclear changes precede degradation of the side

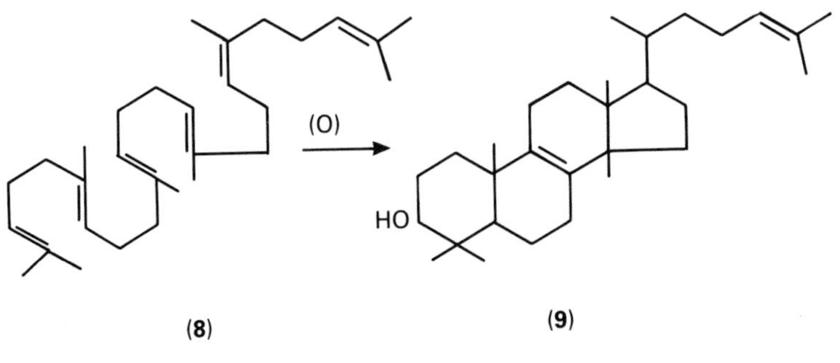

(2)

(8)   (9)

Absorption, Function and Metabolism

Cholesterol → Cholic acid (3)

Table 5. Rates of sterol synthesis by tissues of the monkey and rat (brain=1·00)[a]

Tissue	Monkey	Rat
Liver	1226·0	358·0
Ileum	208·0	228·0
Colon	144·0	112·0
Stomach	38·0	72·0
Oesophagus	138·0	34·0
Jejunum	62·0	30·0
Testes		18·0
Ovary	30·0	
Lung	8·0	14·0
Adrenal	2·0	10·0
Skin	20·0	10·0
Kidney	12·0	8·0
Spleen	6·0	8·0
Marrow	12·0	
Adipose tissue	10·0	
Smooth muscle		1·80
Heart muscle		1·40
Skeletal muscle	0·60	1·00
Brain	1·00	1·00

After Dietschy and Wilson.
[a] Measured as incorporation of exogenous [^{14}C]acetate. Synthesis measured as nanomoles per gram of tissue in 2 h.

chain. The initial (and rate limiting) step in conversion of cholesterol to bile acids is the hydroxylation at C7. The hydroxylations at positions 7 and 12 are carried out in the liver mitochondria but steps leading to epimerization of the C_3 hydroxyl group and reduction of the double bond take place in the microsome and cytosol. Degradation of the side chain takes place in the mitochondria with trihydroxy coprostane being oxidized at the terminal carbon atom to a hydroxyl then a carboxyl derivative. This acid is then cleaved by mitochondrial preparations to yield propionyl-CoA and, presumably, cholyl-CoA.

As with cholesterol, bile acid synthesis is regulated by a feedback mechanism. The bile acid reacts with glycine or taurine to yield amides (called bile salts) called glyco and tauroderivatives. The ratio of glycine/taurine (G/T) conjugated bile acids differs among species and is influenced by thryoid status.

Current work indicates that there is a direct correlation between cholesterol synthesis and cholesterol 7α-hydroxylase activity and that this is regulated by availability of newly synthesized cholesterol. It has been suggested that these complex interrelationships are governed by phosphorylation and dephosphorylation of four enzymes, namely HMG-CoA reductase and acyl-CoA-cholesterol acyltransferase (ACAT), which are active in the unphosphorylated state and cholesterol 7α-hydroxylase and cholesterol ester hydrolase which require phosphorylation. Several factors (glucocorticoids, glucose refeeding, thyroid hormone) increase both HMG-CoA reductase and cholesterol 7α-hydroxylase activity whereas adrenalectomy, thyroidectomy or fasting decrease activity of both enzymes.

It is estimated that 85–95% of newly synthesized cholesterol is converted to bile acids. Newly synthesized bile acids (about 600 mg day^{-1}) enter the small bowel via the common bile duct. Some of the bile acid is secreted into the colon and excreted but most of it (95%) enters the portal vein and re-enters the liver. A 2–4 g pool of bile acid cycles 4–12 times daily so that a total of 12–36 g of bile acids recycle daily.

Bibliography

Gibbons GF, Mitropoulos KA and Myant NB (1982) *Biochemistry of Cholesterol*. Amsterdam: Elsevier.

Kritchevsky D (1985) Nutrition and cardiovascular disease. In: Sidransky H (ed.) *Nutritional Pathology*, pp 127–160. New York: Marcel Dekker.

Kritchevsky D (1991) Bile acids: biosynthesis and functions. *European Journal of Cancer Prevention* 1(suppl. 2): 23–28.

Mead JF, Alfin-Slater RB, Howton DR and Popjak G (1986) *Lipids: Chemistry, Biochemistry and Nutrition*. New York: Plenum Press.

David Kritchevsky
The Wistar Institute, Philadelphia, USA

Factors Determining Blood Cholesterol Levels

Dietary cholesterol mixes with endogenous cholesterol in the intestine and is absorbed in the form of free cholesterol as part of a micelle containing bile salt, lysolecithin and 2-monoglyceride. After digestion the cholesterol is re-esterified and enters the circulation as a chylomicron particle, which is particularly rich in triglyceride. Via a series of lipolytic reactions, exchanges of surface protein and addition of cholesterol, the absorbed cholesterol appears in very low-density lipoprotein (VLDL), intermediate-density lipoprotein (IDL), low-density lipoprotein (LDL) and high-density lipoprotein (HDL). Some physical and chemical characteristics of the lipoproteins are detailed in Table 1. Lipoproteins are not true compounds but rather are aggregates of lipid and protein which are defined by their hydrated density and can be separated by their patterns of flotation in the ultracentrifuge, by electrophoresis or by column chromatography. Since they are described by their physical properties it stands to reason that their actual composition may not always be the same despite the similar hydrated densities of the aggregates. Thus, two aggregates with similar densities may differ in relative amounts of free and esterified cholesterol or in fatty acid composition. Workers in the field are beginning to recognize these possibilities and the future may provide better understanding of how different diets affect lipoprotein composition as well as lipid spectrum. *See* Lipoproteins

Among the lipoprotein classes LDL is the one which transports the greatest amount of cholesterol and its levels in the plasma correlate positively with cardiovascular risk. HDL levels appear to correlate with relative 'protection'. Data relating to total cholesterol, LDL cholesterol, HDL cholesterol or the LDL/HDL cholesterol ratio have all been studied and there are arguments regarding the superior validity of one analytical value over another. About 30–40 years ago triglyceride levels were also considered to be an indicator of risk. Their predictive ability was then downgraded but recent reports are again beginning to invoke the diagnostic importance of plasma triglyceride levels.

Since cholesterol is a fat most of the studies relating to effects of diet on plasma cholesterol have involved dietary fats. However, other dietary components, such as protein, carbohydrate and fibre, also exert their influence on plasma cholesterol. Two other aspects of the diet–cholesterol question are important but have received little attention to date. One of these is the use of mixed fats or proteins rather than single representatives of each class. Thus many studies have involved substitution of all of one component for all of another. This type of experimental design makes for easy interpretation of results but it is not a reflection of reality. The other aspect of dietary studies which has been largely overlooked is interaction among dietary components.

The ensuing discussion will present data derived from studies in humans and animals. Many of the animal studies have been designed to permit assessment of experimentally induced atherosclerosis, and the influence of diet on plasma cholesterol – which may influence severity of human atherosclerosis – is the reason for the vast amount of research in this field. *See* Atherosclerosis

Fats

No fat found in nature is composed totally of saturated or unsaturated fatty acids. Table 2 lists the names, formulae and shorthand notations for the more com-

Table 1. Physical and chemical properties of human plasma lipoproteins

Physical properties	Chylomicron	Lipoprotein class VLDL	IDL	LDL	HDL
Density (g ml^{-1})	<0·95	0·95–1·006	1·006–1·019	1·019–1·063	1·063–1·210
Molecular weight (daltons)	10^9–10^{10}	5×10^6	$4·5 \times 10^6$	2×10^6	$0·2 \times 10^6$–$0·4 \times 10^6$
Chemical composition (%)					
Protein	2	10	15	20	53
Triglyceride	85	55	30	10	4
Phospholipid	10	15	22	20	26
Free cholesterol	1	7	8	9	3
Esterified Cholesterol	4	13	22	37	15

Factors Determining Blood Cholesterol Levels

Table 2. The common dietary fatty acids

Name	Carbon atoms	Double bonds	Numerical notation
Lauric	12	0	12:0
Myristic	14	0	14:0
Palmitic	16	0	16:0
Stearic	18	0	18:0
Oleic	18	1	18:1
Linoleic	18	2	18:2
Linolenic	18	3	18:3
Arachidonic	20	4	20:4
Eicosapentaenoic	20	5	20:5
Docosahexaenoic	22	6	22:6

Table 3. Percentage fatty acid composition of selected fats and oils

	12:0	14:0	16:0	18:0	18:1	18:2	18:3
Butter oil[a]	2·9	10·8	26·9	12·1	28·5	3·2	0·4
Chicken fat	0·1	0·8	25·3	6·5	37·7	20·6	0·8
Cocoa butter	—	0·1	26·3	33·8	34·4	3·1	—
Coconut oil	47·1	18·5	9·1	2·8	6·8	1·9	0·1
Corn oil	—	0·1	10·9	2·0	25·4	59·6	1·2
Cottonseed oil	0·1	0·7	21·6	2·6	18·6	54·4	0·7
Lard	0·1	1·5	26·0	13·5	43·9	9·5	0·4
Olive oil	—	—	9·0	2·7	80·3	6·3	0·7
Palm olein	0·2	1·0	39·8	4·4	42·5	11·2	0·2
Peanut oil[b]	—	0·1	11·1	2·4	46·7	32·0	—
Safflower oil	—	0·1	6·8	2·3	12·0	77·7	0·4
Soya bean oil	—	0·1	10·6	4·0	23·2	53·7	7·6
Tallow	0·1	3·2	24·3	18·6	42·6	2·6	0·7

[a] 11·5% as 6:0+8:0+10:0.
[b] 7·3% as 20:0+20:1+22:0+24:0.

mon fatty acids. As Table 3 shows, even the most unsaturated fats contain a few per cent of saturated fatty acids and vice versa. So that when we refer to unsaturated fats it should be clear that we really mean fats whose component fatty acids are predominantly unsaturated. There is a tendency to stigmatize fats of animal origin as 'bad' because they may be more saturated than fats of plant origin but we must remember that the most saturated fat in common use, coconut oil, is a plant fat. It is more reasonable to regard each fat individually with regard to its fatty acid composition. *See* Fatty Acids, Properties; Fatty Acids, Dietary Importance

In the 1950s, studies of human populations revealed that those whose diets contained a large portion of saturated fat exhibited a higher average plasma cholesterol level and a higher incidence of coronary disease. At the same time studies carried out using cholesterol-fed rabbits showed that rabbits fed unsaturated fats exhibited less severe atherosclerosis than their counterparts fed more saturated fats. Later, it was shown that this saturated–unsaturated difference was also manifest in rabbits fed semipurified, cholesterol-free diets.

In an effort to systematize the research findings, Keys and Hegsted and their colleagues independently arrived at formulae which could be used to predict changes in plasma cholesterol in subjects who were switched from one dietary fat to another. The formulae took into account energy contributions from various fatty acids as well as the cholesterol content of the diet. In general, changes in plasma cholesterol appeared to depend on the dietary content of polyunsaturated fat, palmitic and myristic acids and cholesterol. Hegsted suggested that about two-thirds of the cholesterol-raising effect of dietary saturated fat could be attributed to myristic acid.

There were anomalies. Cocoa butter, a very saturated fat high in stearic acid, was not as cholesterolaemic in humans or as atherogenic for rabbits as one might predict. These findings were due to the fact that stearic acid is not well absorbed. It was also shown that fats rich in oleic acid (which had been considered 'neutral' in the cholesterol equation) lowered LDL cholesterol but not HDL cholesterol, thus reducing the LDL/HDL ratio. More unsaturated fats had been shown to lower both LDL and HDL cholesterol.

Dietary cholesterol can raise plasma cholesterol levels to a small extent but the principal influence on cholesterolaemia is that of the extent of saturation of the dietary fat. McNamara *et al.* conducted a study in which subjects were fed low or high levels of cholesterol together with fat that was mainly saturated or unsaturated. The influence on plasma cholesterol of going from low to high levels of dietary cholesterol was small when the cholesterol doses were fed with the same type of fat. Going from unsaturated to saturated fat was effective in raising cholesterol levels significantly even when low levels of this sterol were fed. They also were able to measure cholesterol synthesis under the various dietary conditions and found that two-thirds of their subjects could compensate for increased dietary cholesterol by reducing endogenous cholesterol synthesis.

The structure of a fat may have an influence on its utilization and biological properties. Since the fat is absorbed as a 2-monoglyceride, the fatty acid in the 2-position may affect absorption and subsequent metabolism. Although this observation was approached experimentally a number of years ago, interest in pursuing it ebbed and it is only very recently that investigators are reinvestigating the possible different effects of fats with different fatty acids in the 2-position. An example is peanut oil, which is unexpectedly atherogenic for rabbits but whose atherogenicity is significantly moderated when the oil has been autointeresteri-

Factors Determining Blood Cholesterol Levels

fied (randomized). While a native fat may have different proportions of its component fatty acids in different positions of the glycerol molecule, in a randomized fat every fatty acid appears in every position of glycerol at one-third of its total concentration.

Another issue that keeps surfacing is that of *trans*-unsaturated fatty acids (TFAs). The double bonds of most, but not all, naturally occurring fats are in the *cis* configuration:

$$\begin{array}{cc} H & H \\ | & | \\ -C & = C- \end{array}$$

In the course of hydrogenation of these fats, whether it be by cattle rumen bacteria or commercially as in the manufacture of margarine, some of the double bonds are inverted to give a *trans* configuration:

$$\begin{array}{c} H \\ | \\ -C = C- \\ | \\ H \end{array}$$

Is this change harmful? Research on TFAs has been going on since 1960. In general, TFAs are cholesterolaemic compared to *cis* fats but not more atherogenic. They have been described as 'quasi-saturated fatty acids'. The question to be resolved is if they pose any special threat when ingested at current levels. Most scientists think not, but research continues. In studies where the fatty acid composition of tissues from persons who had died of coronary disease were compared with those of subjects who had died from other causes the TFA content was similar for the two sources.

Fish oil is another type of fat which has figured prominently in the cholesterol literature recently. The predominant polyunsaturated fatty acid of seed oils such as corn oil or safflower oil is linoleic acid. Linoleic acid contains 18 carbon atoms and two double bonds. The double bonds occur between the 9, 10 and 11, 12 carbons. The second double bond is six carbon atoms removed from the terminal or ω end of the fatty acid chain and linoleic acid is classified as an ω-6 or *n*-6 fatty acid, referring to the distance between the double bond furthest from the carboxyl end of the fatty acid and the terminal end of the fatty acid. Fish oils, especially those from fish living in colder waters, contain appreciable quantities (10–25%) of fatty acids whose chain length is longer than 18 carbon atoms, which contain more than two or three double bonds and whose double bond furthest from the carboxyl end is only three carbon atoms removed from the terminal carbon atom of the chain. These are known as ω-3 or *n*-3 fatty acids. Common plant fats contain small amounts of linolenic acid, which is an 18 carbon atom *n*-3 fatty acid. The two most common fish oil fatty acids are eicosapentaenoic (20 carbon atoms, five double bonds) and docosahexae-

noic (22 carbon atoms, six double bonds). Because few Eskimos exhibit heart disease (but many die of stroke) it was thought that fish oil fatty acids might offer exceptional protection against coronary disease and for a while fish oils were very popular and, while we have gone back to more conventional dietary modalities, it should be noted that most recipes for healthful diets suggest that fish be eaten several times each week. *See* Fish Oils, Dietary Importance, Vegetable Oils, Dietary Importance

Protein

Although there are some analyses of the literature that suggest that protein of animal origin is better correlated with risk of coronary disease than fat of animal origin, this line of investigation has never been too popular, possibly because in most diets animal fat and animal protein occur together. Interest in the effects of animal protein on experimental atherosclerosis dates to 1909 but the observations of the role of cholesterol made a few years later put the protein work into eclipse. About 50 years ago it was shown that soya bean protein was less cholesterolaemic and atherogenic for rabbits than casein. Carroll has shown that generally plant-derived protein is less cholesterolaemic for rabbits than animal protein. However, within both types of protein there is a wide variation in effects. So that in rabbits casein (fed as 30% of the diet) gives cholesterol levels of 200 mg dl^{-1} (5·17 mmol l^{-1}) and egg white gives levels of 100 mg dl^{-1} (2·58 mmol l^{-1}) while wheat gluten (80 mg dl^{-1}; 2·07 mmol l^{-1}) and fava bean protein (30 mg dl^{-1}; 0·78 mmol l^{-1}) give equally disparate effects. Most research has compared the proteins most readily available, casein and soya bean protein, and neither may be the best example of its class. Thus, there are no data on a wide variety of proteins. *See* Protein, Chemistry; Protein, Quality

Interest has turned to the possibility that specific amino acids or amino acid patterns may be responsible for the observed protein effects. For instance, one of the differences in amino acid composition between casein and soya bean protein is in the ratio of lysine to arginine, which is higher in the former than the latter. Addition of lysine to soya bean protein in a semipurified rabbit diet increases cholesterol levels by 33%, triglyceride levels by 17% and the severity of atherosclerosis by 49%. Addition of arginine to casein does not influence lipidaemia but reduces atherosclerosis by 16%. A diet in which the ratio of casein to soya bean protein is 1 is no more cholesterolaemic or atherogenic for rabbits than one containing only soya bean protein – an example of why mixed diets should be studied. *See* Hyperlipidaemia

What of vegetarians? True vegans, persons who eat nothing of animal origin, have lower levels of plasma cholesterol than lacto-ovo vegetarians, persons who do not eat meat but do eat other foods of animal origin such as cheese or eggs. Cholesterol levels of lacto-ovo vegetarians are not much different than those of the general public. *See* Vegan Diets; Vegetarian Diets

Carbohydrate

There are few studies relating to the effects of carbohydrates on lipid levels in humans. In general, high-carbohydrate diets may be hypertriglyceridaemic. Diets high in fructose have been shown to be hypertriglyceridaemic in humans as well as in rats, baboons and monkeys. In rabbits fed a semipurified diet containing 40% carbohydrate, fructose was more cholesterolaemic but less triglyceridaemic than either sucrose or starch. *See* Carbohydrates, Classification and Properties; Carbohydrates, Requirements and Dietary Importance

Fibre

Fibre has been defined as that part of the plant cell wall that is impervious to mammalian digestive secretions. It is efficiently fermented by the colonic microflora, however. All of the plant materials that we call fibre, except for lignin, are carbohydrate in nature although they have different chemical structures, different physical properties and different physiological effects. The term 'fibre' has recently been applied to other naturally derived materials such as agar and to modified substances such as methylcellulose (Table 4). *See* Dietary Fibre, Properties and Sources

Interest in dietary fibre goes back to Hippocrates and possibly earlier, but the current preoccupation dates to the observation by Burkitt that populations subsisting on diets higher in fibre are relatively free of Western diseases such as diabetes or atherosclerosis. Initial attempts to reduce cholesterol levels by adding fibre to the diet involved the use of wheat bran, but it has virtually no effect on plasma lipids. A simple, but somewhat inaccurate means of characterizing fibre is as soluble or insoluble fibre. Most brans and cellulose are considered to be insoluble fibres. They reduce intestinal transit time but have no effects on lipids. Soluble fibre such as guar gum, pectin or psyllium are really gel-forming fibres. They all have cholesterol-lowering properties. Oat bran can lower cholesterol because it contains an appreciable amount of oat gum, which is a soluble fibre. The fibre hypothesis suggest that we ingest fibre-rich foods and not that we use fibre as a pharmacological agent, which is what we do when we add isolated or purified fibre to the diet. Among fibre-rich foods,

Table 4. Classification of dietary fibre

Cell wall polysaccharides (structural)

Cellulosic
  Cellulose
  Cellulose derivatives

Noncellulosic polysaccharides
  Hemicellulose
  Pectin
  Gums

Structural nonpolysaccharides
  Lignins

Nonstructural polysaccharides
  Guar gum
  Locust bean gum
  Gum Arabic
  Gum Ghatti
  Karaya gum
  Xanthans

Nonplant substances
  Agar
  Chitosan

Manmade substances
  Polydextrose
  Methylcellulose

beans and apples have been reported to lower plasma cholesterol levels. *See* Dietary Fibre, Physiological Effects; Dietary Fibre, Effects of Fibre on Absorption

Trace Minerals

The effects of trace minerals on cholesterol metabolism or cardiovascular disease have not received the attention that other elements of the diet have. Most of the available literature describes experiments conducted in animals, usually rats. As we learn more about trace mineral requirements, attention will turn to lipid metabolism. In general, it has been shown that deficiencies of calcium, magnesium, copper, chromium or iron can lead to elevated cholesterol levels. There have been studies in which water hardness is correlated negatively with coronary disease in humans. *See* Minerals, Dietary Importance *See* also individual minerals

Interactions

There are not many examples of interactions among nutrients which may influence lipidaemia. One has already been alluded to, namely, animal protein is more cholesterolaemic than plant protein, but a diet containing equal amounts of the two gives the same result as does plant protein alone. In rabbits fed different proteins in a diet containing cellulose, casein is more cholesterolaemic and atherogenic than is soya bean

Factors Determining Blood Cholesterol Levels

protein, but when the fibre is alfalfa the two proteins give the same levels of cholesterol and the same severity of atherosclerosis. More experiments in which the nutrients are mixed rather than being from a single source should be carried out. Such studies would present a much more accurate picture of nutrient effects.

Bibliography

Grundy SM (1979) Dietary fats and sterols. In: Levy RI, Rifkind BM, Dennis BH and Ernst ND (eds) *Nutrition, Lipids and Coronary Heart Disease*, pp 89–118. New York: Raven Press.

Kritchevsky D (1979) Dietary interactions. In: Levy RI, Rifkind BM, Dennis BH, Ernst ND (eds) *Nutrition, Lipids and Coronary Heart Disease*, pp 229–246. New York: Raven Press.

Mead JF, Alfin-Slater RB, Howton DR and Popjak G (1986) *Lipids: Chemistry, Biochemistry and Nutrition*, New York: Plenum Press.

Tso P and Weidman SW (1987) Absorption and metabolism of lipids in humans. In: Horisberger M and Bracco V (eds) *Lipids in Modern Nutrition*, pp 1–15. New York: Raven Press.

David Kritchevsky
The Wistar Institute, Philadelphia, USA

Role of Cholesterol in Heart Disease

Cholesterol is essential for life. All human and many animal body cells need a continuous supply of this molecule for the synthesis of new membranes; it is also essential for biosynthesis of bile acids and steroid hormones. Homeostasis of cholesterol involves a complex series of mechanisms including synthesis, metabolism, transport and catabolism. In common with all steroids, cholesterol is a derivative of a condensed ring system named cyclopentanoperhydrophenanthrene. Various groups are introduced into the nucleus in the form of methyl, hydroxyl, keto and branched side-chains. The cholesterol molecule contains one hydroxyl group (OH) and is therefore able to form esters, e.g. with fatty acids. Cholesterol was recognized as a specific substance at the beginning of the nineteenth century. At that time the main component of gallstones was found to be a waxy, white substance. The French name 'cholesterine' was assigned to indicate its biliary origin (*Chole*) and its solid nature (*stereos*). The name was changed to cholesterol when it was found to have a hydroxyl group. *See* Bile; Hormones, Steroid Hormones

Evidence for the Role of Cholesterol in Heart Disease

Despite its essential role in the body the significance of cholesterol is particularly linked to the study of athero-sclerosis and to its relationship with coronary heart disease (CHD) and ischaemic heart disease (IHD). In the early part of this century a high content of cholesterol in atheromatous aortas was recorded; soon after, it was shown that cholesterol was present in the parietal wall – mainly as cholesteryl esters. Severe atherosclerosis was recorded in rabbits fed milk and egg yolk, and some years later atherosclerosis was induced in rabbits fed a cholesterol-enriched diet. *See* Atherosclerosis

A Norwegian physician Carl Müller was the first doctor to identify a relationship between plasma cholesterol level, the presence of xanthomata and the high prevalence of CHD. He studied 17 families with a total of 76 family members and showed that the disease was heritable. It was only some years after the end of World War II that a series of studies were performed including both cross-sectional studies, which compared different populations, and longitudinal studies, which followed prospectively the outcomes of subjects who were enrolled when they had no signs or symptoms of CHD. One example of the first kind of study is the *Seven Countries Study* and the *Framingham Study* is the most well known of the latter type. All studies were intended to identify the relationship between certain risk factors, namely the plasma levels of cholesterol, other lipids and lipoprotein, and dietary habits. *Risk factors* are those factors associated with an increasing risk of CHD. Genetic and familial factors are not modifiable, whereas other factors can be modified. Four which can be altered are (1) high dietary intake of cholesterol and saturated fats, (2) hypercholesterolaemia, (3) hypertension, and (4) smoking; these are considered the major risk factors. Among the several plasma lipids, plasma cholesterol is the most widely studied parameter and to date shows the strongest positive association. The data collected have enabled definition of the *relative risk*, i.e. the ratio of risk for a man in a higher quintile of serum cholesterol level compared to one in the lowest, the *absolute excess risk* or the absolute excess in probability of experiencing a heart attack in any given year for a man in a higher quintile compared to one in the lowest quintile of risk, or the former minus the risk of the latter. Moreover, serum cholesterol level is predictive of risk of dying even in people who have survived from a previous myocardial infarction (MI). *See* Hyperlipidaemia

The main target of the epidemiological studies was to explore correlations between dietary habits of populations, plasma cholesterol and morbidity and/or mortality for CHD. Data from the *Seven Countries Study*, still the most comprehensive study, showed clearly that plasma cholesterol is higher in populations with a high intake of cholesterol and saturated fats, whereas the values are significantly lower in countries characterized by a low intake of cholesterol and saturated fats and by a high intake of polyunsaturated fatty acids. A strong positive relationship was observed between the popula-

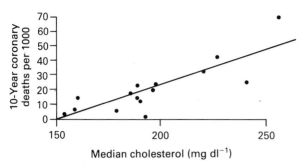

Fig. 1 Relationship between 10-year coronary deaths and serum cholesterol.

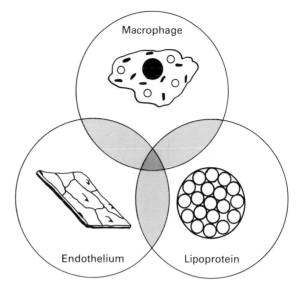

Fig. 3 Interrelation among macrophages endothelium and lipoproteins.

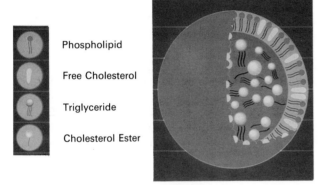

Phospholipid

Free Cholesterol

Triglyceride

Cholesterol Ester

Fig. 2 General structure of a lipoprotein.

tion median for serum cholesterol and 10 years' CHD mortality with a correlation coefficient of 0·8. It was therefore possible to propose some formulae (such as those of Keys and Hegsted) from which the value of plasma cholesterol and the incidence of CHD may be extrapolated after calculation of the intake of saturated and unsaturated fatty acids. However, some discrepancies have emerged: populations having the same plasma cholesterol can have twice the mortality – comparing Australia with France – or a threefold higher mortality, as is the case with Scotland and Sweden. The *Oslo Heart Study* has provided further information: the relationship between serum cholesterol and the extent of autoptically verified coronary atherosclerosis was strikingly linear. *See* Coronary Heart Disease, Intervention Studies

Importance of Low-density Lipoproteins (LDLs)

Cholesterol is synthesized in the body at a rate of 10 mg per kg bodyweight per day. The liver is considered to be the principal site of synthesis, providing 25% of the total amount, but every body organ is able to produce

cholesterol. Endogenous synthesis is negatively correlated with the degree of intestinal absorption of cholesterol. Cholesterol moves out of the liver incorporated in very-low-density lipoproteins (VLDLs), partly as 'free' cholesterol in the membrane and partly esterified in the 'core' of lipoprotein. In the plasma, owing to the lipolytic effect of lipoprotein lipase, VLDL is converted to intermediate-density lipoprotein (IDL), or 'remnant lipoprotein, and then to LDLs. Low-density lipoprotein delivers cholesterol to the peripheral tissues. From the periphery, cholesterol is transported back to the liver and incorporated in high-density lipoproteins (HDLs). *See* Lipoproteins

Low-density lipoproteins have a range of hydrate density from 1·006 to 1·063 g ml^{-1}. The class with a density of 1·006 g ml^{-1} includes chylomicrons and VLDLs, mostly consisting of triglycerides, minor amounts of other lipids (cholesterol, phospholipids), and a series of apoproteins including apo C, apo A-I, apo A-II, apo A-IV, apo B and apo E. The density of IDL ranges from 1·006 to 1·019 g ml^{-1} and IDL contains less triglycerides and more cholesterol, protein and phospholipids than VLDL; it is characterized by the presence of apoproteins B and E. The LDLs are the major carriers of cholesterol, and contain only the apolipoprotein B-100. As apo B-100 is the ligand with the cell receptor for LDL, and owing to the higher cholesterol content, LDL is considered the most atherogenic of the lipoproteins. Varius epidemiological studies have assessed the predictive value of LDL as a risk factor of CHD. The *Cooperative Lipoprotein Phenotyping Study* demonstrated a positive correlation between levels of LDL-cholesterol (LDL-C) and coronary risk. In the *Framingham Offspring Study*, plasma levels of

Cholesterol-rich lipoproteins

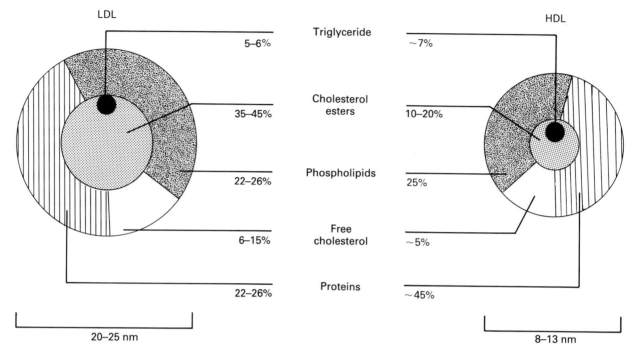

Fig. 4 Chemical composition of LDL and of HDL.

LDL-C were higher in probands with CHD than in probands with no CHD. The *Framingham Prospective Epidemiological Study* has stressed a positive correlation for LDL-C and a negative one for HDL-C and coronary risk in both men and women over a period of 4 years. In addition, LDL-C was presumed to be the major single discriminator between patients affected by CHD and controls. This opinion is no longer supported; in subsequent studies the same *Framingham Study* group has indicated that the best discriminator is total cholesterol, followed by LDL-C, the ratio LDL-C:HDL-C and then HDL-C. Since the 1950s, comparison with data obtained through use of ultracentrifuge techniques has failed to show any advantage in measuring the level of lipoprotein with flotation coefficient (S_f) 0–12 and 12–20. As LDL is the major carrier of cholesterol, it appears obvious that serum cholesterol and LDL-C (S_f, 0–20) are equal predictors of CHD. The combination of all the 'low-density' lipoproteins (VLDL, IDL, LDL) is not a better predictor of cholesterol, especially when the predictive power of total cholesterol is enhanced by adding LDL-C, HDL-C, non-HDL-C and cholesterol ratios such as total-C: LDL-C, total-C:HDL-C, or LDL-C:HDL-C.

It has been recently proposed that evaluation of apo B (the major protein of LDL) is a better discriminator than LDL-C; 14·5% of 200 MI patients had values of LDL-C higher than the 95th percentile, whereas 35% of

patients had values of apo B beyond the 95th percentile. This opinion has not been accepted by other authors: 'since the combination of VLDL, IDL and LDL contains cholesterol which accumulates in the arterial wall it appears that all apo-B-linked cholesterol is as predictive of CHD as apo B'.

The atherogenic power of LDL is a problem not simply of quantity but also of quality. When chemical or biological substances induce modification in composition and physicochemical and immunological behaviour, LDL seems to acquire a strong atherogenic property.

Lp(a) and Apo-a

Low-density lipoprotein is the lipoprotein class characterized by density between 1019 and 1063 g ml^{-1}, electrophoretic velocity β, and the presence of an exclusive protein, apo B, plus scanty traces of apo E. Very close to LDL there is another lipoprotein, characterized by a density of 1050–1081 and the presence of two apoproteins: apo B and a small one, apo a, linked together by a disulphide bridge. This peculiar lipoprotein is called Lp(a) or 'sinking lipoprotein' because in a density gradient solution it sinks like HDL. A first series of studies stressed that higher than normal values of Lp(a) are significantly higher in patients affected by

CHD. More recently, it has been found that the protein part of Lp(a), namely apo a, is an autonomous risk factor with a special relationship with the parental presence of CHD. The meaning and the role of Lp(a) are not completely understood, but some peculiarities have been found in recent years which have clarified the role of Lp (a). The structure is very similar to the plasminogen structure, suggesting that it represents a mutation of the same gene; analogies in structure make Lp(a) an antagonist of plasminogen as it binds to fibrin aggregates and inhibits fibrinolysis, thus promoting thrombus formation. Lp(a) is thus the lipoprotein which establishes a link between the lipids and thrombosis. Moreover, it was found that apo a increases as plasma triglycerides increase and this could represent a pathogenic mechanism for a lipoprotein class (VLDL, density $1\cdot006$ g ml^{-1}) which up to now has appeared as a poor risk factor. Apo B and apo a colocalize in the raised lesions of the parietal wall, forming complexes with glycoaminoglycans and promoting formation of cholesterol esters in peritoneal macrophages. There are many isoforms of Lp(a), fast or slow: the plasma concentration is a function of the electrophoretic mobility, the greater concentration being related to the lower molecular weight. Up to now there are no available drugs which can reduce the level of this peculiar lipoprotein which probably represents one of the major risk factors for CHD. Dietary treatment has no influence, nor is there any benefit from treatment with cholestyramine, bezafibrate and HMG-CoA reductase inhibitors. Recently, it has been stressed that a mild reducing agent, N-acetylcysteine, is effective in decreasing Lp(a) plasma levels through a specific mechanism of dissociation of the two apolipoproteins, apo B and apo a.

Role of LDL Receptors, Foam Cells and Macrophages

Not only are all major organs of the body able to synthesize cholesterol but they are also able to take up lipoproteins containing cholesterol. Chylomicrons, VLDL and IDL are bound and taken up mostly by the liver through B/E receptors – so-called for their affinity for the two apolipoproteins, apo B-100 and apo E. The same receptors specifically bind LDL and internalize LDL-C. The expression of LDL receptors is determined by the cholesterol content of the cell: they are up-regulated by cholesterol deprivation and down-regulated when cholesterol is in abundance. Increasing number and activity of LDL receptors enhances clearance of LDL, thus reducing its plasma level and its penetration in the parietal wall. The efficiency of the 'receptorial line' is genetically determined; however, a large intake of cholesterol and saturated fatty acids over the lifetime suppresses LDL receptors, thus increasing

levels of LDL-C. The LDL-receptor mechanism, when saturated, accounts for nearly 65% of the total cholesterol cell uptake. The remaining cholesterol is taken up through an independent, not saturable receptor pathway which is unable to down-regulate cholesterol uptake by the cell. This alternative pathway is also called the 'scavenger pathway', and it is the only route when there is a complete absence of receptors, as in familial monogenic hypercholesterolaemia or in Watanabe rabbits. The LDL receptor is a single-protein chain which spans the plasma membrane. The outer position of the LDL receptor contains the binding site for LDL. The inner portion of the receptor is projected into the cytoplasm and contains the signal mechanism that allows LDL to be carried into cells; this is by way of the *coated pit*, which contains receptors, invaginates and pinches off to form an endocytic vesicle. The vesicle fuses with a lysosome, wherein the LDL is degraded. The receptor escapes degradation and returns to the surface, where it binds another particle of LDL and initiates formation of another endocytic vesicle. Each receptor migrates into and out of the cell every 10 min. One in every 500 newborns possesses one mutant gene for LDL receptor (*familial hypercholesterolaemia heterozygotes*) whereas 1 in every 1 000 000 inherits two copies of a mutant LDL receptor (*homozygotes*). The former have an average of twofold more plasma cholesterol and characteristically develop CHD between the ages of 40 and 60. The latter have up to 10 times higher values of plasma cholesterol and characteristically develop CHD before the age of 20. Mutations of the gene for LDL receptor are remarkably different and have been numbered up to 16. In the majority of mutations no receptor protein is synthesized; in the second most common class of mutations no receptor protein is synthesized; in the second most common class of mutations the receptor is synthesized but folds improperly and cannot be transported to the cell surface; in the third class the receptor contains abnormalities in the LDL-binding site and therefore does not bind LDL; in the fourth class the receptor reaches the surface and binds LDL but defects of the cytoplasm inhibit the movement of the receptor into the coated pits. *See* Fatty Acids, Metabolism

Four types of cells are fundamental to the pathogenesis of atherosclerosis and the formation of parietal lesions: platelets, endothelial cells, smooth muscle cells (SMCs), and monocytes–macrophages (M-M). The role of the last group has been outlined in recent years and appears to be the most complex. This group shares with SMCs the formation of 'foam cells', usually a cluster of cells present both in fatty streaks and in raised lesions. The term 'foam cells' refers to the appearance of the cells which are engulfed with cholesterol and its derivatives, mainly esters. As already stated, LDL penetrates into the cells via the receptors for normal

LDL; this mechanism is down-regulated when a sufficient amount of cholesterol has been taken up by the cells and the entrance of LDL is inhibited. Moreover, LDL may be damaged during the passage through the endothelium in the matrix of the parietal wall by a series of chemicals (aldehydes, metals), biological cells or substances (e.g. proteoglycans, SMCs macrophages), thus acquiring many chemical, physicochemical and immunological aspects that extensively modify the native LDL. The LDL which undergoes this modification is no longer recognized by receptors for normal LDL but it is recognized, bound and taken up by specific macrophage receptors (scavenger receptors) which are not down-regulated and thus do not inhibit endogenous cellular synthesis of cholesterol. Some recent observations support the hypothesis that these modifications occur *in vivo* and that a small amount of modified LDL may circulate in plasma.

The role of macrophages is not limited to receiving modified LDL but includes a striking range of potent secretory products. All these secretory products may severely influence atherogenesis and include factors of protein origin, such as neutral and acid hydrolases, complement components, coagulation factors, binding proteins and some mitogens, comprising angiogenesis factor, factor stimulating collagen production, and macrophage-derived growth factor (MDGF). Some macrophage products are nonprotein in origin, e.g. reactive metabolites of oxygen and bioactive lipids. The broad spectrum of hydrolytic and proteolytic enzymes may modify some components of the arterial wall, including collagen, elastin and proteins of the matrix. The secretion of MDGF may mediate proliferation of SMCs and endothelial cells, and vascular angiogenesis. The generation of oxygen metabolites may be responsible for cellular injury and endothelial ulceration. Finally, the phagocytic action and the lymphocyte activation are consistent with a role as inflammatory components of macrophages in the atheromatous plaques.

Beneficial Effects of HDL

Atherosclerosis was initially considered to be a 'one way process', in which cholesterol was carried by LDLs into the interior of the parietal wall. In recent years atherosclerosis has been recognized to be a dynamic 'two-way process', during which cholesterol is internalized to form cholesterol esters in the cells of the parietal wall (SMCs and M–M) and then carried out in the plasma to the liver. The efflux of cholesterol from the body pool, especially from the arterial walls, is accomplished by a special class of lipoproteins, the HDLs, which are therefore considered to be an 'antirisk' factor' in CHD. Using various procedures, HDL may be subdivided into

a large number of subclasses. For practical reasons there are two subclasses named HDL_2 (density 1·063–1·121 g ml^{-1} and HDL_3 (density 1·121–1·210 g ml^{-1}). They are mostly comprised of apolipoproteins (50·55% of total mass), the most important being apo A-I (prevalent in HDL_2) apo A-II (prevalent in HDL_3), apo C-I, apo C-II, and apo E. Phospholipids constitute the second relevant component (20–30%), with a minor presence of cholesterol esters (14–18%), free (4%) and triglycerides (3–6%). The efflux of cholesterol from the parietal cells is accomplished by an interaction between apo A-I, the enzyme lecithin-cholesterol acyltransferase (LCAT), and phospholipids. The role of HDL as an antirisk factor was stressed for the first time by analytical ultracentrifugation in the 1950s. In the following years, both clinical and epidemiological observations confirmed the hypothesis of HDL as a beneficial protector for IHD. Some families have been discovered whose members show normal or high levels of plasma cholesterol owing to a high level of HDL-C. The condition was named *hyperalphalipoproteinaemia*; families with this condition are apparently free from cardiovascular events. Other observations have concerned an opposite condition, named *hypoalphalipoproteinaemia*, families with this condition having normal plasma levels of lipids but with some members showing low or absent levels of HDL-C and/or apo A-I. Zonal ultracentrifugation has shown that the subclass defective or absent is HDL_2. Some studies performed in elderly people aged more than 80 years have led to the conclusion that high levels of HDL-C constitute a major trait of a condition called *longevity syndrome*. Others could not confirm these data and considered low levels of apo B as the major stigmata of the elderly. Epidemiological studies have supported the protective role of HDL. An inverse relationship has been found between levels of HDL-C and the prevalence in various populations of IHD. The data have been lately confirmed by several epidemiological studies. The list includes the *Framingham Study*, the *Lipid Research Clinics Study*, the *Lipid Research Clinics–Coronary Primary Prevention Trial (LRC–CPPT)*, the *Multiple Risk Factor Intervention Trial* (MRFIT) and *The PROCAM Study*. All studies have shown an inverse relationship between levels of HDL-C and the incidence of CHD. The regression coefficient analyses have stressed that there is a 2–3% decrease in CHD for each mg increase in HDL-C. Contradictory results have been produced by one study performed in the UK by the *British Regional Heart Study* and by a cooperative work between Russian and American Scientists (*USSR-LRC*).

Several studies performed in recent years have stressed the beneficial role of HDL in a large series of clinical conditions. Plasma levels of HDL are usually higher in fertile females than in men (which partly explains the lower incidence of CHD in females), in people who take regular physical exercise, in people with a low alcohol intake, and in subjects following insulin therapy. Low levels of HDL are common in obese people, in cirrhotic-type liver diseases, in untreated diabetics or diabetics not receiving oral hypoglycaemic drugs, in smokers, and in subjects with a high intake of carbohydrates, especially when this kind of diet induces hypertriglyceridaemia. A special problem is linked to the inverse relationship existing between VLDL-triglycerides and HDL-C; when the former are high the latter is low. Which is the more important risk factor of the two? This relationship obscures the real importance of HDL as an 'antirisk factor'; many studies have lately confirmed an autonomous role of HDL, independent from VLDL-triglyceride values. Moreover, it is possible that there is coexistence of two morbid conditions in which two metabolic defects are present. According to the data coming from the *PROCAM Study*, HDL-C is a better discriminator for IHD than the ratio LDL-C:HDL-C or the ratio apo B:apo A-I. *See* Fatty Acids, Dietary Importance

Bibliography

Avogaro P, Bittolo Bon G and Cazzolato G (1988) Presence of a modified low density lipoprotein in humans. *Arteriosclerosis* 8: 79–87.

Goldstein JL and Brown MS (1983) Familial hypercholesterolemia. In: Stanbury JB, Wyngaarden JB, Fredrickson DS, Goldstein JL and Brown MS (eds) *The Metabolic Basis of Inherited Disease*, pp 672–712. New York: McGraw-Hill.

Goldstein JL, Ho YK, Basu SK and Brown MS (1979) Binding site on macrophages that mediates uptake and degradation of acetylated low density lipoproteins, producing massive cholesterol ester deposition. *Proceedings of the National Academy of Sciences of the USA* 76: 333–337.

Haberland ME, Fong D and Cheng L (1988) Malondialdehyde-altered protein occurs in atheroma of Watanabe heritable hyperlipidemic rabbits. *Science* 241: 215–218.

Kannel WB, Castelli WP, Gordon T and MacNamara PM (1971) Serum cholesterol, lipoproteins and the risk of coronary heart disease: The Framingham Study. *Annals of Internal Medicine* 74: 1–12.

Keys A (1980) *Seven Countries. A multivariate analysis of death and coronary heart disease.* Cambridge; Massachusetts: Harvard University Press.

Miller GJ and Miller NE (1975) Plasma high-density lipoprotein concentration and development of ischaemic heart disease. *Lancet* i: 16–19.

Müller C (1939) Angina pectoris in hereditary xanthomatosis. *Archives of Internal Medicine* 64: 675–700.

Stamler J (1974) The primary prevention of Coronary Heart Disease: *Miocardium: Failure a. Infarction.* E. Braunwald (ed). p 219. New York: HP Publishing.

Thannhauser SJ (1958) *Lipidoses.* New York: Grune and Stratton.

Pietro Avogaro
Regional General Hospital, Venice, Italy

CHOLINE

Contents

Properties and Determination

Choline is an important component of a number of biological compounds, such as the neurotransmitter acetylcholine and the phospholipid lecithin (phosphatidylcholine). This article will briefly discuss the occurrence of choline in foods and its use in fortification. The physical properties and methods of analysis of the many and various choline-containing compounds are beyond the scope of this article; instead, the discussion will focus on those of choline itself.

Occurrence in Foods/Use in Food Fortification

Choline occurs widely in plant and animal foods. It is often present in the form of lecithin and rarely as the free base. Choline is also found in many processed foods and sold as supplements. In the form of lecithin, it is used as an emulsifying agent and additive in commercial foods such as mayonnaise and chocolate products.

Table 1 presents the average choline contents of common foods. Choline occurs in highest concentration in animal organ foods such as liver, brain and kidney.

Wheat germ is one of the richest sources of choline. Other vegetable and animal tissues also contain a considerable amount. It is estimated that the average daily intake of choline in the USA is 400–900 mg.

The choline content of milk varies widely, at least in part, due to seasonal factors. Nonfortified whole-milk powders in particular vary widely: 40–360 mg per 100 g (105 mg per 100 g average). Skim milk values are similar to those of whole milk. In the USA, infant formulae are recommended to contain at least 7 mg of choline per 100 kcal, based on the choline content in human milk. Since formulae provide about 65–95 kcal per 100 ml, the average of 5 mg per 100 g in Table 1 is close to this desired amount. However, the few studies to date have shown that levels vary widely and are sometimes lower than the amounts stated on the label. *See* individual foods

Properties

Choline (trimethyl(2-hydroxyethyl) ammonium hydroxide; hydroxide form $(CH_3)_3N-CH_2CH_2OH)^+OH^-$, M_r 121) usually occurs as a colourless, syrupy liquid. This quaternary amine is a strong base ($pK_b = 5$) and absorbs carbon dioxide from the atmosphere. It crystallizes with difficulty and is very soluble in water and alcohol, but insoluble in diethyl ether. While choline is stable in dilute solutions, at high concentrations and temperatures of 100°C it decomposes to ethylene glycol, polyethylene glycol and trimethylamine.

Choline occurs most commonly as the chloride salt or as a component of the phospholipid lecithin (phosphatidylcholine). Choline chloride is a white crystalline deliquescent salt with a slight odour of trimethylamine and a brackish taste. Like the free base, it is soluble in water and alcohol, but not diethyl ether. Aqueous solutions are stable and neutral in pH. Choline chloride is hygroscopic at room temperature and has a relative humidity greater than 20%. Phosphatidylcholine is a fatlike substance consisting of a glycerol backbone, two fatty acids and choline attached by a phosphoryl ester link. Commercial forms of lecithin are actually mixtures of phosphatides, containing as little as 20% phosphatidylcholine; therefore, use of the latter term is preferred over 'lecithin', except when referring to the commercial product. *See* Phospholipids, Properties and Occurrence

Analysis

Choline may be assayed by a wide variety of techniques. The selection of the method should be based on the detection level required, the type of sample and equipment available. Sample preparation is also often important, especially when levels of different choline metabolites are being measured. For example, because acetylcholine is rapidly hydrolysed to free choline and acetate in animal brain tissue following sacrifice, accurate assessments of choline and acetyl choline were once difficult to obtain. The more recent use of head-focused microwave radiation minimizes this post-mortem hydrolysis.

This section provides a brief description of the major methods of choline analysis, the principal reactions involved, and their advantages and disadvantages. A summary of most of the methods discussed below is presented in Table 2.

Gravimetric Methods

A number of salts form insoluble precipitates with choline, including potassium triiodide, platinum chlor-

Table 1. The choline content of some animal and plant foods (mg per 100 g)

High (> 200 mg per 100 g)		Medium (100–200 mg per 100 g)		Low (< 100 mg per 100 g)	
Egg yolk	1713	Infant formula powder (choline added)	203	Kale	89
Calf liver	650	Skim and whole-milk powder (lecithin added)	154	Trout muscle	84
Beef liver	630	Rolled oats	151	Cauliflower	78
Defatted wheat germ	423	Peanut butter	145	Cabbage	46
Beef brain	410	Wheat bran	143	Potatoes	40
Beef kidney	333	Barley	139	Leeks	29
Spinach	238	Asparagus	128	String beans	21
Soya beans	237	Rice polish	126	Lettuce	18
		Pork ham	120	Liquid skim and whole milk	11
		Skim and whole-milk powders (nonfortified)	105	Carrots	9
				Human milk	9
				Infant formula (liquid)	5

Sources: Woollard DC and Indyk HE (1990); Zeisel SH *et al.* (1986); Wurtman JJ (1979); Sebrell Jr WH and Harris RS (1954).

ide, gold chloride and phosphotungstic acid. Relatively pure choline chloride is assayed by mixing it in solution with aluminium chloride and tetraphenylborate, then filtering, drying and weighing the precipitate. While these methods can be useful in measuring choline in chemical and pharmaceutical preparations, they are usually not applicable to biological samples due to the low levels of choline present.

Bioassays

Mutant 34486 *Neurospora crassa* and *Torulopis pintolopessi* require choline for growth and have been used to estimate choline in various tissues. Mutant 34486 also responds to choline-related compounds such as methylaminoethanol, acetylcholine and phosphorylcholine. Since these methods are less sensitive than many other techniques they are rarely used today.

Various biological assays for choline are based on its conversion to acetylcholine, which causes muscle contraction. A number of standard tissues have been used in these kymographic assays, including the frog rectus abdominis, leech dorsal muscle, clam heart, guinea-pig ileum and rabbit intestine. These methods are generally rapid, convenient, inexpensive and sensitive. However, they are subject to interfering substances such as drugs, and the response of the tissue weakens over successive assays. The additional step of converting choline to acetylcholine is also inconvenient. For these reasons, and because more reliable methods have been developed, bioassays are rarely used nowadays.

Spectrophotometric Methods

The classical reineckate method was once a widely used procedure for quantitatively assessing choline. In this technique, choline is precipitated as an insoluble reineckate complex, extracted in acetone and spectrophotometrically determined at 505 nm. However, this method is usually of insufficient sensitivity for most biological applications.

A simple, relatively sensitive enzymatic/colorimetric assay has been used to measure choline in a wide variety of tissues and foods. Choline is hydrolysed from phospholipids by phospholipase D, then oxidized by choline oxidase to produce betaine and hydrogen peroxide. Oxidation of the latter by peroxidase couples 4-aminoantipyrine and phenol to yield a red chromogen that absorbs at 500 nm. The method has been modified for use with various samples, including various organ tissues, plasma, bile, milk, food and vitamin products. The main drawback to the technique is possible colour

interference as a result of light-absorbing substances in the sample. Another more sensitive technique follows the same initial sequence of reactions to yield hydrogen peroxide, which then produces chemiluminescence in the presence of luminol and horseradish peroxidase. *See* Spectroscopy, Visible Spectroscopy and Colorimetry

In a fluorometric method, choline is phosphorylated by choline kinase. The resultant ADP converts phosphoenolpyruvate to pyruvate, which oxidizes NADH. NAD^+ maximally absorbs at 340 nm and fluoresces in the region of 465 nm. The major advantages of this technique are its usefulness for crude tissue extracts and its sensitivity. These coupled reactions are also the basis for a commercial kit to assay lecithin; the production of NAD^+ is spectrophotometrically monitored at 340 nm. However, methods that rely on choline kinase and acetylcholine esterase may not be sufficiently selective in certain applications, since these enzymes are not highly specific for their substrates. *See* Spectroscopy, Fluorescence

Radioenzymatic Methods

A number of radioenzymatic techniques have been developed to measure choline and acetylcholine in biological samples, especially brain and nervous tissues. These methods rely on some enzyme to create a radioactive species of choline, which is then measured by scintillation spectrometry. The two most commonly used enzymes are choline kinase and choline acetyltransferase, which generate [^{32}P]phosphorylcholine and [^{14}C]acetylcholine, respectively. *See* Enzymes, Use in Analysis

When these methods were first developed, these enzymes had to be prepared from biological materials (e.g. brewer's yeast). However, both are now commercially available with increased purity, hence increasing the sensitivity of the methods. Most assays require 1–2 days to complete and some method of separating the radioactive species for scintillation counting, e.g. by electrophoresis, ion exchange or paper chromatography, or solvent extraction. The basic methods have been adapted to assay for other choline species, such as phosphatidyl choline, and choline in a variety of tissue samples. In one method, both choline kinase and acetylcholine esterase are used to measure choline and acetylcholine in the same sample. The chief disadvantages are the expense of radiolabelled substrates and the relative low specificity of enzymes. *See* Electrophoresis

Amperometric Methods

More recently, a number of sensitive, reproducible methods have been developed to measure choline and

Table 2. Methods for choline analysis of biological samples

Method	Principle/reactions involved	Sensitivity	Advantages/disadvantages
Bioassay			
(1) Microbiological	Measure growth of Ch-requiring organisms, mutant 34486 *Neurospora crassa* or *Torulopis pintolopessi*	50–150 nmol	Inexpensive, simple; assay takes days; growth affected by other substances
(2) Kymographic	Convert to ACh, measure contraction response of a standard tissue (e.g. leech dorsal muscle) on a kymograph	10 pmol	Simple, convenient, inexpensive; converting Ch to ACh somewhat inconvenient; tissue responses to ACh vary by species, season and number of assays; sensitive to interfering substances (e.g. drugs)
Spectrophotometric			
(1) Enzymatic/ colorimetric	Ch→betaine+H_2O_2 (Ch oxidase) 4-Aminoantipyrine+phenol+H_2O_2→red chromagen, 500 nm (peroxidase)	nmol range	Colour-absorbing substances may interfere with assay
(2) Chemiluminescent	Ch→betaine+H_2O_2 (Ch oxidase) H_2O_2+luminol→oxidized luminol (peroxidase) Measure with luminometer	10 pmol	Some substances can interfere with assay
(3) Fluorometric	Ch+ATP→P-Ch+ADP (Ch kinase) ADP+PEP→ATP+pyruvate (pyruvate kinase) Pyruvate+NADH→lactate+NAD^+ (lactate dehydrogenase) Fluorometer measures absorption/ fluorescence of NAD^+ (340/465 nm)	100 pmol	Can be used with crude tissue extracts. Ch kinase not highly specific for Ch; glucose, ethanolamine may interfere with enzyme
Radioenzymatic assay			
(1) Choline kinase	Ch+^{32}P-ATP→ADP+^{32}P-Ch (measured by scintillation spectrophotometry)	pmol range	Ch kinase not highly specific for Ch; ^{32}P-ATP has short half-life; cost of radiolabelled substrate
(2) Choline acetyltransferase	[^{14}C]Acetyl-CoA+Ch→CoA+[^{14}C]ACh (measured by scintillation spectrophotometry)	pmol range	Salts must be extracted from samples to avoid interference with electrophoresis; cost of radiolabelled substrate
Amperometric			
(1) Ch/ACh microelectrode	Ch and ACh complexed with dipicrylamine, detected by ion-selective microelectrode	pmol range	Some substances (e.g. cholinergic drugs) can interfere with assay
(2) Ch oxygen electrode	Ch→betaine+H_2O_2 (Ch oxidase, immobilized on nylon net; electrode detects H_2O_2)	pmol range	Some substances (e.g. betaine aldehyde) can interfere with assay

continued

Table 2. *continued*

Method	Principle/reactions involved	Sensitivity	Advantages/disadvantages
Chromatographic			
(1) GC and GCMS	Ch and ACh are extracted from sample and converted to volatile, demethylated form by pyrolysis or benzenethiolate	GC: nmol–pmol range 1–5 pmol	Large numbers of samples can be processed. Requires rigorous extraction steps and expensive equipment
(2) Ion exchange chromatography	Ch and ACh extracted with anion (e.g. dipicrylamine) into organic phase (e.g. dichloromethane), isolated by liquid–liquid chromatography in a microcolumn with an anionic solid phase, detected by spectrometric absorption at 254 nm	nmol range	Method is rapid and simple. Microcells require special handling. Dipicrylamine preparation requires purification and cautious handling
(3) RP-HPLC	Ch and ACh separated on RP-HPLC, measured by (a) detection of H_2O_2 by platinum electrode (Ch oxidase immobilized in postcolumn reaction coil), (b) UV spectrometer (UV-absorbing ionic agents in mobile phase), or (c) scintillation spectrophotometry (of labelled Ch)	1–2 pmol	Requires HPLC and additional equipment

ACh, acetylcholine; ADP, adenosine diphosphate; ATP, adenosine triphosphate; Ch, choline; GC, gas chromatography; GCMS, GC with mass spectrometry; NADH, nicotinamide adenine dinucleotide; P, phosphorus; PEP, phosphoenol pyruvate; RP-HPLC, reversed-phase high-performance liquid chromatography; UV, ultraviolet light.

acetylcholine amperometrically. One of the earlier systems was based on an ion-selective microelectrode specific for choline and acetylcholine complexed with the anion dipicrylamine. Later systems were based on an oxygen electrode and choline oxidase, often immobilized on a nylon net. Under the action of the enzyme, choline is oxidized to betaine and hydrogen peroxide, which is detected by the electrode. These latter methods are very sensitive and have been successfully used to assay choline in a variety of biological materials.

Chromatographic Methods

Gas chromatograph analysis methods for choline and acetylcholine have been used for nearly 20 years. These procedures require conversion of either of these amines to a volatile derivative, usually the demethylated form, by pyrolysis or reaction with benzenethiolate. After a number of extraction and separation steps, the samples are injected into the gas chromatograph. These techniques are generally sensitive in the nanomolar to picomolar range and can process a large number of samples. Sensitivity can be greatly increased by combining the gas chromatograph with a mass spectrometer – gas chromatography/mass spectroscopy (GCMS). The time from tissue extraction to gas chromatography or GCMS analysis is usually 1–2 days. Early procedures have been modified for use with various types of samples and greater simplicity. The major disadvantages to

GCMS methods are the expensive equipment and rigorous sample preparation required. *See* Chromatography, Gas Chromatography

Choline and acetylcholine can also be measured through ion pair column chromatography coupled with ultraviolet detection. In this technique, choline and acetylcholine are extracted as ion pairs with an anion (e.g. dipicrylamine) into an organic phase (e.g. dichloromethane). Choline and acetylcholine are isolated by liquid–liquid chromatography in a microcolumn with an anionic solid phase. A spectrometer measures the absorption of the effluent at 254 nm. This method is fairly sensitive; the major drawbacks are the care needed in handling the microcells and dipicrylamine.

A number of methods have been developed employing high-performance liquid chromatography (HPLC) systems. In one system, choline and acetylcholine are first separated by reversed-phase HPLC (RP-HPLC), then mixed with choline oxidase and acetylcholine esterase. The hydrogen peroxide produced is then measured by a platinum electrode. There have been a number of modifications of this method, such as immobilization of the enzymes on postcolumn reaction coil materials and other improvements. The use of ultraviolet-absorbing ion interaction agents in the mobile phase of an RP-HPLC system enables direct measurement of choline metabolites by an ultraviolet detector without the need for derivitization. Other HPLC techniques have been developed that separate radiolabelled choline from a wide range of potentially interfering metabolites. Generally, HPLC techniques are sensitive, specific, relatively fast and simple. *See* Chromatography, High-performance Liquid Chromatography

Choline and its metabolites are important in nutrition, food processing, and a number of biological processes. Methods of choline analysis have evolved over the last 20 years, and today a variety of techniques are available. Selection of a procedure should take into consideration the nature of the sample, equipment available, and sensitivity and selectivity required. While each method has advantages and disadvantages, it would seem that those utilizing HPLC provide a high degree of selectivity and sensitivity, and involve equipment available in most laboratories.

Bibliography

Boehringer Mannheim GmbH (1987) *Methods of Biochemical Analysis and Food Analysis, Method 529362*, pp 76–78. Mannheim: Boehringer Mannheim GmbH.

Campanella L, Carrara D, Cordatore M, Salvi AM, Sammartino MP and Tomassetti M (1987) New methods of analysis and control of biological fluids, drugs and foods. In: Piemonte G, Tagliaro F, Marigo M and Frigerio A (eds) *Developments in Analytical Methods in Pharmaceutical, Biomedical and Forensic Sciences*, pp 19–28. New York: Plenum Press.

Chan MM (1990) Choline. In: Machlin LJ (ed.) *Handbook of Vitamins*, pp 537–556. New York: Marcel Dekker.

Hanin I and Shih T-M (1980) Gas chromatography, mass spectrometry, and combined gas chromatography-mass spectrometry. In: Hanin I and Koslow SH (eds) *Physicochemical Methodologies in Psychiatric Research*, pp 111–154. New York: Raven Press.

Hanin I (1974) *Choline and Acetylcholine: Handbook of Chemical Assay Methods*. New York: Raven Press.

Hanin I (1982) Methods for the analysis and measurement of acetylcholine: an overview. In: Spector S and Back N (eds) *Modern Methods in Pharmacology*, pp 29–38. New York: Alan R Liss.

Jaramillo A, Lopez S, Justice Jr JB, Salamone JD and Neill DB (1983) Acetylcholine and choline ion-selective microelectrodes. *Analytica Chimica Acta* 145: 149–159.

Jukes TH (1979) Choline. In: Grayson M and Eckroth D (eds) *Kirk-Othmer Encyclopedia of Chemical Technology*, 3rd edn, vol. 6, pp. 19–28. New York: Wiley.

Neff NH, Meek JL, Hadjiconstantinou M and Laird II HE (1987) Analysis of choline and acetylcholine in tissue by HPLC with electrochemical detection. In: Parvez H, Parvez S, Bastart-Malsod M *et al.* (eds) *Progress in HPLC*, vol. 2, pp 181–191. Utrecht: VNU Science Press.

Potter PE and Hanin I (1988) Estimation of acetylcholine and choline and analysis of acetylcholine turnover rates in vivo. In: Whitaker VP (ed.) *Handbook of Experimental Pharmacology*, pp 103–124. Berlin: Springer-Verlag.

Sebrell Jr WH and Harris RS (1954) *The Vitamins: Chemistry, Physiology, Pathology*, vol. II, p 766. New York: Academic Press.

Takayama M, Itoh S, Nagasaki T and Tanimizu I (1977) A new enzymatic method for determination of serum choline-containing phospholipids. *Clinica et Chimica Acta* 79: 93–98.

Woollard DC and Indyk HE (1990) The routine, enzymatic estimation of total choline in milk and infant formulas. *Journal of Micronutrient Analysis* 7: 1–14.

Wurtman JJ (1979) Sources of choline and lecithin in the diet. In: Barbeau A, Groden JH and Wurtman RJ (eds) *Nutrition and the Brain*, pp 73–81. New York: Raven Press.

Zeisel SH, Char D and Sheard NF (1986) Choline, phosphatidylcholine and sphingomyelin in human and bovine milk and infant formulas. *Journal of Nutrition* 116: 50–58.

Acknowledgements

The authors gratefully acknowledge the invaluable help of Israel Hanin, PhD, Loyola University, Chicago, in reviewing this manuscript.

Mabel M. Chan and David J. Canty
New York University, New York, USA

Physiology

Choline is ubiquitously distributed in foods where it is present in free and esterified forms (Table 1). It is required to make the phospholipids phosphatidylcholine, lysophosphatidylcholine, choline plasmalogen and sphingomyelin – essential components of all membranes. It is a precursor for the biosynthesis of the neurotransmitter acetylcholine and is also an important source of labile methyl groups.

Chronic ingestion of a diet deficient in choline, or its precursors methionine and folate, can lead to hepatic, renal, pancreatic, memory and growth disorders in animals. In many animal species, including the rat, pig, dog and monkey, choline deficiency results in liver dysfunction. During choline deficiency, hepatocyte turnover is greatly increased, and large amounts of lipid (mainly triglycerides) accumulate in the liver, eventually filling the entire hepatocyte. The term 'lipotropic' was coined to describe choline and other substances that prevented deposition of fat in the liver. Lipid accumulation occurs because triglycerides must be packaged as very low density lipoprotein (VLDL) to be exported from liver. The choline metabolite, phosphatidylcholine, is an essential component of VLDL, and cannot be substituted for by other phospholipids. *See* Folic Acid, Physiology; Liver, Nutritional Management of Liver and Biliary Disorders

Renal function is also compromised by choline deficiency, with abnormalities in the ability to concentrate urine, the reabsorption of free water, sodium excretion, glomerular filtration rate and renal plasma flow; in some cases there is gross renal haemorrhage. Infertility, growth impairment, bony abnormalities, decreased haematopoiesis, and hypertension have also been reported to be associated with diets low in choline and its precursors. *See* Hypertension, Physiology

In the adult human, serum choline concentrations fluctuate over an approximately twofold range when common choline-containing foods are ingested. Individuals in the USA probably ingest at least 6 g of phosphatidylcholine per day (100 mg per day of this amount deriving from addition to foods during processing). Total choline intake in the adult human (as free choline and the choline in phosphatidylcholine and other choline esters) is probably in excess of 6–10 mmol (600–1000 mg) per day. Consumption of choline will be higher in humans ingesting phosphatidylcholine (also called lecithin), a dietary 'health-food' supplement. Human milk contains approximately 200 μmol l^{-1} each of free choline, phosphatidylcholine and sphingomyelin (colostrum and transitional milk have three- to fourfold

higher free choline content than does mature milk; bovine milk and formulae derived from it are similar in choline content to mature human milk; soya-bean-derived formulae can have three- to fourfold higher choline concentration than that of bovine milk). The human mammary gland can achieve choline concentrations in milk that are 60 times those found in maternal plasma. Neonatal animals and humans have exceptionally high blood choline concentrations. The delivery of choline to the neonate appears to be very important for normal brain development. *See* Health Foods, Definition and Dietary Importance; Infant Foods, Milk Formulas; Infants, Breast- and Bottle-feeding

Metabolism of Choline

All tissues accumulate choline, but uptake by liver, kidney, mammary gland, placenta and brain are of particular importance. Most tissues take up choline by a combination of transport processes (diffusion and mediated transport) such as have been described in brain, liver, kidney, erythrocytes, placenta and intestine. Within tissues choline can be acetylated to form acetyl-

Table 1.   Choline content of some common foods

Food	Choline (μmol kg^{-1})	Phosphatidylcholine (μmol kg^{-1})	Sphingomyelin (μmol kg^{-1})
Apple	27	280	15
Banana	240	37	20
Beef liver	5831	43 500	1850
Beef steak	75	6030	506
Butter	42	1760	460
Cauliflower	1306	2770	183
Corn oil	3	12	5
Coffee	1010	15	23
Cucumber	218	76	27
Egg	42	52 000	2250
Ginger ale	2	4	3
Grape juice	475	15	5
Iceberg lettuce	2930	132	50
Margarine	30	450	15
Milk (bovine, whole)	150	148	82
Orange	200	490	24
Peanut butter	3895	3937	9
Peanuts	4546	4960	78
Potato	511	300	26
Tomato	430	52	32
Wholemeal bread	968	340	11

Choline, phosphatidylcholine and sphingomyelin were measured using a gas chromatography/mass spectrometry assay in foods prepared in the form that they would normally be consumed. From Pomfret EA, daCosta KA, Schurman LL and Zeisel SH (1989) Measurement of choline and choline metabolite concentrations using high pressure liquid chromatography and gas chromatography–mass spectrometry. *Analytical Biochemistry* 180: 85–90.

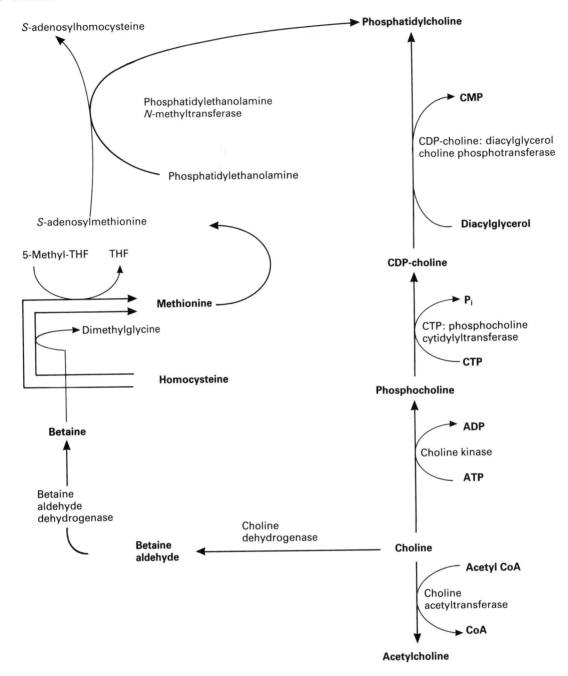

Fig. 1 The three major functions for choline are as a precursor for phosphatidylcholine biosynthesis, as a methyl donor, and as a precursor for acetylcholine biosynthesis.

choline, phosphorylated to form phosphocholine and phospholipids, or oxidized to form betaine which is a methyl donor (Fig. 1). The demand for choline as a methyl donor is probably the major factor which determines how rapidly a diet deficient in choline will induce pathology. The synthesis of acetylcholine within neurons can be enhanced by loading them with choline. This effect has been the basis for using supplements of choline-containing compounds in the treatment of neurological disorders.

Physiology

Choline and Carcinogenesis

Choline-deficient animals (fed diets just adequate in methionine and folate) are much more likely to develop liver cancer spontaneously, or in response to a carcinogen. Several mechanisms have been suggested for this cancer-promoting effect of choline deficiency. These include increased cell proliferation, formation of lipid peroxides, decreased DNA methylation and accumulation of diacylglycerol with resulting perturbations of transmembrane signalling. Choline phospholipids are important modulators of protein-kinase-C-mediated signal transduction. *See* Carcinogens, Carcinogenic Substances in Food

Groups at Risk for Choline Deficiency

Choline and phosphatidylcholine are so ubiquitous in our diet that a deficiency syndrome in humans has not yet been proven. However, there are certain clinical situations which act to increase the demands for choline, and therefore might be more likely to result in organ dysfunction secondary to choline deficiency.

Amino acid and glucose solutions used in total parenteral nutrition (TPN) of humans contain no choline. The lipid emulsions used to deliver extra calories and essential fatty acids during TPN contain choline in the form of phosphatidylcholine. It was observed that malnourished humans, at the time they were referred for TPN therapy, had significantly lower plasma choline concentrations than did those of well-fed control subjects. Plasma choline concentrations in these patients declined further when they were treated with the amino acid and glucose solution lacking choline during the first week of therapy. However, when patients were treated with lipid emulsion as well as an amino acid and glucose solution, their plasma choline concentrations rose slightly. Neither group received sufficient choline to restore plasma choline concentrations to normal. Hepatic complications such as fatty infiltration of the liver and hepatocellular damage have frequently been associated with TPN, often resulting in termination of TPN. It is possible that some of the liver disease associated with TPN is related to choline deficiency.

Conditions that enhance hepatic triglyceride synthesis (such as carbohydrate loading) increase the requirement for the choline-containing lipoprotein envelope used to export this lipid from liver. Thus, treatment of malnourished patients with high-calorie TPN solutions, at a time when choline stores are depleted, might cause hepatic dysfunction. The definitive experiment, in which supplemental choline is administered and found to decrease the incidence of hepatic dysfunction during TPN, has not yet been performed. Until such data are available, it is impossible to state that humans require choline during TPN. The information available to date only suggests that this may be so.

Bypass surgery involving large segments of the bowel (i.e. to produce weight loss in very obese humans) is associated with fatty liver. Similarly, in obese rats which have had 90% of their small intestine bypassed, fatty liver develops as insufficient choline is absorbed. Choline supplementation prevents this, and choline-deficient diets in such patients exacerbate the accumulation of fat in the liver.

Pregnancy is associated with increased requirements for tissue (fetus) biosynthesis. As discussed earlier, a placental transport system withdraws choline from mother into fetus. The hepatic choline concentration falls from a mean of 130 nmol per g in adult non-pregnant rats to 38 nmol per g in late pregnancy. Pregnant women, especially those in their third trimester, are particularly susceptible to development of fatty liver, and it has been suggested that this may be related to an increased choline requirement.

Healthy humans consuming a choline-deficient diet for 3 weeks had depleted stores of choline in tissues, and developed signs of incipient liver dysfunction. These observations support the suggestion that choline is an essential nutrient for humans.

Toxicity

The median (LD_{50}) lethal dose of choline iodide in rats is 1·7 mmol per kg ip (intraperitoneal) and 28·7 mmol per kg orally. Estimates of the oral LD_{50} in rats for choline vary from 24 to 48 mmol per kg. For choline chloride the ip LD_{50} in rats was 3·2 mmol per kg; in mice the ip LD_{50} was 2·4 mmol per kg (when coadministered with 100 mg of morphine per kg, LD_{50} was 1·2 mmol per kg). The iv (intravenous) LD_{50} for choline chloride in rabbits was 0·01 mmol per kg and in cats was 0·25 mmol per kg.

Neither choline nor phosphatidylcholine is mutagenic by the Ames test. Teratogenicity of choline has not been studied; lecithin (phosphatidylcholine) was not teratogenic in mice at dietary levels of 1600 mg per kg per day. High doses of choline (5–30 g per 70 kg of bodyweight) have been associated with 'fishy' body odour, vomiting, salivation, sweating, and gastrointestinal distress. These side-effects are probably dose-dependent, and all but the fishy body odour can be prevented by prior administration of a muscarinic receptor blocker such as methscopolamine.

Bibliography

Newberne PM and Rogers AE (1986) Labile methyl groups and the promotion of cancer. *Annual Review of Nutrition* 6(407): 407–432.

Sheard NF, Tayek JA, Bistrian BR, Blackburn GL and Zeisel SH (1986) Plasma choline concentration in humans fed parenterally. *American Journal of Clinical Nutrition* 43(2): 219–224.

Zeisel SH (1988) 'Vitamin-like' molecules: choline. In: Shils M and Young V (eds) *Modern Nutrition in Health and Disease*, pp 440–452. Philadelphia: Lea and Febiger.

Zeisel SH, daCosta K-A, Franklin PD *et al.* (1991) Choline is an essential nutrient for humans. *FASEB Journal* 5: 2093–2098.

Elizabeth M. Rohlfs, Kerry-Ann da Costa, Melinda Fine and Steven H. Zeisel
Department of Nutrition, The University of North Carolina at Chapel Hill, USA

CHROMATOGRAPHY

Contents

Principles

Chromatography is a physical process in which separation of the components in a mixture is achieved by differential partition between a stationary phase and a fluid phase passing over it. The various techniques used can be divided into gas chromatography and liquid chromatography on the basis of the nature of the mobile fluid phase involved. This article discusses the basic theory of the chromatographic process and the factors that affect separation efficiency, as applied to liquid chromatography. The factors affecting chromatographic separation in gas chromatography are similar, and the theory may be readily extended to gas phase techniques. The apparatus required to realize separations of mixtures in practice is covered in the articles dealing with the various techniques, where specific examples to food analysis will also be found.

Basic Theory

An ideal chromatographic separation would involve separation between molecules in the sample according to their structure, with molecules of the same type staying together. In the case of column chromatography the sample is applied as a narrow band to the head of the column and passes through the column under the influence of the mobile phase; the components in the mixture would separate into individual narrow bands, but these bands would be no wider than the initial sample, assuming no diffusion had taken place. However, in practice this ideal situation does not arise as diffusion is an intrinsic phenomenon and there is significant spreading within the bands. The degree of retention of the components on the column depends on the relative affinity of the compounds for the mobile and stationary phases. This process is essentially under thermodynamic control. However, the degree of band spreading is dependent on a number of kinetic factors.

Chromatographic Retention

The degree of retention of a compound on a column packed with a stationary phase under the influence of a flowing mobile phase depends on the partition (or distribution) of that compound between the two phases. This is characterized by the distribution coefficient (K) for the compound, which is simply the ratio of its concentration in the stationary phase (C_s) to that in the mobile phase (C_m):

$$K = C_s/C_m. \tag{1}$$

In practice this distribution is more commonly characterized by the capacity factor (k'), which is the ratio of the amount of sample in the stationary phase (a_s) to that in the mobile phase (a_m),

$$k' = a_s/a_m. \tag{2}$$

This parameter is used extensively to quantify retention of peaks and is related to retention time as shown in the expression

$$k' = \frac{t - t_0}{t_0}, \tag{3}$$

where t is the retention time of the peak of interest and t_0 is the time in which an unretained compound will emerge from the column. The capacity factor can be used for theoretical studies of the chromatographic process as a thermodynamic model, for example $\log_{10} k'$ is found to be proportional to T^{-1} (temperature in kelvin). More practically, k' is not altered by changes in column geometry, whereas t is. The chromatographic process can only be described by the thermodynamic model under ideal conditions and deviations are to be expected once the distribution coefficient is no longer independent of sample concentration. The most commonly encountered such deviation can be found at high sample concentrations, where peak broadening occurs together with a reduction in retention time.

Band Broadening

In practice band broadening takes place as the sample passes through the column. The smaller the extent of this broadening the more efficient the column and hence the greater its ability to separate similar compounds.

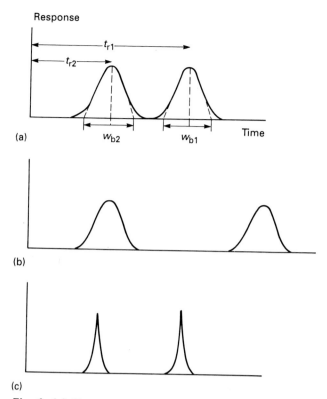

(a)

(b)

(c)

Fig. 1. (a) Chromatographic resolution; increased by (b) increasing $(t_{r1} - t_{r2})$, or (c) decreasing $\frac{1}{2}(w_{b1} + w_{b2})$.

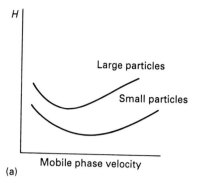

(a)

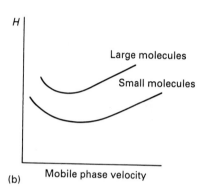

(b)

Fig. 2. Effect of mobile phase velocity on column efficiency for (a) large- and small-particle stationary phases, and (b) large and small sample molecules. Note that small values of H represent efficient columns.

Thus, in the example shown in Fig. 1 the resolution has been increased by decreasing the bandwidths (c). Alternatively the resolution could be increased by increasing the difference in retention times of the two compounds, but this may also lead to an increase in analysis time (b).

The effect of these two changes can readily be seen from the mathematical definition of the term 'resolution' (R_s):

$$R_s = \frac{(t_{r2} - t_{r1})}{\frac{1}{2}(w_{b2} + w_{b1})}, \tag{3}$$

where t_{r1}, t_{r2} are the retention times and w_{b1}, w_{b2} are the peak widths.

A significant advantage in reducing bandwidths is that for a given amount of material a narrower band will yield a taller peak and hence greater sensitivity.

In practice, narrow peaks will only be achieved where there is efficient exchange of sample molecules between the mobile and stationary phases; in other words where there is good mass transfer. Additionally there will be contributions to band broadening as a result of eddy diffusion (multiple paths through the stationary phase, each with differing pathlengths and velocities) and mobile-phase mass transfer (gradation of solvent velocities across a flowing stream). Pools of stagnant mobile phase held within pores can also lead to broadening as sample molecules held within them will be further

delayed. The factors affecting these individual processes are complex but the most important are the particle size of the stationary phase material and the velocity of the mobile phase over it. These two factors are shown in Fig. 2 where it will be noted that the material with smaller particles gives narrower bands, but also that these can be achieved at a higher solvent velocity, so that this will allow more rapid analyses. Another important factor that affects the transfer of sample molecules between the phases is the ease with which they can diffuse in the mobile phase, which in turn will depend on the diffusion coefficient of the solvents involved which will also be influenced by temperature. Solvents with low viscosity will tend to produce narrow peaks and an increase in column temperature will, generally, result in reduced band spreading.

The efficiency of a chromatographic column is expressed by its plate number (by analogy with fractional distillation) which is given by the expression

$$N = 5.54(t_r/w_h)^2, \tag{4}$$

where t_r is the retention time of the peak and w_h is the peak width at half height. Modern microparticulate phases (5 μm) will have plate numbers approaching 100 000 per metre.

Table 1. Modes of liquid chromatography

Mode	Basis of retention
Adsorption	Polarity
Partition	Solubility
Ion exchange	Charge
Size exclusion	Molecular size
Chiral	Stereospecificity
Affinity	Biochemical specificity

Modes of Liquid Chromatography

The mode of chromatography refers to the mechanism by means of which the solute is retained on the stationary phase. The most commonly encountered modes in liquid chromatography are shown in Table 1. The choice of mode of chromatography for a particular group of compounds is far from simple, and although there are some types of compound which are not compatible with a given mode, there are often two or three modes which could be used. The modes available for gas chromatography are discussed in that article.

Adsorption Chromatography

Silica gel is by far the most common material used for this mode of chromatography, in which solute molecules are partitioned between solution in the mobile phase and adsorption on the polar surface of the silica. The activity of the material depends strongly on the degree of hydration of the surface. In the presence of polar solvents such as alcohols, which are often used as polar modifiers in a less polar solvent, the silica surface becomes solvated and the solute (sample) molecules then interact with this solvated surface. The elution power of the mobile phase is related to the solvent polarity and can readily be calculated from a weighted average for solvent mixtures. However, the solvent strength alone does not adequately predict its chromatographic behaviour as different solvents show differing selectivities in relation to their ability to interact with solutes (samples) of particular types. Solvents are therefore further characterized with respect to their ability to interact via hydrogen bonding or dipole effects. This classification of solvents, together with their solvent strength values, then allows significant predictions as to the most suitable solvent for a particular separation. Adsorption chromatography is not extensively used with high-performance liquid chromatography (HPLC) as the columns are slow to equilibrate and can readily be contaminated with highly polar compounds due to irreversible binding.

Partition Chromatography

This mode of chromatography involves partition between the liquid mobile phase and a stationary liquid phase held on a support material. Originally, the stationary liquid was simply adsorbed onto an inert material, but the resulting phases were found to be unstable, since the liquid coating was easily stripped from the column. The logical solution to this problem is to bond the liquid stationary phase covalently to the support material. This may be achieved by esterification of the surface silanol groups of silica, for example, but the resulting silicate esters can only be used with nonaqueous mobile phases. A more robust bonded phase is achieved by silylation of the surface hydroxy groups with chlorosilanes to form siloxanes. Monochlorosilanes give rise to monomeric phases whilst di- and trichlorosilanes lead to polymeric phases. The 'art' of producing good bonded phase materials is to have sufficient liquid stationary phase present for good chromatographic retention yet at the same time having phases with good mass transfer characteristics, which requires a relatively thin bonded layer. It may also prove necessary to remove any residual unreacted silanol groups by 'capping' with a highly reactive reagent such as trimethylchlorosilane.

Bonded phases may be polar in nature, as for example an aminopropyl phase, or they may be hydrophobic, as in the case of an octadecyl-bonded material. Polar phases behave in a similar manner to adsorption materials, with more polar compounds being more strongly retained, and an increase in mobile phase polarity resulting in decreased retention times. Hydrophobic materials, on the other hand, form the basis of reversed-phase chromatography in which compounds of lower polarity are more strongly retained and mobile phases of lower polarity have increased eluting power. Octadecylsilyl phases are often used with aqueous methanol (or acetonitrile) as mobile phase. Reversed-phase materials are extensively used with gradient elution, as they equilibrate rapidly with changes in solvent composition, and in the example cited here a gradient would be run with increasing methanol concentration to yield increasing eluting power. Modern reversed-phase materials are extremely robust and are not prone to contamination with polar compounds since in complex mixtures these are not retained. The materials are therefore widely used with complex samples of food or physiological origins, which often contain highly polar species. The versatility of reversed-phase chromatography can be further extended to ionic compounds by the technique of ion pair chromatography. Here a hydrophobic ionic species of opposite charge to that of the analyte is added to the mobile phase. The resulting ion pair is far more hydrophobic than the initial ionic species and can then be chromatographed under reversed-phase conditions.

Ion Exchange Chromatography

In ion exchange chromatography the mechanism of retention is simply electrostatic, involving opposite charges on the analyte and the stationary phase. The stationary phase may carry a net positive charge and is able therefore to retain anions (anion exchange) or it may be negatively charged and retain cations (cation exchange). Ion exchangers can be classified further as strong or weak exchangers, by analogy to strong or weak bases, depending on the charged groups. Thus, a sulphonic acid group will behave as a strong cation exchanger and a carboxymethyl group as a weak cation exchanger. Similarly, quaternary ammonium groups will form strong anion exchangers and tertiary amino groups will act as weak exchangers. The prerequisite for ion exchange is that the stationary phase, and determinand, must be charged. The charge on weak exchangers will alter gradually over wide pH ranges, whereas strong exchangers will only lose their surface charge at extremes of pH.

Ion exchange chromatography is a two-stage process, adsorption where the determinand displaces the counterion on the exchanger and desorption where the ions of interest are displaced by other counterions. Separation between compounds will only be effected where there is selectivity, in either the adsorption or desorption stages, for particular compounds. The desorption stage is often carried out with gradient elution, either by gradually changing the pH of the mobile phase or by altering the concentration of competing counterions. The most common materials for ion exchange stationary phases are chemically modified cross-linked polymers of styrene and divinylbenzene. The degree of cross linking affects the porosity of the material and hence the accessibility to the charged site, particularly for macromolecules.

Size Exclusion Chromatography

This mode of chromatography differs from those already discussed in that there are no direct interactions between the solute molecules and the stationary phase. Separation is effected between molecules of different sizes due to differential migration into porous material. The molecular size range of compounds that can be separated by this procedure depends on the pore size range of the stationary phase. If the solute molecules are all too large, in relation to the pores present, total exclusion will take place with no separation resulting. On the other extreme if all the solute molecules are small, allowing complete penetration into the pores, they will all be retained to the same extent, also resulting in no separation. Each phase is therefore characterized by a fractionation range between complete penetration and complete exclusion, and a wide range of such phases is commercially available.

Porous soft gels, e.g. Sephadex or Biogel, can only be used under low-pressure conditions, whereas porous glass or cross-linked polymers can be used as small particles under high-pressure conditions, allowing higher mobile phase velocities and shorter analysis times. In practice most size exclusion materials also exhibit secondary interactions, such as hydrophobic bonding or anionic exclusion, so that pure size exclusion is rarely encountered. Stationary phases are available that are compatible with both organic or aqueous mobile phases.

Chiral Chromatography

The enantiomeric form of optically active compounds is of vital importance to their biological activity. There is considerable interest in being able to separate these forms to determine their optical, or enantiomeric, purity as for example with drugs. There are two methods of achieving these separations by HPLC. In the first method a chiral phase is used to distinguish the spatial differences between enantiomeric forms and in the second, or indirect method, diastereomeric derivatives are formed using optically pure derivatizing reagents.

In the direct method the stationary phase may contain the chiral component or a chiral additive may be included in the mobile phase. Both of these methods are effective but where the chiral agent is included in the stationary phase it is preferable to use bonded phases, where the chiral agent is covalently bonded to the base silica. These are exemplified by Pirkle phases. Intrinsically chiral phases such as β-cyclodextrin are also available.

Affinity Chromatography

Affinity chromatography is based on the specific interaction of the determinand with a complementary compound immobilized on the stationary phase. Such specific interactions are commonly encountered in biological systems, e.g. hormone and binding protein, and it is in this field that affinity chromatography is widely used. A prerequisite is that it must be possible to bond covalently the complementary compound to the support material without reducing its binding specificity. Also, the specific binding must be reversible so that the determinand can be subsequently eluted, for example with a pH shift or change in ionic strength. It may also be important that the elution conditions do not cause loss of biological activity, if the material is to be isolated for further studies. For analytical purposes only it is possible to elute the bound compound by using denaturing conditions.

Bibliography

Brown PR and Hartwick RA (1989) *High Performance Liquid Chromatography*. New York: Wiley.

Giddings JC (1991) *Unified Separation Science*. New York: Wiley

Macrae R (1988) *HPLC in Food Analysis*, 2nd edn. London: Academic Press.

Poole CF and Schuette SA (1984) *Contemporary Practice of Chromatography*. Amsterdam: Elsevier.

Ravindranath B (1989) *Principles and Practice of Chromatography*. Chichester: Ellis Horwood.

Snyder LR and Kirkland JJ (1979) *Introduction to Modern Liquid Chromatography*, 2nd edn. New York: Wiley.

Robert Macrae
Hull University, Hull, UK

Thin-layer Chromatography

Outline of the Technique

A solution of sample is applied as a small spot or narrow band to a thin layer of adsorbent (stationary phase) which has been spread uniformly over a supporting plate. A solvent mixture (mobile phase) then passes through the adsorbent by capillary action and the sample is resolved into discrete components. After the solvent has evaporated from the plate the separated components are located either by physical methods or by the use of chemical staining reagents. Depending on the conditions employed, the relative amounts of components may be then quantified.

Apparatus

The basic equipment required for thin-layer chromatography (TLC) is relatively simple although elaborate instrumentation can be employed, particularly for automatic sample application and the quantification of separated components.

Adsorbents and Supports

The main adsorbent types used in TLC are silica gel, cellulose and aluminium oxide. Others include kieselguhr (celite), polyamide and polyethyleneimine (PEI) cellulose. The particle size of the adsorbent is usually in the range 1–25 μm.

TLC plates can be made in the laboratory by coating glass plates with adsorbent using apparatus sold for this purpose. However, more preferable is the use of ready made, precoated plates which are available in a variety of sizes and with various adsorbents. Unlike self-prepared TLC plates, precoated plates are consistently of high quality, but may not be available for every adsorbent. To enhance its adherence to the support the finely powdered adsorbent is mixed frequently with an inorganic binder such as calcium sulphate at around 10% (w/w). Organic binders, including polyacrylic acid, are also used, particularly with precoated plates.

Silica gel is the most commonly employed adsorbent in TLC, particularly that with a pore size of 6 nm. Precoated analytical plates frequently use silica gel of particle size 10–12 μm coated in a layer of thickness 250 μm. Plates coated with this type of silica provide 1000–2000 theoretical plates per 5 cm migration. A recent development is high-performance TLC (HPTLC) which uses silica gel of particle size 5–7 μm in layers of thickness 200 μm. The reduced particle size provides 5000–10 000 theoretical plates per 5 cm of migration distance and increases the separation efficiency. In comparison with conventional TLC, HPTLC allows faster separation of smaller amounts of material over a shorter separation distance and thus has greater sensitivity as well as increased resolving power. HPTLC plates cannot be prepared easily in the laboratory and are usually purchased ready made. The adsorption properties of silica gel can be modified by impregnation with various complexing reagents such as silver nitrate, urea, boric acid and ethylenediaminetetraacetic acid (EDTA) to aid the separation of particular classes of compounds. Kieselguhr, a diatomaceous earth, is used less often than the synthetic silica gel on account of its natural variability. Alumina (aluminium hydroxide) is manufactured in three types, acidic, basic and neutral, according to its pH.

Glass is the support employed most commonly for adsorbents on grounds of rigidity, flatness and inertness. Layers of adsorbents can also be obtained precoated on flexible aluminium or plastic sheets. These have the advantage of being able to be cut to smaller size, but greater care has to be taken in ensuring their compatibility with solvent systems employed and subsequent spray reagents. The standard sizes of TLC and HPTLC plates are 20×20 cm and 10×10 cm, respectively.

Sample Applicators and Development Chambers

The application of the sample solution to the adsorbent layer is usually performed manually using microsyringes or disposable glass capillaries. However, a wide range of instruments, some microprocessor controlled, are available for the automated application of samples either as spots or streaks. Rectangular glass chambers with lids are usually employed for the linear development of chromatograms in solvent mixtures. Sizes are available for standard 20×20 cm plates and 10×10 HPTLC plates. Chambers can be purchased with vertical grooves in the side and end walls to allow the development of several plates simultaneously.

Equipment for Detection and Quantification of Components

Atomizers operated by compressed air or hand bellows are required for spraying developed chromatograms evenly with detection reagents. An oven is necessary for heating plates sprayed with certain reagents. For the quantification of separated components on developed chromatograms, modern scanning densitometers, microprocessor controlled and capable of being linked to microcomputers for data storage and evaluation, are available. The location and quantification of radiolabelled compounds on developed TLC plates can be achieved using specialized radioactivity scanners. Less elaborate equipment is required for the location of radiolabelled compounds on developed chromatograms by autoradiography.

Specialized Systems

Several techniques which rely on the same chromatographic principles as conventional TLC, but which require the use of specialized equipment, have been developed recently. In over-pressured TLC (OPTLC) the TLC plate is held beneath a flexible membrane under hydrostatic pressure, and solvent is forced through the adsorbent using a pump. This system allows compounds to be eluted completely from the TLC plate for collection or detection using detectors associated normally with high-performance liquid chromatography. Centrifugal layer chromatography also involves the forced flow of solvent. In this case solvent is fed into the centre of a rapidly rotating TLC plate and is forced through the adsorbent by centrifugal force.

In radial-development TLC the sample spot is applied to the centre of a plate and the solvent supplied through a hole in the plate via a wick which dips into a solvent reservoir. The most recent advance in this technique is the application of solvent under pressure to HPTLC plates, allowing very short development times. Instruments are also available which permit the automated multiple development of TLC plates in either the same or different solvent systems. This repeated development of TLC plates can improve the separation of components.

A quantitative technique requiring specialized equipment is TLC with flame ionization detection (TLC–FID). In this system samples are applied to silica gel fused to thin quartz rods which are then developed conventionally in a mobile phase. The developed 'chromarods' are passed through a flame ionization detector to quantify the mass of individual components.

Methodology

Sample Application

In conventional TLC and HPTLC the sample is applied as a small volume of solution onto the adsorbent near the bottom of the plate. The point of application is termed the origin. A maximum of about 80 or 10 μg for TLC and HPTLC, respectively, can be applied as a spot on adsorbent layers of silica gel G 0·20–0·25 mm thick. Samples can also be applied as a narrow streak along the origin. Standards are applied as separate spots on the same plate.

Development

The choice of solvent system depends on what is being analysed and the type of adsorbent being used (see Table 1). Regardless of the components, the solvent mixture is placed in the development chamber. In the case of solvent systems containing large proportions of polar solvents the chamber can be lined with filter paper to aid saturation of the atmosphere. The plate is placed within the chamber so that the bottom edge is immersed in the solvent mixture and the chamber sealed with a lid (Fig. 1). When the solvent has migrated to within 1 cm of the top edge of the plate, the plate is removed from the chamber.

Although ascending chromatography as described above is the most common form of TLC, chromatograms can also be developed by descending chromatography using a wick to feed the solvent on to the adsorbent layer.

TLC plates can also be subjected to multiple development in which the plate is developed partially in one solvent system, and removed from the chamber. After evaporation of solvent from the developed plate, the plate is developed fully or partially in another solvent system. Multiple development allows better separation of components. The above form of TLC in which the chromatogram is developed with the mobile phase in only one direction is known as one-dimensional TLC (Fig. 2a). In many instances, one-dimensional TLC/HPTLC does not allow the complete resolution of all the components in a mixture. Improved separation can often be obtained with two-dimensional TLC/HPTLC.

Thin-layer Chromatography

Table 1. Substances separated by selected one-dimensional TLC systems

Adsorbent	Substances separated	Solvent system[a]	Detection reagent[a]
Alumina	Alkaloids	$CHCl_3$	Dragendorff reagent
	Amino acids (dicarboxylic)	2 MHAc	Ninhydrin
	Aromatic hydrocarbons	CCl_4	10% tetracyanoethylene in C_6H_6
	Carotenes	Hexane/C_6H_6/EtOH (100:100:1)	10% $SbCl_3$ in $CHCl_3$
	Food dyes (fat-soluble)	Hexane/EtAc (98:2)	None required
	Food dyes (water-soluble)	H_2O/EtOH/n-BuOH (1:1:5)	None required
	Neutral lipids	Hexane/Et_2O/HAc (94·5:5:0·5)	0·05% 2′,7′dichlorofluorescein in MeOH
	Sterols	C_6H_6/EtOH (95:2)	10% phosphotungstic acid in 90% EtOH
	Steroids	$CHCl_3$/EtOH (99:1)	Anisaldehyde/H_2SO_4/HAc (1:2:100), UV
	Vitamins (fat-soluble)	Toluene	1·3% $FeCl_3$ in 2 M HCl/0·7% K_3FeCN_6 (1:1)
Cellulose	Amino acids	n-BuOH/Me_2CO/Et_2NH/H_2O (10:10:2:5)	Ninhydrin
	Antibiotics (water-soluble)	PrOH/pyridine/HAc/H_2O (15:10:3:12)	Ninhydrin
	Food dyes (fat-soluble)	n-PrOH/EtAc/H_2O (6:1:3)	None required
	Nucleotides	n-BuOH/Me_2CO/HAc/5% NH_4OH/H_2O (4·5:1·5:1:1:2)	20% $SbCl_5$ in CCl_4
	Nucleosides and free bases	H_2O	20% $SbCl_5$ in CCl_4
DEAE cellulose	Amino acids	n-BuOH/HAc/H_2O (4:1:5)	Ninhydrin
	Nucleotides	isobutyric acid/NH_4OH/H_2O (33:1:16)	20% $SbCl_5$ in CCl_4
PEI cellulose	Nucleotides	0·25, 1·0, 1·6 M LiCl in H_2O (successive in each)	20% $SbCl_5$ in CCl_4
Kieselguhr	Sugars	EtAC/iso-PrOH/H_2O (130:57:23)	0·2%naphthoresorcinol in EtOH/ 10% H_3PO_4
	Oligosaccharides	iso-PrOH/EtAc (65:35)	0·2% naphthoresorcinol in EtOH/ 10% H_3PO_4
	Food dyes (fat-soluble)	Cyclohexane	None required
Polyamide	Anthocyanins	HAc/HCl/H_2O (10:1:3)	10% oxalic acid in Me_2CO/H_2O (1:1), UV
	Antioxidants	MeOH/Me_2CO/H_2O (6:1:3)	10% phosphomolybdic acid in EtOH
	Flavonoids	Me_2CO/95% EtOH/H_2O (2:1:2)	25% PbAc in basic aqueous solution
Sephadex	Proteins	0·5 M NaCl	1% naphthalene black in MeOH/ H_2O/HAc (5:4:1)

continued

Thin-layer Chromatography

Table 1. *Continued.*

Adsorbent	Substances separated	Solvent system[a]	Detection reagent[a]
Silica gel	Alkaloids	$CHCl_3/Me_2CO/Et_2NH$ (5:4:1)	Dragendorff reagent
	Amino acids	n-BuOH/HAc/H_2O (4:1:1)	Ninhydrin
	Antibiotics		
	Macrolides	$CHCl_3$/MeOH/H_2O (80:20:2·5)	20% phosphomolybdic acid in EtOH
	Tetracyclines	BuOH/HAc/H_2O (2:1:1)	20% phosphomolybdic acid in EtOH
	Streptomycins	H_2O/Na citrate/citric acid (100:20:5)	20% phosphomolybdic acid in EtOH
	Penicillins	Me_2CO/MeOH (1:1)	20% phosphomolybdic acid in EtOH
	Antioxidants	$CHCl_3$	20% phosphomolybdic acid in MeOH
	Bile acids	Me_3pentane/*iso*-PrOH/HAc (60:20:0·5)	5% phosphomolybdic acid in EtOH/Et_2O (1:1)
	Food dyes (fat-soluble)	Hexane/Et_2O/HAc (70:30:1)	None required
	Food dyes (water-soluble)	HAc/*iso*-BuOH/H_2O (2:5:2)	None required
	Lipids (neutral)	Hexane/Et_2O/HAc (80:20:2)	3% CuAc in 8% H_3PO_4
	Lipids (polar)	MeAc/n-PrOH/$CHCl_3$/MeOH/0·25% aq. KCl (25:25:25:10:9)	3% CuAc in 8% H_3PO_4
	Mycotoxins	$CHCl_3$/Me_2CO (90:10)	p-anisaldehyde/MeOH/HAc/H_2SO_4 (0·5:70:10:5)
	Plasticizers	CH_2Cl_2	4 M H_2SO_4/20% resorcinol (1:1)
	Mono-, di- and trisaccharides	MeCN/H_2O (85:15)	0·5% $KMnO_4$
	Polysaccharides	n-BuOH/MeOH/H_2O (50:25:20)	0·5% $KMnO_4$
	Steroids	$CHCl_3$/EtOH (90:10)	10% phosphomolybdic acid in EtOH
	Synthetic sweeteners	$CHCl_3$/HAc (90:10)	0·2% 2′,7′)-dichlorofluorescein in EtOH
	Terpene alcohols	CH_2Cl_2	0·06% diphenylpicryl hydrazene in $CHCl_3$
	Terpene aldehydes	$CHCl_3$	10% $SbCl_5$ in CCl_4
	Vitamins (fat-soluble)	Cyclohexane/EtAc (75:25)	UV
	Vitamins (water-soluble)	HAc/Me_2CO/MeOH/C_6H_6 (5:5:20:70)	UV

Ac, CH_3CO-; Bu, C_4H_9-; Et, C_2H_5-; Me, CH_3-; Pr, C_3H_7-; DEAE cellulose, diethylaminoethyl cellulose; PEI cellulose, polyethyleneimine cellulose; UV, ultraviolet.
[a] Solvent proportions by volume.

In this technique the sample is applied as a spot at one corner and developed fully in one direction in the first solvent system. The plate is removed from the chamber, the solvent allowed to evaporate and then developed in a second solvent system in a direction at right angles to that of the first development (Fig. 2b).

Identification of Separated Components

Coloured compounds are visible on developed chromatograms, but colourless compounds require detection by physical or chemical means. Detection by chemical means usually involves spraying the adsorbent layer of the developed chromatogram with a derivatizing reagent which reacts with the separated components to produce a coloured derivative *in situ*. Non-specific reagents such as sulphuric acid, iodine and 2′,7′-dichlorofluorescein will detect a wide range of compounds. Specific reagents react with specific functional groups and will only detect compounds containing the group, e.g. ninhydrin for amino groups. The use of specific reagents can be used as an aid to identification and characterization of components.

Physical methods of location commonly involve ultraviolet light. Commercial plates are available coated with adsorbents containing an indicator which absorbs light at 254 nm and re-emits or fluoresces light at the green end of the spectrum. When separated on these plates, compounds which absorb ultraviolet light show up as dark spots on a green fluorescent background. Radiolabelled compounds can be located on TLC plates physically by autoradiography or *in situ* measurement of radioactivity using a radioscanner.

A useful aid to the identification of separated components is the R_f value which is defined as the ratio of the distance travelled by the compound to the distance

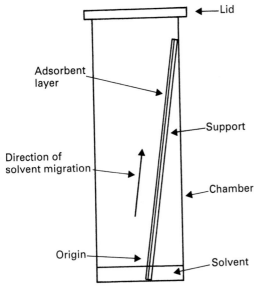

Fig. 1. Schematic side view of a TLC plate in a chamber during ascending development.

travelled by the solvent. Although the R_f value of a given compound in a defined mobile phase and adsorbent is very characteristic, many factors, including the thickness and moisture content of the adsorbent and development distance, affect the reproducibility of the value. For this reason the R_f value is only an indication of the identity of a compound and confirmation of identity should be obtained by other means.

Separated components can be identified by comparison with authentic standards run alongside the samples, if such standards are available.

Quantification of Separated Components

Once located, various methods can be employed for the quantification of separated compounds.

Areas of adsorbent that contain compounds can be scraped from the support and the compound eluted from the adsorbent with suitable solvents. The recovered compounds can then be estimated gravimetrically or by using a specific assay such as the measurement of phosphorus or sugar content.

Developed chromatograms can be subjected to scanning densitometry and the separated components quantified on the basis of transmittance, fluorescence or reflectance intensity, depending on the nature of the compounds and the stain used. As well as locating radiolabelled compounds, radioscanners can also quantify the amount of radioactivity present in individual components. Alternatively, bands of adsorbent that contain compounds can be scraped from the support into scintillation vials and measured directly for radioactivity content by liquid scintillation counting after addition of a suitable scintillation fluid.

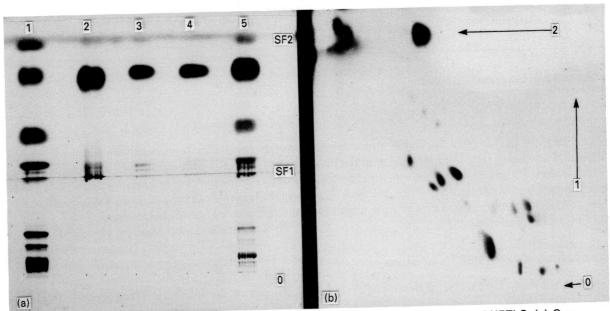

Fig. 2. Typical separations of lipid extracts. by (a) one-dimensional and (b) two-dimensional HPTLC. (a) One-dimensional, double development with methyl acetate/isopropanol/chloroform/methanol/0·25% aqueous potassium chloride (25:25:25:10:9, v/v/v/v/v) as the first solvent system and hexane/diethyl ether/acetic acid (90:10:1 v/v/v) as the second solvent system. O, origin; SF1, first solvent front; SF2, second solvent front. Lipid samples: 1, cod roe; 2, fish oil concentrate; 3 and 4, margarines; 5, salmon fillet. (b) Two-dimensional separation of salmon fillet lipid. The plate was developed in direction 1 using the first solvent system of plate (a) followed by development in direction 2 with chloroform/methanol/7 M ammonium hydroxide (65:35:5, v/v/v). Arrows indicate directions of development. O, origin. Both chromatograms were stained with 3% copper acetate in 8% orthophosphoric acid.

Thin-layer Chromatography

Preparative TLC

Although TLC is mostly used as an analytical technique, one-dimensional TLC can be scaled up to a preparative scale. To this end, sample can be applied as a streak across the origin of an analytical plate, the length of streak being determined by the amount of sample. Specially prepared TLC plates coated with thicker layers of adsorbent can also be obtained which can accomodate large amounts of sample. However, these plates lack the resolving power of the analytical plates. After nondestructive visualization of separated components, the band of adsorbent containing the compound of interest is scraped from the support and the compound eluted with a suitable solvent.

Modes of Chromatography

TLC conforms to the basic principles of liquid chromatography. The most common mode of chromatography used in TLC is adsorption chromatography although other modes can be employed. With silica, celite, kieselguhr and cellulose the separation mechanism is by adsorption chromatography if the adsorbent on the plate is completely free of water and the solvent system is a nonpolar mixture. However, if water is present on the adsorbent or if the solvent system contains a highly polar component then separation will be by partition chromatography as components partition between the liquid mobile phase and stationary liquid phase. Silanized silica gel in which the surface silanol groups of the silica are silylated with chlorosilanes, separates by partition chromatography.

Alumina separates components by adsorption, but depending upon the nature of the surface and the solvent system can also function as an ion exchanger. Modified cellulose such as diethylaminoethyl (DEAE) cellulose can be used for ion exchange separations on TLC. Separation by size exclusion chromatography can be carried out with TLC plates coated with Sephadex gel but is slower and less easy than other forms of TLC. Polyamides such as polyhexamethylenediaminoadipate can be used as the adsorbent to separate components which interact with it by hydrogen bonding.

TLC plates are available precoated with a reversed-phase silica gel which has been impregnated with a chiral reagent and copper ions. These can be used to separate optically active isomers, e.g. amino acids, by chiral chromatography on the basis of ligand exchange.

Applications

The actual method employed for preparing samples from foodstuffs for analysis by TLC depends on the nature of the substances being investigated. Many methods involve the extraction of the food with a suitable solvent followed by precipitation and filtration steps to remove classes of compounds which are of no interest. *See* Analysis of Food

The choice of adsorbent and solvent system used in TLC is dictated by the nature of the sample to be analysed. A broad grouping of TLC systems according to types of substances separated is presented in Table 1.

Bibliography

Ackman RG (1982) Flame ionisation detection applied to thin-layer chromatography on coated quartz rods. *Methods in Enzymology* 72: 205–252.

Jork J, Funk G, Fischer G and Wimmer CJ (1989) *Thin-Layer Chromatography: Reagents and Detection Methods*. Cambridge: VCH.

Kirchener JG (1978) *Thin-Layer Chromatography. Techniques of Chemistry*, vol. XIV, New York: Wiley.

Touchstone JC (1988) Instrumentation for thin-layer chromatography: a review. *Journal of Chromatographic Science* 26: 645–649.

R. J. Henderson
Stirling University, Stirling, UK

High-performance Liquid Chromatography

High-performance liquid chromatography (HPLC) is an instrumental form of liquid chromatography that employs stationary phases consisting of small particles, thereby achieving more efficient separations than those used in conventional liquid chromatography. Since its origin in the late 1960s, it has been known by several different names, including high-pressure liquid chromatography, because of the high pressures required to force the mobile phase or solvent through the stationary phase, and high-resolution liquid chromatography, because of the good resolution achieved using this technique.

This article describes the equipment needed to carry out HPLC and summarizes some of the applications of this method in food analysis. Two techniques related to HPLC, fast-protein liquid chromatography (FPLC) and supercritical fluid chromatography (SFC), are also considered. The basic theory of the chromatographic process and the factors that affect separation efficiency are discussed in the section on Liquid Chromatography.

Instrumental Configurations

Figure 1 depicts the essential components of an HPLC system. The basic equipment consists of a column packed with a stationary phase, a driving force to propel the solvent through the column (pump), a system (injector) for introducing the sample onto the column, a

High-performance Liquid Chromatography

system (detector) for measuring a physical property of the solutes being analysed that differs from the properties of the solvent or a property of the mobile phase which is altered by the presence of the solute, and a system for recording the detector signals and converting them into graphic traces or chromatograms.

A single solvent is often used to carry out the separation (isocratic elution), but differing proportions of various solvents are also often used (gradient elution), in which case a gradient device is needed. A variety of accessories, such as pressure controllers, valves for switching solvents, valves for switching column, ovens for heating the columns, etc., are also commonly employed. Today most chromatographs are controlled by a computer which is also used for data collection.

Solvents

The nature of the solvent will depend upon the mode of chromatographic separation employed, but a series of precautions that are common to all types of HPLC must be taken when preparing solvents. Because the columns have frits at the ends to hold the packing in place, the solvents must be devoid of particles and consequently must be filtered through membranes with a pore size of $0.5\ \mu m$ or smaller, prior to use. Bubble formation must also be avoided, since bubbles may cause variations in the flow rate if they reach the pump, or perturbations in the chromatogram if they reach or form in the detector cell. Solvents must therefore be degassed by immersing the bottle containing the solvent in an ultrasonic bath or by flushing the solvent with a stream of helium or nitrogen before delivering it to the chromatograph. A small stream of helium is commonly bubbled through the solvent during the chromatographic procedure to prevent uptake of air. To prevent bubble formation in the detector cell with depressurization, a restrictor is sometimes attached to the outlet of the detector cell.

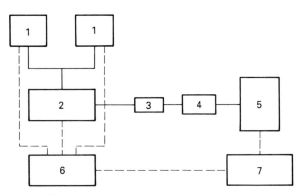

Fig. 1 Diagrammatic representation of HPLC equipment: (1) pump; (2) injector; (3) guard-column; (4) column; (5) detector; (6) controller; (7) recorder.

High-performance Liquid Chromatography

Pumps

The pump is the system for delivering the solvent from the solvent reservoir to the column, through the injector.

Basically, two types of pumps are available: constant-pressure pumps and constant-flow-rate pumps. The latter are more frequently used in HPLC.

Constant-pressure pumps are less expensive and easy to operate, but the flow rate may vary with changes in the viscosity of the mobile phase caused by temperature fluctuations or by the accumulation of undissolved sample components in the column. These variations in flow rate affect retention times, and they may also affect resolution, increasing the difficulty of both qualitative and quantitative analysis.

Constant-flow-rate pumps afford the advantage of maintaining retention times irrespective of changes in solvent viscosity. This type of pump includes syringe pumps, which consist of a cylinder containing the mobile phase, which is expelled by a piston. The piston is driven by a motor, so as to supply a constant flow devoid of pulses. This type of pump can achieve relatively high pressures, but maintenance and changing solvents are complicated.

Reciprocating pumps, also a type of constant-flow-rate pump, are most commonly employed. Their price varies depending on their complexity of design, and their main drawback is that they generate pulses that may cause noise in the detector. Single-piston pumps are the least expensive and have a rotating eccentric cam which drives the plunger, discharging the liquid through a one-way valve. Duplex pumps have two plungers driven by a single motor by means of a shared cam. This arrangement means that while one of the plungers is in the discharge phase, the other is in the intake phase, thereby superimposing the two flow-rate profiles and considerably reducing pulsations. In this type of pump, delivery from the solvent reservoir is stepless and changing solvents is rapid.

Injectors

Introducing the sample onto the column is one of the most critical steps in HPLC. Ideally, the sample should reach the column in the form of a tiny droplet that does not undergo diffusion, which would broaden the chromatographic band width and thus lower resolution.

Several methods are employed to deliver the sample onto the column. In on-column injectors the sample is introduced through a syringe which traverses a septum and enables the desired quantity of sample to be deposited at the column inlet. In this method the mobile phase flows continuously through the column. The stop-flow injector is a variation on this type of injector. In this method the pump is stopped before the syringe is inserted in the injector, and injection is effected when column pressure has dropped to atmospheric pressure. The advantage of these injectors is that they are inexpensive and of simple construction, yet they do not lower efficiency. However, reproducibility is poor, they are not suitable for high working pressures, and they are complicated to operate.

Valve injectors are most commonly used. In these injectors the sample is delivered onto a pressurized column with no appreciable interruption in flow. The sample is deposited by a syringe into an external loop, the valve selector is turned, and the mobile phase passes through the loop on its way to the column. The valve thus has two positions, a load position and an injection position. High injection reproducibility can be achieved with these injectors. The band broadening effect is comparable to or somewhat higher than that obtained using on-column syringe injectors. The drawback afforded by these injectors is that there is a split-second interruption in mobile-phase flow that may damage the column. To avoid this problem, a by-pass may be attached, such that there is always a constant flow of mobile phase from the pump to the column.

Automatic injectors that are capable of running analyses on up to 100 samples without operator attention have been designed on the basis of the same mechanism as valve injectors. There are also injectors equipped with a system of valves connecting them to several columns, which enables columns to be switched without stopping the flow.

Columns

The columns most commonly utilized in HPLC consist of stainless steel, plastic or glass tubes, measuring from 15 to 25 cm in length and packed with small-diameter particles (3–20 μm). Internal column diameter is normally between 2 and 5 mm.

Small-internal-diameter (microbore) columns are of more recent development; they are similar to the columns described above, but their internal diameter is between 0·5 and 2 mm, while they range in length from 10 to 25 cm. Packing particle size normally ranges from 3 to 5 μm. These columns are suitable for use when only small samples are available or when low solvent consumption is required.

The length of both conventional and microbore columns is limited mainly by the pressure needed to drive the solvent through the column, which is inversely proportional to the size of the particles used in the packing. Minimum column diameter is limited by column-wall effects that cause solute molecules flowing next to the wall to move more slowly than those flowing through the centre of the column, resulting in an increase in chromatographic band width.

Open capillary columns similar to those employed in gas chromatography have recently come into use. The column tube is made of glass and is 20–50 μm in diameter and several metres long. The stationary phase is chemically bonded to the wall of the tube. Capillary columns are also prepared by packing a tube with particles 5–30 μm in size and subsequently heating and drawing the tube to an internal diameter of from 50–125 μm.

In addition to the column on which the separation is carried out, two other types of column are also utilized in HPLC to protect the analytical column. These are precolumns and guard columns. Precolumns are placed between the pump and the injector to saturate the mobile phase with the stationary phase and thus prevent dissolution of the stationary phase in the analytical column. Guard columns are placed between the injector and the main column in order to retain components in the sample that might otherwise become permanently adsorbed on the analytical column, thereby affecting column efficiency and permeability. Both precolumns and guard columns are normally made of a material similar to that used in the analytical column.

Chromatography is customarily performed at ambient temperature, but it may be necessary to regulate the column temperature or to carry out the separation at a temperature other than room temperature. In such cases thermostat-equipped compartments (ovens) and systems for heating or cooling the columns are required.

Detectors

In order to be suitable for use in HPLC, detectors must meet a number of requirements. First and foremost, detector design must prevent broadening of chromatographic band width to ensure that the separations achieved on the column do not deteriorate in the detector. In addition, response time must be short, and the response must be linear over a sufficiently broad range of concentrations.

The detectors most frequently employed are the refractive index detector, the photometric detector, and the fluorescence detector.

Refractive index detectors measure the difference between the refractive index of the mobile phase and that of the column eluate. They are universal detectors that are highly sensitive to small changes in the mobile phase and even to small variations in temperature or pressure. This very sensitivity means that to achieve a suitable signal to noise ratio they are only capable of detecting solute concentrations in the order of micromoles. In addition, they are unsuitable for working with gradient conditions.

Photometric detectors measure absorbance in the ultraviolet (UV) or visible regions of all the components in the column eluate. They are less universal than refractive index detectors but by the same token are more specific. This type of detector is normally capable of detecting nanomoles, provided that the compound contains a strong chromophore. The three types of photometric detector most frequently used are fixed-wavelength detectors, variable-wavelength detectors, and diode array detectors. This last type of detector is capable of performing complete spectral analysis of the column eluate on a continuous basis, i.e. without stopping the flow.

Fluorimeter detectors are more specific and more sensitive than photometric detectors, but their linear range is smaller. Detection limits are in the order of picomoles for suitably fluorescent compounds, and they are very useful in trace component analysis.

Electrochemical detectors are also widely employed in HPLC. These come in two types: amperometric and conductometric detectors. Amperometric detectors are highly sensitive but are only applicable to analytes that can be oxidized or reduced; conductometric detectors are moderately sensitive and are applicable for detecting anions and cations. This type of detector is the detector most commonly used in ion exchange chromatography.

Derivatization of the components being analysed may sometimes be employed to increase the detection limit or specificity.

Mass spectrometry (MS) is now being used as an on-line detection system in HPLC. Coupling of MS and HPLC is still in the developmental stage, although several coupled systems are now available commercially. Mass spectrometry has been considered to be the ideal detector, since it furnishes information on component structure. Mass spectrometry in combination with HPLC may become a standard technique in a few years' time. *See* Mass Spectrometry, Principles and Instrumentation

Selected Applications

The use of HPLC in food analysis is growing daily, and it is now routinely applied in many laboratories. The many different types of columns and detectors that are currently available commercially make it possible to apply HPLC in analysing nearly all the nonvolatile components in foods, be they present naturally or added artificially. The techniques employed for certain groups of food components are summarized below by way of example.

Carbohydrates

Nearly all chromatographic modes may be used in separating carbohydrates. For example, ion exchange on strongly or weakly basic anionic resins or on cationic resins, and partition chromatography on ion exchange resins, on chemically bonded cyano, amino, propyl-amino, or combined amino-cyano phases, or on silica gel or gel permeation are all possible. Differential refractometry is the conventional detection system, although direct detection, using short UV wavelengths or by forming derivatives detectable at longer wavelengths or fluorescent derivatives, is also employed. *See* Carbohydrates, Determination

Acids

A variety of chromatographic modes are also applied to this group of components. Certain workers have employed ion exchange chromatography on strongly acid cationic resins or strongly or weakly basic anionic resins. Reversed-phase chromatography and ion pair chromatography have also been used. Detection is carried out by refractometry, photometry using UV or visible wavelengths, as in the case of carbohydrates. *See* Acids, Properties and Determination

Amino Acids and Amines

Most separations of amino acids and amines are performed using reversed-phase chromatography of dansyl chloride, orthophthaldialdehyde (OPA), or phenyl dithioisocyanate derivatives. Detection is carried out by means of fluorescence or UV absorption. Figure 2 shows the chromatogram of the OPA-amino-acids of a wine, as an example of this type of analysis. *See* Amino Acids, Determination; Amines

Peptides

Diverse techniques are used to separate peptides on account of the broad range of molecular weights of these components. Conventional reversed-phase columns are applied for peptides with molecular weights of less than 3000 Da, while reversed-phase columns packed with particles with large pore sizes or size exclusion columns are used for larger peptides. Detection is performed at 214 nm. *See* Peptides

Proteins

Practically all known modes have been used in the separation of proteins, e.g. separations based on molecule size (gel permeation chromatography), on charge (ion exchange chromatography), on hydrophobicity (reversed-phase chromatography and hydrophobic-

High-performance Liquid Chromatography

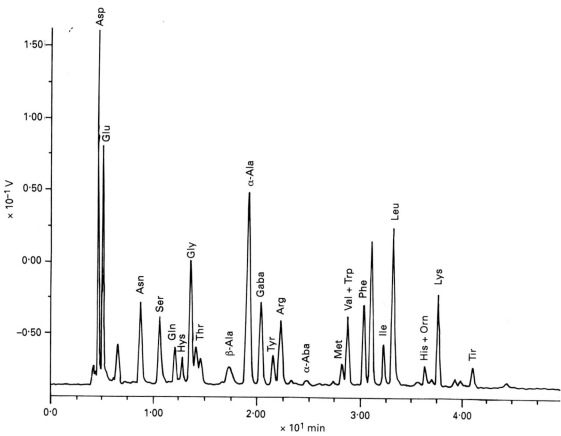

Fig. 2 Chromatogram of the OPA-amino-acids of a wine. Column: Radial Pak C-18, 10 μm. Eluent A: Methanol/10 mmol l^{-1} sodium phosphate buffer (pH 7·3)/tetrahydrofurane (19:80:1). Eluent B: Methanol/10 mmol l^{-1} sodium phosphate buffer (pH 7·3) (80:20). Linear gradient: 0 min (0% B, 1·5 ml min^{-1}); 16 min (30% B, 1·5 ml min^{-1}); 20 min (40% B, 1·5 ml min^{-1}; 32 min (80% B, 1·3 ml min^{-1}); 38 min (80% B, 1·3 ml min^{-1}). Fluorescence detection (λ_{exc}=340 nm, λ_{em}=425 nm).

interaction chromatography), and even combinations of these mechanisms. Detection is carried out at 214 or 280 nm. *See* Protein, Determination and Characterization

In addition to the major groups of food components mentioned above, HPLC has found application in many other areas of food analysis, and details may be found in the relevant articles for the following compounds or groups of compounds: lipid components, phospholipids, triglycerides, vitamins, colours, pesticides, drug residues, polycyclic aromatic hydrocarbons, and nitrosamines. *See* Colours, Properties and Determination of Natural Pigments; Colours, Properties and Determination of Synthetic Pigments; Fatty Acids, Analysis; Nitrosamines; Pesticides and Herbicides, Types, Uses and Determination of Herbicides; Phospholipids, Determination; Polycyclic Aromatic Hydrocarbons; Triglycerides, Characterization and Determination; Vitamins, Determination

Related Techniques

Fast-protein liquid chromatography designates a fast chromatographic method, developed by Pharmacía,

which is similar to HPLC and yields high resolution. Since FPLC needs only a relatively low back-pressure to drive the high flow rates at which the separations are performed, the risk of denaturation caused by shearing forces is reduced. Moreover, the mechanical components are resistant to corrosive buffers, and there is no contamination or inactivation of the components of interest.

Given the range of columns available in the market, a variety of separation modes can be applied using this technique: size exclusion, hydrophobic interaction, chromatofocusing, ion exchange, and reversed-phase chromatography.

This method was developed to separate and purify biomolecules and is very useful in separating isoenzymes and molecular species with similar charge characteristics. It is also used to distinguish between different types of meat or grains.

Supercritical fluid chromatography is another technique, related to HPLC, which uses as the mobile phase a supercritical fluid, i.e. a fluid at a pressure and temperature above the critical point.

The properties of supercritical fluids are intermediate between those of gases and those of liquids. Thanks to

High-performance Liquid Chromatography

their higher diffusivity and lower viscosity as compared to liquids, high efficiencies are achievable with shorter analysis times than those customarily employed using HPLC.

The basic advantage of SFC with respect to gas chromatography (GC) is the possibility of analysing components that span a broad range of volatilities as well as heat-labile components. At the same time, SFC is also compatible with many of the detectors commonly used in GC or HPLC and SFC–MS coupling is easy to carry out.

The critical temperature of the supercritical fluids employed as the mobile phase is between 0°C and 200°C, and the critical pressure of these fluids should not be too high. Carbon dioxide, nitrous oxide, alkanes (such as *n*-pentane), and xenon, all of which are nonpolar, are most often used. Ammonia can be used to elute polar solutes, but mixtures of phases, i.e. a nonpolar mobile phase containing a small quantity of a polar organic solvent, known as a modifier, are normally employed.

Supercritical fluid chromatography can be performed on capillary, packed and micropacked columns. Stationary phases should be cross-linked; otherwise, the supercritical fluids, which are excellent solvents for polymers, could extract the stationary phase. Enantiomers can be resolved using chiral phases.

The equipment used in SFC is similar to that used in HPLC and basically consists of a high-pressure syringe pump, an injector, and a restrictor or postcolumn valve to keep the mobile phase in a supercritical condition inside the chromatographic column.

Fluid density is commonly programmed to adjust mobile phase selectivity, in as much as the physicochemical properties of supercritical fluids (solvation strength, viscosity, diffusion) are all dependent upon density.

This method has been applied in food analysis (oils, cheeses, coffee, etc.). Some of the most interesting applications include separations of acids, alcohols, lipids, carbohydrates, vitamins, and terpenes. *See* Acids, Properties and Determination; Alcohol, Properties and Determination; Analysis of Food; Carbohydrates, Determination; Coffee, Analysis of Coffee Products; Vitamins, Determination

Bibliography

Charalambous G (1984) *Analysis of Foods and Beverages. Modern Techniques.* Orlando: Academic Press.
Gonzalez-Llano D, Polo C and Ramos M (1990) Update on HPLC and FPLC analysis of nitrogen compounds in dairy products. *Lait* 70: 255–277.
Gruewedel D and Whitaker JR (1987) *Food Analysis. Principles and Techniques.* New York: Marcel Dekker.
Henschen A, Hupe KP, Lottspeich F and Voelter W (1985) *High Performance Liquid Chromatography in Biochemistry.* Weinheim: VCH Press.
Macrae R (1987) *HPLC in Food Analysis* 2nd edn. London: Academic Press.
Oliver RWA (1989) *HPLC of Macromolecules. A Practical Approach.* Oxford: IRL Press.
Shaw EP (1988) *Handbook of Sugar Separations in Foods by HPLC.* Boca Raton, Florida: CRC Press.
Smith RM (1988) *Supercritical Fluid Chromatography.* RSC Chromatography Monographs. Cambridge: Royal Society of Chemistry.

M. Carmen Martín-Hernández and M. Carmen Polo
Consejo Superior de Investigaciones Científicas, Madrid, Spain

Gas Chromatography

Gas chromatography (GC) encompasses all chromatographic methods in which the mobile phase is a gas. The 'modes of GC' refer to the mechanism used to retain the solute in the stationary phase. Solid absorbents, or liquid distributed on an inert support in the form of a thin film with a relatively large surface area, may be used. In the former, separation occurs due to an adsorptive mechanism, and this type of chromatography, in which the mobile phase is a gas and the stationary phase is a solid, is known as gas–solid chromatography (GSC). In the latter, separation is based on a partition mechanism between the stationary liquid phase and the mobile gas phase, and this type of chromatography is known as gas–liquid chromatography (GLC). This latter is by far the most frequently employed gas chromatographic method, both generally and in the analysis of foodstuffs.

In GC, samples are volatilized and transported by the mobile phase (the carrier gas) to the column, where separation takes place. The components of the mixture will reach the end of the column more or less separated in time; there they are detected and, if appropriate, recovered.

Samples subjected to GC analysis must be volatile at the analysis temperature to ensure that they remain in the vapour phase, yet they must be sufficiently stable so that they do not undergo alteration during the chromatographic process. In some cases samples must be derivatized in order to enhance their volatility and heat stability.

Equipment

Gas chromatographs consist of three basic parts: the injector or system for introducing the sample; the column, where separation takes place; and the detector. Figure 1 shows the major components of a gas chromatograph.

Injector

The purpose of the injector is to vaporize the sample (in the case of nongaseous samples) and introduce it into the stream of carrier gas so that it will be rapidly transferred to the column inlet, thereby minimizing band broadening. It should also prevent feedback of the sample, since this would result not only in a broader band but also in the appearance of spurious peaks. The injector consists of an easy-to-clean chamber at the column inlet. Its interior volume is small, and it is heated at a temperature sufficiently high to vaporize the least volatile component in the sample. The sample is injected through a rubber septum using a microsyringe. A carrier gas source, normally equipped with a pressure regulator, is connected to the injector. The carrier gas is an inert gas, normally nitrogen, helium, or argon, although hydrogen is sometimes also used to advantage.

In conventional or packed columns the entire sample volume is injected into the column. Some systems allow the sample to be deposited directly at the column inlet, i.e. as on-column injection. Since the sample injected must not exceed column capacity, sample size must be smaller when capillary columns are used, and, consequently, more sophisticated injectors are used with such columns. The injectors most commonly employed are equipped with a flow splitter which, by means of a valve, splits the samples before it reaches the column inlet, so that only a small fraction actually enters the column, the rest being vented out of the system. Depending on their design, however, such injection systems may impede proper quantification of mixtures that contain components spanning a broad range of volatiles, because of preferential selection of certain components with respect to others. On-column injection may also be used with capillary columns.

Another type of injection with a flow splitter makes use of the splitless system, in which injection is initially carried out with the flow splitter closed; after a few seconds, when most of the sample has entered the column, the valve is opened to purge the rest of the sample remaining in the injector.

There is still another injection method designed to avoid the problem of preferential selection referred to earlier, using a programmed temperature vaporizer (PTV), which, as the name itself implies, allows vaporizer temperature to be programmed. The sample may be injected at low temperature, and the injector is then heated to vaporize the sample a few seconds later.

If an inappropriate system is used, precolumn band width will increase, producing wider peaks in the resulting chromatogram and the appearance of reduced column efficiency.

Column

The column consists of a glass or metal tube in a thermostat-equipped oven. Column length may range from 1 to 200 m, with an internal diameter of between 0·1 and 50 mm. This is the part of the chromatograph where separation takes place and it is therefore the most important part of the equipment. During the separation process the sample is adsorbed by or dissolved in the stationary phase, starting at the column inlet, establishing an equilibrium between the stationary and mobile phases. The components of the mixture under analysis are carried through the column by the carrier gas at different rates, which will depend upon the corresponding distribution coefficients at the analysis temperature.

Component separation takes place all along the column length, depending on the differential attraction forces of the stationary phase for the components, in as much as all the components move at the same rate as the carrier gas when they are in the mobile phase.

A variety of different columns have been developed for GLC. Conventional packed columns are filled with a granular support, the surface of which is coated with a film or liquid stationary phase. The lengths of the columns range from 1 to 10 m, with internal diameters of between 2 and 4 mm for analytical columns, or up to 5 cm for preparative columns. Since such columns contain extremely large quantities of stationary phase per unit length, their load capacity is high, but their permeability is low, which constitutes a practical limitation on the development of long columns.

Capillary packed columns are another type of column used in GC. These are similar to the packed columns described above, but their internal diameter does not usually exceed 1 mm. Open capillary columns, in par-

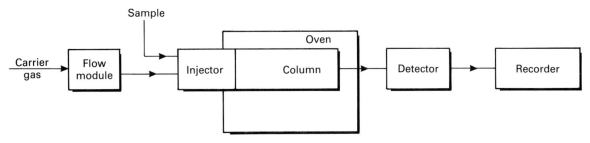

Fig. 1 Schematic diagram of a gas chromatograph.

ticular wall-coated open tubular (WCOT) columns, were first used by Golay in 1957. They consist of a capillary tube with an internal diameter from 0·1 to 0·75 mm. The stationary phase is deposited on or bonded to the inner surface of the column wall itself, which acts as the support. Columns of this type have higher permeability values and can reach lengths of up to 200 or 300 m, although 25–50 m is the range most commonly used. Conversely, load capacity is low because of the high phase ratio, i.e. the small quantity of stationary phase per unit column length.

Capillary columns with a porous layer occupy an intermediate position between WCOT columns and packed columns. These columns have a higher internal surface area in order to lower the phase ratio and hence increase load capacity, whereas they have been used to increase the internal surface area of the columns. In the so-called SCOT (support-coated open tubular) columns, a layer of porous solid support is deposited on the internal column wall, which is then coated with stationary phase. In the so-called PLOT (porous-layer open tubular) columns, the internal wall of the tube is chemically treated to create a porous surface, on which the stationary phase is deposited. The central lumen of the capillary tube is left empty in both types. These two types of column may be used in GSC if the porous layer is not coated with stationary phase.

Detector

The detector is located at the column outlet and maintained by thermostat at a temperature equal to or greater than the column temperature. It continuously measures a physical property (thermal conductivity, ionization current, electronic affinity, etc.) of the carrier gas that is significantly altered by the presence of minute concentrations of the substances being analysed. In general, they give out an electronic signal which is amplified, measured, and finally recorded by any data acquisition system.

Gas chromatography detectors must be suitably sensitive, have a low noise level, and be capable of producing a linear response that will furnish quantitative data. The flame ionization detector (FID) is probably the detector most commonly used in GC. Nevertheless, selective detectors that are extremely sensitive to specific compounds have also been developed, e.g. the electron capture detector (ECD) for sulphur-containing and halogen-containing compounds; thermionic detectors (alkali-bead FIDs) for nitrogen- or phosphorus-containing compounds; and selective flame photometric detectors (FPDs) for sulphur-containing compounds. Since thermal conductivity detectors are non-destructive, the fractions eluted can be assayed and recovered; however, the sensitivity of these detectors is too low for use with capillary columns with small load capacities. Photoionization detectors (PIDs), developed more recently, are also nondestructive and sufficiently sensitive for use with capillary columns.

Identification and Quantification

The purpose of most GC studies is the qualitative and quantitative analysis of mixtures of components.

A variety of procedures have been developed to determine the qualitative composition of mixtures. The simplest procedure involves comparing the retention times of the components of the sample under analysis with those of pure substances analysed under identical chromatographic conditions. However, this information is not sufficient for unambiguous characterization of the mixture components and must be complemented with data obtained using other physicochemical procedures. Another identification route consists of coupling the column outlet to other techniques, such as mass spectrometry (MS) or Fourier transform infrared spectroscopy (FTIR). *See* Mass Spectrometry, Principles and Instrumentation; Spectroscopy, Infrared and Raman

Gas chromatography is a highly appropriate technique for quantitative analysis of complex mixtures. Quantitative measurements are based on peak areas and the relationship between the peak areas and the concentrations of mixture components. Peak areas are influenced not only by sample size but also by other factors that affect detector sensitivity, such as ionization potential, variations in carrier gas flow, and detector temperature. The use of electronic integrators and computers has greatly facilitated measurement of peak areas for individual mixture components.

There are different systems for calculating the results of chromatographic analysis. Normalization is used to compensate for differential component responses, correcting peak area measurements with response factors based on one of the components. The response factors are calculated by injecting known quantities of pure components mixed in a proportion similar to that of the sample and then running an analysis under the same chromatographic conditions. This calculation method is a valid technique for determining the percentage composition of mixtures.

$$P_i = (f_i A_i / \Sigma f_i A_i)100$$

In this equation, f_i is the response factor, P_i (%) is the percentage composition of a component, and A_i is the peak area.

$$f_i = (p_i/p_r):(A_i/A_r)$$

In this equation, p_r is the weight of the reference component of peak area A_r, A_r is the peak area for the reference component, and p_i is the weight of a component of peak area A_i.

Quantification using an internal or external standard is needed to determine the real concentrations of mixture components. When an external standard is used, the peak area for a component in the chromatogram of a sample is compared with that obtained for a known quantity of the external standard. When an internal standard is used, a known quantity of a substance not naturally present in the mixture is added to the sample at the start of the analysis, and the peak area of this substance is compared to those for the mixture components; in this case, the response factors of the different components must be determined.

Selected Applications

This section will discuss some of the more important applications of GC in analysing the major or minor components, flavour, aroma and contaminants in foods.

Food Constituent Analysis

When analysing the major constituent fractions of foods, GC is perhaps applied most frequently to lipids and sugars.

Using GC it is possible to study the degree of lipolysis of fats, by analysing the free fatty acid (FFA) profile, or to examine the genuineness of fats, by analysing the triglyceride fraction, the fatty acid composition, and the different unsaponifiable fractions. Free fatty acids can be analysed using modified polar phases, modifying the carrier gas by saturating it with formic acid (which produces no response in FIDs), so that the formic acid is adsorbed by the active sites on the column and prevents retention of the FFAs, or else by injecting the FFAs in the form of quaternary ammonium salts that are pyrolyzed to methyl esters in the injector. *See* Fatty Acids, Analysis; Triglycerides, Characterization and Determination

Analysis of the composition of the fatty acids in the triglyceride fraction is carried out by standardized GC procedures using volatile derivatives, in particular methyl esters. Direct analysis of triglycerides, which was problematical because of their low volatility, has improved enormously since the development of fused silica capillary columns with bonded phases, and at present very good separations are possible based on the number of carbon atoms or even, for components with the same number of carbon atoms, based on the degree of unsaturation.

Gas chromatography has been used to study the unsaponifiable fraction of fats by analysing the hydrocarbons and aliphatic and terpene alcohols. The most interesting group of compounds from the standpoint of quality control of fats is the sterol fraction. Similar GC conditions are used to analyse the above-mentioned fractions. Different silicones have been tested as the stationary phase at column temperatures of 250–290°C, with excellent results.

Gas chromatography has also been used to analyse carbohydrates in foods. The advantage that GC affords over liquid chromatography (LC) is its greater sensitivity and higher resolution. However, it has the drawback of requiring the formation of volatile derivatives, such as acetates, oximes, methylated derivatives, and, above all, trimethylsilyl derivatives. A range of stationary phases, from polyesters to silicones, have been used in GC. *See* Carbohydrates, Determination

Although GC has been applied in the analysis of amino acids or minor components such as vitamins, flavonoids and phenolic compounds, LC, which does not require derivatization and hence yields shorter analysis times, has now replaced it as the analysis method of choice. However, GC is now widely used for analysis of chiral compounds (sugars, amino acids, flavours). *See* Amino Acids, Determination; Phenolic Compounds; Vitamins, Determination

Flavour and Aroma Compounds

The use of GC in combination with MS has been of fundamental importance in analysing flavour and aroma compounds and has made possible the successful identification of many new compounds. Diverse sample preparation methods have been used: either analysis of fractions obtained by low-pressure distillation or solvent extraction, or separation of headspace (sample vapours) under varying conditions. *See* Sensory Evaluation, Aroma; Sensory Evaluation, Taste

This is without doubt the field in which the greatest advances have been made. Aroma concentrates are extremely complex, because they comprise compounds that span broad ranges of volatility and polarity. No packed column is capable of separating such mixtures satisfactorily, and hence it would be necessary to isolate the different fractions and employ several columns with different stationary phases. New methods of concentrating the volatile components prior to chromatographic analysis, the use of fused silica capillary columns, and headspace analysis (using automatic injectors) have made it possible to determine trace amounts of volatile aroma components present in foods that would otherwise be difficult to analyse by conventional GC. In addition, the use of specific detectors has made possible the detection of components which are present in extremely low quantities in foods, yet, on account of their very low organoleptic detection thresholds, play an important role in flavour development.

Gas Chromatography

Contaminants in Foods

Gas chromatography is the basic method used to detect and analyse the presence of contaminants such as pesticides, polychlorinated biphenyls, polychlorodioxines and polychlorodibenzofurans, polycyclic aromatic hydrocarbons, nitrosamines and mycotoxins. *See* Contamination, Detection; Mycotoxins, Occurrence and Determination; Nitrosamines; Pesticides and Herbicides, Types, Uses and Determination of Herbicides; Polycyclic Aromatic Hydrocarbons

Analysis of chlorinated organic pesticides is carried out following extraction, enrichment and purification. Electron capture detectors are normally used, although alkali-bead FIDs are also used, with columns containing different stationary phases, such as fluorinated and methylated silicones, phenylated silicones, and other silicone derivatives. The use of more than one phase is common.

Polychlorinated biphenyl residues have been identified in foods. Although a number of different methods have been tested, GC using fused silica gel capillary columns, nonpolar phases and ECDs is currently one of the most successful techniques.

Nitrosamines in foods have been analysed by GC on packed or capillary columns. In this and many other fields of food analysis, GC–MS is a very successful combination.

Bibliography

Gruenwedel DW and Whitaker JR (ed.) (1987) *Food Analysis. Principles and Techniques*, vol. 4. New York: Marcel Dekker.

Hachenberg H and Schmidt AP (1977) *Gas Chromatographic Headspace Analysis*. London: Heiden and Son.

Jenning W (1978) *Gas Chromatography with Glass Capillary Columns*. New York: Academic Press.

Knapp DR (1979) *Handbook of Analytical Derivatization Reactions*. New York: Wiley–Interscience.

Lawrence JF (ed.) (1984) *Food Constituents and Residues. Their Chromatographic Determinations*. New York: Marcel Dekker.

Lee ML, Yang FJ and Bartle KD (1984) *Open Tubular, Column Gas Chromatography. Theory and Practice*. New York: Wiley–Interscience.

Sandra P (ed.) (1985) *Sample Introduction in Capillary Gas Chromatography*, vol. I. Heidelberg: Hueting Verlag.

M. Carmen Martín-Hernández and M. Juárez
Consejo Superior de Investigaciones Científicas, Madrid, Spain

CHROMIUM

Contents

Properties and Determination

Physical and Chemical Properties

Chromium is a hard, brittle, white metal of the first transition series, with an atomic number of 24 and an atomic weight of 51·996 amu. Its melting point is $1903 \pm 10°C$.

Chromium is resistant to attack from a wide variety of chemicals at normal temperature, and for this reason it is used to protect other more reactive metals. It reacts, however, with many chemicals at high temperatures.

As a typical transition metal element, chromium forms many compounds that are coloured and paramagnetic. It has oxidation states from -2 to $+6$, but the most common and stable oxidation states are $+2$, $+3$ and $+6$. Since Cr^{2+} is a very strong reducing agent, it is impossible to find it in biological systems. All Cr^{6+} compounds, except the hexafluoride (CrF_6), are oxo compounds; chromium occurs predominantly as either chromate (CrO_4^{2-}) or dichromate ($Cr_2O_7^{2-}$). Cr^{6+} compounds are strong oxidizing agents and, therefore, the Cr^{6+} ion is readily reduced to Cr^{3+} in acidic solutions. The most stable and important oxidation state is $+3$.

One of the outstanding features of Cr^{3+} chemistry is the ability of trivalent chromium to form coordination complexes, most of which are hexacoordinated. In aqueous solution the hexahydrate ion $(Cr(H_2O))^{3+}$ exists in an octahedral configuration. These coordination complexes are relatively inert. In aqueous solution the ligand and displacement reactions have half-lives of several hours.

In biological tissues, the formation of bridges between hydroxyl groups, or olation, occurs. Olation is enhanced by alkalis and temperatures up to 120°C. While oxalate ions and other strong ligands can prevent and reverse olation, weaker ligands can only prevent the reaction. Therefore, the following naturally occurring ligands inhibit olation of Cr^{3+} in biological systems: pyrophosphate, methionine, serine, glycine, leucine, lysine and proline. In such systems, chromium is able to function because its solubility is maintained by weaker organic and inorganic ligands.

Determination in Foods and Beverages

There is a wide range of techniques available for the analysis of trace elements in general and of chromium in particular. Chromium is one of the most difficult elements to determine accurately at the very low levels that occur naturally.

The actual determination of chromium content in biological matrixes has long been a controversial problem because of the many errors that can arise and distort the results. Therefore, much of the earlier work should be viewed critically. Reasons for this scepticism arise from a number of problem areas:

- The low chromium content of normal biological samples. In food samples the content is on the order of nanograms or micrograms per gram and, therefore, it is essential to apply very sensitive measurement techniques.
- Losses by volatilization during sample drying or dry ashing.
- Contamination at any point through sample collection and handling, before the content is measured.
- Errors inherent in the applied analytical method.

The evidence indicates that there is no appreciable volatilization at temperatures up to 450°C and, therefore, inadequate sample collecting and handling, and digestion of the sample, are the major sources of error. In the case of food samples the destruction of organic matter is essential.

Studies should provide precise data on all steps of the analytical procedure, including sample collection, homogenization and matrix reduction. An accurate determination is a challenge because of problems that originate from losses and enrichment by contamination. Interlaboratory assays give rise, in the case of chromium analysis, to very variable results because of significant sources of error of which analysts are, presumably, unaware.

Of all of the proposed analytical methods, atomic absorption spectrophotometry (AAS) is the one most often used for chromium determination in biological samples. When applied with a graphite furnace it is one of the most sensitive techniques, more sensitive than flame atomic absorption spectrophotometry (FAAS) or inductively coupled plasma (ICP) spectroscopy, but it is open to a wide range of interferences, which depend on the matrix and can lead to erroneous results.

On the other hand, determination of total chromium content may not be a valid indicator of the nutritional benefit of a food because not all chromium in foods has activity as a glucose tolerance factor. Some authors point out that the alcohol-extractable fraction of chromium seems to be a more reliable index. The speciation of chromium is of great interest.

Precautions to be Taken in Chromium Determination in Foods

As mentioned above, contamination is one of the main problems encountered in chromium determination in foods. Indeed, it is the explanation why food chromium contents reported some years ago are higher than those obtained now, as measures have been adopted to avoid contaminations.

The possibility that small amounts of chromium can be retained by the surface of vessels makes it necessary to decontaminate the material used, whether glass or plastic. In order to decontaminate the containers, all material used has to be soaked in diluted nitric acid (10–20% v/v), for 12–24 h and then rinsed several times with deionized water. A mixture of 4 M nitric acid and 4 M perchloric acid (1:1, v/v) or a solution of 2,4-pentane-dione or dithizone/carbon tetrachloride has also been proposed.

To avoid losses by adsorption, it is advisable to prepare standard solutions in diluted acid (0.5% nitric or hydrochloric acid). Cr^{6+} solutions are more stable than those containing Cr^{3+}.

Since the acids used in chromium determination, especially nitric acid, are a source of contamination, it is advisable to use reagents of high quality or to distil them previously.

Contact with materials that can give up chromium, i.e. metallic surfaces such as stainless steel and so on, should be avoided. It is preferable to work in a white chamber.

Sample Digestion

The choice of the digestion method is important in trace chromium determination. The use of dry methods carries the risk of chromium losses by adsorption on the walls of the crucible at temperatures higher than 550°C or by volatilization after formation of chromyl chloride, which is often suspected of being a major source of chromium losses during digestion. These losses are minimized when the temperature is increased gradually and does not exceed 450–500°C. Nevertheless, some authors have reported losses of chromium by volatilization at 450°C and obtained better results at lower temperatures together with oxygen plasma. However, in the latter procedure, size is restricted and relatively large amounts of hydrogen peroxide are needed as an ashing aid.

Nitric and sulphuric acids, often together with hydrogen peroxide, have been reported to be useful ashing aids.

Most wet digestion procedures make use of a mixture of acids and oxidizing agents, the most commonly used ones being nitric, sulphuric and perchloric acids with hydrogen peroxide. When foods have a high fat content, mixtures of nitric, perchloric and sulphuric acids, or nitric and sulphuric acids, are recommended.

Nitric acid prevents the coprecipitation of chromium with other major elements as sulphates. The high boiling point of sulphuric acid helps the activity of oxidizing agents and, with the addition of nitric acid, the disadvantage of forming compounds of low solubility is compensated. Digestion, however, with nitric and sulphuric acids requires good refluxing to prevent losses.

Significant losses of chromium during wet ashing occur only when perchloric acid is present; however, they can be avoided by the addition of sulphuric acid. The main risk of wet digestion is contamination through the reagents, especially when high volumes are used. Digestions in closed systems and/or in microwave systems require less time and reagents; therefore, losses by volatilization are reduced and the risk of contamination decreases.

In some kinds of vegetables a lower recovery of chromium is obtained because of the retention of chromium by an insoluble residue of silica. Therefore, treatment with hydrofluoric acid is necessary.

Extreme care must be taken in all wet ashing procedures where strong acids and strong oxidizing agents are used. The formation of explosive nitro compounds has been reported when food samples with high fat contents have been digested with nitric acid.

Determination

Molecular Absorption Spectroscopy

The traditional spectrophotometric method of 520 nm, based on the violet complex formed with 1,5-diphenylcarbazide (DPC), is still widely used for determining chromium in water. Chromium should be present as Cr^{6+} and the diphenylcarbazide is oxidized to the diphenylcarbazone. Iron, copper, molybdenum and vanadium can interfere. To remove interference and to increase the sensitivity of the method, both cation

exchange resins (iron and copper) and cupferron (iron, copper, molybdenum and vanadium) have been used.

Interferences caused by nitrate, free chlorine and organic compounds are eliminated by diluting the sample of water.

This method has been applied to chromium determination in foods after destroying the organic matter and removing the interferences. Detection limits of 10 ng g^{-1} have been reported.

The complex chromium hematoxiline, with a maximum absorbance between 360 and 390 nm, has also been applied to foods, although less often than the diphenylcarbazide method.

Flame Atomic Absorption Spectrophotometry

The low levels of chromium in foods and the complexity of the matrix make it difficult to measure chromium directly in digested samples by FAAS. With an air–acetylene flame and at a wavelength of 357·9 nm it is possible to obtain detection limits of 0·1 $\mu g\ g^{-1}$. It has been well established that chromium atomization is dependent on flame stoichiometry, with higher sensitivity with reducing flames (rich in acetylene).

This determination is not free of interelement interferences. Iron depresses chromium absorbance in fuel-rich air–acetylene flames. It can be separated from the analyte by extraction with acetylacetone/chloroform (1:1, v/v) at pH 1–2, or by extraction, as Fe^{3+}, from 5 M hydrochloric acid into isobutyl acetate or 4-methyl-2-pentanone (MIBK).

Direct chromium determination by FAAS in digested samples is not often applied, owing to interferences and also to the low levels of chromium. For this reason it is more usual to enrich and to remove interference by chelating chromium and then extracting with an organic solvent.

Chromium can be chelated as Cr^{3+} with 2,4-pentanedione at pH 7·5 and heating to nearly 80°C. The chelate is then extracted with chloroform or MIBK. With the former, a back extraction to an aqueous solution should be carried out before measuring by FAAS. To remove metal interferences the same chelating reagent or ammonium pyrrolidinedithiocarbamate (APDC) are added at a lower pH value and then extraction with chloroform is carried out.

Alternatively, chromium can be chelated as Cr^{3+} with APDC (pH 5 at 80–90°C) or as Cr^{6+} (pH 3–9 at room temperature). Therefore, to work under less strict conditions it is advisable to oxidize chromium to Cr^{6+} and to eliminate the excess oxidizing agent. The procedure is not free of interferences, because manganese and tin are also chelated. In order to remove interfering substances and to increase the stability of the element in solution, some authors have proposed that back extraction should be carried out.

Another method that has been applied to chromium determination in foods is based on the formation of a compound by ionic association between Cr^{6+} and the system hydrochloric acid/MIBK ($0°C$). Prior to this, chromium is oxidized to Cr^{6+} with potassium permanganate. This procedure offers the advantage that it is not necessary to remove the excess oxidizing agent.

Electrothermal Atomization Atomic Absorption Spectrophotometry

Electrothermal atomization atomic absorption spectrophotometry (ETA-AAS) is considered one of the best techniques for chromium determination in biological matrices and it is the technique most often used to determine chromium in foods. It is not free of interferences, but it is simpler than FAAS methods, especially when the latter involve chelation and extraction.

If organic matter is present, chromium is found mainly in the form of Cr^{3+}, and in this oxidation state it easily forms refractory oxides during heating in graphite tubes and then reacts with graphite to form a carbide. To avoid the resulting decrease in the signal, pyrolytically or specially coated graphite tubes should be used.

When the furnace temperature reaches $450°C$, breakdown products of chromium complexes are formed. Some of these are volatile and, therefore, there is a risk of losses of the element; other breakdown products can prevent complete atomization of chromium, because of the strong bonding with oxygen, nitrogen or carbon. To achieve complete atomization of chromium, temperatures higher than $2300°C$ should be used.

Diammonium hydrogen phosphate has been used successfully as a matrix modifier.

Since chromium is measured at a wavelength of 357.9 nm, it is better to correct background absorption with the Zeeman effect or a tungsten lamp rather than with a deuterium lamp. The emission intensity of the deuterium arc is low at the chromium resonance line of 357.9 nm. The hollow cathode lamp current has to be reduced to 10 mA from the recommended value of 25 mA in order to balance the source and background beams.

Even when prior digestion of organic matter is carried out, the standard addition method is generally applied. In the case of liquid samples, e.g. beer, it is possible to determine chromium by injecting the diluted sample directly into the graphite furnace and then applying the standard addition method.

Inductively Coupled Plasma Spectrometry

The detection limits of ICP are lower than those obtained by direct FAAS, but they are not much lower than those corresponding to ETA-AAS.

One of the main advantages of ICP is that sample preparation is simpler than in ETA-AAS, because measurement is possible even when organic matter residues are present.

A wavelength of 267.716 nm is usually chosen, though some overlap with emission lines of manganese and phosphorus can be observed.

Polarography

Differential pulse polarography (DPP) is used to measure chromium in water and biological materials (including foods). Chromium is only detectable as Cr^{6+}. A reduction peak is observed at -0.80 V, when sodium citrate is used as a buffer (pH 9–10.5) and ammonia-ammonium chloride as a support electrolyte. Detection limits as low as 0.12 $\mu g\,l^{-1}$ can be obtained.

DPP is mainly used for chromium determination in water. Preparation of the sample depends on its complexity and the expected chromium concentration.

Nitric acid should not be used to acidify the sample, since the formation of nitrous acid can partially reduce Cr^{6+} to Cr^{3+}.

If the water contains sulphites, these can also reduced Cr^{6+} to Cr^{3+}, so Cr^{6+} must be chelated with sodium diethyldithiocarbamate (pH 4, diluted sulphuric acid/potassium acid phthalate) and extracted with MIBK. Sulphuric acid is added and the solution is heated to remove the solvent. Hydrogen peroxide and sulphuric acid are added to ensure that chromium is present entirely as Cr^{6+}.

In the case of samples with a high chloride or organic matter content, sodium sulphite is added to prevent the formation of chromyl chloride.

Samples having chromium levels lower than 1 $\mu g\,g^{-1}$ can be enriched by passing the solution through an ion exchange resin.

Gas–Liquid Chromatography

Since gas–liquid chromatography (GLC) can only be applied to volatile compounds, volatile chromium chelates are formed with fluorine substitutes of acetylacetone derivatives in chromium analyses. Chromium complexes with β-diketones are volatile and stable, and the trifluoroacetyllactone (TFA) is the chelating agent most frequently reported in practical applications. When employing chromium complexes an electron capture detector (ECD) is used. This determination requires a purification step to remove the excess chelating reagent and other interfering substances from the detector. An ion exchange resin can be used for this purpose. *See* Chromatography, Gas Chromatography

The ECD permits the detection of 0.1 pg of chromium injected as $Cr(TFA)_3$ chelate but, at these levels, serious complications arise in the separation of the metal chelate from interfering electron capture impurities. For this reason, several other detectors have been evaluated, among them the nitrogen–phosphorus detector and atomic absorption spectroscopy and mass spectrometry. The last of these techniques provides a positive corroborative identification for the very small amounts of compounds detectable by the ECD. *See* Mass Spectrometry, Principles and Instrumentation

GLC application to foods is more difficult than in biological fluids. For instance, in liver, many of the metals present, such as iron, copper, cobalt and nickel, tend to emerge shortly after the solvent peak in large trailing peaks. These are probably thermal decomposition products, and any chromium peak present is masked. It has been possible to detect 10 ng g^{-1} in liver.

The introduction of the mass spectrometer as a detector meant a substantial improvement over the ECD, in particular the compatibility of monitoring a peak which can be identified with a single metal, and freedom from interferences. The detection limit is around 0·5 pg.

Another useful detector is the atomic absorption spectrophotometer, which provides detection limits of 1 ng.

The great sensitivity of GLC allows the detection of extremely small amounts of chromium. GLC has been applied mainly to chromium determination in biological fluids, such as blood and urine, and to chromium determination in water, when speciation is wanted. It is applied less frequently to foods, because this method requires prior destruction of the organic matter and chromium levels are higher in foods than in biological fluids.

Neutron Activation Analysis

Neutron activation analysis (NAA) is based on the formation of radioactive isotopes, when a sample is irradiated with neutrons from a nuclear reactor or from other neutron sources. The elements of interest are identified and quantified by γ spectroscopy.

It is generally used as a reference method to test the accuracy of other analytical methods, because it is highly specific and accurate. One of its main advantages is that it is a nondestructive method. The chief limitations to widespread use of this technique are the need for a neutron source and the very high cost of the analysis.

Moreover, in the case of chromium, the low abundance of ^{50}Cr (4·31%), a small thermal neutron section (17 barns), a low level of γ decay and a half-life for ^{51}Cr of 27·8 days, make it necessary to apply long irradiations with a high density flux of electrons, especially when chromium concentrations are low. ^{51}Cr is separated by distillation of chromyl chloride.

NAA has also been used to investigate the behaviour of chromium during drying, or when the matrix is subjected to high temperatures in dry ashing, because it allows the direct determination of the sample, without previous destruction of the organic matter.

ETA-AAS appears to be the most useful method for routine determination of chromium in foods. Special precautions should be adopted to avoid sample losses and/or contaminations throughout the period of analysis, i.e. from sampling to measurement. At the moment NAA remains useful as a reference method.

Bibliography

Dean CL and Rains TC (1975) *Elements and Matrices*, Flame Emission and Atomic Absorption Spectrometry, vol. 3, pp 164–167, appendix 635–637. New York: Marcel Dekker.

Fishbein L (1984) Overview of analysis of carcinogenic and/or mutagenic metals in biological and environmental samples. I. Arsenic, beryllium, cadmium, chromium and selenium. *International Journal of Environmental Analytical Chemistry* 17: 113–170.

Hoenig H and De Borger R (1983) Particular problems encountered in trace metal analysis of plant material by atomic absorption spectrometry. *Spectrochimica Acta* 38B: 873–880.

Holzbecher Z, Divis L, Kral M, Sucha L and Vlavic F (1976) *Handbook of Organic Reagents in Inorganic Analysis*, pp 521–529. New York: Ellis Horwood/Halstead Press.

Rollinson CL (1975) In: Trotman-Dickenson AF (ed.) *Comprehensive Inorganic Chemistry*, vol. 3, pp 631–637. Oxford Pergamon Press.

Torgrimsen T (1982) Analysis of chromium. *Biological and Environmental Aspects of Chromium*, pp 65–97. Amsterdam: Elsevier.

R. Farré Rovira and M. J. Lagarda Blanch
University of Valencia, Valencia, Spain

Physiology

Essentiality of Chromium

Chromium is an essential trace element required for normal carbohydrate, lipid and nucleic acid metabolism. Insufficient dietary chromium leads to impaired glucose and lipid metabolism and may ultimately lead to maturity-onset diabetes and/or cardiovascular diseases.

The essentiality of chromium in experimental animals was demonstrated first in rats whose impaired glucose tolerance was restored upon addition of a factor present in brewer's yeast. This factor was called the 'glucose tolerance factor'. The active component of this factor was found to be chromium. Chromium has also been shown to play an essential role in mice, hamsters, squirrel monkeys, chickens, turkeys, sheep and humans. *See* Glucose, Glucose Tolerance and the Glycaemic Index

An essential role of chromium in humans was first documented in a female patient receiving total parenteral nutrition (TPN). The patient displayed overt signs of diabetes, including severe glucose intolerance, weight loss, peripheral neuropathy and impaired energy metabolism. The symptoms were refractory to exogenous insulin but were alleviated upon addition of chromium to her TPN food supply. All other nutrients remained constant.

Function in the Body

The primary physiological function of chromium is in the potentiation of insulin action. In the presence of chromium in a biologically active form, much lower amounts of insulin are required. In the potentiation of glucose breakdown as measured in epididymal fat cells, biologically active chromium complexes increase insulin activity three- to eightfold or more at low concentrations of insulin. Chromium does not replace insulin, so that if the body is not producing insulin, chromium will have little or no effect. These insulin-dependent effects that are improved by chromium are observed in carbohydrate, protein and fat metabolism. Glucose removal from the blood, oxidation in the cell, and incorporation into fat and glycogen are all stimulated by chromium. The incorporation of acetate into fat, which is not an insulin-dependent process, is not stimulated by chromium.

Amino acid incorporation into proteins is also increased by chromium. Incorporation of radioactively labelled amino acids (glycine, serine and methionine) into heart protein was greater in chromium-supplemented animals than in low-chromium controls. *See* Amino Acids, Metabolism

Chromium is also involved in maintaining the structural integrity of nucleic acids and in gene expression by binding to chromatin in rats, causing an increase in the number of initiation sites which leads to enhanced ribonucleic acid (RNA) synthesis. The interaction of chromium and nucleic acids is quite strong since precipitation of beef liver RNA six times from solutions containing metal chelators did not reduce the amount of chromium associated with RNA while the concentrations of other metals tested declined. *See* Nucleic Acids, Physiology

Chromium Requirements

In the USA, the suggested safe and adequate intake for chromium for adults and children over 7 years is 50–200 µg per day; for children aged 4–6 years it is 30–120 µg; for children aged 1–3 years it is 20–80 µg; for infants aged 6 months to one year it is 20–60 µg; and from birth to 6 months it is 10–40 µg. This level of intake for infants is unrealistic since the chromium concentration in human milk is approximately 0·3–0·4 ng of chromium per ml. Assuming a chromium concentration of 0·4 ng per ml, an intake of 25 l of breast milk per day would be required to obtain the minimum suggested daily intake of 10 µg; this is clearly unrealistic. *See* Dietary Reference Values

Normal dietary daily chromium intake for adults in the USA and other Western countries is usually in the range of 20–40 µg. Mean daily intake from diets collected for 7 consecutive days for 22 females was 25 ± 1 µg and that for 10 males was 33 ± 3 µg. Similar values have been reported from England and Finland, with slightly higher values for Canadian subjects.

The chromium content of 22 daily diets designed by nutritionists to be well balanced ranged from 8·4 to 23·7 µg per 4·2 kJ (1000 cal) with mean chromium content of 13·4 µg per 4·2 kJ, SEM (standard error of estimate of mean value) 1·1. Mean chromium content for self-selected diets is 15 µg per 4·2 kJ, SEM 1·4. Thus dietary chromium contents of well-balanced diets designed by nutritionists are similar to those of self-selected diets. However, chromium nutrition is influenced not only by dietary intake and absorption but also by other factors which may enhance chromium losses. One dietary factor that affects chromium losses is intake of simple sugars. Urinary chromium losses are increased with increased intake of simple sugars, such as glucose, sucrose and fructose; complex carbohydrates, such as starch, decrease chromium losses. Experimental animals also absorb and retain more chromium from diets high in starch than from diets high in the simple sugars.

Dietary chromium concentrations of less than 100 ng per g of diet were suggested in early studies as a suitable range to induce chromium deficiency as measured by impaired glucose tolerance in rats. Glucose removal rates of weanling rats are usually 4–5% per min and decrease slightly with age to 3·5–4% per min. Glucose removal rates of rats raised on a low-chromium diet decrease to 2·7% per min, and when rats were raised in a controlled low-chromium environment, glucose removal rates of less than 1% were reported. Similar levels of chromium in the low chromium diet of mice also led to signs of chromium deficiency, as evidenced by the observation that male mice supplemented with 5 µg of chromium per g of water lived a mean of 99 days longer than the nonsupplemented animals.

More recent studies showed that rats raised on diets containing chromium concentrations 50% or less (< 50 µg per g) of those reported in the above mentioned studies demonstrate less marked or minimal signs of

Table 1. Signs and symptoms of chromium deficiency

Function	Animal
Impaired glucose tolerance	Human, rat, mouse
Fasting hyperglycaemia	Human, rat, mouse
Elevated circulating insulin	Human, rat
Elevated blood glucagon	Human
Elevated blood cortisol	Human
Glycosuria	Human, rat
Corneal lesions	Rat, monkey
Impaired growth	Rat, mouse, turkey
Decreased longevity	Rat, mouse
Elevated serum cholesterol	Human, rat, mouse
Elevated serum triglycerides	Human, rat mouse
Decreased HDL-cholesterol	Human
Increased incidence of aortic plaques	Rabbit, rat, mouse
Reduction in aortic intimal plaque areas	Rabbit
Decreased fertility and sperm count	Rat
Hypoglycaemic symptoms[a]	Human
Neuropathy	Human
Brain disorders	Human

[a] Symptoms include drowsiness, shaking, blurred vision and profuse sweating.
HDL, high-density lipoprotein.

chromium deficiency. Whether these differences result from analytical determinations or, more probably, from differences in the composition of the respective diets, remains to be established.

Combined chromium and ascorbic acid deficiency in guinea pigs leads to glucose intolerance and elevated cholesterol in guinea pigs. Guinea pigs, like humans, require dietary ascorbic acid (vitamin C) while rats and mice do not. *See* Ascorbic Acid, Physiology

Deficiency

Glucose intolerance is usually one of the first signs of chromium deficiency, followed or accompanied by impaired insulin function and lipid metabolism (Table 1). All of the signs or symptoms listed in Table 1 are essentially caused by marginal chromium deficiency and those listed for humans are often widespread. Decreased fertility and sperm count are early signs of chromium deficiency in rats but have not been determined in humans. Most of the signs and symptoms of chromium deficiency listed in Table 1 are not specific for chromium and may be related to other factors associated with ageing. However, decreased chromium status is associated with ageing and may play a role in the apparent rapid rate of ageing of some individuals. *See* Ageing – Nutritional Aspects

The last two signs of chromium deficiency listed in Table 1 (peripheral neuropathy and brain disorders) are signs of overt chromium deficiency and have only been observed in patients on total parenteral nutrition. Studies involving patients on TPN have inadvertently led to the establishment of definite requirement for chromium in the control of maturity-onset diabetes in humans. Total nutrient intake in the parenteral nutrition solutions remained constant and the only change was the addition of chromium to the parenteral fluids which alleviated diabetic symptoms. Following 2 weeks of chromium supplementation, diabetic symptoms were eliminated and exogenous insulin requirement dropped from 50 units per day to zero. Chromium is now routinely added to TPN solutions.

Toxicity

Toxicity of trivalent chromium is extremely rare. Trivalent chromium is poorly absorbed, usually less than 2%. Indigestion and vomiting are likely to occur at extremely high levels but with no lasting toxic effects. Feeding up to 1000 mg of trivalent chromium complexes to cats for up to 3 months resulted in no detectable toxic effects. Rats were also unaffected by feeding 100 μg of chromium per g of milk diet. The intravenous median lethal dose (LD_{50}) from chromalum and chromium hexaurea chloride is 100 and 180 mg per kg, respectively. Less than 0·0001% of this amount is required to improve glucose tolerance.

Chromium is a potent allergen and is a common skin sensitizer in allergic eczema. Hexavalent chromium is a common industrial pollutant and has been shown to have numerous toxic effects. Chromium in foods and biological tissues is almost exclusively in the trivalent form since hexavalent chromium is rapidly converted to the trivalent form in the presence of organic matter. *See* Allergens

Role in Diseases and Disorders

Insulin-dependent diabetics excrete threefold more chromium than control subjects. Diabetics are apparently sensitive to an increased need for chromium to improve insulin metabolism, as evidenced by increased absorption. However, once chromium is absorbed it is not converted to a useable form and utilized, but excreted. Genetically diabetic mice also lose the ability to convert chromium to a useable form. Supplementation with inorganic chromium is without effect on glucose and insulin metabolism of diabetic mice, while supplementation with chromium, in a biologically active form, leads to improved glucose and lipid metabolism. Patients with Turner's syndrome, who also have a high prevalence of diabetes, also excrete several-fold more chromium than control subjects.

Proper chromium nutrition leads to significant improvements in the glucose tolerance of most subjects with 90-minute glucose greater than $5 \cdot 5$ mmol l^{-1} (100 mg dl^{-1}). Since the average 2-hour glucose for individuals over age 25 is greater than $5 \cdot 55$ mmol l^{-1}, this applies to a large proportion of the normal US population.

Chromium functions not only in the prevention of maturity-onset diabetes but also in the treatment of individuals who have diabetes. Blood glucose of three of six diabetics improved following inorganic chromium supplementation for more than one week. Insulin requirement of five diabetics whose insulin requirement ranged from 60 to 130 units declined by 20–45 units following supplementation with high chromium yeast. Fasting blood glucose of 13 diabetic patients on either exogenous insulin or oral hypoglycaemic agents dropped from $14 \cdot 4$ mmol l^{-1} (259 mg dl^{-1}) to $6 \cdot 6$ mmol l^{-1} (119 mg dl^{-1}) following 2–4 months' supplementation with 600 μg of chromium as chromium chloride. The amount of oral hypoglycaemic agents or insulin also decreased in 5 of 13 patients receiving chromium, and rose in four of 13 patients taking a placebo. The final fasting glucose of subjects on placebo was unchanged. High-density lipoprotein levels in subjects receiving chromium also increased. Fasting blood glucose, haemoglobin A$_{1C}$, total cholesterol, low-density lipoprotein cholesterol and apolipoprotein of noninsulin-dependent diabetics decreased following supplementation with 200 μg of chromium as chromium picolinate. Severe diabetic symptoms of subjects on TPN were also alleviated following chromium supplementation. Chromium functions as a nutrient, not a therapeutic agent. Only those signs and symptoms caused by chromium deficiency will be alleviated by improved chromium nutrition.

Chromium plays a key role in the control of insulin action. In the presence of suitable amounts of chromium in a useable form much lower amounts of insulin are required. Dietary chromium intake in the USA and other Western countries is suboptimal. Improved chromium intake leads to improved glucose and lipid metabolism of subjects with marginally or elevated blood glucose and lipids. Progressive research over the past three decades continues to strengthen the association of marginal dietary chromium with the increase in factors associated with maturity-onset diabetes and cardiovascular diseases.

Bibliography

Anderson RA (1987) Chromium. In: Mertz W (ed.) *Trace Elements in Human and Animal Nutrition* 5th edn, pp 225–244. Orlando: Academic Press.
Anderson RA (1989) Essentiality of chromium in humans. *Science of the Total Environment* 86: 75–81.
Anderson RA, Bryden NA, Polansky MM and Reiser S (1990) Urinary chromium excretion and insulinogenic properties of carbohydrates. *American Journal of Clinical Nutrition* 51: 864–868.
Mossop RT (1983) Effects of chromium (III) on fasting glucose, cholesterol and cholesterol HDL levels in diabetics. *Central African Journal of Medicine* 29: 80–82.
WHO Task Group (1988) *Chromium*. Geneva: World Health Organization.

Richard A. Anderson
Beltsville Human Nutrition Research Center, Beltsville, Maryland, USA

CIDER (CYDER; HARD CIDER)

Contents

The Product and its Manufacture

A Brief History of Cider

The fermentation of apple juice to produce an alcoholic beverage is believed to have been practised for over 2000 years. Cider is recorded as being a common drink at the time of the Roman invasion of Britain in 55 BC. Celtic mythology revered the 'sacred apple' and in his famous natural history (AD 77) Pliny the Elder refers to a drink made from the juice of the apple. Cider was drunk throughout Europe in the third century, and in the fourth century St Jerome used the term 'sicera' (from whence the name cider was possibly derived) to describe drinks made from apples.

Reputedly, cider was a more popular drink than beer in the eleventh and twelfth centuries in Europe. Cider has been produced throughout the temperate regions of the world where apple trees flourish, including the following localities: the northern coastal area of Spain; France, especially Normandy; Belgium; Switzerland and the FRG; various regions of England; Eire; and, more recently, the USA, Australia and New Zealand.

There are references to cider in many writings from the Middle Ages. The popularity of cider in fourteenth century England was such that William of Shoreham reflected the Church's concern for the niceties of sacramental rites by stating that 'young children were not to be baptised in cider'! William Langdon in *Piers Plowman* and Shakespeare in *A Midsummers Night's Dream* refer to the consumption of cider; Daniel Defoe observed that Hereford people 'boaft the richeft cider in all Britain', and Samuel Pepys noted in his diary that on 1 May 1666 he 'drank a cup of Syder'. From the seventeenth century onwards cider was praised in numerous poems and other literary works as an aid to good cheer and a homely cure for almost every known ailment.

Up to the twentieth century cider was a popular rural drink, cheaper than beer and often more potent, at approximately 7% alcohol by volume (ABV). Farm workers often had part of their wages paid as truck (i.e. in kind) and every farmer would make his own cider for consumption by his workers and his own family and guests, although it is recorded that the best ciders were retained for his personal use. Most farms in the west of England and the West Country had their own cider presses, or used the services of a travelling cider press which was hauled by horse from farm to farm. My own cider mill and press (dated 1717) stand outside my window as I write this account!

Commercial cider production commenced during the nineteenth century in England (e.g. Weston & Sons, 1880; HP Bulmer of Hereford, 1887; Whiteways Cyder of Whimple, in Devon, 1894), although a few farms produced cider commercially from as early as 1727 (Symonds Cider and English Wine Co. Ltd, Stoke Lacey, England). Cider production in England was estimated as 250×10^6 l (55×10^6 gal) in 1900. By 1920, the level of cider production had decreased significantly; although some 73×10^6 l (16×10^6 gal) were still produced on farms, only 23×10^6 l (5×10^6 gal) came from factory producers. By the 1980s, cider sales had risen to over 273×10^6 l (60×10^6 gal) per year and, in the 12 months to September 1991, a total of 343×10^6 l (75.5×10^6 gal) had been produced by members of the National Association of Cider Makers, a trade association formed originally in 1920.

Recent years have seen a significant increase in the volume of cider produced commercially. This growth, which had been inhibited by the imposition of Excise Duty in 1976, results both from the introduction of new cider products, linked to increased marketing activity, and from changes in drinking habits especially of younger adults. In 1992 it is possible to obtain cider either on draught or prepackaged in glass and Polyethyleneterephthalate (PET) bottles and in cans. Products range in alcoholic strength from less than 0.5% to 8.4% ABV, and in sweetness from very dry to sweet. In addition, cider products now include 'white' ciders (using decolorized apple juice or decolorized after fermentation), pink ciders and naturally coloured ciders. Some cider, made from apples of a single crop, may be sold as a defined-year vintage cider; whilst others are made from a single apple cultivar, e.g. Kingston Black.

Cider Fruits

Traditional European ciders are made from the juice of cider apples believed to have been imported into the UK by the Normans, although it is recorded in Gaulmier's *Traite du Sidre* (1573) that a Spaniard named Dursus de l'Etre brought apple trees into France in 1486! *See* Apples

Traditional cider apples are of four main types: bitter sweet (low in acidity but high in tannin); bitter sharp (high acidity and high tannin); sharp varieties (high acidity but low tannin); and sweet varieties (low acidity and low tannin). Some of the more common cultivars are listed in Table 1. *See* Tannins and Polyphenols

In some areas of the UK, especially Kent, Suffolk and Norfolk, cider is made primarily from culinary fruit varieties, such as the Bramley, although blends of bittersweet and culinary juices are frequently used to develop particular flavour profiles in commercial cider blends.

Cider Orchards

The traditional farm orchard of standard trees still exists and, although generally declining in area, many hundreds of such orchards provide both an apple crop and grazing for sheep.

Modern cider apple orchards are largely intensive bush orchards, where the selected cultivar is grafted onto a suitable rootstock. Such trees are frequently planted as closely as 2.4 m apart in rows some 5.5–6 m apart. After planting, staking and protecting against rabbits using a wire guard, the grass under the trees is treated with a suitable herbicide to reduce competition for nutrients and water. Some growers cover the herbicide strips with a mulch of straw or other suitable material to ensure maximum retention of moisture.

Table 1. Characteristics of cider apple varieties

Type	Typical varieties	Typical composition	
		Acidity[a] (g per 100 ml)	Tannin (g per 100 ml)
Sweet	Northwood Sweet Alford Sweet Coppin	< 0·45	< 0·2
Bitter sweet	Ashton Brown Jersey Dabinett Michelin Yarlington Mill	< 0·45	> 0·2
Bitter sharp	Bulmer's Foxwhelp Dymock Red Kingston Black	> 0·45	> 0·2
Sharp	Brown's Apple Frederick Reinette O'bry	> 0·45	< 0·2

[a] As malic acid.

Although it has become standard practice to retain the herbicide strip into the productive years of an orchard, this practice is currently the subject of research to assess whether a grass sward may be better in relation to the quality of harvested fruit.

During the growing season it may be necessary to spray the trees against pests, e.g. red spider mite, mildew, canker and other conditions. In addition, in years of heavy potential cropping, chemical thinning (e.g. using carbaryl/NAA) is frequently recommended. The objective is to reduce stress on the tree in order to minimize the risk of biennialism, a condition which has occurred significantly in English cider fruit orchards in recent years.

Harvesting

In traditional orchards, fruits are generally allowed to fall naturally, or are shaken from the trees using long poles (lugs), and are then picked up either by hand or by machine. Traditionally, fruit from standard trees would be raked into piles or filled into sacks which were stored under the trees until the fruit was in a suitably ripe condition to be milled and pressed.

In intensive bush orchards it is normal to shake the trees mechanically in order to cause the fruit to fall. Such shaking does not harm the tree and permits fruits to be harvested mechanically immediately after falling, so reducing the risk of rots which may occur if fruit are left for any length of time on a herbicide strip. The collected fruit will normally be washed mechanically in the orchard and then transferred by road to the cider mill where, after weighing, the fruit is tipped into a fruit canal or onto a concrete pad for holding prior to milling and juicing.

Processing the Fruit

Milling and Pressing

The fruit is generally transferred into the mill using either a water flume, which provides additional washing, or on other suitable belt or screw conveyors. Detritus such as twigs, leaves and stones are removed mechanically and the fruit is milled generally using a grater, slicer or hammer mill. The apple pulp is then conveyed to a mechanical press where the juice is extracted.

For many years the presses consisted of a frame containing a slatted board covered by a cloth into which a measured amount of the pulp was transferred. The corners of the cloth were folded over to form an envelope, the frame was removed and the next slatted board added, together with the frame and another cloth. This procedure was repeated some 10 to 20 times to build a cheese which was then pressed hydraulically to remove the juice, under a ram pressure of some 14 MPa. (approximately 2 MPa on the cheese). This method removes up to 80% of the juice. Sometimes the pomace residue (see below) would be soaked in a small volume of water and repressed to remove further quantities of fermentable sugar.

Since such processes are very labour-intensive they have now been replaced largely by automatic presses such as the Bücher–Guyer, a horizontal cylinder press, the Ensink, or the Bellmer continuous belt press. Such presses are more efficient, often permit countercurrent extraction of the first pomace with warm water and have little demand for labour once properly set up. Processes such as the electroacoustic dewatering have been claimed to release a higher yield of juice by passing an electric current through the pulp prior to pressing, but have not found application in the UK.

The Product and its Manufacture

Pomace

Apple pomace can be used for the extraction of the natural gelling agent pectin, used in the manufacture of jam, dairy products and other foodstuffs; and in certain medical applications.

Pomace, either before or after depectinization, can be fed to animals either as a wet slurry or after drying, or it can be spread onto agricultural land as an organic mulch or fertilizer. Whilst it aids the breakdown of clay soils, its acidity often poses problems in such applications.

Apple Juice

The extracted juice will be rich in acid, tannins and sugar; it will also be contaminated with a variety of microorganisms derived from the fruit itself, from the orchard floor and from the environment of the cider mill. Immediately after pressing, juice is treated with sulphur dioxide which acts both as an antioxidant to prevent browning of the juice (owing to polyphenol oxidase and chemical browning reactions) and to destroy the wild yeasts and bacteria. The sulphited juice will normally be stored for some 24 h before being pumped into fermentation vessels. *See* Antioxidants, Synthetic Antioxidants

In general, the juice will not be clarified prior to fermentation. However, if the juice is to be concentrated for storage, generally by thermal evaporation, it will be treated with a mixture of enzymes (pectinases and amylases) and then clarified prior to concentration. Failure to destroy pectins and starch results in a thick, viscous mass which does not concentrate effectively or store adequately.

Fermentation of Cider

Fermentation Vessels

Traditionally, the apple juice is fermented in oak vats; although many such vats are still in use, vats of mild steel with a ceramic or resin lining, bitumen-lined concrete vats and, more recently, stainless steel or even lined fibreglass-resin vats are used.

A few cidermakers use redundant brewing vessels such as conicocylindrical vats. However, there is little evidence that tall vats are beneficial. The fermentation of cider is more akin to the fermentation of wine, and the Unitank-style vessel has the benefit of reducing hydrostatic pressure stress on the fermentation yeast.

Fermentation Substrate

Traditional cidermaking used whole juice, often with much of the apple solids remaining. Such solids included the pips, which contain glycosides; hence the cider would contain small quantities of cyanide derivatives. In countries such as France, where the production of cider is constrained by legislation, only fresh apple juice or fresh juice reinforced with secondary juices, can be fermented into cider. In other countries the process of chaptalization has become increasingly common.

Chaptalization is the process whereby the basic juice is supplemented by a suitable fermentation sugar (e.g. brewers' dextrose) which permits the production of cider with alcohol contents up to 11·5–12% ABV. By comparison, fresh juice fermentations, depending upon the sugar content, will rarely exceed 5·5–6·0% ABV.

In the preparation of cider, the apple juice may be fresh or reconstituted from an apple juice concentrate; pear juice (fresh or reconstituted) may be added to a maximum of 25% of the apple juice content. Other than fermentation sugars, the only other primary addition will be a suitable yeast culture. In fermentation brews originating wholly or largely from concentrate, it is normal to add ammonium phosphate and sodium pantothenate and/or thiamin as yeast nutrients. *See* Yeasts

The juice for cidermaking is rarely sterile, but the wild yeasts and other naturally occurring microorganisms are largely constrained by adjustment of the sulphur dioxide level to provide some 10–30 mg of free sulphur dioxide per litre, this level being directly related to the sulphur-dioxide-binding capacity and the pH of the fermentation medium.

Fermentation Process

The fermentation process consists of partially filling the vat with juice, followed by inoculation with a specific starter culture of yeast (frequently a wine yeast capable of growth at elevated alcohol levels). Once fermentation has started, additional substrate is added from time to time until the vat is filled. Although most cider vats are typically of 45×10^3–9×10^5 l (10 000–200 000 gal) capacity, much larger vats do exist. At HP Bulmer Ltd, UK, the world's largest fermentation and storage container for alcoholic beverages holds some $7·27 \times 10^6$ l ($1·6 \times 10^6$ gal) of product.

The fermentation typically continues without control of temperature, pH or other parameters until all the fermentable sugar has been metabolized into alcohol. Depending upon conditions, this process can take from 4 to 12 weeks. There is no doubt that better control of temperature can give more consistent fermentation profiles and products. Whilst ambient temperature fermentation occurs widely, some makers can control temperature to a limited extent and, in France, cider is often fermented at a temperature of 15–18°C.

Maturation

When fermented to dryness, the cider is frequently left for a few days on the lees to permit the yeasts to autolyse, thereby adding cell constituents, such as enzymes and amino and nucleic acids, to the brew. The cider will be separated from the lees (or tank bottoms) and transferred either directly, or after clarification or filtration, into storage vats (usually made of oak). The actual process of maturation is generally uncontrolled. Little is known scientifically about the maturation process, its various chemical markers or the influencing factors. Judgement as to the extent of maturation and the suitability of the cider for use is still an art vested in the cidermaker, who will have many years of experience in judging the quality of the product.

Final Processing

When required for use, different batches of cider, generally made from mixtures of different juices, will be blended by the cidermaker to provide specific flavour attributes. The raw cider will be fined using fining agents, such as bentonite, gelatin or chitin, and filtered to give a bright product with no haze. Recent processing refinements include the use of cross-flow microfiltration systems to obviate the need for fining, and reduce the processing time and labour requirement.

If the cider has a high alcohol content it may be 'broken back' to final product strength using water or dilute apple juice. Other ingredients may be added, e.g. sugars, intense sweeteners (e.g. saccharin), colours and/ or additional preservative (in the UK this will normally be sulphur dioxide, although in other countries benzoic or sorbic acids are frequently used). The finished blend will often be treated with filter aids, such as Kieselguhr (diatomaceous earth), to give an optically bright product. *See* Colours, Properties and Determination of Synthetic Pigments; Preservation of Food; Sweeteners – Intense

Cider Packaging

Although a small market still exists for 'live cider', i.e. cider in a wooden or plastic barrel, to which a small quantity of sugar is added together with a further yeast inoculum, the majority of commercial cider is carbonated and pasteurized, or sterile-filtered, prior to filling into kegs, bottles or cans. *See* Barrels

Keg Cider

The cider is carbonated and pasteurized in line, through a continuous-flow plate heat exchanger. It is filled into stainless steel kegs in a plant which rinses, washes and sterilizes the kegs prior to filling. The filled kegs are despatched to on-trade outlets and dispensed using either carbon dioxide or carbon dioxide and nitrogen overpressure via a cooling system designed to deliver the product into the glass at a temperature of $10 \pm 0.5°C$. This process is analogous to that used for dispensing keg beer.

Bottled Ciders

Cider to be filled into glass bottles may either be carbonated and flash-pasteurized, or carbonated and pasteurized after filling. Since it is generally not possible to pasteurize PET bottles, the product will be flash-pasteurized prior to filling. Bottles will be sealed using either crown closures or tamper-evident metal or plastic screw caps. Glass bottles range in size from 25 cl to 1·13 l; PET bottles from 50 cl to 5 l. Carbonation pressures generally range from 2·5 to 3·5 bar, the higher initial pressures being used in PET bottles which, owing to gaseous diffusion, lose carbonation during storage.

Can Cider

Cider cans are always lacquered to prevent the acidity of the product from attacking the metal. Cans are either of extruded aluminium or mild steel, generally with a retained tag. Since sulphur dioxide is very corrosive to metal, especially if minute pinholes occur in the lacquer, cider for canning is generally prepared with little (< 35 mg l^{-1} total) sulphur dioxide. Such products must, of necessity, be prepared in much more controlled conditions than general-blend ciders, since at these low sulphur dioxide levels microbial contamination can lead to the formation of undesirable flavours. Cider filled into cans is always bed-pasteurized, generally at a process level of 30–40 pasteurization units (PUs). Control of dissolved oxygen levels for can ciders is also most important to prevent the development of oxidation flavours.

Secondary Packaging

Bottles and cans are increasingly packaged using trays and shrink wraps, although the higher value products (e.g. vintage and high-strength cider in glass bottles) cardboard boxes with or without dividers are frequently used.

Special Ciders

Vintage Ciders

Vintage ciders may be made only from fresh juice from a named year. Some vintage ciders are also made from single apple cultivar juices.

The Product and its Manufacture

Sparkling Ciders

Sparkling ciders are generally carbonated to a level of 3·0–4 vols carbon dioxide (equivalent to >3 bar pressure). Such products are generally filled into 'champagne-style' bottles with wired closures (generally plastic-mushroom stoppers). The products are normally sterile-filtered prior to bottling. Traditionally, sparkling ciders received a secondary 'in-bottle' fermentation (*méthode champenoise*), but such processing is rarely seen nowadays. Under EEC law it is illegal to refer to sparkling ciders as 'champagne cider'.

White Cider

White cider is prepared either by using very pale-coloured juices or decolorized by treatment with activated charcoal or other suitable decolorizing agent. In some instances, white cider is prepared by fermentation of decolorized apple juice.

Dealcoholized and Low-Alcohol Ciders

Dealcoholized and low-alcohol ciders are prepared either by using a stopped fermentation process to give a product with an alcohol content not in excess of 1·2% ABV, or by removing the alcohol from strong cider by thermal evaporation, by reverse osmosis or by other suitable technologies. Dealcoholized cider generally lacks body and flavour. It will be fortified with apple juice and other ingredients to provide a product with a flavour and aroma close to that of normal alcoholic cider.

While the flavour of low-alcohol beer bears little relationship to that of the parent product, low-alcohol ciders are very similar to the higher-alcohol products, other than in alcohol content.

Bibliography

Beech FW (1972) English cidermaking: technology, microbiology and biochemistry. In: Hockenhull DJD (ed.) *Progress in Industrial Microbiology*, vol. 11, pp 133–213. Edinburgh: Churchill Livingstone.

Beech FW and Davenport RR (1983) New prospects and problems in the beverage industry. In: Roberts TA and Skinner FA (eds) *Food Microbiology: Advances and Prospects*. SAB Symposium Series No. 11, pp 241–256. London: Academic Press.

Charley VLS (1949) *The Principles and Practice of Cider-Making*. London: Leonard Hill.

Williams RR (ed.) (1991) *Cider and Juice Apples: Growing and Processing*. Bristol: University of Bristol.

B. Jarvis
HP Bulmer Ltd, Hereford, UK

Chemistry and Microbiology of Cidermaking

The fermentation of apple juice to cider can occur naturally through the metabolic activity of the yeasts and bacteria present on the fruit at harvest which are then transferred into apple juice on pressing. Other organisms, arising from the milling and pressing equipment and the general environment, can also contaminate the juice at this stage. Unless such organisms are inhibited, e.g. through the use of sulphur dioxide, the mixed fermentation which results will yield a product which varies considerably from batch to batch, even if the composition of the apple juice for fermentation is identical.

Hence control of the indigenous and adventitious microorganisms, followed by deliberate inoculation with a selected strain of yeast, is the preferred commercial route for the production of cider. However, even in this situation, the transfer of fermented juice from the lees into different maturation and storage vessels may result in a secondary fermentation by those microorganisms which occur naturally in the traditional oak vats that are frequently used for this purpose. Such organisms may produce beneficial or detrimental changes in the chemical and organoleptic properties of the final cider.

Microbiology of Apple Juice and Cider

Freshly pressed apple juice will contain a variety of yeasts and bacteria, many of which will be incapable of growth at the acidity of the juice. Examples of organisms often present in juice are shown in Table 1, together with an indication of their susceptibility to sulphur dioxide.

The Role of Sulphur Dioxide in Apple Juice

The use of sulphur dioxide as a preservative in cidermaking is controlled by legislation; in most countries the maximum level permitted in the final product is 200 mg l^{-1}.

The addition of sulphur dioxide to apple juice results in the formation of so-called sulphite addition compounds through the binding of sulphur dioxide to carbonyl compounds. When dissolved in water, sulphur dioxide or its salts set up a pH-dependent equilbrium mixture of 'molecular sulphur dioxide', bisulphite and sulphite ions (Fig. 1). The antimicrobial activity of sulphur dioxide is believed to be due to the molecular sulphur dioxide moiety of that part which remains unbound (the so-called 'free' sulphur dioxide). Less sulphur dioxide is needed in juices of high acidity; for example, 15 mg of free sulphur dioxide per litre at pH 3·0 has the same antimicrobial effect as 150 mg l⁻¹ at pH 4·0. *See* Preservation of Food

The binding of sulphur dioxide is dependent upon the nature and origin of the carbonyl compounds present in the juice. Naturally occurring compounds which bind sulphur dioxide include glucose, xylose and xylosone. If the fruit has undergone some degree of rotting, other binding compounds will be present, including 2,5-dioxogluconic acid and 5-oxofructose (2,5-D-threohexo-diulose). Such juices will require increased additions of sulphur dioxide if wild yeasts and other microorganisms are to be controlled effectively.

The addition of sulphur dioxide to a fermenting juice results in rapid combination with acetaldehyde, pyruvate and α-oxoglutarate, produced by the fermenting yeasts. Consequently, all additions must be completed immediately after pressing the juice although, provided that the initial fermentation is inhibited, further additions to give the desired level of free sulphur dioxide can be made during the following 24 h.

Fermentation Yeasts

The fermentation process is carried out by strains of *Saccharomyces* spp., especially *S. cerevisiae* and *S. uvarum*, which are added to the sulphited juice as a pure culture. The starter culture will be prepared in the laboratory from freeze-dried or liquid-nitrogen-frozen cultures which are resuscitated in broth and then

Table 1. Typical microorganisms of freshly pressed apple juice

Type	Typical species	Sensitivity to sulphur dioxide
Yeast	*Saccharomyces cerevisiae*	± or −
	S. uvarum	± or −
	Saccharomycodes ludwigii	−
	Kloeckera apiculata	+ + +
	Candida pulcherrima	+ + + +
	Pichia spp.	+ + + +
	Torulopsis famata	+ +
	Aureobasidium pullulans	+ + +
	Rhodotorula spp.	+ + + +
Bacteria	*Acetobacter xylinum*	+ +
	Pseudomonas spp.	+ + + +
	Escherichia coli	+ + + +
	Salmonella spp.	+ + + +
	Micrococcus spp.	+ + + +
	Staphylococcus spp.	+ + + +
	Bacillus spp.	− (spores)
	Clostridium spp.	− (spores)

− Insensitive; ± relatively insensitive; ++, +++, ++++ increasingly more sensitive.

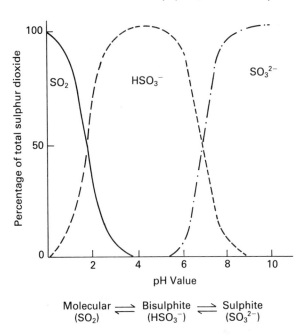

Fig. 1 Percentage of sulphite, bisulphite and molecular sulphur dioxide as a function of pH in aqueous solution. (From Hammond and Carr, 1976.)

Table 2. Higher alcohols in apple juices and ciders

| | Concentration range (mg l⁻¹) | |
Constituent	Apple juices	Ciders
n-Propanol	0·2–2	4–200
n-Butanol	3–24	4–32
iso-Butanol		14–74
iso-Pentanol	0·1	42–196
sec-Pentanol	0·1–2	16–39
n-Hexanol	1–2	2–17
2-Phenylethanol		7–260

cultivated through increasing volumes of a suitable culture medium to give an inoculum for use in a starter propagation plant. The nature of the cultivation medium used will vary, but it is often based on sterile apple juice supplemented with appropriate nitrogenous substrates (e.g. yeast extract) and, sometimes, with vitamins such as pantothenate and thiamin. Increasingly, commercially produced dried or frozen yeast cell preparations are being used, either for direct vat inoculation or as inocula for the yeast propagation plant. *See* Pantothenic Acid, Properties and Determination; Thiamin, Properties and Determination

The choice of culture is dependent upon many criteria, such as flocculation characteristics, ability to ferment efficiently at subambient temperatures, alcohol and sulphur dioxide tolerance, and lack of ability to produce hydrogen sulphide. One desirable characteristic is the ability to produce fusel oils (e.g. higher alcohols)

Chemistry and Microbiology of Cidermaking

which affect both the flavour and aroma of the cider (Table 2). *See* Sensory Evaluation, Aroma; Sensory Evaluation, Taste

The fermentation process typically takes some 3–8 weeks to proceed to dryness (i.e. specific gravity 0·990–1·000), at which time all fermentable sugars have been converted to alcohol, carbon dioxide and other metabolites (Table 2). After inoculation, the starter yeast, together with those sulphur-dioxide-resistant wild yeasts selected from the juice, will increase in numbers from an initial level of about $2 \times 10^4 - 2 \times 10^5$ to $2 \times 10^6 - 5 \times 10^7$ colony forming units (cfu) ml^{-1}. Following an initial aerobic growth phase, the resulting oxygen limitation and high carbohydrate levels in the media trigger the onset of the anaerobic fermentation process.

In controlled fermentations, a maximum temperature of 25°C will generally be permitted, although fermentations controlled at 16–18°C are not uncommon in many countries. Because of the exothermic nature of the fermentation process, temperatures of 30°C or above can be attained during periods of high ambient temperature. In Australia, it is not uncommon for temperatures as high as 35–40°C to occur in the vat, in the absence of a cooling facility.

Such high-temperature processes are generally undesirable, since activity of the desirable yeast strain may be inhibited, leading to 'stuck' fermentations and the growth of undesirable thermoduric yeasts and spoilage bacteria. Stuck fermentations can sometimes be restarted by addition of nitrogen (10–50 mg l^{-1}), usually as ammonium sulphate or diammonium phosphate and thiamin (0·1–0·2 mg l^{-1}). *See* Spoilage, Bacterial Spoilage; Spoilage, Yeasts in Food Spoilage

At the end of fermentation, the yeast cells will have flocculated and settled to the bottom of the vat. During this process a certain amount of cell autolysis occurs, thereby liberating cell constituents into the cider. The raw cider will be drawn (racked) off the lees as a cloudy product and transferred to storage vats for maturation. In some plants the cider may be centrifuged or rough-filtered at this time. If the cider is left too long on the lees the extent of autolysis may become excessive, leading in particular to a build-up of nitrogenous materials which will act as substrates for subsequent undesirable microbial growth and the development of off-flavours in the product.

Maturation and Secondary Fermentation

The maturation vats are filled with the racked-off cider and either provided with an 'over-blanket' of carbon dioxide, or otherwise sealed to prevent ingress of air, which will stimulate the growth of film-forming yeasts (e.g. *Brettanomyces* spp., *Pichia membranefaciens*, *Candida mycoderma*) and aerobic bacteria (e.g. *Acetobacter*

xylinum). Growth of the former will produce precursors for the development of defects such as 'mousey' flavour (e.g. 1,4,5,6-tetrahydro-2-acetopyridine), whilst the latter will acetify the cider through the production of acetic and other volatile acids which impart a vinegary note to the product. Of course, deliberate acetification of cider can be used to produce cider vinegar. *See* Acids, Properties and Determination; Vinegar

During the maturation process, growth of lactic acid bacteria (e.g. *Lactobacillus pastorianus* var. *quinicus*, *L. mali*, *L. plantarum*, *Leuconostoc mesenteroides*, etc.) can occur extensively, especially if wooden vats are used. The 'malo-lactic fermentation' process results in the conversion of malic to lactic acid. Such secondary fermentation will reduce the acidity of the cider and impart subtle flavour changes which are generally considered to improve the flavour of the product. However, in certain circumstances, metabolites of the lactic acid bacteria may damage the flavour and result in spoilage, e.g. excessive production of diacetyl (and its vicinal-diketone precursors), the 'butterscotch-like' taste of which can be detected in cider at a threshold level of about 0·6 mg l^{-1}. *See* Lactic Acid Bacteria

Spoilage and Other Microorganisms in Cider

Bacterial pathogens such as *Salmonella* species, *Escherichia coli*, and *Staphylococcus aureus* may occasionally occur in apple juice; they are derived from the orchard soil, farm and process equipment or human sources. However, the acidity of the product prevents growth and such organisms do not survive for long in the fermenting product. Bacterial spores from species of *Bacillus* and *Clostridium* can survive for long periods and are frequently found in cider but do not create a spoilage threat because of the pH, although their presence may be indicative of poor plant hygiene. *See* *Bacillus*, Occurrence; *Clostridium*, Occurrence of *Clostridium perfringens*; Enterobacteriaceae, Occurrence of *Escherichia coli*; *Staphylococcus*, Properties and Occurrence

The juice from unsound fruits and juice contaminated within the pressing plant may show extensive contamination by microfungi, such as *Penicillium expansum*, *P. crustosum*, *Aspergillus niger*, *A. nidulans*, *A. fumigatus*, *Paecilomyces varioti*, *Byssochlamys fulva*, *Monascus ruber*, *Phialophora mustea*, and by species of *Alternaria*, *Cladosporium*, *Botrytis*, *Oospora* and *Fusarium*. None are of particular concern in cidermaking, except that thermoresistant species (e.g. *Byssochlamys* spp.) can survive pasteurization and can grow in cider if it is not adequately carbonated. Suggestions that the occurrence of mycotoxins such as patulin in mould-rotted apples will lead to carry-over into the cider are unwarranted, since patulin is destroyed during the fermentation process. *See* Mycotoxins, Occurrence and Determination

Reference has been made above to the role of organisms such as *Brettanomyces* species and *Acetobacter xylinum* in the spoilage of ciders during the latter stages of fermentation and maturation. Of equal concern is the yeast *Saccharomycodes ludwigii*, which is often resistant to sulphur dioxide levels as high as 1000–1500 mg l^{-1}.

Saccharomycodes ludwigii can grow slowly during all stages of fermentation and maturation and is often an indigenous contaminant of cidermaking premises. Its presence in bulk stocks of cider does not cause overt problems. However, if it is able to contaminate the 'bright' cider at bottling, its growth will result in a butyric flavour and the presence of flaky particles which spoil the appearance of the product. Although the organism is sensitive to pasteurization processes, it is not unknown for it to contaminate products at the packaging state, either as a low-level contaminant of clean but nonsterile bottles, or from the packaging plant and its environment.

Environmental contamination of final products can also result from other yeasts, such as *Saccharomyces cerevisiae*, *S. bailii* and *S. uvarum*, which will metabolize any residual or added sugar to generate further alcohol and, more importantly, to increase the concentration of carbon dioxide. Strains of these organisms are frequently resistant to sulphur dioxide. In bottles of cider inoculated with such fermentative organisms, carbonation pressures up to 9 bar have been recorded. For this reason it is essential to maintain an adequate level of free sulphur dioxide in the final product, particularly in multiserve containers which may be opened and then stored with a reduced volume of cider; alternatively, a second preservative, such as benzoic or sorbic acid, can be used where permitted by legislation. This precaution is less important for product packaged in single-serve cans and small bottles which receive a terminal pasteurization process after filling.

Special Secondary Fermentation Processes

'Conditioned' Draught Cider

Traditional 'conditioned' draught cider results from a live secondary fermentation process. After filling into barrels, a small quantity of fermentable carbohydrate is added to the cider followed by an inoculum of active, alcohol-resistant yeasts. The subsequent growth is accompanied by a low-level fermentation, during which sufficient carbon dioxide is generated to produce a *pettilance* (sparkle) in the cider, together with a haze of yeast cells. Such products have a relatively short shelf life in the barrel. *See* Barrels

Double-fermented Cider

Double-fermented cider is initially fermented to a lower than normal alcohol content (e.g. 6% alcohol by volume; ABV) by restricting the amount of chaptalization sugar added. The liquor is racked off as soon as the cider has fermented to dryness and is either sterile-filtered or pasteurized prior to transfer to a second sterile fermentation vat. Additional sugar or apple juice is added and a secondary fermentation is induced following inoculation with a different yeast strain, e.g. an alcohol-tolerant strain of *Saccharomyces* species. Such a process permits the development of very complex flavour modifications in the cider.

Sparkling Cider

Sparkling ciders are normally prepared nowadays by artificial carbonation to a level of 2·5–4·5 bar. Traditional sparkling ciders were prepared according to the *méthode champenoise*. After bright filtration of the fully fermented dry cider it was filled into bottles containing a small amount of sugar and an appropriate champagne yeast culture. The bottles were corked and wired and laid on their side for the fermentation process, which lasted for 1–2 months at 18–15°C. Following this stage the bottles were placed in special racks with the neck in a downwards position. The bottles were gently shaken each day to move the deposit down towards the cork, a process which could take up to 2 months.

The disgorging process involved careful removal of the cork and yeast floc, without loss of any liquid (sometimes, the neck of the bottle was frozen to aid this process). The disgorged product was then topped up using a syrup of alcohol, cider and sugar prior to final corking, wiring and labelling. It is not difficult to understand why this process is rarely used nowadays!

Chemistry of Cider

The chemical composition of cider is dependent upon the composition of the apple juice, the nature of the fermentation yeasts, microbial contaminants and their metabolites, and on the nature of any additives used in the final product.

The Composition of Cider Apple Juice

Apple juice is a mixture of sugars (primarily fructose, glucose and sucrose), oligosaccharides and polysaccharides (e.g. starch), together with malic, quinic and citromalic acids, tannins (i.e. polyphenols), amides and other nitrogenous compounds, soluble pectin, vitamin C, minerals and a diverse range of esters which give the

Chemistry and Microbiology of Cidermaking

juice a typical applelike aroma (e.g. ethyl- and methyl-iso-valerate). The relative proportions are dependent upon the variety of apple, the cultural conditions under which it was grown, the state of maturity of the fruit at the time of pressing, the extent of physical and biological damage (i.e. mould rots) and, to a lesser extent, the efficiency with which the juice was pressed from the fruit. *See* Ascorbic Acid, Properties and Determination; Carbohydrates, Classification and Properties; Starch, Structure, Properties and Determination; Tannins and Polyphenols

Treatment of the fresh juice with sulphur dioxide results in the complexing of carbonyl compounds to form stable hydroxysulphonic acids. If the apples contained a high proportion of mould rots then appreciable amounts of carbonyls, such as 2,5-dioxogluconic acid and 2,5-D-threohexodiulose, will occur. Sulphur dioxide is also important in the prevention of enzymatic and nonenzymatic browning reactions of the polyphenols. *See* Browning, Nonenzymatic

Products of the Fermentation Process

The primary objective of fermentation is the production of ethyl alcohol from monosaccharides with the associated formation of carbon dioxide. The biochemical pathways which govern this process are well recognized (Embden–Meyerhof–Parnass pathway).

It is essential to recognize that various intermediates in this metabolic pathway can also be converted to form a diverse range of other metabolites, including glycerol (up to 0.5%). Diacetyl and acetaldehyde may also occur, particularly if the process is inhibited by excess sulphite and/or uncontrolled lactic fermentation occurs. Other metabolic pathways will also operate simultaneously with the formation of long- and short-chain fatty acids, esters, lactones, etc. Methanol will be produced in small quantities ($10–100 \text{ mg l}^{-1}$) as a result of demethylation of pectin in the juice. Table 3 illustrates some of the volatile compounds found in normal and spoiled cider blends.

If other organisms are also present in the fermentation (e.g. lactic acid bacteria), these can convert the fruit acids, malic and quinic acids, to lactic and dihydroshikimic acids, respectively, thereby reducing the acidity of the cider by about 50%. These reactions are accompanied by further diverse but not widely understood chemical changes, which result in subtle, yet important flavour changes in the final product. Lactic and acetic acids can also be formed directly from residual sugars, and great care needs to be taken to avoid excessive production of volatile acids in cider.

The tannins in cider do not change significantly during fermentation although the chlorogenic, caffeic and *p*-coumaryl quinic acids may be reduced to dihydroshikimic acid and ethyl catechol.

The nitrogen content of cider juice comprises a range of amino acids, the most important of which are asparagine, aspartic acid, glutamine and glutamic acid; smaller amounts of proline and 4-hydroxymethylproline also occur. Aromatic amino acids are virtually absent from apple juices. With the exception of proline and 4-hydroxymethylproline, the amino acids will be largely assimilated by the yeasts during fermentation. However, leaving the cider on the lees for an appreciable

Table 3.   Volatile compounds in a normal and a diacetyl-spoiled cider

Compound	Normalized peak area[a]	
	Normal	Spoiled
Ethyl acetate	86.1	89.2
Diacetyl	0.00	3.42
Ethyl-2-methylbutyrate	10.3	12.9
2-Methylpropanol	35.4	97.3
iso-Amyl alcohol	305	213
2- and 3-Methyl-butan-1-ol	503	456
Ethyl hexanoate	233	179
Hexyl acetate	1.95	6.25
Octanol	0.67	1.19
Ethyl lactate	45.9	37.9
Hexan-1-ol	35.7	29.5
Nonanol	0.79	0.86
Unknown ester or acetal (relative molecular mass 172)	25.6	77.7
Ethyl octanoate	280	226
Heptan-1-ol	1.26	0.75
Ethyl octanoate	3.39	11.5
Decan-2-one	3.58	0.90
Benzylaldehyde	1.42	1.41
Ethyl-2-hydroxy-4-methyl pentanoate	4.19	7.03
Ethyl decanoate	57.6	53.4
Decenal	7.52	0.36
Ethyl benzoate	4.70	5.66
Diethyl succinate	5.23	2.88
Unknown ester	3.19	4.93
Methionol	1.29	0.55
Undecanal	2.16	1.23
2-Phenylethyl acetate	11.4	6.42
Hexanoic acid	12.6	12.6
Ethyl dodecanoate	2.10	1.04
2-Phenylethanol	69.0	61.6
Heptanoic acid	0.00	3.39
d-Decalactone	4.39	3.39
Ethyl guaiacol	2.47	4.53
Octanoic acid	34.6	29.4
Nonanoic acid	1.01	1.21
4-Ethylphenol plus eugenol	1.86	1.52

[a] Based on GC–MS (gas chromatography linked to mass spectroscopy) analysis of headspace volatiles.

Chemistry and Microbiology of Cidermaking

length of time will significantly increase the amino nitrogen content as a consequence of release of cell constituents during autolysis. *See* Amino Acids, Properties and Occurrence

Inorganic compounds in cider are derived largely from the fruit and will depend upon the conditions prevailing in the orchard. These levels will not change significantly during fermentation. Small amounts of iron and copper may also occur naturally, but the presence of more than a few milligrams per litre will result in significant black or green discolourations and flavour deterioration. The discolourations are caused by the formation of iron or copper tannates from traces of metal ions, derived from equipment and/or from use of rotten fruit.

Cider Maturation

Maturation will result in further changes in the composition of the cider, but the nature of the changes is poorly understood. A recent doctoral thesis on the subject has been presented in France and this may provide more detailed information, but the thesis is not currently 'in the public domain'!

Commercial Ciders

A final blending of ciders will be made to attain specific characteristics of sweetness, dryness, alcohol content, flavour and aroma. At this stage, sugars, or intense sweeteners such as saccharin, may be added, together with artificial colours, ascorbic acid (as an antioxidant) and additional chemical preservative (e.g. sulphur dioxide or sorbic acid). Prior to, or during, final packaging the cider will be carbonated to give the product a *petillance*, or sparkle. *See* Antioxidants, Synthetic Antioxidants; Colours, Properties and Determination of Synthetic Pigments; Sweeteners – Intense

Bibliography

Beech FW (1972) English cidermaking: technology, microbiology and biochemistry. In: Hockenhull DJD (ed.) *Progress in Industrial Microbiology*, vol 11, pp 133–213. Edinburgh: Churchill Livingstone.

Beech FW and Davenport RR (1983) New prospects and problems in the beverage industry. In: Roberts TA and Skinner FA (eds) *Food Microbiology: Advances and Prospects*. SAB Symposium Series No. 11, pp 241–256. London: Academic Press.

Charley VLS (1949) *The Principles and Practice of Cider-Making*. London: Leonard Hill.

Hammond SM and Carr JG (1976) The antimicrobial activity of SO_2 – with particular reference to fermented and non-fermented fruit juices. In: Skinner FA and Hugo WB (eds) *Inhibition and Inactivation of Vegetative Microbes*. SAB Symposium Series No. 5, pp 89–110. London: Academic Press.

Williams RR (ed.) (1991) *Cider and Juice Apples: Growing and Processing*. Bristol: University of Bristol.

B. Jarvis
HP Bulmer Ltd, Hereford, UK

CIRRHOSIS AND DISORDERS OF HIGH ALCOHOL CONSUMPTION

It is well documented, that heavy drinking of alcoholic beverages carries an increased risk of morbidity and mortality from diseases affecting many organs and may lead to psychic and physical dependence on alcohol. The risks depend on the amount of alcohol consumed, the drinking pattern, and the individual sensitivity. For these reasons, no generally valid threshold value for a safe alcohol consumption can be given. Most authors agree that an upper limit of 80 g of ethanol per day should not be exceeded. A moderate drinker is considered as one who consumes 5–25 g of ethanol per day and a light drinker as one who consumes 0·2–5 g per day (Special Report of the US Congress on Alcohol and Health, 1981).

Alcoholism

Three main patterns of chronic alcohol abuse are described in the *Diagnostic and Statistical Manual of Mental Disorders of the American Psychiatric Association* (1980):

- Regular drinking of large amounts.
- Regular heavy drinking but limited to weekends.
- Episodic binges of heavy daily drinking lasting weeks or months, interrupted by long periods of sobriety.

These criteria for the diagnosis of alcoholism also include an impairment in social or occupational functioning. *Alcoholism* is further distinguished from *alcohol abuse* by tolerance and physical dependence. *Tolerance* is defined as the 'need for markedly increased amounts of alcohol to achieve the desired effect, or a markedly diminished effect with regular use of the same amount'. *Dependence* is defined as 'the development of alcohol withdrawal syndrome after cessation of or reduction in drinking'. *See* Alcohol, Metabolism, Toxicology and Beneficial Effects; Alcohol, Alcohol Consumption

Excessive alcohol intake is often associated with malnutrition. This results from the limited intake of nutritionally adequate foods and from the impairment of digestion, absorption, transport, storage, metabolism and excretion of many nutrients by direct or indirect action of ethanol. The role of nutrient deficiencies in the initiation and progression of the medical complications of alcoholism is still controversial.

Protein malnutrition (kwashiorkor-like) and *protein–energy malnutrition* (marasmus-like) are frequent in alcoholic patients with liver disease and, in some studies, the prevalence of the malnutrition correlates closely with the severity of organ failure. On the other hand, many patients who drink to excess are clearly not protein–energy-malnourished. Ethanol has appreciable effects on amino acid metabolism. Intestinal absorption and transport of isoleucine, arginine and methionine are impaired by high concentrations of ethanol. Branched-chain amino acids and α-amino-*N*-butyric acid are increased in the plasma of alcoholics. *See* Protein, Deficiency

Vitamin deficiencies are frequent in alcoholics and especially in those with liver disease. Most common is an insufficient *folate* supply, characterized by megaloblastic anaemia and macrocytosis of the intestinal epithelium. Many factors contribute to folate deficiency in alcoholics. These include dietary deficiency, intestinal malabsorption, impairment of uptake and/or storage in the liver and increased urinary excretion. Poor dietary intake is undoubtedly the major cause, with the exception of heavy beer drinkers: 2 l of beer contain nearly 50% of the recommended daily allowance of folate for an adult man. The combined effect of low folate concentration in the diet and heavy alcohol drinking leads to damage of intestinal mucosal epithelial structures, often associated with diarrhoea, and results in malabsorpton of folates and other nutrients. Symptoms of *vitamin B12* deficiency are much less common than those of folate deficiency in alcoholics. This is probably attributable to the large stores of vitamin B_{12} in the body and the reserve capacity for absorption. In most studies the circulating levels of vitamin B_{12} in alcoholics are no different from normal controls. *See* Cobalamins, Physiology; Folic Acid, Physiology

As with folate, poor dietary intake and an impairment of absorption are the main causes for unsufficient *thiamin* supply in alcoholics. Alcohol inhibits active transport of thiamin across the intestinal mucosa, whereas the passive transport remains unimpaired. In addition, hepatic storage of thiamin may be reduced owing to fatty infiltration of the liver, hepatocellular damage, or cirrhosis in chronic alcoholic patients. Extreme thiamin deficiency is responsible for the Wernicke–Korsakoff syndrome, beriberi and polyneuropathy in alcoholics. *See* Thiamin, Physiology

The incidence of *pyridoxine* deficiency in alcoholic patients, as defined by low plasma levels of its circulating form, pyridoxal-5-phosphate (PLP), is more than 50% in different studies. Clinical data indicate that malnutrition, rather than the amount and duration of alcohol abuse, is the major determinant of pyridoxine deficiency. Pyridoxine absorption is primarily passive and is affected only by very high concentrations of ethanol. Pyridoxal 5-phosphate in erythrocytes and liver is more rapidly destroyed in the presence of acetaldehyde, the first metabolite of ethanol oxidation, perhaps by displacement of PLP from protein and its exposure to phosphatases. This results in high pyridoxic acid excretion in the urine. Clinical signs of pyridoxine deficiency in alcoholics are infrequent. Sideroblastic bone marrow changes often occur in alcoholics with low plasma PLP values, but most of these patients also suffer from liver disease and folate deficiency. *See* Vitamin B6, Properties and Determination

Studies of *vitamin A* deficiency in alcoholism have mainly concerned patients with established cirrhosis, which may have impaired storage or transport of vitamin A because of an inadequate synthesis of retinol-binding protein. Most of them also have inadequate dietary intake. Other complications of alcoholism, e.g. pancreatic and biliary insufficiency, lead to malabsorption of vitamin A because this fat-soluble vitamin requires for its absorption adequate quantities of pancreatic lipases and bile salts in the small intestine. Another possible mechanism for low hepatic vitamin A level is increased hepatic metabolism of retinoic acid to polar metabolites through the action of microsomal enzymes, which are inducible by ethanol consumption. The clinical consequences of insufficient vitamin A supply in alcoholics are increased incidence of night blindness, follicular keratosis and corneal ulcerations. Alcoholics with these complications often require both vitamin A and zinc treatment to correct visual dysfunction, because of an association between zinc and vitamin A metabolism. *Zinc* is an essential cofactor in the conversion of retinol to retinaldehyde in the retina. Alcohol appears to stimulate the release of zinc from hepatic stores, and its urinary excretion. Zinc levels in plasma and red blood cells are often reduced in humans after chronic alcohol ingestion. *See* Retinol, Physiology; Zinc, Physiology

Vitamin D intake, absorption and metabolism seem to be impaired in alcoholics, and there are abnormalities of *phosphorus*, *calcium* and *magnesium* homeostasis. Alcoholic patients often suffer from decreased bone mass and an increased incidence of fractures. *See* Calcium, Physiology; Cholecalciferol, Physiology; Magnesium

Alcoholic Cirrhosis

Alcohol is the most common cause of cirrhosis in Western countries. The incidence of this disease in alcoholics depends upon the mean daily intake of alcohol and the mean duration of alcohol consumption. However, only about 20% of heavy drinkers develop cirrhosis, and liver disease may progress to cirrhosis after cessation of ethanol ingestion. This fact suggests that other factors superimposed on alcohol drinking are involved in the pathogenesis of this severe form of liver injury. These include gender, genetic or immunological variables, other hepatotoxins, nutrition, viral hepatitis and others. Individual predisposition is an important physiological factor in the development of this disease. *See* Liver, Nutritional Management of Liver and Biliary Disorders

Morphologically, cirrhosis of the liver is a diffuse process, characterized by an excessive proliferation of connective tissue and the deposition of structurally abnormal nodules. Alcoholic cirrhosis is mostly micronodular in type, with a size of nodules from 1 to 5 mm. Macronodules with a size ranging from 5 to 50 mm may occur, especially in the late phases of the disease. The loss of normal liver architecture, with separation of the portal tracts and the central zones of the liver by septa of fibrotic tissue, results in alterations of the vascular supply and a disturbance of the intrahepatic blood circulation.

Morbidity and mortality resulting from alcoholic cirrhosis are related principally to the loss of liver cell function, to derangements in the vascular system of the liver, or to both. The onset of cirrhosis is often insidious and associated with nonspecific symptoms such as fatigue, anorexia, weight loss, nausea and abdominal discomfort. As the disease progresses, signs of hepatocellular failure became prominent. The most severe complications are iron overload, hepatic encephalopathy and portal hypertension with ascites and bleeding from oesophageal varices.

In association with cirrhosis of the liver, hepatocellular carcinoma may develop. The pathogenesis of the carcinomatous transformation is still unclear, especially because these tumour forms may also occur in noncirrhotic livers.

Ethanol leads to a number of metabolic and structural alterations in the liver that predispose this organ to derangements in its functional integrity. These are as follows: an increase in the ratio of NADH (the reduced form of nicotinamide adenine dinucleotide, or NAD) to NAD; interactions of ethanol with lipid and protein metabolism; stimulation of fibrosis with deposition of collagen; inhibition of liver cell regeneration; humoral and cellular immunological alterations; and others. Acetaldehyde, the first oxidation product of ethanol metabolism, may exert some toxic effects of its own in liver tissue.

All stages of liver injury can be produced in the baboon fed high-protein and vitamin-supplemented diets. This evidence suggests that toxic effects of alcohol, and not malnutrition, are the principal causes for the development of cirrhosis in chronic alcoholics. But alcohol abuse establishes only the conditions for the generation of cirrhotic lesions, which require the addition of some independent factors emerging over time.

Abstinence from alcohol is the essential factor for prevention and treatment of alcoholic cirrhosis. If irreversible liver damage is already established, some complications of cirrhosis can be alleviated by nutritional treatment. Portal-systemic encephalopathy, for example, often responds to an application of amino acid mixtures, enriched with branched-chain amino acids, whereas ascites responds favourably to sodium restriction.

Wernicke's Encephalopathy and Korsakoff's Syndrome

Wernicke's encephalopathy and Korsakoff's psychosis are diseases of the central nervous system (CNS) secondary to alcoholism. They represent a continuum of the same neuropathological process and develop in about 2–3% of alcoholics. Wernicke's disease is often followed by Korsakoff's syndrome. Severe alcoholics may have both diseases, but some of them show Korsakoff's psychosis without preceding Wernicke's encephalopathy. Wernicke's disease is an acute or chronic encephalopathy with a triad of clinical abnormalities: ophthalmoplegia, ataxia, and mental confusion. Korsakoff's syndrome is a psychosis with marked abnormalities in cognitive function: the cardinal symptoms are anterograde amnesia, disorientation, learning deficits, and confabulations. The relationship between the two diseases is not entirely clear. The neuropathological changes seen in autopsy materials of Wernicke–Korsakoff patients consist of circumscribed, symmetrical lesions in the diencephalon and brain stem. Most affected are the mammillary bodies and the dorsomedial nuclei of the thalamus. In acute cases the lesions are widespread and severe. In chronic cases the lesions are more restricted and show great variations in extent and severity within the affected area. There are corresponding variations of the clinical symptoms.

Extreme deficiency of thiamin, induced by malnutrition and interaction of ethanol with thiamin absorption and metabolism, is regarded as the primary cause of this syndrome. Patients with Wernicke's disease often have a high energy intake, consisting mainly of ethanol and/or carbohydrates, without sufficient protein and vitamins. Beyond that a direct toxic effect of alcohol on the brain has also been implicated. The Wernicke–Korsakoff's disease is not confined to alcoholism, but is also present in other conditions associated with thiamin malnutrition, e.g. hyperemesis gravidarum, Hodgkin's lymphoma, carcinoma of the stomach, and anorexia nervosa. Thiamin application can reverse Wernicke's syndrome in many but not all patients, at least when administered early in the course of the disease. In contrast, Korsakoff's patients often show poor response to thiamin therapy. Additional factors, of as yet unknown origin, seem to be necessary for the full development of Korsakoff's psychosis. There is evidence to suggest that a genetic predisposition is involved in the aetiology of the Wernicke–Korsakoff syndrome. In some patients a variant form of transketolase with a low affinity for its coenzyme thiamin pyrophosphate has been diagnosed. This isoenzyme requires much larger amounts of thiamin to function than the normal enzyme. Some authors suggest that a variant transketolase and thiamin deficiency together contribute to the pathogenesis of the brain damage of the Wernicke–Korsakoff syndrome. In other studies this hypothesis has not been confirmed. *See* Anorexia Nervosa

Alcoholic Polyneuropathy, and Beriberi in Alcoholics

Symmetric and predominantly distal polyneuropathy is probably the most common sequela of chronic alcohol abuse. It occurs in about 20% of all alcoholics. First symptoms include paraesthesia, dysaesthesia and pain sensations affecting primarily the lower extremities, accompanied by reduced or absent reflex activity. These symptoms are usually followed in the more advanced stages of the disease by marked motor impairments, such as weakness and atrophy of the anterior tibial muscles. Electrophysiological slow-down of the sensory and motor conduction velocities of the peripheral nerves, as well as myopathic changes, are usually observed. The predominant pathological abnormalities are distal pronounced axonal degenerations, mainly of the large fibres with a gradient of changes toward the extremities ('dying-back degeneration'). Segmental demyelination appears as a secondary phenomenon. Alcoholic polyneuropathy is clinically indistinguishable from beriberi ('dry beriberi') neuropathy. As in the Wernicke–Korsakoff syndrome, thiamin deficiency is regarded as the primary cause. Besides that, a long-lasting low protein–energy supply seems to be one of the main pathogenic factors for the development of the

typical lesions of peripheric nerves. In addition, insufficient intake or absorption of pyridoxine, folates, B_{12} and other B-vitamins contribute to the development of the disease, and direct toxic effects of ethanol and its metabolites are involved in the destruction of nerve ultrastructure and function. Recovery from alcoholic peripheral neuropathy is slow and often incomplete. The most important therapeutic factors are abstinence from alcohol and improvement of the overall nutritional status. Additional supplementation with high doses of B-complex vitamins is necessary. With this therapeutic schedule a slow diminution of symptoms may be expected in many but not all cases.

Pancreatitis

The association between alcohol consumption and pancreatitis is well recognized. In general, about 60–90% of all cases of chronic pancreatitis are alcohol-related. As with alcoholic cirrhosis, there has been an increasing prevalence of alcoholic pancreatitis in industrialized countries in the last 30 years. This disease often develops without obvious clinical symptoms. However, in autopsies of patients with a history of alcoholism, marked pancreatic lesions are frequently observed. Patients with severe or complicated forms of this disease may rapidly develop marked generalized malnutrition. *See* Gall Bladder

A favoured hypothesis regarding the mechanism of action of chronic alcohol consumption on the pancreas is the observation, that ethanol increases the protein content of pancreatic juice, with a concomitant decrease in water and electrolytes. This induces a precipitation of protein plugs within the pancreatic ducts, followed by retraction and calcification, resulting in pancreatic stones, atrophy of the duct epithelium and proliferation of the connective tissue. The consequences are stenosis or dilatations of the ducts, cysts and pseudocysts, and progressive disappearance of the pancreatic exocrine tissue which is replaced by fibrosis. Pathologically, the gland is oedematous and haemorrhagic. Besides chronic overconsumption of alcohol, both a high-fat, high-protein diet and, paradoxically, malnutrition have been implicated in the pathogenesis of the disorder.

Alcoholic pancreatitis tends to be recurrent and progressive and to result in pancreatic exocrine insufficiency. One or two per cent of alcoholics suffer from an acute form. This complication can be quite severe, with violent epigastric pain, nausea and vomiting. Cases of sudden death from acute attacks have been reported.

Effect of Chronic Alcohol Consumption on the Brain

Ethanol – in common with other centrally acting agents – rapidly diffuses across the blood–brain barrier and equilibrates in brain tissue. Its concentration depends upon the plasma concentration, vascularization, local blood flow and water content of the concerned brain area. Chronic ethanol consumption is associated with a variety of deficits in brain function over a wide range of doses and is often followed by clinically obvious brain damage.

Alcoholic Dementia

Alcoholics often suffer from disorders in cognitive processes, varying from a relatively slight memory reduction to deep dementia. The deficits in cognitive function are similar to those seen in patients with Alzheimer's disease or multiinfarct dementia. Histopathologically, the possibly involved brain structures do not show any lesion or atrophy, but there is considerable evidence that alcoholic dementia may potentially result from progressive loss of some neurons, synapses and/or their associated receptors. Prolonged abstinence has a considerable reducing effect on dementia symptoms, but in most subjects the reversibility is only partial.

Alcohol Tolerance and Dependence

Functional tolerance and physical dependence are inexorably linked phenomena reflecting adaptive changes in the brain which compensate for the inhibition of functions by ethanol. Functional tolerance means a decrease in the sensitivity of the CNS produced by chronic alcohol intake. Physical dependence means hyperexcitability of the CNS following alcohol withdrawal after adaptation. The molecular mechanisms underlying both phenomena are as yet unknown. Possibly the effects are primarily related to changes in the microorganization and physical state of brain membranes.

Brain Shrinkage

Cerebral shrinkage seems to be one of the most frequent brain lesions induced by chronic alcohol consumption. It can be demonstrated by computerized tomography (CT) scanning in patients with alcoholism and even in 'social drinkers'. Cerebral shrinkage relates to a loss of white matter rather than of grey matter. In alcoholics the shrinking results in a lower brain weight compared to age- and sex-matched controls. After cessation of alcohol drinking cerebral shrinkage is often partially reversed.

Cerebellar Atrophy

Many alcoholics show cerebellar atrophy with progressive ataxia of stance and gait and, occasionally, an impairment of speech and ocular motility. This cerebellar degeneration is characterized by great uniformity of the clinical and pathological manifestations. In the majority of cases the disorder develops over several weeks or months, followed by years of stability. The pathological changes consist of degeneration of neuronal elements of the cerebellar cortex, particularly of the Purkinje cells. The dendritic networks of these cells show alterations in length parameters under the influence of ethanol in rats. Topographically, the lesions of the cerebellum are restricted to the anterior and superior vermis and to the hemispheres.

Although cerebellar atrophy is most frequently encountered in chronic alcoholic patients, it has also been reported in old people and in malnourished individuals, who allegedly did not drink. It has been postulated that alcohol and the ageing process superimposed upon malnutrition may be responsible for the damage caused to the cerebellum.

Fetal Alcohol Syndrome

Prenatal exposure to alcohol produces various morphological, physiological and behavioural abnormalities in the newborn, termed fetal alcohol syndrome (FAS). It has been observed in 1 in every 300 children born to alcoholic mothers, and is the most common known cause of mental retardation. *The Fetal Alcohol Study Group of the Research Society on Alcoholism* has defined three criteria for diagnosis of FAS:

- Growth retardation.
- Abnormalities of the CNS.
- Abnormal facial features.

The mechanisms by which alcohol produces these effects are not yet elucidated, and the minimum level of alcohol consumed during pregnancy that causes FAS has not been established. Animal models have demonstrated conclusively that ethanol can cross the placenta and is teratogenic in several species. The effect is dose-dependent and the type of malformation observed depends upon the stage of development when the exposure occurred. Besides the toxic effects of ethanol, another potential cause of FAS is maternal and/or fetal malnutrition induced by impaired placental transfer of essential nutrients.

Among the neuroanatomical alterations observed in humans and animal models with FAS are decreased brain weight, delays in dendritic development, decreased numbers of pyramidal neurons in the hippocampus, and sprouting in the dentate gyrus. The clinical symptoms of the CNS dysfunction are mental retardation, hyperactivity and learning disabilities. Despite nutritional rehabilitation, the physical and mental development of the children remains impaired. To date, a safe intake of alcohol for pregnant women has not been established. *See* Pregnancy, Safe Diet

Bibliography

Bitsch I (1983) Perspektiven der Alkoholforschung. *Ernäh-rungs-Umschau* 30: 132–135.

Bitsch R (1987) Alkohol und Vitaminstoffwechsel. *Ernäh-rungs-Umschau* 34: 161–166.

Brown ML (ed.) (1990) *Present Knowledge in Nutrition* 6th edn. Washington, DC.

Eriksson K, Sinclair JD and Kiianmaa K (eds) (1980) *Animal Models in Alcohol Research*. London.

Kalant H, Khanna JM and Israel Y (1991) *Advances in Biomedical Alcohol Research*. Oxford.

Lindros KO, Ylikahri R and Kiianmaa K (1987) *Advances in Biomedical Alcohol Research*. Oxford.

Majchrowicz E and Noble EP (eds) *Biochemistry and Pharma-cology of Ethanol*, vols I and II. New York.

National Research Council (1989) *Diet and Health: Implica-tions for Reducing Chronic Disease Risk*. Washington, DC.

Shils ME and Young VR (eds) (1988) *Modern Nutrition in Health and Disease* 7th edn. Philadelphia.

The Surgeon General's Report on Nutrition and Health. (1988) Washington, DC.

Torvik A (1987) Brain lesions in alcoholics: neuropathological observations. *Acta Medica Scandinavica Supplementum* 717: 47–54.

Victor M, Adams RD and Collins GH (1989) *The Wernicke-Korsakoff Syndrome* 2nd edn. Philadelphia.

Irmgard Bitsch
Institut für Ernährungswissenschaft, Giessen, FRG

CITRIC ACID CYCLE

See Tricarboxylic Acid Cycle and Oxidative Phosphorylation

CITRUS FRUITS

Contents

Types on the Market

Citrus is the main fruit tree crop grown throughout the world. It is made up of many species that vary in importance due to different climatic zones. The large production has significance in both local and world trade for both fresh and processed products.

Classification

The taxonomic classification of the *Citrus* species is complex and not universally agreed upon, but that used by Swingle and Reece (1967) will be followed in this article.

Citrus trees belong to the plant family Rutaceae, subfamily Aurantioideae, which comprises 33 well-known and well-described genera and 203 species. In addition, many natural and man-made hybrids have resulted in new edible cultivars or rootstocks. Many genera contain unusual or remote relatives of citrus that have nonedible fruit, but are of ornamental value, such as *Merrillia* and *Murraya*, or have genetic importance in breeding programmes, e.g. *Poncirus* and *Severinia*.

True citrus fruit trees, which have a berry fruit called a hesperidium, belong to six genera: *Citrus*, *Fortunella*, *Poncirus*, *Microcitrus*, *Eremocitrus* and *Clymenia*. Only the *Citrus* and *Fortunella* genera have fresh fruit culti-vars of commercial importance. Both these genera are evergreen and unifoliate, and the genus *Citrus* provides nearly all of the commercial cultivars grown throughout the world.

The main types of citrus fresh fruits on the export or main local markets are normally broadly grouped as oranges, mandarins, lemons and limes, and grapefruit. There is also a wide range of other minor or lesser known species and types that may have regional or local significance. Some of these are mentioned in a later section. The following brief comments are on the classification of the main citrus types.

Sweet Oranges

The sweet orange types (*Citrus sinensis* [L] Osbeck) are the most widely grown citrus throughout the world and provide the greatest fruit marketing production. The many known cultivars can be subdivided into three main groups as the acidless or sugar oranges do not contribute to world trade:

- Common oranges (also known as blond or white oranges)
- Navel oranges
- Blood or pigmented oranges.

Mandarins

Mandarins are also referred to as 'tangerines' in some countries. The mandarin group, with related hybrids, is very diverse but can be classified into four main groups, some of which contain a large number of subgroups and cultivars:

- Satsuma mandarins (*C. unshiu* Marcovitch) (also know as Unshiu mikan in Japan and China)
- King mandarins (*C. nobilis* Loureiro)
- Mediterranean mandarin (*C. deliciosa* Tenore) (also knownn as Willowleaf)
- Common mandarins (*C. reticulata* Blanco), including the clementines and two hybrid groups, have commercial cultivars that are available in world markets, i.e. tangors which are hybrids of the mandarin and orange, while tangelos are hybrids of the mandarin and grapefruit or pummelo.

Lemons

The lemon (*C. limon* [L] Burm. f.) is an important fresh fruit group in world markets. Even though not eaten fresh, they are widely used for their fresh acid juice content, in slices and for processing. A minor related group of sweet or acidless cultivars and hybrids also exists.

Limes

Limes are also a varied group that consist mainly of two broad subgroups:

- Acid limes – small-fruited (*C. aurantifolia* Swing) and large-fruited (*C. latifolia* Tan)
- Sweet limes (*C. limettiodes* Tan), also known as the Palestine or Indian sweet lime.

Grapefruit

Grapefruit (*C. paradisi* Macfadyen) is one of the newer types of citrus. It contains two distinct natural groups:

- Common or white-fleshed
- Pigmented, where the older cultivars were considered 'pink'-fleshed, while newer selections, mutations or cultivars bred in the USA are now classified as 'red'-fleshed, due to deeper pigmentation in both the rind and flesh.

A recent breeding programme in California, where an acidless pummelo was crossed with a white seedy grapefruit, has resulted in the selection and release of two new, low-acid grapefruit type cultivars – Melogold and Oroblanco.

Growing Regions and Conditions

Production regions are located in a wide range of climatic conditions, including the humid tropics, arid subtropics and intermediate climates. Commercial production tends to be located in two narrow belts in the sub-tropics and between 20° and 40° latitude north and south of the equator.

Citrus grows best in cooler, frost-free, Mediterranean-type climates, provided soils are suitable and rainfall is at least 1200 mm, distributed evenly throughout the year or supplemented by irrigation. Climate can significantly affect fruit quality and tree health. In particular, minimum temperatures and degrees of frost restrict commercial production within many countries of the world.

Some cultivars have been bred or selected to extend production into marginally cooler climates, e.g. satsuma mandarins. Limes and pummelos grow well in tropical areas where the normal rind colour of oranges does not develop. High-quality grapefruit tend to be grown in hot desert areas.

Commercial citrus production is recorded by the Food and Agriculture Organization (FAO) in 100 different countries and throughout six regions – Africa, North America, South America, Asia, Europe and Oceania.

Types on the Market

The largest growing areas are located in the northern hemisphere, where 69% of world production occurs, and include the important Mediterranean region and the USA. The southern hemisphere (31%) includes the largest producer in the world – Brazil. Some countries, such as Japan, China, Mexico and Southeast Asia, have important local markets for fresh citrus fruits, while others, such as Spain, Israel, Cuba and South Africa, depend on exports as a major outlet for much of their production.

In the two largest producing countries (Brazil and the USA) a large percentage of the production is processed into frozen concentrated orange juice and then exported throughout the world. Details of the relative importance of the main citrus producing countries in respect to world citrus production in 1989–1990 are shown in Fig. 1.

Production Statistics

The world's citrus production has been gradually increasing from an average for 1976–1981 of $53\,014 \times 10^3$ t to a total of $64\,489 \times 10^3$ t in 1989–1990. The production trends and percentage of the main citrus types grown are shown in Fig. 2. For the 1988–1989 season, other citrus types totalled only 1257×10^3 t, with 52% of this production recorded in Asia.

Information on fresh citrus crop utilization and percentages exported and processed by producing countries for the three crops 1987–1988, 1988–1989 and 1989–1990 are shown in Table 1. World citrus production by types in 1989–1990 is given in Table 2.

Utilization of Lesser Known Types

Some minor and lesser known citrus fruit types which have fresh or processing uses and which have some market importance in different parts of the world are listed in alphabetical order. In many situations local names exist for some of these types.

ˉergamot (*C. bergamia* Risso)

·rgamot appears to be a variant of the sour orange and is mainly grown for rind oil in the coastal region of Calabria, a province of Italy.

Calamondin (*C. madurensis* Loureiro)

Resembles the mandarin and is grown extensively in the Orient, China, Taiwan, Japan and the Philippines. The fresh fruit is sour, but widely used for processing and as an ornamental tree.

Types on the Market

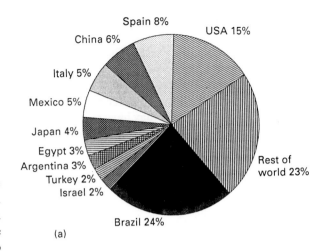

(a)

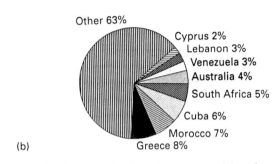

(b)

Fig. 1 World citrus production, 1989–1990: (a) major producers; (b) rest of world (percentages shown are of rest of world component only). (Reproduced from FAO (1989) with permission.)

Citrons (*C. medica* L.)

Like the other members of the acid group of lemons and limes, citrons also have two classes, the acid and the sweet, each with several cultivars. The etrog citron is used in Jewish religious ceremonies.

Citrus hystrix

Citrus hystrix belongs to the subgenus *Papeda*, is also known as the Kaffir lime and is widely grown in Indonesia and Asia. It has unusual looking leaves (with a large winged petiole) and is used as a seasoning for food and in cooking, as the fruit is normally not eaten.

Kumquats (*Fortunella* spp.)

Also known as cumquats, these have the smallest size of the true citrus fruits. Several distinct cultivars that bear edible fruits are known:

- *Nagami* or oval kumquat (*F. margarita* [Lour.] Swing)
- *Marumi* or round kumquat (*F. japonica* [Thumb.] Swing)

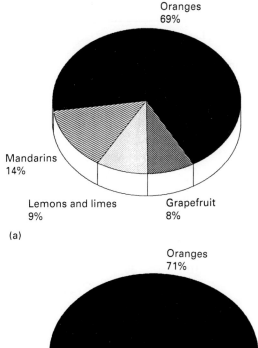

Oranges
69%

Mandarins
14%

Lemons and limes
9%

Grapefruit
8%

(a)

Oranges
71%

Mandarins
13%

Lemons and limes
10%

Grapefruit
6%

(b)

Fig. 2 World citrus production trends by major type: (a) average, 1976/1977–1980/1981; (b) total, 1989–1990. (Reproduced from FAO (1989) with permission.)

Table 1. Fresh citrus crop utilization and percentage exported and processed

Year	Total production ($\times 10^3$ t)	Exported ($\times 10^3$ t)	Processed ($\times 10^3$ t)
1987–1988	61 842	7500 (12%)	19 751 (32%)
1988–1989	63 067	7577 (12%)	24 085 (38%)
1989–1990	64 489	7052 (11%)	21 197 (33%)

Source: FAO (1991).

- *Meiwa* or large round kumquat (*F. crassifolia* Swing).

Several minor kumquats are also grown mainly for ornamental purposes, e.g. Hong Kong (*F. hindsii* Swing) and Malayan (*F. polyandra* Tan).

Pummelo

Also known as shaddock or pomelo (*C. grandis* [L] Osbeck), the pummelo is the largest of the citrus fruits. The pummelo hybridize very readily, and this has resulted in acid, acidless or sweet, pigmented or nonpigmented cultivars being grown. This citrus type is common in some Asian countries, e.g. Thailand, China and Indonesia, but is not common in Western countries or on world markets.

Sour Oranges (*C. aurantium* L.)

Also known as bitter oranges, sour oranges have only minor uses as fresh fruit and are normally used for processing (marmalade or rind oil) or rootstocks. Most cultivars can be classified into three groups:

- Common, bitter or sour oranges, of which the Seville is the most important
- Bitter sweet orange
- Variant bitter oranges.

Industrial Uses of Citrus Crops

Citrus fruits are principally consumed in two forms:

1. As fresh or dessert fruits – sweet oranges, mandarins (eaten out of hand), grapefruit or pummelo (spooned). Slices and segments are also used to garnish food.
2. As processed juice – fresh, chilled, frozen, canned, blended or concentrated. There has been an increasing trend, particularly among the common orange types, for large volumes of fruit to be processed mainly into frozen concentrated orange juice throughout the world. Of the two largest producing countries, Brazil is reported to have processed 67% of their total 1989–1990 production and the USA 63%.

After the juice is extracted, there remain residues which can be a source material from which over 300 valuable by-products can be produced.

Whole Peel or Rind (pericarp)

Whole peel is used for such products as marmalade, candied, brined or dried peel, bioflavonoids, tangeretin, limettin and peel seasonings. Combined with the pulp residue, it becomes feed for animals, molasses, syrups, alcohols and distilled oils.

Flavedo (exterior yellow peel, epicarp)

Flavedo contains the oil glands or vesicles (sacs) from which the cold-pressed and distilled oils and essences are extracted for the aromatic and flavouring industries.

Table 2. World citrus production by types, 1989–1990

Country/region	Oranges ($\times 10^3$ t)	Mandarins ($\times 10^3$ t)	Lemons and limes ($\times 10^3$ t)	Grapefruit ($\times 10^3$ t)
Mediterranean region				
Greece	932	76	189	—
Italy	2170	524	740	7
Spain	2651	1457	720	22
Israel	855	155	44	405
Algeria	—	111	6	2
Morocco	793	243	10	10
Tunisia	175	32	17	50
Cyprus	172	—	61	102
Egypt	1450	155	212	—
Lebanon	270	—	—	—
Turkey	797	331	316	36
Others	271	124	167	71
Subtotal (Mediterranean)	10 536	3208	2482	705
Northern hemisphere				
US	7143	269	633	1772
USSR	350	—	—	—
Japan	239	2379	—	—
Cuba	520	30	70	400
Mexico	2200	169	709	100
China	3715	378	148	235
Others	4788	1134	892	457
Subtotal (northern)	29 491	7567	4934	3669
Southern hemisphere				
Argentina	750	240	500	170
Brazil	14 150	482	614	25
Chile	—	—	60	—
Uruguay	111	43	48	—
Venezuela	432	—	—	—
Australia	486	42	35	30
South Africa	640	—	61	130
Others	149	—	—	8
Subtotal (southern)	16 718	807	1318	363
Total (world)	46 209	8374	6252	4032

Source: FAO (1991).

Natural carotenoids may also be produced and are used in the preparation of colour concentrates for juice and beverage products.

Albedo (interior white spongy peel, mesocarp)

Rich in pectin, albedo is used extensively in commercial gelling agents for jams, jellies, desserts, candies and in the pharmaceutical industry as a suspension material in medicines. *See* Pectin, Food Uses

Pulp (principal edible portion, endocarp)

The juice vesicles of the segments, and the cell contents of the juice vesicles are commercially extracted by mechanical methods to produce the raw juice. The juice is then 'finished' by screening and is ready for preparing and packaging. The material screened from the raw juice is available for products such as clouding agents for juices. This residue from the screening process is also called pulp and is usually combined with other residues to produce many by-products.

Pulp Residue

Pulp residue consists of the fraction screened from the pulp: cores, segment walls or membranes, juice vesicles and seeds. The juice vesicles are sometimes used for

Types on the Market

drying into flours or powders. The pulp residue, or rag, is usually combined with the peel residue for the manufacture of by-products. From the lime-treated mass of peel and pulp residues, citrus processors produce such products as stripper (distilled) oil, press liquor, citrus molasses, pressed peel, citrus pulp, citrus meal, citric and lactic acids, citrus wine, citrus alcohol, citrus vinegar, bland syrup, butylene glycol, brandy spirits and feed yeast.

Seeds

Sometimes separated from the rag to produce seed oils, seed meals and dried seed pressed cake, high in protein for animal feeds.

Waste Waters (aqueous effluent emulsions) from Processing Plants

The waste waters have potential uses for producing methane, activated sludge and yeast.

In addition, the leaves and blossoms can also be utilized for valuable products such as edible fresh or dried leaves, oils for perfumes, and honey.

Bibliography

FAO (1989) *Production Annual Yearbook*, 43: 214–217. Rome: Food and Agriculture Organization.

FAO (1991) *Citrus Fruit Fresh and Processed, Annual Statistics*, pp 22–26. Rome: Food and Agriculture Organization.

Reuther W, Webber HJ and Batchelor LD (eds) (1967) *The Citrus Industry*, vol. 1. University of California, Berkeley: Division of Agricultural Science.

Saunt J (1990) *Citrus Varieties of the World*. Norwich: Sinclair International.

Sinclair WB (1984) *The Biochemistry and Physiology of the Lemon and other Citrus Fruits*, pp 711–718. University of California, Berkeley, Division of Agricultural and Natural Resources.

Swingle WT and Reece PC (1967) The botany of citrus and its wild relatives. In: Reuther W, Webber HJ and Batchelor LD (eds) *The Citrus Industry*, vol. 1. University of California, Berkeley: Division of Agricultural Science.

Young RH (1986) Fresh citrus cultivars. In: Wardowski WF, Nagy S and Grierson W (eds) *Fresh Citrus Fruits*, pp 110–125. Westpoint, Connecticut: AVI Publishing.

USDA (1990) Fresh citrus: production, exports and processing. *Horticultural Products Review* June: 22–23.

Hugh Cope
Adelaide, Australia
J. B. Forsyth
NSW Agriculture, Sydney, Australia

Composition and Characterization

Citrus fruits, with a total world production of about 65 million tonnes (1989), are the second largest fruit crop, surpassed only by grapes (cereal crops are even larger, but it is not usual to consider grains as fruits). About 30% of citrus fruits are processed to obtain various products, mainly juice. Similarly, the citrus industry is also the second largest fruit-processing industry, surpassed again by the grape industry, which mainly produces wine. Neither orange juice nor wine can be considered essential foods but they do have an important role in our lives.

Although citrus fruits have been consumed since ancient times, citrus processing, as it is known today, was not possible until thermal treatment (to inactivate enzymes and microorganisms) and concentration processes were commercially available. Since then, the citrus industry has developed rapidly, becoming prominent among food industries.

Although consumption of fresh citrus fruits is popular in all producing countries, processed products must still be considered almost as luxury products. Breakfast with orange juice is only common in developed countries. Thus, citrus industries process value-added products whose quality, nutritional characteristics, and purity are appreciated. Since these three aspects are closely related with composition, the analysis of citrus constituents is a frequent subject of research work, supported by governments and industries.

This article covers the most important aspects of citrus fruit composition, its relationship to nutritional value, and its importance for product authentication. Several books have been published on these subjects and the Bibliography lists some of them as well as published composition tables.

Constituents

The genus *Citrus* has many species and the differences among them are of great interest to specialists. However, from a general point of view, the similarities are greater than the differences, which is not surprising when considering species of the same genus. The economic importance also differs among species and compositional studies of the main species are more frequent. Thus, data from *Citrus sinensis* (sweet orange) are more extensive than from *C. reticulata* (tangerine), *C. limon* (lemon) or *C. paradisi* (grapefruit), and data from these species are more comprehensive than from other *Citrus* species. Within each species some varieties are better known than others. Valencia orange is the best studied sweet orange, since it is the most important variety for juice extraction, the main citrus product. Thus, most information given here will refer to the juice rather than to the fruit, since juice, accounting for about half of the total weight of an orange, is the most important part of the fruit, and is the part of the fruit mainly consumed by humans.

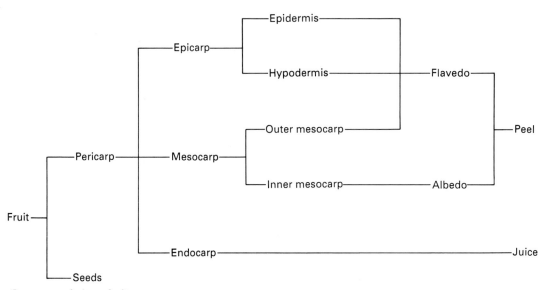

Fig. 1 Structure of citrus fruits.

Orange peel constitutes most of the other half of the fruit, but peel is of much less importance than juice. Although some by-products (cattle feed, molasses) are obtained from peel, it is more a question of removing residues and avoiding pollution than of economic interest. Only peel oil (obtained before or during juice obtention) and pectins (obtained only from suitable species and varieties) are important peel products for human consumption, perfumery and cosmetics.

Our knowledge of the chemical composition of juice and fruits is being continuously improved. The efficiency of instrumental methods of analysis allows the rapid identification of more and more minor constituents. But the basic, major constituents have been well known since the application to citrus research of classical methods of analysis, which are still of interest for some rapid determinations. Both types of methods will be considered in this article, but it must be pointed out that analysis is a dynamic discipline and methods (mainly instrumental) are continuously being improved. Many of them seeming almost perfect today will look old-fashioned tomorrow.

Citrus fruit parts are represented schematically in Fig. 1, and the approximate constitution of oranges is shown in Table 1. Juice vesicles, located in the endocarp, contain the juice, which constitutes about 50% of the total weight of a typical orange fruit. The peel is formed by the flavedo (epicarp and outer mesocarp) and the albedo (inner mesocarp). Flavedo and albedo account, respectively, for about 10 and 25% of the whole fruit. The flavedo contains peel oil in the oil sacs and the albedo most of the pectins. After juice extraction, rag, pulp and seeds account for the rest of the total fruit weight. Most of the fruit, almost 90%, is water. The rest is mainly formed by sugars and acids. Minerals, amino acids, aroma compounds and pectins are present in

Table 1. Approximate composition of oranges

Overall composition (%)	
Juice	40–50
Flavedo	8–10
Albedo	15–25
Rag, pulp and seeds	Rest

Main constituents (%)	
Water	85–90
Sugars	6–9
Acids	0·5–1·5
Pectins	0·5–1·5
Minerals	0·5–0·8
Essential oils	0·2–0·5
Fibre	0·5–1·0
Protein	0·5–0·8
Fat	0·1–0·2

smaller proportions. These percentages vary greatly in other citrus fruits, but they also vary within orange fruits, depending on variety, ripeness, area and culture practices. Concentrations, distribution and methods of analysis of these constituents will be discussed in more detail in the following sections.

Sugars and Acids

Soluble solids of citrus juices consist mainly of sugars and acids. Sugars are more abundant (70–80% of total solids) in oranges, tangerines and grapefruits, whereas citric acid is predominant in ripe lemons and limes. Soluble solids are usually expressed in degrees Brix (for easy and rapid evaluation with refractometers), referring to all juice solids as sucrose. Total acidity is expressed in grams of citric acid per 100 ml of juice, approximately equivalent to percentage.

The total solids increase with ripeness in all citrus species. In most cases, this is due to the increase in sugar content but, in lemons, citric acid increases with ripeness. Ranges from 9 to 14°Brix and from 1·5 to 0·5% acidity can be considered usual in orange juices processed in citrus plants. Commercial juices, prepared by blending juices of different varieties at different degrees of ripeness, show less variations: from 11 to 12°Brix and from 0·8 to 0·9% acidity are normal ranges. *See* Ripening of Fruit

The degrees Brix-to-acidity ratio, also called the maturity index, is a fundamental measure of quality of citrus juices. In commercial orange juice it usually has values from 12 to 14 and no orange juice is considered of high quality if it shows a ratio lower than 11. The importance of the degrees Brix-to-acidity ratio as a quality index lies on its relationship with the equilibrium between sweetness and sourness, one of the most appreciated sensory characteristics of citrus fruits. As discussed above, degree Brix value depends mainly on sugars.

Only three sugars are important in citrus fruits, sucrose, glucose and fructose, which produce juice (or fruit) sweetness. Other sugars such as galactose, heptulose, mannose, rhamnose, xylose or trehalose have only been detected as traces. *See* Carbohydrates, Classification and Properties; Fructose; Sucrose, Properties and Determination

The analysis of citrus sugars has been approached by many different methods. A classical standard method is the determination of reducing sugars (fructose and glucose) by copper reduction, followed by the inversion of sucrose to fructose and glucose, which can then also be determined as reducing sugars. By this method, the concentrations of the main citrus sugars (reducing and nonreducing) are determined. When the sugar composition must be known in more detail, separative (chromatographic) methods are used. Numerous analyses of citrus sugars have been performed by paper chromatography, gas chromatography, and high-performance liquid chromatography. Traces of the different minor sugars mentioned above have been detected by these techniques. The analyses of citrus sugars have shown that the typical ratios of sucrose to glucose to fructose are 2:1:1 in orange juice, 1:4:4 in lemons and 1:3:3 in limes. Typical contents of total sugars are 8% of total weight in orange and grapefruit juices, and 2% in lemon juice, although these percentages can vary greatly with variety and ripeness. *See* Chromatography, Principles; Chromatography, High-performance Liquid Chromatography; Chromatography, Gas Chromatography

The major acid in citrus fruits is citric acid. Total acidity, which is determined by titration, is expressed as grams of citric acid per 100 ml of juice. Malic acid is the second most important acid, present in variable but in much lower amounts than citric acid. Other organic acids such as succinic, malonic, lactic, oxalic, phosphoric, tartaric, adipic, isocitric, etc., are present in even smaller amounts and have been detected by separative methods, such as gas chromatography of methyl ester derivatives. *See* Acids, Properties and Determination

Acid content, like total solids, varies greatly with ripeness. Ranges from 0·5 to 1·5% in orange juice, from 0·8 to 2·5% in grapefruits, and from 4 to 8% in lemons and limes are usual.

Polysaccharides

Citrus fruits contain cellulose, hemicelluloses and pectic substances, mainly in the peel. The juice contains only small amounts of these compounds, although they play an important role. From the nutritional point of view, they provide dietary fibre. Concerning quality, pectin acts as a colloidal stabilizer, protecting juice cloud. Pectins are polymers of galacturonic acid and exist in juices at levels of about 0·5%. In the form of the methyl ester, polygalacturonic acid maintains juice turbidity. If de-esterification occurs, the colloid degrades and the juice clarifies. The main reason for thermal treatment of commercial juices is not only to destroy microorganisms, but to inactivate the enzyme pectinesterase, which produces pectin degradation. Citrus peel, mainly from lemon, is an important source of commercial pectins, of great interest in the food industry because of their gelling power. *See* Dietary Fibre, Properties and Sources

Nitrogenous Compounds

About 0·7% of citrus juices consist of nitrogenous compounds. Free amino acids are the most important part of the nitrogenous fraction (70%), the rest consisting of vitamins, proteins (mainly enzymes) and inorganic compounds. Although not important as nutrients due to their low concentration, amino acids are extensively used for characterization purposes and to detect adulteration in fruit juices. Total nitrogen determination (closely related to total amino acid content) is a standard method of purity control. Nevertheless, the nitrogen content can be easily manipulated by adding inorganic salts. For this reason, separative techniques allowing the determination of individual amino acids are of considerable interest. Gas chromatography of volatile derivatives has often been used for this purpose, as has ion exchange chromatography. Reversed-phase

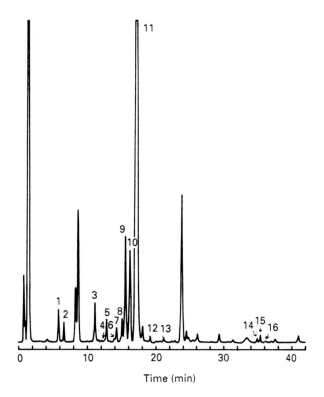

Fig. 2 Liquid chromatogram of orange juice amino acids: 1, aspartic acid; 2, glutamic acid; 3, asparagine; 4, glutamine; 5, serine; 6, threonine; 7, glycine; 8, alanine; 9, arginine; 10, γ-aminobutyric acid; 11, proline; 12, valine; 13, methionine; 14, ornithine; 15, lysine; 16, histidine.

liquid chromatography is an increasingly accepted technique. Figure 2 shows chromatograms obtained by this method from the dansyl derivatives of orange juice amino acids. *See* Amino Acids, Determination; Chromatography, Thin-layer Chromatography

Bitter Compounds

Two main types of bitterness, caused by two different types of compounds, occur in citrus fruits. Flavanone neohesperidosides, as naringin in grapefruit and neohesperidin in sour oranges, produce the typical bitterness of fruits and juices from these species. The other type of bitterness, which constitutes an extremely negative quality factor in some orange juices, is produced by limonin, a triterpene derivative of the limonoid group. Limonin bitterness is known as 'delayed bitterness' since it is not detected in fresh fruits or freshly extracted juices, but develops during juice storage or with heat treatment. The reason is that fresh fruits do not contain limonin, but a nonbitter precursor which converts into limonin after juice preparation. Limonin is detected by taste at concentrations of about 6–8 mg l^{-1} in orange juice. Citrus industries avoid exceeding these concentra-

tions in commercial juices by using only proper fruits or by blending different raw materials to obtain the desired final products. The limonin content of orange juice depends on variety and ripeness. It is extremely high in Navel varieties (still about 15 mg l^{-1} at a degrees Brix-to-acidity ratio of 12) which make them very unsuitable for juice processing. Generally speaking, early varieties produce more bitter juices than late varieties but country/region of origin can also affect limonin contents. Problems of bitterness are worse in temperate areas (California, Australia, Spain) than in tropical or subtropical regions (Brazil, Florida). *See* Flavour Compounds, Structures and Characteristics

Reduction of bitterness has been attempted by many means, involving changes in cultivation practices (rootstock, fertilization) and juice treatments. Debittering of processed juices seems to be the most promising approach and some citrus industries are already equipped with debittering devices.

Limonin analysis is essential in quality control. Thin-layer chromatography or immunoassay methods as well as liquid chromatography techniques are used in its determination.

Minerals

Amounts and proportions of minerals contained in citrus juices are interesting for nutrition. Total mineral content, referred to as 'ash', is about 0·4% of juice weight. Ash composition varies in relation to the species, ripeness, growth area and methods of cultivation. Generally, the major inorganic components of citrus juices are potassium and nitrogen, each accounting for about 40% of the total. Calcium, magnesium and phosphorus are less abundant (about 5% each). Sodium, iron, sulphur and chlorine are also important. About 20 more minerals have been detected in smaller proportions or only as traces. Some of these minor constituents have been proposed for ascertaining the geographic origin of orange juice. Minerals are very satisfactorily determined by atomic absorption spectrometry, or plasma emission techniques, where available. *See* individual minerals

Aromas

The typical citrus aroma depends on many minor constituents. Their individual contribution and relative proportions, as well as interactions among them, give the characteristic odour to each species. These constituents are present in juice vesicles of the endocarp and, in larger amounts and different proportions, in the oil sacs of the flavedo. When extracting the juice, oil sacs break and part of the oil joins the juice. Peel oil is also

Table 2. Composition of the volatile fraction of orange juice

Types of compound	Approximate number of identified constituents of the type	Examples
Alcohols	54	Linalool α-Terpineol[a] 4-Vinylguaiacol[a] Citronellol Nerol Octanol Geraniol Methanol Ethanol
Aldehydes	41	Acetaldehyde Hexanal[a] Citronellal Geranial Neral
Ketones	16	Carvone[a] Nootkatone[a] Acetone
Esters	39	Ethyl butyrate Methyl butyrate Ethyl acetate Linalyl acetate
Hydrocarbons	51	α-Pinene Terpinolene[a] Valencene Myrcene Limonene
Acids	10	Acetic Butyric
Others	12	Ethyl butyl ether Linalool oxides

[a] Some constituents producing off-flavour.

obtained as an independent product in citrus plants. One of its principal uses is as a flavouring ingredient for soft drinks.

Odour compounds constitute a part of the volatile fraction of citrus juices, which also contains nonodorous compounds. The distinction between both types of constituents and the evaluation of their relative importance in juice aromas are important research objectives in this field. Table 2 shows the main types of compounds forming the volatile fraction of orange juice. Several examples of individual constituents, including some which cause off-flavours, are listed in the table. Major constituents of the volatile fraction are ethanol (about 0.5 ml l^{-1} in juice) and limonene (0.15 ml l^{-1}). None of

these are important for aroma, since their concentrations are lower than detection thresholds. Chromatography, preferably gas chromatography using capillary columns of high resolution coupled to a mass spectrometer, is the most suitable method for determining either individual compounds or quite large groups of volatile compounds in a single analysis. Due to the low concentrations in the juice of most volatiles, a concentration step may be necessary for detailed studies. This step can be performed by solvent extraction of the juice or of a juice distillate, followed by solvent removal.

For rapid determinations, necessary in routine quality control, the total analysis of recoverable oil or the specific analysis of some groups of constituents, such as alcohols, aldehydes and ketones, or unsaturated constituents, are also used. *See* Alcohol, Properties and Determination; Essential Oils, Properties and Uses

Other Minor Constituents

Juice colour in all citrus fruits is due to carotenoids, with the exception of blood oranges in which anthocyanins, types of flavonoid compounds, are responsible for their typical colour. β-Carotene is present in orange juice in concentrations of about 0.5 mg l^{-1}, representing a small but significant source of vitamin A. Colour is one of the principal quality attributes of citrus juices and several methods, either visual or instrumental, have been used for its evaluation. The Hunter colorimeter must be mentioned since it was specifically developed for citrus fruits. Basically it determines three parameters: L, a and b, respectively related to lightness, green to red, and blue to yellow preponderance. *See* Colours, Properties and Determination of Natural Pigments

Lipids constitute about 0.07% of orange juice and consist mainly of fatty acids, 90% of them being palmitic, palmitoleic, oleic, linoleic and linolenic acids. The rest of the lipid fraction includes a range of both polar and nonpolar compounds. Lipids can be partially responsible for off-flavour development, since, even though they contribute little to flavour, they are precursors of malodorous compounds. Independently, lipids are important for taxonomy because each different species has its own profile of lipid components. *See* Fatty Acids, Analysis

Fully methoxylated flavones, belonging to the flavonoid group, are considerably more abundant in the peel than in the juice, where their concentration increases with extracting pressure. Consequently, these compounds can be considered as a potential index of extractor performance. Figure 3 shows chromatograms obtained by liquid chromatography of fully methoxylated flavones of orange and tangerine juices.

Vitamins are very important minor constituents of citrus fruits, and will be discussed in the following section.

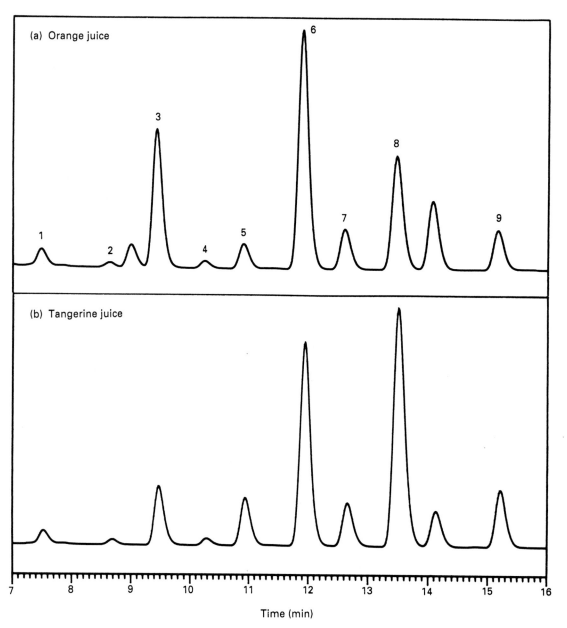

Fig. 3 Liquid chromatogram of fully methoxylated flavones of (a) orange juice and (b) tangerine juice. 1, isosinensetin; 2, gossypetin; 3, sinensetin; 4, isoscutellarein; 5, quercetagetin; 6, nobiletin; 7, scutellarein; 8, heptamethoxyflavone; 9, tangeretin. Sendra JM *et al.* (1988).

Nutritional Value

Although citrus fruits cannot be considered as basic foods, they are excellent complementary foods to appropriate diets. During the 18th century, citrus fruits were the only known source of vitamin C able to prevent scurvy on long sea journeys, but this was a long time ago. Nevertheless, the contribution to the diet of vitamins, minerals and dietary fibre from citrus fruits is still significant. *See* Scurvy

Orange juice is an important source of vitamins. Composition tables show that it contains (per 100 ml) about 100 μg of thiamin, 30 μg of riboflavin, 40 μg of

vitamin B_6, 20 μg of vitamin E, 300 μg of niacin, 200 μg of pantothenic acid, 300 μg of folacin and 50 mg of vitamin C. Thus, a glass of orange juice covers the daily requirements of vitamin C, about 25% of those for folacin and 5% for vitamin B_6. This contribution to dietary needs increases in interest if the low energy content of orange juice (about 50 cal per 100 ml) is considered as this allows higher consumption of orange juice than of other foods richer in vitamins (but also in energy). On the other hand, commercial orange juice needs less heat treatment for microorganism inactivation than other less acid foods, so vitamin losses are lower. *See* individual vitamins

Composition and Characterization

Lemon juice contains similar amounts of vitamins C and B$_6$, but less folacin (100 μg per 100 ml), whereas tangerine juice is poorer in vitamin C (30 mg per 100 ml), and grapefruit juice has a lower content of all these three vitamins.

Concerning minerals, citrus juices are rich in potassium (150–200 mg l^{-1}) but low in sodium (1–2 mg l^{-1}), which makes them very suitable for people receiving treatment with diuretics.

Finally, cellulose, hemicelluloses and pectins contained in citrus fruits are a source of dietary fibre, but which will only make a small contribution to daily intake for most people. *See* Dietary Fibre, Properties and Sources

Authentication

Citrus processing is an important world industry and some products reach high prices, which may make the idea of adulteration attractive. Although typical adulteration of citrus juices (by dilution, addition of sugar, blends of juices from different species without declaration) is not harmful to health, the consumer is paying for a substandard product, and unfair competition against honest producers is always involved. *See* Adulteration of Foods, Detection

The methods for detecting adulteration generally consist of comparing the values of some selected characteristics (i.e. constituent concentrations) of suspicious samples with the known ranges of values in pure products. The effectiveness of the method will depend mainly on the success in selecting those characteristics specific to the pure product, easy to determine accurately, and difficult to mask. For a sound knowledge of the characteristics of pure products, sufficient data, representative of the possible raw materials, must be collected. Data variability is usually high due to ripeness, area or fruit variety. Consequently, values show wide ranges, which complicates the detection of adulteration. Mean values and ranges of several characteristics of Spanish orange juices are presented in Table 3.

Detection methods may be based on the determination of one, few or many characteristics. Instrumental analysis, computers and statistics are useful in all cases but essential where multiple data must be obtained and processed from each sample.

Several types of adulteration are possible in citrus products. The most important will be mentioned and the methods developed for their detection discussed.

Since water, sucrose and citric acid are the main constituents of juices and can be obtained from cheaper sources, an easy type of adulteration consists of their addition to the juice in proportions that keep the solid content and acidity at normal juice levels. In this simple method, the adulteration should be easy to detect, since

Table 3. Mean values and ranges of some characteristics of Spanish orange juices (values in mg l^{-1}, except for absorbances)

	Mean	Minimum	Maximum
Aspartic acid	165·6	26·9	412·8
Glutamic acid	86·5	18·9	205·8
Asparagine	434·0	113·2	933·4
Glutamine	33·3	5·3	132·1
Serine	124·9	33·4	272·4
Threonine	20·9	8·8	50·0
Glycine	26·8	12·4	57·6
Alanine	89·5	49·7	182·6
Arginine	408·0	88·9	953·2
γ-Aminobutyric acid	250·7	83·4	470·4
Proline	1549·0	617·8	3973·0
Valine	14·8	3·4	62·4
Methionine	15·3	1·8	42·2
Ornithine	11·9	3·1	96·8
Lysine	32·8	11·1	62·4
Histidine	8·4	3·0	42·5
Acidity	11 000·0	5090·0	18 400·0
Absorbance at 280 nm	1·46	0·44	3·07
Absorbance at 325 nm	0·960	0·295	2·23
Absorbance at 443 nm	0·131	0·015	0·487
Sucrose	36 920·0	17 900·0	46 300·0
Glucose	20 880·0	13 190·0	29 240·0
Fructose	24 620·0	15 000·0	44 160·0
Potassium	1296·0	562·4	1872·0
Magnesium	98·4	74·6	146·7
Calcium	118·8	62·2	212·0
Ash	3165·0	2100·0	4248·0
Isocitric acid	117·1	40·6	207·2
Isosinensetin	0·129	0·02	0·61
Gossypetin	0·059	0·0	0·22
Sinensetin	1·62	0·07	7·15
Isoscutellarein	0·042	0·0	0·39
Quercetagetin	0·359	0·01	1·77
Nobiletin	2·24	0·0	9·12
Scutellarein	0·569	0·1	2·95
Heptamethoxyflavone	1·01	0·15	4·4
Tangeretin	0·321	0·02	2·81

concentrations of the remaining constituents decrease with dilution level. However, these concentrations can also be manipulated. Detection methods have increased in complexity by successively determining minerals, individual sugars, total nitrogen, nitrogen from amino acids, specific amino acids, and so on. Masking procedures also increased in their complexity by successively adding inorganic salts, blends of sugars, ammonium salts, glycine, amino acid blends, and so on. The ideal final situation to prevent adulteration will be achieved when masking procedures are either more difficult or more expensive than producing pure products.

The methods mentioned above work on the basis that all artificially added constituents, even from external

Composition and Characterization

sources, are normal constituents of juices. So, only through the modification of the natural proportions between added and nonadded constituents can fraud be detected. A different approach is to consider that raw materials from extraneous sources must show some differences. For example ratios of carbon ($^{13}C:^{12}C$) or oxygen ($^{18}O:^{16}O$) isotopes can be used to determine if any sugar or water comes from sources other than the citrus fruit.

Blends of juices from different species can be detected through the knowledge of the pattern distribution of certain compounds in each species. A method of detecting the addition of grapefruit juice to orange juice consists of analysing the profiles of flavanone glycoside concentrations.

Finally, ultraviolet absorption is useful for determining the addition of pulpwash solids to orange juice.

Bibliography

Feinberg M, Favier JC and Ireland-Ripert J (eds) (1991) *Répertoire Général des Aliments. Table de Composition.* Paris: Institut National de la Recherche Agronomique.

Nagy S and Attaway J (eds) (1980) *Citrus Nutrition and Quality.* Washington, DC: American Chemical Society.

Nagy S, Shaw P and Veldhuis M (eds) (1977) *Citrus Science and Technology.* Westport: AVI.

Nagy S, Attaway J and Rhodes M (eds) (1988) *Adulteration of Fruit Juice Beverages.* New York: Marcel Dekker.

Sendra JM, Navarro JL and Izquierdo L (1988) C_{18} solid-phase isolation and high-performance liquid chromatography/ultraviolet diode array determination of fully methoxylated flavones in citrus juices. *Journal of Chromatographic Science* 26: 443–448.

L. Izquierdo and J. M. Sendra
Consejo Superior de Investigaciones Científicas, Valencia, Spain

Oranges*

Of all the various fruits in the world, the sweet orange (*Citrus sinensis* Osbeck) is perhaps the most cherished. The refreshing natural flavour of orange juice or flesh from mature fruit is characterized as uniquely pleasing, with just the right mix of sweetness and tartness. Much effort has been expended in the attempt to imitate orange flavour.

The orange is the most important citrus species worldwide. Its origin is believed to be the tropical and subtropical regions of Asia. Oranges were grown in

China long before being introduced to Europe about 1400. Continental America probably received its first oranges in the early-to-mid 1500s with the arrival of the explorers, Bernal Diaz in Mexico and Ponce de Leon in Florida. Brazil probably received its first oranges with the coming of the Portuguese in the mid-1500s. In the USA, it was not until the early 1800s that oranges entered interstate commerce with the shipping of fruit, usually in barrels, from coastal Florida locales to northern cities. Today oranges and orange products are shipped all over the world from areas of production. Per capita consumption of fresh oranges on a fresh-weight basis in the USA for 1989 was 5·7 kg.

Global Distribution

Oranges are grown in the tropical or subtropical regions of six of the seven continents. World production in 1988–1989 amounted to 36×10^6 t. Of all the countries in the world, Brazil and the USA produce the lion's share of oranges (Table 1). Some lesser-producing countries not listed include Cyprus, Chile, Gaza, Uruguay, Japan, Lebanon, Belize, Venezuela, Tunisia and Jamaica. The USA and Brazil process the bulk of their crops, while countries like Egypt, Spain and Turkey process very little of their crops. About 57% of the world's orange production is consumed fresh. Countries such as Mexico, Egypt and Turkey utilize most of their orange production internally as fresh fruit. Spain is the world's largest exporter of fresh oranges, while Brazil is the largest exporter of processed orange juice.

In Brazil, the state of Sao Paulo accounts for most of the total orange juice produced there. In the USA, the major producing states are Florida and California, with much smaller quantities being produced in Arizona, Texas, and Louisiana. A typical orange grove in the central interior of Florida is illustrated in Plate 6. During the 1989–1990 season, according to the US Department of Agriculture (USDA) February 11 1991 Citrus Estimate, the following number ($\times 10^6$) of 40·8-kg (90-lb) boxes were produced: 186·0 for the USA; 110·2 for Florida (68·1 early season Hamlins and mid-season primarily Pineapple oranges, with 42·1 late-season Valencias); 73·0 34·0-kg (75-lb) boxes for California (44·0 navels and miscellaneous with 29·0 Valencias); 1·6 34·0-kg boxes for Arizona (0·4 navels and 1·2 Valencias); 1·2 38·5-kg (85-lb) boxes for Texas (1·0 early and 0·2 Valencias). Only about 8% of Florida's orange production, on average, is marketed fresh, compared with about 65% for California.

The on-tree value of the 1988–1989 US orange crop was 1471 million dollars. Of that total, the value of Florida oranges was 1086 million dollars, California 361 million dollars, and Texas and Arizona 12 million dollars each. In Florida, the average on-tree price per

---

* The colour plate section for this article appears between p. 1146 and p. 1147.

40·8-kg (90-lb) box was $7·41, the fresh price being $7·61, and the price for processing oranges being $7·40. For California, the average price per 34·0-kg (75-lb) box was $6·12, the fresh price being $8·37, and the processing price $1·15.

Varieties

Oranges may be classified as sweet or bitter (sour), the latter having generally little commercial importance for the fruit, but great importance for use as a rootstock. Sweet orange varieties are further classified, as follows: (1) common orange, represented by many important varieties, including Valencia (perhaps the major variety worldwide), Hamlin (important in Florida and Brazil), Pera and Natal (both of importance in Brazil), Pineapple (important in Florida), Parson Brown, Shamouti (of importance in Israel and several other Middle Eastern countries); (2) sugar or acidless orange, possessing a bland flavour; (3) blood or pigmented orange, important in the Mediterranean area of Europe, especially Spain; and (4) navel orange, especially Washington navel (of great importance in California). The Temple orange, a natural tangor, has economic significance in Florida. A promising new variety, the Ambersweet orange, with half of its parentage coming from *C. sinensis*, is being planted in quantity in Florida.

Table 1. Major sweet-orange-producing countries and amount ($\times 10^3$ t) exported and processed for 1988–1989

Country	Production[a]	Fresh[b]	Fresh export[a]	Fruit processed
Brazil	14 150	3460	91	10 690
USA	8269	1884	367	6385
Mexico	2269	1925	8	344
Spain	2216	2051	998	165
Italy	2170	1370	128	800
Egypt	1199	1189	178	10
Morocco	994	705	463	289
Greece	770	646	225	124
Turkey	700	625	90	75
South Africa	604	423	336	181
Argentina	580	430	77	150
Israel	546	205	205	341
Australia	524	212	35	312
Cuba	520	395	300	125

[a] For the 1987–1988 season, China produced 3 395 000 t of oranges, of which 14 700 t were exported. Source: FAO (1989) *Citrus Fruit, Fresh and Processed*. Annual Statistics, 1989. Rome: Food and Agriculture Organization.
[b] As calculated from production amount less the amount of fruit processed.
Source: Citrus Administrative Committee (1990) *Annual Statistical Report*. Lakeland, Florida: Citrus Administrative Committee.

Commercial propagation of citrus is usually accomplished by bud grafting a desired variety onto a suitable rootstock. Major rootstocks currently used in Florida for sweet orange varieties are Carrizo, sour orange, Swingle, Cleopatra, Volkameriana, and Milam.

Anatomy

An orange is botanically classified as a berry, and develops from an ovary with axil placentation. Oranges are generally round, in contrast to the various shapes of many other citrus species. Generally, grapefruit are larger than oranges, while mandarins (especially tangerines), lemons and limes are smaller. The major structural features of an orange from the outside to the centre of an equatorial section are as follows: peel composed of the epidermis (outer layer of cells), flavedo and albedo; flavedo, a layer of tissue containing chromoplasts (generally orange to light green when the fruit is mature and dark green when immature), and oil glands dispersed throughout; albedo, a white pulpy material surrounding the segments which in turn hold the individual juice vesicles or juice sacs; seeds (if any) arranged around the pulpy core. Each segment is encased by a rather tough segment membrane or wall which, along with the juice vesicles, is ruptured when the fruit is extracted for the juice. Examples of seedy orange varieties are Pineapple and Parson Brown; Hamlin, Washington navel and Valencia are seedless or nearly seedless.

Proximate Analysis

Orange juice is composed (per 100 g) of about 88·3 g of water, 0·7 g of protein, 0·2 g of fat, 10·4 g of total carbohydrate, 0·1 g of fibre and 0·4 g of ash; the food energy is about 45 kcal.

Chemical Composition

The chief soluble solids in orange juice are the soluble carbohydrates or sugars (*c*. 10%), while citric acid is the main soluble solid in lemons and limes. The chief carbohydrates in orange juice – glucose, fructose and sucrose – occur in the approximate ratio of 1:1:2. Total sugars (especially the sucrose fraction) generally increase with advancing maturity, and the stylar half of the fruit possesses more than the stem half. *See* Fructose; Sucrose, Properties and Determination

Pectin or pectic substances, made up of complex carbohydrate derivatives or polysaccharides, are important in terms of juice quality for imparting body or viscosity and the cloudy appearance. Pectic substances are a major component of the primary cell wall and middle lamella in all fruits; in the orange, up to 30% of the albedo on a dry-weight basis may be pectin, but only 0·01–0·13% occurs in the juice. Without heat stabilization to inactivate pectinesterase enzyme, clarification or loss of cloud may occur in single-strength orange juice due to the settling out of pectins and other solids, while in concentrate a pectin gel may form, resulting in a nonpourable product.

The acidity of orange juice is due primarily to the organic acid, citric acid and, to a much lesser extent, malic and succinic acids. Orange juice with about 0·5–1·0% acid (pH of about 3·5) is less acidic than that of grapefruit, and much less acidic than lemon and lime. Perhaps more so than any other quality factor, it is the favourable ratio of sugar to acid (sweetness to tartness), along with the unique orange flavour, which gives orange juice its universal high consumer acceptance.

Orange essential oils are found primarily in the peel, with significantly less in the juice vesicles. In a large 3-year study in Florida of the major orange varieties, the proportion of oil in the fruit ranged from a low of 0·29% in Hamlins during 1969–1970 to a high of 0·94% in Valencias during 1968–1969. Orange oil contains at least 112 volatile essential oil components. Of these, D-limonene is most abundant, comprising about 95% by weight of orange oil, but it is the oxygenated aldehydes and esters that are considered the most important contributors to orange flavour. Many oxygenated alcohols are present in orange oil but not ketones. Coumarins and flavonoids comprise most of the 1% of the nonvolatile constituents in orange oil. Generally, total yield of orange oil decreases with increasing maturity. *See* Flavour Compounds, Structures and Characteristics

The most abundant mineral in orange juice is potassium, with other minerals of significant quantity being calcium, iron, sodium, phosphorus, and sulphur. Other elements of note are chlorine and nitrogen. *See* individual nutrients

Most of the lipid content of oranges occurs as fatty acids, with most being in the seeds. The five major fatty acids are palmitic, palmitoleic, oleic, linoleic, and linolenic. Phosphatidylcholine and phosphatidylethanolamine comprise the bulk of the phospholipid fraction of Florida and California orange juice. *See* Fatty Acids, Properties

About 70% of the nitrogen in citrus juices occurs in free amino acids which constitute about 0·1% (w/w) in oranges. Proline is the major amino acid with less quantities of asparagine, aspartic acid, arginine and gamma-aminobutyric acid. *See* Amino Acids, Properties and Occurrence

In addition to the very important pectinesterase enzyme system in orange juice, numerous other enzymes have been identified, including 13 oxidoreductases, 7 hydrolases, 7 lyases, 3 transferases and single isomerase and ligase enzymes. *See* Enzymes, Functions and Characteristics

An unusually large number and quantity of flavonoids, C_{15} compounds, occur in citrus. Compounds have been identified in oranges representing the three major flavonoid types: (1) flavanones (including flavanonols) generally occurring as glycosides e.g. hesperidin, the major flavanone glycoside in oranges, (2) flavones (including flavonols), and (3) anthocyanins, of importance in citrus only as red pigments in blood oranges.

Limonin, a highly oxygenated triterpene derivative, is an important constituent in certain citrus fruits, such as navel orange and grapefruit, because of its bitter nature. Limonin exists in the major sweet orange varieties (Hamlin, Pineapple and Valencia) but generally in low enough levels so as not to produce significant bitterness problems. However, in the navel orange, of great significance in several large citrus producing areas around the world, the extracted juice takes on a noted bitterness, especially if heat-processed. A large California commercial citrus operation is currently employing styrenedivinylbenzene adsorbent resin to debitter navel orange juice.

The orange colour in peel generally associated with mature fruit is due primarily to carotenoids, chiefly β-citraurin, while the green peel colour generally associated with immature oranges is due to chlorophyll. The main pigment in orange juice producing the orange colour is the carotenoid, β-cryptoxanthin. *See* Carotenoids, Properties and Determination; Colours, Properties and Determination of Natural Pigments

Fresh Oranges and their Utilization

Harvesting is accomplished primarily by hand, and the fruit is placed in a picking bag or other container. A considerable effort has been expended on developing mechanical harvesting methods, especially with fruit in Florida which is destined for processing. Most mechanical harvesting is still in the experimental stage. Bough shaking has provided for 80–90% removal of Hamlin and Pineapple oranges in Florida, while pulsating air blasts, used in conjunction with abscission chemicals, has resulted in 85–95% removal. In most of the heavy citrus-producing areas, oranges harvested for the fresh market are placed in pallet boxes (a standard pallet box in Florida holds 408·2 kg or 900 lb of oranges) for transport to the packing houses. Otherwise, fruit may be loaded onto semitrailer trucks for bulk transport to the processing plants.

In most citrus-producing areas, maturity standards, some of which are complex, must be met prior to the fruit being utilized in the fresh or processed market. In the USA, the USDA and various state agencies develop

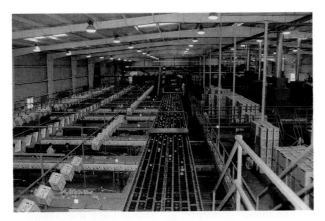

Fig. 1 Modern fresh citrus packing house in south Florida (courtesy of A. Duda and Sons, LaBelle, Florida; photograph by M. Ismail).

and oversee the maturity standards. Internal standards generally consider a minimum ratio of °Brix to percentage of acid (below which the juice will taste too acidic or tart), total soluble solids, total acid and juice content. External grade standards include skin colour, texture, discoloration and blemishes; fruit form, and firmness.

Most fresh oranges are marketed in the USA in fibreboard boxes holding 14·5–19·0 kg (32·0–41·9 lb) net weight of fruit. Preparation of oranges for market may include degreening, washing, applying fungicides, grading, waxing, and sizing. Figure 1 depicts a modern fresh citrus fruit packing house. Some early season oranges in Florida, such as Hamlins and Washington navels, may be degreened if the external fruit is showing greenish or patchy green. Ethylene gas, a natural plant hormone is generally applied at about 5 ppm to fruit held for 72 h or less in a room at 29–30°C, 90–97% relative humidity, with an hourly change of air. In Florida, (but not California and many countries outside the USA) pale (yellowish) oranges including Temples may be colour-enhanced through immersion in a tank containing Citrus Red No. 2, with 2 ppm residue being allowed. Fruit may be treated with fungicides to control post-harvest decay, and waxed to prevent moisture loss and enhance appearance. There are numerous formulations of waxes and waxlike materials available for application on oranges, but the most commonly used are water waxes, either emulsion-based or as a resin solution. Important post-harvest fungal diseases are stem-end rot caused by *Diplodia natalensis* or *Phomopsis citri*, green mould caused by *Penicillium digitatum*, and sour rot caused by *Geotrichum candidum*. Fungicides, each with its own mode of application, used to control decay include sodium *o*-phenylphenate (SOPP), thiabendazole (TBZ), and imazalil. Oranges to be exported from the USA to other citrus-producing areas are either fumigated with methyl bromide or subjected to cold treatment at 1·1°C for 17 days to rid the fruit of potentially harmful fruit fly larvae and eggs. *See* Fungicides; Spoilage, Moulds in Food Spoilage

Cold storage of oranges at 0–1°C for Florida fruit, and 3–9°C for California fruit, will generally provide several weeks of marketability; otherwise, fruit held at room temperature has a shorter shelf life. Controlled-atmosphere storage, using increased carbon dioxide and decreased oxygen at cool temperatures, does not work for citrus fruit. *See* Controlled Atmosphere Storage, Applications for Bulk Storage of Foodstuffs

Freshly squeezed orange juice is enjoyed around the world, but the shelf life is minimal at ambient temperature. In recent years, Florida has developed a significant freshly squeezed orange juice market in which juice is packed and marketed chilled at 0–4°C in 0·946- or 1·892-litre (generally polyethylene) bottles. Shelf life is about 14–18 days. If this product is frozen after packing and marketed in frozen condition at about −18°C, shelf life is increased to more than a year. Thawing may be accomplished in a matter of minutes (about 20 min for a 0·946-litre container) in a microwave oven, with negligible loss of flavour or vitamin C.

Nutritional aspects of orange juice are discussed in the following article. Nutritional data for freshly squeezed orange juice are very similar to those for the processed product shortly after processing. Freshly squeezed orange juice packed in plastic containers and held at −1 to 4°C loses somewhat less than 1% ascorbic acid per day. The loss of ascorbic acid in the juice of whole oranges during the normal marketing life is expected to be less than 10%.

Acknowledgement

Florida Agricultural Experiment Station Journal Series No. N-00413.

Bibliography

Fellers PJ (1985) Citrus: sensory quality as related to rootstock, cultivar, maturity and season. In: Pattee H (ed.) *Evaluation of Quality of Fruits and Vegetables*, pp 83–128. Westport, Connecticut: AVI Publishing.

Hassee G (ed.) (1987) *The Orange, a Brazilian Adventure 1500–1987.* Sao Paulo: Duprat and Iobe Publishing.

Kefford JF and Chandler BV (1970) *The Chemical Constituents of Citrus Fruits.* New York: Academic Press.

Nagy S and Attaway JA (eds) (1980) *Citrus Nutrition and Quality.* Washington DC: American Chemical Society.

Nagy S, Shaw PE and Veldhuis MK (eds) (1977) Citrus Science and Technology, vols 1 and II. Westport, Connecticut: AVI Publishing.

Reuther W, Batchelor LD and Webber HJ (eds) *The Citrus Industry*, Vol. 1 (1967), Vol. 2 (1968). University of California, Berkeley: Division of Agricultural Science.

Saunt J (1990) *Citrus Varieties of the World.* Norwich: Sinclair International.

Oranges

Seelig RA and Bing MC (1990) Oranges. In: *Encyclopedia of Produce*. Alexandria, Virginia: United Fresh Fruit and Vegetable Association.

Sinclair WB (ed.) (1961) *The Orange, its Biochemistry and Physiology*. University of California, Riverside: Division of Agricultural Science.

Wardowski WF, Nagy S and Grierson W (eds) (1986) *Fresh Citrus Fruits*. Westport, Connecticut: AVI Publishing.

Paul J. Fellers
Florida Department of Citrus, Lake Alfred, USA

Processed and Derived Products of Oranges

Prior to the 1948 invention of the 'Cinderella' product, full-flavoured frozen concentrated orange juice, by Florida Department of Citrus researchers MacDowell, Moore and Atkins, the primary processed orange product in the world was canned, single-strength orange juice. This canned product, first packed in volume in Florida in 1929, was most often made from packing-house eliminations or culls from the fresh-fruit industry. In the mid-1930s, Florida began producing significant quantities of blended, canned grapefruit and orange juice generally containing 50–60% grapefruit juice and 50–40% orange juice. Other early processed orange products were canned orange sections and canned citrus salad, the latter being a combination primarily of grapefruit and orange sections, and a small quantity of hot-pack concentrated orange juice. From this beginning emerged the huge and diversified present-day citrus processing industry, utilizing oranges chiefly as orange juice, and lesser amounts of other orange and orange-based products, and by-products.

Processed Orange Juice

The processed products, orange juice and concentrated orange juice, had international 'Recommended Standards' from 1972 to 1981, at which time they became known as 'Codex Standards' by the United Nations Food and Agriculture Organization/World Health Organization (UN FAO/WHO) Codex Alimentarius Commission. Of the greatest significance are the sections dealing with standards for natural soluble orange solids exclusive of added sugar in orange juice of not less than 10% by weight, as determined by refractometer at 20°C, uncorrected for acidity, and in reconstituted concentrated orange juice of not less than 11% by weight. Also of importance are the sections allowing the use in orange juice or concentrate of 10% by weight of mandarin (*Citrus reticulata* Blanco) juice with proper label declaration.

Regulation of the US citrus-processing industry is accomplished through federal Standards of Identity, issued by the Food and Drug Administration (FDA) and US Standards for Grades, as overseen by the United States Department of Agriculture (USDA) (voluntary outside of Florida, mandatory in Florida). Producing states have their own grades which must conform to federal grades, but which may be stricter than federal grades. The several orange juice products covered by US Standards for Grades of Orange Juice include canned, frozen concentrated, reduced-acid frozen concentrated, canned concentrated, dehydrated, and pasteurized orange juices; concentrated orange juice for manufacturing; and orange juice from concentrate. For all of these products, there is a 100-point grading system in which flavour and colour each constitute 40% of the grade, and absence of defects 20%. To attain minimum grade A, flavour and colour must be no less than 36, with 32 for grade B; absence of defects, 18 for Grade A, 16 for Grade B. A limiting rule applies to the grading system stating that the lowest score of any single factor determines the grade, even though the total product score might place it in a higher grade. USDA inspectors grade flavour when requested by a processing plant outside the state of Florida. Plants inside Florida must be continuously inspected. Colour is determined objectively through use of a colorimeter such as the Hunter-Lab D45-2 citrus colorimeter (Hunter Associates Laboratory, Reston, Virginia). Juice defects may include seed or membrane fragments, dark-coloured extraneous matter, etc. Depending on product type, other quality factors included in the grading system include appearance, reconstitution, coagulation and separation.

Important analytical factors utilized in the US federal grading system for orange juice include minimum °Brix*, minimum and maximum values for the ratio of °Brix to percentage acid, and maximum percentage by volume of recoverable oil. For most citrus products, Florida Standards for Grades incorporate stricter requirements than those required by federal standards. Major examples for frozen concentrated orange juice (FCOJ) are a Florida maximum 12% by volume of sinking pulp (reconstituted basis) versus no requirement out-of-state; a 13:1 minimum °Brix:percentage acid ratio for Florida Grade A or B versus 11·5 or 12·5 out-of-state for US Grade A, and 10 for Grade B, depending on the fruit source; a minimum 0·010% by volume recoverable oil for Florida product (reconstituted basis) versus no out-of-state minimum requirement; and disallowing use of pulpwash (that product obtained after washing extracted and finished pulp) in Florida juice versus possible use out-of-state of the approximately

---

*The term 'Brix' refers to the percentage by weight of soluble solids, chiefly sugars, in the product and is expressed in degrees.

3·8% pulpwash recovered from the fruit used to make the juice.

In the USA, canned and chilled orange sections (often packed with other citrus fruit sections and packed in water, juice or light sugar syrup) and blends of orange juice with other fruit juices (e.g. grapefruit or pineapple) have lost their importance.

Production and Economic Considerations

Brazil produced 1305×10^6 42° equivalent Brix litres of FCOJ during the 1989–1990 season; of that total, 1207×10^6 l were exported, with most going to the USA (about 40%) and Western Europe (about 48%). Florida, which suffered a significant freeze in December 1989, produced $341\cdot8 \times 10^6$ 42° equivalent Brix litres of FCOJ during the 1989–1990 season, but with greatly improved prospects for the 1990–1991 season, production of $674\cdot9 \times 10^6$ l is estimated. US orange juice consumption of all types was estimated at 2619×10^6 single-strength litres during 1989. In 1989–1990, about $1004\cdot9 \times 10^6$ l of FCOJ (single-strength basis) were sold in the USA, about 40·3% of retail orange juice sales, at an average \$1·12 per litre; sales of chilled orange juice were $1426\cdot6 \times 10^6$ l. There are about 250 plants in the world producing FCOJ; about 80 produce single-strength orange juice. In the USA, contracts for future delivery of concentrated orange juice for manufacturing are traded actively on the New York Cotton Exchange. A contract is for 6803 kg (15 000 lb) orange solids for up to 18 months. Important points are that product must be US Grade A with a minimum score of deliverable juice being 94, have a Brix value of not less than 51°, and have a °Brix:percentage acid ratio of not less than 14:1 and not more than 18:1.

General Manufacturing Operations

Oranges meeting at least minimum maturity standards are transported to the processing plant, often in bulk, where they may be stored for a short period of time in wooden holding bins, in the trailer itself (in bulk or in pallet boxes), or utilized immediately. In preliminary grading, debris, decayed fruit and green fruit may be removed. Washing with detergent is accomplished generally with brush washers. Fruit is given a final grading, then sized before going to the juice extractors. Two extractor types account for most of the orange juice production in the world – the FMC citrus juice extractor (FMC Corporation, Lakeland, Florida) (Fig. 1) and the Brown International Corporation citrus juice extractor (Covina, California) (Fig. 2). The FMC machine features instantaneous peel-oil separation from the juice stream; the preferred Brown International

method is to use the Brown oil extractor which de-oils the fruit prior to juice extraction by utilizing needlelike points to penetrate the flavedo, causing the oil to be released from the cells. FMC has recently introduced an extractor with the primary advantage of producing a juice with about half the amount of peel oil and less bitterness than in other models. The chief use for this juice in the USA is in the manufacture of pasteurized orange juice. Many extractor (juice) rooms in processing plants are highly automated. Juice rooms may have just a few extractors in the small processing plants, and more than 200 in the largest (in Brazil). For the 1989–1990 season in Florida, a 40·8 kg (90 lb) box of oranges yielded an average of 19·4 kg of juice, somewhat lower than normal, presumably because of a major freeze during December 1989. Extraction pressure is important in that too much pressure will cause off-flavours (especially bitterness due to limonin) to occur in the juice, while too little pressure will cause undue economic loss. Following extraction, juice is commonly directed through a screw-type finisher which reduces pulp and

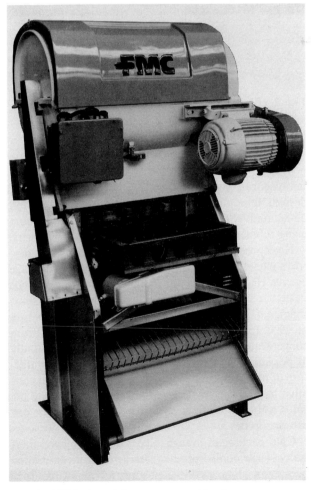

Fig. 1 FMC citrus juice extractor with oil recovery capability. (Courtesy of FMC Corporation, Citrus Machinery and Services Division, Lakeland, Florida.)

Processed and Derived Products of Oranges

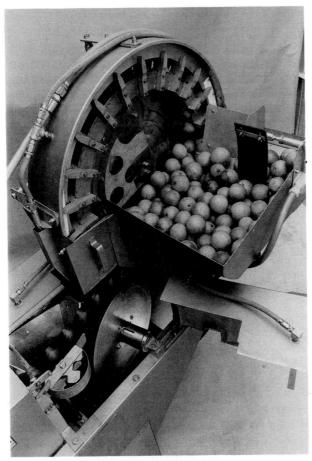

Fig. 2 Brown International Corporation Model 700 citrus juice extractor showing the fruit being fed in with the inspection door open. (Courtesy of Brown International Corporation, Covina, California.)

removes rag, membrane, seed and peel fragments. If desired, juice may be de-oiled (up to 90% removal) and de-aerated by flashing the heated product in a vacuum using tubular, plate or steam-infusion heat exchangers.

Heat processing inactivates pectic enzymes and destroys bacteria, yeast and mould – all potential spoilage agents. Heat processes using either plate or tubular type pasteurizers are all HTST (high temperature–short time), e.g. in Florida, orange concentrate manufacture at 99°C for 6 s and production of orange juice from concentrate at 85°C for 1 s. Product is cooled as rapidly as possible following heat processing. In the manufacture of hot-pack canned juice, the filled and sealed cans must be inverted to sterilize the lid, before cooling the can's contents to about 38°C in order to allow the can exterior to dry.

Cold-packing of orange juice is done using commercially sterile cooled product, sterile containers, aseptic hermetic sealing, sterilized closure and microorganism-free filling atmosphere. There are many methods (all complex) available for aseptically packing orange juice. Marketing this type of product at ambient temperature, however, may result in browning and development of excessive heated-type off-flavours in the juice.

Frozen Concentrated Orange Juice

In the manufacture of concentrate, the common evaporator is the steam-utilizing, energy-efficient 'thermally accelerated short-time evaporation' (TASTE) evaporator which has eight stages, seven effects and a flash cooler. Initial juice temperature may be 100°C, dropping to 10°C in the final concentrate. An evaporating capacity of 36 000 kg of water per hour is common in evaporators. A high °Brix of 65 is usual in concentrate for storage in 'tank farms', 208·2-l (55-gallon) drums or other holding containers. Tank farms, which are common in the USA and Brazil, are operations where concentrate is stored in large stainless steel tanks with capacities of 378 500—567 750 l, the tanks themselves being in large, insulated rooms kept at between −13°C and −8°C. FCOJ of 41·8° Brix is often a blend of the juice from more than a single variety to achieve product uniformity for degree of flavour, especially sweetness and tartness, and colour. Flavour is augmented by addition of a number of substances: (1) cold-pressed peel oil to allow about 0·015% by volume in the reconstituted juice, (2) orange essence (aqueous and oil-phase mixtures of volatile compounds), or (3) about 10% of either heat-stabilized or unheated, good, single-strength juice (known as cut-back juice). Natural essence is recovered during the concentration process, normally at the beginning. During this process, essence is generally concentrated or folded using a series of condensers. Much of the FCOJ manufactured today contains added essence. Almost all FCOJ manufactured around the world is 100% orange juice, with only negligible amounts having added sugar. In the USA and many other countries, if sugar or other sweeteners are added, their presence must be clearly disclosed on the label. The international Codex Standards allow up to 50 g per kg of added sugars in reconstituted 11·0° Brix product, but addition of anything more than 15 g per kg requires a label declaration. To satisfy a demand for a reduced-acid FCOJ, one US company developed a method utilizing anionic exchange to produce such a product, for which there now exist US federal and Florida Standards for Grades. A recent innovation in the USA has been the marketing of calcium-supplemented FCOJ, in which about 20% of the US Recommended Daily Allowance (RDA) of calcium is supplied in the form of the lactate, carbonate or tribasic phosphate in a standard US 6 fl oz (177 ml) serving. *See* Calcium, Physiology

A major problem worldwide in producing processed navel orange juice is the development of bitterness due to often excessive, naturally occurring limonin. Very recently developed technology allows for the debittering of citrus juices, including excessively bitter orange juice. Most debittering systems use neutral resins, such as styrenedivinylbenzene adsorbent resin, which have been approved for use in food in the USA.

FCOJ will maintain its excellent flavour and nutritional value for a year or longer, provided that storage is at −18°C or lower. Long periods of frozen storage above this temperature will probably result in stale or oxidized off-flavours with some browning.

The most common container size for retailing FCOJ in the USA (about 75% of the market) is the 354 ml (12 fl oz) composite fibreboard, plastic-lined can with metal ends, followed by the 473 ml (16 fl oz), 177 ml (6 fl oz), and 946 ml (32 fl oz) sizes.

Processed Chilled Single-strength Orange Juice

Ready-to-serve (RTS) orange juice, the most popular form of retail orange juice in the USA, is marketed primarily as chilled product. About 68% of this juice is packed in 1·89-l (64 fl oz) plastic-lined, fibreboard cartons with lesser quantities in polyethylene containers and glass. About 75% of the juice is marketed in 1·89-l containers with the balance in 3·78-l (1-gal), 2·84-l (96-fl-oz), 0·95-l (1-qt) and other miscellaneous containers. Of all of the chilled RTS juice produced, the current trend in the USA is for increased amounts of the product, pasteurized orange juice (about 22% of the market in 1988), primarily at the expense of FCOJ. However, the product, orange juice from concentrate, is by far the chief RTS chilled juice.

Storage of chilled RTS orange juice in fibreboard cartons or polyethylene containers at −1°C to 3°C will result in a normal shelf life of about 5–6 weeks, whereas above this temperature will result in reduced shelf life with the possibility of fermentation and spoilage. With the advent of a new multi-ply high-oxygen-barrier plastic bottle, at least two Florida companies are placing a 3-month shelf life on their chilled RTS juice.

Processed Canned Orange Juice

Some canned orange juice is packed in nearly every citrus-producing region of the world. Most of this product is hot-filled, sealed, the can inverted for a short while to sterilize all the interior, cooled to about 38°C and stored at ambient temperature. Unfortunately, this product is very susceptible to off-flavours resulting from excessive heating – first during the rather severe heat processing, then in ambient storage.

Microbiological Aspects of Processed Juices

Primarily because of its low pH (about 3·0–3·5), most types of bacteria, including pathogens, cannot grow in orange juice. However, *Leuconostoc* and *Lactobacillus* can grow, and at low temperatures, which may result in diacetyl (buttermilk flavour) in the juice without gas formation. Some *Lactobacillus* species can grow at relatively high temperatures. Yeast in the juice generally manifests itself in fermentation with gas. Mould growth in juice generally appears as filamentous growth on the product surface. Every effort should be made to discourage growth of microorganisms, especially by careful grading out of spoiled or decayed fruit, ensuring proper heat treatment of the juice, and practising good overall sanitation. *See* Lactic Acid Bacteria; Spoilage, Bacterial Spoilage; Spoilage, Moulds in Food Spoilage; Spoilage, Yeasts in Food Spoilage

Additional Uses of Oranges

The major by-products and specialty products of oranges include the following: dried pulp and meal, and molasses; cold-pressed peel oil; distilled oil; D-limonene; essences; fermented products such as alcohol, wines, vinegar, citric and lactic acids, riboflavin, feed yeast, methane and 2,3-butylene glycol; pulpwash solids; and pectin. Other uses are as orange jellies and marmalades, frozen heat-stabilized pulp or juice sacs, brined and candied peel, citrus purées, frozen orange juice bars, and nonalcoholic squashes and cordials (these last two products generally being consumed in the UK and in countries having close ties with the UK).

In 1989–1990, Florida produced 542 150 t of dried pulp and meal (having about 10% final moisture) and 25 767 t of molasses (about 72° Brix) for cattle feed supplements. About 75% of the dried pulp and meal is exported.

The most important use of the essential oils (primarily cold-pressed peel oil) of the orange is to augment the flavour of processed orange juice, but the oils are also used in a host of other products requiring natural orange bouquet and taste. In a concentrating or folding process, D-limonene, which constitutes about 95% of orange oil but which does not contribute significantly to orange flavour, may be 'stripped off' from the oil using steam. However, the principal source of D-limonene is as a by-product in the manufacture of citrus molasses. About $6·9 \times 10^6$ kg of D-limonene was produced in Florida in 1989–1990 for various uses, including (1) raw material for syntheses of terpene resins and various other compounds, (2) a solvent, (3) a substitute for chlorofluorocarbons, which have been found hazardous to the ozone layer, (4) penetrating oil, and (5) a base for

Processed and Derived Products of Oranges

flavourings such as L-carvone and L-menthol. *See* Essential Oils, Properties and Uses

Production in Florida in 1983 of natural orange essence, composed of an aroma or aqueous fraction and oil fraction, was about 4.5×10^6 kg, and 0.3×10^6 kg, respectively; most was used for adding back to processed orange juice for flavour enhancement.

Pectin made from the orange peel (de-oiled) is the least desirable of the citrus-based pectins, the most desirable pectin being that extracted from lemons and limes. Pectin manufacture from citrus using any of several processes is very complicated. A book entitled *Citrus Pectin* (Sunkist Growers, Ontario, California) is devoted to the subject and presents recipes for numerous foodstuffs requiring pectin.

Orange pulpwash, which is also known as water-extracted soluble orange solids (WESOS), is the product obtained after washing the finisher pulp, and amounts to about 3–8% additional solids from the fruit. The flavour and colour quality of WESOS is generally poor, with few characteristics of good orange juice. Florida disallows use of WESOS in any of its pure juice products, but it can be used in certain other products, such as drinks. WESOS produced in the USA outside Florida may be used in the manufacture of FCOJ and concentrated orange juice for manufacturing, provided that it is the WESOS removed from the excess pulp of the same juice used in the making of those particular concentrates. For the 1985–1986 season in Florida, 10.8×10^6 kg of WESOS was produced.

Nutritional Aspects

Orange juice is one of the most important dietary sources of ascorbic acid (vitamin C), especially in citrus-producing countries. A 177 ml (6 fl oz) serving of orange juice in any form will normally supply at least 100% (60 mg) of the US RDA of this water-soluble vitamin which is required daily. With orange juice being about 88% water, it supplies significant liquid; a 177 ml (6 fl oz) serving of orange juice supplies approximately 90 cal, 1 g of protein, 21 g of carbohydrate, less than 1 g of fat, 1 mg of sodium, 250 mg of potassium and the following proportions of the US RDA of the following vitamins and minerals: 110% ascorbic acid, 8% thiamin, 8% folic acid, 4% vitamin B_6, 2% phosphorus, 4% magnesium, 2% copper, and less than 2% protein, vitamin A, riboflavin, nicotinic acid, calcium and iron. The ratio of high potassium to extremely low sodium is a very positive factor for large numbers of consumers for health reasons. *See* individual nutrients

Ascorbic acid retention is excellent in all forms of orange juice during processing. FCOJ retains 91–94% of its ascorbic acid after a year in frozen storage at $-20°C$; chilled juices in plastic or cartons lose about 1.4–2.0%

ascorbic acid per day; single-strength juice packed in glass held at 4.4°C for 8 months retained 87% of its ascorbic acid, and about 67% at 26.7°C.

Dietary fibre has been found in quantities of 0.01–0.13% in orange juice. The role of dietary fibre in lowering serum cholesterol in humans is well established. *See* Dietary Fibre, Fibre and Disease Prevention

Acknowledgements

This paper was reviewed at the Education Center, Lake Alfred, Florida, USA and was given the following assignment, Florida Agricultural Experiment Station Journal Series No. N-00414.

Bibliography

Carter RD (1985) *Reconstituted Florida Orange Juice: Production, Packaging, Distribution.* Lakeland, Florida: Florida Department of Citrus.

FAO/WHO (1982) *Codex Standards for Fruit Juices, Fruit Nectars.* Joint FAO/WHO Food Standards Programme, Codex Alimentarius Commission. Rome: Food and Agriculture Organization of the United Nations.

Fellers PJ, Nikdel S and Lee HS (1990) Nutrient content and nutrition labeling of several processed Florida citrus juice products. *Journal of the American Dietetic Association* 90 (no. 8): 1079–1084.

Kesterson JW and Braddock RJ (1976) *By-Products and Specialty Products of Florida Citrus.* Technical Bulletin 784. Institute of Food and Agricultural Sciences, University of Florida, Gainesville.

Kimball DA (1991) *Citrus Processing, Quality Control and Technology.* New York: Van Nostrand Rheinhold.

Lopez A (1987) *A Complete Course In Canning,* book III, pp 225–227. Baltimore: The Canning Trade.

Nagy S and Attaway JA (eds) (1980) *Citrus Nutrition and Quality.* Washington DC: American Chemical Society.

Nagy S, Shaw PE and Veldhuis MK (eds) (1977) *Citrus Science and Technology,* vols I and II. Westport, Connecticut: AVI Publishing.

USDA (1983) *United States Standards for Grades of Orange Juice.* Washington DC: US Department of Agriculture, Agricultural Marketing Service, Fruit and Vegetable Division, Processed Products Branch.

US FDA (1990) *Code of Federal Regulations.* Title 21, Part 146. Washington DC: US Food and Drug Administration.

Paul J. Fellers
Florida Department of Citrus, Lake Alfred, USA

Lemons

Origin and Distribution

Citrus fruits were probably among the most delectable fruits of primitive man living in northeastern India and the adjoining areas, where primitive citrus fruits are thought to have originated. In prehistoric times these fruits might have been carried to different oriental countries, where they delighted the local inhabitants and became established. The lemon was one of these fruits. The commercial lemon (*Citrus limon* (L.) Burm. F.) is believed to have originated as a bud sport from a native lemon in the eastern Himalayan region of India.

Known as *limón* in Spanish, *citroen* in Dutch, *citron* or *citronnier* in French, *zitrone* in German, *limao* in Portugese, *limone* in Italy and *lembu* in India, the lemon is the third most important citrus fruit today.

Lemon trees grow from 3 to 5 m tall and are covered with spines; the leaves have prominent winged petioles. The fruit matures throughout the year, and the trees have a tendency to overbear, resulting in varying sizes and appearance of fruit on the tree. The fruits are generally, ovoid to elliptical, with characteristic necks and nipples. The peel is light yellow at maturity, of varying thickness and surface texture, with prominent oil glands. The pulp is the colour of pale straw, very acid and slightly bitter.

Although not eaten fresh, as are oranges or mandarins, lemons constitute an important fresh fruit group. Lemons, appropriately called 'the fruit of many uses', are used primarily for drinks and fresh juice, baked goods, confectionery, perfumes, cosmetics, pharmaceuticals and lemonade. The principal by-products obtained from the fruit are citric acid from the juice, and pectin and lemon oil from the rind.

Commercial lemon cultivation is concentrated in the mild sub-tropical regions between 40°N and 40°S. The USA and Italy produce most of the world's lemons. Other major producers are Argentina, Brazil, Spain, Greece, Turkey, Israel, Lebanon and Chile. Lemons are also produced in Australia, Cyprus, South Africa, Algeria, Tunisia, Morocco and India. The annual world lemon production is about 5×10^6 t. The world lemon trade figures – exports worth 381×10^6 and imports worth 450×10^6 – indicate the economic importance of this fruit.

Soil

Lemon trees show enormous adaptability to different soil types; they grow in any type of soil if it is sufficiently aerated and penetrable. Soils which are light to medium, well aerated, deep, loose, and free from moisture stagnation are ideally suited. A hard substratum is detrimental, and a high water table should be avoided. Lemon plants lack fine root hairs, so that humus is essential for soil improvement. Some cultivars adapt to certain soil conditions better than others.

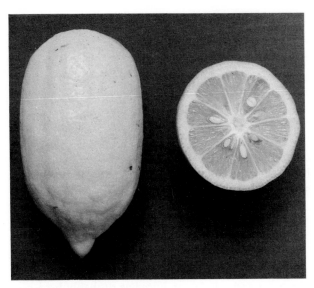

Fig. 1 Eureka lemon fruit.

Propagation

Commercial citrus is a vegetatively propagated crop. Vegetative propagation is mostly performed by budding the desired lemon cultivar onto a selected rootstock. The most commonly used rootstock for lemon cultivars is the Rough lemon, which has a very positive influence on the growth, yield and fruit quality of the lemon. The rootstock plays a major role in lemon cultivation, along with other cultivation practices such as planting distance, fertilization, irrigation, pruning and plant protection.

Cultivars

The lemon cultivars are broadly grouped into two categories – Eureka and Lisbon. Eureka (Fig. 1) originated as a seedling from an Italian cultivar, in Los Angeles, and is the major lemon cultivar grown throughout the world. Most of the lemon cultivation in California is in the Eureka category. The fruits are medium to small with a yellow, medium-thick rind, ridged longitudinally. The fruits are harvested in the late winter, spring and early summer, and have excellent storage and shipping qualities. The other popular Eureka cultivars are Femmenello, Inter-donato and Monachello lemons in the Mediterranean countries, Villafranca lemon in California, Ponderose lemon in the USA and Mediterranean countries, and Nepali Oblong and Pat lembu in India.

The Lisbon lemon originated in Portugal. It is grown in the USA, Italy and the Mediterranean countries. The fruits are medium-sized, with a large prominent nipple and a medium-thick, finely pitted rind. The main crop matures in winter and spring. The other popular cultivars in the Lisbon group are Bears lemon in Florida, Berna in Spain, Algeria and Morocco, Mesero in the Mediterranean countries and Meyer in Florida, Texas, China, New Zealand, South Africa and the Mediterranean countries.

Processing

Most of the lemon crop is processed, lemon juice being the most important product. Lemon juice has many uses in the food industry. Large quantities of lemon juice are used to enhance food flavour, and to develop and balance the flavours of many food items, seafood being an outstanding example. Lemon juice has a distinct composition, different from other citrus fruits. It has varied uses and it is no exaggeration to say that, except for sugar and salt, lemon juice has probably been used more extensively than any other food item to enhance and develop inherent food flavour. The major constituents of lemon juice (per 100 g of juice) are as follows:

- Citric acid, 6 g
- Ascorbic acid, 45 mg
- Soluble solids, 9 g
- Total sugars, 2 g
- Reducing sugars, 1·6 g
- Ash substances and minerals, 250 mg
- Potassium, 100 mg
- Calcium, 10 mg
- Phosphorus, 9 mg
- Magnesium, 7 mg
- Sodium, 2 mg

The following are minor constituents of lemon juice (per 100 g of juice):

- Protein, 0·4 g
- Fat, 0·2 g
- Malic acid, 0.3 g
- Iron, 0·2 g
- Thiamin (B_1), 0·04 mg
- Riboflavin (B_2), 0·02 mg
- Nicotinic acid, 0·09 mg
- Inositol, 65·0 mg
- Flavanones, 45·0 mg

The demand for lemon-flavoured, powdered soft drink mixes, fruit drink mixes, as well as the carbonated and noncarbonated soft drinks, is increasing steadily, giving a new impetus to the lemon processing industry. *See* Flavour Compounds, Production Methods; *See* individual nutrients.

By-products

One of the most important aspects of lemon industry is the manufacture of a variety of by-products. In fact, in some countries the by-products are more important than lemon juice. Citric acid from the juice, and pectin and lemon oil from the fruit rind, are the most important by-products from lemon.

Citric acid is by far the most important single constituent of the lemon. It is used extensively in the food industry to develop and balance the flavour of food items. Concentrated juices are standardized on the basis of the acidity, in which citric acid plays an important role. Lemon fruits can yield citric acid up to 1% of the fruit weight, and most of the world's citric acid requirements are met by lemon.

Lemon peel and the albedo, or inner skin of fruit, contain abundant sources of pectin. Commercial pectins have their principal applications in food as gel-formers, or thickeners for suspending solids, and as body-producing agents, emulsifiers, etc. They are also used in pharmaceuticals, cosmetics and creams, and as a blood plasma substitute. Several processing steps are required for the commercial production of pectin from lemon. Processing economics are a major factor in determining the extent of the commercial recovery of pectin. *See* Pectin, Food Uses

Lemon oil is one of the oldest citrus by-products. It is mostly obtained from the oil glands present in the flavedo, or outer skin of the fruit. The lemon oil, a mixture of essential oils, is composed of several compounds, including terpenes, aldehydes, esters, sterols and alcohols. Most of the lemon oil is consumed by the food and beverage industries for flavouring food and soft drink items. Lemon oil is used in soap, perfume, cosmetics, fruit cordials, flavours, liqueurs, pharmaceuticals, etc. The essential oils from lemon peel, leaves and seeds are used in the production of germicides and in the paper industry. *See* Essential Oils, Properties and Uses

Secondary Products

Several secondary products are produced from the lemon crop. Animal feed is produced from the waste pulp after juice extraction; after drying, 10% of the pulp is available as an animal feed. Molasses from fruit, and lactic acid, citronade and alcohol from peel are also produced. Oil from the seeds is used for commercial margarine production.

Nutritional and Medicinal Aspects

Lemons are an important source of several vitamins, minerals and trace elements, as well as some essential oils, which are extensively used in the pharmaceutical industry. Vitamin C is an important constituent of lemon. Vitamins B and E are also present. Vitamin C is supposed to be involved in increasing tissue resistance to respiratory viruses. Pectin is associated with the property of lowering blood cholesterol. Minerals such as potassium, sodium, calcium, magnesium and phosphorus are present in lemon juice, in substantial amounts. Potassium is recommended as a supplement for people taking diuretic medicines. Copper, zinc, iron and manganese are the important trace elements in the juice. *See* Tocopherols, Physiology

Bibliography

FAO (1983) *FAO Production Year Book 1982*, vol. 36. Rome: Food and Agriculture

FAO (1983)*FAO Trade Year Book 1982*, vol. 36. Rome: Food and Agriculture Organization.

Fritz WD (1970) *Citrus Cultivation and Fertilization*. Bochum, FRG: Ruhr-Stickstaff.

Nagy S and Attaway JA (1980) *Citrus Nutrition and Quality*. Washington, DC: American Chemists Society.

Nagy S and Shaw PE (eds) (1977) *Citrus Science and Technology*, vol. 2. Westport, Connecticut: AVI Publishing.

Reuther W, Webber HJ and Batchelor LD (eds) (1967) *Citrus Industry*, vol. 1. Riverside: University of California.

Ting SV and Rouseff RL (1986) *Citrus Fruits and their Products – Analysis and Technology*. New York: Marcel Dekker.

Wardousi WF, Nagy S and Grievson W (eds) (1986) *Fresh Citrus Fruits*. Westport, Connecticut: AVI Publishing.

M. B. N. V. Prasad and M. M. Mustaffa
Indian Institute of Horticultural Research, Bangalore, India

Grapefruits

Grapefruit is one of the most popular and desired citrus fruits. It has many unique qualities, including a distinct, pleasant aroma, a piquant taste which is characteristic of the citrus essential oils, and typical colours that arise from the presence of various carotenoids in the plastids. Most citrus fruits, but especially grapefruit, have a combination of sour and sweet which delights the palate of people of all ages. Everything from grapefruit is utilized, from the seed to the aroma which is recovered as essence.

Citrus fruit is considered to be one of the most important sources of vitamin C. Citrus fruits and their products supply a major portion of the vitamin C requirement for a large percentage of the population of the developed countries. Grapefruit and citrus products provide nearly 60% of the US Recommended Dietary Allowance of vitamin C in the American diet. *See* Ascorbic Acid, Physiology

Grapefruit is considered a distinct species (*Citrus paradisi* Macf.), and appears to have arisen as a mutant of shaddock (*Citrus grandis* Osbeck.) in the West Indies during the eighteenth century. It was first heard of in Barbados in 1750 under the name 'forbidden fruit'; hence the origin of grapefruit is not known with certainty. In 1789, the forbidden fruit or smaller shaddock was reported to be common in Jamaica, and in 1814 it was called 'grapefruit' because the fruit hung in small clusters, like some grapes, instead of one on a twig. *Pomelo* is still the common name in Brazil, although *toronja* is the common name in Spanish; it is popularly called 'grapefruit' in the USA.

Grapefruit originated in the Western hemisphere and is little cultivated anywhere in the Old World, although Israel and South Africa have commercial plantings for export. The USA produces about 90% of the world crop: Florida state produces more than 50% of the world crop, with Texas a good second, and much smaller production in California, Arizona and Puerto Rico. The major production areas are the USA, Israel, West Indies, Cuba, Argentina and South Africa.

The grapefruit tree is large, with a rounded or conical head and dense foliage. A few, relatively small thorns are present. New growth is nonpubescent and the twigs are angular when young. The leaves are glabrous, ovate, dark glossy green, leathery, petiole-less, and broadly winged. The flowers are large, solitary in cymose clusters of 2–20 or more, and sweet-scented. The fruits are large, globose or pyriform, light lemon or orange coloured, and borne in clusters. The rind is medium thick, yellow and smooth, the flesh yellow in colour, and the flavour a blend of sweet and sour with a trace of bitterness. The juice sacs are large and closely packed; the core is open at full maturity. The seeds are wedge-shaped, and the cotyledons white and highly polyembyronic.

Fruit Morphology

Grapefruit is composed of three distinctly different morphological parts. The epicarp consists of the coloured portion of the peel and is known as the flavedo. In the flavedo are cells containing the carotenoids which give the characteristic colour to the fruit. The oil glands, also found in the flavedo, are the raised structures in the skin of the fruit that contain the essential oil, naringin, characteristic of grapefruit. *See* Carotenoids, Properties and Determination; Essential Oils, Properties and Uses

Immediately under the epicarp is the mesocarp, or albedo. This is typically a thick, white, spongy layer. The albedo consists of large parenchymatous cells that are rich in pectic substances and hemicelluloses. It completely envelops the endocarp, the usual edible portion of the citrus fruits. The combined albedo and flavedo are called the pericarp, commonly known as the rind or peel. *See* Hemicelluloses

The edible portion of the citrus fruit or the endocarp is composed of many carpels or segments. A fruit gener-

Table 1. Distribution (percentage fresh weight) of the component parts of two varieties of grapefruit

	Duncan Seedy	Marsh Seedless
Peel	27·2	44·1
Segment membrane	10·3	3·5
Juice vesicle	59·4	52·4
Seeds	3·4	—

Table 2. Proximate composition (g per 100 g fresh weight) of grapefruit

	Whole fruit	Juice	Segment
Moisture	88·9	90·2	91·3
Protein	0·5	0·5	0·6
Fat	0·1	0·1	0·1
Carbohydrates			
Soluble	10·1	9·0	7·6
Insoluble	0·2	—	0·2
Ash	0·4	0·2	0·4

ally has 9 to 13 segments. Inside each segment are located the juice vesicles, which are attached to the segment membrane by the vesicle stalk. Juice vesicles have relatively strong membranes and many thin-walled juice cells.

The many chemical constituents are distributed among the various tissues. Some are more concentrated in one tissue than in another. Flavanose glucosides are found in higher concentration in the albedo than in either the juice vesicle or the flavedo, and the level of bitter naringin is highest in the albedo and membrane. Sugars are well distributed in the cells of all tissues, but the juice cells store the greatest quantity of sugars in the vacuoles, which also contain the acid. Pectin occurs as calcium pectate in the cell walls or as protopectin. It is most abundant in the albedo, and lesser amounts occur in other parts of the fruit. Over 400 different constituents have been isolated from grapefruit. The principal components of a fruit are carbohydrates, which include mainly sucrose, glucose and fructose, plus trace amounts of several other sugars. These constitute about 75% of the total soluble solids (TSS) in juice. Organic acids, mainly citric and malic with traces of others, constitute less than 10% of the TSS, and free amino acids, plus nitrogenous bases and glutathione, about 6%. The remaining components include inorganic ions (about 3%), vitamins (2·5%), flavonoids and volatiles (1·2%), and lipids (1·2%). The distribution of different fruit components, the proximate composition, different sugar fractions, and the composition of fresh and canned grapefruit are given in Tables 1 to 4. *See* individual nutrients

Table 3. Average sugar composition (g per 100 g) of grapefruit

	Juice	Peel
Glucose	1·6	11·6
Fructose	1·75	12·80
Total reducing sugar	3·41	24·40
Sucrose	2·56	14·30
Total sugar	5·97	38·70

Table 4. Composition of fresh and canned fruit

	Fresh	Canned (fruit and syrup)
Edible matter (%)	0·48	1·0
Water (g)	90·7	81·8
Sugar (g)	5·3	15·5
Dietary fibre (g)	0·6	0·4
Energy value (kcal)	22	60
Protein (g)	0·6	0·5
Minerals (mg)	258	113
Vitamin C (mg)	40	30
Thiamin (μg)	40–100	10–50
Nicotinic acid (μg)	200–220	80–200
Folic acid (μg)	80–180	10–220
Pantothenic acid (μg)	290	70–190

Varieties

Grapefruit was introduced to Florida in 1823 by Dr Odette Philippe, a French count, who settled near Safety Harbour on Tampa Bay. All present varieties descended from this introduction by seedling variation, mutation or hybridization. The relationship of the mutants to their parents is shown in Table 5.

Duncan

Duncan is the oldest grapefruit variety, introduced and propagated by AL Duncan of nearby Dunedin around 1892. The fruits are large, broadly obovate, seedy, medium early in maturity, and harvested during January to March. They have excellent flavour and white

Table 5. Relationships of mutant varieties of grapefruit

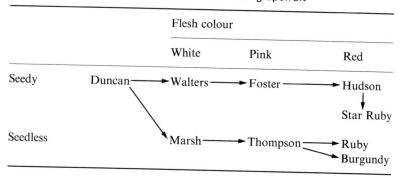

flesh. Duncan is probably the most cold-resistant grapefruit.

Foster

Foster was the first pink-fleshed variety to be discovered. It arose as a bud sport of the Walters variety. The rind is also flushed pink, and the maturity season is November and December. Quality is good but the number of seeds is large.

Marsh

The original Marsh tree was a seedling planted from Duncan variety. The fruit is smaller than Duncan and Foster, and matures later; it can be held longer on the tree without excessive dropping. Flesh colour is white and the number of seeds ranges from zero to six.

Thompson

Thompson originated as a pink-fleshed bud sport of a Marsh tree. It is seedless and pink-fleshed. It matures earlier than Marsh and it can be held longer on the tree, for several months, without dropping, although the pink colour fades out with age.

Ruby

Ruby was the first grapefruit with deep red flesh, originated as a bud sport on the Thompson variety. The fruits are similar to Thompson fruits, except that the flesh colour is more deeply pigmented and the rind has a crimson blush with some pigmentation in the albedo.

Triumph

Triumph is one of the best varieties for home planting, because of its unusually fine flavour and freedom from bitterness. It is very seedy but very juicy.

Burgundy

Burgundy is a bud sport of Thompson with red flesh. The fruit is seedless and late ripening, with a white albedo, like that of Thompson.

Star Ruby

Star Ruby was developed from an irradiated seed of the Hudson variety in Texas. The fruit is red-fleshed, seedless, and late maturing. Used in the 'sectionizing' industry, since the segments hold together well, it is also suitable for juicing because at single strength it retains its colour well.

Climate

Grapefruit trees require dry and arid conditions for the production of excellent quality fruits. They can stand a maximum temperature of 50°C and a minimum temperature below freezing point. Grapefruit thrives in frost-free subtropical and semi-tropical climate, and can be grown in two belts, 20–40°N and 20–40°S.

Soil

Grapefruit grow well on deep, well-drained, free-working sandy loams and silt or clay loams, with a preference for loose sandy loams. Heavy soils, containing a high percentage of clay and with insufficient aeration, are not suitable. Ideal pH of the soil is between 5·5 and 7·5.

Production

Grapefruit is polyembyronic and can be successfully propagated from seeds. The other means of propagation are by budding, grafting, layering or cutting. Grapefruit stems are difficult to root; hence budding has to be done on the selected rootstock; patch budding is the commonly adopted method. Sour orange and Rough lemon are the common and popular rootstocks for grapefruit. The bud wood should be selected from disease-free, high-yielding, certified trees. The trees are planted at 10 m spacing and should not be interplanted with oranges or tangerines. The major insect pests are scales, mealy bug, leaf-eating caterpillars, leaf miner and aphids. The major fungal diseases are *Phytophthora* and powdery mildew, and the virus diseases are tristeza, greening and psorosis. The trees will start bearing after 4 or 5 years and can become commercially productive within 10 to 12 years, with a potential yield of 400 fruits per tree.

Harvest

Grapefruit if unique among citrus fruits because it stores well on the tree and may be harvested nearly year-round. The varieties may mature early, in midseason, or late, when allowed to develop normally. Some of the seedy varieties naturally develop a pleasing ratio of sugar to acid by November, while the seedless varieties and other good seedy varieties are not naturally mature enough for good eating quality until February or March. The fruits can be held on the tree for up to 7 or 8 months, as a result of very slow physiological changes at maturity. Optimum palatability for grapefruit, which has an unusually long harvest season, tends to coincide with the onset of the next bloom, after which keeping quality deteriorates. The maturity standards for grapefruit vary in different countries depending on the usage. *See* Ripening of Fruit

Fruits should have a rind which is smooth and uniformly yellow or blushed, without any green. Seedless fruits are preferred, and pink or red flesh colour is usually an advantage over white flesh colour. Desirable fruit sizes are large to medium. The fresh fruit and gift box shippers demand a regularly oblate shape which can be cut into two symmetrical halves for serving at the table.

Processing

Most grapefruit is consumed as fresh fruit, but the fruits from Florida and Brazil are used mainly for processing. The processed products are canned grapefruit juices, chilled and pasteurized juices, concentrated juice and reconstituted juice, and grapefruit segments.

The canned sections and salads should have pleasant tasting fruit, and segments which are intact after processing. Pink and red flesh colours do not usually look attractive after canning, and seedy fruit has better section stability than seedless, as well as higher solid content; thus seedy varieties with white flesh are used

generally. For canned juice and frozen concentrate, attractive juice colour, high juice content, high solids, a fair degree of acid and low bitterness are required. The seedy, white-fleshed varieties are preferred but the Star Ruby variety is also processed. *See* Canning, Quality Changes During Canning

Volatile Compounds

The most characteristic property of grapefruit is their unique aroma. The volatile compounds of the oil are produced by the ductless oil glands located in the flavedo layer of the peel. The grapefruit oil contains 20 alcohols, 12 aldehydes, 13 esters, 14 hydrocarbons, 3 ketones and 2 miscellaneous compounds. The characteristic aroma is caused by nookatone, and the main constituent is limonene. The oil is widely used in flavouring juice drinks, citrus-flavoured soft drinks and carbonated drinks. The essential oil is used both in the pharmaceutical and food industries as an aroma and/or flavouring agent.

Pigments

The red colour of pink and red grapefruit is caused by lycopene, whereas that of blood orange is caused by anthocyanins. The red and pink grapefruit juice contains 1500 iu of carotene. *See* Colours, Properties and Determination of Natural Pigments

By-products and Speciality Products

During processing, more than 50% of the fruit is lost in the peel, rag, pulp and seed which are not generally used as human food. Specialized products, such as candied peel, marmalades and essential oil, are made and used in food preparation. The peel, membrane, pulp and seeds have been used as animal feed in the form of dried citrus pulp. Citrus molasses is used in the production of vinegar, bland syrup and alcohol. The peel is used for commercial pectin production, and in the manufacture of fruit jam and marmalades. The dried seeds contain 30–45% lipid. Seed oil is a desirable dietetic substitute becausde of the high percentage of unsaturated fatty acids. Bioflavonoids are extracted from the waste and used for pharmaceutical purposes. The seed residue is useful as animal feed.

Nutritional and Medicinal Aspects

Grapefruits are an important source of vitamin C and, to a lesser extent, vitamins A, B and E. The most important nutrients of grapefruit are the carbohydrates. The polysaccharides of the fruit provide a good source of dietary fibre, which has been recognized for its ability to decrease the transit time of food through gastro-intestinal tract of man and cattle. Pectin has been associated with the property of lowering the serum cholesterol level in mammals. Grapefruit is abundant in potassium and low in sodium. People who take diuretic medicines are known to need a supplemented intake of potassium, and those with high blood pressures are usually placed on a low-sodium diet. The sodium and potassium levels in the juice can be utilized to restore the electrolytic balance in the humans. Calcium, magnesium and phosphorus are also present in the juice. *See* Calcium, Physiology; Dietary Fibre, Physiological Effects; Magnesium; Potassium, Physiology; Retinol, Physiology; Tocopherols, Physiology

It is clear that grapefuit is one of the most important citrus fruits, with a wide range of products and uses.

Bibliography

Chan HT (ed.) (1983) *Handbook of Tropical Food.* New York: Marcel Dekker.

Nagy S, Shaw PE and Veldhins MK (eds) (1977) *Citrus Science and Technology.* Westport, Connecticut: AVI Publishing.

M. B. N. V. Prasad and M. M. Mustaffa
Indian Institute of Horticultural Research, Bangalore, India

Limes

Limes are known worldwide for their tart, tangy flavoured juice and especially for their unique flowery, characteristic aromas. They were introduced to many parts of the world through the explorations of the British navy, where they were probably first used for clinical and nutritional purposes. Their extensive use on-board ship to prevent or treat attacks of 'scurvy' (caused by vitamin C deficiency) earned British sailors the distinctive name 'Limeys', which is still used. Most evidence indicates that limes probably originated in northeastern India and migrated via the trade routes into the Middle East and on to the Western world through sailing vessel trade markets. *See* Ascorbic Acid, Physiology; Scurvy

The juice of most types of limes is too strong to be consumed undiluted. However limes are popular for use in juice-mixtures, -ades (mixes with sugar, water and/or other juices), carbonated beverages and as a component of alcoholic drinks and mixes. In some countries they are used in pickling, culinary and medical applications. A main economical value of limes comes from the highly valued lime oil, used in products as diverse as cosmetics (shave lotions, perfumes, colognes) and household cleaning products (washing powders, soaps, furniture polish and bathroom deodorants). The trees are extremely cold-sensitive and can only be grown in the mildest subtropical to tropical climates.

Limes are the most acid of all citrus fruits and lower in vitamin C content than lemons. Like lemons, they are highly valued for their juice and its acid content. Most limes consist of 40% or more juice by weight or volume. The remainder consists of seeds, vascular bundles, parts of albedo adhering to the skin or flavedo, and parts of fruit segments, collectively referred to as 'rag'. The juice of most cultivars consists of about 90–91% water, 0·2–0·3% protein, 0·7% (in acid types) to 9·0% (in sweet types) sugars, 0·1% fat, and 0·3% minerals (ash). The juice (100 ml) supplies 110–140 kJ (26 kcal) of energy, 50 mg of ascorbic acid (vitamin C) and a trace of dietary fibre. A wide range of vitamin C levels has been reported and, as with most citrus fruits, the level is higher in the peel or rind (63–121 mg%) than in the fruit or juice (30–70 mg%). *See* Dietary Fibre, Properties and Sources

Quite different from the basis of value for other types of citrus, the value of limes (and lemons) is based primarily on the weight of acid (as citric, although there are traces of many others) per unit volume of juice. This is in contrast to the ratio of sugar to acid used for oranges, grapefruits, tangerines, etc. Computer programs and automatic titrator instruments are available to perform such determinations at a high rate in citrus processing plant quality control laboratories. The values reported for lime juice acid content (as citric) have ranged from 6·10% to 8·32% (average 7·20%).

Cultivars, Fruit Types

The small-fruited, acid lime (*Citrus aurantifolia* Swingle) is the most predominant type. It is widely grown in India, Mexico, Egypt, the West Indies, China, California and the southern tip of Florida and the Keys (USA), where it is known as the 'Mexican' or 'Key' lime. Although found in Brazil as the 'Gallego' lime, it is not as well known there. The fruit are small, round, somewhat short-elliptical, and bright to greenish-yellow when mature. Moderately seedy, it has a thin rind, (smooth and leathery) and the flesh is very juicy and acid and has a very distinctive flowery aroma.

The large-fruited, acid limes (main cultivar *Citrus latifolia* Tan.) are more oblong in shape, light to dark green at maturity, and two to five times larger, on average, than the small-fruited limes. These limes, often called Tahitian or Persian, were brought to California from Tahiti, but do not seem to have any connection with Persia. They may be a hybrid of the citron and/or the lemon, but parentage and true source are not definite. This lime is grown mostly in South Florida (and to some extent in Australia and California) because of its better tolerance of cold and its lower requirement for heat to reach maturity. Other types of lime – the Bearss, from California, as well as the Sahesli of Tunisia and the Pond of Hawaii – seem certain, from horticultural evidence, to be the same as the Persian. The juice has a good, characteristic lime flavour and the aroma is typical of that commonly described as 'limelike' throughout most of the world.

The sweet lime (*Citrus limettioides* Tan.) is well liked in India, the Middle East and Latin America. It is known as the Palestine or Indian sweet lime, and is used in those countries for medicinal purposes. Fruit, medium in size and round to slightly oblong, is greenish-yellow to orange-yellow at maturity. The flesh is yellowish; the rind has a distinctive, slightly medicine-like aroma, and the juice is so nonacid as to be insipid to most tastes.

Lime Juice

Lime juice can be prepared and concentrated in the same general manner as orange and grapefruit juice, using similar equipment. For juice extraction, smaller (than usual for oranges) cups are used on one type of extractor which individually cuts and presses each fruit. Another type of extractor presses and disrupts the whole fruit between rotating converging discs, and the fruit, pulp, rag and juice mixture is then separated in a screw press/screen finisher. The juice can be concentrated on a Thermal Accelerated Short Time Evaporator (TASTE), widely used throughout the world citrus processing industries. However, since lime juice contains a higher percentage of organic acids than of carbohydrates, the degree of concentration is determined as grams per litre (GPL) of acid rather than the degrees Brix (approximate percentage of sugars) commonly used for other citrus concentrates. Even so, Brix measurements with a commonly available Brixometer are necessary, to determine the bulk density from which the GPL can be calculated. Computer programs and automated instrumentation make dependable determinations possible at a high rate. Most lime concentrates are evaporated to about 400–500 GPL. The uncorrected, observed, desired Brix value (that is roughly analogous to the acid concentration desired) must be known by the evaporator controller since the control is based on in-line Brixometers. The approximate desired Brix value must be determined based on the acid and Brix of the incoming single strength juice, and standard methods are available for this.

Lime Oil

Lime oil, a major commercial product is, in most processes, more valuable than the juice, which may be considered a by-product of the lime oil process. It may be prepared by allowing the liquid, separated from the pressed mixture of fruit parts described above, to stand until the oil 'layers' off at the top, and then decanting or distilling off the layer. The character and composition of the decanted oil vary considerably from those of the distilled oil. As a by-product of this process, the bottom juice layer is a clarified, sparkling clear, light-green-coloured juice. Special clarifying additives are often used in this process to enhance clarity of the resultant juice. This product is distributed widely around the world, especially in the UK and the Caribbean area as a mixer base for alcoholic and soft drinks.

Lime oil may also be prepared by the conventional 'cold-pressing' process, whereby the flavedo and adhering fruit parts are passed into a conical pressure filtration press. The 'peel juice' is pressed through a steel screen and the oil is separated in a high-speed centrifuge. This process produces a clear, green-coloured oil with fine aromatic quality and stability of aroma and flavour. The juice or concentrate resulting from this type of process has a stable, well-suspended 'cloud' and is used in bases for juice drinks, -ades and soft drinks.

The oil is located in oval-shaped oil sacs situated rather evenly throughout the flavedo or outer layer of the peel. The oil sacs function as a natural toxic barrier to microorganisms and insects which might otherwise attack the fruit. The oil is composed of a base sesquiterpene hydrocarbon (D-limonene, more than 50%) and a mixture of other mono- and sesquiterpenes. From lime oil analyses the following organic components have been identified: 12 alcohols, 7 aldehydes, 4 esters, 1 ketone, and 22 hydrocarbons, with 7% nonvolatiles (mainly coumarins).

To control and classify quality and value of citrus oils, the National Research Council, officially recognized by the US Food and Drug Administration, has published and regularly updates the *Food Chemicals Codex* (FCC). Lime oil FCC standards are summarized in Table 1.

Storage

Because of their extreme high acidity and low pH, limes are more stable than many other citrus fruits. However, problems are encountered at certain temperatures and humidities with growth of acid-tolerant surface fungi. Control has been accomplished using biological growth-regulators. In Persian limes 2,4-dichlorophenolindophenol (24D) and gibberellic acid (GA) have been successful in reducing growth of *Penicillium*-type moulds, yellowing, mottling and discoloration of the rinds during storage. Such problems have not been solved through use of controlled-atmosphere storage, but can be greatly controlled through use of optimum storage conditions for fresh fruit, i.e. 10°C and 90–95% relative humidity,

Table 1. Summary of lime oil specifications according to the *Food Chemical Codex* (1981)

Cold pressed	Mexican	Persian	Distilled oil
Aldehydes percentage citral	4·5–8·5	3·2–7·5	0·5–2·5
Optical Rotation (+ degrees)	35–41	38–53	34–47
Refractive index	1·482–1·486	1·476–1·486	1·474–1·477
Specific gravity	0·872–0·881	0·858–0·876	0·855–0·863
UV absorption (315 nm)	0·45	0·24	—
Evaporative residue (%)	10·0–14·5	5·0–12·0	—

where storage life of up to 4 weeks or longer has been reported without notable injury, pitting or discoloration of fruit. *See* Controlled Atmosphere Storage, Applications for Bulk Storage of Foodstuffs; Spoilage, Moulds in Food Spoilage

Value

Because by far the majority of limes in the world are produced in India, Indonesia and Mexico, predominantly for the local fresh fruit markets, any statistical data on value and extent of the crop and the fresh market are unavoidably biased. Few dependable agricultural statistics are available for local fresh markets in those geographic areas. Although the USA is a notable and important producer of limes and lime products, it is not the major world producer of the fresh fruit, but the most dependable statistics on production and value of products are those for the USA. The total annual production of all types of limes in the USA from 1980 to 1990 ranged from about 52 to 72×10^3 t. In general, the amount of those processed has been about 40–50% of the total crop. Annual value of the US crop has ranged from around $\$16 \times 10^6$ to $\$20 \times 10^6$. Almost all significant production has been in Florida. During the same period the USA imported 15 000 to 30 000 and exported 3000–4500 t per year. During the 1970s and 1980s, the total US annual crop was about equal to 25% of the world crop. Extrapolating that to the present, the annual crop worldwide would be in the range of 200 000 t, with an approximate value in the range of $\$64 \times 10^6$ to $\$80 \times 10^6$.

Bibliography

Hicks D (ed.) (1990) *Production and Packaging of Non-carbonated Fruit Juices and Fruit Beverages*. New York: Van Nostrand Reinhold.

Kimball DA (1991) *Citrus Processing Quality Control and Technology*. New York: Van Nostrand Reinhold.

Pattee HE (ed.) (1985) *Evaluation of Quality of Fruits and Vegetables*. Westport, Connecticut: AVI Publishing.

Sinclair WB (1984) *The Biochemistry and Physiology of the Lemon and Other Citrus Fruits*. Oakland: University of California, Division of Agriculture and Natural Resources.

US Department of Agriculture (1988) *Agricultural Statistics 1988*. Washington, DC: US Government Printing Office.

Wardowski WF, Nagy S and Grierson W (eds) (1986) *Fresh Citrus Fruits*. Connecticut: AVI Publishing.

Robert E. Berry
Institute of Food Technologists, Florida, USA

CLAMS

See Shellfish

CLEANING PROCEDURES IN THE FACTORY

Contents

Types of Detergent
Types of Disinfectant
Overall Approach
Modern Systems

Types of Detergent

Cleaning within the food industry has traditionally been as much an art as a science. This can be accounted for by the need to develop detergents before the processes of soiling, cleaning and disinfection were fully understood or analysed in a scientific manner. Early detergents and their method of application were, therefore, by design, aimed at providing a satisfactory performance. As the function of specific chemicals and the contribution of other factors were researched and, as improvements in plant design, detergent handling and control came about, detergents gradually improved, leading to the high standards expected and obtainable today.

The determination of the correct detergent for any cleaning process in a food or beverage factory is subject to a number of selection criteria. These criteria include plant design and construction, the result required, cleaning techniques available, the type of soil present, the manner in which the soil is formed, the nature of the production process and the chemical composition of water supplies. This article assesses these selection criteria, specific detergent types and their function.

Selection Criteria

A successful cleaning application is reliant on consideration of a number of selection criteria. These criteria will vary according to the food product and process concerned, but the following criteria are common to all applications.

The Result Required

In all cases, the result required must be considered before detergents are selected. There are three commonly used classifications for the level of cleanliness: physically clean, chemically clean and microbiologically clean.

A physically clean surface is one which is visually clean to a satisfactory standard. Within the food processing environment, this standard is limited to nonfood contact areas and covers such applications as floor cleaning in warehouse areas, yards and so on. At the basic level, this standard may not require the use of a detergent, with a satisfactory result obtained using physical means only; other applications may require the use of light-duty detergents.

A chemically clean standard is applied to all applications within the food processing area. In this instance, plant is cleaned to a standard at which anything in contact with the cleaned surface suffers no contamination. This standard is sometimes referred to as 'water-break-free', indicating that the cleaned surface is easily wetted by water. The materials used to provide this standard are numerous, varying from acidic, through neutral to alkaline detergents.

A microbiologically clean standard is required for all direct and indirect food contact surfaces. This standard involves the creation of a water- and break-free surface with the elimination of food spoilage and food poisoning microorganisms and a reduction in total viable colonies to an acceptable level. The acceptable level is determined by legislative standards, set in the UK by the Ministry of Agriculture, Fisheries and Food (MAFF), by food retailers' 'own label' standards, or by process-generated standards (i.e. commissioning and adaptation of plant and processes create their own standards). The materials used to achieve the microbiologically clean standard are again numerous, and include those used to achieve a chemically clean surface.

For a microbiologically clean surface, the detergents are used in conjunction with disinfectants to achieve the desired result. Alternatively, combined detergent and disinfectant products, known as sanitizers, may be used.

Soil Type and Manner of Generation

Soil may be defined as any unwanted material on a surface. In general, soils may be categorized as organic (derived from living matter) or inorganic (derived from minerals). The former are removed primarily by alkaline

Table 1. Variations in milk soil compositions

	Fat	Protein	Mineral	Total deposit
Milk soil on cold surfaces				
Average	Major	Average is 17–25% of amount of fat	Very minor	
Fresh milk	Increases			
High bacteria	Phospholipids interact with some bacteria	Increases		Increases More tenacious
Increased milk temperature	Decreases	Increases	Increases	More tenacious
Milk soil on heated surfaces				
Average	Minor	Denatured Major amounts	Calcium phosphate Major amounts	
Increased temperature		Increases or decreases (depends on temperature range)	Increases	More compact soil
Milk held in holding section before heating to high temperature		Decreases	Increases	More compact soil
Aged milk				Decreases

materials whilst the latter require the use of acids. In reality, the soils encountered are a combination of both inorganic and organic components. Soils vary substantially in composition, which is dependent on processing parameters, including the foodstuffs produced, the processing temperature, the age of the soil and water hardness conditions.

Soils produced on heated surface differ significantly from those produced on nonheated surfaces. These variations can have a number of origins. The high temperatures of heat exchange units can cause the denaturation of proteins, caramelization of sugars, and precipitation of mineral salts which readily plate out on heat exchange surfaces. In general, oils and fats enter soil residues unaltered, but excessively high temperatures may lead to polymerization of these components.

Food soils obviously vary from one food processing industry to the next. Components of soil types in different applications are determined by the raw materials used during processing; hence meat and poultry soils have a major fat component, whilst bakery soils may contain carbonized starch and sugar deposits.

To further complicate the matter, a combination of processes involved in the manufacture of the food product will modify the raw materials used and, consequently, the soil composition. The effect of processing on soil composition is illustrated in Table 1, in which the wide range of composition of milk soil is shown as a function of the conditions under which it is formed and the age of the milk which formed it.

Some generalizations can be made, as Table 1 shows. Mineral content of soils increases as the temperature is raised. Fat deposits tend to decrease with an increase in

temperature but also depend on the history of the milk. Interestingly enough, fresh milk tends to give greater amounts of soil, in particular fat, than milk which has been aged.

Heat exchanger surfaces, such as those found in HTST (high temperature, short time) pasteurizers, usually have only a small amount of fat present which is presumed to be entrapped by other soils such as proteins. It has also been shown that air drying (as opposed to steam drying), turbulence of the flow of milk products, the microbial quality of the milk, and the acidity of the milk can all affect the nature of milk soils.

Plant Design and Construction

The compatibility of the materials used in construction of a process plant with the detergents used to clean that plant is of utmost importance. Any detergent used should not detrimentally affect the construction materials. Limitations due to this factor should be determined at the earliest opportunity to prevent costly damage to capital items. The majority of modern plant is constructed of stainless steel, which is generally resistant to corrosion by detergents and disinfectants; however, in older production plants or in areas where specific materials are required for processing reasons, incompatibility may occur. *See* Plant Design, Designing for Hygienic Operation

A major concern with respect to compatibility is the effect of sodium hydroxide (caustic soda)-based detergents on aluminium, galvanized and other soft metal surfaces. Contact with such materials will lead not only to rapid corrosion, but also to the release of hydrogen gas which can form an explosive mixture with air.

Plant design will restrict the detergent selection and method of application. Electrical installations and moisture-sensitive processes require the minimal use of water; hence the need for detergents which contain nontoxic and nontainting alcohols. Intricately designed plant which is both difficult and time-consuming to clean by hand may require the use of foam- or gel-cleaning techniques which, through longer contact times and greater coverage, can achieve the desired result more rapidly and with a minimum level of manual input. With regard to automated cleaning techniques, such as cleaning-in-place (CIP) and bottle-washing, even the equipment used to clean the process plant may dictate detergent selection.

Available Cleaning Techniques

More often than not, cleaning within the food and beverage industries is automated through the use of CIP techniques. In these instances, powerful materials are used, leading to greater reproducibility of results. CIP techniques provide greater control, in terms of temperature, contact time and detergent strength, when compared with manual cleaning.

However, there are areas in which manual cleaning or a degree of manual input is necessary. The use of such aggressive materials in this instance should be avoided on health and safety grounds. In manual cleaning applications, the use of neutral or near-neutral materials is recommended.

Water Supplies

The chemical composition of the local water supply will affect the selection of detergents. Water, falling as rain, dissolves gases and becomes mildly acidic. As it percolates through soil and flows over various strata, minerals are dissolved in the water. These dissolved minerals are collectively termed 'water hardness' and are measured in parts per million of calcium carbonate (ppm $CaCO_3$). The quality and quantity of water hardness will vary according to the composition of the rock strata. Within the UK, water hardness varies from less than 20 ppm $CaCO_3$ in and around Glasgow to more than 350 ppm $CaCO_3$ in the East Midlands.

Water hardness may be broken down into temporary hardness, which is precipitated by heat, and permanent hardness, which is precipitated by high alkalinity. In any application where alkaline detergents are used at elevated temperatures, there is then the potential for scale deposition on plant surfaces. The result is unsightly and, if it occurs on a direct or indirect food contact surface, it may become a source of physical and microbial contamination. In order to prevent scale deposition, sequestering and dispersing materials are used in alkaline formulations. The function of these materials is covered later in this article (see *Sequestrants*).

In addition to the criteria listed above, there are factors specific to individual applications which affect detergent selection. Fermentative applications, for example, will generate carbon dioxide which will rapidly break down sodium hydroxide to sodium carbonates, these will subsequently precipitate as process-generated scale.

As can be seen, there is no such entity as the universal detergent and these various selection criteria require the formulation of specific detergents. Not only is the ability of the detergent to clean important, its ease of dispensing, rinsability, chemical stability and other factors, which include safety and cost, must also be given serious consideration. Formulated detergents are a direct response to these challenges.

Detergent Components

Formulated detergents are based on acids, alkalis or neutral materials. These materials have inherent properties which are desirable within a detergent formulation. Acids are effective in dissolving mineral salts and in the hydrolysis of proteins, whilst caustic alkalis will break down carbonized deposits and saponify fats and oils. The effect of neutral materials, such as sequestrants and surfactants, is discussed later in this article.

It may be argued that since these raw materials have desired properties, there is no need for formulated detergents; however, the drawbacks, in terms of comparatively high use rates, poor rinsability, lack of soil suspension, a reliance on more than one material to achieve the required result, and the time required to clean, far outweigh any advantage. Furthermore, modern process plant demands the use of high-performance formulated detergents and there are certain applications (e.g. bottle-washing) in which raw materials alone will not achieve the required result.

Formulated detergents combine the inherent properties of the raw material with those of other components to produce the following required physical and chemical interactions:

1. Wetting of the surface to allow intimate contact between detergent and soil.
2. Chemical reaction with the soil. At least three distinct interactions may occur: saponification by caustic reaction with oils and fats; hydrolysis reactions to solubilize proteins; acidic dissolution of mineral salts.
3. Dispersion of large soil particles into finely divided ones.
4. Suspension of removed soil in the detergent solution.

Types of Detergent

Table 2. Detergent types

Detergent type	pH range	Commonly used components in order of importance	Typical applications
Caustic	13+	Caustic soda or potash Sequestrants Surfactants	CIP, HTST, cleaning, bottle-washing
Alkaline	10–13	{ Carbonates Silicates Phosphates Caustic soda Sequestrants Surfactants	CIP, tray- and crate-washing, floors
Neutral	5–10	Surfactants Phosphates Solvents	Manual hand-cleaning of plant surfaces, utensils, etc., janitorial applications, personal hygiene products
Acidic	0–5	Phosphoric acid Nitric acid Sulphamic acid Hydrochloric acid Surfactants Microbiocide	Descalants, formulated acid detergents for low-pH (fermentative) applications, formulated detergents for use in light soil areas (e.g. raw milk applications in dairies)
Nonaqueous	5–10	Alcohol Surfactant Microbiocide	Moisture-sensitive areas
Gel	1–14	Dependent on application	Specialist applications where a long contact time is require to produce a satisfactory result. Materials are either self-gelling on dilution with water or are supplied as gel to be used neat
Foam	1–14	Dependent on application	Specialist applications. Contact times not as long as gel but better visibility. Air required to generate foam either as secondary injection or by venturi action
Additives	1–14	Dependent on application	Added to existing detergent or rinsing applications. Categories include scale control, foam control, microbiostatic control (preservative)

Table 2 shows detergent types frequently used within the food and beverage industry and an indication of typical applications. The list of applications is by no means exhaustive. The commonly used components are discussed below.

Sequestrants

Sequestrants are used to prevent precipitation of water hardness salts in hot or alkaline solutions. There are two types of sequestrants, divided by their mode of action.

Stoichiometric sequestrants work by chemically combining with water hardness salts, forming complexes which are water-soluble and not precipitated. They have to be present in sufficient quantities to combine with metallic cations, thereby forming the soluble complex. This process is known as chelation.

Threshold sequestrants work at extremely low concentrations (typically 1–5 ppm). They do not function by solubilization but by changing the physical structure of the precipitate such that they do not form scale. This type of sequestrant is said to be a 'crystal growth modifier'. An alkaline material employing threshold sequestration will be cloudy in hard water, but no scale will be deposited on plant surfaces.

The most commonly used sequestrant types are listed below.

Hydroxycarboxylic Acids

Gluconic acid is the most commonly used of this type of sequestrant. It is very soluble in caustic soda and has good long-term and high-temperature stability. To be fully effective as a chelating agent sodium gluconate needs to be used in the presence of free caustic alkali.

Around pH 11, for example, 1 g of sodium gluconate will only chelate about 25 mg of calcium carbonate, whereas in the presence of 3% caustic soda solutions (pH 14) 1 g of sodium gluconate will chelate 325 mg of calcium carbonate. Sodium gluconate also appears to be an effective sequestrant for ferric iron over quite a wide pH range.

Glucoheptonic acid or sodium heptonate, when in caustic solution, has similar properties to sodium gluconate. However, some isomers are better able to break down mineral scales, whilst other isomers are effective at lower pH levels than gluconate.

Citric acid is less widely used. It is more expensive than the other acids mentioned and less effective in chelating calcium at high pH.

Aminocarboxylic Acids

The two main members of this class of sequestrant are ethylene diamine tetracetic acid (EDTA) and nitrilotriacetic acid (NTA); both are normally used as their sodium salts in alkaline and caustic detergent formulations. The solubility of these sequestrants is very limited in high caustic levels, so that they are normally to be found in medium-to-low free caustic formulae. EDTA is able to form a more stable chelate than NTA and is favoured if some descaling ability is required. For softening water over neutral to mildly alkaline pH, both products are very effective, although NTA usually works out to be slightly more cost-effective. Both sequestrants are also effective for iron control in slightly acidic and neutral conditions.

Both the hydroxycarboxylic acids and the aminocarboxylic acids behave only as *stoichiometric sequestrants*, i.e. they form chelates in a fixed ratio with the metallic ions.

Phosphates

The phosphates form a very versatile sequestrant group but, because of limited solubilities and stability in liquid caustic, polyphosphates are more commonly found in powdered detergents.

The polyphosphates not only behave as stoichiometric sequestrants at high concentrations, but also have a threshold effect. Furthermore, they help to build the detergency of formulations by improving dispersion and rinsing properties. Their use in liquid formulations is mainly restricted to alkaline and neutral products.

Phosphonates

Phosphonates retain most of the advantages of the phosphates, have better solubility in caustic and are stable in solution. There is always a cost to pay for progress, and phosphonates are significantly more expensive than their phosphate counterparts. Phosphonates can operate by stoichiometric or threshold effects, and are thus very versatile for use in CIP and bottle-washing products.

Other Sequestering Materials

A number of polymers with both water-conditioning and building properties* have recently become available. The most notable of these materials belong to the polyacrylic acid group. Depending on the molecular weight range chosen, these polyacrylics can behave as threshold sequestrants, dispersing or suspending agents. They have reasonable solubility and stability in caustic solution, and are being used more and more to functionally replace polyphosphates.

Surfactants

Surfactants are widely used in detergent formulations for wetting of soil, soil penetration, soil suspension and to aid rinsing by reduction of surface tension. Surfactants are also used for specific high and stable foam creation or, at the other extreme, for defoaming. All surfactant molecules have a water-liking (hydrophilic) and a water-hating (hydrophobic) structure. When added to water the molecules concentrate at the surface in an attempt to have as much of the hydrophobic portions out of the liquid. Above a certain concentration the molecules which cannot find space at the surface form structures called 'micelles' in the bulk solution. These micelles are capable of holding soils in suspension and even dissolving them.

Surfactants are classified according to the charge on the dissociated species, the anionic being negatively charged and the cationic being positively charged molecules. When there is no net charge, the surfactants are called nonionic, and the amphoteric group may carry either charge depending on pH.

Soaps are the most original of the anionic surfactants, although there is now a wide range of petroleum-derived anionics. Examples include alkyl sulphonates and sulphates, which are used in high-foaming 'neutral' detergents, such as washing up liquids; they all have good detergency and are all high-foaming.

Cationic surfactants include fatty amine salts, which

---

* Building properties: The principles of wetting/penetrating, lifting, dispersing, suspending and rinsing that an effective detergent should possess cannot be provided by any single chemical. Consequently it is necessary to mix together one or more raw materials to provide a product that fulfils all these requirements. Such products are called 'Built detergents'.

Types of Detergent

Table 3. Relative properties of various alkalis

Alkali	Organic detergent	Inorganic detergent	Water tolerance	Soil suspension	Bactericidal properties	Corrosion[a] acceptability	Formulatibility
Sodium hydroxide	+ + +	+	+	+	+ +	+ + +	+
Potassium hydroxide	+ + +	+	+	+	+ +	+ + +	+ +
Sodium carbonate	+ +	+	+	+	+	+ + +	+
Alkaline silicates	+ +	+	+	+ +	+	+ + +	+
Phosphates	+ +	+	+ +	+ +	+	+ + +	+

[a] Towards stainless steels, grades 304, 316.
+, Poor; + +, fair; + + +, good.

are used as corrosion inhibitors, especially in water treatment applications. Quaternary amonium compounds have limited detergency and are usually high-foaming; they are therefore mainly used for their biocidal properties. Some cationic salts based on alkyl imidazoline salts form the active ingredients in fabric softeners.

Nonionic surfactants are petroleum-derived from alcohol, with ethylene oxide or propylene oxide condensates. Nonionic surfactants have a wide range of detergent properties and may be high-foaming, non-foaming or defoaming. Defoaming surfactants work by the cloud point effect, whereby the molecules become insoluble above a fixed temperature and separate from solution.

The amphoteric group is a versatile if somewhat expensive group of surfactants. Certain members are biocidal, whilst others are used for their 'mildness' in personal hygiene products.

Alkalis

Table 3 shows the relative properties of a range of alkaline materials. By far the most commonly used alkali is sodium hydroxide (caustic soda), which denaturates and dissolves proteins, saponifies fats and is, to an extent, bactericidal. In common with all the alkalis listed, it is acceptable in terms of corrosion towards stainless steels; however, as mentioned earlier, it is corrosive towards soft metals. Potassium hydroxide (caustic potash) is occasionally used when product stability is a problem. In terms of mode of action, corrosivity and bactericidal performance, it is similar to sodium hydroxide.

Carbonates are almost exclusively used as the sodium salt, Na_2CO_3. It is a very cheap material and contributes to the total alkalinity of a formulation, but its detergency is limited.

Alkaline silicates are widely used for two properties. They contribute to soil penetration and aid soil suspension, preventing re-deposition. Silicates also inhibit the attack of alkaline materials on certain metals, especially aluminium, and are often included in detergent formulations for this reason. The most commonly used silicate is sodium silicate (Na_2SiO_3), although the more expensive potassium salt is occasionally used for stability reasons.

There is a potentially serious problem in using silicated formulations in low-pH atmospheres in that, if the solution falls to acid pH, a virtually insoluble silica scale is precipitated.

Phosphates are also used as sequestrants, as indicated earlier, but as alkalinity sources they are used in two forms: orthophosphates – the most common in use is trisodium phosphate (TSP) – and condensed or complex phosphates. Phosphates make a significant contribution to detergency in that they aid wetting, soil suspension and, especially, rinsability. The condensed phosphates, particularly sodium tripolyphosphate, also react synergistically with anionic surfactants to aid detergency. Phosphates are commercially available as mixtures of complex phosphates and are widely used.

Acids

Acids have existed as detergents for many years. Originally used mainly for descaling, their use has spread to include CIP applications. Fully formulated products will never totally replace caustic cleaning, but will certainly complement it in a much wider sense than we see today. From a purely chemical view point, acids offer different possibilities to the formulation chemist in terms of what is compatible, and this is leading to new biocide and surfactant options being used.

The most commonly used acid in detergent applications is phosphoric acid. Blended with suitable surfactants this can form the basis of a satisfactory CIP detergent. When blended with nitric acid the mixture is somewhat more aggressive but offers some bacteristatic properties if sufficient nitric acid is present. Nitric acid is cheaper than phosphoric acid and has a passivating effective on stainless steeels. It is, however, totally destructive to any copper, brass or phosphor–bronze in the system.

In its raw form, sulphuric acid is corrosive towards

stainless steel and should be formulated with a corrosion inhibitor if regular use is envisaged. Sulphuric acid is the cheapest source of acidity but its inherent detergency is poor and hence not cost-effective. It is used in some sanitizer formulations in which low pH is a prerequisite for effective use of the biocide present.

Hydrochloric acid can be effectively inhibited from attacking mild steel with the use of cationic corrosion inhibitors. When formulated in this way the products are used mostly for removing water hardness scales.

Sulphamic acid is available as a powder and has good descaling properties. It can be formulated into liquid products but tends to hydrolyse, forming sulphuric acid. It is quite expensive and does not offer significant advantages over phosphoric acid; hence it has limited application.

Other Components

Sodium hypochlorite has notable detergent-building functions in addition to biocidal properties, but needs to be used with caution. In alkaline and caustic conditions the oxidizing power of hypochlorite is useful in solubilizing protein films. Hypochlorite products form effective detergents but there are problems associated with their use. These include the possibility of taint pick-up with certain plastics, and pitting corrosion on stainless steel. The use of over-strength solutions and neutralization of alkalinity by acid environments can aggravate these problems.

Solvents are rarely used in detergent formulations since the misuse of low-volatility solvents can lead to product taint in terms of taste and smell. Those solvents which are used are of high volatility and, except in nonaqueous formulations, are used primarily to solubilize other detergent components.

Diluents and fillers are inert and contribute little or nothing to detergency. However, they are not necessarily present merely to cheapen a product. They may be present to ensure the stability of a liquid product, or to ensure that a powder remains free-flowing. They may be present to lower the freezing point of a liquid product, or to make the measurement of a powder more easy. They may aso inhibit the corrosive nature of other components.

Effluent Problems

Problems associated with effluent and the use of detergents are often misconstrued. The blame for foam in effluent is frequently put on the detergent in use. The argument takes the form that a detergent foams in use; hence it is that which caused the foam in the effluent. This is rarely the case.

However, there are problems associated with effluent which may arise from the misuse of detergents and disinfectants. The various water authorities have specific effluent discharge consent limits in terms of pH, typically 6–10. The majority of detergents used in the food and beverage industries are alkaline, so that there is a potential for exceeding the upper pH limit. In practice, the degree of dilution in effluent and the contribution of other components will considerably reduce the excess alkalinity of effluent samples. If, however, high alkalinity occurs through excessive discharge of alkaline materials, as in spillage of neat caustic detergent, the limit may be exceeded. In many operations, the use of acidic detergents will complement the use of alkali and hence the effluent will stay within consent limits. This is of particular value in the brewing, soft drink and dairy industries. *See* Effluents from Food Processing, Composition and Analysis

The perceived problem of foam associated with detergent use arises from the use of non-biodegradable materials in the past. Biodegradable organic materials are broken down into smaller units by the action of microorganisms. The use of biodegradable anionic surfactants was introduced by the UK detergent industry in 1963. Comparatively recent European and UK legislation now dictates that anionic and nonionic surfactants must exceed 80% biodegradation under specified test conditions. In practice, in excess of 80% biodegradation is achieved, and removals of over 95% are observed in efficient sewage treatment plants.

The change to rapidly biodegradable surfactants has virtually eradicated foaming problems in effluent caused by detergent use. However, the contribution of other materials used within food production environments, and the combination of detergents with these materials in effluent, may very well lead to foam. The saponification of fats by alkaline materials producing soaps is one example of a situation in which foam-generating materials may occur. The biodegradability of such by-products is unpredictable.

Other detergent materials may on occasions be highlighted as causing specific effluent problems. The effects of eutrophication, resulting from the action of phosphates in conjuction with nitrates under ideal environmental conditons, are well known. The contribution of phosphate from industrial users (detergents and other sources) is minimal ($\sim$3% of total phosphate); the major contribution comes from agricultural sources ($\sim$80% of total phosphate); hence the benefits of the inclusion of phosphates in detergent formulae far outweigh any perceived effluent problems. Any changes to detergent formulae must be shown to provide real advantages without detrimentally affecting the standards currently achievable.

Types of Detergent

Bibliography

Davies RA (1978) Cost effective cleaning and hygiene. *Dairy Industries International* April, 15–20.

Romney AJD (1990) *CIP: Cleaning in Place* 2nd edn. Cambridge: The Society of Dairy Technology.

Sedgwick A (1989) Cleaning and disinfection at the dairy. *Society for Applied Bacteriology Colloquia.*

SDIA (1989) *Detergent Phosphate and Water Quality in the UK.* Hayes, UK: Soap and Detergent Industry Association.

Swisher RD *Surfactant Biodegradation* 2nd edn. New York: Marcel Dekker.

Andrew Sedgwick
Diversey (FB) Ltd, Northampton, UK

Types of Disinfectant

In food factories the detergent stage is normally followed by a disinfecting stage. The detergent stage is required to remove all the soil, leaving a chemically clean surface. The disinfectant stage is used as an extra guarantee of cleanliness and to prevent recontamination in some cases. It does not compensate for a bad detergent stage or badly designed process or cleaning equipment.

Disinfection

The definition of disinfection taken from BS5283 (1986) says 'The destruction of microorganisms, but not usually bacterial spores. It does not necessarily kill all microorganisms but reduces them to a level acceptable for a defined purpose, for example a level which is harmful neither to health nor to the quality of perishable goods'. The acceptable level of microbial contamination on a surface or piece of equipment has to be determined; obviously, no pathogens should be found. *See* Spoilage, Bacterial Spoilage; Spoilage, Moulds in Food Spoilage; Spoilage, Yeasts in Food Spoilage

The state of sterility is defined as free from all living microorganisms. This is not achievable in the food factory by using acceptable chemicals ('acceptable' meaning safe for humans, plant materials and products).

Disinfectants are used after the detergent application in cleaning-in-place (CIP) operations where the term 'terminal sterilant' may be used. They are also used after hand cleaning. Equipment should be left in a soak bath until it is ready to be used, thus ensuring that it remains free from recontamination.

There are a wide range of disinfectants available. The choice of disinfectant depends on the user's requirements, the type of processing and cleaning equipment, the method of use and, to some extent, the personal preference of the user.

Types of Disinfectant

Disinfectants can be split into two broad groups, oxidizing and nonoxidizing. Oxidizing disinfectants include the halogens, chlorine, iodine, bromine and chlorine dioxide, and oxygen-releasing materials such as peracetic acid and hydrogen peroxide. Nonoxidizing disinfectants are as follows: quaternary ammonium compounds, amphoterics, biguanides, and acid anionics.

Physical and Chemical Properties

Oxidizing Disinfectants

Halogens

Chlorine and iodine have been used as terminal disinfectants for many years. More recently, bromine and chlorine dioxide have been introduced.

Chlorine Chlorine was first used as a gas for fumigation in hospitals in 1791, but this application has one obvious drawback – chlorine gas is toxic. Active chlorine is available from two types of material:

1. Inorganic compounds containing hypochlorite ions either as a liquid, e.g. sodium hypochlorite (NaOCl), or as a powder, e.g. chlorinated trisodium phosphate $((Na_3PO_4.11H_2O)_4NaOCl, NaCl)$.

2. Powdered organic chlorine release agents, e.g. trichloroisocyanurate (Fig. 1).

In solution, both types hydrolyse to produce hypochlorous acid and/or hypochlorite ions, depending on pH.

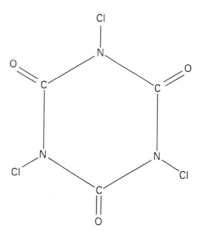

Acid

$$Cl_2 \;\rightleftharpoons\; HOCl \;\rightleftharpoons\; OCl^-$$

Alkaline

Chlorine gas   Hypochlorous acid   Hypochlorite ion

Fig. 1. Trichloroisocyanuric acid.

In the food industry, sodium hypochlorite is used as a general-purpose disinfectant. It is most stable in a slightly alkaline solution, and it is for this reason that the concentrate is supplied stabilized with sodium hydrocide at a pH of up to 12. An in-use solution of between 50 and 300 ppm will have a pH between 7 and 9. The optimum pH for disinfection is pH 5·0 but the solution is less stable. Below pH 5·0, chlorine gas will be produced.

Applications for sodium hypochlorite in the food industries are CIP, soak and spray. Sodium hypochlorite has many advantages: it is nonfoaming; it is not affected by water hardness; it does not leave an active residue, and it has a wide antimicrobial spectrum which includes activity against bacterial spores and viruses. It is also fast-acting and cheap.

However, sodium hypochlorite has numerous disadvantages: it can be corrosive to a wide range of components, including stainless steel; it is irritating to the skin and eyes; the in-use solution is unstable; it is inactivated by organic materials, and it may give rise to taint problems.

Chlorine dioxide Chlorine dioxide (ClO_2) is an unstable and toxic gas which is soluble in water. When chlorine dioxide is generated in solution, as shown below, it is a very effective water disinfectant at point of use.

$$5NaClO_2 + 4HCl \rightleftharpoons 4ClO_2 + 5NaCl + 2H_2O$$

Chlorine dioxide at use concentrations (0·5–1 ppm) overcomes some of the disadvantages of hypochlorite in that it is nontainting, noncorrosive and nontoxic. Its sole use at present is in water disinfection.

Iodine Iodine itself is not very soluble in water, and the vapour is irritating to the eyes, making it difficult to handle. Iodine is a very reactive element, and it is this reactivity which makes it a good disinfectant.

Iodine compounds used in the food industry contain iodine complexed with polyvinylpyrrolidone and other surface active agents, usually in an acid solution. These are known as iodophors and were first introduced in 1949.

The complexes formed between iodine and carrier molecule are water-soluble and overcome the handling difficulties of iodine whilst retaining the disinfecting power. On dilution the iodophors release iodine gradually, and it is the free iodine which acts as the disinfecting agent. The optimum pH for microbial activity is pH 5·0.

Acid			Alkaline
$I_2 \rightleftharpoons$	$HOI \rightleftharpoons$	$OI^- \rightleftharpoons$	IO^-
Greatest activity	Some activity	Inactive	Inactive

The surface-active agents provide better wetting and organic soil penetration, thus making iodophors less affected by soil than hypochlorite. The choice of surface-active agent may lead to foam generation in applications such as CIP.

Iodophors have a broad antimicrobial spectrum which is similar to hypochlorite, although they are less active against bacterial spores. In common with sodium hypochlorite, they are fast-acting but are more expensive. Iodophors are used in soak baths and spray application at up to 10 ppm available iodine. In solution, iodophors are yellow-brown in colour. This colour can be an advantage: in a soak bath application the colour indicates the presence of iodine; the in-use solutions are unstable, so that as the iodine dissipates the solution will become colourless.

Staining may be a problem, especially with some plastics, and this may also result in taint problems. Iodophors can be corrosive; it is therefore necessary to ensure that the correct dilution is used; otherwise, damage to plant and personnel may occur.

Bromine Bromine itself is not used as a disinfectant, mainly because of its handling difficulties. Bromochlorodimethylhydantoin is supplied as a powder or a solid. In solution it releases hypobromous and hypochlorous acids.

Oxygen-releasing Compounds

Peracetic acid Peracetic acid was introduced in 1955. The material is supplied as an equilibrium mixture:

$$\underset{\text{Peracetic acid}}{CH_3C(\!=\!O)OOH} + \underset{\text{Water}}{H_2O} \rightleftharpoons \underset{\text{Acetic acid}}{CH_3C(\!=\!O)OH} + \underset{\text{Hydrogen peroxide}}{H_2O_2}$$

It is soluble in water and is completely biodegradable, breaking down to harmless products:

$$2CH_3C(\!=\!O)OOH \rightarrow 2CH_3C(\!=\!O)OH + O_2$$

As supplied, peracetic acid is corrosive and has a very irritant smell, similar to vinegar; because of these properties it is unpleasant to handle and manual use is not recommended. It is suitable for CIP as it is nonfoaming.

Peracetic acid is a highly reactive material. As an in-use solution is it not very stable and will react with organic materials. Peracetic acid may attack plant materials, such as rubber gaskets, and at higher concentrations corrosion may be a problem.

Peracetic acid has a wide antimicrobial spectrum which includes bacterial spores and viruses. This activity is fast and is maintained at temperatures lower than ambient.

Hydrogen peroxide Hydrogen peroxide (H_2O_2) was introduced as a disinfectant in 1887. It is supplied in solution which has a tendency to decompose:

$$2H_2O_2 \rightarrow 2H_2O + O_2$$

Manual use of hydrogen peroxide is not recommended,

but it is used in spray applications such as aseptic packaging. Hydrogen peroxide is both bactericidal and fungicidal. Some bacteria and fungi are less sensitive because of catalase activity which destroys H_2O_2. Hydrogen peroxide is slow-acting, so that a long contact time or elevated temperature is required for effective disinfection.

Nonoxidizing Disinfectants

Quaternary Ammonium Compounds

Quaternary ammonium compounds (QACs) were first introduced in 1917 and are probably the best known cationic surface-active agents. Their general formula is as follows:

$$\left[\begin{matrix} R_1 & & R_2 \\ & N & \\ R_4 & & R_3 \end{matrix} \right]^+ \qquad X^-$$

X is usually a halide but sometimes a sulphate ion. R_1, R_2, R_3 and R_4 may be a variety of alkyl or aryl groups.

QACs are generally poor detergents but good wetting agents. In solution they ionize to produce a cation, the substituted nitrogen part of the molecule, which provides the surface-active property. The length of the carbon chain in the R groups affects the disinfectant ability; usually C_8 to C_{18} are the most effective.

The surface-active nature of these molecules tends to make them too high-foaming for CIP use, but they can be used for soak and manual cleaning at 200–400 ppm active. The optimum activity is around neutral pH, but QACs are active between pH 3·0 and 10·0. Activity may be inhibited by water hardness.

QACs are noncorrosive and are stable at in-use dilution. Their major disadvantages are that they are affected by organic soil, and that they tend to cling to surfaces, so that they may be difficult to rinse off, resulting in possible taint problems.

The antimicrobial range of QACs is less than that of the oxidizing disinfectants. They are less effective against Gram-negative bacteria than against Gram-positive bacteria. They also have limited activity against bacterial spores and very little activity against viruses. To be effective against yeasts and moulds, a higher concentration is required.

Biguanides

Biguanides with antimicrobial activity were first reported in 1933. The biguanides are derivatives of guanidine, a naturally occurring substance found in vegetables such as turnips and cereals:

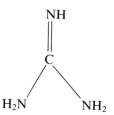

Biguanides are usually supplied as polymers in the salt form, mostly as the hydrochloride. Optimum activity lies between pH 3·0 and pH 9·0. Below pH 3·0, activity is suppressed, whilst above pH 9·0 they are precipitated.

They are cationic in nature but are not regarded as surface-active. Biguanides do not foam and are, therefore, suitable for CIP; they may also be used for soak and manual cleaning. They are noncorrosive but taint may be a problem if not properly rinsed. The in-use solution is stable, but is affected by organic soil and, to some extent, by hard water.

Most biguanides have equal antibacterial activity against Gram-positive and Gram-negative microorganisms. They are less effective against moulds and yeasts, and are ineffective against bacterial spores and viruses.

Amphoterics

Amphoterics have been in use as disinfectants since the early 1950s. They are based on a substituted amino acid, usually glycerine. The term ampholyte is often used to describe them because in solution they ionize to produce cations, anions or zwitterions, depending on pH:

$$R—\overset{+}{N}H_2—CH_2—CH_2—C(=O)OH$$
Acid cation

$$R—\overset{+}{N}H_2—CH_2—CH_2—C(=O)O^-$$
Zwitterion

$$R—NH—CH_2—CH_2—C(=O)O^-$$
Akaline anion

Only certain amphoterics have disinfecting ability and surface activity. The disinfecting ability appears to increase with the increase of basic groups.

Amphoterics tend to be viscous liquids that are freely soluble in water. They are generally too high-foaming for use in CIP, but are suitable for soak, spray and hand use. Amphoterics are equally effective against Gram-negative and Gram-positive bacteria; they are less effective against yeasts and moulds, and have very little effect against bacterial spores and viruses. Optimum activity lies between pH 3·0 and 9·0.

Properties such as soil tolerance and corrosion vary with the amphoteric concerned. Corrosion is not usually a problem. The in-use solution, usually 1000 ppm active, is stable.

Acid Anionics

The active molecule in acid anionics varies considerably. There are two main types: those based on carboxylic acids, which include fatty acids and derivatives, and those based on anionic surfactants combined with mineral acid.

Acid anionics tend to be formulated products with additions to aid activity or solubility. Properties will vary with product, but they tend to have some detergent and wetting ability. The higher-foaming products are unsuitable for CIP, so that their general use is for spray. They are not suitable for hand use since a pH of 2 is required for optimum antimicrobial activity.

The antimicrobial activity is against Gram-negative and Gram-positive bacteria, but they are less effective against bacterial spores and viruses. Certain carboxylic acid types are active against yeasts and moulds. Both types are affected by organic soil and water hardness but, again, both properties will vary with the product. The in-use solutions are stable.

Effluent Problems

The oxidizing disinfectants are degraded very easily by organic soil to ineffective products. Peracetic acid and hydrogen peroxide break down to the products that have been described earlier.

The breakdown products from the halogens will vary with pH of the effluent but in general, halide ions will be produced. The halogens should not be mixed with acid products as chlorine will react with organic chemicals to produce organo-chloro compounds which may be carcinogenic. The nonoxidizing disinfectants in modern products tend to consist of biodegradable compounds. The cationic products will adsorb onto organic material. The biguanides are incompatible with alkaline chemicals and will form a precipitate. See Effluents from Food Processing, On-site Processing of Waste; Effluents from Food Processing, Disposal of Waste Water; Effluents from Food Processing, Composition and Analysis

Analysis of Disinfectants in Waste Water

Obviously, detection will tend to depend on the concentration of disinfectant present. The oxidizing disinfectants are unlikely to be detected. Halide ions can be detected but cannot be identified as coming from the disinfectant.

Using an available chlorine probe, chlorine may be detected up to 200 ppm but, because of the presence of organic material and other chemicals, the presence of available chlorine may not be detected. As with chlorine, available iodine can be detected using a probe but iodine is converted very quickly to iodide. The breakdown products of peracetic acid and hydrogen peroxide are unlikely to be detected.

For the quaternary ammonium compounds, the biguanides and the amphoterics, it would be necessary to know the specific active molecule to be able to quantify these activities in effluent. The active content could then be determined by HPLC.

Acid anionics can be detected in the effluent by determining the anionic content.

Comparison with Steam

There is no chemical suitable for use as a disinfectant in the food factory that can compete with steam. It is effective against bacteria, moulds, yeasts, bacterial spores and viruses. It is not affected by soil and hard water. There are no corrosion or stability problems and it leaves no residues. The drawbacks are that it cannot be used with heat-sensitive plant materials, and it needs careful use to avoid human contact.

Bibliography

Block S (1977) *Disinfection, Sterilisation and Preservation.* Lea and Febiger.

Hugo WB (1971) *Inhibition and Destruction of the Microbial Cell.* Academic Press.

Hugo WB (1991) A brief history of heat and chemical preservation and disinfection. *Journal of Applied Bacteriology* 71: 9–18.

Sykes G (1972) *Disinfection and Sterilisation* (ICMSF) International Commission on Microbiology Specification for Foods. Chapman and Hall.

Jackie Fisher
Diversey Ltd, Northampton, UK

Overall Approach

In considering the overall approach to cleaning procedures in the factory, a number of aspects are significant, and these can be grouped under three main headings: general factory and environmental hygiene; process equipment, and cleaning and sanitation; training, monitoring and audits.

Legislation, in the form of the Food Safety Act 1990, has focused attention on the rights of the consumer. The legal implications of failure to comply with the law are extensive, should the product not meet the expectations of the consumer, the Environmental Health Officer or the Office of Fair Trading. Demonstration of 'Due Diligence' under the terms of the law could rely on effective cleaning methods, monitoring of performance, clearly defined controls of the procedure and accurate records. See Legislation, International Standards

General Factory and Environmental Hygiene

Design Parameters

During the design phase of a plant or process, the environment in which the product is to be processed is a significant element. Hygienic floors, walls, ceilings, drainage, ventilation and air conditioning must be included in the design specification. Careful selection of materials and the surface finishes is required to ensure compatibility with processing requirements, together with the cleaning and sterilizing materials and methods that will be used. *See* Plant Design, Designing for Hygienic Operation

The layout and installation of equipment, pipework, services and electrical cables, should be designed with the objective of cleanliness. The equipment design should prevent product spillage and dust emissions, with the arrangement of horizontal surfaces planned to minimize the build-up of dust and airborne contamination, which could subsequently drop into processing equipment. This also facilitates the free draining of cleaning solutions during external cleaning. At the same time, covers, guards and acoustic hoods, should be designed to ensure that they do not constitute a separate hazard, by creating areas that are not accessible for inspection and cleaning.

In the early stages of the design, access and activity of the operators should be considered, with adequate provisions of suitable hand-washing stations at the entry points to the area. The design should also encompass the requirements of raw and finished materials, including access, temporary storage, and exit from the process area. Special attention should be given to any trucking or handling that may be required, in order to ensure that the effect of contamination from external sources (e.g. road vehicles) does not introduce a further hygiene hazard.

Where high-risk products are to be processed or packaged, clean areas must be designated. For a clean area, the standards of hygiene are more rigorous and the access restricted to key and authorized personnel only. Entry into the area is through changing, washing and sterilizing areas. The clothes, overalls, hats, hairnets, boots, shoes and gloves, together with the physical health of the operators, are strictly controlled to ensure that contamination from the operator and other processing areas is curtailed. In addition, the condition of any mobile or temporary equipment that enters the area would be required to meet the standards for the clean area.

Environmental Cleaning and Sanitation

The cleaning and sanitation of the processing environment is influenced by the process and product processed, the cleaning equipment and materials available, and the quality of the labour. *See* Sanitization; Sterilization of Foods

Process and Product Processed

The effect of the process and the product processed on the cleaning and sanitation regimes will depend on whether the process is wet or dry, the type of product and the processing 'shelf life' of the various ingredients.

For dry processes, the cleaning is with vacuum cleaner and a self-contained floor cleaner or scrubber. Washing of the walls and external surfaces is often limited to the major, periodical, clean-up routine. For wet processes, routine wash-down procedures are used. These include the regular washing of walls, floors, drains and external equipment surfaces, as part of the end-of-production procedures.

With sensitive processes, such as yoghurt manufacture, cheese starter vats and yeast propagation, the equipment usually encloses the product. However, as access is required during production, the environmental cleaning frequency is similar to the equipment cleaning frequency and includes monitoring of bacteriological levels.

Cleaning Equipment and Materials

The equipment that is available to improve cleaning efficiency includes vacuum cleaners, floor cleaners, mops, and brushes for dry areas, and mops, brushes, hoses, steam and water mixers, boosted-pressure systems, and foam cleaning equipment for wet areas.

The use of boosted-pressure systems, as opposed to high-pressure systems, has become the accepted method, as a result of health and safety legislation with respect to potential injury to operators, containment of aerosol fog (thus preventing the contamination of areas that have already been cleaned), and reduction of danger and damage caused by jet cutting power.

With more sophisticated equipment the provision for controlled addition of detergents and sterilizing products can be included.

For the cleaning materials that are used in systems, formulated or 'built' detergents and sterilants will usually produce superior results over commodity chemicals, such as caustic soda, owing to the inclusion and properties of the various additives. The formulated cleaning material can be purchased as a proprietary product or 'built' *in situ* by the correct dispensing of a proprietary additive into a commodity chemical.

Procedure

Prior to all cleaning procedures, food and packaging materials should be removed. If hoses or boosted-

Overall Approach

pressure systems and foam cleaning methods are used, all electrical switches, motors and control panels should be correctly rated against the ingress of water, i.e. IP65 standard.

Manual Method

A suitable cleaning solution at the required temperature and detergent strength is prepared in a bucket or container. During use the solution should be replaced regularly or when soiled. Prior to brush washing, all the surfaces are rinsed with clean water.

The surfaces that are to be cleaned are brush-washed using a brush designated to the duty, working in small areas at a time. Different colours can be used to define the duty of the brushes, ensuring that different brushes are used for finished and raw product areas. Before the surfaces are allowed to dry, they are rinsed with cold water.

After the entire area has been cleaned and rinsed, it is sanitized by spraying with a sterilant solution at the required strength. The surfaces are then allowed to dry.

Foam Methods (5–15 bar plus inlet pressure)

All the surfaces are foamed with a suitable product(s), and the foam is allowed to remain on the surface for appropriate time (5–10 min) without drying. Whilst rinsing is carried out from the top downwards, the foam should be built from the bottom upwards to minimize collapse of the foam and increase the contact time on the surface.

All surfaces are then rinsed with cold water. When the entire area has been cleaned and rinsed, it is sanitized by spraying with a sterilant solution at the required strength and the surfaces are then allowed to dry.

Boosted-pressure Method (15–25 bar pressure)

The boosted-pressure method is similar to the foam method; the detergent solution is injected into the boosted-pressure system, sprayed onto the surface and rinsed off with clean water after a suitable residence time. This method would also be followed by spraying with sterilizing solution after the whole area had been cleaned.

Floor Cleaner and Scrubber

Loose debris should be removed and the area swept thoroughly; heavy build-up may have to be scraped loose and then removed.

The tanks on the cleaner should be thoroughly cleaned before and after use. The detergent tank is charged with detergent and water to the required concentration and temperature.

After the entire area has been cleaned and rinsed, it is sanitized by spraying with a sterilant solution at the required strength and the surfaces allowed to dry.

Cleaning Frequency

High-risk products and surrounding areas should be cleaned every 2 h. All food processing and handling areas should be cleaned daily. Nonprocessing and dry storage areas should be cleaned weekly.

Additional Precautions

During the process operation, all spillages and blockages from the process plant should be cleaned and cleared up immediately.

After breakdowns and maintenance, the equipment and area should be cleaned and sterilized prior to restarting the process.

Damage to the surfaces of walls, floors and drains (e.g. poor grouting, cracks, porosity and puddling) should be reported and repaired immediately.

Process Equipment Cleaning and Sanitation

In the modern food processing plant, the equipment used is generally constructed from stainless steel, type 304 or type 316.

Processing of dry products or drying processes is usually operated for extended periods and the equipment then washed. Under these conditions, the equipment often has an extraction system for collection of fines and dust, for recycling and/or removal. At the end of the process period, the equipment is isolated from the extraction system and wet-cleaned, after which the dust collection bags are changed. The dust collection system is wet-cleaned only after extended periods of use.

In the selection of process equipment, the hygiene factors that should be considered include the following: materials of construction; surface finish; freedom from crevices; effective distribution of cleaning solutions; containment of cleaning solutions; free draining construction; adequate ground clearance to enable the floor under the equipment to be cleaned; access for manual cleaning and inspection.

In the first instance the equipment manufacturer's cleaning procedure and performance guarantees should be examined, together with experience of other users of the equipment.

The methods, procedures and performance guarantees that are available from specialist cleaning equipment and detergent suppliers will often provide an effective alternative. The correctly chosen specialist will have a broader base of technical knowledge and appli-

Overall Approach

cation experience of cleaning the same or similar equipment.

Cleaning Tanks and Vessels

The cleaning of tanks and vessels is usually accomplished with a spray device. The spray device can be a sprayball, sprayring, spraybar (high-volume, low-pressure) or a rotating spray (low-volume, medium-pressure). Spray devices can be permanently installed, or installed for cleaning only. Spray units are used singly or in combination to distribute the cleaning, sterilizing and rinse solutions to the product contact surfaces.

For the most effective spray cleaning, the inside of the vessel should be smooth, with dished or conical tops and bottoms, rounded corners between the vertical and horizontal surfaces and no internal projections. The vessel outlet should be accessible, at an adequate height to provide the minimum static head requirements for the product and cleaning-in-place (CIP) scavenge pumps.

In practice, the tank and vessels often include agitators, manway, viewing and lamp ports, contents gauges, thermometer pockets, level gauges, hypodermic sample points, sample cocks, heating coils, pipework connections, and pressure and vacuum protection. These items should be analysed individually to ensure that they are crevice free, that the cleaning solution will make contact adequately, that there are no shadow areas caused by projections, and that that the surfaces will drain freely. The CIP supply may need to be split to clean sight glasses and sample points, with suitable velocity.

If agitators and baffles are fitted, more than one spray device may be required to prevent 'shadowing' or inadequate coverage. If complex agitators are fitted in the vessel, or bottom bearings are installed to support the agitator, the cleaning solution volume should be increased to flood or cover these components. During the cleaning operations the agitator should be run continuously or pulsed to ensure coverage. Complicated equipment may require a combination of spray devices, with the routes controlled by automatic valves, to ensure that all the items are adequately cleaned.

Pipework

Pipework is cleaned by passing the rinse, cleaning and sanitizing solutions through the pipework. The velocity required would normally be in the range of 1.5–2.5 m s^{-1} for pipe sizes up to 100 mm in diameter. The velocity for a particular route is determined by the largest diameter. Where pipe diameter reductions are unavoidable, a suitable bypass should be installed to maintain the velocity in the largest diameter.

During the design phase of the pipework installation,

Table 1. Summary of typical methods for cleaning equipment

Plant	Method of cleaning	
	Manual process	Automatic
Small vessels	Foam/Man/Circ	Circ/CIP
Large vessels	Circ/CIP	CIP
Mixing vessels	Circ/CIP	CIP
Heat exchangers	Circ/CIP	Circ/CIP
Positive pumps	Man/CIP	CIP
Centrifugal pumps	Circ/CIP	CIP
Centrifuge	Circ/CIP	CIP
Screw conveyors	Foam/Man/CIP	CIP
Conveyors	Foam/Man/CIP	CIP
Cookers	Man/CIP	Man/CIP
Driers	Man/CIP	Man/CIP
Extruders	Man/CIP	Man/CIP
Evaporators	Circ/CIP	CIP
Fillers	Foam/Circ/CIP	Foam/Circ/CIP
Spray drier	Man/CIP	Man/CIP
Aseptic processes	CIP	CIP
Pasteurizers	Circ/CIP	Circ/CIP
Blenders	Man/CIP	CIP
Brewhouse	Circ/CIP	Circ/CIP

Man, manual (require the plant operator to provide the method and mechanical action); Circ, circulation (involves the use of the production equipment, i.e. pumps, vessels and pipework, to recirculate the cleaning solutions); CIP, cleaning-in-place (cleaning solutions would be provided by the external system); Foam, foam or boosted-pressure systems.

the following factors should be considered: maximum use of continuously welded (orbital or hand) pipework (installed with Argon purging); sanitary fittings and unions to the approved international standards where dismantling for access or maintenance is required; rigid supports; CIP routes which enable the pipework to be cleaned without dismantling; and pipework fall, pitched with a minimum slope of $1:200$ to allow adequate drainage. Dead ends or pockets should be avoided but if required should be horizontal, not longer than 1.5 times the pipe diameter, with the flow of the CIP solution directed into the pocket or 'dead-leg'. Valves, pumps, filters, inline mixers and other equipment that is installed in the pipework should be of hygienic design, i.e. with suitable surface finishes and crevice-free.

Methods

The cleaning and sanitation of process equipment can be carried out in a number of different ways including manual, circulation and CIP systems (see the following article). Table 1 shows a summary of the typical methods used to clean equipment.

Overall Approach

Manual Cleaning

The food industry still has many operations that involve manual cleaning; these applications include small-scale equipment, low-risk product processing plant with minimal bacteriological risk, unhygienic plant which is unsuitable for CIP, complex plant that requires dismantling to clean, low-value product and/or labour-intensive processes and dry processing plant.

For manual cleaning the equipment is dismantled, cleaned, and placed in a soak tank containing a suitable sterilant until the plant is reassembled prior to production start-up. In the case of some gear-type pumps, the pump head is opened, and the gears are removed, cleaned, and placed in a soak tank. The front plate is replaced and the body of the pump cleaned by CIP with a pipework circuit.

Large or complex equipment should be opened or dismantled and cleaned with hose, boosted-pressure systems or foam systems. Sterilant is provided by the hose or boosted-pressure system or with a hand-spray. Where tanks are manually cleaned, the operative with an abrasive pad, hose pipe and buckets of detergent and sterilant (or pressure hose and foam cleaner) is rare, but still used. It is more usual for a spray device to be installed for cleaning, or for a permanently installed spray device to be utilized. A suitable pump delivery connects to the spray device inlet to provide required flow rate and pressure. The suction of the pump is connected to a water supply and the vessel outlet to provide the prerinse, detergent recirculation and final rinse operations. Detergent is then added through the manway, but sterilant applied with a hand spray. To provide a heated detergent solution, a hot water supply is required; if the vessel is fitted with a heating jacket, this is often used to heat the detergent solution.

Circulation Cleaning

The process plant and equipment are used to recirculate the rinse detergent and sterilant solutions. Water is added to one of the tanks or vessels and distributed to the various parts of the plant. Typically, small-scale process plant, filters, pasteurizers, brewhouse and complex mixing plant are cleaned by this method, particularly if at the end of the cleaning routine the detergent is heavily soiled.

Training, Monitoring and Audits

Training

Training in the methods, practices and operations of hygiene is an essential part of the general hygiene procedures. It is an opportunity to explain the method and requirement of the procedures, and the individual operator responsibilities. Monitoring and audits will demonstrate the effectiveness of the cleaning programmes and identify any retraining that may be required.

Monitoring

Parallel to the development of the Food Safety Act 1990, British Standard BS 5750 (EN 29000 and ISO 9000) was published and 'total quality management' techniques were developed. Together these items provide the legislation, procedural accreditation, documentation and management objectivity for food manufacture. Within this structure the monitoring of cleaning procedures is a significant factor in the quality assurance controls of performance. *See* Quality Assurance and Quality Control

The quality control department normally prepares a procedure for checking the hygiene programmes. The starting point is often a checklist, confirmed and signed by the cleaning staff. Key areas are then checked by immediate supervision. Laboratory staff should carry out the bacteriological checks on a regular basis, and the results should be published with the figures for the target levels indicated. Copies of the results are usually circulated to senior management for review and action as required.

Equipment should be swabbed regularly using recognized procedures. The points for swabbing should be identified and used each time the equipment is tested. For sensitive and high-risk products and areas, the swabs should be taken after each cleaning operation, and other equipment swabbed at random. If the bacteriological counts for a particular area or piece of equipment are above the required level, the cleaning, sterilizing and sampling should be increased until the results are below the target level.

Auditing

The British Standard which provides the guidance on auditing quality systems, BS 7229, also formalizes procedures that have been used for a number of years to assess and report on the performance of a manufacturing plant, department or process against defined financial, manufacturing, process, CIP and hygiene procedures and practices. Traditionally, this activity has been carried out by a team of experienced personnel from other plants and departments, normally on an annual basis.

Within the guidelines set down in the British Standard, effective mechanisms are provided to set up audits of the hygiene operations as part of the total quality management programmes. The audit team can be made up of internal staff or specialist external organizations. Audits provide the opportunity to review methods, procedures and performance against defined objectives. The report that is issued following an audit is used for modifying and updating the methods and procedures, identifying training and retraining needs, and demonstrating general improvements that need to be made.

Bibliography

British Standard BS 5750 (1987) Quality Systems parts 1,2 & 3. Milton Keynes: BSI.

British Standard BS 7229. (1989) Quality Audit Systems. Milton Keynes: BSI.

Campden Food and Drink Research Association (1987) *Hygienic Design of Liquid Handling Equipment.* Technical Manual 17, pp 1.3–1.6, sect. 3 and sect. 5. Chipping Campden, Gloucestershire: Campden Food and Drink Research Association.

Flagg PL and Thompson RP (1986) Dedicated CIP Control for Better Informed Manager. *Brewing and Distillery International* September: 40.

Institute of Food Science and Technology (1989) *Food and Drink Manufacture – Good Manufacturing Practice. A Guide to its Responsible Management,* pp. 4–26. London: Institute of Food Science and Technology.

Tamplin TC (1990) *Designing for Cleanability CIP: Cleaning In Place,* pp. 41–105. Huntingdon, Cambridgeshire: Society of Dairy Technology.

Vinson HG (1990) Hygienic design of a dairy. *Journal of the Society of Dairy Technology* 43(2): 39–41. pp39–41.

P. J. Purnell
Henkel-Ecolab Ltd., Swindon, UK

Modern Systems

As processing equipment in the modern food processing plant has increased in size and complexity, the need for systems has increased. Automated plants usually include an automated system to ensure that predictable and reproducible cleaning and bacteriological standards are achieved. At the same time, the increase in safety aspects and diminishing social acceptability of entering tanks and equipment with 'brush, mop and bucket' means that the use of systems will continue to increase.

Aims of Cleaning-in-place (CIP) Systems

Primary Aim

The primary aim can be defined as the removal of the residues of the manufacturing process or soil, without significant dismantling of the processing equipment, and the establishment of an environment which will not contaminate the next process operation.

Secondary Aim

The secondary aim can be defined as the cleaning of the process equipment to the required standard in the available time, with a detergent at a suitable concentration that will remove the process residues without damaging the process equipment, at an efficient and cost-effective temperature, using an optimum mechanical action provided by the CIP system and its associated components.

In setting the particular cleaning philosophy for a process plant or production process, each of the parameters of time, temperature, detergent concentration and mechanical action must be considered, together with an assessment of the interaction between them.

Time

Availability

During the processing programme there may be a suitable pause or logical interval. If such a 'cleaning window' is not available the CIP procedures will have to be carried out post- or preproduction. Cleaning preproduction may require more rigorous regimes if the residual contamination has been allowed to dry onto the surface or harden. Equipment or plant that is cleaned during production requires a secure and effective separation of the CIP solutions and the product.

Duration

The CIP programme used has a finite time to complete each of the required operations. Rinsing, detergent recirculation and sterilizing operations have an optimum time. In the case of complex equipment, such as automatic routeing valves, the time required to operate and pulse these items has to be included in each of the operations.

Temperature

The water and detergent solubility of the soil can generally be improved by raising the temperature during the cleaning operations. In deciding on the cleaning temperature, the following factors must be considered: resistance of the product to heat denaturing, the ability of plant and equipment to accommodate temperature changes, the most effective detergent solution, the availability of a heating source, and energy costs.

Raising the temperature during rinsing and detergent recirculation can reduce the duration of cleaning programmes, provided that the time required for heating does not extend the CIP programme.

Detergent Concentration

The nature and quantity of the soil, and the materials of construction of the plant and equipment dictate the *type* of detergent used, whereas the *concentration* is determined by the temperature, contact time, and mechanical action. Most products have a minimum effective concentration; use at higher concentrations should only be necessary when the other parameters are reduced, or to meet a short cleaning window. *See* Sanitization

Mechanical Action

The mechanical action is usually provided by the CIP system. Pipework that is designed for effective cleaning requires solutions with a velocity of $1\cdot5$–$2\cdot5$ m s^{-1} to be passed through it. Hygienically designed vessels and processing equipment are normally fitted with spray devices to effectively distribute the solutions to the surfaces that require cleaning. *See* Plant Design, Designing for Hygienic Operation

The frequency of cleaning is decided by the effective processing life and the level of soiling that accumulates during the processing period. High-risk product is cleaned at short intervals, and low-risk product at longer intervals. Equipment that is used for heat treatment and mixers should be cleaned at short intervals to prevent excessive build-up on the equipment surfaces. Cleaning-in-place is most effective when applied 'little and often'.

Types of CIP System (Fig. 1)

Traditionally, CIP systems are one of three types: single-use systems; recovery systems; combination systems. In considering modern systems the boosted-pressure and foam system has a rightful place which has developed significantly.

Single-use Systems

The basis of the single-use system is a compact package of equipment that enables an economical combination of rinses and detergent solutions to be prepared to suit the individual cleaning duties. Fresh detergent is used each time a detergent recirculation is needed, with the appropriate blend of cleaning compounds that the

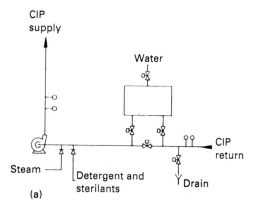

(a)

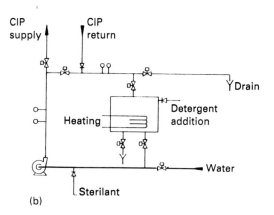

(b)

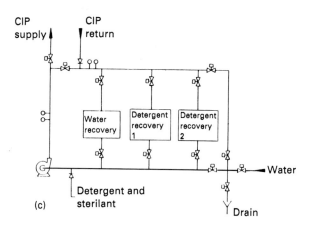

(c)

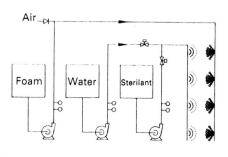

(d)

Fig. 1   Cleaning-in-place (CIP) systems. (a) Simple single-use CIP system; (b) simple detergent recovery system; (c) tank combination CIP system; (d) foam system.

Modern Systems

process requires. The operation of the system components is usually controlled automatically.

Recovery Systems

The basis of recovery systems is a package of equipment that includes a number of tanks, for detergent and water recovery. The space required is much greater, depending on the tank sizes and number. The strength of the cleaning solutions is controlled to suit the most arduous cleaning circuit. In its simplest form the recovery system can be manually operated.

Combination System

As the name implies, combination systems combine the best features of single-use and recovery. This allows the storage of dilute detergents at the most economical strength and the facility for increasing the strength on arduous cleaning duties. In addition, where the cleaning solution is severely contaminated it is possible to discharge the solution to drain or, for sensitive cleaning programmes, use fresh detergent.

Foam and Pressure Systems

In the design of the modern food processing plants, provision is often made for a system to provide a central source of water, detergents and sterilant for the environmental cleaning. Using this equipment, the opportunity for using both fixed spray devices installed on process equipment and a sequence controller provides an effective CIP system.

CIP Routine

The routine that is used to clean a process plant includes all or part of the following operations.

Prerinse

The function of the prerinse is to remove gross and loose soil or contamination and prepare the surface for the detergent wash. Effective prerinsing will reduce the 'cleaning load' on the detergent. For recovery-type CIP systems an effective prerinse is essential to reduce the build-up of contamination, carry-over and sludge in the detergent tank. This increases the life of the detergent tank between full and partial dump operations.

Depending on the nature of the soil and the CIP system, the prerinse can be hot, cold or recovered from previous cleans. After the rinse solution has passed through or over the plant, the solution is usually discharged to drain.

Detergent Wash

Detergent solutions of the required formulation, strength and temperature are recirculated through the process plant. For single-use systems, the solution is prepared each time, to suit the application; in recovery systems, the detergent solution is of a strength to suit the most arduous duty. After a suitable recirculation period, the used detergent is returned to the detergent recovery tank, rinse recovery, or discharged to drain. Depending on the application, the detergent recirculation may be repeated or the type of detergent changed. If a number of recirculations are required, each operation is followed by intermediate rinses which may be hot, cold or recovered.

Intermediate Rinse

Following the recirculation, the detergent residues are removed by rinsing. These rinses can be discharged to the rinse recovery tank for use as the prerinse of subsequent cleans.

Acid Wash

The acid wash operation is similar to the detergent wash operation but using an acid-based product. This operation can be used to remove residual detergent from the surface, to remove and prevent scale build up, and to passivate the stainless steel. If used during all cleans, the acid wash can be used at low concentrations and can leave the surface with a pH of 4 to 5, which reduces the possibility of bacteriological growth.

Intermediate Rinse

Following the recirculation, the detergent residues are removed by rinsing.

Sterilant Recirculation

The sterilant recirculation is similar to the detergent recirculation and is used to achieve the required bacteriological standard. It is preferable to use fresh sterilant to prevent any cross-contamination caused by recovery of sterilant from a plant that has not been adequately rinsed or cleaned by the detergent. Depending on the chemical nature of the sterilant, a final rinse may be required to remove residual sterilant from the process plant. Caution is recommended as the source of the final rinse must be of suitable quality, filtered to less than $5\,\mu$m, and treated with an ultraviolet source to a minimum of $30\,\text{mW s cm}^{-2}$ to prevent contamination.

Instrumentation

Fundamental Requirement

For a basic CIP system, the instrumentation may simply consist of pressure and temperature indicators in the supply pipework, and a sight glass, temperature and detergent concentration indicators in the return pipework. If cleaning at ambient temperatures, the temperature indicators are not required. This equipment provides no documentation for records unless readings are recorded manually during CIP operations.

Definitive Requirement

The definitive requirement for instrumentation that is expected with a modern CIP system is as follows:

- Supply pressure indication and records.
- Supply temperature probe or switches to provide the control of heating equipment and temperature alarms.
- Supply flow meter.
- Return flow switch.
- Return temperature probe or switches to provide the monitoring of actual temperature in the process equipment.
- Chemical strength probe and monitor, to control and monitor the strength and addition of detergents.
- Chemical addition flow meters, as some of the products (sterilants in particular) that are used are not easy to detect, within the range of standard probes and controllers.

Control

Control for modern systems has developed as the production requirement has become more sophisticated. With the range of computer, microprocessor and programmable logic controllers (PLC) available, the control opportunities are really only limited by the intellect and experience of the author(s) of the functional specification and software.

The modern system controller is required to control, monitor and report on a number of parameters, including the following:

1. The sequence and duration of rinses, draining, scavenging, detergent wash, acid wash and sterilant operations and recirculations.
2. Chemical formulations and concentrations.
3. Temperatures of rinses and washes.
4. Pressures to achieve desired flow rates and spray patterns.
5. Flow rates through pipework, spray devices and process equipment.
6. The operation of ancillary process plant, such as process pumps, agitators, mixers, and process valves.

Since it is not yet possible to monitor microbiological results on-line or to obtain reliable results quickly, the function of the automatic controller is to carry out the cleaning of a designated route to a preset routine. Feedback of operation of the individual plant items is then used to confirm that the desired sequence has been accomplished using the preset parameters.

Data can be collected from temperature, pressure, flow and chemical transmitters and sensors on valves, pumps, and route selector plates. The operator can be given confirmation, in the form of a visual display and a print-out, of the CIP operations that have been carried out. These data would normally include the date and times of each operation, the plant reference, any alarm conditions and the action taken.

Management Information

Because of the importance of effective CIP on the ultimate product, management must be advised that CIP has been satisfactorily completed. If not, production management must be advised of the reasons for any failure, the immediate remedial action taken, and the actions necessary to prevent recurrence. Depending on the severity of a shortcoming on any particular CIP circuit, management may well wish to delegate the decision-making to supervisory or even operator level. For example, if temporary loss of steam pressure prevents the system achieving the desired temperature, the supervisor could be empowered to do one of the following:

- Increase chemical strengths or wash cycle times to compensate.
- Proceed at low temperature.
- Abort until steam pressure is restored.

In any event, senior management should be made aware of the failure, and action should be taken by the operator or supervisor. It is therefore essential that the CIP control system produces a printed management report, either whilst events are happening, or at the request of management at a later time.

Modern Systems

Review of Manual Operations

The single most significant factor for manual operation of cleaning is the quality, ability and conscientiousness of the cleaning personnel. Even with high-quality personnel, the supervision, monitoring procedures and methods of operation must be thorough and rigorous.

During cleaning, personnel are required to provide the mechanical action of the clean, the detergent of the correct type, concentration and temperature, and to allow the required contact time. Where a sterilant is used this must be of the correct type, concentration and temperature, with a suitable contact time.

Within the quality control aspects of hygiene, the keeping of records is required. The records of manual systems are more difficult to collect, collate and interpret without error. Where records are used to provide the historical data to demonstrate 'Due Diligence', the accuracy and credibility of the records could be called into question.

Bibliography

British Standard BS 5750 (1987) Quality Systems parts 1,2 & 3. Milton Keynes: BSI.

British Standard BS 7229. (1989) Quality Audit Systems. Milton Keynes: BSI.

Campden Food and Drink Research Association (1987) *Hygienic Design of Liquid Handling Equipment*. Technical Manual 17, pp 1.3–1.6, sect. 3 and sect. 5. Chipping Campden, Gloucestershire: Campden Food and Drink Research Association.

Flagg PL and Thompson RP (1986) Dedicated CIP Control for Better Informed Manager. *Brewing and Distillery International* September: 40.

Institute of Food Science and Technology (1989) *Food and Drink Manufacture – Good Manufacturing Practice. A Guide to its Responsible Management*, pp 4–26. London: Institute of Food Science and Technology.

Tamplin TC (1990) *Designing for Cleanability CIP: Cleaning In Place*, pp 41–105. Huntingdon, Cambridgeshire: Society of Dairy Technology.

Vinson HG (1990) Hygienic design of a dairy. *Journal of the Society of Dairy Technology* 43(2): 39–41. pp 39–41.

P. J. Purnell
Henkel-Ecolab Ltd., Swindon, UK

CLOSTRIDIUM

Contents

Occurrence of *Clostridium perfringens*

Clostridium perfringens is probably the most widespread of all pathogenic bacteria. There are several toxigenic types: A, B, C, D and E. Type A is primarily associated with human illness. The other types are associated with diseases of domestic animals. In very specific situations, type C is occasionally involved in human illness. *Clostridium perfringens* is an anaerobic, spore-forming organism commonly found in fresh meat and poultry products. Spores of the organism can survive many food processing procedures. Because of its ability to grow over a wide temperature range it is often implicated in human food poisoning. With regard to human illness in general it should be noted that, historically, *C. perfringens* have been most closely associated with gangrene and wound infections. In this article, discussion will be limited to its role in human food poisoning.

Occurrence in Humans, Foods and the Environment

Clostridium perfringens is part of the normal intestinal flora in humans and animals and also occurs widely in soil. It is the most commonly found *Clostridium* in clinical specimens. Because of its abundance in faeces the organism is also found in sewage-polluted water. Water authorities in certain localities use its presence as an index of water quality.

Clostridium perfringens has also been found in the intestinal tract of virtually every animal examined, with wide variation within and between species. Although the levels of *C. perfringens* in healthy adults are relatively small compared to other strict anaerobes, *C. perfringens* can be isolated from virtually all humans. In infants, adult levels are established by 6 months of age.

Early studies on the incidence of *C. perfringens* focused on the isolation of so-called heat-resistant strains (those whose spores could survive – and be activated by – heating at 100°C for 60 min) since it was thought that this group was more likely to survive cooking than less heat-resistant, i.e. 'heat-sensitive' spore strains. By the mid-1960s it became apparent that heat-sensitive strains were equally capable of causing outbreaks of food poisoning. In epidemiological investigations no distinction is now made between the two groups.

There is wide variation in the total *C. perfringens* count in human faeces. However, in healthy adults the values are usually between 10^3 and 10^5 per g (Table 1). Patients in outbreaks carry 10^6–10^8 per g. The level of spores of this organism in faeces is within one log of the total count. The procedure used to obtain the spore count – heating the sample at 75–80°C for 10–20 min – also eliminates competing microflora. The faecal spore count is one of several laboratory criteria for investigating outbreaks caused by this organism (see below).

It has become apparent that the elderly, although healthy, often carry relatively high (total or spore) numbers of *C. perfringens*, often above 10^6 per g. This phenomenon is not attributable to ingestion of elevated levels of *C. perfringens* since surveys have been conducted in extended-care facilities where the daily intake was monitored. Such high levels in asymptomatic elderly people limit the usefulness of examining stools of patients for elevated levels of *C. perfringens*. In such situations other criteria for confirming outbreaks, discussed below, are available.

Early studies on the incidence of *C. perfringens* in raw foods focused on heat-resistant strains, thus understating true levels of the organism. Representative results of many market and slaughterhouse surveys, conducted over the years, are presented in Table 2. No distinction is made between vegetative cells and spores. The latter would obviously be more able to withstand subsequent cooking procedures. The data for meat and poultry were from surveys conducted in North America and the UK. Results from Japan are consistently lower. It should also be noted that such surveys have been carried out using a variety of methods for enrichment, heat selection, selective plating, and confirmation. It is clear from Table 2 that the organism is abundant in raw, protein-rich foods. The source of the organism is the intestinal contents of these animals. As noted above, the faeces of all animals examined, domestic and wild, contain *C. perfringens*. In the case of fish and shellfish, wide fluctuations in isolation rates occur, presumably depending on the degree of water pollution. Such products are rarely involved in outbreaks of *C. perfringens* food poisoning.

The organism is also found in virtually all types of processed foods, although at a low level. However, in some cases, such as soups and sauces, only short heating times are required for preparation. Other items, such as herbs and spices (well known for their high general bacterial spore levels, including *C. perfringens*) are often added to large amounts of cooked foods. Slow cooling or inadequate reheating of such foods can result in the large numbers of *C. perfringens* necessary to cause food poisoning. Oxygen is driven off during cooking, creating ideal conditions for growth of this organism.

Table 1. Representative surveys of *C. perfringens* cells and spores in faeces from various populations of various countries

Population	Country	Cell type	Levels (per g)
Healthy adults	USA, UK	Total viable count	10^3–10^4
Young patients	UK	Total viable count	3 of 6, $\geq 10^4$
			0 of 10, $\geq 10^6$
Elderly adults	Japan	Total viable count	5 of 30, $\geq 10^7$
Elderly patients	UK	Total viable count	10 of 11, $\geq 10^4$
			5 of 11, $\geq 10^6$
Elderly mental patients	UK	Total viable count	6 of 10, $\geq 10^4$
			3 of 10, $\geq 10^6$
Healthy adults	Canada	Spore count[a]	10^3–10^4
Food poisoning patients	UK	Spore count[a]	56 of 66, 10^6–10^8
Food poisoning patients	USA	Spore count[a]	2.0×10^4–4.0×10^8
			Mean, 10^7
Food poisoning patients	USA	Spore count[a]	$< 10^3$–2.2×10^{5b}

[a] Faecal samples heated 80°C for 10 min.
[b] 30 days after illness.

Occurrence of Clostridium perfringens

Table 2. Results of surveys of the incidence of *C. perfringens* in foods and feeds

Raw food types	Incidence (%)
Meat and poultry	
Poultry carcass	58
Frozen chicken	63
Beef carcass	26
Pork carcass	66
Lamb carcass	85
Ground beef	50–70
Beef liver	26–50
Veal	82
Pork	37
Pork sausages	39
Lamb, mutton	52
Fish and shellfish	
Fish, body surface	84
Fish, alimentary tract	82
Vacuum-packed fish	67[a]
Oysters	100
Trout	0
Miscellaneous	
Spices and herbs	42
Dehydrated soups and sauces	18
Animal feeds	35

[a] Incidence of *Clostridium*; predominant species is *C. perfringens*.

Clostridium perfringens is part of the microflora of soil and is present at levels of 10^3–10^4 per g. Even in Antarctica, most soil samples examined contained this organism. In view of its widespread presence in soil, its presence in air and dust (including kitchen dust) is not surprising. In the case of marine sediments there is a close relationship between the amount of faecal pollution and the numbers of *C. perfringens*.

Food Poisoning

Food poisoning attributable to *C. perfringens* usually occurs 8–24 h after the ingestion of temperature-abused food containing large numbers of vegetative cells. Symptoms last 1–2 days and generally include diarrhoea and severe abdominal cramps. Vomiting is not uncommon and fever is rare. Type A cells are usually responsible. A more severe type of illness, caused by type C, occurs among young adults of the highlands of New Guinea. It is necrotizing (necrosis: death of areas of tissue surrounded by healthy parts), haemorrhagic jejunitis (inflammation of the jejunum, the second portion of the small intestine extending, from the duodenum to the ileum) which is often called pig-bel (enteritis necroticans) because it follows traditional pig feasting.

It should be noted that ingestion of low levels of microbial spores, including *Clostridium botulinum* and *C. perfringens*, is a common occurrence and not a public safety issue for adults. Only when these spores have been allowed to germinate and grow in food products do they pose a health threat.

Mechanisms of Entry into Food Chain

The vegetative cells and spores of *C. perfringens* are common surface contaminants of fresh meat and poultry carcasses. This is not surprising in view of the common occurrence of the organisms in the intestine of these animals. They can be easily disseminated during processing steps such as evisceration and scalding. Unlike the case for *Salmonella*, the absence of this organism from fresh meat and poultry is an unreasonable expectation. Furthermore, the mere presence of *C. perfringens* (as spores) surviving cooking will not cause outbreaks of foodborne illness. For the latter to occur, gross mishandling and temperature abuse must always be involved. *See* individual meats and poultry

Fate during Processing and Storage

Temperature is the single most important determinant of the survival and multiplication of *C. perfringens* subsequent to slaughter and packaging. Generation times as low as 8–10 min have been reported for this organism at its optimum growth temperature. Other considerations affecting growth include absence of oxygen, water activity, pH and salt content. However, alterations of these usually involve further processing steps and epidemiological investigations have consistently implicated fresh meat and poultry as sources of the organism. *See* Meat, Preservation

The fate of *C. perfringens* during processing and storage depends on the form of the organism, i.e. vegetative cell or spore. Both are present in fresh meat and poultry, but each require different considerations with regard to immediate or potential hazard.

Vegetative cells can grow over the temperature range of 15–50°C, with optima between 43°C and 46°C. Even between 60°C and 70°C, viability may be maintained, but vegetative cells are rapidly inactivated at 75°C. Considering the short generation time of the organism the slow attainment of a safe interior temperature can actually increase the initial number of organisms and permit more cells to survive. Thus the rate at which the interior temperature is attained may also influence the thermal survival of vegetative cells. For example, rump roast cooked to an internal temperature of 77°C in 2·25 h has been shown to retain significant numbers of viable *C. perfringens* cells. On the other hand, experiments with chicken breast and thigh have shown complete killing of 10^8 vegetative cells when the pieces were cooked in water at 82°C and the internal temperature of 77°C was attained in 20 min or less. The standard dictum that cooked meat should be kept above 62·8°C or below 10°C will ensure safety of properly heated food.

Most *C. perfringens* spores isolated from meat and poultry are the heat-sensitive variety. These are killed in a few minutes at 100°C. Unfortunately, spores of the heat-resistant variety are also present in lower numbers. These have D_{100} (decimal reduction value at 100°C) values of 6–17 min and can survive cooking procedures (which themselves drive off oxygen), germinate and resume vegetative cell growth given the proper conditions, principally suitable temperature.

The effect of low-temperature storage on *C. perfringens* cells is important because food safety with regard to this organism is based largely on proper refrigerated holding. *Clostridium perfringens* vegetative cells are sensitive to low temperature, e.g. refrigerated storage. Slow die-off occurs under these conditions. Similarly, long-term (several weeks) freezing slowly inactivates vegetative cells. The initial freezing step reduces the population approximately 10-fold. Surprisingly, vegetative cells die more rapidly at $-5°C$ than at $-20°C$. As one would expect, spores are considerably more resistant. They are virtually unaffected by refrigerated storage and only somewhat inactivated by freezing. Indeed, frozen storage in the spore state is routinely used for culture carriage.

Before spores can resume vegetative cell growth they must germinate. Proper nutrients must be available and these are readily available in meat and poultry products. Viable bacterial spores are traditionally measured by heating a culture at an elevated temperature (75–80°C, depending upon the strain) for 10–20 min and performing routine plating procedures. This procedure 'activates' the spore population (and inactivates any vegetative cells). In the case of raw food this function is effectively achieved by routine cooking procedures. Optimal temperatures for germination are similar to those for vegetative cell growth, in a pH range of 5·5–7·0.

It is difficult to specify the time required for cells of *C. perfringens* to multiply in foods to attain toxic numbers, but it has been observed that meats stored at a 'warm' temperature for at least 2 h after cooking were common factors in many outbreaks. The hazard is magnified when such food is allowed to cool slowly for several hours, e.g. overnight at room temperature, as has occurred with large turkeys or large bulks of other meats.

The multiplication of bacteria is a logarithmic function. The rate at which a product may accumulate harmful numbers of cells will depend to a large extent on the size of the inoculum. The temperature at which cooked foods is held or stored is the other highly dependent variable. As mentioned above, this is especially true with *C. perfringens* in view of its ability to grow at relatively elevated temperatures.

Bibliography

Labbé R (1989) *Clostridium perfringens*. In: Doyle M (ed.) *Foodborne Bacterial Pathogens*, pp 191–234. New York: Marcel Dekker.

Labbé R and Harmon S (1991) *Clostridium perfringens*. In: Vanderzant C and Splittstoesser D (eds) *Compendium of Methods for the Microbiological Examination of Foods* 3rd edn, pp 469–478. Washington, DC: American Public Health Association.

McClane B (1988) *Clostridium perfringens* enterotoxin. *Microbial Pathogenesis* 4: 317–323.

McDonel J (1980) *Clostridium perfringens* toxins (type A, B, C, D, E). *Pharmacology and Therapeutics* 10: 617–655.

Smith L and Williams B (1984) *The Pathogenic Anaerobic Bacteria* 3rd edn. Springfield, Illinois: Charles Thomas.

Stringer M (1985) *Clostridium perfringens* type A food poisoning. In: Borriello S (ed.) *Clostridia in Gastrointestinal Disease*, pp 117–141. Boca Raton, Florida: CRC Press.

Stringer M, Watson G and Gilbert R (1982) *Clostridium perfringens* type A: serological typing and methods for the detection of enterotoxin. In: Corry J, Roberts D and Skinner F (eds) *Isolation and Identification Methods for Food Poisoning Organisms*, pp 111–135. London: Academic Press.

Ronald G. Labbé
University of Massachusetts, Amherst, USA

Detection of *Clostridium perfringens*

Laboratory Criteria for Confirming Outbreaks

Laboratory confirmation of an outbreak of *C. perfringens* food poisoning is based on one of five criteria: (1) more than 10^5 of the organism per gram of food; (2) more than 10^6 spores of the organism per gram of the faeces of ill persons; (3) the presence of the same serotype in most of the ill patients; (4) the presence of the same serotype in the incriminated food and faeces of the patients; and (5) detection of enterotoxin in faeces. Detailed procedures for serotyping are available from citations in the *Bibliography*, at the end of the next article.

Detection in Raw and Processed Foods

Detection of *C. perfringens* in raw and processed foods is performed by similar methods. Such foods, properly handled, would not normally contain more than 100 *C. perfringens* cells or spores per gram, usually much less. In such situations, most probable number (MPN) test tube procedures can be used for enumerating low numbers in foods. Iron-containing milk (iron milk medium, or IMM, i.e. 10 ml of homogenized milk containing 0·2 g of iron powder) has been used for this purpose. When incubated at 46°C, *C. perfringens* produces a typical 'stormy fermentation' in IMM. This is defined as the production of an acid curd (caused by lactic acid fermentation) with subsequent disruption of the curd by large volumes of gas. Non-MPN enrichment media (Trypticase–glucose–yeast-extract broth), with incubation at 37°C followed by selective plating on Trypticase–sulphite–cycloserine (or neomycin blood agar) agar plating, can also be used for enumeration of very low numbers. Confirmation (see below) is required in either method.

Detection of Cells in Suspected Food Poisoning

Foods implicated in outbreaks of human food poisoning would normally contain large numbers of vegetative cells and relatively few spores. Such food should be chilled and processed rapidly because of the susceptibility of the cells to cold shock. For delayed analyses, highest counts are obtained when foods (finely chopped if necessary) are mixed 1:1 with 20% glycerol and kept at −20°C or, if shipping is necessary, placed in a container of dry ice. *See* Food Poisoning, Tracing Origins and Testing

Selective plating methods are used for enumeration of viable cells. Enrichment techniques are unnecessary for examination of food containing large numbers of cells. Most plating media depend on the ability of *C. perfringens* to reduce sulphite to sulphide which, in the presence of an iron salt, results in formation of black colonies owing to ferrous sulphide. Collaborative analyses have indicated that pour-plated Tryptose Sulphite Cycloserine (TSC) without egg yolk is the medium of choice. More consistent blackening of surface colonies can be obtained by overlaying plates with sterile media. Tryptose Sulphite Cycloserine is commercially available from Unipath (Oxoid). After anaerobic incubation for 24 h at 37°C, representative black colonies (usually 10) must be confirmed. This is achieved by inoculating a liquid medium, such as Trypticase Peptone Glucose Yeast Extract Broth (TPGY) or Fluid Thioglycollate medium, and incubating at 46°C for 4 h or overnight at 37°C. Tubes of lactose–gelatin and motility-nitrate are inoculated from each and incubated at 37°C for 24 h. *Clostridium perfringens* is nonmotile, ferments lactose, liquefies gelatin, and reduces nitrate to nitrite. The number of *C. perfringens* per gram is determined by multiplying the presumptive plate count by the ratio of colonies confirmed as *C. perfringens*. Faecal spore levels are determined in the same manner, except that the sample is heated at 75°C for 20 min. The elevated-temperature MPN methods mentioned above are not recommended for quantification of *C. perfringens* in outbreak stools.

Surface-plated neomycin blood agar plates are often used in the UK and can be prepared well in advance. This medium also provides information on the haemolytic activity of isolates. However, because recovery of certain heat-resistant strains may be no more than 10% on this medium, its use is limited to outbreak stools or food samples containing large numbers of *C. perfringens*. Neomycin blood agar is not recommended for examining normal food samples in which the organism is present in low numbers.

Detection of Enterotoxin in Suspected Food Poisoning

The ingestion of large numbers of vegetative cells in incriminated food is followed by multiplication of the cells in the small intestine. When they sporulate there is an accompanying formation of enterotoxin. Lysis of the sporangia to release the mature spore also results in the release of enterotoxin.

Serum values of antienterotoxin are of little value in the diagnosis of *C. perfringens* food poisoning, and enterotoxin detection in foods is not a practical approach. However, detection of the enterotoxin in stools is of significant diagnostic importance since the toxin is not detectable in the faeces of healthy adults. Of the criteria listed above there are occasions when only detection of enterotoxin in faeces is conclusive; for example, when no food is available, when the strains are not typeable or when the incidents concern geriatric patients who may carry large numbers of the same serotype or spores without symptoms of food poisoning. Most faecal specimens from food poisonings incidents have enterotoxin concentrations exceeding 1 μg per g of faeces.

Two procedures for detection of enterotoxin in faeces have found widespread use and are effective when used within 2 days of onset of symptoms. They are enzyme-linked immunosorbent assay (ELISA) and the reversed phase latex agglutinations assay (RPLA). The latter is available as a kit from Unipath (Oxoid). Although expensive (if obtained commercially) for multiple samples, the RPLA method is the simpler one. In it, latex beads which have been sensitized (treated) with enterotoxin antiserum are exposed to serial dilutions of enterotoxin-containing material. After overnight incubation the agglutination titre is determined. Expensive equipment, such as a microplate reader (needed for

Table 1. Incidence of confirmed *C. perfringens* foodborne illness in selected countries

Year	Canada[a] Outbreaks	Cases	USA[b] Outbreaks	Cases	England and Wales[c] Outbreaks	Cases	Japan[d] Outbreaks	Cases	Scotland[e] Outbreaks	Cases
1975	12	556	16	419	70	2418				
1976	18	598	6	509	87	2924				
1977	13	498	6	658	83	2576				
1978	6	215	9	617	42	1042				
1979	11	495	20	1110	56	1607				
1980	18	753	25	1463	55	1054	13	5178	7	171
1981	15	399	28	1162	46	918	23	3482	10	364
1982	18	1420	22	1189	69	1455	11	896	6	95
1983	14	324	5	353	68	1624	16	4571	5	185
1984	20	891	8	882	68	1716	9	971	8	164
1985	15	270	6	1016	64	1466			5	84
1986	11	174	3	202	51	896	22	3258	6	108
1987			2	290	51	1266	9	288	5	149
1988					57	1312	19	2671	11	234
1989					54[f]	901[f]	24	3316	5	75

[a] Todd (personal communication).
[b] Centers for Disease Control, Atlanta, USA, yearly annual summaries.
[c] R Gilbert (personal communication).
[d] T Uemura (personal communication).
[e] J Sharp (personal communication).
[f] Provisional.

ELISA), is unnecessary. On the other hand, nonspecific agglutination can occur at very low (near the detection limit) dilutions. The ELISA method is preferable when more than occasional samples are to be assayed. Some half-dozen different ELISA procedures have been proposed with sensitivities of 2–5 ng per g of faeces. *See* Immunoassays, Radioimmunoassay and Enzyme Immunoassay

Statistics

As mentioned above, meat and poultry products are invariably involved in cases of human food poisoning attributed to *C. perfringens*. The organism has complex nutritional requirements which are easily satisfied by such foods. On the other hand, cured meats are rarely implicated. Bacon and ham, for example, are seldom involved, presumably owing to the presence of curing salts and the lowered water activity, both of which inhibit vegetative cell growth. *See* Food Poisoning, Statistics

Mass feeding establishments are consistently cited as the source where implicated food was eaten. Examples of these have included restaurants, cafeterias, prisons, schools and hospitals. All such sites prepare large amounts of food well in advance of serving. Opportunities for mishandling of food in such settings are plentiful.

As with other agents of human food poisoning, the number of outbreaks of food poisoning attributable to *C. perfringens* is greatly underreported. This is particularly true with *C. perfringens* because of the relatively mild and short-lived nature of the symptoms. In addition, in some countries, e.g. the USA, medical personnel are not required to report incidences of outbreaks to central public health officials. Thus the data in Table 1 represent only a fraction of the true number of cases and outbreaks. In Western countries the organism ranks second or third behind *Salmonella*, *Campylobacter* or *Staphylococcus aureus* in terms of number of cases of human food poisoning caused by bacteria. *See* Campylobacter, Properties and Occurrence; *Staphylococcus*, Properties and Occurrence

Bibliography

Labbé R (1989) *Clostridium perfringens*. In: Doyle M (ed.) *Foodborne Bacterial Pathogens*, pp 191–234. New York: Marcel Dekker.

Labbé R and Harmon S (1991) *Clostridium perfringens*. In: Vanderzant C and Splittstoesser D (eds) *Compendium of Methods for the Microbiological Examination of Foods* 3rd edn, pp 469–478. Washington, DC: American Public Health Association.

McClane B (1988) *Clostridium perfringens* enterotoxin. *Microbial Pathogenesis* 4: 317–323.

McDonel J (1980) *Clostridium perfringens* toxins (type A, B, C, D, E). *Pharmacology and Therapeutics* 10: 617–655.

Smith L and Williams B (1984) *The Pathogenic Anaerobic Bacteria* 3rd edn. Springfield, Illinois: Charles Thomas.

Detection of Clostridium perfringens

Stringer M (1985) *Clostridium perfringens* type A food poisoning. In: Borriello S (ed.) *Clostridia in Gastrointestinal Disease*, pp 117–141. Boca Raton, Florida: CRC Press.

Stringer M, Watson G and Gilbert R (1982) *Clostridium perfringens* type A: serological typing and methods for the detection of enterotoxin. In: Corry J, Roberts D and Skinner F (eds) *Isolation and Identification Methods for Food Poisoning Organisms*, pp 111–135. London: Academic Press.

Ronald G. Labbé
University of Massachusetts, Amherst, USA

Food Poisoning by *Clostridium perfringens*

Clinical Features and Characteristics

It is now well established that an enterotoxin is responsible for the symptoms of *C. perfringens* food poisoning. The symptoms are typically diarrhoea and severe abdominal cramps (fever and vomiting are unusual) which occur 8–24 h after ingestion of food containing large numbers of vegetative cells. Sufficient numbers of cells survive stomach passage and sporulate in the small intestine.

The sequence of events can be duplicated in the laboratory by inoculating vegetative cells into a suitable sporulation medium. Many different types of sporulation media have been developed for this but no single one is suitable for all strains. Figure 1 shows that about 3 h after inoculation of the sporulation medium, heat-resistant spores develop, followed closely by the intracellular accumulation of enterotoxin. Maximum numbers of spores are obtained after 7 h and free spores can be detected after 10–12 h. With the liberation of the mature spores from the sporangia, enterotoxin is released and the concentration of enterotoxin in the cell extract therefore decreases. The concentration of extracellular enterotoxin increases in parallel with the increase in free spores. In humans this corresponds to the release of enterotoxin into the lumen of the small intestine.

Site and Mode of Action

The enterotoxin of *C. perfringens* causes fluid accumulation in ligated small intestinal loops (sections), and overt diarrhoea in a large number of experimental animals. The colon is not affected by the enterotoxin since, at least in rabbits, there is no change in the transport of fluid or electrolytes in this tissue. To determine the mode of action of the toxin, rabbit small intestines have been perfused with various electrolytes and nutrients after exposure to the toxin. The effects on intestinal transport and structure were determined. These procedures indicate that the enterotoxin causes a net secretion of water, sodium and chloride. Glucose

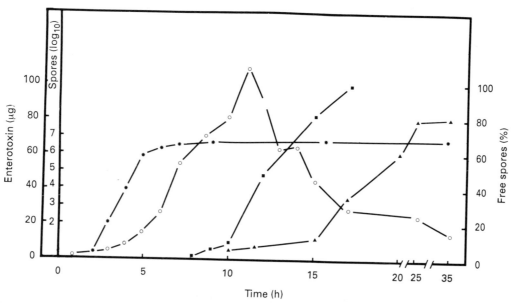

Fig. 1 Time course of intracellular enterotoxin formation and release during sporulation of *C. perfringens* type A. ○ Content (μg) of biologically active enterotoxin per mg of cell protein extract; ■ μg of biologically active enterotoxin per ml of culture filtrate; ∗ heat-resistant spores per ml; ▲ percentage of refractile spores free from sporangia. Adapted from Labbé R (1989) and reprinted with permission of Marcel Dekker, New York.

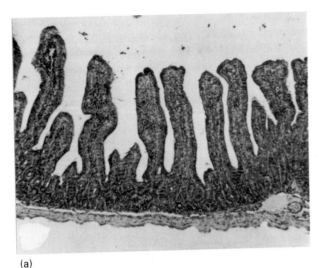

(a)

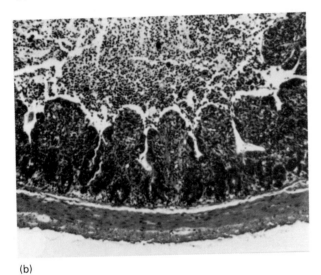

(b)

Fig. 2 Effect of *C. perfringens* enterotoxin on rabbit ileum. (a) Control showing typical villous morphology. (b) Ileum treated with enterotoxin for 90 min showing shortened villi denuded of epithelial cells. (Reprinted with permission from Laboratory Investigation, Baltimore, USA).

absorption is inhibited, whereas potassium and bicarbonate absorption are unaffected. The sensitivity of the rabbit's small intestine to the toxin increases from the upper duodenum downward, with the terminal ileum being the most responsive. Histological studies indicate that there is destruction of intestinal epithelial cells at the tips of villi (Fig. 2). Intestinal brush border membranes lose their characteristic folded configuration and large quantities of membrane and cytoplasm are lost to the lumen. Similar morphological changes occur after intravenous injection of the enterotoxin. The brush border (microvillus membrane) of villus tip epithelial cells is considered the primary site of action of the enterotoxin.

In contrast to the effects of cholera toxin and *Escherichia coli* heat-liable enterotoxin, *C. perfringens* enterotoxin does not increase levels of cyclic adenosine monophosphate (cAMP) in intestinal mucosa that is actively secreting fluid.

Our understanding of the mode of action of the enterotoxin at the molecular level has been greatly facilitated by the use of *in vitro* model systems using various cell lines. Vero (African green monkey kidney) cells are particularly sensitive to the toxin. Rat liver, HeLa, small intestinal epithelial cells, and other cell lines have also been used as models.

The enterotoxin causes rapid membrane bleb formation in cultured Vero cells (Fig. 3). Total inhibition of amino acid transport and deoxyribonucleic acid (DNA), ribonucleic acid (RNA), and protein synthesis occurs within 30 min of exposure. Within 40 min, 75% of the Vero cells detach (from the plastic culture flask) and nearly 50% are nonviable.

Disruption of the plasma membrane is the specific action of the enterotoxin in Vero cells. Binding to the cell membrane must occur and is an early event. This does not occur in naturally resistant cell lines or in cells selected for resistance to the toxin. A protein of molecular weight 50 000 has been extracted from rabbit intestinal brush border membranes. This protein inhibits biological activity of enterotoxin in Vero cells, suggesting that it has a role in enterotoxin binding. No role has been found for ganglioside GM_1 (gangliosides constitute a family of acidic glycolipids which are important membrane components) from rabbit intestinal brush border membranes in binding *C. perfringens* enterotoxin. This is in contrast to the role ganglioside GM_1 plays in binding cholera toxin.

The enterotoxin causes functional holes of defined size in Vero cell membranes. The result is an alteration of membrane permeability, causing rapid water and ion flux changes immediately after binding. Osmotic stabilizers protect against such enterotoxin-induced morphological and permeability changes, further suggesting the membrane as the site of action. With a net influx of water and ions, the membrane stretches and bleb formation results. This is followed by the loss of essential precursors through leakage. With the interruption of macromolecular synthesis the cell eventually dies. While such specific events in an *in vitro* cell model cannot be directly extrapolated to the effects of the enterotoxin in human intestinal cells, such evidence is highly suggestive that the membrane of the human small intestine is the primary site of action of *C. perfringens* enterotoxin.

Treatment of Illness

As in most cases of enterotoxin-mediated human food poisoning, symptoms are self-limiting. In the case of *C.*

Prevention and Control

The factors contributing to outbreaks of foodborne illness by *C. perfringens* were identified long ago. Those most frequently cited are (1) preparation of food too far in advance, (2) inadequate cooling, (3) storage at ambient temperature, and (4) inadequate reheating. Multiple factors are frequently cited, but failure to refrigerate properly large portions of previously cooked foods, especially in institutional settings, invariably summarizes the events leading to an outbreak.

Spores on raw meat and poultry can survive cooking which effectively heat-activates the spores to promote germination when the product reaches a suitable temperature during cooling. Rapid, uniform cooling is therefore imperative. Gravies, broths and large pieces of meat should be cooled to 10°C within 2–3 h. The organism can multiply rapidly in the slowly cooling masses of meat and poultry. Cooking also drives off oxygen and thereby promotes anaerobic conditions; this is especially important in liquid foods, and in rolled meats where the contaminated outside surface is rolled into the middle. Cooked, chilled foods should be reheated to a minimum internal temperature of 75°C immediately before serving, in order to destroy vegetative cells. As noted in the preceding article, cooked meat should be kept above 62·8°C or below 10°C.

Human carriers are not a danger. It is impossible to prevent human carriers from handling food because most people harbour *C. perfringens* in their intestinal tract. Similarly, the organism is present in a wide variety of foods. Hence preventative measures depend largely on knowledge of proper food preparation and storage techniques, especially temperature control. Certain trade organizations related to the food service industry offer short courses dealing with proper food handling procedures. Clearly, education of food handlers is a key aspect in prevention of human food poisoning in general, and that caused by *C. perfringens* in particular.

Bibliography

Labbé R (1989) *Clostridium perfringens*. In: Doyle M (ed.) *Foodborne Bacterial Pathogens*, pp 191–234. New York: Marcel Dekker.

Labbé R and Harmon S (1991) *Clostridium perfringens*. In: Vanderzant C and Splittstoesser D (eds) *Compendium of Methods for the Microbiological Examination of Foods* 3rd edn, pp 469–478. Washington, DC: American Public Health Association.

McClane B (1988) *Clostridium perfringens* enterotoxin. *Microbial Pathogenesis* 4: 317–323.

McDonel J (1980) *Clostridium perfringens* toxins (type A, B, C, D, E). *Pharmacology and Therapeutics* 10: 617–655.

Smith L and Williams B (1984) *The Pathogenic Anaerobic Bacteria* 3rd edn. Springfield, Illinois: Charles Thomas.

Stringer M (1985) *Clostridium perfringens* type A food poisoning. In: Borriello S (ed.) *Clostridia in Gastrointestinal Disease*, pp 117–141. Boca Raton, Florida: CRC Press.

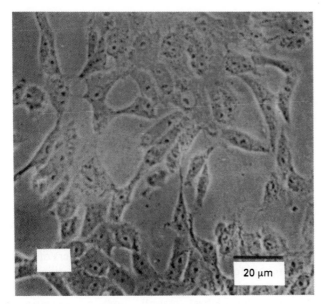

(a)

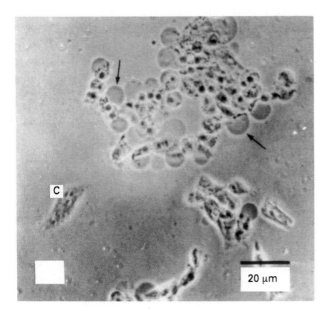

(b)

Fig. 3 Effect of enterotoxin on morphology of Vero cells. (a) Control culture showing typical Vero cell morphology. (b) Vero cells after 30 min of exposure to enterotoxin. Note spherical morphology and formation of blebs (arrows). Reprinted, with permission of John Wiley, New York, from McClane B and McDonel J (1979) The effects of *Clostridium perfringens* enterotoxin on morphology, viability and macromolecular synthesis in Vero cells. *Journal of Cellular Physiology* 99: 193.

perfringens, symptoms subside within 1 or 2 days. Death is uncommon but has occurred in institutionalized individuals, especially the elderly. In such cases fluid and mineral replacement therapy is essential.

Stringer M, Watson G and Gilbert R (1982) *Clostridium perfringens* type A: serological typing and methods for the detection of enterotoxin. In: Corry J, Roberts D and Skinner F (eds) *Isolation and Identification Methods for Food Poisoning Organisms*, pp 111–135. London: Academic Press.

Ronald G. Labbé
University of Massachusetts, Amherst, USA

Occurrence of *Clostridium botulinum*

The *Clostridium botulinum* species is made up of gram-positive, anaerobic, rod-shaped, spore-forming bacteria. They are distinguished by the production of the most potent biological toxin known, botulinum neurotoxin. This article will discuss the distribution of botulinum spores in the environment and in foods, the different factors affecting growth in foods, and the methods to detect the organism and its neurotoxin in foods.

Strains of *C. botulinum* are separated into seven types, A through G, based on the serological specificity of the toxin produced. Human botulism, including foodborne, wound and infant botulism, is associated with types A, B, E, and, very rarely, F. Types C and D cause botulism in animals. To date, there is no direct evidence linking type G to disease. Based on physiological differences, the species is also divided into four groups: (I) all type A and proteolytic strains of types B and F; (II) all type E and nonproteolytic strains of types B and F; (III) type C and D strains; (IV) type G strains. The emphasis here will be on groups I and II since they are involved in human illness.

Presence of *C. botulinum* in the Environment

Spores of *C. botulinum* are commonly present in soils and sediments, but their numbers and types vary, depending on the location (Table 1). The possibility of contamination of food with *C. botulinum* depends on the distribution and incidence of spores in the environment.

C. botulinum spores are widely distributed in North America, but the spore load varies considerably, as does the predominating type. Soils in the USA east of the rise of the Rocky Mountains usually contain type B spores, while type A spores predominate in the western USA. Most US type B strains are proteolytic. Type C spores are localized in soils along the Gulf of Mexico coast. Overall, type E is found infrequently, and only in damp to wet locations. However, in the region around the Great Lakes, and particularly around Green Bay of Lake Michigan, high numbers of type E are found in shoreline and sediment samples. Type E is also found in the coastal areas of Washington and Alaska. The distribution of types on the Pacific coast changes with latitude; south of 36°N, the prevalent types shift from E to A and B.

Type B predominates in the terrestrial environments of Britain, Ireland, Iceland, Denmark and Switzerland. It is associated with most botulism outbreaks in Spain, Portugal, Italy, France, Belgium, Germany, Poland, Czechoslovakia, Hungary and Yugoslavia, indicating wide distribution of this type in the European environment. Type B also predominates in the aquatic environments of the UK. Most European type B strains are nonproteolytic. The predominant serotype from other aquatic environments is E. The highest numbers of type E spores are found in Scandinavian waters, particularly in the Sound and Kattegat, between Denmark and Sweden. The highest overall spore concentrations detected in Europe were reported in the Netherlands, where a mixture of types was found.

Type E spores also predominate in most parts of the USSR, except for the central portion, where type B spores predominate. In general, surveys of Asia report lower numbers, with the exceptions of a high incidence of type E spores around the Caspian Sea, and a high incidence of all types in the Sinkiang district of China.

Fewer surveys have been carried out in the southern hemisphere. Spores of all types have been detected in South America; type E has been found in fish, oyster and shrimp samples taken off the Brazilian coast. Type A spores predominate in Brazilian and Argentine soils. In the tropical regions of Asia, types C and D replace type E as the predominant type in aquatic environments.

The distribution of spore types in fish and shellfish is similar to that in the sediments from their respective areas. Because the methods of sampling fish and shellfish differ widely, it is difficult to compare numbers.

In summary, type A spores predominate in soils in the western USA, China, Brazil and Argentina, and type B spores in the eastern USA, the UK, and much of continental Europe. However, most US type B strains are proteolytic, while most European strains are nonproteolytic. Type E is the predominant type in northern regions, and in most temperate aquatic regions and their surroundings. Types C and D are found more frequently in warmer environments. The reasons for this distribution pattern are not well understood. Type A appears to be favoured by neutral to alkaline soil with low organic content, consistent with its virtual absence in the highly cultivated soils of the eastern USA and Europe. Type E is psychrotolerant, which undoubtedly plays a role in its prevalence in the north and in many aquatic environments. Similarly, the higher optimum growth temperature for types C and D is consistent with their presence in warmer environments.

Table 1. Quantitative soil and sediment surveys for *C. botulinum*[a]

Location	Sample size (g)	Positive samples (%)	MPN per kg[b]	Type (%)[a] A	B	C/D	E	F
Eastern USA soil	10	19	21	12	64	12	12	0
Western USA soil	10	29	33	62	16	14	8	0
New York–Florida coast	1	4	36	8	17	42	33	0
Florida–Texas coast	1	6	62	12	4	38	46	0
Great Lakes sediment	1	2	24	0	0	0	100	0
Green Bay sediment	1	72	1280	0	0	0	100	0
Washington coast	5	71	250	1	3	0	96	0
Alaska coast	1	49	660	0	0	0	100	0
California coast north of 36°	5	16	29	5	5	0	90	0
California coast south of 36°	5	10	20	44	50	0	0	6
Britain miscellaneous soil	50	10	2	0	100	0	0	0
Britain coast	2	4	18	0	100	0	0	0
Ireland miscellaneous soil	50	18	4	0	100	0	0	0
Iceland soil	10	3	3	0	100	0	0	0
Faroe Islands coast	10	1	1	0	0	0	100	0
Greenland coast	10	37	46	0	0	0	100	0
Skagerrak, Kattegat sediment	6	100	>780	0	0	0	100	0
Norway coast	5	7	7	0	0	0	100	0
Sweden miscellaneous soil	6	29	30	0	5	0	95	0
Sweden inland	6	47	110	0	4	0	96	0
Sweden coast	3–6	84	410	0	0	1	99	0
Danish coast	10	67	110	0	0	0	100	0
Denmark miscellaneous soil	10	13	15	0	93	7	0	0
Netherlands soil	0·5	94	2500	0	22	46	32	0
Poland, Baltic coast	5	32	76	3	0	0	97	0
Czechoslovakia soil		42		0	0	100	0	0
Switzerland soil	12	44	48	28	83	6	0	27
Italy, Rome soil	7·5	1	2	86	14	0	0	0
USSR soil								
Northeastern		2		0	14	0	86	0
Southeastern		13		8	17	0	73	0
Central		14		16	77	0	6	0
Northwestern		4		14	0	0	86	0
Far East		14		0	8	5	87	0
Iran, Caspian Sea sediment	2	17	93	0	8	0	92	0
China, Sinkiang soil	10	70	25 000	47	32	19	2	0
Taiwan soil	10	78	30	34	37	4	20	5
Japan, Hokkaido soil	5–10	4	4	0	0	0	100	0
Japan, Ishikawa soil	40–50	56	16	0	0	100	0	0
Brazil, cultivated soil	5	35	86	57	7	29	0	7
Paraguay soil	5	24	10	14	0	14	0	71
Argentina soil		34		67	20	0	0	5
Kenya soil	5	25	33	89	0	11	0	0
South Africa soil	30	3	1	0	100	0	0	0
Bangladesh sediment	10	37	19	0	0	100	0	0
Thailand, Hua-Hin sediment	10	3	3	0	0	83	17	0
Indonesia sediment	50	21	5	0	0	100	0	0
Java coast	10	13	14	0	33	67	0	0
Auckland New Zealand sediment	20	55	40	0	0	100	0	0

[a] From Hauschild AHW (1989).
[b] MPN calculated using the Halvorson–Zeigler equation $\log_e(n/q)$, where n=the total number of samples analysed and q=the number of nontoxic samples.
[c] As percentage of the types identified.

Presence of *C. botulinum* in foods

The sequence of events resulting in foodborne botulism begins when *C. botulinum* contaminates a food. This often occurs during growth or harvesting, and is most likely to occur when a product originates in an environment with a high incidence of spores. However, contamination can also occur during or after processing. There have been considerably fewer surveys of foods for contamination with *C. botulinum* than environmental surveys, and they have focused primarily on fish, meats and infant foods, particularly honey.

Fish may become contaminated with spores of *C. botulinum* in their environment, or during processing and handling. The presence of *C. botulinum*, mostly type E, in fish is readily demonstrated, although the incidence is lower than in environmental surveys. The average level of contamination of prepared fish in the USA

($\sim$263 spores kg^{-1}, 22% of all samples positive) appears to be higher than in Europe and Asia ($\sim$57 spores kg^{-1}, 10% of all samples positive). The highest contamination level reported was in salted fish from the Caspian Sea.

The level of contamination of meats is generally low. It appears lower in North America, where the average most probable number (MPN) is about 0·1 spore kg^{-1}, than in Europe, where the average MPN is about 2·5 spores kg^{-1}. The types most often associated with meats are A or B. *See* Fish, Spoilage

C. botulinum may be present on fruits and vegetables, particularly those in close contact with the soil. Types A or B are usually identified. One product of particular concern is cultivated mushrooms, in which up to $2\cdot1 \times 10^3$ type B spores kg^{-1} have been detected.

Spores in honey and other infant foods pose a unique hazard because, in some infants, the spores are able to colonize the intestines, produce toxin and cause infant botulism. By 1984, honey had been implicated as the likely source of botulinum spores in 20 cases of infant botulism in California. Surveys for the presence of *C. botulinum* spores in honey suggest that the botulinum spore level in random samples of honey is in the order of 1–10 spores kg^{-1}. However, in honey samples associated with infant botulism the level is approximately 10^4 spores kg^{-1}. Other infant foods have also been examined. While *C. botulinum* has been detected in samples of corn syrup and rice cereal, exposure of infants to botulinum spores via these foods seems to be minimal. The spore levels are low, and spores are unlikely to multiply during manufacture and storage.

Other foods examined, including dairy products, vacuum-packed products and convenience foods, show a very low incidence of *C. botulinum* spores.

Factors Affecting Growth and Toxin Production in Foods

The main factors affecting growth of *C. botulinum* in foods are temperature, pH, water activity (a_w), redox potential, added preservatives and other microorganisms. The growth of types A, B, E and F, of groups I and II, has been intensively studied. Traditionally, food microbiologists have established maximum and/or minimum limits for these parameters which would permit growth of *C. botulinum* (Table 2), and these limits have often been used in the control of *C. botulinum*. However, these factors seldom function independently; usually, they act in concert, often having synergistic or additive effects.

Temperature

Because foods are generally stored at low temperatures, studies have focused on determining the minimum

Table 2. Properties of group I and II *C. botulinum*

Property	Group I	II
Toxin types	A, B, F	B, E, F
Minimum temperature for growth (°C)	10	3·3
Maximum temperature for growth (°C)	48	45
Minimum pH for growth	4·6	5·0
Inhibitory [NaCl] (%)	10	5
Minimum a_w for growth	0·94	0·97
$D_{100°C}$ of spores (min)	25	<0·1

temperatures permitting growth. The established lower limits are 10°C for group I and 3·3°C for group II. However, these limits apply to relatively few strains and depend on otherwise optimum growth conditions. Production of toxin generally requires several weeks at the lower temperature limits. The optimum growth temperature is in the range 35–40°C for group I organisms, and in the range 25–30°C for those of group II. The upper temperature limits for group I and group II organisms are approximately 45–50°C and 40–45°C, respectively.

pH

It is generally accepted that the minimum pH permitting growth of *C. botulinum* group I is 4·6, and many regulations worldwide use this limit. For group II, the limit is about pH 5·0. The upper pH limits for growth are in the pH range 8–9, but are of no practical consequence. Many fruits and vegetables are sufficiently acidic to inhibit *C. botulinum* by their pH alone, while other products, such as marinated mushrooms, are preserved by added acidulants. Several factors influence the acid tolerance of *C. botulinum*, including strain, substrate, temperature, nature of the acidulant, the presence of preservatives, a_w and redox potential. The growth of acid-tolerant microorganisms such as yeasts and moulds may raise the pH in their immediate vicinity to a level that permits growth of *C. botulinum*. *C. botulinum* can also grow in some acidified foods if excessively slow pH equilibration occurs. While high concentrations of proteins in laboratory media appear to protect *C. botulinum* and permit growth at pH levels below 4·6, this does not occur in foods preserved by acidity. Current regulations stipulating a minimal acidity of pH 4·6 for the control of *C. botulinum* are therefore valid.

Salt and a_w

Salt (NaCl) is one of the most important factors controlling *C. botulinum* in foods. Its inhibitory effect is primarily due to the depression of a_w and consequently to its concentration in the aqueous phase, also called the brine concentration (% brine = % NaCl × 100/ (% H_2O + % NaCl)). Under otherwise optimal conditions, the growth-limiting brine concentrations are about 10% for strains of group I and 5% for strains of group II. These concentrations correspond well to the limiting a_w of 0·94 for group I and 0·97 for group II in foods where NaCl is the main a_w depressant. The type of solute used to control a_w may influence these limits. Generally, NaCl, potassium chloride, glucose and sucrose show similar patterns, while the use of glycerol reduces the growth-limiting a_w level by up to 0·03 units. The limiting a_w may be raised significantly by other factors, such as increased acidity or preservatives. *See* Water Activity, Effect on Food Stability

Redox Potential

C. botulinum grows optimally at an E_h of −350 mV, but growth initiation may occur in the E_h range of +30 to +250 mV. The presence of other inhibitory factors lowers this upper limit. Once growth is initiated, the E_h declines rapidly.

Modified atmosphere packaging is being used increasingly to extend the shelf life and improve the quality of foods. Depending on the atmosphere and the food, growth of *C. botulinum* may be inhibited or stimulated. Many studies have shown that *C. botulinum* will grow as well in foods packed in air as in vacuum-packed foods; the presence of oxygen in the package headspace does not necessarily inhibit *C. botulinum*. The safety of different atmospheres with respect to *C. botulinum* should be carefully investigated before use. *See* Chilled Storage, Packaging Under Vacuum

Preservatives

Nitrite is important in producing the characteristic colour and flavour of cured food products, but its most important role is the inhibition of *C. botulinum*. It is more effective with decreasing pH, increasing NaCl content, and addition of ascorbate or isoascorbate to the food product. Nitrite reacts with many cellular constituents and appears to inhibit *C. botulinum* by more than one mechanism, one of which is probably its reaction with essential iron–sulphur proteins to inhibit the phosphoroclastic system which supplies the cell with energy. The reactions of nitrite, or nitric oxide, with secondary amines in meats to produce nitrosamines, some of which are carcinogenic, has led to regulations limiting the amount of nitrite used. *See* Curing; Nitrosamines

Other compounds which are active against *C. botuli-num* include sorbates, parabens, nisin, phenolic antioxidants, polyphosphates, ascorbates, ethylenediaminetetraacetic acid (EDTA), metabisulphite, *n*-monoalkyl maleates and fumarates, and lactate salts. The use of natural or liquid smoke has a significant inhibitory effect against *C. botulinum* in fish, but appears insignificant in meats. *See* Smoked Foods, Applications of Smoking

Other Microorganisms

Other microorganisms have a very significant role in the control of *C. botulinum* in foods. Acid-tolerant yeasts and moulds may make the environment more favourable for growth of *C. botulinum*. Other microorganisms may inhibit *C. botulinum*, either by changing the environment, or by producing specific inhibitory substances, or both. Lactic acid bacteria, including *Lactobacillus*, *Pediococcus* and *Streptococcus* spp., can inhibit growth of *C. botulinum* in meat products, largely by reducing the pH, perhaps also by the production of bacteriocins. The use of lactic acid bacteria and a fermentable carbohydrate, the 'Wisconsin process', has been permitted for producing bacon with a decreased level of nitrite in the USA. The growth of other microorganisms may also protect the consumer by causing spoilage that would make a toxic product less likely to be consumed. *See* Lactic Acid Bacteria

Thermal Inactivation

C. botulinum spores of group I are very heat-resistant. D values (the time required to inactivate 90% of the population at a given temperature) vary considerably among *C. botulinum* strains and depend on how the spores are produced and treated, the heating environment and the recovery system. Spores of types A and B are the most heat-resistant, having $D_{121°C}$ values in the range 0·1–0·2 min. These spores are of particular concern in the sterilization of canned low-acid foods, and the canning industry has adopted a D value of 0·2 min at 121°C as a standard for calculating thermal processes. Z values (the temperature change necessary to bring about a 10-fold change in the D value) for the most resistant strains are approximately 10°C, which has also been adopted as a standard. Actual Z values may vary by several degrees. Despite the variations in D and Z values, the adoption of a 12D process as the minimum thermoprocess applied to commercial canned low-acid foods by the canning industry has ensured the production of safe products. *See* Canning, Principles

Although strains of group II are considerably less heat-resistant ($D_{100°C}$ < 0·1 min) than those of group I, their survival in pasteurized, refrigerated products is of

Occurrence of Clostridium botulinum

concern because of their ability to grow at refrigeration temperatures. $D_{82°C}$ values of type E in neutral phosphate buffer are generally in the 0·2–1·0 min range. While the D values are often higher in foods, the Z values are essentially the same. The pasteurization of products such as crabmeat and processed fish should achieve a 10 $\log_{10}$ reduction of type E strains.

Inactivation by Irradiation

C. botulinum spores are probably the most radiation-resistant spores of public health concern. D values (irradiation dose required to inactivate 90% of the population) of group I strains at −50 to −10°C are in the range 2·0–4·5 kGy in neutral buffers and in foods. Spores of type E are only marginally more sensitive, having D values in the range 1–2 kGy. The goal of radappertization is to reduce the number of viable spores of the most radiation-resistant *C. botulinum* by 12 $\log_{10}$ cycles. D values are affected by any pretreatment of spores, the presence of oxygen, irradiation temperature, and irradiation and recovery environments. Generally, spores are more sensitive in the presence of oxygen or preservatives and at temperatures above 20°C. *See* Irradiation of Foods, Basic Principles

Detection of *C. botulinum* and its Toxins in Foods

It is not necessary to isolate *C. botulinum* in pure culture from foods in order to demonstrate its presence. Usually, the sample is inoculated into a nonselective enrichment medium. If the neurotoxin is present in the culture after incubation, the toxin-producing organism must have been present originally.

Botulinum neurotoxins are recognized by their lethal action in mice and neutralization with specific antisera. While several *in vitro* tests have been developed, they are generally less sensitive and less specific than the mouse bioassay which remains the standard. The sample, or an extract prepared by homogenizing it in a slightly acidic buffer, is clarified by centrifugation and normally filter sterilized. Trypsin treatment may be required to activate low levels of toxin from nonproteolytic strains. The prepared sample is injected intraperitoneally into mice with and without neutralization with antitoxin. Typical signs of botulism are ruffled fur, pinched waist, laboured breathing, limb paresis, and general paralysis before death. Definitive results are obtained if mice injected with untreated sample die within 72 h, while mice injected with neutralized sample survive. Several investigators have developed enzyme-linked immunosorbent assay (ELISA) protocols for detecting the neurotoxin but, as yet, reagents are not commercially available. *See* Immunoassays, Radioimmunoassay and Enzyme Immunoassay

Common enrichment media for detecting viable *C. botulinum* are cooked meat medium (CMM), CMM glucose, chopped meat glucose starch (CMGS) medium, and trypsin–peptone–glucose–yeast extract (TPGY) broth to which trypsin may be added (TPGYT). Trypsin is necessary to activate the toxin produced by group II organisms, and may also inactivate potential inhibitors of *C. botulinum* such as boticins in mixed cultures. While foods may be inoculated directly, the sediments of centrifuged samples are preferred because potential growth inhibitors are removed. At least two tubes of media are inoculated. One is heated at 75–80°C or 60°C, depending on whether the suspected type belongs to group I or II, to select for spores. Or spores of group II may be selected by holding samples in 50% alcohol for 1 h before inoculation. The other tube is incubated without any heating to allow development of vegetative *C. botulinum* cells in case few or no spores are present. Adding lysozyme to the medium may increase recovery of heat-injured spores. *C. botulinum* is identified after incubation of the enrichment medium by toxin analysis of the supernatant fluid as outlined above.

Bibliography

Hatheway CL (1990) Toxigenic Clostridia. *Clinical Microbiology Reviews* 3: 66–98.
Hauschild AHW (1989) *Clostridium botulinum*. In: Doyle MP (ed.) *Foodborne Bacterial Pathogens*, pp 111–184. New York: Marcel Dekker.
Hauschild AHW and Dodds KL (1992) Clostridium botulinum: *Ecology and Control in Foods*. New York: Marcel Dekker.
Lewis GE (1981) *Biomedical Aspects of Botulism*. New York: Academic Press.
Simpson LL (1989) *Botulinum Neurotoxin and Tetanus Toxin*. Toronto: Academic Press.
Smith LDS and Sugiyama H (1988) *Botulism: The Organism, its Toxins, the Disease*, 2nd edn. Toronto: Academic Press.

K. L. Dodds
Health and Welfare, Ottawa, Canada

Botulism

Human botulism is currently classified into four categories. Foodborne botulism, the most common form worldwide, is caused by ingestion of food contaminated with preformed botulinum neurotoxin, usually type A, B or E. Wound botulism is very rare and is due to infection of a wound with spores of *Clostridium botulinum* which grow and produce toxin *in situ*. Infant botulism, first recognized in 1976 and now the most

Table 1. Recorded outbreaks of foodborne botulism

Country	Period	No. of outbreaks	No. of cases[a]	Predominant type[b]	Predominant food type[c]
Poland	1984–1987	1301	1791 (3)	B	Meats
China	1958–1983	986	4377 (13)	A	Vegetables
USA[d]	1971–1988	261	574 (11)	A	Vegetables
Italy	1979–1987		310	B	Vegetables
France	1978–1989	175	304 (2)	B	Meats
Japan	1951–1987	97	479 (23)	E	Fish
USSR	1958–1964	95	328 (29)	B	Fish
Iran	1972–1974		314 (11)	E	Fish
Canada	1971–1989	79	202 (14)	E	Meats[e]
Spain	1969–1988	63	198 (6)	B	Vegetables
FRG	1983–1988	63	154 (4)	B	Meats
Alaska	1971–1988	48	117 (6)	E	Fish
GDR	1984–1989	33	52 (8)	B	Meats
Hungary	1985–1989	31	57 (2)	B	Meats
Portugal	1970–1989	24	80 (0)	B	Meats
Norway	1961–1990	19	42 (7)	B, E	Fish
Czechoslovakia	1979–1984	17	20 (0)	B	Meats
Argentina	1980–1989	16	36 (36)	A	Vegetables
Yugoslavia	1984–1989	12	51		Meats
Belgium	1982–1989	11	25 (4)	B	Meats
Denmark[f]	1984–1989	11	16 (12)	E	Meats

[a] Fatality rate shown in parentheses.
[b] Of outbreaks with type identified.
[c] Of outbreaks with the food vehicle identified. Vegetables includes fruits.
[d] Includes Alaskan data.
[e] Mostly traditional Inuit meat dishes.
[f] Greenland data included.

common form of botulism in the USA, is caused by ingestion of viable spores which colonize the intestinal tract of infants under 1 year of age and produce toxin locally. The environment appears to be the most common source of spores. Honey is the only food which has been associated with infant botulism. The fourth category, unclassified, includes cases of unknown origin, and adult cases which resemble infant botulism. This entry will discuss the epidemiology, clinical aspects, and prevention of foodborne botulism, and give a brief overview of the structure and mode of action of the neurotoxin.

Epidemiology

Because of the severity of its symptoms, botulism is more likely to be detected and reported than other, milder forms of food poisoning. Hence, the epidemiological data for botulism are probably more complete than for most other foodborne illnesses. Table 1 shows the data for countries with relatively frequent outbreaks. Unrecognized and misdiagnosed cases of botulism do occur, as shown by a 1985 outbreak in Vancouver, Canada, where the initial diagnoses for 28 patients included psychiatric illness, viral syndrome, laryngeal trauma, overexertion and a variety of other maladies. As well, in large areas of the world, particularly where botulism occurs infrequently, epidemiological data are scarce.

Incidence in North America

In Canada, most botulism outbreaks have occurred in northern native communities. The foods involved were mainly native dishes, and type E was usually implicated. These foods included raw and parboiled meats from sea mammals, fermented meats such as muktuk (meat, blubber and skin of the beluga or white whale), and fermented salmon eggs. Toxin production in raw and parboiled meats can occur because the meats are often held at ambient temperature for some time. The problem with the so-called fermented products is that the level of fermentable carbohydrates is too low to ensure a sufficiently rapid pH reduction to prevent growth of *C. botulinum*. Commercial products have been implicated in three incidents in Canada since 1971: bottled marinated mushrooms imported from the USA; bottled garlic in oil, also imported from the USA but temperature-abused locally; and in-house bottled mushrooms.

In Alaska, the situation is similar to that in northern Canada. All of the Alaskan outbreaks have involved native Alaskans; they involved raw or fermented native foods, and type E was usually implicated.

In the continental USA, the situation is quite different. Most of the implicated foods were home-preserved vegetables. The relative prevalence of type A and type B outbreaks was about equal in the east, but type A outbreaks were much more prevalent in the west, where type A spores predominate in the environment. Commercially processed foods have seldom been involved, but five outbreaks were associated with commercial eating establishments, involving 130 cases from 1977 to 1989. Temperature abuse of either food ingredients or the final product was often the problem.

Incidence in Europe

Poland reported by far the highest number of cases on an annual basis. This probably reflects both a high local incidence of botulism and a very thorough surveillance system. In Poland and several other European countries, including Italy, France, Spain, Germany, Hungary, Portugal, Czechoslovakia and Belgium, the predominant type involved was B. The foods most frequently implicated, except in Italy and Spain, were home-preserved meats, such as ham, fermented sausages or canned products. A significant number of implicated foods were of commercial origin in Poland (25%), GDR (27%) and Belgium (38%). Of the implicated foods in France, 12% were of commercial origin, but the manufacturers were generally small, local establishments. In Italy and Spain, the most commonly implicated foods were home-preserved vegetables, most of which in Italy had been preserved in oil; in Spain, all of the incriminated vegetables had been canned. Scandinavian countries recorded fewer outbreaks, and these were mainly associated with fish and type E. In Greenland as well, type E was usually involved, but the incriminated food was more often meat. Botulism outbreaks have been rare in the UK; however, a major outbreak in 1989 involved 27 cases with one death. Type B toxin had been produced in a hazelnut purée which was then used to flavour a yoghurt produced by a local dairy. Other European countries either reported few or no botulism outbreaks.

Incidence in the USSR

There is no recent summary on botulism outbreaks in the USSR because epidemiological work on botulism there was discontinued. During the period for which information was available, types A, B and E were implicated in approximately equal numbers of outbreaks, with a slight predominance of type B. The type B outbreaks occurred mostly in the western region of the USSR, and usually involved meats, nearly always home-cured ham, very similar to the situation in central Europe. Incidents associated with fish occurred mainly in regions around the Black Sea, the Sea of Azov, the Caspian Sea and Lake Baykal. Surprisingly, type A was involved in as many outbreaks from fish as type E.

Incidence in Asia

Only a few other countries in Asia report outbreaks of foodborne botulism. Israel reported an outbreak in 1987 which affected six people with one fatality. The incriminated food was kapchunka (salted, uneviscerated whitefish) contaminated with type E toxin. It had been bought in New York City and transported to Israel unrefrigerated. Iran reported a high incidence of botulism. Of the 314 cases recorded between 1972 and 1974, 170, comprising 63 outbreaks, were investigated. The majority of outbreaks (97%) were associated with type E and with fish or fish products. However, fleshy portions of fish were responsible for only 10% of the outbreaks; the other 90% were caused by fish eggs. These eggs (ashbal) are salt cured for several months and then eaten without further treatment. China recorded almost 1000 outbreaks from 1958 to 1983. Most were associated with type A, followed by types B and E. The northwestern province of Xinjiang (Sinkiang) recorded the majority of outbreaks (approximately 80%), which were usually type A. Typically, the incriminated food was fermented bean curd. In the northern provinces of Ningxia, Shanxi and Hebei, outbreaks associated wtih type B predominated. The few incidents reported from the northeastern region were all associated with type E. The majority of Japanese outbreaks occurred in northern areas and were associated with type E and fish or fish products. Izushi was the food most often implicated. To prepare izushi, fleshy pieces of fish are soaked in water for a few days, and then packed tightly into a tub with cooked rice, vegetables, salt, vinegar and spices and left to ferment, often for 3 weeks or longer. Izushi is eaten without further cooking. Two outbreaks in Japan were associated with commercial food. A type A outbreak was caused by vacuum-packaged, stuffed lotus rhizome and involved 36 cases with 11 deaths. An outbreak caused by imported bottled caviar with 21 cases and three deaths was due to type B toxin. Taiwan has also reported a few botulism outbreaks, but reports from other Asian countries are rare.

Incidence in Other Areas

Argentina is the only country in the southern hemisphere which reported a substantial number of botulism outbreaks. These occurred mostly in the provinces of Mendoza and Buenos Aires, and at a latitude between 30° and 40° S. Most outbreaks were associated with type A and the implicated foods were usually vegetables. Mexico, Guatemala, Venezuela, Peru, Brazil and Chile have all reported few outbreaks. Chad, Kenya, Madagascar and Rhodesia are the only African countries with reported outbreaks. In Kenya, two outbreaks were caused by native foods; one by sour milk prepared in a gourd, and one by consumption of raw termites. One of the two outbreaks reported from Madagascar was unusual; the numbers involved were high, and type E toxin was associated with a meat product. About 60 people were involved, with 30 deaths, and locally manufactured bologna was the vehicle. Since 1942, Australia has recorded only five outbreaks of foodborne botulism, and none since 1983. One outbreak of type A botulism was recorded in New Zealand, caused by home-bottled fermented mussels and watercress, a traditional Maori dish.

Conclusions Regarding Epidemiology

Most botulism outbreaks have occurred in the northern hemisphere, particularly in countries north of the Tropic of Cancer. Argentina is the only country in the southern hemisphere which has reported a substantial number of outbreaks. Seasonal trends in outbreak frequencies are apparent in some areas. In Canada, Alaska, Poland, the USSR and Iran, most outbreaks occur from May until October, whereas, in China, most outbreaks occur in the winter and early spring. There is a strong association between the prevalent outbreak type and the prevalent environmental type, as well as the implicated food. In colder regions, Canada, Alaska, Greenland, Scandinavia, parts of the USSR, Iran and northern Japan, type E causes most botulism outbreaks and is the prevalent environmental type. The implicated foods are usually fish or marine mammals. In central Europe, type B causes most outbreaks and is the prevalent environmental type. Meats, particularly home-cured smoked ham, are the major cause of botulism. In the western USA, Argentina and China, type A causes the majority of outbreaks and is the prevalent environmental isolate. In these areas, the most frequently implicated foods are vegetables.

Clinical Aspects

Symptoms

The disease may vary from a mild illness which may be overlooked or misdiagnosed, to a serious disease which may be fatal within 24 h. The onset of symptoms typically occurs 12–36 h after ingestion of toxin, with a range from a few hours to 14 days. In general, the earlier symptoms appear, the more serious the disease. The first symptoms are generally nausea and vomiting. Mainly neurological signs and symptoms appear next, including visual impairments (blurred or double vision, ptosis, fixed and dilated pupils), loss of normal mouth and throat functions (difficulty in speaking and swallowing, dry mouth, throat and tongue, sore throat), general fatigue and lack of muscle coordination, and respiratory impairment. Other gastrointestinal symptoms include abdominal pain, diarrhoea and constipation. Diarrhoea occurs relatively early in the course of the disease, whereas constipation persists in the advanced stages. Nausea and vomiting appear more often in cases associated with type B and E than with type A. Dysphagia and muscle weakness are more common in outbreaks of types A and B than of type E. Dry mouth, tongue and throat are observed most frequently in type B cases. Respiratory failure and airway obstruction are the main causes of death. Fatality rates in the first half of the century were about 50% or higher, but with the availability today of antisera and modern respiratory support systems, they have decreased to about 10%.

Treatment

Initially, treatment of botulism is directed towards removing or inactivating the toxin by (1) neutralizing circulating toxin with antiserum, (2) enema or treatment with cathartics to remove residual toxin from the bowel and (3), in the absence of vomiting, gastric lavage or treatment with emetics. Treatment with antiserum is most effective in the early stages of the illness. The impact of antiserum is obvious from the Chinese data; prior to the availability of antisera in 1960, the death rate in China was approximately 50%, but it was only 8% in the nearly 4000 patients who received antitoxin. Subsequent treatment is mainly to counteract the paralysis of the respiratory muscles by artificial ventilation.

Diagnosis

The initial diagnosis of foodborne botulism is based on the patient's signs and symptoms, and perhaps food history. It must be confirmed by detecting toxin or viable *C. botulinum* in a suspect food or clinical sample, or by epidemiological association with a laboratory-confirmed case. Serum, faeces, enema fluid, stomach contents, and autopsy sections of the small and large intestines, and of the liver, are suitable specimens for toxin detection. Except for serum, these specimens are also suitable for detecting viable *C. botulinum*. The methods for detecting the toxin and *C. botulinum* are given in the previous article. Other than neutralizing any acidic samples, little special treatment is required. Occasionally, extracts prepared from faeces cannot be filter sterilized. In that case, tetracycline should be added to 200 ppm to control infections.

Case History

One of the most severe, nonfatal cases of botulism was documented in a patient in the UK. Within approximately 10 h of eating the suspect food, he had blurred and double vision followed by nausea and vomiting, difficulty in swallowing and talking, dryness of the mouth, and arm weakness. He suffered a respiratory arrest on arrival at the hospital and was intubated. A progressive flaccid paralysis ensued. He was given polyvalent antitoxin, a tracheostomy was done and total parenteral nutrition (TPN) was started. There was little change in his condition for 100 days. His ptosis did not resolve until 46 days after onset of symptoms. TPN was stopped on day 158, and respiratory support was withdrawn after 173 days. He was not discharged until after 237 days.

Prevention

In most cases, the preservation of high-moisture foods is geared towards control of *C. botulinum*, which usually involves inhibition rather than destruction. Such control generally also ensures control of other foodborne pathogens and of many spoilage microorganisms. The effects of different factors on the growth of *C. botulinum* in foods are described in the previous entry. Control of *C. botulinum* in foods is generally achieved by one of the following methods:

(1) low-acid shelf-stable canned foods are preserved by a full thermoprocess *See* Canning, Principles;
(2) shelf-stable canned cured meats are preserved by a combination of thermoprocessing and addition of salt and nitrite *See* Curing;
(3) canned acid foods are preserved by a pasteurizing thermoprocess and acidity;
(4) products such as dry fermented sausages are preserved by reduced water activity (a_w) and pH, and added nitrite *See* Water Activity, Principles and Measurement;
(5) packaged raw or cooked meats or fish and shellfish are preserved by refrigeration alone;
(6) many meat and fish products are preserved by a combination of added salt and refrigeration;
(7) a number of cured meat products are preserved by a combination of added salt and nitrite, and refrigeration;
(8) vacuum-packaged smoked fish are preserved by a combination of thermoprocessing, added salt, smoking and refrigeration *See* Smoked Foods, Principles;
(9) a few perishable products such as processed cheese, caviar, pickled fish and acidified meats are preserved by decreased a_w and pH, and refrigeration.

An effective botulinal toxoid is available from the US Centers for Disease Control for immunization. Immunization of high-risk populations, such as Alaskan and Canadian Inuits, has been repeatedly proposed, but never implemented. At present, only laboratory workers at risk are immunized.

Neurotoxin

As previously stated, seven serologically different neurotoxins are produced by various strains of *C. botulinum*. In general, the designation of the strain is that of the toxin it produces. Strains of subtypes AB, AF, BA and BF are rare and produce, in addition to the first toxin type, lesser amounts of toxin of the second type. Type C and D strains often produce small amounts of D and C toxin, respectively. They may also produce a toxin, C_2, which is distinctly different from the neurotoxin and will not be discussed here.

Structure

The neurotoxins are all very similar proteins with a molecular weight of approximately 150 kDa. They are synthesized as a single-chain protein with relatively low toxicity, which is activated when it is 'nicked' by a number of proteases, including proteases of group I *C. botulinum*, into a double-chain molecule which is held together by a disulphide bond. The two components of the nicked toxin, a light (L) and heavy (H) chain, have molecular weights of approximately 50 and 100 kDa, respectively. Individually, the two components are not toxic, but toxicity can be restored by reestablishing the disulphide bond.

The neurotoxins exist as complexes of four molecular sizes: 7S, 12S, 16S and 19S, designated S (small), M (medium), L (large) and LL (extra large) toxins, respectively. The molecular weights range from 150 to 900 kDa. The M form is the most common natural form, found in foods and cultures, along with the L form. It is a complex of the S form with an atoxic component. In the L form, a haemagglutinin is also part of the complex. The LL form is only known for type A, and was the first form of the botulinum toxin to be purified and crystallized. It has not been found in cultures and is probably an artificial aggregate. The M and L forms are referred to as progenitor toxins. They dissociate under mild alkaline conditions into the S, or derivative, toxin, which is the single-chain protein.

Mode of Action

The neurotoxins cause paralysis by blocking transmitter release at neuromuscular junctions. Cholinergic systems are affected the most, but adrenergic systems may also be affected by high concentrations of toxin. Paralysis appears to be caused by a three-step process. First, the toxin binds to a type-specific receptor on the presynaptic membrane. This step is mediated by the carboxy terminus of the H chain. Secondly, the toxin or a portion of it is internalized into the nerve cell by an initial receptor-mediated endocytosis, followed by pH-dependent membrane penetration. The amino terminus of the H chain is believed to create channels in the membrane which permit the L chain to enter. After this step, the toxin can no longer be neutralized. Finally, the internalized portion of the toxin acts to prevent acetylcholine release, the actual poisoning step, which is probably enzymatic in nature.

Inactivation

The most effective means of inactivating botulinum toxins in foods is by heat. Heat inactivation curves are biphasic, with an initial steep decline that levels off with time. Foods, especially those high in protein, colloidal components or ionic strength, have a protective effect. The toxin is most stable between pH 4 and 5. For the safe thermal inactivation of toxin at concentrations up to 10^5 LD_{50} per gram, time/temperature combinations of 20 min at 79°C or 5 min at 85°C have been recommended. Other means of toxin inactivation include treatment with chlorine or ozone. *See* Heat Treatment, Chemical and Microbiological Changes

Bibliography

Hauschild AHW (1989) *Clostridium botulinum.* In: Doyle MP (ed.) *Foodborne Bacterial Pathogens*, pp 111–184. New York: Marcel Dekker.
Hauschild AHW and Dodds KL (1992) Clostridium botulinum: *Ecology and Control in Foods.* New York: Marcel Dekker.
Lewis GE (1981) *Biomedical Aspects of Botulism.* New York: Academic Press.
Simpson LL (1989) *Botulinum Neurotoxin and Tetanus Toxin.* Toronto: Academic Press.
Smith LDS and Sugiyama H (1988) *Botulism: The Organism, its Toxins, the Disease*, 2nd edn. Toronto: Academic Press.

K. L. Dodds
Health and Welfare, Ottawa, Canada

COBALAMINS

Contents

Properties and Determination

Vitamin B_{12} (cyanocobalamin), the most recent vitamin discovered, is the most potent of the vitamins. It is best known for its association with Addisonian pernicious anaemia. The history of vitamin B_{12} development involves widely divergent investigations into the human deficiency diseases, animal nutrition, and metabolism of microorganisms.

Two crystalline 'vitamin B_{12}' preparations were isolated from cultures of *Streptomyces aureofaciens*. The first of these had an absorption spectrum similar to that reported for vitamin B_{12}; the second had a different spectrum and was termed vitamin B_{12b}. Unlike vitamin B_{12}, vitamin B_{12b} did not contain cyanide and was named hydroxocobalamin. Hydroxocobalamin was indistinguishable from cyanocobalamin in biological activity, including effectiveness against pernicious anaemia. The cyanide in cyanocobalamin apparently originated from charcoal used in the preparation process.

The isolation of the coenzyme forms of vitamin B_{12} led to the further recognition that cyanocobalamin is not the naturally occurring form of the vitamin but is, rather, an artefact that arises from the original isolation procedure. The two *coenzyme* forms of cobalamin found in animals are adenosylcobalamin and methylcobalamin. Humans and other animals contain three main cobalamins: hydroxocobalamin, adenosylcobalamin and methylcobalamin. Cyanocobalamin, however is the most widely used form of cobalamin in clinical practice because of its relatively greater availability and stability.

Most of the metabolic studies utilized cyanocobalamin. *See* Coenzymes

Structure

Soon after cyanocobalamin was crystallized, structural studies were initiated by classic degradation experiments and by X ray crystallography. Considerable knowledge was obtained by degradation studies, but the molecular structures of cyanocobalamin and its coenzyme forms were not definitely established until the brilliant work of Hodgkin and her colleagues using X ray crystallography.

Cyanocobalamin consists of a fundamental portion containing four pyrrole nuclei joined in a large ring containing six conjugated double bonds, a structure very similar to that of the iron porphyrins. One of the four pyrrole nuclei is completely saturated. The cyano group is attached to the cobalt atom, which in turn is linked coordinately to a nitrogen of the 5,6-dimethylbenzimidazole group. As with nucleic acids, vitamin B_{12} contains a nucleotide. However, the base consists of 5,6-dimethylbenzimidazole rather than the various purine or pyrimidine bases of the nucleic acids, and the sugar, ribose, has an α-glycosidic linkage, unlike the β linkage in the nucleic acids. The D-1-amino-2-propanol moiety of one molecule is esterified to the nucleotide and joined in amide linkage to the porphyrinlike nucleus. The structure of cyanocobalamin, based on the work of Hodgkin is shown in Fig. 1.

Physical Properties

Cyanocobalamin forms red, needlelike, hygroscopic crystals. Its empirical formula is $C_{63}H_{88}N_{14}O_{14}PCo$, and its molecular weight is 1355.

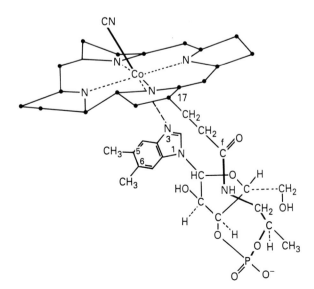

Fig. 1 Sketch of the structure of vitamin B_{12} (cyanocobalamin). Based on the work of Hodgkin.

Properties and Determination

Cyanocobalamin is a neutral, odourless, tasteless compound that is soluble in water (1·2% at 25°C). It is also soluble in alcohol and phenol but is insoluble in acetone, chloroform and ether. Advantage is taken of its insolubility in acetone for crystallization from water–acetone solutions.

The red crystals of cyanocobalamin darken at 210–220°C and melt above 300°C. It is laevorotatory and, although difficult to measure accurately because of its colour, its reported optical activity at 656 nm is −59° and at 643 nm, −100°.

The absorption spectrum of cyanocobalamin shows three characteristic maxima that are relatively independent of pH. The extinction coefficients ($\varepsilon_{1\,cm}^{M}$) are: $\varepsilon_{278} = 16·3 \times 10^3$; $\varepsilon_{361} = 28·1 \times 10^3$; and $\varepsilon_{550} = 8·7 \times 10^3$.

Chemical Properties

The chemical reactions and properties of cyanocobalamin are numerous and detailed, and some good reviews on this subject have been presented (see Bibliography). Some of the most important properties are given below.

The cyanide group of cyanocobalamin can be replaced by other ions to form hydroxocobalamin, chlorocobalamin, nitrocobalamin, thiocyanatocobalamin and others. All the above-mentioned cobalamins are readily converted to cyanocobalamin after treatment with cyanide. A purple compound formed on addition of excess cyanide to alkaline solutions of cyanocobalamin is called dicyanocobalamin. This compound, which contains two cyanide molecules coordinated to the cobalt atom, is quite unstable. Cyanocobalamin is slowly decomposed by ultraviolet or strong visible light. The cyano group is split off, yielding hydroxocobalamin. Prolonged exposure to light causes irreversible decomposition and inactivation.

Mild acid hydrolysis of cyanocobalamin induces the removal of the nucleotide, whereas more vigorous acid hydrolysis liberates ammonia, 5,6-dimethylbenzimidazole, D-amino-2-propanol and cobyrinic acid. Hydrolysis with dilute acids splits the amide group off the sidechains, resulting in mono- and polycarboxylic acids.

Stability

Cyanocobalamin is stable in air and, in dry form, is relatively stable at 100°C for a few hours. Aqueous solutions at pH 4–7 can be autoclaved at 120°C. Cyanocobalamin appears to be the most stable of the various analogues studied to date. Crystalline cyanocobalamin is compatible with a wide variety of therapeutic and nutritional substances. In solution, thiamin and nicotinamide, or nicotinic acid, destroy cyanocobalamin slowly, whereas the addition of small amounts of iron or thiocyanate appear to protect it.

Table 1. Dietary sources of cobalamins

High (50–500 μg per 100 g)	Medium (5–50 μg per 100 g)	Low (0·2–5 μg per 100 g)
Kidney	Kidney	Fish
Lamb	Rabbit	Cod
	Beef	Flounder
		Haddock
Liver	Liver	Sole
Lamb	Rabbit	Halibut
Beef	Chicken	Lobster
Calf		Scallop
Pork	Heart	Shrimp
	Beef	Swordfish
Brain	Rabbit	Tuna
Beef	Chicken	
	Egg yolk	Beef
	Clams	Lamb
	Oysters	Pork
	Crabs	Chicken
	Sardines	Egg (whole)
	Salmon	Cheese
		American
		Swiss
		Milk (cow)

Sources of Cobalamins

Until 1962, the occurrence in nature of cobalamin was considered to be limited to bacteria and animal tissues. In 1962, it was reported that peas, cultivated under aseptic conditions, produced corrin that supported the growth of the B_{12}-requiring organisms, *E. coli* (strain 113–3), *E. gracilis* and *Goniotrichum elegans*. In 1964 low amounts of cobalamins were detected in several plants. In 1967, slices of potato tubers were shown to catabolize labelled proprionate in a manner consistent with the participation of the coenzyme B_{12}-dependent enzyme methylmalonyl-CoA mutase. Vitamin B_{12} was detected by microbiological assay in bean plants in 1969. The presence of coenzyme B_{12}-dependent leucine 2,3-aminomutase in beans, ryegrass and potato tubers was also shown. Excellent sources of cobalamins are animal organ meats, especially the liver, kidney and heart. Table 1 gives the dietary sources of cobalamin. Cobalamins originate from the ingestion of vitamin-containing tissues of animals and from an animal's own digestive tract. Herbivorous animals obtain all their cobalamins from that produced by the intestinal flora, and by coprophagy. In carnivorous animals and humans, intestinal synthesis of cobalamins is not sufficient, and dietary cobalamins are required. *See* individual foods

Methods of Determination

Clinical

Before cyanocobalamin was first isolated and crystallized, the antipernicious anaemia factor (APA), as it was then called, was assayed with difficulty and with only semiquantitative precision in human subjects with pernicious anaemia. Potency of APA was determined by the magnitude of the increase in red blood cell count, haemoglobin, and the rise in reticulocyte percentage.

Doses of crystalline cyanocobalamin are now expressed in terms of weight. The unit of weight generally used is the microgram because of the very low levels needed in clinical use. Human serum levels of cobalamins are measured in picograms per millilitre ($1 \text{ pg ml}^{-1} = 10^{-12} \text{ g ml}^{-1}$). The normal values range from 200 to 900 pg ml^{-1}, and values below 100 pg ml^{-1} are diagnostic of cobalamin deficiency.

Chemical

Spectrophotometric

This rapid and accurate method for the assay of cyanocobalamin depends upon the absorption of cyanocobalamin at 361 nm. As little as 25 μg ml^{-1} can be determined. Many of the cobalamin analogues have absorption maxima at 361 nm also, and therefore the usefulness of the assay is limited for the most part to pure samples of cobalamin. *See* Spectroscopy, Overview

Vitamin B_{12}

Colorimetric

A sensitive assay method for cyanocobalamin is based on the cyanide content. Cyanide is liberated by reduction or by photolysis and is measured by a sensitive colorimetric procedure. Of course, this technique does not differentiate cyanocobalamin from other analogues containing cyanide. An alternate method has been proposed based on the difference in the spectrum of cyanocobalamin and its purple dicyanide complex.

Other colorimetric methods are based on the presence of 5,6-dimethylbenzimidazole and on the hydrolysis products resulting from treatment of cyanocobalamin with strong hydrochloric acid. *See* Spectroscopy, Visible Spectroscopy and Colorimetry

Microbiological

Microbiological assays for cyanocobalamin are sensitive and can be applied to crude materials. They have been widely used, principally for determining the vitamin content in a large number of blood and other tissue samples. However, there is a problem of specificity, since cobalamin analogues give varying responses in microorganisms.

Lactobacillus spp.

The first microbiological assay for cyanocobalamin utilized *L. lactis*. This assay was very difficult to carry out, and a more stable organism, *L. leichmannii* 313 (American Type Culture Collection (ATCC) 7830) was found to respond well. Another strain of this organism (ATCC 4797) has also been used. In the approved technique of the US Pharmacopoeia, ATCC 7830 is used.

Lactobacilli respond to various cobalamin analogues, as well as to thymidine and other deoxyribonucleosides. For many problems, particularly serum analyses, response to deoxyribonucleosides is not serious, since *L. leichmannii* requires about 1000 times more deoxyribonucleosides than cyanocobalamin for growth.

Escherichia coli

Several assays based on the use of this organism (strain 113-3) have been used successful. This organism is slightly less sensitive than *L. leichmannii* and responds to many analogues, but it does not respond to deoxyribonucleosides. Methionine at comparatively much higher levels will substitute for cobalamins.

Euglena gracilis

Of all the organisms tested, *E. gracilis* appears to offer the greatest sensitivity in assaying for cyanocobalamin. The conditions of this assay have been improved and further developed by Hutner and associates. The disadvantage of this organism is that it grows slowly, requiring about 5 days for optimal growth.

Microbiological assays are painstaking procedures that require sterile technique and several days to perform and cannot be used if patients are taking drugs such as antibiotics that interfere with the growth of the organism.

Ochromonas malhamensis

Ochromonas malhamensis, a chrysomonad, was discovered by Hutner *et al.*; the assay method was subsequently developed. The response of this organism to cobalamin analogues, which is one of the most specific, parallels the discrimination shown by humans toward cobalamins. This organism is also a slow grower.

Biological

Cyanocobalamin assays involving higher animals are somewhat more difficult and time-consuming than microbiological assays. The large stores of cobalamins found in young, growing animals reared from normal mothers present the biggest problem. Some of these objections have been overcome by including stress factors to intensify depletion or by feeding diets that increase the requirements for cobalamin. The chick assay has been the most widely used of the biological assays.

Isotope Dilution

Radioisotope Dilution

The development of radiodilution assays, particularly for the measurement of serum cobalamin levels, has met the need for a rapid and simple method and has made the determination of blood levels in humans more generally available. Radiodilution assays of blood involve extraction of bound cobalamin from a sample of serum, the conversion of the cobalamin to cyanocobalamin, and, after mixing with a known quantity of radioactive cyanocobalamin, association with a cobalamin ligand with high affinity for the vitamin. Dilution of the radioactive cyanocobalamin by endogenous cobalamin allows calculation of the concentration of the vitamin extracted from the serum.

The specificity of the cobalamin ligand (binding protein) is crucial to the accuracy of the assay. The ligand, or binder, is usually intrinsic factor. It is important to use purified intrinsic factor as the binder when performing radiodilution assay for serum cobalamin, since human plasma contains cobalamin analogues that may mask cobalamin deficiency. These biologically inactive analogues are present in serum in sufficient concentrations to interfere substantially with a radiodilution assay for cobalamin when nonpurified intrinsic factor is used as the binding protein. The less purified preparations of intrinsic factor contain, in addition to intrinsic factor, proteins that can bind the inactive cobalmin analogues. In the absence of pure intrinsic factor, nonradioactive cobinamide (a vitamin B_{12} analogue) can be added to saturate the non-intrinsic-factor proteins prior to addition of cobalamin.

The isotope dilution methods for the assay of cobalamins have been replacing the microbiological methods in the past few years, and at present they are more widely used than most other methods.

Over 90% of cobalamin assays are performed by radiodilution. As a result of earlier reports of unreliable results, the US National Committee for Clinical Laboratory Standards (NCCLS) published a standard, which was ratified by the US Food and Drug Administration earlier in 1980, recommending that all radiodilution kits for cobalamin should contain purified intrinsic factor as the cobalamin-binding protein.

Bibliography

Lenhert PG and Hodgkin DC (1961) *Nature (London)* 102: 937.

Ellenbogen L and Cooper BA (1991) Vitamin B_{12}. In Machlin LJ (ed.) *Handbook of Vitamins*, 2nd edn. New York: Marcel Dekker.

Folkers K (1957) In: Heinrich HC (ed.) *Vitamin B_{12} und Intrinsic Factor 1, Europaiches Symposium, Hamburg, 1956* Stuttgart: Enke.

Smith EL (1965) *Vitamin B_{12}.* London: Methuen.

Zagalak B and Friedrich W (eds) (1979) *Vitamin B_{12}.* Berlin: Walter de Gruyter.

Acknowledgements

This article contains material extracted from a chapter on Vitamin B_{12} written by the authors in *Handbook of Vitamins*, edited by LJ Machlin, and published by Marcel Dekker in 1991, by kind permission of the publishers.

Leon Ellenbogen
American Cyanamid Company, Lederle Laboratories, New York, USA
Bernard A. Cooper
McGill University, Royal Victoria Hospital, Montreal, Canada

Physiology

The importance of vitamin B_{12} in human nutrition has been dominated by the potentially fatal disease, pernicious anaemia, which results from a failure of secretion of the specific cobalamin-binding protein, intrinsic factor, by the parietal cells of the stomach. This protein is essential for the subsequent recognition, binding and transport of vitamin B_{12} at the ileal wall. Transcobalamin II then carries it to the portal circulation. The treatment of the disease with massive amounts of dietary liver, followed by the isolation, characterization, and X-ray crystallographic structure determination of vitamin B_{12}, are classical and major achievements of the first half of this century. During the past few years, new evidence has been accumulating to suggest that more subtle, insidious and easily overlooked forms of vitamin B_{12} deficiency may occur in modern-day western society, and that the challenges of their determination and treatment are by no means entirely solved. The fact that prolonged vitamin B_{12} depletion can lead to irreversible neural damage, coupled with the prediction that defects of absorption can arise slowly and remain entirely unnoticed as people grow older may, if correct, be of special relevance at a time when the quality of life in old age is becoming a major priority issue. *See* Anaemia, Megaloblastic Anaemias

Dietary intake by omnivores is much greater than by vegetarians or vegans (who depend to a large extent on 'contamination' sources, unless they deliberately take B_{12} supplements). There is controversy at present over B_{12}-like corrinoids in certain seaweeds and their possible usefulness in vegetarian and macrobiotic diets that lack B_{12}. Some authorities believe these to be useful sources; others consider most of them to be biologically inactive. *In vitro*, vitamin B_{12} may be destroyed by contact with vitamin C (ascorbic acid), but *in vivo* this probably does not occur, which suggests that the catalysis of destruction may depend on free transition metal ions, not present in living tissues. *See* Macrobiotic Diets; Vegan Diets; Vegetarian Diets

Although B_{12} intakes are much lower in Third World countries than in western countries, overt dietary deficiency is surprisingly rare in the Third World except in relatively strict vegetarians. Nevertheless, fully breast-fed infants of mothers with very low intakes, or of mothers with vitamin-B_{12} malabsorption syndromes (usually pernicious anaemia), may develop overt B_{12} deficiency. Older omnivores usually accumulate considerable amounts in their tissues, and in these subjects the effects of a switch to diets with low contents or the onset of impaired absorption only become apparent long after the B_{12} supply to the internal milieu has virtually ceased.

There are still some problems with the assay of vitamin B_{12} levels in food, and 5–30% of the reported B_{12} content may be biologically inactive corrinoids. Small amounts of B_{12} arising from bacteria in the ileum can be absorbed, but B_{12} produced by bacteria in the colon is not. An efficient enterohepatic circulation of B_{12} occurs in normal people, and if this cycle is interrupted, as it is in cases of impaired intestinal absorption, this results in an additional source of losses for subjects with impaired B_{12} absorption. *See* Microflora of the Intestine, Role and Effects

Large-scale industrial production of vitamin B_{12} makes use of the capacity of organisms such as *Propionibacterium* spp. to synthesize as much as 40 mg B_{12} per litre of growth medium. World consumption was around 5000 kg in the early 1980s.

Absorption and Tests of Status

The key stages in vitamin B_{12} utilization from food sources are: (1) enzymatic release of B_{12} from protein in food, with transfer to both intrinsic factor and gastric juice 'R' binders; (2) transfer of the B_{12} on non-specific 'R' binders to intrinsic factor secreted in the stomach, after their digestion by pancreatic enzymes; (3) interaction of specific B_{12}–intrinsic factor complex in the presence of calcium ions; and (4) transfer of the B_{12} to transcobalamin II binder in the enterocyte and then from the enterocyte to the plasma, whence it is carried to the tissues and taken up by endocytosis into the cells.

In addition to classical pernicious anaemia (lack of secretion of intrinsic factor due to atrophy of gastric mucosa), there are several other medical conditions that can result in impaired absorption, as well as a variety of congenital abnormalities of transport of the vitamin, which require both specialized detection procedures and specialized therapeutic measures. These include (1) surgical procedures such as total gastrectomy, removal of ileum or blind loops of the small gut producing an abnormal bacterial flora there, (2) the effects of certain parasites, drugs or substances like nitrous oxide, (3) the Imerslund-Grasbeck syndrome which appears to result from lack of ileal receptors, and (4) lack of circulating transcobalamin II. The classical procedure for the recognition of impaired absorption, specially designed to detect pernicious anaemia, is the urinary excretion (Schilling) test. Around 57% of people with pernicious anaemia also have circulating antibodies to intrinsic factor in their blood, and their detection can provide further corroborative evidence of the presence of pernicious anaemia. In conjunction with a macrocytic anaemia and a standard assay of circulating plasma vitamin B_{12}, the measurement of these antibodies can be a useful screening procedure to be performed before the more complex Schilling test is undertaken.

Serum vitamin B_{12} levels are usually measured nowadays by radioisotope dilution assay, preferably using intrinsic factor as the specific binder. Normal levels are above $200\ \mathrm{pg\ ml^{-1}}$, and levels below $100\ \mathrm{pg\ ml^{-1}}$ are strongly indicative of deficiency. Until recently, there have been serious difficulties in obtaining comparable results by microbiological and by the newer radioisotope dilution assays, and caution is urged in comparing values obtained in different laboratories, especially if they are using different assay procedures. Many commercial kits are now available for the radioisotope dilution assay. *See* Immunoassays, Radioimmunoassay and Enzyme Immunoassay

Another diagnostic test is the deoxyuridine suppression test, usually performed *in vitro* on bone marrow aspirates. This looks directly at the cells' ability to synthesize thymidine from deoxyuridine. For B_{12}-deficient cells, B_{12} cofactor is the only addition which will partially overcome the block in conversion, whereas formyl tetrahydrofolate will reverse it in both folate- and B_{12}-deficient cells. This test has the potential advantage of being a functional test and of probing a specific tissue site, but a disadvantage is the complexity of performance. *See* Coenzymes

Another functional test involves the metabolism of an oral load of valine: if B_{12} deficiency is present, then methylmalonic acid accumulates, and large amounts of this by-product are excreted. Some recent studies have demonstrated that raised plasma levels of methylmalonic acid can arise in subjects with marginal vitamin B_{12} status, even without the loading dose, so that it may become a useful screening procedure. Detection methods are, however, rather complex and expensive. Circulating levels of homocysteine can provide further evidence, but both folate and vitamin B_6 status can also affect homocysteine economy, so the evidence in this case is somewhat less specific.

Biological Functions of Vitamin B_{12}

The most important biochemical reaction catalysed by vitamin B_{12} in man and animals is the conversion of homocysteine to methionine. However, the most obvious result of deficiency *in vivo* is a block in DNA synthesis, leading characteristically to megaloblastosis, and macrocytic anaemia, which is indistinguishable, at least at the cytological level, from the megaloblastosis and anaemia of folate deficiency. A good test for response of a probable case of pernicious anaemia, or other B_{12}-deficiency syndrome, is an increase in circulating reticulocyte numbers following treatment. *See* Amino Acids, Metabolism; Anaemia, Megaloblastic Anaemias

One popular explanation for the connection between B_{12} deficiency and the failure of cell division leading to anaemia is the 'methylfolate trap hypothesis', in which methylene tetrahydrofolate polyglutamate, the intracellular cofactor for thymidine synthesis, becomes depleted by excessive conversion (i.e. reduction) to methyltetrahydrofolate polyglutamate. The latter is unable to transfer its carbon unit (methyl group) to homocysteine and thus complete the folate cycle back to the methylene form, because of the absence of B_{12} cofactor (methylcobalamin). At the same time, short-chain methylfolate glutamates from the diet are poorly utilized and therefore excreted, so that intracellular folate levels decline. *See* Folic Acid, Physiology

An alternative interpretation, the 'formate starvation hypothesis', maintains that because B_{12} deficiency causes a reduction in methionine levels, an important consequence of its deficiency is a reduced conversion of methionine to active formate. Active formate in turn is needed for synthesis of intracellular formyltetrahydrofolate, which is a good precursor of folate polyglutamates and hence of active methylene groups for thymidine synthesis. In the absence of vitamin B_{12}, formate accumulates in blood, liver and brain, and there is increased formate excretion in the urine. In support of this hypothesis, formylfolate, but not tetrahydrofolate, can correct the functional evidence of B_{12} deficiency, and the organism is still able to oxidize the methyl group of methylfolate to methylene- and formyl-folates. Clearly there is a need for further studies of these pathways and control mechanisms. One very useful tool has been the use of nitrous oxide, which can chemically inactivate vitamin B_{12} in vivo, e.g. in experimental animals. This procedure has permitted the rapid induction of tissue B_{12} deficiency, without the tedious and protracted use of B_{12}-deficient diets.

The second important functional result of vitamin B_{12} deficiency is the failure of maintenance of nerve tissue myelin, which accounts for the irreversible neurological damage seen after prolonged B_{12} deficiency. This lesion may also be connected biochemically with the block in methionine formation (and hence in phospholipid metabolism), but its aetiology has not yet been fully elucidated. There may also be other disturbances in lipid metabolism in B_{12}-deficient subjects.

Human Vitamin B_{12} Requirements

In the absence of the metabolic abnormalities that can affect B_{12} absorption and utilization, human dietary requirements for the vitamin are small. A purely nutritional deficiency may, however, occur in lifelong vegetarians such as strict Hindus who have very low intakes because they do not eat animal products. Studies of the amount of B_{12} needed to cure this, together with studies of populations with low intakes who, nevertheless, do not show deficiency signs, have indicated that the requirement is generally less than 1 μg per day for adults, and is probably in the range 0.1–1 μg per day. There is little firm evidence for a major increase in requirement during pregnancy and lactation, but modest increments in the RDAs (Recommended Dietary Allowances) are usually applied to these physiological states. The amount secreted in breast milk ranges from 0.1 to 3 μg per day. At least 12 examples of infants have been observed with B_{12}-responsive megaloblastic anaemia, who were breast-fed by mothers who were themselves deficient and were secreting milk with a very low content of the vitamin. *See* Lactation

Elderly people generally have similar requirements to younger adults, but efficient screening for incipient pernicious anaemia or other malabsorption syndromes in elderly people is clearly an important public health service, which needs to be supported and encouraged. Likewise, the early recognition of B_{12} deficiency in certain immigrant vegetarian groups, especially Asians, merits attention, at least in the UK.

Typical B_{12} intakes by omnivorous people in Western countries are 3–30 μg per day.

Food table values of B_{12} contents of foods have been obtained mainly by microbiological assays and some verification is needed of values obtained using organisms which have been insufficiently specific in their requirements. Vitamin B_{12} is stored mainly in the liver (60%) and muscles (30%). Methylcobalamin is the most abundant form in human plasma, whereas in most human tissues, deoxyadenosyl cobalamin is the most abundant, with aquacobalamin coming second.

At high intakes, there is little evidence of toxicity, and injections of as much as 3 mg per day have been used in an attempt to treat fatigue and neurological disorders. However, there is no evidence that such high doses can have any benefit for normal subjects and they may occasionally result in allergic reactions. Degradation of B_{12} to B_{12} antagonists in multinutrient preparations has been claimed.

The RDAs from the WHO (World Health Organization) currently stand at 1 μg per day for adults, except in pregnancy (1.4 μg) and lactation (1.3 μg), and at 0.1 μg per day for infants. A typical treatment schedule for pernicious anaemia would be 500 μg by injections every two to three months. It was suggested by the WHO working group that there is still a need for better methods to measure cobalamins in food and in biological materials, to investigate human requirements and to develop new procedures for the early detection of functional deficiency states.

Bibliography

Chanarin I (1987) Megaloblastic anaemia, cobalamin and folate. *Journal of Clinical Pathology* 40: 978–984.

Chanarin I (1990) *The Megaloblastic Anaemias*, 3rd edn. Oxford: Blackwell.

Doyle JJ, Langerin AM and Zipursky A (1989) Nutritional vitamin B_{12} deficiency in infancy: three case reports and a review of the literature. *Pediatric Hematology and Oncology* 6: 161–172.

Food and Agriculture Organization of the United Nations (1988) Requirements of vitamin A, iron, folate and vitamin B_{12}. *Report of a Joint FAO/WHO Expert Consultation*. Geneva: Food and Agriculture Organization.

Friedrich W (1988) Vitamin B_{12}. In: *Vitamins*, chap 13, pp. 837–928. Berlin: Walter de Gruyter.

Herbert V (1987) Recommended dietary intakes (RDI) of vitamin B_{12} in humans. *American Journal of Clinical Nutrition* 45: 671–678.

Woodson RD (ed) (1990) New frontiers in vitamin B_{12} metabolism. *American Journal of Hematology* 34: 81–139.

Zittoun J and Cooper BA (eds) (1989) *Folates and cobalamins*. Berlin: Springer-Verlag.

C. J. Bates
MRC Dunn Nutrition Unit, Cambridge, UK

COBALT

Cobalt was first isolated by a Swedish chemist, Brandt, in 1735 and more fully characterized by Bergman in 1780. It had, however, been used as its ores for millenia to give a bright blue colour to Egyptian pottery and Iranian glass from 2600 and 2250 BC, respectively. The name is derived from the German word *kobold*, meaning an evil spirit or gnome, as copper miners working in the Harz mountains believed that these spirits delighted in exposing ores that looked like copper, but which yielded none when smelted.

Cobalt is widely distributed in the earth's crust but only 30th in order of abundance and thus less common at 25 mg kg^{-1} than all other elements in the first transition series with the exception of scandium (22 mg kg^{-1}). There appears to be some overall loss of cobalt during soil formation as the world mean value is quoted as 12 mg kg^{-1} and Scottish soils at 8 mg kg^{-1}.

The metal itself is silvery in appearance with a bluish tinge and considerably harder than iron. It has only one naturally occurring isotope, ^{59}Co, but this can be converted to radioactive ^{60}Co by bombardment with thermal neutrons. This has a half-life of 5·271 years and decays to nonradioactive ^{60}Ni. The radioactive isotope ^{60}Co is used medically in cancer therapy and also as a concentrated source of radiation for research purposes. ^{57}Co is used in the assay of vitamin B_{12} by radioisotope dilution. Like iron, cobalt is a ferromagnetic element, but is considerably less chemically reactive. It is stable to oxygen and the range of oxidation states is considerably fewer than for earlier members of the first transition series. The commonest are +2 and +3 but, as the latter is a strong oxidizing agent, it decomposes rapidly in aqueous solution with the production of oxygen. As a result only a few Co^{3+} salts exist and these tend to be unstable. On the other hand, Co^{3+} forms a large number of coordination complexes, particularly with nitrogen donor ligands, and this is important in its biological role as a structural component of vitamin B_{12}. This structure is characterized by a 'corrin' ring where the cobalt is coordinated to four coplanar nitrogen atoms with another (imidazole) nitrogen in the fifth position. The sixth position, however, makes vitamin B_{12} unique as here the cobalt is bonded to carbon, making it to date the only naturally occurring organometallic vitamin. *See* Vitamins, Determination

The incorporation of cobalt into the corrin ring affects its reduction potential and gives it the three consecutive oxidation states shown in eqn [1]. The reduced Co^+ species is a highly reactive compound and can liberate hydrogen from water. Both vitamin B_{12r} and vitamin B_{12s} are very labile in the presence of air and are instantly oxidized to the Co^{3+} compound cobalamin. The sixth coordination site is crucial to the biological role of vitamin B_{12}, where it is involved as a hydrogen carrier in substitution reactions of the type shown in eqn [2].

$$\begin{array}{ccccc}
H & R & & R & H \\
| & | & & | & | \\
- C & - C & - \rightleftharpoons - C & - C & - \\
| & | & & | & | \\
\end{array} \tag{2}$$

Occurrence in Soil

This is primarily dependent on the geological nature of the parent material from which the soil is derived. Thus, soils formed from old red sandstone, granitic and other acid igneous, limestone and predominantly sandy rocks are liable to be cobalt-deficient. The availability of soil cobalt and hence its uptake by pasture and crops is affected by the natural drainage conditions of the soil, being greatest where this is poorest. Consequently, cobalt deficiency is most likely to be found on freely drained soils. Improvement of upland pasture by the removal of heather and the introduction of more productive grass species, raising of the soil pH by liming and improvement of the drainage tends to lower the availability of soil cobalt and so produce cobalt deficiency in the grazing animal where none existed previously. Soil maps have been produced based on the total cobalt content of the B horizon and these categorize the concentrations (in mg kg^{-1}) as follows: low < 5, medium 5–15 and high > 15. Areas falling into the 'low' category have the highest risk of cobalt deficiency. Soils which have a high content of secondary manganese or iron oxides adversely affect cobalt availability as they strongly absorb native cobalt.

$$\text{Vitamin B}_{12}(Co^{3+}) \underset{O_2}{\overset{NaBH_4, H^+}{\rightleftharpoons}} \text{Vitamin B}_{12r}(Co^{2+}) \underset{O_2}{\overset{NaBH_4, OH^-}{\rightleftharpoons}} \text{Vitamin B}_{12s}(Co^+) \tag{1}$$

Red   Brown   Blue-grey green

Table 1. Range of cobalt concentrations in foods

Food	Co (mg kg^{-1})[a]	Co (mg kg^{-1})[b]	Co (mg kg^{-1} FW)[c]
Green leafy vegetables	0·20–0·60	<0·02–0·02	
Dairy products	0·01–0·03		<0·01–0·01
Liver and kidney	0·15–0·25		
Muscle meat	0·06–0·12	<0·02–0·02	<0·01–0·03
Cereal grains	0·01–0·04	<0·02–0·06	0·03
Sugar	0·01–0·03	<0·02–0·04	
Fish	<0·10–0·03	<0·02–0·04	0·03
Milk	0.50 μg l^{-1}	<0·01–0·01	<0·01
White bread			0·01
Wholemeal bread			0·03
Fruit		<0·02–0·04	0·02–0·03
Eggs			0·01
Peas/beans			0·01–0·02
Root vegetables		<0·02–0·04	0·01–0·02

[a] Values (dry matter) from Underwood EJ (1977) *Trace Elements in Human and Animal Nutrition*, 4th edn. London: Academic Press. (NB: these data are quoted unchanged by Smith RM (1987).)
[b] Data (fresh weight) from Ministry of Agriculture, Fisheries and Food (1985) *Food Surveillance Paper*, No. 15. London: HMSO.
[c] Data (fresh weight) from Barbera R and Rosaura F (1986) Teneur en cobalt des aliments dosage par spectrophotometrie d'absorption atomique. *Annales des Falsification et De l'Expertise Clinique et Toxicologique* 79: 209–214.

Concentrations in Food and Dietary Intakes

Cobalt, like other trace elements, tends to be concentrated in the young actively growing parts of plants, with green leafy material often having the highest concentrations. Concentrations tend to be lower in stems, roots, tubers and cereal grains and also to diminish as maturity is reached. Typical values for some foods are given in Table 1, but data are scarce and a recent dietary and nutritional survey of British adults published in 1990 contained no reference to it. This is understandable since it did contain a significant amount of data on vitamin B$_{12}$ status, but a similar lack of reference to selenium is less easily understood.

There is, however, a wide margin of safety between the cobalt concentration of ordinary diets and toxic levels which are around 250–300 mg kg^{-1} and thus more than 1000 times normal dietary concentrations. High cobalt levels have, however, been implicated as a triggering factor in cases of severe cardiac failure in heavy beer drinkers (up to 12 litres daily). Cobalt had been added as a foaming agent in concentrations of 1·2–1·5 mg l^{-1}. The high alcohol and cobalt intakes, together with poor quality diets, combined to produce a distinctive cardiomyopathy. This practice has been discontinued. Cardiomyopathy has also been reported in humans following industrial exposure to cobalt. Recent (1990) work in the FRG has suggested that solutions used for total parenteral nutrition (TPN) are

Table 2. Reported values for mean daily cobalt intake

Country	Year	Co intake (mean or range)
Japan	1963	10
USA	1966	160–170
USA	1967	140–580
USA	1971	297–1767
USSR	1972	31
USA	1973	150–600
UK	1977	11–27
New Zealand	1978	242
UK	1979	14–28
UK	1980	1–110

virtually all contaminated with cobalt but, despite that, several preparations include supplemental cobalt in addition. Serum cobalt concentrations in preterm babies on TPN at 1·44±0·48 ng l^{-1} were significantly higher than those (0·67±0·47 ng l^{-1}) of age-matched controls. No toxic consequences were reported, but any clinical consequences of long-term cobalt surplus have yet to be studied systematically. Most species studied have a high tolerance to cobalt with sheep being particularly so, although recent evidence suggests that this does not extend to lambs <6 weeks old. Cattle are more susceptible to toxic effects from excess cobalt intakes.

Cobalt is present in very low concentration in body

fluids and tissues with the total content of an adult human body being < 1·5 mg, with liver, heart and bone containing the highest concentrations. Reference levels are said to be 0.22, <0·16, 0·06, 0·11 and <0·08 mg of cobalt per kilogram (dry matter) in liver, spleen, kidney, heart and pancreas, respectively. Cobalt deficiency in ruminants has been diagnosed on the basis of liver concentrations of <0·06 mg kg^{-1} (dry matter) with values >0·1 mg kg^{-1} being regarded as adequate. Deficiency during pregnancy will result in the offspring being born with inadequate concentrations and this has an adverse effect on their viability. Supplementation of the dams diet or by direct treatment overcomes this problem.

Cobalt differs from all other essential trace elements in that it is required by the body in a preformed compound, vitamin B_{12}, whereas the other elements, are required in ionic form and then converted into their metabolically active species. Animals and humans are unable to synthesize vitamin B_{12}. This ability is found only in some bacteria and algae. Some of these occur in ruminants so that, provided there is an adequate dietary supply of cobalt salts (>0·1 mg kg^{-1}, dry matter), vitamin B_{12} is synthesized in the rumen and then absorbed lower down the intestinal tract. Humans derive their essential vitamin B_{12} through the consumption of animal-related foods. It has been thought that plants do not produce or require these cobalt-related compounds and strict vegetarians – vegans – have been at risk from pernicious anaemia unless they take synthetic supplements. Some recent evidence suggests that this may not be strictly true, but it remains practically so, as the amounts involved would be of little nutritional significance. *See* Vegan Diets; Vegetarian Diets

The cobalt atom in vitamin B_{12} catalyses the reactions of two B_{12} coenzymes – adenosyl cobalamin and methyl cobalamin – which are essential cofactors in the activity of methylmalonyl-coenzyme A mutase and methionine synthetase. The unique nature of the cobalt–carbon bond in adenosylcobalamin means that it can undergo reversible homolytic splitting with the production of free radicals which are stabilized by the cobalt atom. This allows the intramolecular rearrangements of the type referred to earlier to take place. Methylcobalamin has a similar cobalt–carbon bond which is involved in the synthesis of methionine. The mechanism has not yet been fully established, but it is thought that vitamin B_{12s} (in the Co^+ form) is involved as it can undergo rapid addition and substitution reactions.

Analytical Methods

Sample Preparation

Since many of the available analytical methods require cobalt to be in solution, solid samples such as foods or clinical and biological materials need to be subjected to a primary dissolution process. Most commonly this involves either acid digestion or dry-ashing procedures which mineralize cobalt through destruction of the organic matter present. The most frequently used ashing technique is by muffle furnace at temperatures within the range 450–550°C. Alternatively, there are low-temperature ashers which operate between 100 and 200°C under low pressure using a gaseous oxidant, usually oxygen or an oxygen/tetrafluoromethane mixture; the oxidant is activated by a high frequency electromagnetic field. Dissolution of cobalt from the ashed material is usually achieved using dilute acid.

There are a number of different combinations of acids and oxidizing chemicals which have proved to be effective digestion mixtures, namely nitric acid/perchloric acid, nitric acid/perchloric acid/sulphuric acid, and sulphuric acid/hydrogen peroxide. These operations have been traditionally performed in open Kjeldahl-type flasks; however, much more rapid digestion procedures have recently been developed using Teflon bomb vessels and microwave heating.

Dissolution of cobalt from soils and related materials can be performed using strong acid digestion, normally hydrofluoric acid or a hydrochloric acid/nitric acid mixture (aqua regia), while the more readily available fractions of cobalt are extracted with dilute acetic acid. Water samples and biological fluids such as urine and blood plasma can be analysed directly using one of the more modern sensitive techniques such as electrothermal atomization atomic absorption spectrometry (ETA-AAS).

Where limited sample preparation of solid material, other than drying and milling is required, solid sample presentation can be made using direct-current arc emission spectrometry (DCarcES), direct current plasma atomic emission spectrometry (DCP-AES) and ETA-AAS; presentation in slurry form can also be made with the latter two techniques. Nondestructive analysis can be performed using X ray fluorescence (XRF).

Analytical Techniques

Traditional gravimetric and titrimetric methods have much poorer levels of detection for cobalt than modern instrumental techniques, they are also subject to interferences. Two of the more commonly used precipitating reagents are 1-nitroso-2-naphthol (interference from copper and iron) and anthranilic acid (interference from iron, nickel and zinc). Typical titrants are potassium cyanide (interference from copper, mercury and zinc), potassium hexacyanoferrate (interference from manganese), and ethylenediaminetetra-acetic acid (EDTA) (interferences from nickel, zinc and copper).

Prior to the rapid expansion of flame atomic absorption spectrometry (FAAS) in the 1960s, the analysis of cobalt at the microgram level was performed routinely by colorimetric techniques using spectrophotometry in the ultraviolet and visible wavelength range (300–700 nm). However, this technique is also subject to chemical interference from a wide range of other elements. These have to be eliminated either by the addition of masking agents or buffers, or by solvent extraction of the cobalt complex. The more widely used complexing agents are ammonium thiocyanate (interferences from iron and copper), nitroso-R-salt (interferences from iron, chromium, nickel, vanadium and copper), 1-nitroso-2-naphthol (interferences from iron and copper) and sodium diethyldithiocarbamate (interferences from iron, aluminium, chromium, titanium, manganese, copper and nickel. Recently, sensitive spectrophotometric methods have been developed which depend on the catalytic effect of the cobalt ion on the oxidation reaction between hydrogen peroxide and o-dihydroxybenzene derivatives such as tiron (disodium 1,2-dihydroxybenzene-3,6-disulphonate), catechol, quinizarin, quinalizarin and gallocyanine; detection limits at the picogram level are obtainable.

The following spectroscopic techniques have been used for the analysis of cobalt, approximate detection limits are quoted to an order of magnitude: (FAAS, detection limit, 0·01 $\mu g\ g^{-1}$), ETA-AAS (detection limit, 0·0002 $\mu g\ g^{-1}$), inductively coupled plasma atomic emission spectrometry (ICP-AES, detection limit 0·01 $\mu g\ g^{-1}$), inductively coupled plasma mass spectrometry (ICP-MS, detection limit 0·0002 $\mu g\ g^{-1}$), DCarcES (detection limit 0·3 $\mu g\ g^{-1}$), spark source mass spectrometry (SSMS, detection limit 0·005 $\mu g\ g^{-1}$), DCP-AES (detection limit 0·01 $\mu g\ g^{-1}$). *See* Mass Spectrometry, Principles and Instrumentation

FAAS has been the most extensively used technique for the routine determination of cobalt at the microgram level in food, agricultural and biological materials. The technique is relatively free from chemical and spectral interferences and a large number of preconcentration chemical procedures have been developed to improve detection levels. Ammonium pyrrolidinedithiocarbamate and sodium diethyldithiocarbamate are the two principle chelating agents which have been used for multitrace element complexation prior to solvent extraction, although a more cobalt specific chelate is 1-nitroso-2-naphthol. A range of different organic solvents have been used for extraction of the chelated cobalt compounds, the two most common are methyl isobutyl ketone and chloroform. Ion exchange resins such as chelex-100 have also been widely used as a method of preconcentration. These are capable of being used for in-line preconcentration in automatic flow injection systems for AAS.

ETA-AAS has proved to be sufficiently sensitive for the determination of cobalt at the nanogram level in clinical and biochemical samples. The technique is more susceptible to sample matrix interferences than FAAS, but these have been significantly reduced by using FAAS-type preconcentration techniques as separation procedures for the removal of major elements. Alternatively, matrix modifiers such as palladium, magnesium, or certain inorganic salts such as ammonium phosphate have proved effective. The resonant absorption wavelength for cobalt lies in the ultra-violet region at 240·7 nm. Measurements are therefore subject to background interferences which occur to a greater degree in electrothermal rather than flame atomization. All modern AAS instruments have automatic background correction; there are four different types Zeeman, deuterium continuum, Smith–Hieftje and xenon continuum in the simultaneous multielement atomic absorption continuum instruments (SIMAAC). The nominal detection limit for cobalt as determined by ETA-AAS has been further improved through the coupling of laser technology with electrothermal atomization. This is either in the form of laser-excited atomic fluorescence spectrometry (LAFS) or with the laser-enhanced ionization technique (LEI). *See* Spectroscopy, Fluorescence

The 1980s has seen a rapid growth in the number of commercial ICP-AE spectrometers being used for multielement analysis. Since the detection limit for cobalt by ICP-AES is similar to that for FAAS, similar preconcentration techniques have been applied. The two most prominent emission lines are almost equal in sensitivity; however, since the line at 238·9 nm is subject to strong spectral interference from iron, the cobalt line at 228·6 nm has been preferentially used, but this suffers from a significant spectral interference from titanium, and slight spectral interference from nickel and iron. The exact magnitude of the interfering spectral overlap depends on the spectral resolution of each particular type of spectrometer. Interfering elements which produce strong spectral overlap need to be removed by chemical separation prior to instrumental analysis while those which exhibit a small degree of spectral overlap can be corrected for by appropriate interelement spectral subtraction procedures.

Since the mid-1980s there has been a steady growth in the application of ICP-MS to multielement ultra-trace analysis of clinical and biochemical samples. Detection limits are about the same as for ETA-AAS and, therefore, cobalt can be determined at the nanogram level. Interferences occur from the production of polyatomic ions within the plasma which have the same atomic mass as ^{59}Co, e.g. calcium–oxygen and argon–sodium. These are corrected for by measuring the background levels of such ions in simulated blank solutions.

DCarcES, SSMS and XRF have mainly been applied to the direct analysis of cobalt in solid samples such as soils and related materials, with these techniques matrix matching of samples with calibration standards and choice of internal standards are the most critical aspects of the determination. The application of DCarcES to plant and agricultural materials has been largely superseded by AAS and ICP-AES.

Electrochemical techniques have proved to be very effective in the determination of cobalt at the microgram and nanogram levels in food, biological and environmental samples. It is one of the most sensitive techniques for the determination of cobalt in natural waters. During the 1980s the technique of adsorptive stripping voltammetry has been developed as the most sensitive of the polarographic methods for trace metal analysis. For the determination of cobalt the square wave stripping mode is more sensitive than the differential stripping mode. Electrolytic preconcentration of cobalt at the mercury electrode is made with chelated cobalt since the free cobalt ion would be irreversibly adsorbed. The most widely used chelating agent has been dimethyl glyoxime; adsorption of the cobalt dimethyl glyoxime occurs at -0.7 V, and the voltammetric peak at -1.12 V in a cell system using a silver/silver chloride/potassium chloride electrode as the nonworking electrode. Interference from zinc can be masked by the addition of nitrilotriacetic acid or sodium iminodiacetate; nickel interferes if present in large excess, but this is reduced by using alternative chelating agents such as 1,2-cyclohexanedione dioxime or α-furil dioxime for complexing the cobalt.

High-performance liquid chromatography (HPLC) has been successfully applied to the determination of cobalt and other trace metals in plant materials, natural waters and environmental samples and detection levels of nanogram quantities are obtainable. The use of disubstituted dithiocarbamates such as sodium diethyldithiocarbamate, ammonium pyrrolidinedithiocarbamate and ammonium bis(2-hydroxyethyl)dithiocarbamate has been favoured since they rapidly form stable complexes with a wide range of trace metals. These metal complexes can be separated chromatographically using alkyl-bonded silica columns and quantitatively determined with ultraviolet/visible diode array detectors or electrochemical detectors. Precolumn derivatization can be made off-line using solvent extraction for water-insoluble complexes or in-line using a preseparation column loaded with an appropriate ion pair reagent such as cetyltrimethylammonium bromide–dithiocarbamate. On-column derivatization can be performed by inclusion of the dithiocarbamate reagent in the mobile phase, usually a water/methanol mixture or an acetonitrile/water mixture; however, this process is less sensitive than precolumn derivatization. Other complexing chelating agents which can be used include ethylenediaminetetraacetic acid or 4-(2-pyridylazo)resorcinol. Metal ion chromatography can be applied to cobalt analysis using an appropriate complexing chelating agent such as pyridine-2-carboxyaldehyde phenylhydrazone as a stationary phase immobilized on a silica matrix. *See* Chromatography, High-performance Liquid Chromatography

HPLC can be interfaced to a number of spectroscopic instruments, e.g. FAAS, ETA-AAS and ICP-AES, to provide a powerful technique for speciation studies. For instance, the distribution of cobalt as cyanocobalamin can be determined by HPLC–ICP–AES coupling in a range of biological fluids, e.g. blood serum, seminal fluid and milk serum.

Neutron activation analysis (NAA) can be used for the determination of cobalt in biological and environmental samples; typical detection levels are 0.03 $\mu g\ g^{-1}$. This technique usually requires a postirradiation period of around 3 weeks before γ ray emission from the ^{60}Co isotope can be measured; radiation flux levels are usually around $10^{12}–10^{13}$ neutrons cm^{-2}s^{-1}. Concentration techniques using dithiocarbamate complexation are usually applied to improve detection levels.

Bibliography

Brown S and Savory J (1984) *Chemical Toxicology and Clinical Chemistry of Metals.* New York: Academic Press.

Schneider Z and Stroinski A (1987) *Comprehensive B_{12}.* Berlin: Walter de Gruyter.

Smith IC and Carson BL (1981) *Trace Metals in the Environment. Cobalt,* vol. 6, pp 1202. Ann Arbor: Ann Arbor Science Publishers.

Smith KA (1990) *Soil Analysis, Modern Instrumental Techniques,* 2nd edn. New York: Marcel Dekker.

Smith RM (1987) Cobalt. In: Mertz W (ed.) *Trace Elements in Human and Animal Nutrition,* 5th edn, vol. 1, pp 143–183. San Diego: Academic Press.

A. MacPherson and J. Dixon
The Scottish Agricultural College, Auchincruive, UK

COCKLES

See Shellfish

Cobalt

COCOA*

Contents

Chemistry of Processing

The particular flavour of cocoa is due not only to its genetic makeup but also to chemical reactions which take place during processing and manufacturing. The unprocessed cocoa seed would not give the characteristic flavour when roasted unless it was first fermented and dried. The sequence of raw cocoa processing and then manufacturing is essential since reactions during processing depend on water and enzymes of the living seed, whilst manufacturing comprises nonenzymatic reactions in a dry lipid phase. Reactions during fermentation and drying are described in this article. The end product of processing is dried raw cocoa beans. Reactions taking place during manufacturing are also considered in this article. Thus, raw cocoa beans are the link between processing (normally in the tropics) and manufacturing (normally in the consuming countries). The quality of raw cocoa is of considerable interest in assessing its value. For grading raw cocoa, visual descriptors are used which reflect previous processing. While accepted analytical criteria for beans are lacking, cocoa products are judged by means of analytical methods and organoleptic tests. A large number of essential constituents of cocoa flavour are produced during roasting of raw cocoa from flavour precursors formed during processing. Thus, this first article describes both the formation of flavour precursors and the subsequent formation of flavour compounds.

Chemistry of Processing

Both the seeds and the pulp are essential components in raw cocoa processing. However, the reactions which are essential for raw cocoa quality take place within the seeds alone and not in the pulp. Enzymes of the seeds are directly involved but microorganisms only indirectly, in that bacteria and fungi are responsible for the degradation of the pulp, and their metabolites, especially acetic acid, are instrumental in the subsequent changes in the seeds. Organisms participating in the direct attack on

the nibs during the late stage of fermentation and overfermentation are also important.

Processing depends on the chemical composition and physiological state of the pods and beans, the anatomy and cytology of the living seeds and their post-mortem status of subcellular structures and enzymes. Therefore, chemical and cell-biological aspects are involved and experimental results on the formation of specific cocoa flavour precursors during fermentation and drying greatly affect the final product quality.

Biology of the Seed

Two commercially exploited types of the species *Theobroma cacao*, Criollo and Forastero, are distinguished on the basis of fruit morphology and geographic origin. Criollo gives fine flavour cocoas, although in low yields, while the more vigorous, high-yielding Forastero subtypes and hybrids predominate in plantations worldwide. Cocoa pods contain 35–45 seeds consisting of the embryo and the shell, which is covered when ripe by a mucilagenous pulp, the endocarp (Fig. 1). The main parts of the embryo are two folded cotyledons connected by a small embryonic axis. A rudimentary, skin-like endosperm covers the surface of the embryo. After fermentation the shell, covered with residues of pulp, comprises about 12–16% of the seed dry weight, depending on bean size and pulp degradation during fermentation. The dry weight of a seed varies considerably, but is approximately 1·0–1·2 g. Only the cotyledons are used for cocoa and chocolate manufacturing and in these the leaf mesophyll is the dominating tissue, consisting of two types of cells which differ in composition.

About 80% of the cells store lipid and protein, the major volume of which is occupied by a large number of individual lipid bodies of constant size (about 2 μm) surrounding one or more branched protein storage vacuoles and amyloplasts. The remaining 20% of the cells are polyphenol storage cells. Their lumen is almost entirely occupied by one central vacuole containing all the stored polyphenols and purines.

Subcellular structures in the lipid and protein storage cells control pre- and post-mortem reactions during fermentation, which are not the same as in cell free systems. On the subcellular level, *in vivo*, the situation

* The colour plate section for this article is between p. 1146 and p. 1147.

can roughly be described as a dispersed lipid phase (lipid bodies) in a continuous water phase (cytoplasm) (Fig. 2). During fermentation, the cells are killed by heat and acetic acid, but post-mortem structures are maintained. In the cell lumen, with low concentrations of acetic acid, the lipid bodies fuse *in situ*, and they form, more or less, a continuous lipid phase which separates cytoplasmic inclusions as a hydrophilic dispersed phase. In contrast, in the presence of a high concentration of acetic acid, fusion of the lipid bodies is more extensive, causing complete segregation of the lipid in the cell centre (Fig. 2). In the first case, intracellular diffusion of water-soluble compounds is reduced by lipid barriers. In the latter case, diffusion is not restricted. Proteolysis, browning reactions, acid diffusion and flavour precursor formation mutually depend on these structures. *See* Lipids, Classification

Composition of Unfermented Cocoa Seeds

The prominent secondary compounds are flavonoids and purines (theobromine and caffeine). The storage reserves include predominantly cocoa butter but also protein and starch. The composition of ripe seeds is

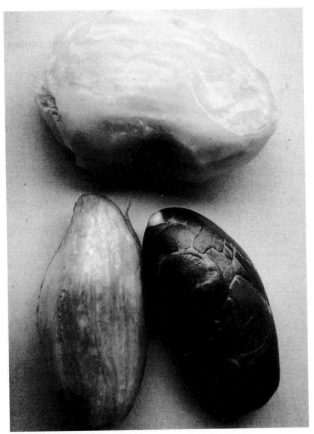

Fig. 1 Unfermented cocoa seeds showing the pulp, the testa and the cotyledons.

Chemistry of Processing

shown in Table 1. Genetic differences of cocoa butter, proteins and pigments are found between Forastero and Criollo types.

Cocoa Butter

Fat, the main storage component, comprises 52–57% of the cotyledon dry weight. It contains 95% triglycerides, 2% diglycerides, <1% monoglycerides, 1% polar lipids and 1% free fatty acids, (as percentages of lipids). Triglycerides consist of 37% oleic (O), 32% stearic (S), 27% palmitic (P) and 2·5% linoleic (L) acids (as percentages of total fatty acids). Other saturated and monounsaturated fatty acids do not contribute more than about 2% of the fatty acids. These values are typical of fermented beans but do vary between samples, and between genetic and geographic origins. This is also true of the complex fatty acid composition in triglycerides. Since the melting temperature of cocoa butter at 31–34°C is an essential characteristic, differences of fat hardness are of interest. POS, SOS and POP are by far the predominant triglycerides. South American cocoas are the softest, containing more POO and SOO. The ambient temperature during pod growth, climate, ripeness and time of harvest affect the composition of triglycerides, and thus the melting and crystallization characteristics. *See* Fatty Acids, Properties; Triglycerides, Structures and Properties

Polyphenols

Flavanols are the major components. The order of quantities in Forastero types is (approximate weight percentages of total polyphenols): leucocyanidins (58–65%), catechins (29–38%), then anthocyanins (1·7–4·0%). Specific compounds detected include: anthocyanins (3-α-L-arabinosidyl cyanidin and 3-β-D-galactosidyl cyanidin); catechins ((−)-epicatechin, (+)-catechin, (+)-gallocatechin, (−)-epigallocatechin); leucocyanidins (5,7,3′,4′-tetrahydroxyflavan 3,4-diol, a (−)-epicatechin dimer); and, in addition, seven less well-characterized isomers and polymers. Three flavonols have been found as minor constituents: quercitin, quercitin-3-glucoside and quercitin-3-galactoside. Up to 17 phenolic acids and esters have also been reported. The total amount of seven of them comprise not more than 23 ppm of the seed dry weight (phloroglucinol, protocatechuic acid, vanillic acid, *o*-hydroxyphenylacetic acid, *p*-coumaric acid, caffeic acid, ferulic acid). *See* Tannins and Polyphenols

Anthocyanins and their aglyca are lacking in Criollo-type seeds but provide the characteristic colour of Forastero seeds. They are also taken as an indicator of the 'degree of fermentation'. Leucocyanidins and catechins are strongly astringent and are effective tannins. Their enzymatic oxidation causes browning reactions

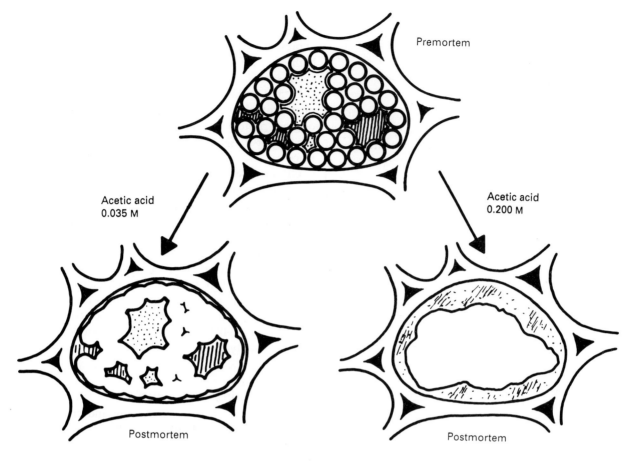

Fig. 2 Schematic representation of electron microscopic aspects of post-mortem changes in mesophyll cells caused by different concentrations of acetic acid during fermentation-like seed incubation. Spherical lipid globules in the living cell fuse *in situ* (left) or form a central bulk of lipid (right). Hydrophilic compartments are indicated by dots or dashes.

during drying after fermentation. *See* Colours, Properties and Determination of Natural Pigments

Alkaloids

The composition of methylxanthines in cocoa seeds is genetically variable but characteristic of cocoa. Theobromine (1–2%, dry weight) and caffeine (0·2%, dry weight), together with traces of theophylline and 7-methylxanthine, are found. They are not metabolized during fermentation. Theobromine plays a role in the bitter taste of cocoa. Several phenolic amines and alkaloids derived from tyrosine and tryptophan have been detected at very low levels (3–40 μg^{-1} g) in both unroasted and roasted cocoas. *See* Alkaloids, Toxicology

Sugars and Acids

Besides a total of around 12% (dry weight) of polysaccharides (Table 1), the free sugar content in cocoa seeds is not more than 2–4% (dry weight). Sucrose is the major component (about 90% of total sugars) followed by fructose plus glucose (about 6%). In addition, galactose, raffinose, melobiose, mannotriose, xylose, arabinose, mannitol and inositol have been detected by several investigators, in minor quantities. *See* Carbohydrates, Classification and Properties

Volatile acids are not found in fresh cocoa beans, but nonvolatile acids are found in low concentrations. Phosphoric, lactic, malic plus tartaric acids were found to make up 0·32% (dry weight), oxalic acid 0·35% and citric acid 0·73%. These acids in unfermented seeds are not metabolized during processing nor contribute to cocoa quality.

Proteins and Amino Acids

The protein content varies in ripe cocoa seeds between 10 and 16% (dry weight). Criollo cocoa seeds have been reported to contain less protein than Forastero seeds. Using sodium dodecyl sulphate–polyacrylamide gel electrophoresis, the proteins of Forastero seeds reveal about 16 peptide bands, three of which are present in

Table 1. Analyses of unfermented West African Cocoa

Constituent	Dried beans (%)	
Cotyledons	89·60	
Shell	9·63	
Embryonic axis	0·77	
Fat	53·05	
Water	3·65	
Ash (total)	2·63	
Nitrogen		
Total nitrogen	2·28	
Protein nitrogen	1·50	
Ammonia nitrogen	0·028	
Amide nitrogen	0·188	
Theobromine	1·71	
Caffeine	0·085	
Carbohydrates		
Fructose		(0·09)
Glucose	0·30	(0·07)
Sucrose	0	(2·48)
Starch	6·10	
Pectins	2·25	
Fibre	2·09	
Cellulose	1·92	
Pentosans	1·27	
Mucilage and gums	0·38	
Tannins (total phenolics)	7·54	(13·5)
Acids		
Acetic (free)	0·014	
Oxalic	0·29	

After Rohan TA (1963) with permission of the Food and Agriculture Organization of the United Nations, except data in parentheses for sugars in Bahia from Berbert PRF (1979). Total phenolics from Swain (1954) as cited by Rohan TA (1963) assuming 55% fat.

large amounts. Two of them (44–46 and 26–31 kDa) are part of the vacuolar storage globulin, which has now been found to be a vicilin-type glycoprotein. The third one is an albumin of 19 kDa not found in the protein vacuoles. The solubility of the vacuolar storage protein is almost zero at pH ≤5·0. This protein is enriched in hydrophobic amino acids. The fresh cotyledons contain about 5 mg g^{-1} (dry weight) of free amino acids. Acidic amino acids dominate both the total protein and the free amino acids in unfermented seeds. *See* Amino Acids, Properties and Occurrence

Enzymes

Various enzymes have been identified in fresh cocoa seeds which are active during post-mortem fermentation or drying, including glycosidases, proteases and polyphenoloxidase. The proteolytic activity in fresh, recalcitrant cocoa seeds is surprisingly high, compared to orthodox seeds. Results in the author's laboratory revealed that one endopeptidase, an aspartylproteinase, is present in ungerminated cocoa seeds. Its activity is highest at pH 3·5. The exopeptidase of ungerminated cocoa seeds is a serylpeptidase with its highest activity at pH 5·5. It reveals some substrate specificity. Among the final proteolytic products, oligopeptides (75% of the original protein nitrogen) dominate over amino acids (about 25%). *See* Enzymes, Functions and Characteristics

Glycosidases are responsible for hydrolysis of anthocyanins. Their highest activity in cocoa beans was found between pH 3·5 and 4·5. Invertase was detected in early investigations. Polyphenoloxidase (o-diphenol: O_2 oxidoreductase) in unfermented seeds displays a high activity, which is strongly reduced after anaerobic fermentation. However, the residual activity, which is due to a modified form of the original enzyme, is sufficient to induce browning reactions during drying. Under a wide range of pH optima reported by several authors, pH 6·0–6·4 is the most probable range of highest activity.

Changes During Fermentation

Reactions start in the living seeds and proceed to postmortem reactions. Little is known about reactions prior to seed death, which is caused by heat and diffusion of acetic acid. An extended initial period at low temperatures (≤40°C) has been found to increase subsequent post-mortem proteolysis and flavour potential during both seed incubation and fermentation. Acidic amino acids are metabolized before post-mortem acidic hydrolysis.

The subsequent uptake of acetic acid controls the post-mortem activity of acidic hydrolases (proteases, glycosidases) under anaerobic conditions. An acetic acid gradient slowly moves from the cotyledon surface into the mesophyll. Temperature increase and change in pH also controls the subcellular structure (Fig. 2). Once the plasma membranes and tonoplasts are destroyed, proteins, polyphenols and other compounds are released from their compartments and come into contact with enzymes. At this stage the nib pH drops to pH 5·0–4·0, depending on the concentration of acetic acid.

As a result of cell destruction and enzymatic degradation, variable amounts of soluble constituents, flavonoids, amino acids, purines and sugars are lost from the seeds due to exudation. A loss of 10–40% of soluble substances modifies the original composition of cocoa seeds. Reported changes in the content of fat are in accordance with this loss of soluble substances. Sucrose disappears to a very large extent from the seeds during fermentation, probably due to invertase activity. However, the amount of fructose plus glucose in the

Table 2. Amino acids in cocoa seeds

Fraction	Free amino acids in fermented seeds (mol % of total free amino acids)		Protein-bound amino acids in unfermented seeds (% of total protein-bound amino acids)[b]	
	After shallow box fermentation[a]	After laboratory seed incubation[b]	Total seed protein	Storage globulin (enriched)
Acidic amino acids	15·9	20·5	31·5	26·0
Hydrophobic amino acids,	58·3	58·6	33·5	41·3
including Leu, Ala, Phe, Tyr	45·3	50·4	22·0	28·7
Other amino acids	25·8	21·0	35·0	32·7
Total amino acids	38·2[c]	25·0[c]	11·3[d]	4·5[d]

Data from Kirchoff P-M, Biehl B and Crone G (1989) Peculiarity of the accumulation of free amino acids during cocoa fermentation. *Food Chemistry* 31: 295–311.
[a] Ghanaian and [b] Malaysian seeds analyses. Aseptic seed incubation at pH 4·5 in acetic acid containing media for 20 h at 40°C and 40 h at 50°C simulates fermentation with respect to known reactions in the seeds. Storage globulin was enriched by chromatography on sephadex G 150. Protein was hydrolysed in hot concentrated hydrochloric acid. Determination of amino acids by reversed phase high-performance liquid chromatography.
[c] μmol g^{-1} (dry weight).
[d] % of dry weight; the amount of proteins is calculated from nitrogen determination and sodium dodecyl sulphate–polyacrylamide gel electrophoresis.

fermented beans is not more than 50% of the original amount of sucrose. Since their proportions are variable, they obviously undergo further reactions.

The cyanidin glycosides are hydrolysed by glycosidases. The aglycon cyanidin subsequently undergoes bleaching by nonenzymatic transformation to a colourless pseudobase. Leucoanthocyanidins are transferred nonenzymatically to more complex forms. Although no reactions of the catechins have been established, the loss of more than 50% suggests nonenzymatic oligomerization. These strongly tanning compounds are released from polyphenol storage cells but they do not prevent proteolysis.

Proteolysis in the beans starts after uptake of acetic acid and is mostly completed within a few hours. The decrease in the rate of proteolysis during fermentation is not due to tanning since it is also found during acetone–dry powder autolysis.

Since oligopeptides and amino acids are precursors of cocoa flavour, the accumulation of leucine, alanine, phenylalanine and tyrosine among free amino acids after proteolysis is interesting. Their proportions are significantly higher than in the proteins (Table 2). The splitting site of the aspartyl endopeptidase (hydrophobic amino acids), and the finding that the exopeptidase of the cocoa seed reveals some substrate specificity, may be responsible. Furthermore in well fermenting seeds, the storage globulin is the only protein attacked by the proteases during proteolysis under mild acidification (pH $\geq$ 5·0). In contrast, all seed proteins are degraded after strong acidification of seeds. The subcellular structures shown in Fig. 2 are probably responsible for this difference. During acetone–dry powder incubation, all seed proteins are degraded at pH 5·5 and 4·5. Although the extent of proteolysis is less, the flavour potential was found to be higher at pH 5·5 than at pH 4·5.

The liberated amino acids and peptides do not seem to be metabolized unless the seed takes up oxygen, but they are changed in amount during drying and microbial attack.

Changes During Drying

Reactions during drying are an oxidative continuation of fermentation. They are important for quality. Polyphenols are oxidized by oxygen itself, the resulting quinones undergo polymerization to give brown products. Oxidation is brought about by residual activities of the polyphenoloxidase. However, in view of its optimum at pH 6, in acidic beans (pH 4·0–5·0) browning is impaired during drying. At pH > 7·0 polyphenols are oxidized nonenzymatically. Thus, overfermented cocoa easily turns brown, giving the incorrect appearance in the cut test of perfectly fermented cocoa beans. Since enzymatic browning requires high oxygen concentrations, browning does not take place before drying. A consequence of polyphenol oxidation and quinone polymerization is the reduction of the astringent flavour, which is due to the tanning property of catechins and leucocyanidins, especially of dimeric forms. Oxidation and polymerization transfer these mono- and oligomeric flavonoids to nonastringent, brown polymers. *See* Browning, Nonenzymatic

Thus, the extent of these polymerizations is controlled

by the nib pH, the permeability of the shell to oxygen and by the destruction of subcellular compartmentation. Roughly, the internal colour of raw cocoa beans is related to astringency. Slaty beans reveal a strongly astringent taste while entirely brown beans and, especially, overfermented beans give an insipid taste.

The extent of the browning reaction also affects the residual seed proteins. Free amino and sulphhydryl groups of proteins readily react with quinones and thus participate in the production of brown polymers. Amino acids and oligopeptides are less reactive. However, they participate in the formation of Maillard products during drying. The spontaneous reaction of proteins and quinones is also responsible for toxic effects of quinones on bacteria and fungi. Therefore, overfermentation is suppressed during browning reactions in the course of drying. However, the resulting polymers are not toxic and would not impair microbial growth on brown raw cocoa beans during storage and on fully brown beans in particular.

Microbiology

The events taking place during pulp fermentation correspond to a succession of microorganisms metabolizing the pulp. The wide range of organisms in the wild inoculum is quite similar in different cocoa-growing countries. When starting fermentation the low pH value and the high sugar content of the pulp allow anaerobic fermentation by yeasts and lactic acid bacteria. The size of the population of lactic acid bacteria is subordinate, and is further repressed when acetic acid bacteria subsequently become active after exhaustion of pulp sugars. *See* Lactic Acid Bacteria

Several authors have isolated more than 30 species from 13 genera of yeasts, some of which reveal pectolytic activity and help in pulp drainage. Several homofermentative and heterofermentative lactobacilli have been isolated. A number of species of the genus *Acetobacter* which have been found in fermented cocoa not only oxidize ethanol to form acetic acid but also oxidize this acid. Additionally, *Gluconobacter* spp. were found. The size of these populations correlates with the amount of products formed (ethanol, lactic acid, acetic acid). However, the various species reveal different substrate specificities, and temperature and pH requirements. There is no information available about the more detailed succession, competition and significance of all these individual species. Following the detailed review of Lehrian and Patterson (see Bibliography), the available data are questionable with respect to the methods of isolation.

The last aerobic stage of pulp fermentation is characterized by the development and dominance of aerophilic bacteria. Up to 14 species of the genus *Bacillus* have been isolated, which, in part, are facultative anaerobes. Further species of other genera have been reported. There is no direct evidence as to how they contribute to cocoa fermentation in detail. Most probably they participate by increasing the shell permeability and later on in overfermentation. *Bacillus stearothermophilus*, *B. subtilis*, *B. circulans*, *B. licheniformis* and *Streptococcus thermophilus* have been found as dominating organisms. Species like *B. megaterium*, *B. subtilis*, *B. coagulans*, *B. cereus*, *B. polymyxa* or *Enterobacter aerogenes* have been isolated, which metabolize carbonic acids, proteins and amino acids, producing low-molecular-weight fatty acids. Propionic, butyric and isovaleric acids are increased to $0.1–1.0\%$ of dry weight each in overfermented cocoa beans compared to $0–0.02\%$ in the controls. These findings strongly indicate bacterial degradation of amino acids (and flavour precursors) during overfermentation. *See Bacillus*, Occurrence

A large number of different filamentous fungi develop on the seeds in well-aerated niches, especially when less acidic and strongly aerated during the later stages after a steep pH increase. They may develop further during drying when the humidity is high. Xerophilic fungi like *Aspergillus fumigatus* as well as *A. glaucus*, *Penicillium* spp., *Mucor* sp., *Paecilomyces* sp. and *Geotrichum* sp., which have been found to develop during late stages of fermentation, have also been reported to occur on stored raw cocoa beans.

Flavour Precursors

The precursors are formed during fermentation and drying and they are subjected to Maillard reactions on roasting. In view of the large number of volatile components, no particular aroma precursors are known, but the classes are identified. Methanolic extracts from raw cocoa beans develop cocoa aroma when roasted. Reducing sugars, amino acids and oligopeptides have been found in fractionated extracts to be essential. There is no agreement with respect to the importance of flavonoids as direct precursors of cocoa aroma, but they participate in flavour and have been found to enhance cocoa aroma.

Since the amino acid sequence of proteolytic peptides results from particular proteins and the specificity of proteases, peptides among aroma precursors may be responsible for the plant specificity of cocoa aroma. A large number of oligopeptides in fermented cocoa have been found. They differ in composition depending on the acidity in the beans during fermentation. The composition of free amino acids in fermented cocoa is characteristic. Predominantly, hydrophobic amino acids (leucine, alanine, phenylalanine) and tyrosine are accumulated (Table 2). Derivatives of phenylalanine are prominent volatiles after roasting. The reaction during drying of quinones with amino acids or peptides and its significance for aroma formation is still speculative. In contrast to amino acids, glucose and fructose are consumed to a very large extent during roasting (up to 90%). Minor sugars resulting from hydrolysis of, for example, anthocyanins or glycoproteins may therefore be important.

In addition to aroma formation, oligopeptides and theobromine are flavour precursors. During roasting, N-terminal amino acids of several hydrophobic peptides produce diketopiperazines which give the characteristic cocoa bitter principle in a 1:2 complex with theobromine. There is no experimental information about the role of acids as flavour precursors. When present in high concentrations acids resulting from fermentation are believed to reduce the impression of cocoa aroma.

Chemistry of Manufacturing Processes

Cocoa flavour is chemically very complex because it arises from fermentation and roasting and is influenced by further processing steps. The flavour of plain chocolate is modified but chemically very similar to cocoa. The flavour sensations of cocoa products and chocolates are based on a great number of volatile aroma compounds and their interaction with nonvolatile constituents which affect taste and tactile characteristics.

Cocoa Flavour Development

Flavour of Unroasted Cocoa

Raw cocoa has an acid taste and a flat but characteristic aroma. As a result of the fermentation process it contains aroma precursors, mainly free amino acids, monosaccharides and their first reaction products (Amadori compounds), peptides, monomeric flavonoids and methylxanthines. The first aroma compounds were developed in an early Maillard reaction during the drying of the fermented seeds or absorbed from the fruit pulp. The major volatiles in the concentration range $0.1–1$ mg kg^{-1} are aldehydes (produced via Strecker degradation of amino acids), alcohols, acetates and acids, which derive from valine, leucine, isoleucine and phenylalanine (Table 3). Tetramethylpyrazine is formed by microorganisms. Special flavour-grade cocoas, mainly harvested in Venezuela, Trinidad and Ecuador (Arriba), reveal a flowery and tea-like aroma and contain significant concentrations ($0.5–2$ mg kg^{-1}) of linalool and further terpenoids which contribute to this valuable note. On the other hand, basic cocoas from West Africa, Malaysia or Brazil (Bahia) carry a fairly strong inherent flavour and have very low concentrations of linalool. The sharp acidity of raw cocoas arises from acetic acid, the astringency and bitterness from soluble polyphenols (mainly epicatechin), tannins, theo-

Table 3. Typical aroma compounds in unroasted cocoas and some of their precursors (Val, valine; Leu, leucine; Ile, isoleucine; Phe, phenylalanine)

Acids		Carbonyls	
Acetic		Acetone	
2-Methylpropanoic	(Val)	2,3-Butandione	
3-Methylbutanoic	(Leu)	Acetophenone	
2-Methylbutanoic	(Ile)	Dihydrohydroxymaltol	
Benzoic	(Phe)		
Phenylacetic	(Phe)		
Aldehydes		**Heterocyclic Compounds**	
2-Methylpropanal	(Val)	Tetramethylpyrazine	
3-Methylbutanal	(Leu)	2-Acetylpyrrole	
2-Methylbutanal	(Ile)		
Benzaldehyde	(Phe)		
Phenylacetaldehyde	(Phe)		
Alcohols		**Terpenes**	
2-Methylpropanol	(Val)	Linalool	
3-Methylbutanol	(Leu)	Linalool oxides	
2-Methylbutanol	(Ile)		
Benzyl alcohol	(Phe)		
2-Phenylethanol	(Phe)		
Acetates			
2-Methylpropyl acetate	(Val)		
3-Methylbutyl acetate	(Leu)		
2-Methylbutyl acetate	(Ile)		
Benzyl acetate	(Phe)		
2-Phenethyl acetate	(Phe)		

bromine and caffeine. A smoky flavour, a flavour defect of some cocoas, is produced by the absorption of volatile phenols from the smoke of the firewood used for drying.

Roasting and Aroma Formation

The entire cocoa aroma is formed by careful roasting of fermented and dried seeds at temperatures between 120 and 140°C. Using modern technology, cocoas can be roasted at different particle sizes, such as whole beans, as nibs, which are coarsely ground and broken beans, or as liquid cocoa mass, which is produced by a fine grinding of cocoa and liquefying within its own fat. The roasting of smaller particles has the advantages of better controlled roasting, partial exhaustion of abundant acetic acid and reduced roasting time (beans about 30 min, nibs 12 min, mass 2 min). Since the intensity and quality of the cocoa aroma increases with decreasing initial water content during roasting, modern roasters are subdivided into predrying and actual roasting zones.

About 500 compounds have been separated in cocoa aroma, of which the greater proportion has been identified, but some of these only tentatively. In common with all roasting aromas there is a large number of carbonyl and heterocyclic compounds. The main carbonyl groups are acids and esters (each about 50 compounds), alcohols, aldehydes and ketones (each between 30 and 40 derivatives). The main heterocyclic compounds are pyrazines and chinoxalines (together about 80 compounds), furans, pyrones and lactones (together 40 compounds), diketopiperazines, phenols, pyrroles and oxazoles (each group about 10 compounds). As a result of the Maillard reaction, pyrazines, pyrroles, phenylacetaldehyde, phenylalk-2-enals, pyrones, furanones and furans are increasing during cocoa roasting, whereas alcohols, esters and acids remain more or less unchanged.

Simple aldehydes arise by Strecker degradation of free amino acids. Their immediate flavour characteristics are not very striking, but they act as most important reactants. Some phenylalk-2-enals are generated via the aldol condensation, for example, which carry a typical flowery odour fairly reminiscent of chocolate or cocoa. Many pyrazines with different substitutes and chinoxalines with desirable flavour properties contribute to the roasted note. It was found that methylpyrazines are formed during roasting according to a specific rate depending on substitution. Some pyrones and furanones arise from degradation of monosaccharides and reach remarkable concentrations in roasted cocoas. Dihydrohydroxymaltol, hydroxymaltol, furanol and cyclotene are of great importance for the aroma intensity because they carry caramel tastes and have enhancing properties. Characteristic of cocoa aroma are abundant phenyl derivatives which arise from phenylalanine and contribute to the intensive sweet aromatic note. Besides the action of the Maillard reaction, several volatiles are produced via thermolysis of nonvolatile substances, e.g. thiazoles from thiamin, 1,2-benzenediol from epicatechin and diketopiperazines from peptides. The typical intense bitterness of roasted cocoa is to a great extent induced by adducts of such diketopiperazines with theobromine and caffeine. By increasing the roasting time, monosaccharides react to the extent of about 60%, free amino acids only about 20%. Therefore, in several roasters the unroasted nibs or masses are treated with aqueous sugar solutions to increase the concentration of the carbohydrate precursors and to improve the aroma yield. *See* Caffeine

Technologically Influenced Flavour Changes

Roasted cocoa nibs and mass are important semimanufactured goods and are used for the production of cocoa powder, cocoa butter or chocolate mass. The cocoa flavour is modified and improved by the subsequent processing, mainly by alkalization of nibs, degassing of cocoa mass or conching of chocolate mass.

Conching of Chocolate The conversion of the bitter cocoa flavour to the finer chocolate flavour occurs in the conche. There, a mixture of cocoa mass, sugar, cocoa butter and milk powder (for milk chocolate production), fine ground in rolling mills, is stirred vigorously and treated for about 8–36 h at 50–75°C. In addition to the aroma improvement, this process gives the desired consistency to the chocolate by covering all the solid particles with fat. Aroma and consistency are important for the flavour of the finished product. There are two main functions of the conche: degassing and mechanical–thermal treatment of the chocolate mass. Low-boiling volatiles are removed together with steam. Acetic, propionic, isobutyric and isovaleric acids are reduced by about 30%. About 20–40% of the unspecified aroma compounds, such as abundant aldehydes and alcohols, as well as of aroma-damaging substances like volatile phenols, are also removed. As a result the typical and slightly volatile aroma becomes more pronounced.

However, the long period of time needed for the aroma improvement suggests further chemical reactions that proceed slowly. A small decrease (between 0 and 10%) in free amino acids has been reported, as has a decrease in furans and pyrones, which have a high chemical reactivity. No reaction products could be identified. The absorption of oxygen during conching has also been observed but no change in soluble polyphenols has been detected so far. Sorption phenomena of aroma materials at particle surfaces of the heterogeneous chocolate mass of fat and fat-free portions obviously have considerable influence on the flavour.

Thin-layer Treatment of Cocoa Mass During modern chocolate processing the cocoa liquor is degassed before being put into the chocolate recipe. By application of special equipment, degassing can be performed more effectively than in the conche. Thin-layer vaporizers are used generally, which may shorten the remaining conching time considerably. The process conditions have to be coordinated with the quality of the cocoa liquor, so that the valuable aroma is not removed together with the more volatile unknown materials, thereby flattening the taste of the product. A reduction of 10–30% of acids and low-boiling compounds seems to be optimal.

Alkalization of Cocoa Alkalization ('Dutching') is mainly used to intensify the colour, to modify the flavour and to improve the dispersability of cocoa powder in water or milk. In this process, beans, nibs or mass are treated with solutions or suspensions of alkali, usually potassium or sodium carbonate, sometimes hydroxides or ammonia. The permitted maximum is generally 2·5–3 parts of potassium carbonate (or equivalent alkali) per 100 parts of cocoa. The pH of a natural cocoa is about 5·5, whereas the pH of commercially available Dutch process cocoas will fall between 6·8 and 8·0.

Colour and flavour changes during alkalization are mainly based on modifications of polyphenolic substances. Dutch processing results in a milder and altered flavour, and a darker colour. Under alkaline conditions, soluble monomeric flavonoids (mainly epicatechin) are oxidized and condensed to give polymer tannins and phlobaphenes. Red and brown pigments are developed and the astringency is reduced. Changes within the volatile compound are a partial breakdown of oxygen-containing heterocyclic compounds (furans, furanones, pyrones), an intensified generation of 1,2-benzenediol from epicatechin, chemical reactions of amino compounds and partial neutralization of acids.

Cocoa Aroma Analysis

The 500 or so cocoa aroma volatiles only occur in milli- or microgram per kilogram quantities. They are dissolved in the fat phase or physically bound to a heterogeneous matrix of constituents of differing polarity. Isolation and enrichment techniques are necessary to obtain the flavour volatiles in sufficiently high concentrations. Distillation methods, headspace techniques, and extractions, or combinations of these techniques are used. The separation of the volatiles is performed by means of capillary gas chromatography (GC) or high-performance liquid chromatography (HPLC). *See* Chromatography, Gas Chromatography; Chromatography, High-performance Liquid Chromatography

Isolation and Analytical Techniques

Extraction Extraction techniques have several disadvantages (time-consuming and the possibility of introducing artefacts) but have the advantage of quantitatively isolating volatiles independent of their boiling points. Usually, cocoa is defatted with petroleum ether and the residue is extracted with a polar solvent such as water, ethanol, acetonitrile, ethyl ether or subcritical carbon dioxide. By means of extraction, specific high-boiling compounds have been isolated from cocoa: diketopiperazines, pyrones, amines, amides, aromatic acids and phenols (these compounds mainly for subsequent GC separation), and theobromine, caffeine and monomeric flavonoids (for HPLC measurement).

Distillation Most of the known aroma volatiles have been isolated from cocoa by means of distillation (steam distillation, vacuum condensation, simultaneous steam distillation–extraction (SDE), headspace enrichment). Nonvolatile impurities can thus be avoided and a defatting step is not necessary, but high-boiling compounds are partially lost and one has to be aware of possible reactions during the heat treatment.

The aqueous distillates are usually extracted with small portions of ethyl ether for performing GC or may be injected directly into an HPLC system.

Table 4 shows typical volatiles of roasted cocoa. The flavour chromatograms of different cocoas are rather similar, but the quantitative distribution of the single constituents and their total amounts vary distinctly with origin, fermentation, drying, roasting, degassing, alkalization or conching. Distillates of chocolate contain similar compounds in lower concentration and altered distribution.

Analysis of Key Compounds

Objective analytical data are necessary to relieve the industrial quality control of time-consuming sensory tests. For that purpose suitable indicators are needed to evaluate the flavour. The concentration of these compounds may be correlated with the cocoa flavour character. Several examples of indicative compounds in cocoa aroma follow, together with methods suitable for their estimation (GC; HPLC; UV, ultraviolet detector; ELCD, electrochemical detector): Fermentation degree – epicatechin (HPLC–ELCD), tetramethylpyrazine (GC or HPLC–UV); flavour grade cocoas – linalool (GC); roasting intensity – ratios of 2,5-dimethyl- to tetramethylpyrazine or trimethyl- to tetramethylpyrazine (GC or HPLC–UV), ratio of 5-methyl-2-phenyl-hex-2-enal to 2-phenylethanol (GC), dihydrohydroxy-maltol (GC or HPLC–ELCD–UV); intensity of degassing of cocoa masses – 3–methylbutanal (headspace GC). All the compounds with exception of epicatechin and 3-methylbutanal may be isolated by steam distillation.

Sensory Evaluation

Sensory evaluation is extremely important for cocoa process control and for the quality assurance of cocoa and chocolate products. Based on a tasting panel, which consists of trained and selected members, different sensory tests (flavour profile, difference and scoring tests) are used and the results statistically evaluated. *See* Sensory Evaluation, Taste

The Flavour Profile Test

This test is essential to obtain an assessment of the development of taste and flavour within the mouth as a result of individual sensory perceptions. The varying intensities of the specific characteristics are observed and evaluated. An evaluation plan is used which considers the flavour and texture characteristics and is completed by a numeric scale. Some characteristics of cocoa mass are raw, acid, flavourful, typical cocoa

Table 4. Selected aroma compounds identified in extracts of roasted cocoas. Usual concentration range (mg kg^{-1}): I, <0·1; II, 0·1–0·5, III, 0·5–2; IV, 2–10; V, >10. Succession of gas chromatographic retention times on a DB–Wax capillary column

Compound	Concentration range
3-Methylbutanal	IV
2,3-Butandione	III
3-Methyl-butan-1-oe	IV
Acetone	II
2-Methylpyrazine	III
2,5-Dimethylpyrazine	III
2,6-Dimethylpyrazine	II
2-Ethylpyrazine	I
2,3-Dimethylpyrazine	II
Methyltrithiomethane	I
2-Ethyl-5-methylpyrazine	II
2-Ethyl-3-methylpyrazine	II
Acetic acid	V
Trimethylpyrazine	III
Linalool oxide (*cis*-furanoid)	I
2,5-Dimethyl-3-ethylpyrazine	II
2-Furfural	II
Linalool oxide (*trans*-furanoid)	I
Tetramethylpyrazine	IV
Pyrrole	I
Benzyaldehyde	III
Linalool	II
2-5-Diethyl-3-methylpyrazine	I
5-Methyl-2-furfural	I
3-Methyl butanoic acid	V
Phenylacetaldehyde	IV
Acetophenone	III
Furfuryl alcohol	I
1-Phenylethanol	I
2-Phenethyl acetate	II
2-Hydroxy-3-methyl-2-cyclopenten-1-one (cyclotene)	II
Guajacol	I
Benzylalcohol	II
2-Phenylethanol	III
2-Phenylbut-2-enal	III
2-Phenethylamine	II
2-Acetylpyrrole	III
4-Methyl-2-phenylpent-2-enal	II
Phenol	I
3-Hydroxy-2-methyl-4-pyrone (maltol)	II
4-Hydroxy-2,5-dimethyl-3-(2*H*)-furanone (furanol)	III
5-Methyl-2-phenylhex-2-enal	III
2-Pyrrolecarbaldehyde	II
5-Methyl-2-pyrrolecarbaldehyde	II
2,3-Dihydro-3,5-dihydroxy-6-methyl-4-pyrone (dihydrohydroxymaltol)	IV
3,5-Dihydroxy-6-methyl-4-pyrone (hydroxymaltol)	II
5-(2-Hydroxyethyl)-4-methylthiazole	III
1,2-Benzenediol	III
Benzoic acid	II
2-Phenylacetic acid	IV
2-Phenylacetamide	IV

bitterness, burnt/bitter, astringent, off-taste (cooked, mouldy, smoky, ham, chemical, etc.). In addition, descriptors for plain chocolate are sweetness, aromatic, cocoa intensity, harmonic, persistent, caramel, vanilla, off-taste (cardboard, metallic, rancid, etc.). Intensities range from 0 to 4: absent, barely perceptible, weak, medium, strong. Texture descriptors are sticky/neat, coarse/smooth, dry/mellow, snappy/soft. *See* Sensory Evaluation, Descriptive Analysis

Difference Tests

These are preference tests to compare a sample against a control, in the simple form a 'paired test' or, with one sample duplicated, a 'triangular test'. Preferences and the intensity of deviations are reported. Triangular tests are used to check samples which have slight deviations from the standard.

Scoring Test

This test is used for production quality control and for assessing chocolate samples after periods of storage under different conditions. Sensory evaluation: 9–7, optimal to good; 6–4, satisfactory to sufficient; 3–1, lacking to unsatisfactory. *See* Sensory Evaluation, Sensory Rating and Scoring Methods

Tasting Method

Solid cocoa masses are chopped and tasted with a spoon. Cocoa powders are suspended to 10% in warm water, plain chocolates are broken into pieces and tasted.

Bibliography

Berbert PRF (1979) Contribuicao para o conhecimento dos acucares componentes da amendoa e do mel de cacau. *Revista Theobroma (Brasil)* 9: 55–61.
Biehl B (1989) Biochemie und Technologie der Kakaoaufbereitung: pH-kontrollierte Proteolyse und Fermentation; 47. Diskussionstagung, Forschungskreis der Ernährungsindustrie e.V., Kiel, April 1989. Forschungskreis der Ernährungsindustrie, Lavesstrasse 67, 3000 Hannover 1.
Carr JG (1982) Cocoa. *Economic Microbiology* 7: 275–292.
Fincke A (1989) Analytische und technologische Entwicklungen auf dem Gebiet der Kakaoerzeugnisse. *Lebensmittelchemie und gerichtliche Chemie* 43: 49–55.
Forsyth WGC and Quesnel VC (1963) The mechanism of cocoa curing. *Advances in Enzymology* 25: 457–495.
Holden M (1959) Processing of raw cocoa III: Enzymic aspects of cocoa fermentation. *Journal of the Science of Food and Agriculture* 12: 691–700.
Kirchhoff P-M and Biehl B (1989) Kinetics of the formation of free amino acids in cocoa seeds during fermentation. *Food Chemistry* 34: 161–179.
Lehrian DW and Patterson GR (1983) Cocoa fermentation. In: Rehm HJ and Reed G (eds) *Food and Feed Production with Microorganisms. Biotechnology*, vol. 5, pp 529–575. Weinheim: Verlag Chemie.
Martin Jr RA (1987) Chocolate. *Advances in Food Research* 31: 211–342.
Rohan TA (1963) *Processing of Raw Cocoa for the Market. FAO Agric. Stud.*, No. 60. Geneva: Food and Agriculture Organization.
Ziegleder G (1991) Composition of flavor extracts of raw and roasted cocoas. *Zeitschrift für Lebensmittel Untersuchung und Forschung* 192: 521–525.
Ziegleder G and Biehl B (1988) Analysis of cocoa flavour components and flavour precursors. In: Linskens HF and Jackson JF (eds) *Analysis of Nonalcoholic Beverages. Modern Methods of Plant Analysis*, new series, vol. 8, pp 321–393. Berlin: Springer-Verlag.

B. Biehl
Technical University, Braunschweig, FRG
G. Ziegleder
Fraunhofer-Institute, Munich, FRG

Production, Products and Uses

This article describes raw cocoa processing and the nature, the technologies and the use of cocoa powder and chocolate. These are made from defatted and non-defatted raw cocoa beans, respectively, which come from the fermented seeds of the tropical tree *Theobroma cacao* L. 'Cocoa' here is used as the overall term covering the finished products (cocoa powders and chocolate), the semifinished product (the raw cocoa beans) and the original seeds in the pods on the tree. In some countries 'cacao' is also used as this overall term.

Although cocoa products contain valuable nutrients, their special nature lies in the unique flavour which is not obtained from other plants. The unprocessed seeds, however, do not have this desired flavour, but instead an astringent unpleasant taste. Hence the unique genetic potential of the cocoa seeds is profoundly changed by processing and production techniques, and these are responsible for realizing or destroying the flavour potential.

'Processing' covers the total of all steps from harvesting the pods up to the stage where the raw cocoa beans come to the industrial manufacturer's plant for 'production' of the final goods.

Raw Cocoa Processing

General Outline

Processing usually includes the harvesting and breaking of the pods, extraction of the wet beans, transport (of pods or wet beans), fermentation in covered heaps, wooden boxes, or other containers for some days,

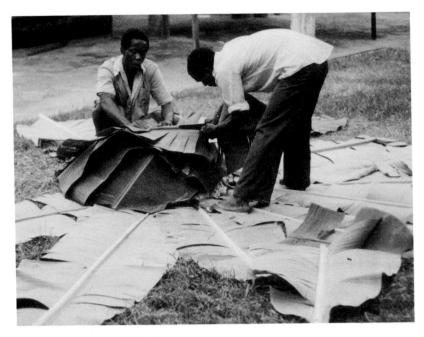

Fig. 1 Preparing a heap fermentation (CRIG, Ghana).

drying of the fermented beans, sorting, grading, sacking and storage. 'Beans' is a traditional term used commercially for seeds of cocoa at any stage of their processing. Wet beans are the seeds covered by the mucilaginous, sweet and acidic pulp or its remainder during fermentation. Raw cocoa beans are fermented and dried. The term 'fermentation' is used to describe the overall process of heaping wet cocoa beans for several days, the microbial pulp degradation, and also the endogenous post-mortem reactions, both enzymatic and nonenzymatic, that take place, in the seeds, which are induced by the pulp fermentation. They are responsible for the formation of flavour substances and flavour precursors.

At the cocoa plantations, fermentation and drying may primarily be looked upon as a curing process in order to stabilize the fresh beans by microbial degradation of the firmly adhering, perishable pulp, and by drying.

From this point of view the resulting qualities, especially the flavour potential, may be subordinate aspects. However, the quality is essential for subsequent manufacture of finished products. Raw cocoa quality may vary considerably depending on the manner of processing. First grades command an extra premium. However, since grading takes into account defects of raw cocoa, but not flavour intensities or flavour notes, there is no way of providing an extra premium for raw cocoa with superior flavour potential. Certain raw cocoa origins are given preference (and a higher price) by the industry and the market in virtue of experienced quality differences compared to less desirable origins. Some experts assume these differences to be due to climatic, geogenic or plant genetic particularities in the cocoa-growing countries. However, these differences may partially or even predominantly be due to traditional processing practices which are not uniform in the various producing countries. Handling and care during processing significantly affect raw cocoa quality and flavour. Nothing is known about the genetic influence on flavour potential of raw cocoas except for a difference between Criollo and Forastero types. There is inadequate knowledge about the genetic diversity, the variability of the planted cocoa trees and the heterogeneity of clonal plantings with respect to their influence on flavour quality.

For improving raw cocoa quality, attempts have been made to modify the methods of fermentation in several cocoa-growing countries, based on empirical or scientific concepts. Few have been applied to commercial fermentation. They will not be described in this article. Instead, representative processing methods as practised in Brazil, Ghana and Malaysia, variable courses of fermentation, and effective modifications will be described. The reader is referred to earlier reviews cited below for detailed information. Since cocoa is processed in traditional ways, earlier reviews still give valuable information.

Practice of Fermentation

The different methods of cocoa fermentation are mostly developed from local traditions in the various cocoa-growing countries. Most of the common practices correspond to the description in the following sections. Heap fermentation and box fermentation as the prevailing methods will be described briefly (Figs 1 and 2):

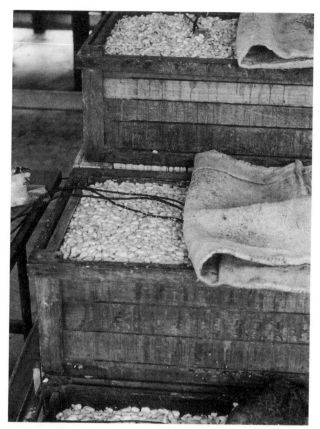

Fig. 2 Experimental shallow box fermentation (MARDI, Malaysia).

compared to boxes, the bottom layer and the surface layer are large, which promotes not only aeration but also cooling. Thus, at least one turning after 48 h is necessary. The highest temperature may normally be found 5 cm beneath the surface.

Box Fermentation

Boxes are placed under roofs and are made from locally indigenous timbers. They are jacked up and their bottom (sometimes also the walls) are perforated to allow drainage. On large plantations the fermentary would consist of batteries of several open boxes ($1.0 \times 1.0 \times 1.0$ m) which facilitate turning from one box to the next. Alternatively, long boxes (e.g. 10 m length) can be divided by partitions. Depending on the harvest, the cocoa is filled up to 100 cm in depth.

Compared to average-sized heaps (about 50–80 cm top height), the 'deep box' (100 cm) depth requires a longer time for fermentation because of reduced aeration (almost exclusively from the top).

In Malaysia, shallow boxes have been introduced to overcome the lack of uniformity (see below and Fig. 2). Cascades of shallow boxes are used in large estates, each of which may have a capacity of several tonnes, but a height not exceeding 35 cm. Alternative fermenters have been subdivided by vertical or horizontal slits for improving aeration. However, the cocoa cannot be turned, and niches of fungal growth develop near to the cold corners. Revolving barrels which are provided with perforations for aeration and with some device for effective mixing during gentle rotations allow quite uniform fermentations. Aeration, pulp loss and water evaporation are significantly increased by frequent turnings.

Standardized methods – such as the heap and box fermentations described here – are used at well-established farms or estates but they are not in common use elsewhere. Any kind of box or other receptacle such as troughs, frames, baskets, boats or bags can be found to serve for curing widely varying quantities of wet cocoa. Alternatively, the wet cocoa is left on the ground or on a drying platform where a partial 'fermentation' may occur, depending on the depth of the layer, occasional heaping and weather conditions. These irregular types of curing probably play a subordinate role in most of the raw cocoa-producing countries, but they contribute to the non-uniform low-quality cocoas as they appear on the market. However, among those procedures which create low-quality products when performed without care, some are used for producing high-quality cocoas, as is reported from Ecuador, where in some estates the wet beans are spread at day but heaped overnight. This reminds us that cocoa fermentation is still basically an empirical procedure.

In both cases, ripe pods are harvested and the husks are opened by means of a cutlass or wooden billet. The wet seeds are removed from the husk and placenta and are collected for transport. Abnormal, black, infested or clustered beans and foreign matter are removed. The wet cocoa is piled up in heaps or boxes of variable capacity allowing drainage of sweatings through the bottom. Care is taken that mixing can be carried out by turning the fermenting cocoa upside down and inside out. The wet cocoa is covered with banana leaves or jute bags and is left by itself for 5–7 days, interrupted by one or more turnings after 24, 48 or 72 h. After a given time, or following an assessment of its appearance and odour, the fermented cocoa is transferred to a dryer.

Heap Fermentation (Fig. 1)

The typical succession of microbial pulp degradation as described below occurs whenever wet cocoa is piled up for several days. Heap fermentation is used in West Africa. The heap is prepared outdoors on banana leaves layered on wooden sticks to allow better drainage. The cocoa is covered by the same leaves by folding up the peripheral ends in such a way that rain is kept off. The amount of wet cocoa (80–1000 kg) depends on the harvest. Due to the flat, conical shape of the heap

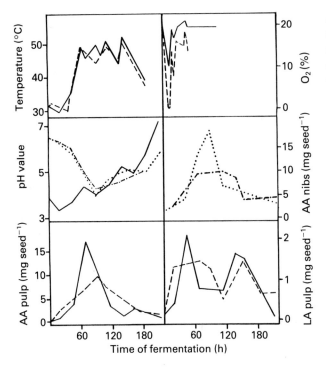

Fig. 3 Shallow box fermentation (simplified). Course in the pulp (——, top layer; – – – –, middle layer) and nibs (· · · · ·, top layer; – · – · – ·, middle layer). AA is acetic acid, LA is L-lactic acid. Turning after 44 h, 92 h and 139 h. (From Meyer B *et al.*, 1989).

Standard Course of Fermentation

The progress of fermentation is characterized by visual changes and changes of odour. Most typical are colour changes and the accumulation of a red sap in the beans beyond the shell. The internal appearance of dried beans taken at regular stages from the fermenter also indicates the progress of fermentation. Seeds appear slatey as long as anthocyanins have not yet been released from their intact storage cells. After seed death they would dry to compact beans, violet in colour, with the shells sticking strongly to the nibs. When fermentation is completed the nibs would turn brown and the beans retain a plump, porous structure, with a loosened shell. This is the type of bean required for marketing. For grading on the market, the internal appearance of beans is taken to estimate the so-called 'degree of fermentation' in a cut test. *See* Colours, Properties and Determination of Natural Pigments

After breaking the harvested pods the wet cocoa is inoculated by spores of an ubiquitous range of airborne microorganisms. The course of fermentation may be subdivided into four stages (I–IV). The succession of events generally is as follows (Fig. 3):

I. Pulp. In the mucous, acidic (pH 3·5–4·0) pulp, anaerobic, microbial metabolism of sugars starts immediately, with alcoholic fermentation first dominating over the lactic acid fermentation. Pulp is drained off. Carbon dioxide is produced which displaces air from the box.

Seeds. The majority of seeds at this stage are still alive (germination test).

II. Pulp. As more pulp has been drained off and sugar metabolized, less carbon dioxide is produced. Consequently, more air is taken up by the pulp, giving rise to oxidative formation of acetic acid, an exothermic process heating up the cocoa from the ambient temperature to 45–52°C. Aeration would now be randomized and accelerated by turning.

Seeds. Both, the temperature increase to ≥ 45°C and the uptake of acetic acid kills the seeds. A maximum level of acetic acid produced in the pulp is followed by a maximum amount of acetic acid absorbed in the beans. The average pH value in the nibs drops from 6·4 to, mostly 4·0–4·7. Oxygen is quantitatively consumed in the fermenting pulp, keeping the nib under anaerobic conditions and allowing post-mortem reactions in the absence of oxygen.

III. Pulp. As acetic acid production slows down because of exhaustion of substrate, bacterial oxidation of acetic acid causes a slow increase of the pulp pH. The temperature may drop because of lack of substrates and reduced microbial activity in the pulp, which is still acidic (pH 5·0). Lactic acid formation, which has been suppressed during stage II, may increase once more.

Seeds. Most of the post-mortem enzymatic and non-enzymatic reactions in the seeds have been completed by this time. However, stage III and stage IV seem to be important to ensure browning of the beans during subsequent drying. Although no experimental explanation is available, it is probable that developing aerophilic organisms may now help to increase shell permeability. This stage (up to stage IV) has also been found to be necessary to produce maximum levels of flavour precursors in the resulting raw cocoa. *See* Lactic Acid Bacteria

IV. Although this fourth stage cannot clearly be distinguished from the foregoing one, it merits special attention for correct termination of fermentation to avoid subsequent overfermentation. Now, after pulp degradation, a buoyant air flow from the bottom to the top of the hot cocoa provides the beans with access to air. A second temperature increase indicates a new aerobic microbial activity on the shells, which will spread to the nibs if drying is delayed.

Overfermentation subsequent to stage IV is characterized by a steep increase of the pH value first at the surface of the beans and later in the nibs. It is accompanied by a pronounced darkening or even blackening of the beans and a characteristic hammy off-flavour which persists in the raw cocoa to an extent which depends on how severely this process took place before drying. Overfermentation may be looked upon as a direct aerophilic microbial attack on the nibs, destroying the cocoa flavour potential. Depending on the bean surface moisture at stage IV, the transition to overfermentation may be slow or very rapid. Wet beans may turn black overnight and may evolve a typical strong hammy off-flavour.

Variables in the Course of Fermentation

Rate of Fermentation

The above description may give the incorrect impression of a uniform process running on a constant timescale. The stages described in the previous section and illustrated in Fig. 3, however, are not bound to a fixed time but may be considerably shorter or longer.

The main reason is aeration: the more the wet cocoa is aerated in stages I and II, the quicker the temperature increases, the quicker the peak of acetic acid appears and the pH value of the nib decreases. The described succession of events is not changed. Wet cocoa containing ≥ 1.0 ml of pulp per seed would pass through an ethanol fermentation even under continued aeration during stage I. In contrast, if no aeration is allowed at stage I, the pulp of wet cocoa may appear unchanged for several days. Lactic acid fermentation would slowly acidify the seeds at a low temperature. Forced aeration at stages III or IV causes a quick pH increase in the nibs.

Thus, if fermentations are terminated at a prefixed time, e.g. after six days, the cocoa may be at stage III, stage IV or overfermented, revealing a low or a high pH value in the nibs, respectively. In practice, aeration is intensified by turning, batch size, type of fermenter and pulp volume per seed: the smaller the batch size, the larger the specific surface for air uptake. The surface area is also influenced by the type of fermenter. A small conical heap (e.g. 250 kg) is much more aerated than a deep box (100 cm depth). A shallow box (30 cm depth) helps to increase surface aeration. The influence of pulp volume on aeration is described below.

Nonuniformity in the Course of Fermentation

Not only variation in rates of fermentation but also local differences in the fermenting heaps or boxes are due to inhomogeneous aeration. At stage I, oxygen is accessible only at the surface layer, where the process shown in Fig. 3 is accelerated, while the lower layers are still under a carbon dioxide atmosphere. The hot zone of pulp oxidation and acetic acid production slowly moves down to the bottom. If pulp volume is large and the cocoa is not turned, the anaerobic, cold situation (stage I) in the bottom layer may persist during the time the top layer goes through stages I to IV. After drying, the bottom layer would produce slatey or violet beans, whereas the top layer would consist of properly fermented or overfermented brown beans. Turning after 24 and 48 h reduces this inhomogeneity but not enough to eliminate this effect entirely. While this type of non-uniformity is typical for fermentation of wet cocoa beans with a fully developed pulp layer, the situation may be different with beans from overripe pods covered by a thin layer of pulp. Too many turnings would reduce the capacity of the pulp to fulfil the entire sequence of stages I to IV and a premature overfermentation would result. Additionally, beans in unturned, aerated niches of the batches in boxes or heaps may undergo abnormal changes due to heat loss, drying out or fungal attack.

Effect of Harvest and Postharvest Treatment on Fermentation and Raw Cocoa Quality

Controlled aeration is helpful in overcoming nonuniformity but does not help in avoiding strong nib acidification and low flavour quality. The minimal pH value in the beans during enzymatic reactions at stage II is essential for the formation of flavour precursors rather than the final nib pH. With the large pulp volume per seed, an excess of aeration during the first stages accelerates acidification, but does not limit acetic acid production. However, the composition and the volume of the pulp depends on harvest and postharvest treatments, and pulp preconditioning allows a reduction in nib acidification and an increase in flavour potential. Ten days of open-air 'postharvest pod storage' or several hours of 'bean spreading' for pulp drying after breaking the pods significantly reduces pulp volume, pulp water and pulp sugar per seed (Table 1). The pulp surface layer is considerably reduced from ≥ 1.0 to ≤ 0.6 ml of pulp per seed. After proper preconditioning, subsequent shallow box fermentation proceeds aerobically in stage I and, correspondingly, there is an early steep temperature increase, but the formation and the accumulation of acetic acid in pulp and nibs in the course of fermentation is considerably reduced (Fig. 4). It is assumed that early aeration of a thin pulp surface layer enhances respiration of sugars by yeasts and reduces alcoholic fermentation beneath the surface in the voluminous pulp containing $\geq 10\%$ of sugars.

The important pulp/seed relation depends on both genetic and physiological parameters: large seeds bear less pulp per seed surface area than small seeds. However, seed size does not depend only on genetics. Pods and seeds may be considerably smaller than usual when growing under adverse conditions, e.g. during severe drought. Furthermore, the pulp:seed ratio is

Table 1. Changes in the pulp during pod storage and bean spreading

Wet beans	Pulp volume (ml seed^{-1})	Pulp water (g seed^{-1})	Sucrose + glucose (mg seed^{-1})[e]	Reducing sugars (mg seed^{-1})[f]
Malaysia, ripe (from unstored pods)[a]	1.19 ± 0.14	0.95 ± 0.12	121.3 ± 57.1	
Malaysia, ripe (from pods stored for 10 days)[b]	0.74 ± 0.06	0.58 ± 0.05	39.9 ± 5.4	
Malaysia (from unstored pods after spreading)[c]	0.46 ± 0.06	0.34 ± 0.12	79.2 ± 32.3	
Ghana, ripe (from unstored pods)[d]	0.84	0.69		91.2
Ghana (from pods stored for 7 days)[d]	0.55	0.41		68.6

Mean values and standard deviations from samples of [a] 10, [b] four experiments with 1000 pods each.
[c] Samples from four experiments with 130 kg of wet cocoa, each of different ripeness, sun spreading and surface drying for several hours.
[d] From one experiment with 10 pods each.
[e] Estimated polarographically.
[f] 3,5-dinitrosalicylic acid (DNSA) method (Biehl B *et al.*, 1989).

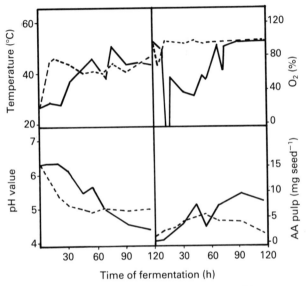

Fig. 4 Shallow box fermentation with spread beans (– – – –) and unspread beans (——). AA is acetic acid. One turning after 66 h. From Biehl B, Meyer B, Mamot Bin Said and Samarakoddy RJ (1990) Bean spreading: a method for pulp preconditioning to impair strong nib acidification during cocoa fermentation in Malaysia. *Journal of the Science of Food and Agriculture* 51: 35–45, with permission of the Society of Chemical Industry, London.

significantly reduced during ripening. Large pulp volumes per seed from unripe seeds cause badly aerated slimy fermentations. In overripe pods the pulp volume is reduced as with stored pods, leading to well-aerated, rapid fermentations. Raw cocoa flavour characteristics with particular origins may depend to a large extent on these physiological stages of wet cocoa due to local traditions in postharvest treatments. The ripeness of pods harvested in Malaysia or in Ghana are quite different.

Seasonal effects on fermentation and raw cocoa quality are often due to these differences in the pulp.

Finally, delay of fermentation after pod breaking causes loss of pulp. If wet cocoa is exposed to rain, subsequent fermentation may lack sugar for heating and acetic acid production, and would proceed in an erratic way.

Drying

Enzyme-controlled browning reactions which do not occur before drying are essential for quality.

For sun drying, the beans are spread on the ground, on mats or on wooden floors raised from the ground and protected against rain. Care is taken to move the drying cocoa. The layers of cocoa are made shallow or high to regulate the time of drying. Five to seven days are usually necessary for reducing the water content to less than 7.0%, a limit for fungal growth. *See* Drying, Drying Using Natural Radiation

For artificial drying, wood fires or oil burners are connected to a flue under a floor of closely spaced slats. There are many devices of this type for passing a stream of hot air, but not of smoke, through the layer of cocoa beans. The industry rejects smoky beans but the smell of smoke may be confused with a hammy off-flavour of overfermented beans. On large estates, different types of industrial driers are used for effective, short-time drying. *See* Drying, Theory of Air Drying

The first stage of drying should be effective in order to avoid overfermentation or fungal growth on the wet cocoa, if the internal pH value is high. At this stage, there is no danger in using hot air (e.g. 100°C), although the temperature of the beans should not exceed 40–60°C. In a shallow layer of cocoa beans, water evaporation will keep the beans cool. However, hot air flow through a deep layer (≥ 10 cm) would heat the beans excessively. After external dryness of the beans has been attained, the second stage of drying can be continued slowly to facilitate enzymatic browning in the nibs and to allow moisture equilibrium in the beans from the wet core to the dry surface. Artificial drying may be interrupted for a while by a resting period. In a third stage, the cocoa should effectively be dried <7·5% water (w/w), preferably in a stream of warm (<60°C) but not hot air.

Rewetting, polishing and drying raw cocoa is practised locally to improve the external appearance, especially of mouldy beans, but shell breaking and reinfection of the nibs may result. Rewetting also increases browning of violet beans.

After drying, the raw cocoa is sorted by removing flat, broken, externally mouldy beans and foreign matter and by sieving (in the case of nonuniform bean size) to meet the quality standards. Locally, batches from different origins may be blended to reach the maximum percentage of the particular visible bean defects which are allowed in the official grading system.

Storage

Provided good storage conditions, properly processed raw cocoa can be stored for years without any unwanted, serious sensory or analytical indication of loss of quality or of spoilage. However, once processed, raw cocoa usually travels a long way from the tropical origin to the final manufacturing plant, being subjected to several risks underway. These risks are primarily water and high air humidity, insect infestation and consequences of improper processing. *See* Storage Stability, Parameters Affecting Storage Stability

In addition to general rules for storage in tropical and temperate climates, the hygroscopy of raw cocoa beans must be considered. Dry raw cocoa containing <7·5% water will not be attacked by fungi. According to moisture absorption isotherms this bean moisture would not be exceeded at <80% relative humidity. However, at a high level of air humidity, any reduction in air temperature (e.g. during shipping) would cause damage by condensation and mould growth. Residual humidity from fast drying must be considered. Repeated moisture determinations are necessary in every lot. Fungal spores are ubiquitous. However, mouldy beans resulting from fermentation and drying increase the danger of fungal growth at a critical level of moisture. Thermophilic and xerophilic fungi such as *Aspergillus glaucus*, *A. fumigatus*, *Penicillium* spp. and *Mucor* sp. have been found to occur during both processing and storage. Internal mould is further facilitated on broken beans and on injured shells. Brittle shells, particularly from overfermented or rewetted cocoa, not only increase the danger of mould but also increase the amount of broken beans during transport and stacking of bags. *See* Spoilage, Moulds in Food Spoilage

Out of nine insect species, listed by Rohan (see Bibliography), four were mentioned to be important threats to stored raw cocoa in the tropics: *Cadra*

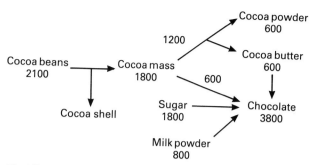

Fig. 5 Products derived from cocoa beans. The figures are approximate and in 1000 tonnes.

cautella, *Lasioderma serricorne*, *Araecerus fasciculatus* and *Tribolium castaneum*. *Ephistia elutella*, the cocoa moth, is only found in temperate climates. In tropical countries, insects are controlled by fumigation of raw cocoa using the gases methyl bromide or phosphine applied to stacks of stored cocoa under a gas-proof and water-proof polythene sheet for 1·5 h. The gas is then extracted by fans. The sheets are left to protect the cocoa against uptake of moisture and insects. *See* Fumigants; Insect Pests, Problems Caused by Insects and Mites

Production of Cocoa Powder and Semifinished Products

Cocoa Products

Basically two products are derived solely from cocoa beans: chocolate and cocoa powder. These products are interrelated, and two intermediate products play an important role, namely cocoa mass and cocoa butter. This relationship is made clear in Fig. 5. The system shown in Fig. 5 is not fully in balance. The chocolate industry needs a certain quantity of cocoa butter and this implies that a fixed quantity of cocoa powder is also produced. However, the demand for cocoa powder does not always meet this volume. As a result, the price of cocoa butter is usually substantially higher than that of cocoa powder. The relatively high price of cocoa butter has made it attractive to lipid chemists to look for cheaper fats which could replace cocoa butter. This is not easy as cocoa butter has unique properties, especially hardness and melting behaviour. In the course of time, cocoa butter substitutes (CBSs) were developed, mostly based on palm kernel fat. These are used in combination with cocoa powder for manufacturing imitation chocolate, or coatings (for biscuits, cakes, ice cream, etc). Recently, ways have been found to separate the desired triglycerides from other fats and to put them together in the right proportion, thus obtaining a fat that closely resembles cocoa butter. Such a fat is called a cocoa butter equivalent (CBE) and can replace cocoa

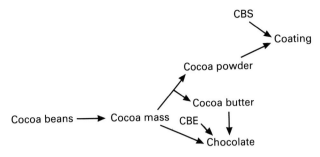

Fig. 6 The use of alternative fats to cocoa butter.

butter in chocolate. There use is not legally permitted in important chocolate markets like the EEC, USA and Canada. The use of alternative fats is shown in Fig. 6. *See* Lipids, Classification

Concentration and specialization have taken place in the cocoa processing industry on a large scale since the World War II. In the past, each chocolate factory produced its own cocoa butter. Thus, it also produced cocoa powder as a by-product. However, cocoa powder of a quality meeting the standards required by industrial users is such a specialized product that today it is mainly manufactured by a small number of very large companies, most of them located in the Netherlands. Thus, cocoa powder is by no means a by-product any more. The cocoa pressing industry considers both cocoa butter and cocoa powder as main products, each with strict quality specifications. The cocoa butter is supplied to the chocolate industry. The pressing industry also supplies the chocolate industry with cocoa mass. Again, this is a very specialized business. Each chocolate factory has its own very tight specifications for flavour and other quality aspects. For a chocolate factory, receiving cocoa mass and cocoa butter in bulk from outside manufacturers contributes highly to the sanitation in its plant. Instead of the crude, dusty cocoa beans, clean materials arrive now. Specialization and bulk delivery is also undertaken by the chocolate industry itself, supplying chocolate in large slabs, or even as a liquid in tank lorries, to confectionery or biscuit manufacturers.

Quality Aspects

Cocoa powder is sold in retail packages to consumers. However, most cocoa powder reaches the consumer as a colour and flavour in other products, like dessert powders, sterilized chocolate milk, chocolate cake, ice cream, etc. Most of the cocoa powder produced is sold as an ingredient to other food manufacturers. Such a product should obviously have the necessary quality aspects to meet the needs of the user, regarding microbiology, consistency, purity and other factors. In the case of cocoa powder this can be fulfilled only when

maintaining strict good manufacturing practices, the reason being that there are a number of problems which put cocoa powder in a high-risk catogory:

● Cocoa beans undergo a fermentation process, which leaves very high bacteria counts on the bean shell.
● During the fermentation the temperature goes up to 50°C, which leaves thermoresistant spores on the bean. These may interfere with the sterilization process of chocolate milk.
● The cocoa beans, after fermentation, are dried in the open air, allowing contamination with bird droppings, etc. Salmonella bacteria can thus be found on crude cocoa beans.
● Bacteria which are present in cocoa mass are surrounded by fat during the grinding process. The fat gives them good protection and it has been shown that Salmonellae can live for months in chocolate. Also, the bacteria will be protected in the stomach against its natural acidity, when chocolate is eaten.
● Cocoa powder is used in many different foodstuffs, made with different manufacturing processes, requiring different shelf lives, having different moisture contents, etc. As the cocoa manufacturer does not always know how the powder will be used, all of the product must meet the strictest hygiene specifications. *See* Spoilage, Bacterial Spoilage

Environment

The cocoa-processing industry is not one of the major polluters of the environment. The raw materials and the products are simply too expensive to be discarded. Of course, there are the general problems of each factory like noise and high, ugly buildings. How these can be avoided is well known and is taken into consideration when new chocolate factories are built. The main problem comes from the smell of exhaust gasses: air blown through the grinding systems and combustion gas from the roasters. These gases also contain dust. To collect the dust, cyclones are used on a large scale in the cocoa industry. Biological filters are being tested for the removal of odours but they have not been completely successful. The present method of solving the problem is to build high chimneys. Cocoa bean processing gives one waste product: the shell, about 10% of the weight of the beans. This loose material is usually ground to reduce its volume and sold to fertilizer or cattle feed manufacturers. Burning the shell could be worthwhile when energy costs are high, but introduces the problem of removing large quantities of dust from the combustion gas.

Production of Cocoa Mass

All cocoa beans are initially turned into cocoa mass. The necessary processes are illustrated in Fig. 7. The word

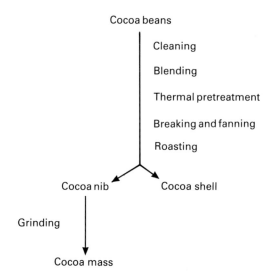

Cocoa beans
— Cleaning
— Blending
— Thermal pretreatment
— Breaking and fanning
— Roasting

Cocoa nib   Cocoa shell

Grinding

Cocoa mass

Fig. 7 The production of cocoa mass.

'nib' is used in all languages to indicate the broken pieces of the kernel of the cocoa bean. Cocoa mass contains approximately 55% cocoa butter. The fat is liquid after the roasting and grinding procedures, which makes the whole mass liquid. It can be pumped and transported in tank lorries.

Cleaning

Cocoa beans, from silo storage or directly from their burlap bags, first pass through cleaning machines: screens, magnets and controlled air streams. Extraneous materials removed include sticks, stones, string and metal objects.

Blending

Substantial variety in flavour exists among cocoa beans from different producing countries. It is seldom that one batch of beans will be used exclusively in a formula. One reason is that the blending provides the opportunity to obtain a certain flavour. Another reason stems from the inconsistency of cocoa beans in flavour and other quality aspects. Batches of cocoa beans show variations from one locality to another, due to differences in the weather during growth and ripening, from differences in fermentation and other variations in processing conditions. Blending will contribute to uniformity.

Thermal Pretreatment

An important quality aspect in cocoa bean processing is the removal of the cocoa shell. The shell, as the covering of the kernel, is always greatly polluted with sand, high bacteria counts and pesticide residues. Depending on the fermentation, the shell, however, often sticks to the kernel, which prevents easy removal. Recently machines have been introduced which loosen the shells by means of a thermal shock. This is achieved with hot air, saturated steam or infrared radiation.

Breaking and Fanning

To remove the shell, the beans are first broken between adjustable toothed rollers. The broken pieces are subsequently separated in fractions by sieving. Each fraction is treated with a stream of air which carries away the light shell pieces. This breaking and fanning process is often referred to as 'winnowing'.

Roasting

The roasting process is needed for the development of the typical flavour of cocoa. The time–temperature conditions are critical for obtaining the desired flavour. These depend very much on the type of roasting machine used, so it is not possible to give exact conditions. In the literature, temperatures from 70 to 200°C are mentioned. The amount of heat applied is considerably less than is used in roasting coffee. The roasting conditions also depend on the use that will be made of the beans. Certain types of milk chocolate require beans with a very mild roasting. On the other hand, when the pressing process is involved, a high roast will be used in order to obtain a sufficient reduction in the bacteria count and, in particular, a good reduction in the thermoresistant spores.

There are many types of roasting equipment, and new developments appear frequently. The latest method involves roasting the mass instead of the beans or nib. This is done continuously in thin-layer columns and gives very good control over the roasting conditions. However, a never-ending discussion is going on regarding whether it is better to roast whole beans or nibs. One of the arguments is the need to have particles of a uniform size, to obtain uniform heating. It may seem that pieces of broken kernel are not very uniform, but whole beans also differ considerably in size. Another argument relates to microbiological aspects. The bacteria present are on the shell and by removing the shell first the material enters the roasting (=sterilization) process with a lower initial bacteria count.

Grinding and Refining

The next step is grinding of the cocoa nib particles. The nib consists of 55% cocoa butter and 45% solid material coming from the plant cells. The latter must be ground very finely. When eating chocolate or drinking chocolate milk, no grittiness should be felt in the mouth. For both cocoa powder and chocolate it is important that the final particle size distribution is narrow. This facilitates the pressing operation and improves the

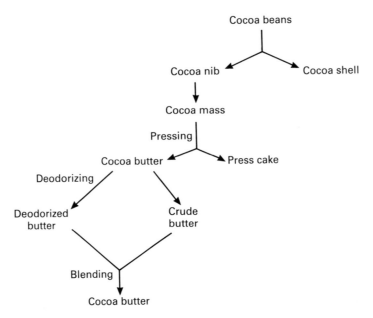

Fig. 8 The production of cocoa butter.

rheological properties of chocolate. The desired fineness (15–70 μm) and particle size distribution are reached in several successive grinding steps. Pregrinding of the large and hard nib particles is done in disc mills, hammer mills or pin mills. To reach the ultimate fineness, mass for pressing is refined in modern versions of the triple stone mill, or in vertical ball mills (attrittors). In the chocolate industry, roller mills with five rolls are most commonly used for refining the mass. These are also used to grind the chocolate mass, after adding pre-ground sugar and milk powder. *See* Milling, Characteristics of Milled Products

Types

Cocoa mass may be used for the production of chocolate, or for pressing, i.e. the production of cocoa butter and cocoa powder. The difference between these two types of cocoa mass are the bean blend, fineness, microbiological condition, among others.

For chocolate, many manufacturers prefer beans from Ghana and Nigeria on account of their desirable flavour attributes. For the highest qualities, South American, so-called flavour beans, may also be added to the blend.

Although mass for all purposes needs to be completely safe from the bacteriological point of view, cocoa powder requires, moreover, that thermoresistant spores are absent. This condition must already have been reached in the mass, which tolerates higher temperatures than cocoa powder.

Mass for pressing is also already alkalized. This process will be discussed below.

Packaging and Shelf Life

When cocoa mass has to be stored or transported, it is usually packed into 30 kg cardboard boxes with a plastic liner or bag inside. In Europe and the USA most of the transport takes place in liquid form.

Cocoa mass has a very good shelf life. The solid particles are protected by a fat with a high degree of saturation. Moreover, cocoa contains powerful natural antioxidants. These conditions also apply to cocoa beans. If the moisture content of the beans is well under control, their shelf life will be several years. *See* Antioxidants, Natural Antioxidants

Production of Cocoa Butter

Cocoa mass contains 55% cocoa butter. Part of this can be extracted by mechanical pressing. The solids which stay in the press contain 22% fat, or even as low as 10%. These press cakes are ground to cocoa powder. The cocoa butter is filtered and part of it is deodorized. The production process is illustrated in Fig. 8.

Pressing

The cocoa mass is pumped to horizontal hydraulic presses, with pots lined up face to face, each equipped with very fine mesh metal filter screens. When all the pots are filled with mass at a temperature of 90°C, the hydraulic ram is set in motion and the cocoa butter begins to flow through the screens on both sides of each pot. The pressure then increases to 400 bars. The hard cocoa cakes remaining are then discharged from the press. The cocoa butter collected from the press is not 'clean', having carried with it a small amount of tiny nonfat particles. It is therefore filtered through filter paper.

Deodorization and Blending

Crude cocoa butter has a strong flavour. This is desirable in dark chocolate. However, in milk chocolate much more cocoa butter is used and the cocoa flavour would become too strong, suppressing the milk flavour. Thus, buyers are stipulating a cocoa butter with a weak flavour, or no flavour at all. This is reached by steam deodorization of the cocoa butter and blending crude and deodorized butter to the desired flavour. This is controlled by sensory testing, or a chemical method, the determination of the flavour profile. Crude cocoa butter, being a natural product, has a rather inconsistent flavour strength. Even if crude cocoa butter is asked for, some blending with deodorized butter is performed to standardize the flavour. *See* Sensory Evaluation, Taste

Properties

Cocoa butter is one of the most expensive natural fats. This is due to its unique melting behaviour. Cocoa butter has a much narrower melting range than any other fat. This quality is fundamental to chocolate. Chocolate should be hard – even in hot weather – and it should not stick to the fingers. On eating, the cocoa butter in the chocolate should melt completely in the mouth. If this does not happen – even if only a few per cent of the fat does not melt – a waxy sensation is noticed (this occurs, for instance, with cocoa butter substitutes made from hydrogenated oils). At room temperature, a substantial part of the triglycerides in cocoa butter are solid (about 60%), whereas all become liquid in the mouth. The melting takes up a considerable amount of heat, causing a cooling in the mouth which greatly contributes to the pleasant taste sensation when eating chocolate. The narrow melting range of cocoa butter is also important in the production of chocolate. When the chocolate is cooled and the fat solidifies, a considerable decrease in volume takes place. This contraction makes it easy to release chocolate articles from their moulds.

Types

The above discussion has been restricted to the processing of sound cocoa beans, from which the shell has been properly removed. The fat derived from this raw material is called prime pure pressed cocoa butter. In practice, not all cocoa beans that are harvested are of a good quality. Even if the beans are unripe, mouldy or smoky they contain a fat that can be made fully fit for human consumption by refining. When processing

subgrade cocoa beans, it is difficult to remove their shells. Such beans are processed whole in continuous expeller presses. The resulting press cake still holds another 10% of fat, which can be obtained by solvent extraction. The remaining solids are, of course, not edible and are best put back on the land as a fertilizer. Although the fat will be edible after refining, the quality is inferior to the prime pure pressed butter. It is less hard and shows a smaller volume contraction. The following types of subgrade cocoa fat are recognized by the Codex Alimentarius:

(1) Expeller cocoa butter: the fat extracted by means of mechanical pressing from material which has approximately the composition of whole cocoa beans.
(2) Solvent-extracted cocoa butter: the fat obtained from cocoa beans or cocoa waste materials by means of extraction with permitted solvents.
(3) Refined cocoa butter: any of the fats obtained in the ways mentioned above and afterwards fully refined according to the standard processing techniques for edible oils and fats.
(4) Cocoa fat: fat extracted from waste materials and having a quality below certain standards.

The above processing options are summarized in Fig. 9.

Packaging, Transport and Shelf Life

Much like cocoa mass, cocoa butter is packed in 30 kg slabs or transported and stored in a liquid form. The shelf life of cocoa butter is good, due to its high degree of saturation and the shelf life of solid cocoa butter is several months to a year, if properly packed and stored.

Production of Cocoa Powder

The press cakes are ground to powder, which is packed after complete cooling. The alkalizing process can be used to create many types of cocoa powder with differing colours. The production of cocoa powder is shown in Fig. 10.

Alkalizing

The alkalizing process was invented in the first half of the last century in Holland. It improves the quality of cocoa powder in two ways:

(1) It takes away the slight acid taste of cocoa.
(2) It makes the colour darker. This is due to condensation reactions forming high-molecular-weight coloured products. Careful control of the reactions can lead to different shades of colour: orange, red, brown and even black is possible.

Alkalizing consists of treating the cocoa with a solution

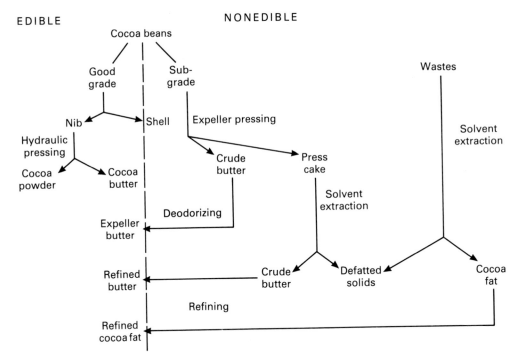

EDIBLE   NONEDIBLE

Fig. 9 Types of cocoa butter.

of an alkali, mostly potash. Legally, the maximum amount of potash which may be used is 3%, calculated on the nib. The treatment can be performed with the nib, mass, press cake or powder. The specific colour is reached by choice of the reaction conditions: temperature, time, amount and concentration of the alkaline solution, and other factors.

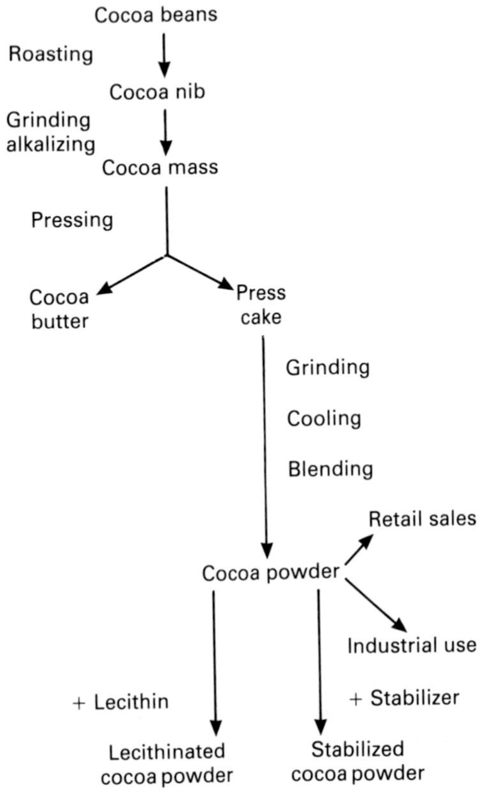

Grinding, Cooling and Blending of Cocoa Cake

The press cakes are broken and then ground to powder in pin or other mills. The cocoa powder leaves the mill hot. It should be completely cooled before packing, otherwise the setting fat will turn it into hard lumps inside the package.

Blending of pieces of broken cake before grinding allows standardization of the colour, or the preparation of blends with intermediate colours.

Types

Variations in the two main processes leads to the formation of hundreds of different types of cocoa powder. The pressing can be performed to a fat content in the cake of 20% (giving cocoa powder) or to 10% (giving low-fat cocoa powder), while the alkalizing process creates many different colours. Cocoa powder with 20% fat is the common household type. The food industry uses mostly low-fat cocoa powder (10%), in many different colours.

For use in certain cocoa-flavoured products, some special types of cocoa powder have been developed. Lecithinated cocoa powder contains 5% of soya lecithin. Owing to its fat content, cocoa powder is difficult to wet and to disperse in water. Even in hot

Fig. 10 The production of cocoa powder.

Production, Products and Uses

water or milk, lumps will be formed easily. Lecithin can improve these properties by its action as a wetting agent. Five per cent of soya lecithin is intensively mixed with cocoa powder and the resulting lecithinated powder is agglomerated with sugar. This gives the so-called instant cocoa, which can be put directly into cold milk. *See* Emulsifiers, Organic Emulsifiers

Stabilized cocoa powder contains about 2% carrageenan. This is a polysaccharide derived from seaweed. It prevents the cocoa powder from settling in sterilized chocolate milk. *See* Stabilizers, Types and Function

Packaging, Transport and Shelf Life

Paper or tin retail packaging is well known. For bulk deliveries, 25 kg (or 50 lb) multiple paper bags are commonly used. Loose bulk delivery or storage of cocoa powder is difficult. The fat-containing fine powder tends to stick and to block pipelines for pneumatic transport. Only large users, in cooperation with large suppliers, have developed workable bulk systems. The shelf life of cocoa powder is excellent. Even after 10 years the flavour is good when packed in air- and moisture-proof containers. Only some fading of the colour may be noticed, comparable with fat bloom on chocolate. This disappears when the cocoa is used in milk.

Production of Chocolate

The major ingredient of chocolate is cocoa mass, which is mixed with sugar and, in the case of milk chocolate, also with milk powder. The conching process then follows, which is very important for the development of the full chocolate flavour. Melted cocoa butter is added, the chocolate mass becomes liquid, and is cooled, tempered and poured into moulds to form chocolate products.

Mixing of Ingredients and Refining

Sugar, cocoa mass and milk powder are intensively mixed, forming a dry powder. This powder is preground in various types of mills and then finely ground in a five-roll roller refiner. Small operators also use vertical ball mills. The sizes of particles in chocolate are between 15 and 70 μm.

Conching

The flavour which has been formed during roasting, is rounded off into the typical chocolate flavour by the conching process. This process also contributes to the physical properties of the chocolate, and hence its eating

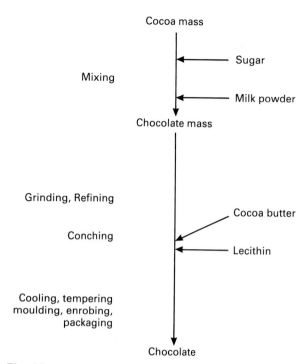

Fig. 11 The production of chocolate.

characteristics. Conching is a mechanical treatment of the chocolate mass in large containers fitted with rollers, paddles or a variety of other devices. Chemical and physical changes take place under the influence of air which is brought into the mass, at a temperature of about 60°C, and of rubbing and shearing forces. The result is the formation or liberation of flavour components which give the delicate chocolate note. The chemistry of this process is largely unknown. Physically the dry, crumbled mass is converted into a flowable liquid suspension. The sharp edges of the sugar particles are rounded off, which will give the chocolate a smooth feeling in the mouth. Three phases can be distinguished in conching:

(1) Dry phase. The powdered chocolate mass loses moisture and less desirable volatile flavour components like acetic acid.
(2) Pasty phase. During dry conching the mass becomes pasty. Flavour development takes place under the influence of shearing forces.
(3) Liquid phase. The last component – cocoa butter – is added. The chocolate mass becomes liquid. Homogenizing takes place under the influence of intensive stirring and shearing.

The final degree of viscosity is very important: the melted chocolate must be sufficiently thin to fill all cavities of the moulds. The melted cocoa butter is the liquid phase. However, this is the most expensive component of chocolate. A substantial saving of butter can be obtained by using an emulsifier. Soya lecithin

Table 2. Indicative composition of some types of chocolate

	Cocoa mass (%)	Cocoa butter (%)	Milk powder (%)	Sugar (%)
Dark chocolate	40	10	—	50
Milk chocolate	10	20	15	55
Enrobing chocolate	40	15	—	45
White chocolate	—	25	25	50

(0·3%) is the most commonly used emulsifier which is added during the third conching phase.

A special way to produce milk chocolate is from crumb. The sugar and cocoa mass are brought into liquid milk and the whole is dried. During the lengthy drying a caramel flavour is developed. Dry milk chocolate crumb has a good shelf life, due to the natural antioxidants of cocoa. To make chocolate only cocoa butter has to be added. Crumb is much used in the UK.

Cooling and Tempering

Critical to the appearance, gloss, shelf life and mouth feel of chocolate is the way it is cooled before solidifying in moulds. Cocoa butter triglycerides can set in several polymorphic forms. Some are unstable and recrystallization into the stable form will occur after some hours or days. This will result in a loss of gloss and the formation of white fat crystals on the surface of the chocolate, the so-called fat bloom. To obtain stable crystals, stable seed crystals must be formed first. This is done in a process called tempering. The liquid chocolate at a temperature of 45–50°C is cooled to 32°C, then to 27–27·5°C. Stable and unstable crystals are formed during this cooling. The temperature is now raised to 29–31°C, causing the crystals of unstable forms to melt. The exact temperatures required for this process depend on the type of chocolate. After tempering, the chocolate is still liquid, ready to be poured into the moulds.

Moulding and Enrobing

Chocolate articles are made in two distinct ways.

In moulding, the chocolate is poured into a mould, which then moves on a belt through a cooling tunnel. After setting, the mould is turned upside down and as a result of the volume contraction of cocoa butter, the article will easily fall out of the mould. Solid bars are then ready for packaging. It is also possible to partly fill the mould. After filling, the mould is immediately emptied, and a thin layer remains on the bottom and wall of the mould. The mould is then cooled, and a filling is poured in. After cooling, a further chocolate layer is put on the filling: this becomes the bottom of the candy when the mould is turned. Large filled bars are made this way, as also is smaller confectionery.

To make easter eggs and other hollow products, a small quantity of chocolate is poured into a split mould. The mould is then closed and put in a shaking machine to cool. The chocolate sets against the inner wall.

In enrobing, the liquid chocolate is poured over a solid centre. Many different products are made this way, like candy bars, biscuits, cakes and ice cream. The viscosity of the chocolate determines the thickness of the layer. This can be controlled with the fat content of the chocolate, which is usually a bit higher than that of moulding chocolate (Table 2).

Packaging, Storage and Shelf Life

Packaging should protect chocolate products against moisture and against odours, which can easily be picked up by the chocolate fat. Furthermore, of course, the outside of the packaging must radiate the delicacy and luxury which is the image of chocolate. Up to now these requirements have resulted in multiple packages: aluminium foil first, paper or heat-sealed foil, finally a cardboard box. Often, the combination of materials prevents reuse and it is foreseeable that less complicated packaging will be developed in the near future.

Chocolate, with its very low moisture content (below 1%) and natural antioxidants, has a very good shelf life. However, rats, insects and moulds like it just as much as humans. Thus, proper storage is important. Another danger arises from high and irregular storage temperatures. The latter causes the formation of fat bloom. Although the white colour of the fat resembles mould growing on the product, the phenomenon is completely harmless.

Food Uses of Cocoa Products

Uses of Cocoa Powder

Cocoa powder is used as a natural colour and flavour in a wide variety of sweet foodstuffs. These may be solid, semisolid or liquid, and consumed frozen or hot. These products can be grouped in the following way:

(1) Aqueous systems – consumed frozen. This is the category to which ice cream belongs. The cocoa powder used is mostly low fat (10%). A great variety of colours is used to attain effects resembling dark or milk chocolate.

(2) Aqueous systems – consumed at room temperature. Examples are milk products like chocolate milk drinks and desserts. Lightly alkalized cocoa with 10% fat is used mostly.

(3) Aqueous systems – consumed hot. Hot chocolate is the product in which lightly alkalized cocoa powder with 20% fat is used most frequently.

(4) Fat systems. These are coatings based on cocoa butter substitutes, made with 10% fat cocoa and often not alkalized (real chocolate is also not alkalized). Cocoa butter substitutes may be used for the sake of economy and, indeed, their use may be unavoidable for technical reasons. The latter is the case with coatings on ice cream. At the low temperature of ice cream, chocolate becomes too brittle and softer fats are needed.

Uses of Chocolate

Chocolate can be consumed as such, but it is also much used as an ingredient on or in other foodstuffs. Enrobing of biscuits and other items has already been mentioned. Chocolate drops go into biscuits, and chocolate is used in between wafers. The latter is an example of the possible use of chocolate in tropical or subtropical countries. Even if the chocolate melts, it does not spoil the outside appearance of the product, nor does it stick to the fingers.

It is interesting to notice the different taste of the public for different types of chocolate or cocoa-flavoured products. Children prefer milk chocolate while adults more often prefer the dark types. However, there are also great differences in preference in different countries. In the UK milk chocolates with the typical crumb caramel note is predominant. In Germany and, especially, in France, adults prefer dark chocolate. In Germany a very strong, dark type of chocolate is marketed, called 'Herrenschokolade'. In North America, chocolate is the most popular flavour for desserts, ice cream, cakes and many other products. Much fantasy is used in creating cocoa-flavoured items in many tastes and colours. Here, advantage is taken from the fact that the cocoa flavour combines very well with many others. The most popular combinations are vanilla, peppermint, coffee and orange. Fruit flavours are common, but many others such as nuts, cardamon, etc., are used.

Legislation of Cocoa Products

General directives, serving as a guideline for national food laws, are laid down by the Codex Alimentarius. Based on this the EEC has developed harmonized directives for the member countries. The Food, Drug and Cosmetics Act in the USA gives similar rules. In most of these countries the name 'chocolate' may only be used if no other fat is present but cocoa butter. Cocoa butter equivalent fats, up to 5% of the total chocolate content, may be used in the UK, Ireland, Denmark and Sweden. In Japan three types of chocolate are distinguished: pure chocolate, chocolate and semichocolate. Only the first of these may not contain fats other than cocoa butter. *See* Legislation, International Standards

Bibliography

Beckett ST (1988) *Industrial Chocolate Manufacture and Use.* London: Blackie.

Biehl B and Adomako D (1983) Die Kakaofermentation (Steuerung, Acidation, Proteolyse). *Lebensmittelchemie und gerichtliche Chemie* 37: 57–63.

Biehl B, Meyer B, Crone G, Pollmann L and Mamot B Said (1989) Chemical and physical changes in the pulp during ripening and post-harvest storage of cocoa pods. *Journal of the Science of Food and Agriculture* 48: 189–208.

Burle L (1962) *Le Cacaoyer.* G. P. Maisonne uve et Larosse 11, Paris.

Chatt EM (1953) *Cocoa, Cultivation, Processing, Analysis.* London: Interscience.

Cook LR and Meursing EH (1982) *Chocolate Production and Use.* New York: Harcourt Brace Jovanovich.

Fincke A (1965) *Handbuch der Kakaoerzeugnisse.* Berlin: Springer-Verlag.

Knapp AW (1973) *Cacao Fermentation: A Critical Survey of its Scientific Aspects.* London: Bale and Curnow.

Martin RA (1987) Chocolate. *Advances in Food Research* 31.

Meursing EH (1983) *Cocoa Powders for Industrial Processing.* Koog aan de Zaan, The Netherlands: Cacao de Zaan.

Meyer B, Biehl B, Mamot B Said and Samarokoddy RJ (1989) Post-harvest pod storage: a method for pulp preconditioning to impair strong nib acidification during cocoa fermentation in Malaysia. *Journal of the Science of Food and Agriculture* 48: 285–304.

Roelofsen PA (1958) Fermentation, drying and storage of cocoa beans. *Advances in Food Research* 8: 225–296.

Rohan TA (1963) *Processing of Raw Cocoa for the Market. FAO Agriculture Studies,* No. 60. Geneva: Food and Agriculture Organization.

Wood GAR and Lass RA (1985) *Cocoa,* 4th edn. Harlow: Longman.

B. Biehl
Technical University, Braunschweig, FRG
E. H. Meursing
Cacao De Zaan (retired), Koog aan de Zaan, The Netherlands

COCONUT PALM

The coconut palm (*Cocos nucifera* L.) is 'the tree of life', with 'a thousand and one uses' or with 'as many uses as there are stars in the sky', yet for the last 150 years one use has dominated all others – the production of copra. This is the dried kernel of the nut, from which coconut oil is extracted. The residual cake is used for animal feed. Coconut oil was once the most important vegetable oil. It is no longer, but it remains important because it is a lauric oil and commands a premium price on world markets when not oversupplied.

Coconut oil competes directly with palm kernel oil from the oil palm. That crop, which also produces palm oil, has taken over the plantation role of the coconut which is now almost entirely grown by smallholders. Harvesting either of these tropical tree crops is laborious. Their future may be at risk from *Cuphea*, a lauric-oil-producing shrub which is being bred for mechanization, or from recombinant DNA biotechnology which is used to convert oil crops such as rapeseed into lauric oil producers. Nevertheless, should copra and coconut oil become less dominant, other uses of the palm may gain or regain value. Nutritional uses are as follows: the immature fruit for drinking; the mature fruit for fresh endosperm processed to cream, or food grade oil and flour; the sap to produce toddy, sugar, alcohol or vinegar; and the palm heart as a vegetable. Non-nutritional uses include the following: fibre and coco-peat from the husk; flour, charcoal and activated carbon from the shell; and timber from the trunk. Coconut oil can even be used directly to fuel unmodified diesel engines. These options mean that farmers and processors must be equally flexible and not limit their production to copra and oil. *See* Vegetable Oils, Oil Palms

Economic History

The original importance of the coconut palm was to coastal communities. With fish and shellfish to eat, coconut provides refreshing, sweet and uncontaminated drinking water in an otherwise saline environment. No tools are needed to obtain it, and daily consumption of the water contained in one or two coconuts is enough to ensure good kidney function. Domestication of the coconut enhanced the drinking qualities in particular. The wild-type coconut spread without human interference, the domestic type depended on human activity for its survival and dissemination. Both types were eventually taken into cultivation and introgressive hybridization produces the wide range of variability seen today.

The coconut has a historical social importance in the successful human settlement of uninhabited Pacific and Indian Ocean islands. The presence of the wild coconut encouraged settlement by supplying water, food and fuel whilst the crops brought by the settlers were planted and harvested. Settlers would have to wait several years for any introduced domestic coconut to come into production, but established wild coconuts provided material for building shelters and boats, as well as supplies for inter-island expeditions. For obvious reasons, the coconut has a significant role in religious and family ceremonials connected with birth, marriage and death. It is commemorated in folklore throughout Asia and the Pacific.

The coconut assures tolerable subsistence. For thousands of years, on the tropical coasts and islands of the Pacific and Indian oceans, there has always been strong and continual demand for fresh fruit and for nonedible products, particularly coir fibre from the husk. Canoes built and provisioned by the coconut took Polynesians into the Pacific. The hulls of Arab dhows which sailed the Indian Ocean were sewn with coconut fibre. In contrast, the coconut has been known for less than 500 years on the Atlantic coasts of Africa and America, including the Caribbean, or the Pacific coast of Central and South America. It was taken to those shores by captains of Portuguese caravels and Spanish galleons who realized the value of the coconut even before they circumnavigated the globe. At that time the coconut was a curiosity to Europeans, but the fibre from the husk of the fruit made coir ropes that became essential to sailing ships of all nations. The coconut became established at every important trading post in the tropics along the sea routes of the world. In the nineteenth century, maritime trading companies took advantage of this fact. Coconut trade, which had previously been inter-island or from coast to hinterland, became tropical to temperate.

Trading in coconut products, between the coastal coconut groves and the inland, upland, drier or cooler districts where the palm would not flourish, used the surplus coconuts. These fall, or are cut from the palm, often drying naturally to produce edible (ball) copra inside the shell; alternatively, they are split and dried to copra in the sun or over an open fire. Copra is merely a convenient way to process, store and transport surplus coconuts. Traders collected copra from wherever they anchored in the tropics to meet a growing demand in Europe and North America for a cheap source of oil, first for lighting (stearine candles), then for cooking (deep frying and margarine), more importantly for hygiene (soap) and most significantly for explosives (glycerine). Coconut plantations were planted to provide European industries with raw materials and war materials for economic and political competition. The coconut boomed on the stock market about the time of World War I in Europe. All attention was given to one product – copra – until this was superseded by other vegetable oils and, eventually, by petrochemicals. It is for this reason that coconut is common everywhere, generally over-aged and nowhere as productive as it should be. Coconut is now mainly a smallholders' crop. It remains to be seen how well it will move into the twenty-first century.

Agricultural Botany

The coconut palm is found throughout the lowland humid tropics, bearing fruit all the year round. It grows in well-drained, well-aerated soils. On shallow sands it responds to fertilizer application. On deep loams it may be intercropped successfully with high-value food or fruit crops. The roots will not tolerate compacted soils and will not penetrate hardpans. The coconut palm flourishes where the average temperature is 25–30°C. It requires 100 mm or more of rain every month but not so much cloud cover that the number of sunshine hours is below 2000 per annum. Dry periods longer than 3 months reduce yields; after 6 months there is premature loss of leaves; more than 9 months and the palms die. Nevertheless, coconuts are known to grow very well where precipitation is marginal but groundwater is constantly present. The coconut palm tolerates salinity but only when rain or freshwater irrigation prevent salts accumulating. It withstands short periods of flooding and a high but fluctuating water table, but not a permanently high and static water table or prolonged waterlogging. Latitude north or south of the equator and altitude above sea level both limit successful growth and development, as a function of low seasonal temperatures. For example, they grow without setting fruit at 1000 m, and established coconut palms survive frost and snow in subtropical winters. In latitudes where hurricane-force winds occur, the coconut palm will bend rather than snap, grow up again from a prone position, or regenerate from fallen fruit.

Botanically, there is only one species of coconut (*Cocos nucifera* L.) with two plant habits (tall or dwarf) and three basic colour forms (yellow, red and green), but the actual range of intermediate palm habits, fruit sizes, shapes and colours, exhibits every possible combination. There are very many named varieties, particularly in the Asia-Pacific region. This extensive area represents the centres of domestication and diversity rather than the centre of origin. In effect, a geographical location for the primordial coconut is not on any of the continental landmasses but on their margins. Specifically, on the coasts and islands of the Gondwanaland super-continent, from which the major continental landmasses are derived. The original wild coconut dispersed between islands in the Indian and Pacific oceans, but not the Atlantic.

The coconut grows from a seed which is the entire fruit, including the husk. The number, size and weight of the fruit depends on variety, and differs from palm to palm and from season to season. Some weigh as much as 5 kg. Even a small coconut can weigh 500 g. Size is in proportion, some are as big as a head, others about the size of two fists. When the palm is in full production it may produce more than 100 nuts, depending on the different seasonal effects during the 11–15-month development period. In some varieties, ripe fruit fall and lie on the ground before germinating. In other varieties, ripe fruit germinate on the bunch.

The energy for early seedling growth comes from the oil-rich endosperm. This is converted to sugars through enzymatic activity of the placenta-like haustorium which develops to fill the nut cavity. There are sufficient reserves for about 15 months. This enables the seedling to survive through dry periods in the first year, when its roots may not have grown far enough or the rainfall is deficient. Roots are produced adventitiously from the base of the stem, or from any part of the stem that comes into contact with the ground. In this way, fallen palms may continue to grow. Abnormal coconut palms may sucker at the base, may branch or twist, or may produce plantlets instead of flowers. No practical method of vegetative propagation is possible. Tissue culture methods continue to be researched but coconut has proved less amenable than date or oil palm. Hardly any clonal coconuts have reached the field. Culture of zygotic embryos is possible and has research and direct commercial application.

The growth of the seedling becomes self-supporting as photosynthesis takes over. The energy generated goes into producing longer leaves with more leaflets and larger leaf bases. The increasing size of the leaf base corresponds to the increasing size of the stem. Coconut is a monocotyledon, with no secondary thickening, and the stem morphology is such that the older basal part increases in density as the ground tissue lignifies. There is a high silica content. Immediately below the crown of green leaves which surround the growing point, and in the centre of the stem, the tissue is softer.

The single major vegetative growing point produces a spiral succession of leaves throughout the life of the palm. Each green leaf may last about 2 years before it falls to reveal the stem internode. In this way the stem grows vertically, often with a characteristically graceful curve. When a large enough growing point has developed, flowering is initiated. From then and throughout the life of the palm until senility, each leaf has an inflorescence in its axil. Flowering may be affected by poor growing conditions, when flower initials abort. Eventually, the stem grows too high. Then the fruit get smaller, no more set, female flowers are no longer produced, inflorescences abort completely, leaves get very short, the trunk tapers (known as pencilling) and the palm dies. The palm may live 80–100 years before this happens, or less in poor growing conditions.

Precocity of flowering depends on variety and environment and may be delayed or prevented by poor growing conditions. Inflorescences, with both male and female flowers, begin to emerge from leaf axils after the third year. Successive inflorescences are produced every 25–35 days, leading to the generalization that the coconut will flower and fruit every month of the year. About 6–7 months after flowering, the immature nuts are full size. By about 12–15 months, these are mature and they fall or are reaped. Allowing for season and climate, the palm carries a range of fruit in every stage of development from the small, fertilized, postreceptive female flower, through the full-sized, immature nut which is filled with water and very heavy, to the slightly smaller, fully mature, ripe nut in which weight and size has decreased due to the nut cavity forming and the fibrous husk becoming drier and shrinking.

The most interesting morphological character of the palm is the development of the large cavity within the seed. The endosperm or kernel is laid down inside a hard shell, which in turn is protected within a thick husk. To produce this cavity the developing fruit fills with an increasing amount of liquid. This is unmatched in any other plant and is the key element in the plant's successful evolution and dissemination – both naturally and under human influence. The husk and cavity combined gave the primordial wild coconut the ability to disseminate by floating long distances at sea. The liquid in the immature nut was the reason for the coconut's early domestication by man.

Food Uses

From the Germinated Seed

Coconut 'Apple' (Haustorium)

The haustorium begins to develop at the earliest stage of germination, before the shoot or roots emerge through the husk. Coconuts that are in this condition are used for domestic purposes or for second-grade copra, but generally not for desiccated coconut. On these occasions the apple may be put to one side for eating. It is slightly sweet and slightly oily, with a cotton-wool-like texture. As the endosperm lasts for up to 15 months during germination, a large apple is also to be found in well-developed seedlings. To obtain this, children uproot sprouted seednuts and swing them by the leaves to split the nut against the trunk of the nearest mature palm.

From the Palm before or after Flowering

Heart of Palm, Millionaire's Salad, or Coconut Cabbage

Farmers are often unwilling to cut down coconut palms, even from stands that are too densely planted or where palms are over-aged and unproductive. Yet to do so provides a gourmet's treat – heart of palm. This is called millionaire's salad, on the mistaken assumption that only the very rich can afford to cut down a whole palm for the comparatively small edible part. In fact, the yield of the remaining palms would benefit from the reduction in competition and the farmer would benefit from selling a luxury item (and also the timber). Palm hearts are eaten fresh or cooked, canned or pickled.

From the Flowering Palm

Tapping for Toddy

Palms are tapped for toddy but not in the same way that the cambium below the bark is tapped in the production of maple syrup or rubber; palms are monocotyledons with many scattered vascular strands through the stem rather than in a convenient subcutaneous layer. Casual observers sometimes think that the coconut palm leaf-stalks are tapped. In fact, it is the palm inflorescence which is used. This is a large structure and when cut in the tapping process it could indeed resemble the cut leafstalk.

There are many flowering stalks within an inflorescence, each capable of exuding sap. They are packed tightly into an enveloping spathe which would normally split to allow pollination. Natural splitting is prevented by binding the spathe tightly. It may also be lightly beaten and flexed to stimulate sap flow. Once ready, the end is cut off to allow the sap to drip into a receptacle. The palm is visited, morning and evening, to decant the accumulated sap from the container before fermentation gets too active. Sap flow continues for many days, and each day a sliver is removed to reopen blocked vascular elements and increase flow. This continues until only a stump remains and the next inflorescence in sequence is prepared. Obviously, tapped bunches do not flower normally and the palm ceases to set fruit. If the sap flow reduces, the palm may be rested. The palm may respond to this with particularly high yields of fruit on the next normal bunches. Excessive tapping followed by high fruit set could shorten the life of the palm. However, the financial return to the farmer would more than compensate for this.

Sugar

After straining, sweet toddy is boiled in shallow pans to crystallizing point, to give a 12–15% yield of jaggery, a rough sugar which is hard, semi-crystalline and golden brown in colour. A lesser degree of concentration gives treacle (or syrup). Syrups and sugar are produced for the local market or domestic use and are unlikely ever to compete economically with cane or beet sugar.

Palm Wine

Toddy produced overnight and collected first thing in the morning contains about 3% alcohol and 10% fermentable sugar. Various additives can be used to slow or stop fermentation. Otherwise, if fermentation continues for 33 h, palm wine is produced with an alcoholic content of 8%. Sweet, unfermented toddy contains 16–30 mg of ascorbic acid per 100 g, and the content changes little during fermentation. The yeast in fermented toddy adds vitamin B. *See* Ascorbic Acid, Properties and Determination

Arrack

Arrack is the product of distilling fermented toddy. Doubly distilled arrack is used as the basis of local gin, rum, etc., by the addition of appropriate flavours.

Vinegar

Fermenting toddy with free access to air produces 45% acetic acid in 10–14 weeks. It is then matured for up to 6 months in closed casks and may be flavoured with spices and coloured with caramel.

From Male and Female Flowers at Anthesis

Honey

Honey bees are often kept in coconut groves to enhance fruit set. The hundreds of male flowers in one inflorescence open over a period of about 3 weeks and each secretes a single drop of nectar. The larger, but fewer female flowers produce a flow of nectar from three nectaries over a period of days when the stigmatic surfaces are receptive. The year-round flowering in a coconut plantation assures a perpetual supply of nectar. It also means that bees are unlikely to store large amounts of surplus honey.

From Male Flowers at Anthesis

Pollen

Coconut pollen is sold in health food shops. It is collected from bees simply by incorporating a trap in the hive entrance which removes the pollen pellets from the insects' leg sacs. A side-effect of research into coconut

breeding is that kilogram quantities of pollen are collected manually for artificial pollination in F_1 hybrid seed production. Here again, the year-round flowering of the coconut means that regular supplies of pollen would be easy to maintain.

Female Flowers (Immature Fruit)

Pickled 'Button' Nuts

It is possible to pickle the very young female flowers, or buttons, using vinegar produced from fermented coconut sap.

From the Fruiting Palm

Edible Husk

The husk is generally bitter and stringy when young, and dry and fibrous when mature. Some individual palms have an edible husk which is less fibrous, spongier, and easily cut. It is sweet and crisp, and chewed like sugar cane.

Endosperm (Kernel)

Although the coconut may be notable for the amount of oil that can be extracted from the endosperm of one nut, its yield per hectare is matched or surpassed by other oil crops. However, two features of coconut endosperm are not found in any other plant – the amount of drinkable water, when young, and the characteristic coconut flavour, when mature.

Immature Fruit

Liquid Endosperm (Coconut Water)

The liquid endosperm is coconut water, not coconut milk (qv). The immature fruit, used for drinking, will not fall naturally but must be cut from the palm. Bunches are selected just as they reach maximum size, when a jellylike endosperm begins to line the cavity of the still thin and soft shell. At this stage each nut is full size, full of water, with no airspace (it does not splash when shaken), and very heavy. Usually, one or two entire bunches of nuts are cut and lowered to the ground on a rope. If they fall, the weight of water would crack or even burst the soft shell inside the soft husk, and the water would drain away and the fruit rot and spoil.

The freshly harvested coconut from a bunch that has been in the sun has a natural effervescence and will hiss with released gas when opened. Nevertheless, the 'packaging' of this 'product' leaves it at a disadvantage against internationally trademarked colas and mineral waters. Young coconuts deteriorate over a few days unless kept cool. Much of the husk may be cut away to reduce size, so that they can be kept in a refrigerated cool store. This extends shelf life considerably. Drinking coconuts are sometimes transported hundreds of kilometres in refrigerated trucks but this occurs only where such a vehicle would otherwise return empty, where the roads are good, and where an affluent urban market has no other access to coconut.

At the proper stage, the water contains about 5% sugar. A large nut may have 25 g of sugar. It also contains minerals, amino acids and vitamin C. It ferments easily, producing alcohol and vinegar. Coconut water has auxinic and plant-growth-promoting properties and is used in plant tissue culture. Historically, various medicinal values have been attributed to it. There is no doubt that it is a perfect oral rehydration fluid for severe diarrhoea in cholera cases and similar situations. Being naturally sterile, it may be used intravenously to substitute for blood plasma in emergency surgery. It provides fluid plus minerals, sugar and protein. In combination with egg yolk it is used as a diluent in artificial insemination.

Makapuno Endosperm

Solid endosperm begins to be laid down inside the shell as a jelly; drinking nuts cut at this stage, before the endosperm begins to go white and firm, are known as jelly nuts. One sort, the makapuno, retains the jelly characteristic into maturity. This is a recessive characteristic which develops in only some fruit of only some palms. Seednuts with this characteristic will not germinate naturally, but the embryos can be rescued and they are now routinely cultured. By this method it should be possible to produce palms on which every fruit is a makapuno type. A favourable market already exists for makapuno coconuts in the Phillippines, and could probably be developed elsewhere.

Aromatic Endosperm

Certain varieties are valued because the normal coconut-flavoured endosperm has an additional aromatic accent. This is usually best appreciated in the immature drinking nut.

Mature Fruit

Residual Liquid Endosperm

The small quantity of liquid that remains inside the nut cavity, after the kernel has finished developing but before germination begins, is little more than insipid water. It has a low sugar content and is not as pleasant to drink as the sweet liquid in the immature fruit. It is

incorrect to call it milk, which it does not resemble. However, in a very-large-fruited variety it provides enough to drink. One of the reasons that coconuts have been widely dispersed is that travellers take such nuts, and those which are not consumed may germinate and be planted.

Normal Endosperm

Normal endosperm from a fully mature nut eaten raw is slightly indigestible. It may be sliced and frozen for sale in urban markets or for export. It is used domestically in cooking, by separating an oil emulsion known as coconut milk or coconut cream (qv). Naturally or artificially dried endosperm, known as copra, is a source of oil and residual cake. Shredding before drying produces desiccated coconut.

Coconut Milk or Coconut Cream

Coconut milk is prepared by squeezing freshly grated endosperm, usually with a little added water, through cloth. On storing, coconut cream forms an upper layer. When either emulsion is heated, clear oil separates. This is the basis of the village method of oil extraction. Coconut cream is also produced industrially in both liquid and spray-dried forms. It is used extensively in all sorts of cookery recipes in the national cuisine of every country where coconuts grow.

Coconut Flour for Human Consumption

Coconut flour produced from fresh processing has been researched for use in breadmaking and other foods. However, it is not superior to other protein sources in the proportions of the various amino acids.

Edible (Ball) Copra

Ball copra may form naturally inside the whole ripe nut, particularly in those varieties which do not germinate quickly. The endosperm dries away from the shell and becomes a ball of copra which rattles loosely inside the nut. This happens when the weather is very dry or if the nuts are kept dry in a store. The husk is not removed, so that the shell will not crack, and the process takes 8–12 months. Fires may be lit to assist drying but the heat and smoke do not come into contact with the endosperm, so that it retains a very high quality.

Copra

Fresh coconut meat contains about 47% moisture and is quite perishable. Since the nut contains about 50% husk, 12% shell, 10% water and only about 28% meat, the husk and shell are removed after harvesting and the moisture content reduced by drying. Commercial copra is prepared by sun-drying, by direct firing over a barbecue, or by indirect hot air in various sorts of kiln. Moisture content reduces from 45–50% to 6–8%, and oil content increases from 35% to 60–65%. Although copra contains 20–25% protein of reasonably good nutritional quality, its food value is limited. For safe storage, the moisture content of copra should be 6%. At first point of sale it often has a much higher level. It dries further during storage but under such conditions can be attacked by moulds. One of these is *Aspergillus flavus*, which produces aflatoxin. The presence of this carcinogen is a stimulus to improve copra quality or to bypass it and process the fresh fruit. *See* Mycotoxins, Occurrence and Determination; Spoilage, Moulds in Food Spoilage

Coconut Oil

In countries of origin, coconut oil is largely used for edible purposes. It is prepared domestically by heating coconut milk (qv), when a clear oil separates. The extraction of oil from copra is one of the oldest seed-crushing industries in the world, although some claim that olive oil is of greater antiquity. Copra is processed by methods ranging from simple village processes to modern high-pressure expellers and prepress/solvent extraction plants. Throughput can be more than 500 t of copra per day. In parts of Indonesia, chopped fresh kernel is cooked in previously extracted coconut oil before pressing. Various commercial methods for wet processing of edible-grade oil and flour from fresh meat have been developed, but none are yet commercially viable. *See* Vegetable Oils, Extraction

Coconut oil is the most important of the small group of commercial fats which contain a high proportion of glycerides of lower fatty acids, in particular lauric acid. The chief fatty acids are lauric (45%), myristic (18%), palmitic (9·5%), oleic (8·2%), caprylic (7·8%), capric (7·6%), and stearic (5%). There is a minute amount of tocopherol (vitamin E). The natural volatile flavour components of fresh meat and of oil are mostly δ-lactones. Lauric oils are characterized by high saponification value, and they have the lowest iodine value of vegetable oils in common industrial use. Coconut oil, as it is ordinarily prepared in tropical countries, is colourless to pale brownish yellow. In temperate climates, or air conditioning, it appears as a greasy, somewhat white or yellowish, solid fat which has a melting point range between 20°C and 26°C. Until refined it has a pronounced odour of coconut. *See* Fatty Acids, Properties; Tocopherols, Properties and Determination

Coconut oil is refined, bleached and deodorized using standard vegetable oil processing technology. If coconut oil is cooled until crystallization, part of the oil produces a semisolid mass and is then separated under hydraulic pressure. The solid fraction, coconut stearine, is a harder fat with a higher melting point. It finds use as a valuable confectionery fat and as a substitute for cocoa butter on account of its brittleness and 'snap' fracture. The liquid fraction, coconut oleine, has a correspondingly lower melting point. The oleine is used in margarine manufacture. If hydrogenated, its unsaturated glycerides are converted into stearic glycerides; thus the product has a melting point higher than coconut stearine and is used as a brittle confectionery fat, even more closely resembling cocoa butter. *See* Vegetable Oils, Refining; Vegetable Oils, Processing

When refined and deodorized, coconut oil is mixed with nonfat milk and used as a replacement for whole milk for many purposes, including the feeding of infants. Other uses include imitation dairy products, filled milk, coffee whiteners, soft-serve desserts, frozen desserts, whipped toppings, milk shake mix, chocolate-filled milk, etc. It is used because it is bland in flavour, resists oxidation, is extremely stable in storage, and possesses a unique liquefying property that contributes to 'mouth feel' of the food of which it is a component.

The main nonedible uses are for soaps, detergent foam boosters, lubricating oil additives, mineral flotation agents, shampoo products, and corrosion inhibitors. The lathering quality of soaps is enhanced by the use of lauric oils, and this makes coconut oil particularly useful for hard water or marine soaps. A feature of soapmaking with coconut oil is the higher yield of glycerol, 14% compared with 10% for most oils. Other nonedible uses include illuminating or fuel oil in rural areas or for lighting in ceremonial lamps. Coconut stearine is also used to advantage in candle manufacture. Coconut oil will directly fuel unmodified diesel engines.

Copra Cake and Copra Meal

After the oil has been extracted from copra, a good-quality residual cake will contain 6–8% oil, with a protein content of around 20%. Copra meal, the solvent-extracted residue, contains 1–3% oil, depending on the efficiencyf of the plant. Both cake and meal are used in cattle or poultry feeds. They are useful for dairy and for fattening, and are said to give firmer butter and harder body fat than other oil cakes. Cake with a high oil content is generally fed to pigs. The deficiency in certain amino acids, notably tryptophan, lysine, methionine and histidine, limits the amounts that can be used in animal feed. If aflatoxin is present in poorly prepared copra it can pass into the cake or meal.

Desiccated Coconut

Desiccated coconut was first manufactured in the early 1880s. It is an important product, sensitive to changes in production costs and easily susceptible to overproduction. Nuts are stored for 3 or 4 weeks before being dehusked in the field and carried to the factory. The shell has to be chipped off when the kernel comes away easily. Damaged or germinated nuts or kernels are rejected to make low-grade copra. The brown testa has to be removed. This is usually pared off by hand, although machines are available. Kernels are then washed and sterilized, to avoid risk of salmonella contamination. After sterilization, disintegrators reduce them to a wet meal, or cutters produce fancy cuts such as threads or chips. Drying is by indirect drier at 75–80°C, or by direct firing at 120°C. The dried product is cooled and graded before being packed. Parings oil and drain oil are by-products. Desiccated coconut should be pure white and crisp, with a fresh taste. It should have less than 2·5% moisture, 68–72% oil (on a dry-weight basis), less than 0·1% free fatty acid (as lauric) and about 6% protein. If there is more than 6–7% sucrose, then sugar has been added. Unavailable carbohydrate content is about 18%, crude fibre about 4%, and there is some mineral content. Desiccated coconut is widely used in sweets, biscuits, cakes and cake fillings.

Other Food Uses Indirectly Related to Coconut

There are two other food uses with a coconut connection which are included here for a sake of completeness. The first is the palm weevil, which is a serious pest of coconut groves, killing palms directly by burrowing in the stem, or indirectly as a vector of the red ring nematode. Nevertheless, under these circumstances, subsistence cultivators collect grubs from fallen or felled palm stems and benefit from the resulting energy-rich diet.

The second example of indirect food use is the coconut crab. The crab climbs coconut palm stems and is reputed to cut off nuts before returning to the ground to eat them. The association between the crab and the coconut is not purely fortuitous. The coconut's ability to spread long distances by interisland floating also accounts for the equally widespread distribution of this otherwise terrestrial crab, which only spends about 30 days of its larval life in coastal waters. On many islands where it was once found the crab has been eaten to extinction.

Health Considerations

Coconut oil is easily digested and absorbed into the system to the extent of 95–98% as rapidly as butter fat. This is attributed to the low molecular weight of the fatty acids. In common with other vegetable oils, coconut oil contains virtually no cholesterol, but there are objections to its food use due to the high saturation of the fatty acids. In the USA, 'tropical oils' have come under attack from pressure groups. Their criticisms overlook the facts that most coconut oil is used for nonedible purposes, that other domestic sources of oils and fats have replaced it for deep frying, and that many of the food uses now are to improve the quality of factory-prepared products. Only in the countries where the coconut grows is it still used extensively for cooking, where it makes lower quality protein and carbohydrates more acceptable and more digestible. In fact, naturally saturated medium-chain coconut oil may be healthier than artificially hydrogenated short-chain vegetable oils. *See* Vegetable Oils, Dietary Importance; Vegetable Oils, Analysis

Bibliography

Banzon J, Gonzales ON, de Leon SY and Sanchez PC (1990) *Coconuts as Food.* Quezon City: Philippine Coconut Research and Development Foundation.
Child R (1974) *Coconuts* 2nd edn. London: Longman.
Coconut Statistical Yearbook (annual publication). Jakarta, Indonesia: Asian and Pacific Coconut Community.
Grimwood BE (ed) (1975) *Coconut palm products: their processing in developing countries.* FAO Agricultural Development Paper No. 99. Rome: Food and Agriculture Organization.
Ohler J (1984) *Coconut: Tree of Life.* Rome: Food and Agriculture Organization.
Thampan PK (1975) *The Coconut Palm and its Products.* Cochin: Green Villa Publishing House.
Thieme JG (1968) *Coconut oil processing.* FAO Agricultural Development Paper No. 80. Rome: Food and Agriculture Organization.
Woodroof JG (1978) *Coconuts: Production, Processing, Products.* Westport, Connecticut: AVI Publishing.

Hugh C. Harries
International Coconut Cultivar Registration Authority, Dar es Salaam, Tanzania

COD

See Fish

CODEX

See Legislation

COELIAC DISEASE

Definition

Coeliac disease is defined as that disease in which there is an abnormality of the small intestinal mucosa, made manifest by contact with the gluten fraction of wheat and other, related cereal grains. This implies that there is a predisposition in the patient to the disease but that the presence of gluten in the diet is necessary to produce the abnormality. The typical abnormality of the small intestinal mucosa is the pathological finding of total absence of villi, crypt hyperplasia and inflammatory cell infiltration (see Figs 1 and 2), although less severe degrees of abnormality have been described.

Aetiology

Wheat Gluten

Wheat gluten, by definition, is an aetiological factor in the development of coeliac disease. Gluten is the insoluble material (a complex mixture of proteins, with small amounts of lipids, sugars and minerals) obtained when flour is washed in tap water to remove the soluble substances (albumins, globulins, starch). Gluten is thus an ill-defined mixture which varies between different flours and is even dependent upon the solubilizing properties of the tap water used. Gliadin is the ethanol-soluble component of wheat flour, usually solubilized in 70% ethanol; the same component can be similarly extracted from gluten. Gliadin, although a complex mixture of proteins, is thus more homogeneous than gluten. Both gluten and gliadin are similarly provocative of coeliac disease, and thus both terms are used interchangeably when referring to aetiological factors in coeliac disease. Despite a great deal of research it is not known which fraction of either gluten or gliadin is responsible for producing the coeliac abnormality, although it is believed to be a relatively small polypeptide, which is common to all wheat varieties and other related cereals. *See* Wheat

Theories of Causation

Not only is the specific cereal peptide responsible for coeliac disease unknown but also the way in which such a peptide produces the mucosal abnormality; the latter is the subject of much debate. There are several theories of causation:

1. An enzyme (a peptidase) may be absent from the small intestinal mucosa of people predisposed to coeliac disease. On exposure to gluten in the diet, the gluten peptide responsible for provoking the disease would then not be digested at the mucosal surface and would accumulate, causing toxic damage directly to the mucosa, resulting in the typical mucosal abnormality. There is little scientific support for this theory.
2. The epithelial cells lining the mucosa of the small intestine may have a cell membrane receptor which specifically binds the gluten peptide, such an interaction then leading to direct or indirect (via pathological mechanisms) damage to the mucosa and the typical abnormality. There is very little support for this hypothesis.
3. There may be a permeability defect of the mucosa in coeliac individuals, allowing the particular gluten peptide access across the mucosa in abnormal amounts, once again producing the typical abnormality via direct or indirect pathological mechanisms. Again, there is little support for this theory.
4. The immunological theory, at the time of writing, attracts considerable support. This theory suggests that the implicated gluten peptide stimulates an excessive immunological reaction against it, the mucosal damage resulting from this reaction. *See* Immunity and Nutrition

None of these theories is mutually exclusive, and all suggest that there is a predisposition to the disease so that the susceptible person inherits either a missing enzyme, or a cell membrane defect, or an abnormal immune responsiveness. In support of such an inherited predisposition are the genetic findings in coeliac disease.

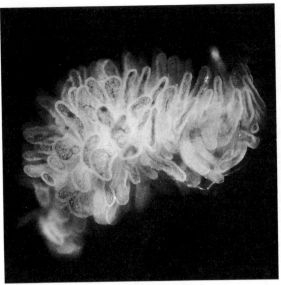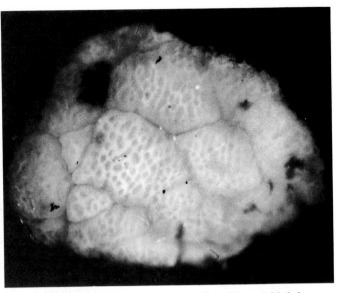

Fig. 1 Dissecting microscopic appearance of (left) normal mucosal biopsy showing finger-like villi, and (right) biopsy from untreated coeliac patient with total absence of villi and a 'flat'-looking mucosal surface.

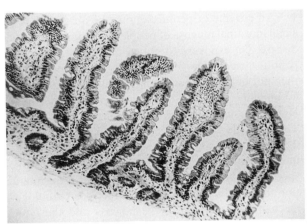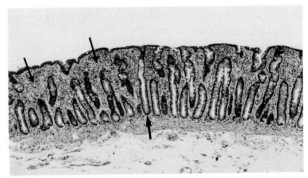

Fig. 2 Light microscopic appearance of (left) normal mucosa with tall finger-shaped villi, and (right) untreated coeliac mucosa with absence of villi, deep crypts (➡) and an increase in inflammatory cells (→).

Ten per cent of first-degree relatives of a coeliac patient are likely to have the disease and certain major histocompatibility locus (MHC) antigens, i.e. B8, DR3 and DQw2, are particularly prevalent in coeliac patients. Such antigens are encoded by genes related to the immune responsiveness of an individual and this finding therefore strengthens the immunological hypothesis of causation. *See* Inborn Errors of Metabolism

Prevalence

Coeliac disease has been described principally in Caucasian peoples, although cases have been diagnosed in all other ethnic groups. This variation may be due to varying MHC genes which are associated with the disease in different populations, but it may also be attributed to the diagnostic facilities available in different areas. Since, by definition, the disease requires gluten, it can only present in wheat-eating populations. Typically, these have been of Caucasian extraction. The prevalence of coeliac disease in the UK is approximately 1:2000, although it is as high as 1:300 in the west of Ireland.

Clinical Features

Coeliac disease can present at any age, in both adults and children. The clinical features are protean, although since it is a disease affecting the small intestine, symptoms of gastrointestinal disease predominate in classical descriptions of the disease. Patients may have diarrhoea, anorexia, nausea, vomiting, abdominal distension and pain, flatulence, a sore tongue or mouth ulcers. As well as these gastrointestinal symptoms, patients commonly have constitutional symptoms of lassitude and malaise, weakness, and weight loss. Children may fail to thrive as infants and be underdeveloped, not reaching their expected height. Apart from these general symptoms, there are symptoms which arise as a result of poor absorption of various vitamins and minerals due to the small intestinal mucosal abnormality which causes 'malabsorption'; such symptoms include features of anaemia (malabsorption of iron and/or folic acid), a bleeding tendency (vitamin K), and cramps, paraesthesiae, rickets, proximal muscle weakness (vitamin D). Finally, there are rarer symptoms which may result from the chronicity of the disease or malabsorption of undiscovered factors; these include disorders of the nervous system, reproductive system, and the skin.

It is important to stress that many of these symptoms are described in untreated patients with coeliac disease and almost all are reversible with treatment. It is also of note that as physicians have become more aware of the disease, the diagnosis is being made more quickly and patients do not nowadays present with such gross features; in fact, the majority of patients are diagnosed with mild symptoms and minor biochemical or haematological abnormalities.

When untreated patients are examined, the findings on physical examination reflect the symptoms referred to above. For example, a patient with major symptoms may be thin and wasted, with muscle weakness, bruising of the skin and a sore tongue, and a distended abdomen. Patients diagnosed at an early stage may be apparently normal on physical examination.

Chemical Pathology

Haematological Investigations

The majority of untreated patients are anaemic. This is caused by iron or folic acid deficiency, or both, and is a result of the malabsorption of these factors. Vitamin B_{12} may be low but rarely causes the features of B_{12} deficiency. Unexplained anaemia may therefore alert the physician to the possibility of coeliac disease. *See* Anaemia, Iron Deficiency Anaemia; Anaemia, Megaloblastic Anaemias; Cobalamins, Physiology

Biochemical Investigations

Similarly, other nutritional factors are often low in the serum of untreated coeliac patients, e.g. the fat-soluble vitamins A, E, D and K, deficiency of the latter two being responsible for the features of osteomalacia and a bleeding tendency referred to above. Calcium and magnesium may be low, also water-soluble vitamins such as vitamin C, although scurvy is rare in coeliac disease. Albumin is often low, owing to loss into the gastrointestinal tract from the blood, rather than malabsorption. This can lead to peripheral oedema in the patient. None of these measurements is specific for coeliac disease and, therefore, they are not used in diagnosis. *See* individual nutrients

Tests of Malabsorption

Apart from finding low levels of various nutrients in the serum, as outlined above, absorption can be assessed more formally. For example, the absorption of fat can be assessed by measuring the dietary intake and faecal output over a period of days. A more indirect method measures the serum levels and urinary excretion of D-xylose, a carbohydrate not normally in the diet. Such tests can indicate malabsorption but are not specific for coeliac disease and are rarely used routinely.

Diagnosis

As the definition of coeliac disease states, there is an abnormality of the small intestinal mucosa. The cornerstone of diagnosis must therefore be the examination of a biopsy of this mucosa. Such a biopsy can be obtained using a biopsy tube or fibre optic endoscope, which the patient swallows, usually under sedation. Careful examination of the biopsy will reveal the typical pathological features. Since there are other, rarer causes of the same abnormality, the diagnosis is only definite when a second biopsy is obtained after a period (usually 6–12 months) on a gluten-free diet and the abnormality has been shown to improve and return towards normal (Figs 1 and 2). If such an improvement in the pathological features is seen, the diagnosis of coeliac disease can be firmly made. Such a scheme for diagnosis is suggested in the definition of the disease since this indicates that the mucosal abnormality must be related to the presence of gluten in the diet.

Other tests have been described to try to avoid the need for intestinal biopsies; for example, serum antibodies to gliadin can now be measured with approximately 90% sensitivity and specificity for coeliac disease. This implies that the test is not always diagnostic, and intestinal biopsies are ultimately necessary to make a firm diagnosis. However, assessment of such antibodies is a useful screening test, especially in children. Similar remarks apply to the assessment of intestinal permeability using a variety of sugar molecules, e.g. lactulose and mannitol.

These screening tests are also useful for the follow-up of patients to monitor the effects of treatment and perhaps to indicate the timing of further intestinal biopsies.

Treatment: a Gluten-free Diet

The cornerstone of treatment is a gluten-free diet, which should be taken for life. Patients should omit foods containing wheat, rye, barley, and probably oats from their diet. In severely symptomatic untreated patients initial treatment may also include replacement of nutritional deficiencies such as iron, folate, and vitamins D and K. Rarely, severely ill patients may require parenteral nutrition.

Once treatment with a gluten-free diet is established, patients begin to respond quickly, and usually note a remarkable improvement within weeks. Patients vary in their sensitivity to gluten in the diet; some can eventually consume some gluten and appear to remain clinically well; others have to adhere strictly to their diet, even to the extent of avoiding Communion wafers. If patients do consume gluten they can produce some damage to the small intestinal mucosa which may take months or years to produce clinical symptoms. Evidence is accumulating, however, that the malignancy which can occur in coeliac disease can be reduced by strict adherence to a gluten-free diet.

If patients are to adhere to a gluten-free diet, they need help from an experienced dietitian. Some patients have problems once dietary treatment has started. Initially, some put on weight, presumably as a result of improved absorption. These patients need advice about weight reduction. In this situation diabetes may be unmasked.

Constipation sometimes becomes a problem, reflecting the fact that bran from most cereals is omitted from the diet. Defatted rice bran or soya bran has been shown to help, and bulking agents such as ispaghula husk or methyl cellulose may also help. The dietitian can help with all these problems and advise about a diet based around fresh meat, vegetables, fish and fruit, with the gradual introduction of other safe foods as the patient becomes more confident about the gluten-free diet.

Prognosis

The prognosis is good for coeliac patients. Nearly all respond clinically and pathologically to treatment with a gluten-free diet, there being an improvement in symptoms and in the small intestinal mucosa. Lifelong treatment with the diet is recommended, as is follow-up in an out-patient clinic with the help of a dietitian. Younger patients, particularly teenagers, need sympath-etic follow-up since they often find the restrictions of the diet quite onerous.

Some physicians recommend further intestinal biopsies (after the first two which are necessary for diagnosis) every few years. This provides an objective assessment of the patient's condition and helps to motivate patients to maintain a strict diet.

Occasionally the mucosa does not respond to a gluten-free diet and the physician must consider the other, much rarer causes of an abnormal small intestinal mucosa. However, by far the most common cause of failure to respond to the gluten-free diet is inadequate dietary gluten exclusion; this may be conscious or inadvertent. Dietary compliance needs to be assessed by a well-informed dietitian. Rarely, other foods, e.g. milk, eggs and soya, need to be excluded as well as gluten, either temporarily or permanently. Other causes preventing a mucosal response to gluten exclusion may be pancreatic insufficiency, or contamination of the small intestine by bacterial overgrowth. Such causes should be sought and treated in this situation. Finally, nonresponse may be associated with serious complications of the disease which, fortunately, occur only rarely. These are the development of ulcers and strictures in the small intestine and also malignancy, particularly small intestinal lymphoma. Such complications may be a cause not only of nonresponse but also of deterioration in a previously well patient who has been adequately treated for some time with a gluten-free diet. As already suggested, there is preliminary evidence that the incidence of malignancy in coeliac disease may be reduced in patients who maintain a strict gluten-free diet.

If no underlying cause is found for non-response to a gluten-free diet and the diagnosis has been carefully considered, patients may be treated with oral steroids in order to induce a remission. This should only be done under careful supervision and there are no long-term studies, but the side-effects of steroid therapy suggest that such a course of treatment has a limited role in coeliac disease.

Apart from the complications reported above, mention should be made of various diseases which occur in association with coeliac disease. In the majority, the association has probably occurred by chance, simply because coeliac disease is fairly common and a lifelong condition. Any significant associations may result, in part, from similarities of MHC genes, or activation of the immune system. Associated diseases include pulmonary disorders, diabetes mellitus, liver abnormalities, thyroid disease, and chronic inflammatory conditions.

Bibliography

Cooke WT and Holmes GKT (1984) *Coeliac Disease*. Edinburgh: Churchill Livingstone.

Davidson AGF and Bridges MA (1987) Coeliac disease: a

critical review of the aetiology and pathogenesis. *Clinica Chimica Acta* 163: 1–40.

Holmes GKT, Prior P, Lane MR and Allan RN (1989) Malignancy in coeliac disease – effect of a gluten-free diet. *Gut* 30: 333–338.

Howdle PD and Losowsky MS (1987) The immunology of coeliac disease. *Bailliere's Clinical Gastroenterology* 1: 507–529.

Howdle PD and Losowsky MS (1990) A review of methods for measuring gliadins in food. *Gut* 31: 712–713.

Scott BB and Losowsky MS (1977) The definition and diagnosis of coeliac disease. *Journal of the Royal College of Physicians of London* 11: 405–411.

Peter Howdle
Leeds University Medical School, Leeds, UK

COENZYMES

Life as we know it is made possible by *enzymes*, highly specific proteins that facilitate biochemical reactions. The term *holoenzyme* refers to an active enzyme complex. An *apoenzyme* is the protein portion of the active unit. The term *prosthetic group* is used to refer to minerals, activated vitamins or other non-protein compounds that are required for full enzyme activity. *Cofactors* are non-protein substances, typically mineral ions and activated vitamins that are required for the function of certain enzymes. Some cofactors are essential at the active site of a reaction, while others help maintain the structural integrity of an enzyme or protein. *Coenzymes* are activated vitamins that participate in reactions with a stoichiometry equal to substrate. *See* Enzymes, Functions and Characteristics

An overview of how vitamins and minerals participate as cofactors in the overall processes of metabolism is illustrated in Fig. 1. Cofactors are essential in numerous biochemical pathways, including the breakdown, or *catabolism*, of nutrients and the synthesis, or *anabolism*, of biological compounds. The vitamin and mineral cofactors complex with enzymes to convert nutrients into usable energy and produce biomolecules that are the basis of life. *See* Vitamins, Overview; Minerals, Dietary Importance; Trace Elements

Nutrients as Coenzymes and Cofactors

Without the required vitamins and minerals, cofactor-dependent enzymes could not regulate metabolism or maintain normal cell function and biological processes that are essential for cell division, differentiation, growth and repair. Nutrient cofactors are also necessary for the structural integrity of certain hormones and regulatory proteins.

Vitamins

All of the water-soluble vitamins and two of the fat-soluble vitamins, A and K, function as cofactors or coenzymes. Coenzymes participate in numerous biochemical reactions involving energy release or catabolism, as well as the accompanying anabolic reactions (Fig. 1). In addition, vitamin cofactors are critical for processes involved in proper vision, blood coagulation, hormone production, and the integrity of collagen, a protein found in bone. *See* Cerebal Palsy – Nutritional Management; Retinol, Physiology

The active coenzyme form of *thiamin*, vitamin B_1, is thiamin pyrophosphate (TPP) (Fig. 2a). TPP is involved in oxidative decarboxylation and transketolase reactions. An example is the decarboxylation (removal of —COO^-) of three-carbon pyruvate to two-carbon acetyl CoA, an important step in carbohydrate breakdown. *See* Thiamin, Physiology

The active forms of *riboflavin*, vitamin B_2, are the coenzymes flavin mononucleotide (FMN; Fig. 2b) and flavin adenine dinucleotide (FAD). These coenzymes serve as hydrogen carriers for oxidation reactions that affect all energy nutrients in the citric acid cycle and in the electron transport system. *See* Riboflavin, Physiology

The coenzyme forms of *nicotinic acid*, are nicotinamide adenine dinucleotide (NAD) and nicotinamide adenine dinucleotide phosphate (NADP). These compounds assist dehydrogenase enzymes in the catabolism of fat, carbohydrates, and amino acids, and in the enzymes involved in synthesis of fats and steroids. *See* Niacin, Physiology

Pyridoxal phosphate (PLP; Fig. 2c) and pyridoxamine phosphate (PMP) are the coenzyme forms of *vitamin B_6*. These are cofactors for approximately 60 enzymes, such as the transaminases, racemases, decarboxylases, cleavage enzymes, synthetases, dehydrases, and desulphydrases. Both PLP and PMP participate in the metabolism of amino acids, including transamination, racemization, deamination and desulphydration, and the conversion of tryptophan to nicotinic acid. *See* Vitamin B_6, Physiology

Pantothenic acid (PA) is a B vitamin that is a

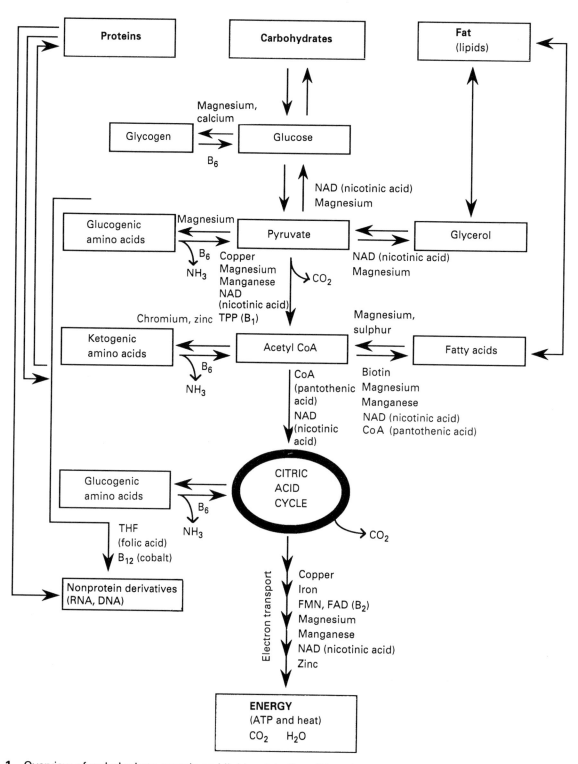

Fig. 1 Overview of carbohydrate, protein and lipid metabolism. Minerals and vitamins play crucial roles as cofactors in both the energy-releasing, catabolic pathways and the anabolic pathways involved in synthesis of proteins, lipids, carbohydrates and nucleic acids. Current estimates of the number of enzymes involved in nutrient metabolism (catabolism and anabolism) requiring just minerals as catalysts or cofactors range well over 300.

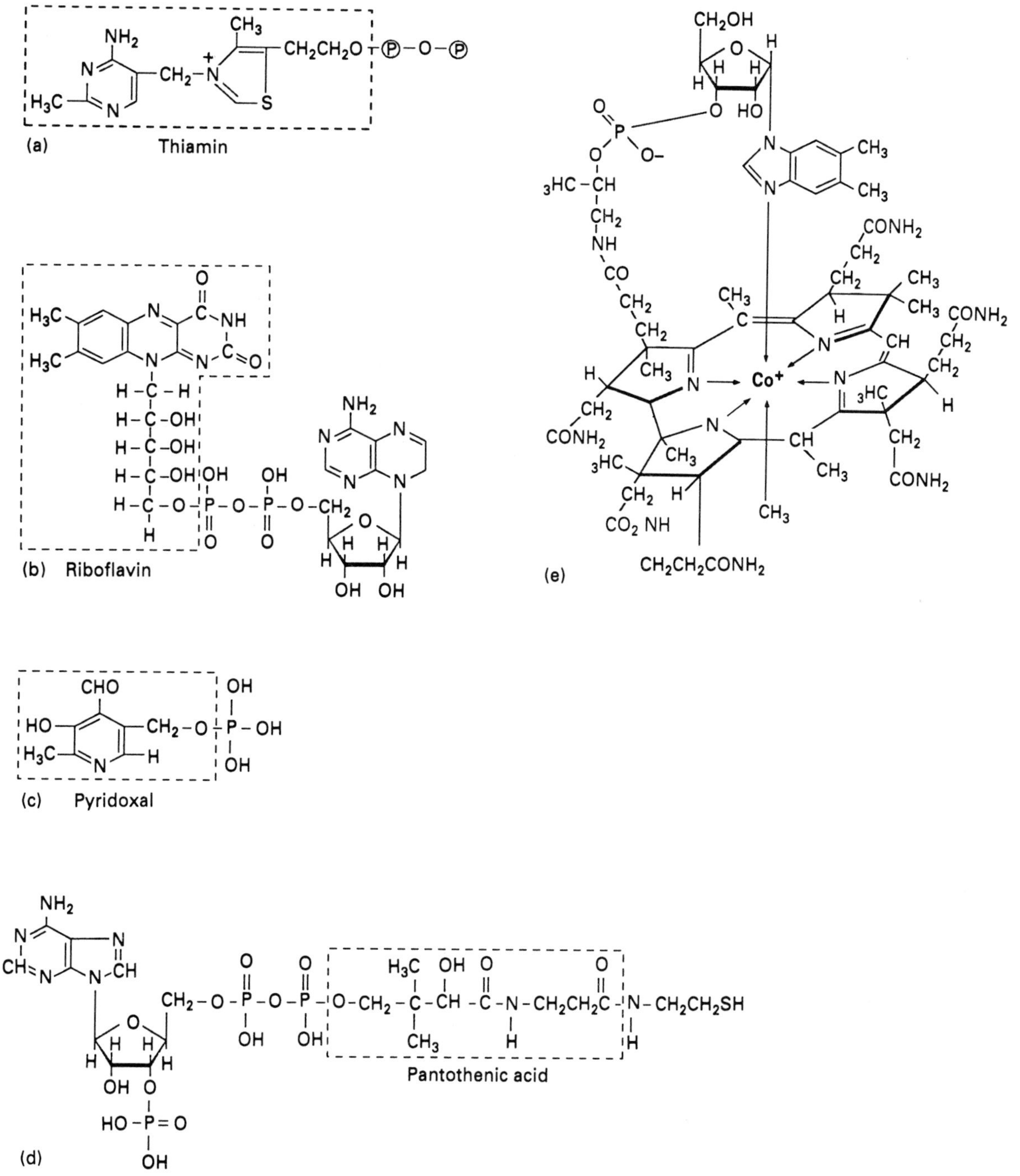

Fig. 2 Selected examples of vitamins as cofactors: (a) thiamin pyrophosphate; (b) flavin mononucleotide; (c) pyridoxal phosphate; (d) coenzyme A; (e) methylcobalamin or coenzyme B_{12}.

component of coenzyme A (Fig. 2d). Coenzyme A is necessary for the metabolism of carbohydrates, amino acids, fatty acids, and other biomolecules. As a cofactor of the acyl carrier protein, pantothenic acid participates in the synthesis of fatty acids. *See* Osteoporosis

The coenzyme forms of *vitamin B_{12}* are methylcobalamin (Fig. 2e) and deoxyadenosylcobalamin. These assist in the conversion of homocysteine to the amino acid methionine, the oxidation of amino acids and odd-chain

fatty acids, and the removal of a methyl group from methyl folate, which regenerates tetrahydrofolate. *See* Cobalamins, Physiology

Biotin as the coenzyme, biocytin, functions in carboxylation reactions that convert odd-carbon-numbered amino acids and fatty acids to even-carbon-numbered compounds, which can then be metabolized. Biocytin also is necessary for the synthesis of pyrimidines and the formation of urea. Some holoenzymes containing biotin act as carboxylases to convert acetyl CoA to cholesterol precursors, and as transcarboxylases, and decarboxylases in other important reactions. *See* Biotin, Physiology

The coenzyme of *folacin* is tetrahydrofolate (THF), a carrier of one-carbon units, such as methyl groups ($—CH_3$). One-carbon units arise primarily from the metabolism of amino acids. They are needed to interconvert amino acids and to synthesize purines and pyrimidines for the formation of RNA and DNA. *See* Nucleic Acids, Physiology

Vitamin A, as retinol, is a cofactor for apoproteins in the eye. These include opsin (rhodopsin) in the rods, which is responsible for dim-light vision; (and iodopsin) in the cone, involved in colour and bright-light vision in the retina.

Vitamin C (ascorbic acid) is a cofactor for the hydroxylases. Some examples are the hydroxylation of proline and lysine to create cross-links that are critical to the structural integrity of collagen, the hydroxylation of cholesterol to form bile acids, and the hydroxylation of tyrosine to form the hormone norepinephrine. *See* Ascorbic Acid, Physiology

Vitamin K acts as a coenzyme for γ-carboxylases, enzymes that transfer CO_2 groups. The resulting carboxylic acid groups are available for calcium-binding. Gamma-carboxylation is necessary for the formation of osteocalcin, a protein important in bone remodelling, and prothrombin, a coagulation factor (II) involved in blood clotting.

Minerals

Minerals participate as both catalysts and cofactors in biological reactions. As catalysts, minerals are not part of an enzyme or substrate, but accelerate the reaction between the two. As cofactors, they become a structural component which is essential for the function of an enzyme or protein. Minerals that play critical roles as cofactors for enzymes include magnesium, manganese, molybdenum and selenium. Other minerals, such as calcium, cobalt, phosphorus and iodine, act as essential cofactors for nonenzymatic proteins. Zinc, copper and iron are cofactors for both enzymatic and nonenzymatic proteins.

Mineral Cofactors in Enzymatic Reactions

Some examples of how minerals serve as cofactors for enzymes involved in metabolism are as follows.

Magnesium (Mg) is required as a cofactor for over 300 enzyme reactions. One critical function is the stabilization of the structure of adenosine triphosphate (ATP). Energy provided by magnesium-dependent ATP hy-

drolysis is required during the catabolism of carbohydrates (glycolysis and the citric acid cycle) and fatty acids (β oxidation) and the anabolism of proteins. Magnesium also plays a cofactor role in enzymes involved in the synthesis of DNA, and it helps maintain the double-helical structure of DNA. *See* Magnesium

Manganese (Mn) has been identified as an essential cofactor for more than a dozen metalloenzymes. Some examples are the glycosyltransferases, which are necessary for the formation of glycoproteins; proline depeptidase, which catalyses the final step in the breakdown of collagen; and pyruvate carboxylase and phosphoenolpyruvate carboxylase, enzymes that participate in carbohydrate metabolism. Manganese also activates superoxide dismutase, a mitochondrial enzyme which catalyses the breakdown of superoxide free radicals to hydrogen peroxide and water, and thereby protects cells from free radical damage.

Molybdenum (Mb) is a cofactor for several oxidation enzymes. Xanthine oxidase is necessary for the production of uric acid from purines; sulphite oxidase converts sulphite to sulphate; and aldehyde oxidase is involved in the hydroxylation of heterocyclic nitrogen compounds, such as nicotinic acid.

Selenium (Se) functions as a component of glutathione peroxidase (GSH). Although the metal is needed for activation, it is not a cofactor since it is bound between amino acids as selenocysteine. GSH prevents oxidative damage of cell membranes from peroxides produced when lipids (fats) are oxidized. *See* Selenium, Physiology

Zinc (Zn) is an essential component for more than 200 enzymes. Examples of zinc-containing enzymes are found in all known classes of enzymes, including transferases, hydrolases, oxidoreductases, lyases, isomerases and ligases. Zinc is a cofactor in key biochemical reactions in the body, such as carbohydrate, lipid and protein metabolism, stabilization of membranes, and synthesis and catabolism of DNA and RNA. Consequently, zinc is an important contributor to the processes of replication (synthesis of new DNA), transcription (synthesis of messenger RNA), and translation (synthesis of enzymatic and non-enzymatic proteins). Some of the general biological functions depending upon the cofactor functions of zinc include cell replication, tissue growth and repair, bone formation, skin integrity and cell-mediated immunity. *See* Zinc, Physiology

Mineral Cofactors in Nonenzymatic Molecules

Minerals also serve as integral structural components of a variety of non-enzymatic proteins, as well as for hormones and vitamin B_{12}.

Calcium (Ca) functions as a cofactor when it forms a

complex with two structurally related proteins – calmodulin and troponin C. Calmodulin is a protein with two globular lobes, each having two binding sites for calcium (Fig. 3a). When calcium ions bind to calmodulin, a variety of calcium-dependent enzymes are activated, including membrane phosphorylase kinases and some forms of cyclic nucleotide phosphodiesterases and adenylate cyclases. These enzymes change the three-dimensional conformation of the target protein and influence activity of signalling pathways whereby cell surface receptors transmit extracellular signals into cellular responses. For example, insulin reacts with its cell surface receptor to signal the cell to synthesize glycogen and to stop breaking down glycogen. These 'signals' ultimately involve the phosphorylation of glycogen synthase, which stimulates the polymerization of glucose molecules into glycogen and the phosphorylation of phosphorylase kinase. When the kinase enzyme is phosphorylated, it is inactivated and no longer stimulates glycogenolysis (glycogen breakdown). *See* Calcium, Physiology

Troponin C is a muscle protein which is structurally similar to calmodulin. When this protein is activated by calcium binding, it enhances interactions between actin and myosin, proteins involved in muscle contraction.

Cobalt (Co) is a central atom in the structure of vitamin B_{12} (Fig. 2e). This vitamin is essential for methylation reactions such as reactions involved in the synthesis of DNA. *See* Cobalt

Copper (Cu) ions play a critical role in the structure of transcriptional regulatory elements. In the presence of copper ions, certain transcription factors acquire a looplike structure which forms a cluster close around the copper ions (Fig. 3b). This complex is called a 'copper fist' since it appears to be similar to a fist clutching a small object. The loop 'knuckles' of the fist are thought to bind to a regulatory (promotor) region of the metallothionein gene. Once the transcription factor–copper complex (copper fist) is bound to the promotor region, another part of the transcription factor stimulates gene transcription. The translated metallothionein protein regulates copper levels and prevents toxicity. *See* Copper, Physiology

Iodine (I) forms part of the thyroid hormones, thyroxine (Fig. 3c) and thyronine. Both hormones help regulate the basal metabolic rate of organisms. *See* Iodine, Physiology

Iron (Fe) is a critical constituent of haem (Fig. 3d), which forms part of the haemoglobin and myoglobin molecules. Haemoglobin transports oxygen to and carbon dioxide away from cells in the body; myoglobin stores oxygen in muscle. *See* Iron, Physiology

Phosphorus (P) forms part of the energy-storage compound, ADP. When a third phosphate group is added, ATP is formed, when the third phosphate group is removed, energy is released. The storage and release of

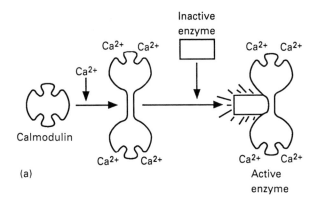

(a)

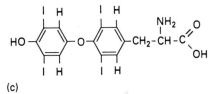

(b)

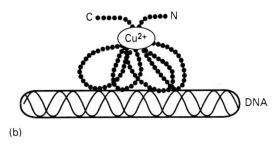

(c)

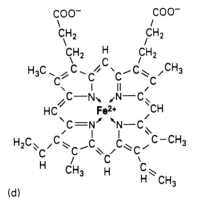

(d)

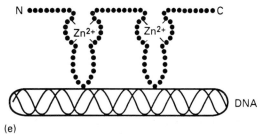

(e)

Fig. 3 Selected examples of minerals as cofactors: (a) calmodulin; (b) copper-fist motif; (c) thyroxine or T_4; (d) haem; (e) zinc-finger motif.

Coenzymes

energy via ADP and ATP is how the major components of food (carbohydrates, fats and protein) generate energy for the body.

Zinc ions are also needed for the structure of some transcriptional regulatory elements. The transcription of certain genes is regulated by DNA-binding proteins that contain important functional domains characterized as 'zinc fingers' (Fig. 3e). Zinc stabilizes the folding of the transcription factor into a 'finger loop' which is capable of site-specific binding to double-stranded DNA. Zinc finger loops are present in the DNA-binding domains of receptors for glucocorticoids, mineralocorticoids, oestrogen, progesterone, thyroid, 1,25-dihyroxy-vitamin D_3, and retinoic acid.

Effect of Nutrient Deficiencies

A primary deficiency of an essential vitamin or mineral cofactor is caused by inadequate amounts of the nutrient in the diet. A secondary deficiency occurs because of something other than diet, such as a disease state or metabolic alteration, which leads to decreased absorption, impaired transportation, or increased requirements, utilization or excretion. If a deficiency of a nutrient continues, body stores begin to diminish.

A continued insufficiency of a nutrient cofactor will impair or inhibit biochemical functions of the dependent enzyme. The lack of a functional enzyme–cofactor complex produces an accumulation of the substrate and a deficit of the enzyme product. At this point, measurements of biochemical parameters may indicate a problem that is not yet evident by a physical examination. This condition is known as a subclinical deficiency state. Eventually, the deficiency state is developed to the point at which it can be observed physically and produces the classical clinical symptoms of a nutrient deficiency.

An example of this process is seen when a dietary deficiency of iron produces iron-deficiency anaemia. Inadequate dietary intake of the mineral leads to declining stores in the body. A sensitive clinical test that measures the amount of the body's iron-carrying protein, transferrin, and the amount of iron it is carrying, can detect a developing iron deficiency before many of the symptoms of anaemia are observed. As body stores continue to be depleted, a lack of sufficient iron impairs the production of haem, a protein necessary for the formation of haemoglobin in red blood cells. The production of red blood cells declines and the reduced cell number can be determined by a simple clinical blood test called a haematocrit. When the decreased number of red blood cells cannot transport enough oxygen to the peripheral tissues, the result is fatigue, a clinical symptom associated with iron-deficiency anaemia. *See* Anaemia, Iron Deficiency Anaemia

Bibliography

Hunt SM and Groff JL (1990) *Advanced Nutrition and Human Metabolism*. West St. Paul, Minneapolis: West Publishing.
Machlin LJ (1991) *Handbook of Vitamins*. New York: Marcel Dekker.
Mertz W (1986) *Trace Elements in Human and Animal Nutrition* 5th edn. New York: Academic Press.
Shils ME and Young VR (1988) *Modern Nutrition in Health and Disease*. Philadelphia: Lea and Febiger.
Spallholz JE (1989) *Nutrition: Chemistry and Biology*. Englewood Cliffs, New Jersey: Prentice Hall.

Jeanne Freeland-Graves and Kimberly Kline
Department of Human Ecology, University of Texas at Austin, USA

COFFEE

Contents

Green Coffee

Green or raw coffee comprises green coffee beans; though, in trading practice, it may also contain small amounts of extraneous matter, derived from the harvested and processed coffee cherry and other foreign matter such as stones.

Classification of Green Coffee Beans

A green coffee bean, as defined in the International Standard, ISO 3509-1989 is 'a commercial term designating the dried seed of the coffee plant'. The coffee plant or tree (not shrub) belongs botanically to the *Coffea* genus in the family Rubiaceae, with subdivisions and some 80 separate species, of which only two species are commercially important for green coffee; these are *C. canephora* (known in the trade as *C. robusta*), and the other *C. arabica* L. In each of these two species, there are a number of true botanical varieties; but also cultivars, developed by horticultural research and used in plantations for various agronomic advantages. In recent years, a number of interspecies hybrids have been developed, notably arabusta in the Ivory Coast, from the crossing of the arabica and canephora (robusta) species, but also with other lesser known species growing wild in the hope of conferring advantage in respect of disease resistance, etc. None of these hybrids have yet developed much commercial success. Two particular 'original' varieties of arabica have been generally recognized, *C. arabica* var. *arabica* (syn. var. *typica*) and *C. arabica* var. *bourbon*. Cultivars are usually intraspecific by breeding/selection, such as caturra, mundo novo and catuai in Central/South America amongst the arabicas. Varieties in the *C. canephora* species are less precise, originally found in Africa; but *C. canephora* var. *kouillensis* is important and planted also in Indonesia and latterly in Brazil (where it is known as *Conillon robusta*); and also *C. canephora* var. *nganda*, especially found in Uganda. Whilst these varietal/cultivar names are not normally used in the trade, the different coffee types will contribute, along with other factors, to differences in flavour quality (after roasting/brewing).

Genetically speaking, most of the coffee species are diploid, as is *C. canephora* but *C. arabica* is tetraploid, that is, arabica has $4 \times 11 = 44$ chromosomes in its genome, unlike *C. canephora* with 22. This phenomenon has given rise to problems in interspecific breeding. Arabica plants are self-pollinating, though they can be crossed; whereas canephora (robusta) plants are self-sterile and require cross-pollinating for seed development. Robusta plants are generally propagated by use of cuttings (Fr. *bouterage*), whereas arabica plants are generally grown from seeds in nurseries, and then transplanted. These two species differ in their optimal environment for growing. Robusta will grow at low altitudes, will tolerate high temperatures and heavier rainfalls and requires a higher soil humus content than arabica, and is generally more resistant to diseases and pests (hence its common name). Whilst arabica is grown at higher altitudes (with quality connotations in respect of height above sea level) the plants are particularly susceptible to frost damage, which can occur from time to time, particularly in Brazil.

In general, coffee plants are only grown in those countries between the Tropics. Arabica is generally believed to have originated in Ethiopia, and first cultivated for large-scale export from the Yemen in about 1600 by the Turks. From the Yemen, seedlings were transported by Europeans to other parts of the world, so that it is now found mainly in Central/South America, and also in India, Kenya, Tanzania and other countries. Robusta derives from the rain forests of Central Africa, but only really discovered and commercialized from about 1880. It is now mainly grown in plantations in West Africa, and also in Uganda and Indonesia.

The flavour quality (after roasting/brewing) of robusta is generally considered to be inferior to arabica. It is certainly less expensive per unit weight of green coffee, and constitutes now about 25% of the world trade (imports into consuming countries). Its particular characteristics have been found favourable in the manufacture of some instant coffees; but robusta is also widely consumed as regular brewed coffee in countries such as France, Italy and Spain, and often features in espresso coffees.

A further classification of coffee beans relevant to both arabica and robusta coffee are into (1) flat beans, a term characterizing the majority of beans produced, with their single flat side with a central cleft, and (2) peaberries, which are small rounded beans resulting from a false embryony within the original cherry. The latter have a speciality roaster interest, as do so-called Maragogype, with an abnormally large-size arabica bean, found in some parts of Brazil.

A further basis of classification is described in the next section.

Green Bean Processing

Since coffee is originally harvested in the various growing countries, as 'cherries' or 'berries' with a fleshy interior usually carrying two seeds, and an outer skin, a sequence of operations is carried out in those same countries, in order to remove their seeds and present them as beans (dried seeds) or the 'clean coffee' of commerce. Figure 1 illustrates the sequences.

Removal of Beans from within Coffee Cherries

Two procedures have been developed; one, called dry processing, and the other wet processing (for washed and pulped coffee). The first, also in historical order, requires the sun drying of the coffee cherries laid out in layers (about 30 mm thick), which need to be periodically turned over during a period of some 3 weeks, until the moisture content is brought down at least below 13% w/w. This time period may be substantially reduced by the alternative use of specialized machine air driers. This type of process is used for nearly all robusta coffee production in the world; but it is still used for most of the

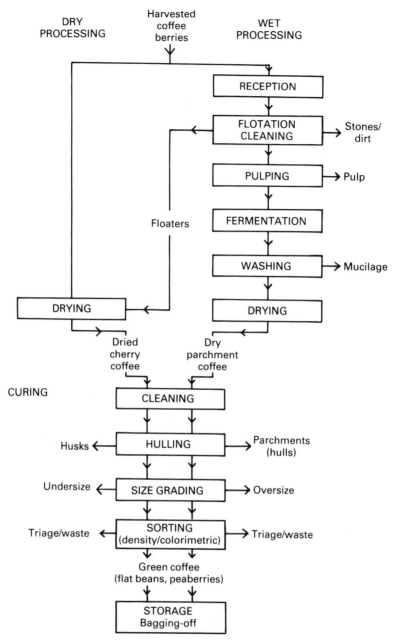

Fig. 1 Flow sheet illustrating the stages of wet and dry processing. Reproduced with permission from Clarke RJ and Macrae R (1987).

arabica coffee in Brazil and also in Ethiopia and Haiti. The product is now in the form of so-called husk coffee, that is, dried coffee cherries, carrying the dried seeds and all outer covering, which await the next stages known as 'curing', usually carried out at a central large-scale curing station, which takes in consignments from various out-lying plantations, both large and small. In curing, after cleaning, the beans are first separated from their outer coverings by dehusking machines, based upon a screw principle of which there are a number of commercial designs. The final presentation as clean coffee is described in a subsequent paragraph. *See* Drying, Drying Using Natural Radiation

The second procedure known as wet processing is more sophisticated than that of the first. In this procedure, it is important that the coffee cherries be first graded for ripeness, preferably by harvesting only those judged to be ripe and of a red skin colour; though water-flotation methods may be used for those overripe and dried on the tree, but not underripe, which are equally if not more undesirable. These cherries are then fed into pulping machines, of various commercial designs, which tear off and separate the skins and fleshy pulps (exocarp and mesocarp, respectively) in the presence of much water. Such machines will, however, leave a portion of the mesocarp, a mucilaginous layer adhering to the

Green Coffee

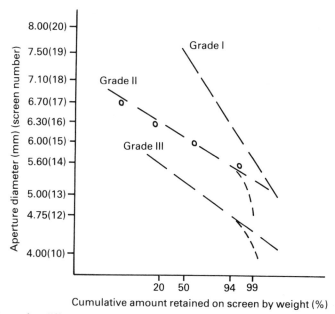

Fig. 2 Typical screen analyses for different size grades of Ivory Coast robusta green coffee beans according to specifications (including allowable tolerances), plotting percentage cumulative amount by weight (probability scale) held at each screen size (aperture diameter, mm) for screens according to ISO 4150. o—o, actual experimental data for grade II sample. Reproduced with permission from Clarke RJ and Macrae R (1987).

pericarp or a parchment layer directly surrounding the beans. The next stage in the process is, therefore, a means of removal by firstly loosening with fermentation, which is carried out in tanks. There are variants of detail of this operation in different countries, according to local 'know-how', climatic conditions and location height above sea level. Fermentation proceeds through the action of microorganisms/enzymes from within the semipulped coffee, over a period of about 24 h under either 'wet' or 'dry' (no added water) conditions. Care has to be taken that excess acidity does not develop, nor that of taints. After a dry fermentation, a water soak has been recommended (Kenya). The loosened mucilage is then complete washed off, by use of large quantities of water as the product is allowed to flow along long concrete channels, after which it is drained of excess water. An alternative system to pulping/fermentation/washing is in the use of the Aquapulper, the manufacturer of which claims will achieve all these operations within one machine. The resulting product is now known as 'wet parchment coffee', which has to be dried. Air drying is usually practised, that is, the parchment coffee is laid out on supported trays, with movable coverings that can be used during the hottest hours of the day, or again during cold nights. The drying time will be between 10 and 15 days to reach a desired moisture content of 11% w/w. Alternatively the parchment coffee may be machine dried in a shorter time, or for part of the time. In either method, great care is necessary for quality reasons, and optimal conditions have been the subject of much study in research stations

in Kenya, Colombia and elsewhere with many published papers. It is now necessary to remove the dry parchment layer to uncover the beans, by hulling machines similar in principle to those used in the dry process, already described, though the percentage amount of dried coverings to be disposed of, is clearly much less.

Preparation of the Clean Coffee for Export

The next stages of curing from either of the two processes above, after cleaning, involve firstly a size-grading stage; that is, by machines with rotating cylinders on a horizontal axis, fitted along their length with punched hole screens, of about three different hole sizes. Size grading is particularly needed for dry processed coffees (Figs 2 and 3). Each of the size-grades are then subjected to a series of sorting operations. The first is a density separation, which enables residual extraneous matter originating from the cherry, such as pieces of husk, parchment, etc. (dependent upon the wet or dry process previously used), abnormally light density beans, and indeed of foreign matter, to be removed as much as possible. Separation methods generally rely on air levitation principles, for which a number of machine types are available. A second sorting based upon the colour of beans has traditionally relied upon hand-picking as the beans move along a travelling belt, which also enables some other defects such as malformed beans and other residual defective matter to be removed. Electronic sorting is, however, becoming very widely

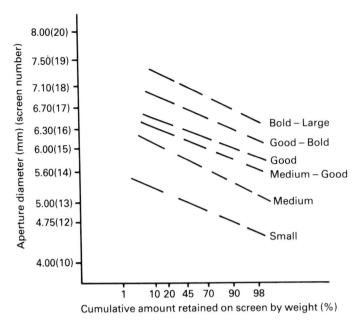

Fig. 3 Typical screen analyses for different size grades of Brazilian arabica green coffee beans according to specifications (including allowable tolerances). Percentage cumulative amount by weight held at each screen size (screens according to ISO 4150) plotted on a probability scale. Reproduced with permission from Clarke RJ and Macrae R (1987).

used, with monochromatic light used to sort out, in particular, 'black beans', regarded as especially unfavourable to quality, which may otherwise be of frequent occurrence in dry processed coffees. The target is to achieve substantially less than 1% by weight of black beans (or less than five per 300 g sample). Electronic sorting may also use multichromatic light, which enables a wider range of discoloured beans to be discarded, though such sophisticated machines are more usual in the consuming countries. For wet processed arabica there has also been a considerable growth in the use of sorters, in the producing countries, based upon fluorescence differences, which are designed to remove any so-called 'stinker beans', difficult to detect easily otherwise but especially undesirable to flavour quality if present, even in very small numbers.

The object of all the foregoing stages is therefore to provide 'Clean Coffee' at the right moisture content, which can then be bagged for export (or internal consumption) and documented according to origin, type and grade. They further subdivide commercial green coffees into wet-processed arabicas, known as 'milds' in the trade, dry-processed arabicas and robustas (dry processed).

Marketing, Grades, Shipping and Storage

The marketing of coffee is a complex commercial operation, with an underpinning by the International Coffee Organization, based in London, which, for example, through international governmental agree-

ments in force from time to time can organize quota systems for price stability. For the various green coffees under their control for export, the marketing authorities in different countries issue specifications, which may be either detailed or brief, without necessarily direct reference to flavour (i.e. when roasted/brewed). Test methods are available, many from the ISO on representative samples from consignments.

Grades/Types of Green Coffee

An important grade criterion is that of bean size (range) as can be characterized by a screen analysis using a number of internationally recognized screens with specific hole diameters (ISO 4150–1980, revised 1991). Different shorthand terms are used to express bean size distribution, e.g. letters such as A, B, C, etc., in Kenya, words (large–small with intermediates) in Brazil, and numbers (1, 2, 3) in robustas from the Ivory Coast. From Colombia, virtually only one size grade (excelso) is exported, defined on all through screen No. 15 (6 mm) and all on No. 18 (7·5 mm hole diameter).

A second criterion is that of type, specifically defining the number of defects present per sample, that is, defective beans of various kinds, extraneous and foreign matter. Different systems are in force, though most adopt a black bean equivalency system, where one black bean per 300 g (or 1 lb) sample equals one defect, and where other kinds of defect are assessed as numbers required to equal one black bean. Total numbers of defects define the type; which may be expressed in

Table 1. Green coffee composition

Component	Typical average content (%, dry basis[a])	
	Arabica	Robusta
Alkaloids (caffeine)	1·2	2·2
Trigonelline	1·0	0·7
Minerals (as oxide ash; 41% K and 4% P)	4·2	4·4
Acids		
Total chlorogenic	6·5	10·0
Aliphatic	1·0	1·0
Quinic	0·4	0·4
Sugars		
Sucrose	8·0	4·0
Reducing	0·1	0·4
Arabinogalactan, mannan and glucan[b]	44·0	48·0
Others[c]	1·0	2·0
Lignin[c]	3·0	3·0
Pectins[c]	2·0	2·0
Proteinaceous		
Protein	11·0	11·0
Free amino acids	0·5	0·8
Lipids		
Coffee oil (triglyceride with unsaponifiables)	16·0	10·0
TOTAL	100·0	100·0

Also small quantity of volatile organic compounds

[a] Data up-dated from Clarke RJ and Macrae R (1987) and Clarke RJ (1987).
[b] Data from Bradbury AGW and Halliday DJ (1987).
[c] Only very limited data available.

words, e.g. supérieure in the Ivory Coast for robusta, or terms, e.g. NY numbers (1–8) in Brazil. Such type numbers are not, however, used for wet-processed coffees from Kenya, Colombia and some other countries, where the number of defects in most of their exported coffee is very small (e.g. < 13 per 1 lb sample). Numbers of particular defects such as mouldy or insect-damaged beans are rigorously controlled in many countries (both importing/exporting); especially in the USA by the Federal Drug Administration with legislative backing, primarily for health and hygiene reasons.

A specification will, of course, refer to country of origin, maybe also growing area/port of embarkation and species/green bean processing method where this may be otherwise uncertain; and whether new crop/old crop. Purchase or otherwise may be primarily on the basis of exchange of samples, where the opportunity of inspecting for flavour quality/appearance is available.

Shipping and Storage

Some storage of green coffee is inevitable at various times from source to roaster, including of course during transit by ship (whether in bags in holds, or now more usually bags or loose in containers). It is generally recognized that green coffee should not be allowed to reach a moisture content in excess of 13% w/w; otherwise, mould growth will start to occur, which increases rapidly with increasing moisture content, causing flavour deterioration and the possibility of mould toxin formation. It should be noted that green coffee at a moisture content of 12% w/w is in equilibrium with ambient air of a relative humidity of about 65% at 28°C. Deterioration is also markedly accelerated by temperature, so that it has been stated that the temperature should not exceed 26°C or even 20°C. For a shelf life of 6 months, the air humidity should also be kept low, and the green coffee at < 11% w/w moisture content. However, there is some evidence that some storage of green coffee is desirable for flavour quality, with enzymatic generation of favourable aroma precursor before roasting. Holding of crop from one harvesting season to another, i.e. from new crop to old crop, even under favourable conditions, will give rise to changes in flavour and also in colour (fading or whitening on long storage), so that the crop year needs to be known. *See* Spoilage, Moulds in Food Spoilage; Storage Stability, Mechanisms of Degradation

Compositional Data. Chemical Changes During Processing

The fully detailed composition of green coffee, which is quite complex, has been gradually unravelled by both classic methods of analysis and the more modern laboratory techniques, such as high-performance liquid chromatography. Green coffee, is, of course, especially characterized by its content of caffeine, trigonelline and of chlorogenic acids; otherwise, its composition is similar to that of other comparable vegetable substances with their protein, carbohydrate, vegetable oil and mineral content. However, the carbohydrate portion consists mainly of polysaccharides, the exact nature of which has only recently been determined. A particular constituent is a mannan (of low degree of polymerization), responsible for the observed physical hardness of green coffee beans. The two main species of the *Coffea* genus, described previously, differ in composition in a number of respects, e.g. caffeine content, on a dry basis, averages 1·2% in arabica and 2·2% in robusta. Like all natural substances, variations from an average can be found, to which can be added those lesser ones accompanying green processing and storage effects. It may be noted, however, that commercial shipments of green coffee of a particular origin often have a surprisingly uniform composition, resulting from bulking procedures over the range of producing centres arranged by marketing authorities in a given country. *See* Caffeine; Carbohydrates, Classification and Properties; Chromatography, High-performance Liquid Chromatography

Table 1 shows the average composition of the two main species, in broad terms.

In finer detail, the quantity of free amino acids, whilst small, may well be of significance as an aroma precursor in subsequent Maillard reaction during roasting. The content of free amino acids and that of reducing sugars may well increase from zero during green processing through storage; though data are not available, primarily on account of difficulties in carrying out the sophisticated types of analysis on site in producing regions. *See* Browning, Nonenzymatic

There are a number of well characterized enzymes present in green coffee, such as the polyphenol oxidases, which may vary in activity according to their denaturation, relatable to quality by some authorities, though discounted by others. *See* Enzymes, Functions and Characteristics

The distribution of these components within the bean has been a subject of study, facilitated by scanning and transmission electron microscopy. A distinction between cell wall polysaccharides and reserve carbohydrates can be observed, and the occurrence of a coffee wax at the surface of the bean can be seen. However, the majority of the lipid material is bound as a globular membrane between the cell walls and the cytoplasm. *See* Lipids, Classification;

Bibliography

Bradbury AGW and Halliday DJ (1987) Polysaccharides in Green Coffee Beans. *Proceedings of the 12th ASIC Colloquium*, pp 265–269 Paris: ASIC.

Clarke RJ and Macrae R (eds) (1985) *Coffee: Chemistry*, vol. 1; (1987) *Technology*, vol. 2. Barking: Elsevier.

Clifford MN and Willson KC (eds) (1985) *Coffee: Botany, Biochemistry, Production of Beans and Beverage*. London: Chapman and Hall.

Clarke RJ (1987) Coffee Technology. In: Herschdoefer SH (ed.) *Quality Control in the Food Industry*, vol. 4. London: Academic Press.

R. J. Clarke
Chichester, UK

Roast and Ground

Green coffee itself has no comestible value for humans, and must first be roasted before use as a flavourful and stimulant aqueous beverage. Furthermore, roasted whole beans must be ground, either by the housewife or the manufacturer, after which brewing in any one of a number of appliances, manual or automatic, is required.

Roasting Processes

Roasting is a time–temperature-dependent process, whereby chemical changes are induced by pyrolysis within the coffee beans, together with marked physical changes in their internal structure. In particular, a whole range of different volatile organic compounds is generated, many of which are responsible for the flavour/aroma of a prepared coffee beverage, and for the headspace aroma of the dry product; though it is still not entirely certain which compounds, either singly or in combinations, are crucial. The required changes will take place with a bean temperature from about 190°C upwards, subsequently needing to be controlled on account of exothermic reactions occurring, so that bean temperatures up to 240°C may be reached in a time which should be less than 12 min. The particular time–temperature chosen will determine the degree of roast from very light to very dark (with intermediate subdivisions) assessed in the first place from visual bean colour.

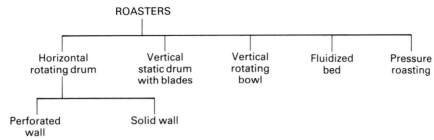

Fig. 1 Mechanical principles in roasting methods.

Choice of degree of roast is primarily a matter of consumer preference, with medium most usual for US and UK tastes.

In commercial roasting practice, green coffee beans under movement are subjected to heat by conduction from hot metal surfaces, or convection from hot air, or more generally a mixture of both methods of heat transfer, together with a contribution by radiation. Roasters may be broadly classified as in Fig. 1. The modern types of roaster maximize use of convective heating, whilst older household machines will rely mainly on conductive heating. The most widely used type has been the batch-operated horizontal rotating drum roaster (with either solid or perforated walls) in which hot air from a furnace/burner is passed through the tumbling green coffee beans. A typical example is shown in Fig. 2. Dependent upon the air (with combustion gases) flow rate, the temperature of the hot gases/air has to be substantially above bean temperatures to effect satisfactory heat transfer. In batch operation, the roasted beans have to be quickly discharged at the end of the required roasting period into a cooling car, or vessel, allowing the upward passage of cold air. In addition, water may also be sprayed from within the rotating drum, just before the end of the roast, so-called water quenching. Not only does this operation assist necessary cooling, but also adds a small percentage of water by weight to the roasted beans, which has been found to assist uniformity of particle size in subsequent grinding. Generated gases, mainly carbon dioxide, from the pyrolysis often carry solid particulate matter (chaff) which have to be continuously vented away and, with current environmental concerns, need to be 'after-burned' before actual discharge to the outside air. After-burning requires very high temperatures (450°C), and therefore further energy consumption, though lower-temperature catalytic convertors are also available. In recent decades there has been a general movement towards incorporation of recirculation methods for the hot gases, in which they are passed back, boosted with additional air, through the furnace, though with controlled partial release to the atmosphere, still including some after-burning or catalytic conversion. A typically sized roaster of this type would hold 240 kg of green coffee, with an out-turn (charging to discharging) of 15 min. The furnace/burner will be either oil or gas fired, and a net energy requirement of about 320 kcal per kilogram green coffee (excluding after-burning). Recirculation techniques provide higher velocities of air flow, increasing heat transfer coefficients, and therefore shortening roast time per unit weight of green coffee; though do not necessarily offer energy savings per unit weight of coffee.

The rotating drum principle was first applied to continuous operation in about 1950 of Jabez Burns 'Thermalo' roasters. Since then roasters based on other mechanical principles have been developed and widely used, e.g. the rotating bowl, vertical drum (with mixing blades) and fluidized air roasters of various designs.

The general improvement in heat transfer rates has now enabled shorter roast times (i.e. of the order of 3–5 min) in many of these roasters, with claimed advantages for the resultant coffee, so-called fast-roasted coffee of lower bulk density and 'high yield' on brewing.

Chemical and Physical Changes Taking Place on Roasting

Green coffee contains sucrose, polysaccharides and proteins together with free amino acids. Considerable potential therefore exists for the occurrence of Maillard-type reactions (essentially between reducing sugars, derived from partial inversion of sucrose during roasting, or already present, and amino acids), leading to the formation of both volatile compounds and high-molecular-weight polymers. Caramelization of sucrose also leads to the production of both volatile and nonvolatile compounds of sensory significance. Under roasting conditions, reactions are necessarily complex and difficult to unravel, with the effect of heat on proteins/carbohydrates in providing reactive centres and molecules to be also considered. *See* Sucrose, Properties and Determination

To date, some 700+ different volatile compounds in roasted coffee have now been identified by modern gas chromatography–mass spectrometry (GC–MS) techniques by numerous investigators since 1960. Many of these compounds have also been quantitatively deter-

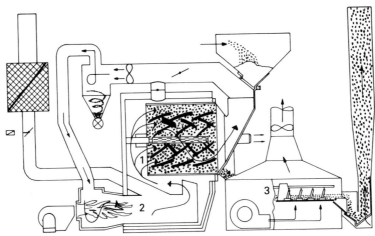

Fig. 2 Probat batch roaster, type R, showing (1) solid-wall roaster drum, (2) furnace, (3) cooling car, and ancillaries. Courtesy of Probat-Werke GmbH.

mined by GC–MS methods, and their total amount found to match closely the actual 700–800 mg per kilogram of roast coffee by steam distillation or other extractive methods. Some 6000 mg of semi-volatile acids per kilogram, e.g. acetic and formic acids, are also present. It is clear that amounts of individual compounds present will be in the milligram or microgram per kilogram range. It has been reported recently that the volatile complex comprises by weight 38–45% furan derivatives, 25–30% pyrazines, 3–7% pyridines, 3–5% benzenoid aromatics, 1% aliphatics, and 0·5 alicyclics and 1% of various sulphur compounds (which may well be particularly important for flavour/aroma) in a medium-roast arabica coffee. The mode of formation can be demonstrated by model heating experiments of selected components. Some compounds may also be generated by straight pyrolysis of single compounds, e.g. trigonelline in forming mainly pyridines, chlorogenic acids in generating phenols and of coffee oil in forming small amounts of aldehydes and hydrocarbons. *See* Chromatography, Gas Chromatography; Flavour Compounds, Structures and Characteristics

After roasting, substantial amounts of the compounds present may be found to be unchanged, dependent upon the degree of roast by direct analytical determinations. However, there is a newly formed residuum of about 25% by weight of the roast coffee, which is of uncertain composition but variously described as melanoidins/humic acids. These are caramelized sugars/condensation products of carbohydrates and proteins, linked with breakdown products of chlorogenic acids or even these acids themselves. The protein content (assessed by hydrolysis into amino acids) holds up quite well, though the term 'protein' is more applicable. Similarly, the polysaccharide content (assessable by hydrolysis into sugars); but the coffee oil is practically unaffected as is the caffeine. Since there is a loss of mass on roasting, which will range on a dry basis

from some 2–3% for a light roast up to about 12% for a very dark roast; indeed, the percentage content of coffee oil and of caffeine will show a slight increase from green to roasted coffee on a per cent dry basis. The change of chlorogenic acid content (together with that of its individual component acids) will be marked on roasting; thus, there is an overall 40% residual content for a medium roast (with differential figures for the individual components), which observations can be used as an analytical measure of degree of roast. The fate of much of the chlorogenic acids destroyed during roasting remains obscure. Table 1 shows a typical average final composition for medium roast coffee. *See* Caffeine

Physical changes in the roasted coffee can be equally significant, including, of course, colour. Scanning electron and light microscopy studies have been undertaken of cross-sections of coffee beans during roasting; cell walls are generally intact, but with a softening of internal structure, and the formation of cavities/cracking of the surface.

There is a marked change in individual bean density through swelling during roasting, which will be reflected in bulk density measurements (both of the whole roasted beans, and of the roast and ground). For a medium-roast bean, the void volume percentage is about 47% compared with virtually zero in the green bean. The cavities are initially filled with gaseous products of pyrolysis, mainly carbon dioxide, which can amount to some 2% by weight of the roasted bean. On standing, this carbon dioxide is slowly released, and of course as a result of subsequent grinding, more rapidly.

Grinding

Grinding of whole roast coffee beans may be conducted either as a small-scale household operation or on a large scale (e.g. typically of the order of 1000 kg h^{-1}). For the

Table 1. Roast coffee composition

Component	Typical average content (%)[a] Arabica	Robusta
Alkaloids (caffeine)	1·3	2·4
Trigonelline (including roasted by-products)	1·0	0·7
Minerals (oxide ash)	4·5	4·7
Acids		
Residual chlorogenic	2·5	3·8
Quinic	0·8	1·0
Aliphatic	1·6	1·6
Sugars		
Sucrose	0·0	0·0
Reducing	0·3	0·3
Polysaccharides (unchanged from green)	33·0	37·0
Lignin[b]	3·0	3·0
Pectins[b]	2·0	2·0
Proteinaceous		
'Protein'	7·5	7·5
Free amino acids	0·0	0·0
Lipids (coffee oil with unsaponifiables)	17·0	11·0
Caramelized/condensation products (melanoidins, etc.) by difference	25·5	25·5
TOTAL	100·0	100·0

Also 0·7–0·8% volatile substances (other than acids)

Data up-dated from Clarke RJ and Macrae R (1987).
[a] Dry basis figure for a medium-roast coffee.
[b] Limited data.

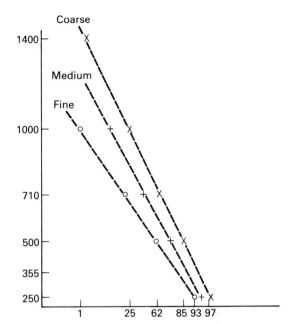

Fig. 3 Screen analyses for different degrees of grind of roast and ground coffee, plotting percentage cumulative amount by weight held at each screen size (aperture in μm) according to the R.20/3 series of screens (ISO 565 or BS 410). x – – – x, coarse; + – – – +, medium; ○ – – – ○, fine. Data from tabulation in BS 3999 part 8 (1982).

first, a variety of single-stage machines, either manually or electrically operated, have been available for some time. The use of a rotating serrated disc against a similar static one with an adjustable gap is the most usual mechanical principle adopted. On the larger scale, however, multistage twin horizontal rollers are employed, primarily to ensure more uniform particle size distribution than would otherwise be possible. Up to four stages may be used, the first two essentially cracking or crushing the beans into smaller units, followed by stages for progressively finer grinding. The type of serrations on the rollers is important; the most successful type was originated and patented in 1905 by Lepage and still features in Gump grinders. The fast roller of each of the first three pairs has slanting U-shaped corrugations running lengthways from end to end, whereas the slow rollers have a straight U-shaped groove, 'ring-around' or helically cut. The gaps are again adjustable. Simpler corrugations are used in the fourth pair as required for fine grinding.

Different degrees of grind are defined from the results of screen or sieve analysis, with three or four different screens in a set or nest. The nests of screens need to be shaken/tapped under standardized conditions for a given time (e.g. 5 mins for a 100 g sample). Especially important is the use of standard wire mesh screens with precisely defined mesh sizes or even certified screens, as described in BS 410-1976 or later, ISO 565-1983 and corresponding other national standards. Relating to roast and ground coffee, the number of different screen sizes numbered by aperture size within the range of about 1400 mm to 250 μm is quite large, so that it will be noted that there are a principal and two supplementary series described in ISO 565, which may result in some confusion. Care is needed in selection of appropriate screen sizes to give suitable weight distributions at each size. In addition, in the USA there is another set of sieve sizes in the Tyler series. Plotting the results of test screenings will show a good straight line relationship between aperture size (plotted on a linear scale) and the cumulative percentage weight at that size (probability scale), except at the ends (Fig. 3). The approximate average size of the particles will be given at the 50% cumulative weight point. More sophisticated statistical methods may be employed to assess average particle size. Newer methods of sizing by laser beams are becoming available.

Grind size required is related to the subsequent method of brewing to be adopted, and whether for home use or subsequent large-scale extraction. Grinds are usually defined as coarse—medium, fine, very fine—though the screen analysis which determines these, may differ in, say, the UK to the USA. Coarse grinds were used for household percolators, when the average particle size will be 850 μm (Europe), 1130 μm (USA), and fine grinds, as used for the now more popular filter machines, are 430 μm (Europe) and 800 μm (USA).

Packaging

Roasted whole coffee beans (RWB) and roasted and ground (R and G) coffee are not really finished products until they have been packaged for sale to the consumer. The type of packaging needed depends upon the time interval between manufacture and sale/consumption. In the case of small speciality retail shops, with in-house roasting, simple packets of paper or plastic are all that is necessary to maintain quality, provided the coffee is freshly roasted and ground and consumed shortly thereafter, say within a week for R and G coffee (or 10–12 days or longer for RWB).

However, packaged RWB and especially R and G coffee from large scale manufacture have been available for some considerable time, accelerated by the advent of supermarkets. There are now twin problems in the inevitably longer time scale (e.g. 3–12 months or more) between manufacture and consumption. The first problem is that roast coffee, especially R and G coffee, deteriorates quite rapidly, in respect of headspace aroma and of flavour, in the presence of air/oxygen/moisture; and the second is that roasted coffee gradually releases substantial quantities of its entrapped carbon dioxide gas (and other minor gaseous components), R and G coffee much more quickly than RWB. In the case of the former, however, about half will be released in the course of grinding. The amount of gas still retained plotted against time is asymptotic in character to zero, which may well show some 1000 h to near completion for RWB but substantially less time for R and G coffee after grinding.

A fully closed package containing freshly ground roast coffee will therefore rapidly develop a high internal pressure, maybe sufficient to cause the package to burst, and is thus dangerous. RWB will cause a similar or greater problem, though the rate of development of internal pressure will be much slower.

In practice, these twin packaging problems have been solved in a number of ways. Firstly, packaging under vacuum, allowing a low percentage oxygen content in the headspace to be established within the package (e.g. 25 mmHg pressure means less than 1% oxygen headspace level), and also accommodating release of carbon dioxide, so that the final pressure in the package may eventually just reach atmospheric. Secondly, by allow-

ing the R and G coffee in bulk to degas over a sufficient period of time to a low level, followed by gas purging whilst individual packages are being filled. In the first method tin cans have been used for many years; and more recently plastic packages, closed by heat sealing and then fitted into cardboard boxes. Such plastic packages have raised a number of additional problems, not least of seal integrity due to the hazard of coffee dust, but also due to a smaller headspace volume than possible in a tin can, to take up residual carbon dioxide, some prior degassing may be necessary. The package must not be allowed to become soft, which restricts the final internal pressure that is tolerable (around 500 mmHg abs. max.). These packages are so-called 'hardpacks', though in fact a package which has gone soft does not necessarily indicate of itself that the coffee has deteriorated in quality.

In the second method, where no vacuum is employed, various packaging materials can be used and heat sealed, to give so-called 'soft packs'. Gas purging is used to ensure that, again, the residual percentage oxygen content in the headspace gas is preferably less than 1%. In both these methods care is necessary in the selection of plastic packaging material (usually laminates) in consideration of gas ingress/egress, both of oxygen and carbon dioxide and also of volatile aroma compounds, and importantly, high resistance to water vapour ingress.

A third method which is especially popular in Europe is in the use of plastic packages to which a non-return valve (e.g. Goglio valve) has been securely attached, which allows release of excess carbon dioxide when the internal pressure exceeds a certain predetermined level. In this way the amount of prior degassing is minimized, and use of vacuum is not necessary.

All of these methods allow a much longer shelf life than is possible with simple air packs, though it will be appreciated that shelf life is shortened once any package is opened. Stability is discussed in the next section.

Deterioration on Storage

As will have been evident from the previous section, both oxygen and moisture are the agents that are primarily responsible for flavour quality deterioration together with the effect of temperature. It should be noted that like all foodstuffs, deterioration is continuously occurring from the time of harvesting and, in the case of roasted coffee, from immediately after roasting. Deterioration of flavour quality is, however, a subjective phenomenon, though accompanying chemical changes, only some of which may be directly related, can be of course be detected by laboratory analytical techniques. Nevertheless, trained panels with statistical treatment of results can be used to assess deterioration in terms of

Table 2. Shelf life of roasted and ground coffee

Storage conditions			Allowable time[a] before reaching quality ratings of			
Headspace oxygen (%)	Moisture content (%)	Temperature (°C)	High 9→8	Medium 6–5 Satisfying	Low 4 Acceptable	Roast coffee type
0·5	<4	21–23	6	12–17	20–25	R and G
1·0	<4	21–23	4	9–17	14–20	R and G
21·0	<4	21–23	—	—	10 days	R and G
21·0	<4	21–23	21 days	41 days	74 days	RWB

Data from sources fully cited in Clarke RJ and Macrae R (1987),
[a] Time in months except where otherwise stated.

rating scales/words. Considerable work has been undertaken at the Munich Technological University and others in recent years to study the deterioration of both RWB and R and G coffee under different conditions. They found it useful to rate on a scale (10→4→1), with word subdivisions of quality as 'high' (close to fresh) 'medium' (satisfying) and 'low' (still acceptable without emergence of stale or off flavours). Table 2 shows some of these findings. Other data are available for different conditions but not directly comparable, showing the markedly increased rate of deterioration at (1) higher moisture contents of the R and G coffee beyond 4%, and (2) percentage oxygen headspace levels beyond 1% (though an air pack is already included in Table 2). The effect of temperature on stability has been estimated by saying that each 10°C decrease doubles the shelf life, and vice versa. The advantages of storing roast coffee in a refrigerator is therefore clearly indicated, provided the moisture content does not rise, even if the package has been opened. *See* Storage Stability, Parameters Affecting Storage Stability

Various attempts have been made to correlate flavour quality changes with determinable compositional parameters. It may be noted that the chemical changes occurring are primarily related to the volatile organic compounds, called staling; only after a very considerable storage time do the changes start to affect the coffee oil by the development of rancidity. Headspace aroma deterioration may be found to be more rapid than detectable flavour deterioration, but does not necessarily mean a corresponding deterioration in the latter.

Domestic and Catering Methods of Brewing

It has already been stated that roast coffee must be ground before brewing. There are three further factors in brewing: coffee-to-water weight ratio, the appliance used and the temperatures employed. Some 14–28% w/w of soluble substances are extractable from roasted coffee by hot or boiling water, so-called 'yield', though the concentration of these solubles in the final brew (which will be between 0·75%–4%, and optimally at 1·2% for US/UK tastes), most markedly affects the flavour. Brewing is not only the extraction of soluble substances contributing only to basic tastes but also of the volatile substances for overall flavour, which also is not necessarily exhaustive (40–80%). The less polar substances will tend to reside in the coffee oil within the roast coffee, and will be more difficult to extract than the more polar substances, but are likely to be the more important for coffee flavour.

Apart from the brewing conditions, the actual flavour quality will be determined by choice of blend used, and the degree of roast. The choice of grind is also important. Different brewing devices or appliances (for home and catering use) have been developed over the centuries, both from the functional and artistic point of view, leading to a present apotheosis in the automatic electric filter machines. The appliances have been ascribed different names, often according to the maker, but the mechanical operation involved essentially is a means of separating the undesired so-called spent coffee grounds from the required brew formed by sufficient contact with water. The brew should contain as little of the spent ground particles as possible. At the same time, the brew must be presented hot (between 50 and 55°C), having been prepared using water at or somewhat below boiling temperatures, ostensibly to minimize loss of volatiles to the air. Two main mechanical principles can be identified: (1) 'steeping' (slurrying) of the R and G coffee with water, with or without agitation, followed by sedimentation or filtration or both, and (2) percolation in fixed beds of R and G coffee held in an open or closed container. In the second method, the water may be passed through either in a single pass under gravity, now perhaps the most popular, or under pressure (including steam, as in espresso making), or in multipass, which water may then include increasing amounts of soluble substances as in so-called household percolators. In the first method, two separate methods can be identified; one is infusion and the other, decoction (using boiling water). Of the components of roasted coffee, only some will be extracted completely with variable amounts of the others to reach about 28% w/w total maximum, and about 21% optimum under household brewing conditions.

Some comparative studies have been carried out on exactly the same blend/roast degree of coffee in different types of appliance, with one study suggesting a flavour advantage for an automatic filter machine.

Bibliography

Clarke RJ and Macrae R (eds) (1987) *Coffee: Technology* vol. 2, Barking: Elsevier.

Clarke RJ (1990) The volatile compounds of roasted coffee. *Italian Journal of Food Science* 2: 79–88.

Silwar R, Kampschroer H and Tressl R (1986) Gaschromatische-massenspektrometrische Untersuchungen des Röstkaffeearomas. *Chemische Mikrobiologie Technologie Lebensmittel* 10: 176.

R. J. Clarke
Chichester, UK

Instant

Instant coffee is the dried soluble portion of roasted coffee, which can be presented to the consumer in either powder or granule form for immediate make-up in hot water; whilst the insoluble part, or spent coffee grounds, are left behind at the factory, for the manufacturer to dispose of. Instant coffee is the name by which this product is now generally known, though there are two synonyms, soluble coffee and dried coffee extract, which names all express in different ways what the product is.

Definitions and Composition

Most countries have made a point of insisting that instant coffee be made from roasted coffee using water only (which includes steam); though allowance is needed for the commercial reality of added aroma oils prepared by mechanical pressing of roasted coffee or by other nonorganic solvent methods. This view is expressed in a standard of the International Standards Organization, ISO 3509–1989 (originated in 1970), which carries a simple definition, 'the dried water-soluble product, obtained exclusively from roasted coffee by physical methods using water as the only carrying agent which is not derived from coffee'. The European Economic Community (EEC) Directive for coffee and chicory extracts, 1977 and as amended 1983, in legislative force in all member countries has a somewhat longer definition, 'coffee extracts are the products in any concentration obtained by extraction from roasted coffee using water only as the medium of extraction and excluding any process of hydrolysis involving the addition of an acid or base and,

(1) containing the soluble and aromatic constituents of coffee
(2) which may contain insoluble oils derived from coffee, traces of insoluble substances derived from coffee, and insoluble substances not derived from coffee or from the water used for extraction.'

Instant coffee is then the dried product of such an extraction, and can only be labelled as such (or with synonyms, or foreign language equivalents) when the product so conforms. Products may of course contain other soluble beverage constituents, but then need to be appropriately labelled and all ingredients declared. Some soluble mineral constituents (e.g. 0–1000 ppm of sodium or calcium ions, etc.) may be present from the water used in the extraction.

Historically, most instant or soluble coffees first contained added carbohydrates (about 50% w/w) such as corn syrup solids, since it was found that a simple aqueous extract of roasted coffee, extracted under atmospheric conditions (100°C temperature) could not be dried (usually spray dried) to a satisfactory free-flowing low hygroscopic powder. It was only from about 1950 that instant coffee at 100% pure coffee solids became commercially available on a large scale. This step forward resulted from the discovery that the desirable carbohydrate (polysaccharide) substances could be obtained from the roast coffee itself, by a further aqueous extraction at temperatures up to 175°C and addition to the simple extract before drying, and thus providing a powder of satisfactory physical properties. *See* Carbohydrates, Classification and Properties

Instant coffees therefore have a higher yield of soluble substances from the roast coffee than that of a normal household brew prepared at 100°C or below. The additional substances, though extracted or solubilized at temperatures above 100°C, are fully soluble in hot or even cold water. It is often asked what is the difference in composition between cups of brewed and of instant coffees, when in fact there is a continuum, since they contain essentially the same substances, though the proportions or percentages of individual components will be different according to solubilization achieved for each. Commercial yields can differ considerably from one instant product to another, and for a short time were subject to legislative control in the European Community, but this was abandoned in 1983. It is now recognized that yield is only tenuously related to

Table 1. Approximate typical composition of brewed and instant coffees[a]

Component	Roast coffee (%, dry basis)	Filter brew[b] R and G basis[a] (%, dry basis)	Filter brew[b] Extract basis (%, dry basis)	Filter brew[b] Per cup (mg)	Instant[c] R and G basis (%, dry basis)	Instant[c] Extract basis (%, dry basis)	Instant[c] Per cup (mg)[e]
Caffeine	1·3	1·1[f]	5·3	11·0	1·3	2·9	58
Trigonelline (including roasted by-products)	1·0	0·9	4·3	90	1·0	2·2	44
Minerals (as oxide ash)	4·5	4·0[g]	19·0	400	4·2	9·3	186
Acids							
Residual							
Chlorogenic	2·5	2·5	12·0	250	2·5	5·5	110
Quinic	0·8	0·8	3·8	80	0·8	1·8	36
Aliphatic	1·6	1·6	7·6	160	1·6	3·5	70
Reducing sugars	0·3	0·3	1·4	30	2·2	4·9	98
Polysaccharides (unchanged from green)	31·0	3·2	15·1	320	12·9	28·7	574
Lignin/pectins	5·0	—	—	—	—	—	—
'Proteins'	10·0	2·0	9·5	200	5·5	12·2	244
Lipids	17·0	0·01	0·04	1	0·02	0·04	1
Caramelized/condensed compounds (by difference)	25·0	4·6	22·0	460	13·0	28·9	578
TOTALS	100	21·0	100·0	2100	45·0	100·0	2000
Volatile compounds (excluding acids)	0·08	0·04–0·07	—	4–7	Variable according to process		

[a] Assumed both made from a medium roast arabica coffee.
[b] Brew prepared using 10 g of roasted and ground coffee per cup (150–170 ml) at 21% yield of soluble solids from roasted coffee.
[c] Extract manufactured at a 45% yield of soluble solids from roasted coffee, both on a dry basis; and instant coffee without added coffee oil.
[d] R and G, roasted and ground.
[e] Beverage made up using 2 g instant coffee per cup (150–170 ml)
[f] Assumed extraction efficiency of 85%.
[g] Assumed extraction efficiency of 90%.

'quality'; the extraction and retention of aromatic substances in the total manufacturing process is much more important in determining flavour quality. The yield (on a dry basis) of soluble solids from roasted coffee will be around 21% w/w in brewed coffee, up to 32% in exhaustive extraction at 100°C, and typically 40–55% for instant coffees, dependent upon blend/roast colour of the originating roasted coffee. A highly water-soluble substance such as caffeine will be extracted to about 85–100% under household brewing conditions, and to 100% in instant coffee manufacture, but the actual percentage content in the soluble solids of the former will be substantially lower in the latter. In a cup of coffee, the quantity present will be determined by its strength, typically from 2 g of instant coffee dissolved in 150–170 ml of water in a cup. Table 1 shows a comparison of approximate composition by the main individual components for a typical filter coffee brew and a corresponding instant coffee beverage. The manufacture of instant coffee is accompanied by some slight hydrolysis of the polysaccharides in the roast coffee,

which is reflected in the slightly increased reducing sugar content (i.e. arabinose, mannose and galactose), and probably assists solubilization of these polysaccharides, not otherwise easily possible at 100°C. The quantity of volatile organic substances present in an instant coffee, which are so important to the flavour of a coffee beverage, will depend upon the particular process used in its manufacture as described below. The moisture content of instant coffee is controlled by the drying stage, which should be less than 5% w/w. *See* Caffeine

Physical Forms of Instant Coffee

In its earlier marketing, instant coffee was almost entirely sold as a spray-dried powder, light-to-dark brown in colour, free-flowing and, importantly, with a bulk free-flow density of between 180 and 220 g l[-1]. The latter two properties enable easy spooning out from a container, such that a typical semiheaped teaspoon would carry about 2 g of instant coffee to a 150–170 ml cup, giving a strength typically representative of average UK and US consumer taste preference.

From about 1965 onwards, instant coffee in granule form became available, though having the same free flow and bulk density characteristics, but generally somewhat darker in colour than the corresponding powder. With improved retention of aromatics also, such products were compared with brewed coffee far more favourably by most consumers than before.

Whilst freeze drying can produce powders from liquid feeds, its use for instant coffee was specially developed to provide a granular product. In a subsequent attempt to match the general appearance of freeze-dried granules, spray-dried powders were granulated by agglomeration methods (either simultaneously with spray drying, or subsequent to it), and now form a high percentage of instant coffees sold in the market place. *See* Freeze Drying, Structural and Flavour Changes

Dilute or concentrated aqueous extracts of roasted coffee would also be 'instant', but their stability at room temperature is poor, not more than 3 days even at refrigerator temperatures. Nevertheless, recent reports show canned coffee liquid to be very popular in Japan. Frozen granules or chunks ($-20°C$) would be quite stable, though they have only been commercialized in a very limited way; spoonable frozen instant coffee has been developed but requires the presence of gel-like additives.

Manufacturing Processes

The initial stages in manufacture, selection of green coffees, roasting and grinding (coarse grind) are as for roasted coffee. The subsequent basic processes needed are extraction, drying and packing; but with ancillary optional processes of concentration of extract, separate handling of aromatics and agglomeration. Know-how and patents are largely in the hands of large international companies. A typical scheme (simplified) is shown in Fig. 1.

Extraction

Percolation batteries with from five to eight interconnected columns holding roast coffee in different stages of exhaustion is the most widely used system for extraction to obtain coffee extracts of an economic soluble solids concentration (20–25% w/w) for subsequent drying. Its operation and variants are fully described in the literature, though it should be emphasized that the operation is intermittent (for draw-off of extract), countercurrent (in respect of water–coffee) and under pressure for all columns except the first (to keep the system hydraulic at temperatures in excess of $100°C$ up to $175°C$). The first

column contains fresh roasted coffee extracted with liquor at $100°C$ from which draw-offs are made; whilst the most spent is contacted with pure feed water at the highest temperature. The operation is outlined in Fig. 2.

Concentration of Extract

The removal of water from a percolated coffee extract is more economically achieved if concentrated extract is fed to the driers. Evaporation is widely used, and again for reasons of heat economy conducted in various types of multistage units. Short contact time evaporators are favoured, such as plate and centrifugal film evaporators, coupled with close attention to operating temperatures to minimize undesirable changes in the extract. However, evaporation of water is always accompanied by evaporation and loss of organic volatile substances contributing to flavour. Certain prestripping techniques are available to overcome this problem.

Freeze concentration can be used alternatively, which has the marked advantage of substantially retaining the volatile substances whilst the water is removed as ice, but has the disadvantage of only allowing a final concentration of about 38% w/w soluble coffee solids, due to high viscosity problems.

Spray Drying

Extracts from a percolation battery as described above can be directly spray dried, though an intermediate filtration stage (centrifuges) may be included. To provide dried particles of an average size around $300 \mu m$, needed for a satisfactory bulk density and flowability, specialized spray driers are used. The main features are:

(1) tall drying chambers, e.g. of height 7·5 m or more;
(2) use of centrifugal pressure nozzles rather than spinning discs for feed spraying, with their inherent narrow angle of discharge;
(3) internal chamber separation arrangements between desired product and dust, though not essential.

Spray drying is conducted also to give powder of desired colour, and a final moisture content of less than 5% w/w.

More concentrated extracts, say up to 60% w/w soluble solids, may also be spray dried, though some controlled foaming of extract with carbon dioxide or nitrogen gas is then generally required, if the desired physical properties are to be maintained. *See* Drying, Spray Drying

Freeze Drying

Freeze drying has been particularly successful for coffee

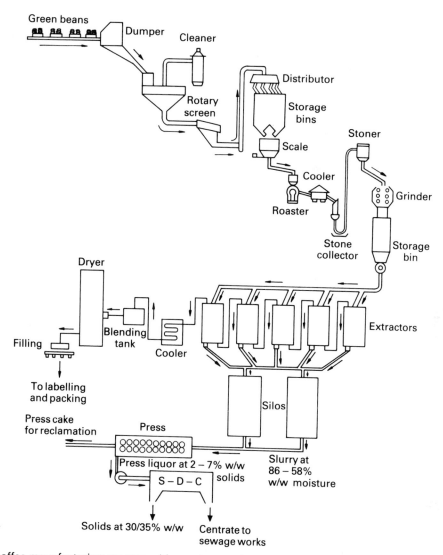

Fig. 1 Instant coffee manufacturing process with spent grounds recovery (omitting volatile compound handling). Reproduced with permission from Clarke RJ and Macrae R (1987).

extracts, when its use for other foodstuff liquids/solids has markedly declined in the last decades. However, a specialized technique has developed, first patented around 1965, whereby the coffee extract is first frozen, and then the slabs are granulated, whilst still frozen, to particles approximately the same size as desired in the finished dried product. Oversize/undersize particles are recycled. There are a number of designs of freeze drier available, which will generally handle the frozen granules in trays resting on heated shelves in a batchwise manner. The time of freeze drying required is up to 7 h under a very high vacuum (approx 0·4 torr), and a carefully controlled supply of heat to the drying granules, either by conduction and/or radiation.

Whilst satisfactory product can be obtained by freeze-drying extracts direct from a percolation battery, it is more usual for economic and other reasons for concentrated extracts up to 40% w/w by freeze concentration (q.v.) or by evaporation (40% w/w or higher) to be

freeze dried. If a favourable bulk density of 180–220 g l^{-1} is required, it is additionally necessary to foam the extract in the slush-frozen form, before full freezing and freeze drying. *See* Freeze Drying, The Basic Process

Separate Volatile Compound Handling

In recent decades, instant coffee manufacture has become increasingly sophisticated, through greater attention to methods of maximizing extraction and retention of volatile compounds responsible for flavour/aroma, which earlier procedures of simple extraction and spray drying could not accomplish. The first method concerns headspace aroma of the finished powder, due to the presence of very highly volatile substances which cannot be retained by any method of spray or freeze drying. A convenient vehicle was found to be coffee oil, which can be sprayed or plated (at a level of about 0·5% or less) onto the powder/granules as

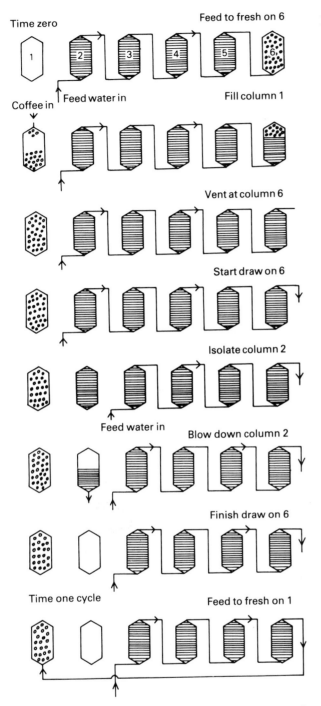

Fig. 2 Typical sequence of events in the operation of a percolation battery for instant coffee. Shape, size and number of columns are diagrammatic. Reproduced with permission from Clarke RJ and Macrae R (1987).

already described, and will give an aroma similar to that of dry roasted and ground coffee when sniffed. The coffee oil can be that obtained by mechanical expression of part of the roast coffee blend to be percolated; or a spent grounds coffee oil purified and enhanced with suitable aromatics from other stages of the manufacturing process. The coffee oil and its aromatics are very susceptible to oxidation, hence the need for gas-packed

product as already described. Its application (so-called 'aromatization') will play only a small role in the flavour of the made-up beverage product, so that other methods are needed, of which there are many available, mostly patented. *See* Oxidation of Food Components

Battery extraction, designed primarily for the extraction of soluble solids, can be fairly successful also for the extraction of volatile compounds, so that, when followed by freeze concentration and freeze drying, a flavourful product is formed. However, volatile compounds can be prestripped by steam from the roasted coffee before aqueous extraction, in the form of an aqueous condensate to be reincorporated later. Similarly, a percolated extract can be stripped of the important volatile compounds by partial evaporation (say 10–20% of the water), again to give an aqueous essence condensate. The stripped extract can then be further evaporated as required, with the condensate discarded.

The final solution after evaporation containing a high concentration of solubles, can then be slightly diluted-back with either or both of the aqueous essence condensates, and used as feed for either spray or freeze drying. The retention of volatile substances in spray drying is known to be very markedly improved when feed extracts of high soluble solids concentration are spray dried. This will be true also of freeze drying; though, additionally, it has been found that parameters of the freezing itself are also very important (e.g. slow freezing to large ice crystals favours subsequent volatile retention).

Agglomeration

Agglomeration was a process first used for dusty skim milk powders to increase average particle size and, more importantly, for ease of rapid dissolution in water, so-called 'instantization'. Whilst the latter is not required for a satisfactory instant coffee powder, a similar agglomeration process, using steam/water to rewet the surface of particles followed by drying, is used to manufacture instant coffee granules which are not in fact freeze dried. Precise details of processes differ, as the numerous patents will indicate. The diminution of volatile compound content from spray drying to granule formation will only be small.

Packing

Instant coffee was originally packed into tins, but since 1960 has now been almost entirely packed into glass jars. Under EEC prescribed weight directives, allowable packed weights for retail sale are 50, 100 and 200 g, and certain multiples, accompanied by the average weight system to be assessed over a stipulated number of containers. Filling machinery is now very high-speed (e.g. 250 per minute for 50 g jars), operating by volumetric fill, and adjustable by vacuum level according to the bulk density of the product being packed. Two other operations may be also incorporated, simultaneous spraying of small amounts of coffee oil into the powder/granules for headspace aroma purposes and a final provision of a carbon dioxide/nitrogen atmosphere within the jar to lower the headspace oxygen level to 4% v/v or preferably less.

General Comments

In recent decades, all these process stages have been investigated fundamentally through the disciplines of chemical (food) engineering by a number of people, especially the late Professor Thijssen of Eindhoven Technical University, to provide very considerable mathematical insight into their mechanisms.

Storage and Stability

Instant coffee is relatively hygroscopic, easily picking up moisture from the atmosphere and caking at about 7–8% w/w moisture content. For example, to keep instant coffee below 5% (dry basis) moisture content, the relative humidity of the air with which it is in contact must be below 35–40%, though the precise value depends upon the nature of the instant coffee in question, primarily due to differences in porosity of the particular particles made. It is necessary therefore that jars of instant coffee are well sealed prior to sale.

A simple spray-dried product, provided the dry matter content is kept above 95% w/w (i.e. <5% w/w moisture content), will have a shelf life of several years. The modern sophisticated products, containing substantial amounts of volatile compounds (especially plated coffee oils), need to be packed in jars also with not more than 4% in-pack oxygen content and preferably less, so that the shelf life to acceptable quality is maintained up to 18 months.

Bibliography

Clarke RJ and Macrae R (1985–1988) *Coffee: Chemistry*, vol. 1, *Technology*, vol. 2, *Commercial and Technico-legal Aspects*, vol. 6. Barking: Elsevier.

Clarke RJ (1987) Coffee technology In: Herschdoefer S (ed.) *Quality Control in the Food Industry*, 2nd edn, vol. 4. London: Academic Press.

Clifford MN and Willson KC (eds) (1985) *Coffee: Botany, Biochemistry, Production of Beans and Beverage*. London: Chapman and Hall.

R. J. Clarke
Chichester, UK

Analysis of Coffee Products

Coffee, like many food materials of plant origin, contains a very large number of different compounds. These range from discrete low-molecular-weight compounds, such as caffeine, to less well-defined high-molecular-weight polymers, such as polysaccharides and proteins. During roasting a diverse set of complex chemical reactions take place which increases the range and complexity of the compounds present. Brewing, or extraction, is essentially a physical process, yet even at this stage further chemical reactions can take place. Analytically, therefore, coffee, particularly after roasting, is an extremely complex mixture of compounds and consequently difficult to characterize completely.

Most analyses of coffee, and its processed products, are carried out with relevance to the determination of quality. For example, the keeping quality of green coffee is influenced by its water content, or the aroma of coffee brew is a direct consequence of the presence of volatile compounds formed during the roasting process. Analyses are also required to ascertain the optimum processing conditions, for instance the progress of roasting can be followed by studying the degradation of thermally labile compounds such as chlorogenic acids or trigonelline. Finally, analyses are often required to ensure that the product has not become contaminated during growth (e.g. pesticide residues), processing (e.g. polycyclic aromatic hydrocarbons contamination during roasting) or storage (e.g. mould growth, or staling).

Analyses for certain compounds, or groups of compounds, can be applied to green, roast and instant coffee but in general the methods need to take into account the differing matrices of these products, and the levels of the compounds to be determined in them. In this article only the major analyses will be discussed and reference will be made to other articles where greater detail of particular methods may be found.

Water Content

The simplest and most straightforward method of determining the water content of foods is by oven drying and this can be applied to green, roast and instant coffee. However, the precise value of the result obtained will depend on the actual conditions employed, due to water formation by the browning reaction or loss of nonwater volatiles. For green coffee, a wide range of conditions have been employed, including a two-stage process involving heating at 130°C for 6 h followed by a rest period in a desiccator for 15 h and then a second drying period for 4 h. The result is computed from the sum of the weight loss in the first stage and one-half of that in the second stage. This is a recognition of the fact that some water will be formed by chemical reaction under these conditions. In practice, many laboratories adopt a simpler overnight drying at 105°C. The water content of coffee beans on the tree is around 50% but this is reduced to 10-12% by processing for storage prior to roasting. *See* Water, Structure, Properties and Determination

Roast and ground coffee, and also instant coffee, has a much lower water content (approximately 2–5%) and this cannot be so accurately determined by oven drying methods, although such methods are still widely used for routine purposes. Alternatively, the Karl–Fischer method is often employed, in which water in the sample is extracted with methanol prior to titration.

Minerals

The ash content of green coffee is about 4% (dry basis) of which about 40% is potassium. The ash content can be determined by dry ashing at 580°C and its potassium content can then readily be quantified by flame photometry or atomic absorption. In addition to potassium, some further 30 elements have been quantified in coffee products by atomic absorption and even neutron activation analysis. Of all these elements only manganese shows a species difference, being somewhat higher in arabica (25–60 ppm) than in robusta coffees (10–33 ppm). The precise values of the elements found depend on both growing and processing conditions, but there is some evidence that trace metal profiles may provide a means of discriminating between coffees. In instant coffees the processing water used adds considerably to the trace metals derived from the actual beans.

Protein and Amino Acids

The protein content of coffee products (10–15% (dry basis)) *per se* is of little value as coffee is never consumed as a protein source. However, much research has been carried out trying to relate desirable features of the final coffee brew, e.g. aroma or mouth feel, with the initial protein contents of the green coffee. To date this research has met with only limited success. On roasting, much of the protein is degraded and reactions with many other components, such as carbohydrates, take place. The protein is therefore no longer in its initial state, as in the green coffee, but it will still contain organic nitrogen and may still yield amino acids on hydrolysis and therefore the 'protein content' of roast coffee products depends widely on the precise definition of protein adopted and on the method of analysis. *See* Amino Acids, Determination; Protein, Determination and Characterization

The crude protein content of coffee products is determined by the Kjeldahl procedure, usually based on the nitrogen content after some allowance has been made for the nitrogen contribution from caffeine. These values will be somewhat elevated in green coffee by other nonprotein nitrogen compounds, such as free amino acids or trigonelline. In roast or instant coffee there is a significant loss of organic nitrogen but it is no longer valid to calculate even crude protein values from the residual nitrogen content, as clearly significant protein degradation has occurred.

A better approach to protein determination is based on amino acid analysis after acid hydrolysis. In green coffee this should lead to accurate protein values but in roasted products the hydrolysis stage will liberate amino acids from proteins condensed in early Maillard products and so will not provide 'true protein' values. *See* Browning, Nonenzymatic

The free amino acids present in green coffee (usually less than 0·5% dry basis) are extremely important as aroma precursors. They are completely lost on roasting by degradation and/or combination with other components and are not found to any significant degree in roast or instant products. Free amino acids can be extracted from ground green coffee with aqueous buffers, although care must be taken to eliminate any proteolytic activity (e.g. by addition of ethanol) and to precipitate proteins (e.g. by addition of sulphosalicylic acid). The individual amino acids may then be determined by amino acid analysis, in a similar manner to protein hydrolysates.

Lipids

Coffee beans contain a significant amount of lipid material (arabica coffees 14–17% and robustas 7–11% (dry basis)). In green coffee the lipid is present within a globular membrane around the cytoplasm and adjacent to the cell walls. The traditional Soxhlet extraction procedure is therefore not effective in extracting lipid unless prior hydrolysis (usually acidic) is carried out to release the lipid from the membrane. On roasting, the lipid is widely dispersed and this, coupled with partial breakdown of the cell walls, allows more facile lipid extraction. The amount of lipid present is not greatly affected by roasting. The triglyceride fraction remains largely unchanged although there are some significant effects on the more polar lipids. *See* Triglycerides, Characterization and Determination

Oil from green coffee is quite different from that of many other beans in that it contains a significant proportion of nontriglyceride components as shown in Table 1. The precise proportions of these constituents will depend on the extraction conditions. In particular, the esters of the diterpene alcohols cafestol and kahweol make up a significant proportion of this fraction. Sterols

Table 1. Composition of lipids of green coffee (percentage of total lipids, average)

Triglycerides	75·2
Esters of diterpene alcohols	18·5
Diterpene alcohols	0·4
Esters of sterols	3·2
Sterols	2·2
Tocopherols	0·04–0·06
Phosphatides	0·1–0·5
Tryptamine derivatives	0·6–1·0

Data abstracted from Maier HG, (1981) *Kaffee*, p 21. Berlin: Paul Parey.

(4-desmethylsterols mainly) are also present at high levels. The fatty acid composition of coffee oil can be determined by conventional transmethylation to form fatty acid methyl esters (FAMEs) followed by quantification by gas chromatography (GC). However, unless the polar lipids (terpene and sterol esters, etc.) are removed, the fatty acids determined will include those liberated from these esters, in addition to the triglyceride fatty acids. If the precise location of fatty acids is required, coffee oil may be fractionated by column chromatography (silica or alumina) prior to FAME determination. Individual terpenes or sterols may be determined, after liberation from their esters, by GC or thin-layer chromatography (TLC). For GC, derivatization is often carried out to produce more volatile compounds, hence reducing the risks of thermal degradation. *See* Chromatography, Thin-layer Chromatography; Chromatography, Gas Chromatography; Fatty Acids, Analysis

In addition to coffee oil, held mainly within the cellular structure, coffee beans are coated with a more polar wax which can be removed by rapid washing with chloroform. This wax (about 0·2–0·3% (dry basis) of the bean) contains high levels of fatty acid esters of 5-hydroxytryptamine. These compounds are claimed to act as mucosal irritants and are removed in some 'health' coffees. 5-Hydroxytryptamine may be determined, after liberation from its esters, by TLC or high-performance liquid chromatography (HPLC). *See* Chromatography, High-performance Liquid Chromatography

Instant coffee is prepared from aqueous extracts of roast and ground coffee and therefore contains very little lipid material, apart from the small amount of coffee oil which may be added for aromatization at the end of the process.

Carbohydrates

Green coffee contains both low-molecular-weight sugars (sucrose) and a wide range of polysaccharides (arabinogalactan, galactomannan and cellulose). On roasting, the sucrose is completely destroyed, by caramelization and other reactions, and the polysaccharides are somewhat degraded and interact with other coffee components. However, the polysaccharide structures are sufficiently intact for sugars to be liberated on hydrolysis. During the severe conditions used industrially for extraction in instant coffee manufacture hydrolysis can take place to yield a wide range of oligosaccharides, mainly polymers of mannose, but also small amounts of mannose, galactose and arabinose monomers. As a result of these changes there is a considerable requirement for sugar analysis in coffee products, including for free sugars (green coffee), oligosaccharides (instant coffee) and monosaccharides (after hydrolysis of polysaccharides in all coffee products).

Free sugars may be extracted from coffee (green, roast or instant) using warm aqueous ethanol (80%) or warm water. However, with green coffee, water alone should not be used as this would allow hydrolysis by the endogenous enzymes present. Aqueous extracts may then be 'cleaned' by precipitation with Carrez solution or, more effectively, by solid phase extraction. Sugars may be determined by HPLC using either an amino partition column with aqueous acetonitrile or ion-moderated partition with water as the mobile phase. Detection is most commonly achieved by refractive index, although the mass detector has been advantageously used in some instances. More recently, ion chromatography has been employed in which the sugars are separated as anions under high pH conditions (0·1 M sodium hydroxide). With this system the highly sensitive pulsed amperometric detector is used. In addition to sucrose (around 6–8% (dry basis) in arabica and somewhat lower in robusta) there have also been reports of very low levels of other sugars in green coffee. However, it is far from clear whether these are formed from sucrose during storage and/or extraction, or whether they are actually present in the living plant. *See* Sucrose, Properties and Determination

The polysaccharide fraction of green coffee has been extensively studied, at least from the point of view of their constituent monosaccharides. Considerably less work has been reported on their precise molecular weight and structures. The first stage, after removal of the free sugars, involves hydrolysis with dilute mineral acids, usually 1 M sulphuric acid. The liberated sugars are then determined using the chromatographic techniques outlined above. In one major study the sugars were determined by GC, after extraction/solubilization of defatted green coffee with 4-methylmorpholine N-oxide to obtain the polysaccharides, with the results shown in Table 2. This particular study also involved some structural analysis and allowed an arabinogalactan to be identified with a galactose backbone and short side-chains of arabinose and galactose mainly termi-

Table 2. Polysaccharide analysis of green beans

	Polysaccharide content (% w/w)[a]				
	Arabinose	Mannose	Glucose	Galactose	Total
India robusta	4·1	21·9	7·8	14·0	48·2
Ivory Coast robusta	4·0	22·4	8·7	12·4	48·3
Sierra Leone robusta	3·8	21·7	8·0	12·9	46·9
El Salvador arabica	3·6	22·5	6·7	10·7	43·5
Colombia arabica	3·4	22·2	7·0	10·4	43·0
Ethiopia arabica	4·0	21·3	7·8	11·9	45·0

Data from Bradbury AGW and Halliday DJ (1987)
12th International Scientific Colloquium on Coffee, Montreux, pp 265–269.
[a] Expressed as anhydro sugars in green beans (dry basis).

nating in arabinose residues. The position of these arabinose residues explains their lability during high-temperature extraction. The presence of a glucose polymer resistant to mild acid hydrolysis also confirmed the absence of starch and the likely presence of cellulose.

Caffeine

Caffeine is undoubtedly the most extensively studied component in coffee, primarily because of the intense interest in its physiological functions. There is a significant difference in the levels found in arabica (about 1·2% (dry basis)) and robusta (about 2·2% (dry basis)) coffees. On roasting, caffeine is unchanged, although there may be small losses due to sublimation. Its percentage concentration may actually increase slightly due to the loss of other components on roasting. During extraction for instant coffee production essentially all the caffeine is solubilized and so the level in resulting coffee powders will depend on the rate of extraction of other components, particularly polysaccharides. Typical caffeine levels in instant coffees cover the range 2·8–4·6% (dry basis). *See* Caffeine

Earlier methods of determination were based on extraction into organic solvents, such as chloroform, followed by purification on columns of Celite or alumina and quantification by absorption measurements at 272 nm. Methods based purely on absorption are likely to be complicated by the presence of interfering species and therefore much effort has been directed into the development of chromatographic methods where the caffeine is completely resolved from other compounds before quantification. At present the preferred methodology is HPLC. A simple aqueous extraction of the coffee may be carried out, followed by precipitation or solid phase extraction before the HPLC stage. Most published methods employ reversed-phase columns (C_{18}) with aqueous methanol as the mobile phase. Detection is achieved by ultraviolet absorption at 272 nm. HPLC methods are also suitable for looking at

the low residual levels of caffeine found in decaffeinated products.

Chlorogenic and Other Organic Acids

The chlorogenic acid fraction in green coffee consists of three major groups of esters of quinic acid, caffeoylquinic acids, dicaffeoylquinic acids and feruloylquinic acids. There are also smaller amounts of other esters, e.g. *p*-coumaroylquinic acids. Each group has three isomers, depending on the point of esterification on the quinic acid ring. All of these compounds are thermally labile and therefore their levels are significantly reduced on roasting (up to 90% loss in a very dark roast). All of the components have an effect on the perceived acidity of coffee brews and the dicaffeoylquinic acids have also been implicated in the perception of astringency. *See* Acids, Properties and Determination

Analytical methods can broadly be grouped into two kinds, colorimetric methods which determine total chlorogenic acid content and chromatographic methods which allow separation and quantification of individual isomers. The first stage of extraction is complicated by the wide range of solubilities of the individual compounds and several suggestions have been made ranging from boiling with water to refluxing with aqueous methanol, ethanol or propanol. Cold water should not be used as this would allow oxidation by the endogenous polyphenol oxidases present. A typical colorimetric method would be that based on the formation of a molybdenum–dihydroxyphenol complex. Quantification is complicated by the different molar absorbance of the complexes formed from the various chlorogenic acids. The preferred chromatographic methods are now based on HPLC although GC after derivatization has been used. A reversed-phase column (C_{18}) is used with a low pH (2·5) aqueous methanol mobile phase. A good degree of selectivity of detection is achieved by using ultraviolet absorption at 320 nm. Gradient elution is normally required to allow complete separation of all

Table 3. Mean chlorogenic acid percentage contents of green coffee (dry basis)

	Caffeoylquinic acids			Dicaffeoylquinic acids			Feruloylquinic acids			
	3	4	5	3,4	3,5	4,5	3	4	5	Total
Arabicas	0·51	0·71	4·79	0·20	0·43	0·29	0·02	0·05	0·28	6·57
Robustas	0·79	0·98	5·49	0·58	0·56	0·69	0·08	0·14	0·84	9·04

Data abstracted from Clifford MN (1985) Chlorogenic acids. In: Clarke RJ and Macrae R (eds) *Coffee – Chemistry* Vol I, pp 186–188. Barking: Elsevier.

the monocaffeoyl- and dicaffeoylquinic acid isomers in a single chromatographic run. *See* Spectroscopy, Visible Spectroscopy and Colorimetry

Some mean levels for chlorogenic acids in green coffees are shown in Table 3. Corresponding data for roast and instant coffees is extremely variable, due to differences in roasting and processing conditions.

Whilst the levels of chlorogenic acids decrease significantly during roasting, the amounts of other organic acids may increase as a result of degradation of polysaccharides and other components. The acidity of resulting coffee brews is an extremely important sensory feature. A crude estimate of the acidity of beverages may be obtained from pH values or preferably by titration with alkali to a predetermined pH. However, in addition to contributing to acidity the individual organic acids influence the perceived flavour and so analyses for each acidic component may be required. The acids are normally isolated by ion exchange and then separated and quantified by ion chromatography or possibly GC, after suitable derivatization. Enzymatic methods are also available for selected acids. In a moderately roasted arabica coffee the following percentage (dry basis) acid levels would be typical; citric, 0·5; malic, 0·2; lactic, 0·1; quinic acid, 1·0; pyruvic, 0·1; acetic, 0·3. However, there are wide variations caused by differences in green coffees, degrees of roasting and, not least, varying analytical techniques.

Trigonelline and Nicotinic Acid

Trigonelline is present in green coffee at levels of around 1% but it degrades rapidly on roasting yielding a wide range of compounds including nicotinic acid:

Trigonelline   Nicotinic acid

Roast coffee contains 10–40 mg of nicotinic acid per 100 g, depending on the degree of roasting, and therefore provides a significant source of this vitamin in the diet. Trigonelline may be isolated and determined using an HPLC procedure very similar to that employed for caffeine. However, nicotinic acid requires the addition of an ion pair reagent to the mobile phase to achieve adequate chromatographic retention under reversed-phase conditions. Determination of these compounds also provides a useful means of assessing the degree of roast to which a sample of coffee has been subjected. *See* Niacin, Properties and Determination

Volatile Compounds

Green coffee has a relatively bland aroma which bears little resemblance to that of roast and ground coffee. The characteristic aroma of the latter is due to the very wide range of chemical reactions which take place during roasting, many of which are still poorly understood. The most important aroma precursors are amino acids (and proteins), sugars (and polysaccharides) and chlorogenic acids. Smaller contributions are made from other compounds such as trigonelline, terpenes, sterols and lipids. The most significant reaction would appear to be the interaction between amino compounds (amino acids) and reducing sugars as in the browning reaction. Direct caramelization is also very important. A wide range of compounds is formed, as shown in Table 4. *See* Essential Oils, Properties and Uses; Phenolic Compounds

The simplest analytical method for characterizing coffee aroma is by direct headspace analysis. In this method a sample of the coffee, as powder or a brew, is equilibrated in an enclosed vessel and warmed (40–50°C). A sample of the headspace is then withdrawn from above the sample with an air-tight syringe *via* a septum. This gaseous sample is then injected directly into a GC to produce an aroma chromatogram. Ideally, if instrumentation is available the GC will be coupled to a mass spectrometer, which will allow identification of many of the separated compounds. This simple head-

Analysis of Coffee Products

space technique will only allow the determination of the major volatile compounds present, e.g. aldehydes and alcohols, yet these may not be the most important in relation to the perceived aroma. For example, many sulphur compounds have an extremely low aroma threshold and therefore are significant at levels well below those which could be detected using the above technique.

Alternative procedures which allow concentration of a wider range of volatile compounds include codistillation techniques, where the coffee volatiles are condensed and trapped in a small volume of a volatile solvent (Likens–Nickerson apparatus), and purge and trap methods where the volatile compounds are swept from the sample and then trapped on a suitable adsorbent prior to desorption and introduction into the GC. Using these methods it is possible to detect and quantify compounds at much lower levels. The power of GC to discriminate between closely eluting compounds can be enhanced by using selective detectors in addition to a universal detector, such as the flame ionization detector. Thus, the very important sulphur or nitrogen compounds can be selectively detected by flame photometric detection and alkali flame ionization detection, respectively. Ideally, these detectors could be used in series to provide the maximum information.

The fact that several hundred volatile compounds have been detected in coffee products can be readily appreciated from a capillary gas chromatogram such as that shown in Fig 1. These methods, however, tend to be based on exhaustive extraction, most suited to total analysis content in dry roasted coffee, which will not reflect the amounts present in actual coffee brews. The latter are necessarily lower, depending on brewing conditions. Accurate determinations from dilute solutions are more difficult, and usually not attempted. Even with analytical sophistication of this degree relatively little progress has been made in the correlation of sensory attributes with instrumental analysis. This is

Table 4. The number of volatile compounds identified in roasted coffee

Hydrocarbons	72	Pyrrols	67
Alcohols	20	Benzopyrrols	5
Aldehydes	29	Pyrazines	71
Ketones	68	Benzopyrazines	11
Acids	22	Pyridines	12
Esters	29	Benzopyridines	4
Ethers	2	Thiophenes	30
Acetals	1	Benzothiophenes	1
Nitrogen compounds (nonheterocyclic)	22	Oxazoles	24
Sulphur compounds (nonheterocyclic)	17	Benzooxazoles	5
Phenols	40	Thiazoles	26
Furans	112	Benzothiazoles	1
Benzofurans	3	Pyrones	4
Pyrans	2	Lactones	9
Anhydrides	3		
Total	712		

Data abstracted from Clarke RJ (1990) The volatile compounds of roasted coffee, *Italian Journal of Food Science* 2: 79–88. The compilation of Clarke is based on work published by Van Straten S, Maarse M and Visscher CA (1986) *Volatile Compounds in Foodstuffs. Coffee: Qualitative Data.* Zeist: TNO.

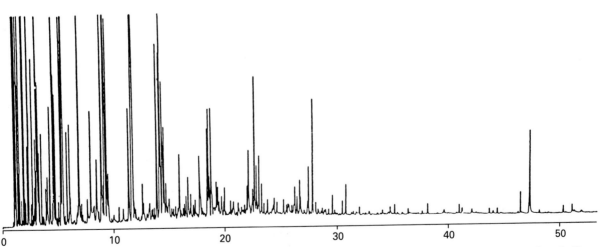

Fig. 1 Chromatogram of a Nickerson–Likens extract of ground roasted coffee. Column, 30 m × 0·32 mm fused silica, coated with a 1·0 μm bonded film of DB-5. One microlitre, ca. 1:100 split injection, 35°C, 2 min; 2°C min⁻¹ to 55°C; 4°C min⁻¹ to 245°C; hold; flame ionization detector. Total run time, 60 min. Extract prepared from approximately 50 g of newly roasted and freshly ground Colombian coffee placed in a 500 ml flask in 200 ml of water, and refluxed against 5 ml of pentane. Extract diluted further. Reproduced from Jennings W, Takeoka G and Macku C (1985) *10th International Scientific Colloquium on Coffee*, Lome, pp 169–180.

Analysis of Coffee Products

Table 5. Possible contaminants of coffee

Contaminant	Source	Method of analysis
Copper	Pesticide residue	Atomic absorption
Iron	Processing equipment	Atomic absorption
Sodium	Softened water	Flame photometry
Lead	Solder	Atomic absorption
Mycotoxins	Fungal contamination	HPLC or immunoassays
Polycyclic aromatic hydrocarbons	Direct-fired roasters	HPLC or GC
Phenols	Disinfectants, sacks	GC
Pesticides	Residues from growing	GC or HPLC

partly due to the fact that a single sensory descriptor, e.g. 'burnt' or 'stale', may be the result of the presence of many compounds. Chemometric techniques (e.g. principal component analysis) have achieved some success but sensory evaluation of aroma quality will not be replaced by techniques such as GC for many years to come.

Contaminants

Coffee, like any other food or beverage, is subjected from time to time to extraneous contamination and therefore is regularly screened for the presence of a wide range of possible compounds. Fortunately, few of these contaminants are found at significant levels and in many instances they are eliminated by the normal processing, e.g. by thermal degradation or by insolubility in water. Table 5 provides a list of some potential contaminants and methods of analysis. *See* Contamination, Detection *See also* individual contaminants

Sensory Analysis

Analysis of coffee should not be confined to determination of chemical content. To some, sensory analysis is the more important, that is, especially assessing brew flavour characteristics in totality, and including colour. Flavour comprises basic taste arising from non-volatile compounds detected by the tongue, plus aroma arising from volatile compounds detected by olfactory organs in the nose, reached from the back of the mouth in drinking or via the nostrils, together with mouthfeel. Expert traditional coffee tasters, panels of experts/nonexperts, and sampled consumers are used for this purpose in different ways. Whilst modern flavour profiling methods are used, often the requirement is merely to confirm expectations or otherwise of a particular coffee type (milds, Brazils, etc.) to a norm, but with reference to any downgrading flavour notes present; or to assess significant difference from a standard by statistical application to triangle tests or similar; or

indeed largely to assess preference between two samples in consumer tests, again using sophisticated statistical methodology. *See* Sensory Evaluation, Sensory Characteristics of Human Foods

Bibliography

Association Scientifique Internationale du Café. *Collection of Colloquia Proceedings (1st to 14th Colloquia, 1963–1991).* Paris: ASIC.

Clarke RJ and Macrae R. (1985) *Coffee – Chemistry*, vol. 1. London: Elsevier Applied Science Publishers.

Clifford MN and Willson KC (1985) *Coffee – Botany, Biochemistry and Production of Beans and Beverage.* London: Croom Helm.

Maier HG (1981) *Kaffee.* Berlin: Paul Parey.

Rothfos B (1986) *Coffee – Consumption.* Hamburg: Gordian-Max Rieck.

Wrigley G (1988) *Coffee.* Harlow: Longman Scientific and Technical.

R. Macrae
University of Hull, Hull, UK

Decaffeination

Decaffeinated roasted coffees have been available since about 1905, especially in Germany and have become a substantial sector in the sales of both roasted and instant coffee in the last two decades.

Definitions and Composition

The International Standards Organization in ISO 3509–1989 (and earlier versions) has defined decaffeinated coffee as 'coffee from which caffeine has been extracted. NB. A maximum residual caffeine content would usually be stated in a specification for decaffeinated coffee'. In fact, there is considerable national legislation specifying this maximum residual amount. In the UK and most other European countries, the maximum caffeine content for decaffeinated roasted coffees is set at 0.1% (dry basis); though in the USA there is no specific legislation but manufacturers generally claim that more than 97% of the original caffeine has been removed. There is no particular market for partially decaffeinated coffees. For decaffeinated instant coffee, in European Community countries, the maximum caffeine content is set at 0.3% (dry basis) by the European Community Coffee and Chicory Products Directive of 1977 (and as amended 1983). This figure is also generally accepted elsewhere in the world, whether by legislation or otherwise; except again in the USA where a 97% elimination figure is usual. It should be pointed out that in commercial practice, both of these figures (0.1% and 0.3%) are in fact higher than those normally obtainable, especially for decaffeinated instant coffee, so that legal enforcement problems rarely arise. The relationship between the maximum figures for roasted and instant coffee was originally based upon a purely nominal extraction yield figure of 33% soluble solids in extracting roast coffee. It can be seen therefore that a cup of brewed coffee (from 10 g of roasted coffee) will contain not more than 10 mg of caffeine; and of instant coffee (using 2 g of product), 6 mg. *See* Caffeine

Decaffeination is the name of the process whereby caffeine is removed. Almost entirely in commercial practice the process is applied to green coffee, after which the decaffeinated green coffee is roasted and ground, or converted to instant coffee exactly as for the corresponding nondecaffeinated products. The composition of these decaffeinated products, apart from caffeine content, will therefore be almost correspondingly identical. However, there will be slight differences, and also of flavour, depending upon the particular decaffeination process employed.

Caffeine is the most studied physiologically active component of coffee. Though this activity is generally weak, it has been the subject of numerous publications and much investigative work. According to the US Food and Drug Administration (1984) 'the evidence received does not suggest that caffeine at present levels of consumption poses a hazard to public health.'

Decaffeination Processes

The various decaffeination processes in use can be classified with subdivisions in various ways. However, the original process, still used, is based upon direct organic solvent extraction of the green beans; subsequent to that an indirect solvent process was devised, in which water is first used to remove the caffeine from the beans, and the aqueous extract then treated with the same kind of organic solvent as before. More latterly,

since 1970, a variant of direct solvent extraction has become available in which the solvent is supercritical carbon dioxide. In all these methods, it is necessary to be able to recover the caffeine from the extracting liquids, and generally to refine it to a pure form for sale. It is also necessary to eliminate all but traces of organic solvent from the decaffeinated coffee beans, which should finally have a normal moisture content of, say, 11% w/w for sale or further processing. In commercial practice, residues of organic solvent will be exceedingly small, less than 1 mg kg^{-1} in decaffeinated green coffee and, in a recent survey by the US Food and Drug Administration of commercial coffees, less in roasted coffee (11–640 μg kg^{-1}) and its brews, and even less in instant coffee (0.49 μg kg^{-1}). No particular legislation for residues has been adopted by European Community countries, though it has been under consideration for a considerable time now, except that of choice of organic solvent which may be used.

Decaffeination processes and their off-shoots have been the subject of much patenting activity, since conventional processes in use can be time-consuming and complex, and furthermore have led to developing environmental concerns. Though it can be seen that residual solvent amounts are negligible in respect of consumer exposure, use of organic solvents at manufacturing sites has to be carefully controlled on account of various potential hazards. This situation has prompted the development of alternative processes, solvents and caffeine adsorbents.

Direct Solvent Decaffeination

The first commercial process was developed and patented in Bremen, Germany, in 1905, and sold as Cafe Hag, which name is still in use. The process used benzene as the solvent upon previously steamed green beans. However, benzene is both flammable and toxic, and became replaced by chlorinated hydrocarbons as they became available, and cheaper. Trichloroethylene was particularly favoured, though in 1976 it became the subject of US Food and Drug Administration investigations and was gradually phased out and replaced by methylene chloride, which was affirmed for use in 1985 by the above regulatory body. A number of other organic solvents have been proposed, though only ethyl acetate and vegetable oils (including coffee oil and purified spent grounds coffee oil) have been or are believed to be used in commercial practice.

It was early found that a dry organic solvent extracted relatively little caffeine, or only very slowly, from green coffee beans, even though the solubility of pure caffeine in methylene chloride is reported, for example, to be 19 g per 100 g of solvent at 33°C or 1.82 g in trichloroethylene at 15°C. By raising the moisture of the green beans,

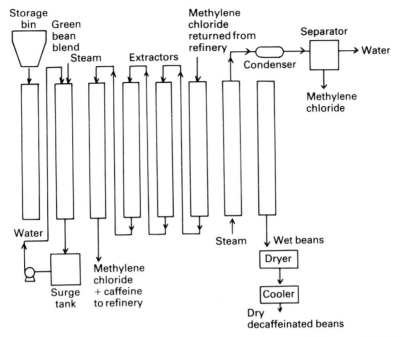

Fig. 1 Solvent decaffeination. Reproduced with permission from Clarke RJ and Macrae R (1987).

first by steaming and then soaking in warm water, to 20–55% w/w (optionally 42% for methylene chloride) at, say, 67°C the transfer of caffeine into the solvent is markedly expedited. The explanation for this effect is twofold; a swelling of the coffee beans to assist diffusion, and destabilization of caffeine–chlorogenate complexes in the coffee bean by heat/water.

The extraction itself is carried out in percolation batteries of five to eight columns (similar to aqueous extraction in the manufacture of instant coffee, though not under pressure), though the time of contact can still be as long as 10 h. About 4 kg of methylene chloride is required per kilogram of coffee. The column containing coffee at the required decaffeination level is then isolated and drained, and steamed to remove traces of solvent for about 1·5 h. The decaffeinated coffee is then dried. The methylene chloride with dissolved caffeine from the most spent column is sent to a refinery, where the caffeine is extracted and the caffeine-free liquid sent back to the battery. A typical operation is shown in Fig. 1.

Methylene chloride is known to be quite selective for caffeine amongst the components of green coffee, e.g. trigonelline is very poorly soluble. There will be some loss of weight in decaffeination, apart from that due to the caffeine, but some of this may be accounted for by normal process losses. No published data are available.

Indirect Solvent Decaffeination or Water Decaffeination

A process was patented in 1941 in which water was used to remove caffeine from the green coffee beans. How-

ever, there are other water-soluble constituents (up to about 20%) present, so to prevent their extraction the extracting water has to contain equilibrium quantities of these noncaffeine solubles, so-called 'green' extract, but little or no caffeine.

The actual decaffeination process is again conducted in a percolation battery. After an initial start-up, the caffeine-rich water extract at about 0·5% caffeine content is contacted countercurrently (e.g. in a rotary disc contactor) with an organic solvent (such as methylene chloride, also described under direct decaffeination) at around 80°C in order to reduce its caffeine content to below 0·05%. This 'green' water extract is then stripped of its residual dispersed and dissolved organic solvent, and is then recycled to the battery to extract further caffeine, and so on. The decaffeinated beans from the most spent column are dropped to a container, after they are washed with water on a screen to remove adhering soluble material, with the wash water being then added to the caffeine-free water extract before actual recycling. The washed decaffeinated beans are then dried. The methylene chloride stream containing the caffeine is evaporated to leave the caffeine which is then refined, and the solvent returned for reuse in the contactor.

This process is somewhat more complex than the direct method, but has the claimed advantages of a faster (about 8 h) and higher extraction rate of caffeine, less heat treatment of coffee, retention of surface waxes and purer recovered caffeine. Though no published data are available, it is probable that there is a slightly higher loss of noncaffeine water-soluble substances, including

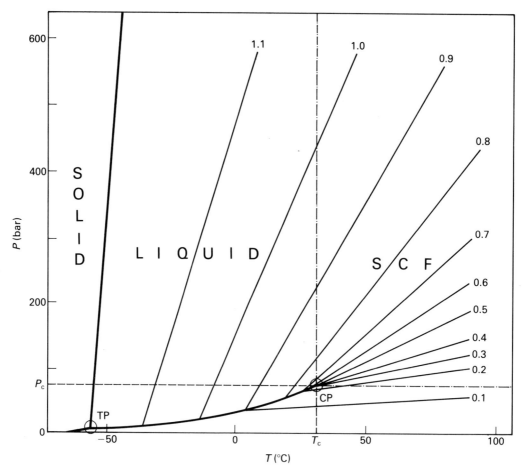

Fig. 2 Pressure–temperature diagram for carbon dioxide, showing liquid, gaseous and supercritical fluid regions (SCF), from P_c and T_c, and isodensity lines.

some aroma precursers like free amino acids, which may affect flavour/aroma on roasting.

Other Water Decaffeination Methods

An important aspect of both of the foregoing processes is the need to separate and recover solvent from the caffeine, usually for low-boiling solvents by multistage evaporation, with a high degree of efficiency. The caffeine itself in an impure form needs to be refined, the subject of a subsequent section.

Recently, methods have been patented and some commercialized based on the removal of the caffeine from the aqueous 'green' extract by adsorbents of various kinds. The Coffex Company of Amsterdam, for example, proposed the use of an activated carbon which is preloaded with other coffee extract substances or with substitute substances of similar molecular structure or size, especially with carbohydrates, so that the charcoal will take up as few extracted substances as possible, other than caffeine.

The caffeine is eventually desorbed, and the charcoal may then be reactivated for reuse or disposed of. These types of processes therefore avoid the use of organic solvents in any way.

Supercritical Carbon Dioxide Decaffeination

Certain fluid substances are known to have superior solvent powers in the supercritical state than when in the liquid state, of which carbon dioxide is perhaps the best known example. The supercritical state, however, is only achieved after reaching a minimum critical pressure (e.g. 75·2 bar for carbon dioxide) and critical temperature (e.g. 31·4°C for carbon dioxide). Numerous diagrams have been published, plotting temperature against pressure indicating in particular the supercritical region for carbon dioxide and other fluids, and incorporating lines of equal density (Fig. 2). Superior solvent powers are associated with increased fluid density, though other factors will also dictate the particular temperature/pressure combination usable and economic in practice.

Zosel, in Mülheim, Germany, from 1970 has published a number of patents relating to the supercritical use of carbon dioxide in extracting caffeine from green coffee beans. The claimed conditions were a temperature range of 40–80°C and a pressure range of 120–180 bar, from which it may be seen that the single fluid phase has a density of the order of $0.5–0.6$ g ml^{-3} compared with a gaseous density below the critical pressure of 0.1 g ml^{-3}. Carbon dioxide, being a nonpolar solvent is quite selective for caffeine. As with organic solvents, it is still necessary to bring the green coffee beans before decaffeination to a moisture content of 30–50% w/w by steaming/wetting for the same reasons. The removal of the caffeine from the enriched supercritical carbon dioxide can be accomplished by a number of methods: (1) reduction of temperature/pressure; (2) adsorption in a closed circulating system onto activated charcoal; (3) washing with water. The second is to be favoured in that a given quantity of supercritical carbon dioxide is loaded into and passed through an extractor vessel holding the moistened green beans; and then through a bed of activated charcoal held in a separate vessel, and recirculation performed in a closed pressure system until the caffeine is sufficiently extracted from the coffee (Fig. 3). At the end of a predetermined time the carbon dioxide is taken out to a holding vessel, and both the decaffeinated coffee beans and adsorbent are discharged. The decaffeinated coffee beans are then dried, whilst the caffeine is removed from the adsorbent, which may be reactivated for further use. A decaffeination process along these lines was commercialized by the Cafe Hag Company, in Bremen, Germany. It can be appreciated that the high pressures necessary involve high capital expense, and the design and running procedures carefully considered to minimize energy and other running costs. Nevertheless, the process and the product have many advantages, especially from the marketing and consumer perception points of view; and, with the high selectivity of this solvent, it is claimed that roasted and soluble products from it are very similar in flavour quality to the corresponding nondecaffeinated products.

There are published and patented variants of this basic supercritical carbon dioxide decaffeination process, including use of other fluid such as nitrous oxide and hydrocarbon gases, and other modified systems of operation.

Decaffeination of Roasted Coffee and Liquid Coffee Extracts

There are a number of patents relating to decaffeination of coffee products, rather than green coffee, including use of organic solvents and supercritical carbon dioxide. It would be necessary to remove first all the organic volatiles which are responsible for aroma/flavour before

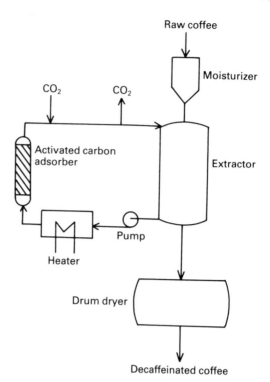

Fig. 3 Carbon dioxide decaffeination process, schematic. Reproduced with permission from Clarke RJ and Macrae R (1987).

decaffeination; as indeed is already widely practised in the manufacture of nondecaffeinated instant coffees, and add back before or after drying.

Effective removal of organic solvent, though not carbon dioxide or vegetable oils, together with emulsification problems are likely to be deterrents to commercialization.

Caffeine Refining

Caffeine represents a valuable by-product of decaffeination, though this substance can be also manufactured by synthetic chemical methods. By-product value may differ in economic terms from time to time. Pure caffeine has an outlet in soft drinks of the cola type, and also for medical purposes.

From the solvent decaffeination processes described, the caffeine will be in a state of 70–85% purity, so that a refining process is required to produce BP or USP grade by eliminating coffee waxes and oils as well as water-soluble or other materials that impart a dark colour. The series of interconnected and recycle steps involve use of activated carbon filtrations, and repeated recrystallizations from water. The final product consists of white, needle-shaped crystals, with a melting point of 236°C but subliming at the much lower temperature of 178°C. Recent studies have shown it to be, when crystallized from aqueous solution, a 4/5 hydrate with 6·95% water content. It has some unusual solubility characteristics in water, in that above 52°C it is anhydrous caffeine which is stable in contact with aqueous solution, and, conversely, below 52°C only the hydrate is stable. However, the interconversion is not very rapid, so that true solubility determinations must be obtained with the appropriate form of caffeine according to temperature. At 40°C, caffeine will have a solubility of 4·6 g per 100 g of water, and at 70°C, 13·50 g. Of especial reference to decaffeination is its reasonable solubility in a number of organic solvents (though very low in carbon tetrachloride and aliphatic/petroleum ethers already described), and its capacity as a weak base for forming unstable salts, such as acetates and chlorogenates. In addition, it can form soluble complexes with polynuclear hydrocarbons, which may be found in roasted coffee and other roasted substances, and which property can be used in their selective extraction.

Bibliography

Clarke RJ and Macrae R, (eds) (1985–1988) *Coffee: Chemistry*, vol. 1, *Technology*, vol. 2, *Physiology*, vol. 3, *Commercial and Technico-Legal Aspects* vol. 6. Barking: Elsevier.

Coughlin JR (1987) *Methylene Chloride: A Review of its Safety in Coffee Decaffeination*, Proceedings of the 12th International Colloquium on Coffee, ASIC, Paris pp. 127–40.

R. J. Clarke
Chichester, UK

Physiological Effects

Consumption Levels in Different Countries

Approximately 1.7×10^9 cups of coffee are drunk each day in the world. The USA is the largest consumer country although the consumption has declined to less than two cups *per capita* per day. The Nordic countries and the Netherlands have the highest *per capita* consumption with four to five cups per day.

Production and consumption figures are shown in Table 1. These data are only indicative as to the quantity and type of coffee and of additives used for preparing a cup of coffee. Patterns of consumption vary widely and evolve in time.

The main coffee brewing techniques are:

- Boiled coffee – brew prepared by boiling coarsely ground light roasted coffee in water (50–70 g l^{-1}); the infusion (1 cup = 150–190 ml) is drunk without separation of the grounds.

- Espresso – brew prepared by extracting very finely ground dark roasted coffee (6–7 g per cup) with water at 92–95°C and 8–12 bar (1 cup = 20–35 ml in Italy, up to 120 ml elsewhere).

- Filter coffee – brew prepared by pouring boiling water over finely ground light to dark roasted coffee (30–80 g l^{-1}) in a paper filter or automatic drip machine (1 cup = 150–190 ml).

- Instant coffee – brew prepared by dissolving 1.5–3.0 g of soluble coffee into 80–190 ml of hot water.

- Liquid coffee – ready-to-drink coffee mixture often containing sweeteners and creamers, consumed either hot or cold, mainly in Japan.

- Percolated coffee – brew prepared by recirculating boiling brew through coarsely ground light or medium roasted coffee (30–60 g l^{-1}) (1 cup = 150–190 ml).

- Mocca coffee – brew prepared by forcing just over-heated water through a bed of very finely ground medium to dark roasted coffee (6–7 g per 40–120 ml cup).

- Turkish/Greek coffee – brew prepared by bringing to a gentle boil extremely finely ground dark roasted coffee (4–6 g) in water (50–60 ml) and sugar (5–10 g per 30–50 ml cup).

Nutritional Value of Coffee/Effect on Availability of Nutrients in Diet

The coffee brew is naturally poor in digestible proteins, fats, carbohydrates and sodium, and is considered a nonnutritive dietary component, drunk for sensory pleasure and for its stimulatory effects. Its use as a vehicle for nutritious additives such as milk and sugar, and its contribution to the total water intake must, however, not be neglected.

Among the micronutrients found in coffee, niacin (nicotinic acid), formed from trigonelline during roasting, present at levels of 1–3 mg per cup, which corresponds to 5–20% of the recommended daily intake, has been shown to play a role in preventing pellagra in populations on marginal diets. Animal studies have indicated that trigonelline itself can be transformed into nicotinic acid. *See* Niacin, Physiology

Amounts of soluble dietary fibre (sum of the indigestible carbohydrate and of carbohydrate-like components formed at roasting) of the order of 10–25% of the total coffee solids present in the brew may explain, on one hand, the protective role of coffee against colorectal cancer, and, on the other, together with chlorogenic acids, the reduction in absorption of non haem iron when coffee is consumed with or just after a meal. *See* Cancer, Diet in Cancer Prevention; Dietary Fibre, Physiological Effects

The hypothesis that the phytate content of coffee

Table 1. Coffee production and consumption, average over period 1986–1990

	10^6 tonnes per year	Green coffee (kg) per person per year	Types of coffee	Trend during last 5 years
Production	5·61			
Local consumption	1·39			Up
Brazil	0·60	4·2	A D f	Stable
Colombia	0·12	4·0	A D f	Up
Mexico	0·10	1·3	A D f/i/id	Up
Indonesia	0·07	0·4	R D f/t	Up
Côte d'Ivoire	Low	?	R D i	Up
Exports	4·22			
Consumption	4·09			Down
Finland	0·06	11·8	A L f/b	Down
Sweden	0·10	11·4	A L f/b	Down
Denmark	0·05	10·7	A L f	Stable
Norway	0·04	10·1	A L f/b	Stable
Netherlands	0·14	9·6	A/R M f	Stable
Austria	0·06	8·3	A M e/f/ed	Stable
Switzerland	0·05	7·3	A M e/f/i	Up
Germany (FRG + GDR)	0·55	7·0	A L f/fd	Stable
Belgium	0·07	7·0	A/R D f	Down
France	0·31	5·6	R/A D e/f	Down
Italy	0·26	4·5	R/A D e	Up
USA	1·09	4·4	A/R L p/f/i/fd/id	Stable
Canada	0·11	4·2	A/R L p/f/i/fd/id	Down
Hungary	0·04	4·0	A/R D i/f	Up
Spain	0·13	3·4	R/A D e/id	Stable
Algeria	0·07	3·1	R D t/e/f	Stable
Greece	0·03	2·9	A D t R D i	Up
Australia	0·04	2·4	R/A L i/l	Stable
UK	0·14	2·4	R/A M i	Stable
Portugal	0·02	2·3	R D e/i	Up
Japan	0·29	2·3	A/R M i	Up
Yugoslavia	0·05	1·9	A/R D e	Up
Ireland	0·01	1·7	R/A M i	Up

A, arabica; R, robusta; L, light; M, medium; D, dark roast; d, decaffeinated; b, boiled; e, espresso and mocca; f, filter; i, instant; l, liquid; p, percolated; t, Greek or Turkish.

(1–20 mg per cup) significantly lowers the gastrointestinal absorption of zinc needs verification. *See* Phytic Acid, Nutritional Impact; Zinc, Physiology

Potassium, present at levels of 80–160 mg per cup, may contribute up to 10% of the daily intake for an adult. The intake of magnesium and of manganese from coffee is significant. *See* Magnesium

The importance of coffee in the calcium balance of the bone is still unclear. *See* Calcium, Properties and Determination

Physiologically Active Components

Coffee is consumed for its characteristic flavour and the mild stimulation produced by caffeine, and all its proven physiological or behavioural effects appear to be related to its caffeine content. *See* Caffeine

Flavour Constituents

Most of the more than 800 volatile constituents identified in the aroma of roasted coffee are common to roasted foods, and none of them alone can explain the aroma of freshly roasted or brewed coffee, so that the organoleptic appeal of the brew is still partially unexplained.

Even the bitter taste of coffee is not due to the presence of caffeine only, itself a bitter substance, but which accounts for no more than 10% of the total bitterness of the brew. The chlorogenic acids, like caffeine, are higher in robusta than in arabica coffees, and participate in the bitter taste. Bitterness increases with the degree of roasting, with the formation of bitter volatile aromatic substances and brown pigments, the melanoidins, from the pyrolysis of carbohydrates, poly-

Physiological Effects

phenols and proteins. *See* Flavour Compounds, Structures and Characteristics

Caffeine

The amount of caffeine present in a cup depends on the type of coffee used and on its mode of preparation, and may vary between 1–5 mg for a cup of decaffeinated coffee, physiologically an insignificant amount, and 50 mg to more than 150 mg for a cup of regular coffee, corresponding to an intake of 1–3 mg per kilogram of bodyweight. These figures are well below those producing a urinary concentration of caffeine of 12 mg l^{-1}, defined by the Olympic Committee as the acceptable upper limit for competing athletes; such a limit could be reached only after a single oral intake of 900–1000 mg.

Ingested caffeine is absorbed and distributed throughout all the tissues in the body within minutes, and is eliminated in a few hours, up to 4% as such in the urine and the rest is metabolized, with a half-life of 2–6 h for a healthy adult. The half-life is increased during pregnancy, and in those with an impaired liver function, like newborn babies and patients suffering from liver diseases.

The variations in the physiological response to the consumption of equivalent levels of caffeine could be explained by different rates of stomach emptying, as a function of the content of the stomach, and by genetic differences in the metabolic clearance of caffeine between slow and fast acetylators.

Consumption of caffeinated coffee increases the time needed to fall asleep and decreases sleep duration, particularly in older subjects. An improvement in visual acuity of as much as 40% in man reported after doses of 180 mg of caffeine needs confirmation. Caffeine shortens reaction time and prolongs the amount of time during which an individual can maintain auditory and visual vigilance, during boring tasks or performing physically exhausting work. The effects of caffeine on short-term memory, if any, is slight. The decrease in hand steadiness (tremor) observed in some people after consumption of caffeine does not affect fine motor control. A link between caffeine consumption and anxiety or panic attacks has not been demonstrated, with the possible exception of psychiatric patients. Mild caffeine withdrawal headaches lasting 1–3 days may be felt by individuals having had a regular consumption of at least 15 g per month after a sudden stop in coffee consumption. The relationship between blood pressor and central stimulatory behavioural effects of caffeine at the concentration of a cup of coffee needs further investigation.

At the doses associated with coffee consumption, caffeine produces a thermogenic effect with an immediate increase of about 10% in the metabolic rate and elimination of carbon dioxide; a delayed lipolytic effect with an increase in the plasma level of free fatty acids has been observed in young lean subjects. Caffeine increases muscular oxygen consumption and glycogen–glucose transformation.

Caffeine in coffee has a rapid and short-lasting diuretic action with increase in urinary volume and sodium in subjects kept on a methylxanthine-free diet.

Epidemiological evidence shows no causal relationship between caffeine consumption and either miscarriages, low infant birth weight or short gestation period, particularly if smoking is taken into account. The US Food and Drug Administration feels that 'there is insufficient evidence to conclude that caffeine adversely affects the reproduction functions in humans'.

Contaminants

Contamination of green coffee beans by low levels of ochratoxin A or, very seldom, aflatoxin B_1 has been occasionally observed; only one laboratory has reported the presence of ochratoxin A in a few commercial roasted samples and in the brew. At the levels encountered in green beans the average intake of these contaminants is, anyway, low compared with that of common staple foods such as maize or peanuts. *See* Mycotoxins, Occurrence and Determination

Formation of polycyclic aromatic hydrocarbons and, in particular, benzo[a]pyrene may occur, especially at nonoptimal roasting conditions. The analysis of brewed and soluble coffee indicates that these strongly lipophilic substances are, anyway, not released, but are retained in the spent grounds, both in home brewing and in industrial extraction. Thus, coffee does not constitute a significant source of dietary intake of polycyclic aromatic hydrocarbons. *See* Polycyclic Aromatic Hydrocarbons

Health Implications of Coffee Consumption

Botanical species (arabica, robusta), roasting degree (light, dark), types of coffee (regular, decaffeinated), modes of consumption (boiled coffee, etc.), or specific constituents (methylglyoxal, dicarbonyls) and contaminants (mycotoxins, benzo[a]pyrene) have been associated occasionally with different adverse symptoms: the only links clearly established, both in epidemiological and clinical studies, are the positive correlation between boiled coffee consumption in the Nordic countries and serum cholesterol levels, and the short-lasting caffeine withdrawal headaches.

Cancer

There is no conclusive evidence from experimental and epidemiological studies that coffee and caffeine are carcinogenic. A doubt still remains on the possibility of a weak link between coffee consumption and cancer of the bladder and urinary tract. Conversely, coffee consumption may have a protective effect on colorectal cancer. In both cases confirmation is considered necessary.

In vitro *Mutagenicity Tests*

Hydrogen peroxide and methylglyoxal present in brewed, instant and decaffeinated coffee are mutagenic in various *in vitro* tests on microorganisms in the absence of the S9 fraction containing mammalian microsomal enzymes. Mutagenic heterocyclic amines related to 2-amino-3,4-dimethylimidazo[4,5-f]quinoline (MeIQ) can only be extracted from roasted coffee beans in laboratory experiments under basic conditions. No MeIQ could be found, however, either in brewed or instant coffees.

Animal Studies

Several lifetime studies in rodents failed consistently to show any correlation between coffee consumption and cancer.

Green, roasted and instant coffee and coffee constituents, the diterpenes cafestol and kahweol, have been shown in animal models to have cancer chemopreventive activity.

Human Studies

There may be a weak positive relationship between coffee consumption and bladder/urinary tract cancer, but the results of the epidemiological studies are inconsistent, and a residual confounding effect of cigarette smoking or another bias cannot be ruled out. Several studies, which had not been planned to verify the hypothesis, have indicated a protective effect on colorectal cancer. The studies on pancreatic cancer have given inconsistent results, and the consensus is now that the protective results of the earlier studies were due to selection biases, and that there is no link between coffee consumption and this form of cancer. All studies showed no correlation between coffee consumption and breast, gastric and upper digestive tract cancers. The marginal increase in relative risk found in a few studies on ovarian cancer has now been attributed to bias from unknown sources or chance on pharmacological arguments.

Cardiovascular Disease

The epidemiological evidence for a direct link between coffee/caffeine consumption and increased risk of cardiovascular disease is inconclusive. This may be explained by the different consumption modes between and within the populations studied or by atherogenic behaviours positively associated with coffee consumption, such as smoking, high dietary fat and cholesterol intakes. Moderate coffee consumption is not likely to be a significant risk factor for cardiovascular disease.

Serum Cholesterol Levels

There is clinical evidence that high coffee consumption is associated with reversible increased levels of total, low-density lipoprotein (LDL) and very low-density lipoprotein (VLDL) cholesterol, while high-density lipoprotein (HDL) cholesterol levels remain unchanged. The responsible factor, which does not appear to be caffeine, is concentrated in the coffee lipid fraction. Lipid concentration depends on the brewing method, and is relatively important in the Nordic-style boiled coffee brew, which would explain why the first data clearly indicating a link between coffee consumption and cholesterol levels originated in Northern Norway. Lipid content is negligible in both regular and decaffeinated filter and instant coffees.

Blood Pressure

Abstention from ingestion of caffeine for a period of several weeks may reduce both systolic and diastolic mean blood pressure by 1–4 mmHg. High single doses of caffeine produce after an abstinence of at least 12 h a 5–10% increase of both systolic and, particularly, diastolic blood pressure for 1–3 h. Tolerance develops rapidly with continued consumption and blood pressure stabilizes slightly upwards in a few days. A contribution of 1–4 mmHg to the increase in systolic blood pressure from components other than caffeine present in boiled coffee, suggested in one study, needs confirmation, and is not supported by current knowledge on the pharmacological properties of coffee constituents. *See* Hypertension, Physiology

Cardiac Arrhythmias

The question of whether caffeine consumption increases the frequency or severity of ventricular arrhythmias is still partially unresolved as there may be particularly sensitive patients: the consensus is now that a 'moderate' coffee consumption, corresponding to 200–500 mg of caffeine per day, is unlikely to increase the frequency of arrhythmias both in healthy subjects and in patients suffering from tachycardia or fibrillation.

Other Health Questions Associated with Coffee Consumption

Effects on the Digestive Tract

An increase in heartburn due to a reduction of the lower oesophageal sphincter pressure and consequent gastric acid reflux has been associated with coffee consumption by sensitive individuals. Both regular and decaffeinated coffee stimulate the secretion of gastric acids in the stomach and the small intestine, and the phenomenon has been linked, without clear proof, to various substances present in the coffee bean. An increase of the distal colon motility within minutes after coffee consumption by about 30% of the subjects has been described in one study. In another study, consumption of two cups of coffee after an overnight fast produced no change in mouth-to-caecum transit time in healthy subjects. Coffee consumption produces contractions of the gallbladder, as is also the case with other foodstuffs. The size of the population suffering gastrointestinal discomfort after drinking coffee, the symptoms themselves and the mechanism remain unclear, with the possible exception of dyspeptic complaints of patients suffering from duodenal ulcer.

Bibliography

Anonymous (1990) *World Coffee Situation*, FCOF 1–90. Washington, DC: US Department of Agriculture.

Anonymous (1991) *IARC Monograph on the Evaluation of Carcinogenic Risks to Humans: Coffee, Tea, Maté, Methylxanthines, Methylglyoxal*, vol. 51. Lyon: WHO-IARC.

Barone, JJ and Grice HG (1990) *Sixth International Caffeine Workshop, Hong Kong 1989. Food Chemical Toxicology* 28: 279–283.

Bättig K. (1985) In: Clifford MN and Wilson KC (eds) *The Physiological Effects of Coffee Consumption*. pp 394–439. London: Croom Helm.

Clarke, RJ and Macrae R (eds) (1988) *Coffee: physiology*, vol. 3. Barking: Elsevier.

Committee on Diet and Health, National Research Council (1989) *Diet and Health*, pp 465–471. Washington, DC: National Academy Press.

Dews PB (ed.) (1984) *Caffeine*. Berlin: Springer-Verlag.

Rousseff RL (ed.) (1990) *Bitterness in Foods and Beverages*, pp 169–182. Amsterdam: Elsevier.

Viani R (1986) *Coffee. Ullmann's Encyclopedia of Industrial Chemistry* A7, pp 315–339. Weinheim: VCH.

R. Viani
Nestec Ltd, Vevey, Switzerland

COGNAC

See Brandy and Cognac

COLE CROPS

See Vegetables of Temperate Climates

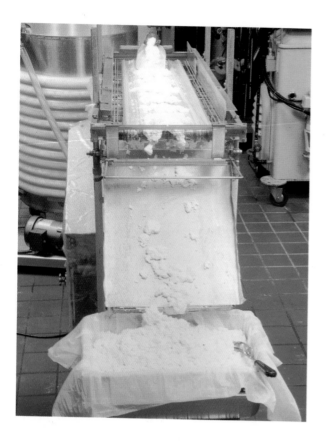

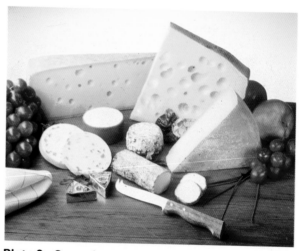

Plate 1 (left) Continuous manufacture of whole-milk Ricotta cheese at the Centre for Food and Animal Research.

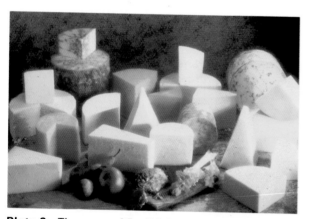

Plate 2 The range of English hard-pressed territorial cheeses. (Courtesy of Dairy Crest.)

Plate 3 Some cheeses from France.

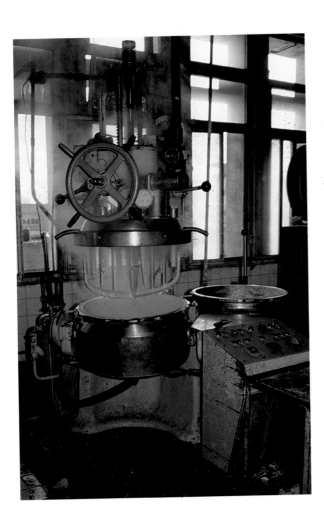

Plate 4 (left) Processed cheeses: processing kettle. (Kustner, Multiform, BF.)

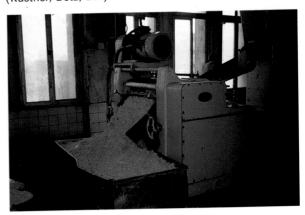

Plate 5 (below) Processed cheeses: shredding machine. (Kustner, Beta, BF.)

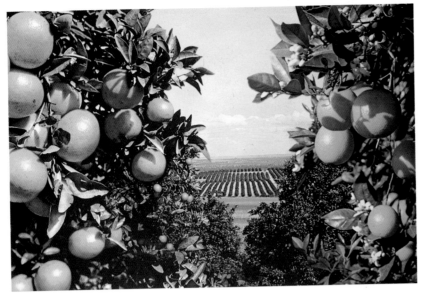

Plate 6 Orange grove in the interior of central Florida. (Courtesy of the Florida Department of Citrus, Lakeland, USA.)

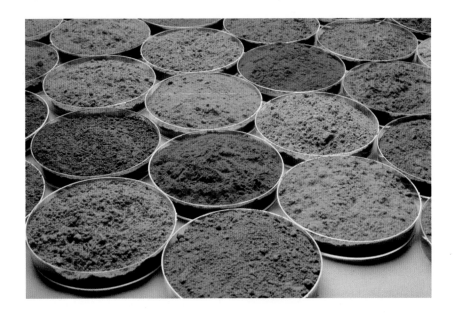

Plate 7 The alkalization process creates cocoa powders in many different colours (Cacao de Zaan).

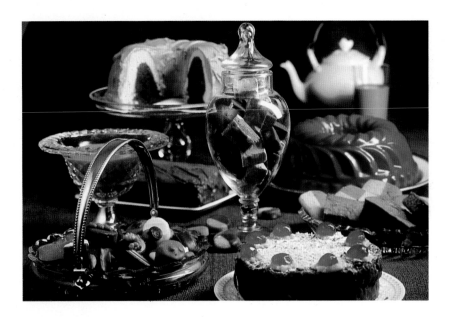

Plate 8 Cocoa brings colour and flavour to foods (Cacao de Zaan).

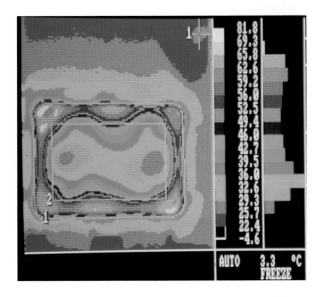

Plate 9 Cooking: Infrared thermography measurement of the temperature distribution in a prepared food packed in a PET container after microwave heating.

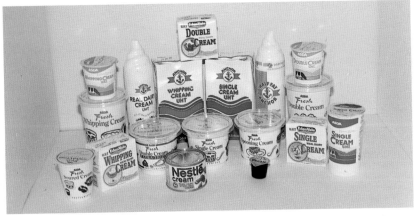

Plate 10 Cream: types on the market.

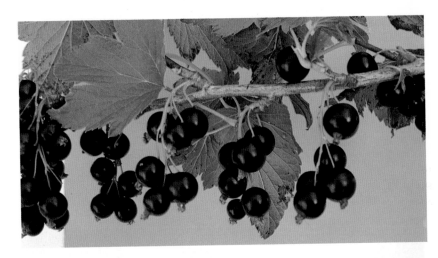

Plate 11 Blackcurrants.

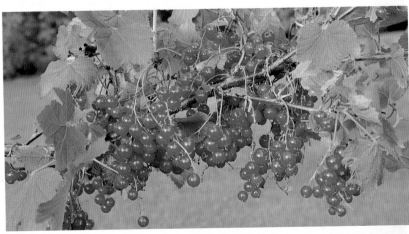

Plate 12 Redcurrants.

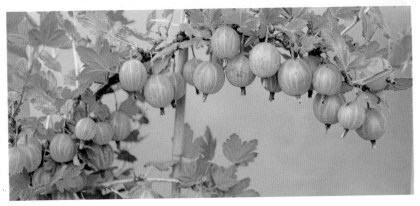

Plate 13 Gooseberries.

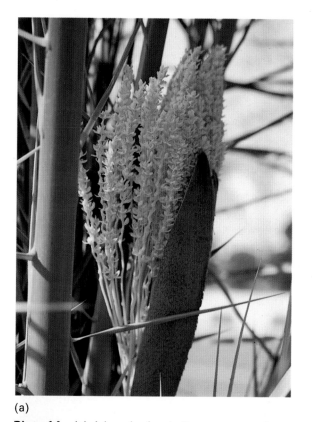

(a)

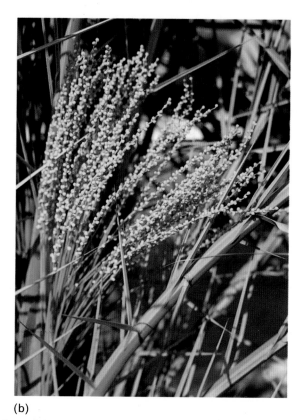

(b)

Plate 14 (a) A bunch of male flowers on a male ornamental variety of date palm. (b) A bunch of female flowers on a female ornamental variety of date palm. Note the difference in shape and colour of the male and female flowers.

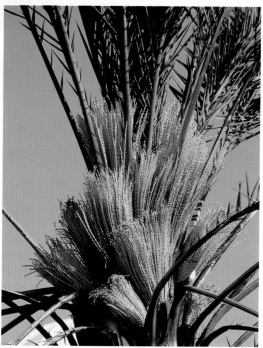

Plate 15 A commercial fruit-producing date palm tree showing a typical exposed arrangement of the female flower bunches.

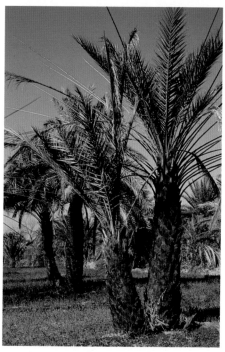

Plate 16 A view of 'cured' date palms. Experienced farmers control the pests which can infect the trunks of old date palms by lightly sprinkling the trunk, avoiding the top green leaves, with an inflammable substance, such as kerosene, and setting it alight. As the dead wood around the trunk burns, the pests either burn or escape. Trees treated in this manner are called 'cured' trees and subsequently flourish and give improved fruit quality and yield.

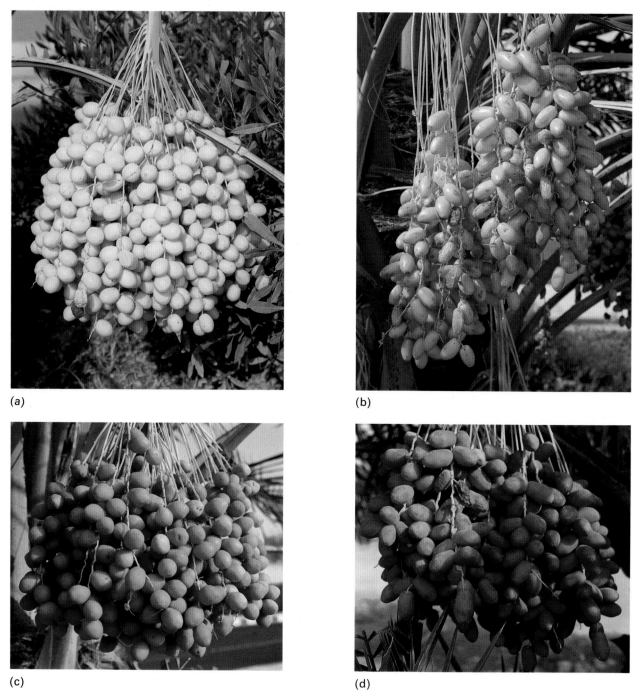

Plate 17 Ripening date fruit colours. After attaining the natural mature fruit size, the fruit colour changes from green to a characteristic colour of the variety. (a) Lemon yellow; (b) deep yellow; (c) light red; and (d) dark red.

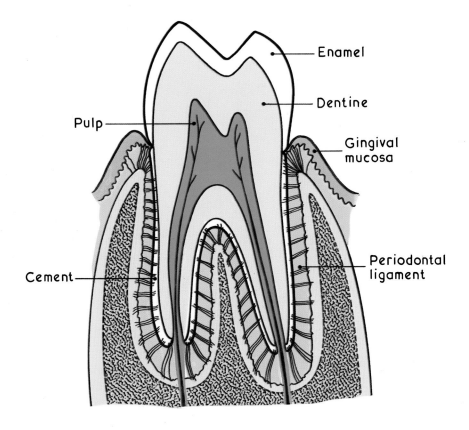

Plate 18 A simplified diagram of tissues making up the tooth structure and its immediate surroundings.

COLLOIDS AND EMULSIONS

Colloids are generally considered to be systems with two or more components (phases) in which one or more of the components has at least one characteristic dimension ζ: 10^{-9} m $\leqslant \zeta \leqslant 10^{-6}$ m. This essentially restricts attention to systems containing large molecules or relatively small composite particles. The lower bound is determined by the constraint that in a dilute suspension the components undergo Brownian motion. Similarly, the upper bound is determined by the requirement not to sediment out. For emulsions where the density difference between the components is small, much larger particles can constitute the colloidal state.

For more complex and concentrated systems, this definition can prove problematical and qualitative criteria based on, for example, symmetry of the properties of the system are increasingly used. However, the quantitative definition has the pragmatic value that it illustrates the ubiquitous nature of colloids. It includes polymer solutions, gels, foams and emulsions, which represent a wide range of food systems.

Colloid science as a field of research has been studied since 1861 when Graham distinguished between colloidal suspension and molecular solutions. In foods, much of the technological interest results from their rheological behaviour. *See* Physical Properties of Foods

Everyday foods such as milk, margarine, cakes, ice cream, mayonnaise, sausages, yoghurt, chilled desserts and drinks (e.g. coffee or more exotic cream liqueurs) all have colloidal structures which control their rheology, texture and, in many cases, colour. *See* individual foods.

Types of Colloids

Macromolecular Solution

Whilst water or oil can form the continuous phase for many colloids, other molecules, especially biopolymers, are often incorporated. The study of such solutions is a field in its own right. For this brief account the significant ability of polymers to modify the continuous phase rheology is noted. The potential of polymers to act as agents able to modify the properties of other classes of colloids is discussed below.

Dispersions

The particles in a colloidal dispersion are usually sufficiently large that they may be considered to have a well-defined surface between themselves and the continuous phase.

Classes of Colloidal Dispersions: Terminology

The various classes of colloidal dispersions are listed in Table 1.

A characteristic of all dispersions is the high surface area to volume ratio of the dispersed phase. The properties of these surfaces plays a key role in influencing the bulk properties of the dispersion. This is the reason for the close relationship between colloid and interface science.

Such colloidal dispersions are not in general thermodynamically stable. Typically after preparation most dispersions will decay into a nondispersed state. The particles may either sediment or cream, depending on the density difference between the particles and the continuous phase. Aggregation of particles, and for liquid drops coalescence, may also occur. In liquid foams, drainage of the thin films responsible for the foam construction can also occur. This decay rate may range from fractions of a second to many years. Most practical food colloids are designed via a combination of ingredients, processing and packaging to be stable over a period which is consistent with both an acceptable shelf life and product microbial safety.

Table 1. Classes of colloidal dispersions

| Continuous phase | Disperse phase | | |
	Solid	Liquid	Gas
Solid	Suspension	Solid suspension	Solid foam
Liquid	Solution	Emulsion	Foam
	Suspension paste		
Gas	Aerosol	Aerosol	

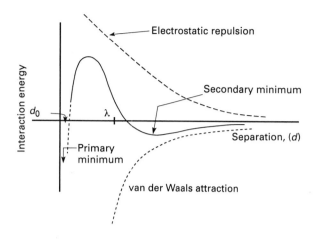

Fig. 1   Schematic of interaction energy versus separation for a pair of colloid particles.

Interactions Between Colloid Particles

A central issue is the origin of 'stability' and its control via practical means. This may be via ingredient modification (chemical means) or process changes (physical modification).

The Derjaguin, Landau, Vervey and Overbeck (DLVO) theory provides the classical description of the force between suspended particles. two forces are assumed to be operating. The van der Waals interaction is always present. This arises from differences in electrical polarizability between the particles and the intervening solvent. For similar particles, the interaction is always attractive; for different particles interacting across some types of solvent the interaction can be repulsive. At its simplest for spherical particles when $d \gg R$ (where R is the particle radius and d is the separation between the particle surfaces) the interaction energy scales as H/d^6. H is the Hamaker constant, which is a function of the various polarizabilities. For $d < R$ the interaction energy scales as R/d. The computation of these forces for complex systems has been exhaustively studied and the reader is referred to the bibliography for further information.

For particles which carry a charge through, say, the presence of ionizable groups at its surface, there is (again for similar particles) an interaction energy due to electrostatic repulsion, proportional to $\exp(-d/\lambda)/d$ where λ is the Debye–Hückel screening length.

For like particles, the addition of these two energies gives an overall potential energy barrier that controls the interaction as the particles diffuse in the colloid displayed schematically in Fig. 1.

If the electrostatic interaction is weak, the repulsive barrier is lowered and the particles may aggregate more readily. When the secondary minimum is weak, particles 'trapped' therein may be separated frequently by simply stirring the colloid (see below). Particles 'trapped' in the

deep primary minimum are much more difficult to separate.

The electrostatic force can be reduced by adding a sufficient amount of salt. Conversely, the weakly aggregated system may be made more stable by the addition of a polymer that adsorbs onto the particle surface. The tails (and loops for long polymers) form a protective layer which prevents the particle surfaces from coming into contact, thus reducing the effect of the van der Waals attraction. This may result in depletion or volume restriction flocculation.

At very close separations $\leqslant d_0$ the interaction energy in Fig. 1 may display a strong oscillatory form. This is a consequence of the molecular nature of the solvent and is referred to as the 'solvation force'. The magnitude and nature of the oscillations depend sensitively on the nature of the solvent and its surface interaction with the dispersion particles. Typically, however, the oscillations operate over 5–10 solvent molecular diameters; their magnitude can be significantly greater than the thermal energy kT (where k is Boltzmann's constant and T is the temperature in degrees kelvin). So two colloid particles in solution are unlikely to reach clean surface-to-surface contact. They will always tend to maintain a few layers of solvent molecules between themselves.

Rheology and Structure

In a dilute colloid, the particles may be observed to undergo Brownian motion and to a first approximation the diffusion coefficient $D = kT/(3\pi \eta R)$, where η is the viscosity of the continuous fluid.

In a more concentrated system the motion of the particles is hindered via collisions with others. This can have a dramatic effect on the overall rheological properties of the colloid. For hard particles all of the same size (monodisperse) the viscosity η_s of the system may be approximated by

$$\eta_s = \eta \, (1 - \phi/\phi_m)^{-1.5}, \qquad (1)$$

where ϕ is the volume fraction of the suspended particles and $\phi_m \sim 0.64$ may be loosely identified with the volume fraction at maximum random packing for hard spheres. Polydispersity introduces added complexity.

In an emulsion, the particles, being liquid, are deformable and formula (1) breaks down at volume fractions $\phi \approx \phi_m$. Similarly for nonspherical particles the situation is more complicated and the reader is referred to the bibliography for further guidance.

Equation (1) takes no account of the influence of shear rate on the viscosity. This becomes important for more concentrated systems containing nonspherical particles and deformable particles (e.g. as in emulsions). It is also important for systems where the particles at zero shear may be aggregated by attractive forces (e.g.

the van der Waals forces noted above). As the shear increases in such systems, the internal stresses which are generated can break up the aggregate, causing marked changes in viscosity. Anyone who has stirred so-called 'set yoghurt' will have noticed the dramatic reduction in viscosity due to the breakdown of the internal network of aggregates.

At high concentrations, the phase behaviour of colloidal dispersions and emulsions can undergo phase transitions similar to those of simple fluids. The thermodynamic parameter that corresponds to the usual gaseous pressure is now the osmotic pressure and it can in principle be calculated via methods of statistical mechanics or measured using standard methods. A related quantity is the radial distribution function, which gives the probability of finding a second particle within a certain distance of a particle chosen at random.

The radial distribution function has been studied for dilute systems using light scattering. Concentrated systems present difficulties from experimental and theoretical points of view. Approximate theories based on analogies with the liquid state have been used to make progress with the latter systems. More recent work uses fractal concepts to characterize their structures. Ultrasound has offered a fruitful way to probe concentrated systems. In this case it turns out that the dynamic behaviour is the simplest property to study. The velocity of ultrasound through a dispersion is dependent on the volume fraction ϕ and hence changes in the velocity reflect changes in ϕ. Using this technique, creaming or sedimentation and flocculation can be detected long before changes become visible to the eye. *See* Flocculation

Emulsions

Dilute emulsions exhibit the features discussed above but, in addition, because of the fluid nature of the particles and mobility of the interfaces, can exhibit a richer and more complex set of features as the volume fraction ϕ increases. As the liquid droplets come into contact and their shape distorts, the thin liquid film separating two regions of similar composition (i.e. the two droplets) can become unstable and break. At high volume fraction this can lead to phase inversion. So, for example, an oil-in-water emulsion may change into a water-in-oil emulsion. The precise conditions for this to occur depend on the details of the phases and the surfactant at the interfaces between the two phases. The nature of the phase change has been extensively studied. Intermediate structures such as interconnected networks may occur and a variety of interesting physical, optical and rheological properties are possible. *See* Emulsifiers, Organic Emulsifiers; Emulsifiers, Phosphates as Meat Emulsion Stabilizers; Emulsifiers, Uses in Processed Foods

In general, food emulsions contain many phases. Ice cream with water, ice and air is typical. Whilst detailed prediction of all their properties may not be possible, the concepts sketched out here have helped greatly our systematic understanding and development of such complex foods.

Bibliography

Bee RED, Richmond P and Mingins J (eds) (1989) *Food Colloids*. London: Royal Society of Chemistry.

Dickinson E (ed.) (1987) *Food Emulsions and Foams*. London: Royal Society of Chemistry.

Dickinson E and Stainsby G (1982) *Colloids in Food*. London: Applied Science.

Everett DH (1988) *Basic Principles of Colloid Science*. London: Royal Society of Chemistry.

Fillery-Travis AJ, Gunning PA and Robins MM (1991) Measurement and simulation of complex colloidal processes. *Advances in Measurement and Control of Colloidal Processes*.

Grimson MJ, Richmond P and Vassilieff CS (1988) Electrostatic interactions in thin films. In: Ivanov IB (ed.) *Thin Liquid Films*, pp 275–326. New York: Marcel Dekker.

Napper DH (1983) *Polymeric Stabilization of Colloidal Dispersions*. London: Academic Press.

Richmond P (1975) The theory and calculation of van der Waals forces. In: Everett DH (ed.) *Colloid Science*, vol. 2, p 130. London: Chemical Society.

Russel WB, Saville DA and Schowalter WR (1989) *Colloidal Dispersions*. Cambridge: Cambridge University Press.

Shaw DJ (1980) *Introduction to Colloid and Surface Chemistry*. London: Butterworths.

Peter Richmond
Cooperative Wholesale Society, Manchester, UK

COLON

Contents

Structure and Function

Structure

The adult human colon is about 100 cm long *in situ* and is divided anatomically into the ascending, transverse, descending and sigmoid colon (Fig. 1). Longitudinal muscle bands (taeniae coli) in its wall cause 'haustrae' – characteristic puckerings and sacculations. Between these, the wall is thrown into crescent-shaped semilunar folds. The lumen is lined by a mucosa of simple columnar epithelium (colonocytes) containing numerous goblet cells. These cells secrete a mucus assumed to act primarily as a lubricant and protectant, allowing the solid and semisolid material to pass easily along the organ without damaging the epithelium. As the mucus contains secretory immunoglobulins IgA it also helps to protect the mucosa from luminal pathogens.

Unlike the small bowel, the colon is devoid of villi but has numerous straight tubular glands or crypts (sometimes called pits) (Fig. 2) with openings onto the near-flat epithelial surface. These crypts are lined with cells similar to the surface colonocytes. At the crypt base, undifferentiated cells form a stem cell population for all the other epithelial cells of the large bowel. These divide by mitosis to replace those shed from the surface. The crypts also contain a few enteroendocrine cells. The lamina propria, containing plasma cells, macrophages, lymphoid aggregates and mast cells, underlies the mucosa and extends down to the muscularis mucosae, a thin layer of inner circular and outer longitudinal smooth muscle fibres. Beneath this is the submucous coat containing areolar tissue and the blood and lymph vessels serving the epithelium. The smooth muscle investing the organ consists of an inner circular and the outer longitudinal layer, the bulk of which is arranged in the three longitudinal bundles (taeniae).

Nervous Innervation

The autonomic supply to the colon has three divisions: the extrinsic (1) sympathetic and (2) parasympathetic nerves link up with (3) the enteric supply in the bowel wall. The latter functions as an integrating system and consists of two ganglionated plexi. One is called the myenteric plexus, positioned between the circular and longitudinal smooth muscle layers and the other the submucosal plexus, lying in the submucosa under the muscularis mucosae. More recently, a third plexus, called the mucosal plexus, has been identified. The mucosal and submucosal plexi are involved in controlling epithelial function but the myenteric plexus inter-

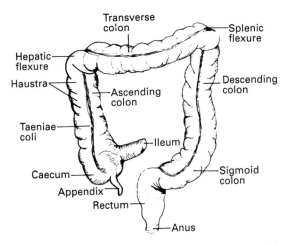

Fig. 1 Diagram showing the anatomical regions of the human large intestine.

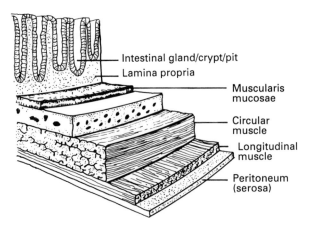

Fig. 2 Schematic diagram showing the various major tissue structures of the human large intestine.

Structure and Function

connects to coordinate motility with absorptive functions by local and extrinsic reflex pathways. Colonic movements include segmentation contractions and peristaltic waves similar to those in the small intestine.

Luminal conditions are probably sensed by afferent nerve endings in the mucosa and the afferent information processed at the enteric plexus, cord or brain level. The efferent output is then fed back via the extrinsic nerves to the muscle and epithelium.

Function

The colon has three major functions: (1) absorption, (2) secretion, and (3) bacterial fermentation.

Absorption

Salt and Water

While the jejunum and ileum are the major sites for the absorption of the salt and water ingested into and secreted by the upper alimentary tract, it is the task of the colon to absorb the remaining fluid. Many authors describe this as the 'salvage' function of the colon. Its efficiency can be judged by the estimate that daily, approximately 1000–2000 ml of the fluid enters the colon at the ileocaecal valve, while less than 100 ml are lost in the faeces. The colon is adapted to extract water and salts from the colonic contents to create initially semisolid and finally solid contents that become the faeces. First, it has a much slower rate of luminal transit than is observed in the small intestine, allowing its contents a greater contact time with the mucosa. Second, the colonocytes can generate very large osmotic forces to extract the fluid from the lumen. Third, the tight junctions between the colonocytes are much less permeable to ions and water than those of the small intestine. Fluid absorptive capacity is determined primarily by sodium ion (Na^+) and chloride ion (Cl^-) absorption. The colonocytes actively transfer Na^+ into the convoluted lateral spaces between the cells and water follows osmotically, mainly through the tight junctions. *See* Sodium, Physiology

Segmental Differences

The mammalian colon is not a single organ with a uniform distribution of electrolyte transport along its length. It is well known that different species exhibit segmental differences in their ion transport and also that the different segments of the colon, in the same animal, display differences in ion transport. The most studied animal colons have been those of the rabbit and rat. Although there are obvious similarities in the colonocyte functions in these two species with human colono-

cytes, neither matches exactly that of the human colon. *In vivo* studies in the human colon indicate that Na^+ and water are primarily absorbed in the ascending and transverse colon, with relatively little or no net absorption in the rectum. The human descending colon (like that of the rabbit) possesses colonocytes with apical membrane channels sensitive to amiloride which abolishes the electrogenic Na^+ absorption (and short-circuit current or net electrogenic ion transfer *in vitro*). In the ascending colon, however, the Na^+ absorption is mainly via an amiloride-insensitive or neutral transfer mechanism(s).

Sodium Ion Absorption Mechanisms

Active Na^+ absorption is accomplished by two mechanisms: (1) electrogenic Na^+ transfer, and (2) neutral NaCl transfer.

Electrogenic Na^+ transfer. The Na^+ ion moves into the colonocyte across its apical membrane through channels (that can be blocked by amiloride) under the influence of a favourable electrochemical gradient as the inside of the colonocyte is negative to the lumen and has a low Na^+ concentration. It is then pumped out of the cell across the basolateral membrane by the agency of a Na^+, K^+-ATPase (the sodium pump or Na^+, K^+ activated adenosine triphosphatase), creating an electric current (rheogenic transfer) and a positive potential difference at the serosa. The ATPase, and thus current and Na^+ transfer, can be inhibited by the cardiac glycoside, ouabain. Mineralocorticoids, especially aldosterone, enhance the entry of Na^+ across the apical membrane by the electrogenic route and thus also increase the absorption of water.

Neutral NaCl transfer. This may represent either coupled Na^+–K^+–$2Cl^-$ cotransport, coupled Na^+–Cl^- cotransport or the coupling of dual ion exchanges such as Na^+ for H^+ and Cl^- for HCO_3^- or OH.

Chloride Ion Absorption Mechanisms

Chloride ions can be absorbed passively or actively.

Passive absorption. This is via an electrical potential difference (pd)-dependent process as the serosal side of the intestine is positive with respect to the lumen.

Active absorption. This occurs either as neutral NaCl absorption (Na^+-dependent process) or as neutral Cl^-–HCO_3^- exchange (Na^+-independent process). It has been estimated that in the human colon *in vivo* the Cl^-–HCO_3^- exchange accounts for about 25% of overall Cl^- absorption, the other 75% being via the favourable electrical pd mechanism via the paracellular route.

Potassium Ion Absorption Mechanisms

Active K^+ absorption has been demonstrated in the distal colon of rat and rabbit. In rat, the mechanism of absorption is electroneutral and independent of Na^+ and Cl^-. In rabbit, it appears that there is a K^+–H^+ exchange which can be unmasked in the presence of ouabain and removal of Na^+. The mechanism for the K^+ uptake across the apical membrane is thought to be a K^+-ATPase. There is no definitive information about the movement of K^+ across the basolateral membrane. Similarly, there are no details about the cellular mechanisms present for K^+ absorption in human colonocytes. *See* Potassium, Physiology

Calcium and Magnesium Absorption

While considerable amounts of these ions are present in the lumen of the colon, most are unavailable for absorption as they are bound to insoluble macromolecules. Moreover, the total removal of the human colon (colectomy) does not upset the balance for these ions. There is evidence from rat experiments that the colon has a Ca^{2+} active transport system sensitive to enhancement by vitamin D and to low calcium intake. In the case of magnesium, other experiments with rats have indicated that the ion is absorbed passively, dependent on the electrochemical gradient and the solvent drag of fluid absorption. *See* Arthritis; Cholecalciferol, Physiology; Magnesium

Secretion

The colon secretes the anions Cl^- and HCO_3^- and the cations K^+ and H^+.

Bicarbonate Secretion

In the human, approximately 70 mmol HCO_3^- leaves the ileum to enter the colon every day and although the organ secretes bicarbonate, only a few mmol appear in the faeces. This is because the secreted HCO_3^- is titrated by the H^+ ions manufactured by the bacterial population of the colon. In diarrhoeal states, when there is an enhanced secretion of bicarbonate, stools can contain an increased amount of bicarbonate.

The mechanisms and control of bicarbonate movements are complex. Other ions move in association with, or in exchange for, bicarbonate. Bicarbonate can come from the plasma, passing between and through cells, and can also come from the intracellular hydration of CO_2. Hydrogen ions, produced from cellular metabolism, can be secreted into the lumen to influence the production and neutralization of bicarbonate ions. Net bicarbonate secretion is accomplished by a combination of bicarbonate and hydrogen ion transport as the blood, cell cytoplasm and luminal contents contain bicarbonate and CO_2. A primary source of HCO_3^- and H^+ ions appears to be from the catalysed hydrolysis of CO_2, as Na^+ and Cl^- absorption is modulated by ambient CO_2. The colonocytes are rich in carbonic anhydrase which can supply bicarbonate and H^+ ions at high catalysed rates. The enzyme may also be directly involved in ion transfer. Inhibition of carbonic anhydrase reduces colonic absorption.

Chloride Ion Secretion

The colon actively secretes Cl^- ions. The intracellular Na^+ and K^+ of the colonocyte are regulated by the basolateral Na^+–K^+ transport ATPase pumping out Na^+ in exchange for K^+. The K^+ can diffuse out across the membrane by a K^+ channel. This mechanism keeps the intracellular Na^+ low and the K^+ high, and produces a negative intracellular pd. The uptake of Cl^- ions is by the coupled Na^+–K^+–$2Cl^-$ cotransport carrier in the basolateral membrane, and is sensitive to loop diuretics such as furosemide and bumetanide. Chloride ions leave the cell via apical Cl^- channels, under the influence of their intracellular–extracellular concentration gradient and the negative intracellular pd. These Cl^- channels are normally closed and are activated to open by increases in the intracellular calcium ion (Ca^{2+}) and/or cAMP (cyclic adenosine monophosphate) levels brought about by a variety of neurotransmitters, secretagogues, hormones and paracrine agents. Because the efflux of the Cl^- ions depolarizes the apical membrane, the movement of Cl^- would gradually cease. To maintain the driving force for the Cl^- exit, an increase in the K^+-conductance of the basolateral membrane occurs shortly (20 s) after the increase in apical membrane Cl^- conductance. The exit of K^+ ions across the basolateral membrane induces a depolarization and, because of electrical coupling between the basolateral and apical membranes, the depolarization maintains the pd across the apical membrane. Thus the stimulation of Cl^- secretion in colonocytes (as in many other Cl^--secreting cells) requires the coordination of four independent systems, the apical Cl^- channels, the basolateral Na^+–K^+–$2Cl^-$ cotransporter, K^+ channels and Na^+,K^+-ATPase. Observations in animals have indicated that secreting cells are located in the crypts.

Potassium Ion Secretion

Although it is known that the colon absorbs and secretes K^+, the cellular sites have not yet been defined. Surface cells of rabbit colon absorb and secrete K^+, but it is not known whether such processes are also found in the cells of the crypts. In rats and rabbits fed high-potassium diets or given aldosterone, K^+ secretion is accomplished first by the active uptake of K^+ at the colonocyte's basolateral membrane by the ouabain-sensitive transport Na^+,K^+-ATPase. Its exit across the apical membrane is then by barium-sensitive K^+ channels that appear to be under the control of cAMP and Ca^{2+}, since raising their cAMP and or Ca^{2+} levels in the colonocytes increases the secretion of K^+. Adrenergic agonists also increase the secretion of K^+, which in rabbit colon is mediated by β_1 receptors. The mechanism involves both increases in the basolateral pump activity and in the conductance of the apical membrane to K^+. In diarrhoea associated with colonic secretion (e.g. colitis) K^+ loss in the stools can be appreciable.

Short-chain Fatty Acids (SCFAs)

Surprisingly, the major anion of the colonic contents comes from SCFAs (acetate, butyrate, propionate, etc.). These originate predominately from the bacterial metabolism of carbohydrate passing into the colon from the ileum. In the human colon, the daily production of SCFAs is estimated to be greater than 300 mmol, while the faecal excretion is only 10 mmol. This indicates that 97% of the SCFAs are removed by the colon. Their absorption is rapid and they enhance the absorption of Na^+. *See* Essential Fatty Acids, Physiology

The SCFAs are weak acids that can exist in solution as two species, the undissociated molecule (acid form HA) and the dissociated anion (A^-). The balance of the species depends on the environmental pH and the pK values of the acid under question. In the colon, the luminal pH is normally approximately 7 and the SCFA pK approximately 4·8, so that the predominant species is the ionized or anionic form. The pathways of absorption of SCFAs across the colon are complex because several mechanisms can operate. These include the following: (1) the generation of luminal CO_2, either from bacteria or from colonocytes, to provide H^+ ions which combine with the anionic form of SCFA (A^-) in an acid microclimate, creating the undissocated acid form (HA) which could diffuse across the apical membrane; (2) luminal H^+ ions from the colonocytes exchange with Na^+ forming the HA; (3) the ionic form, A^-, could diffuse across the tight junctions between the cells; (4) anion exchange mechanisms (e.g. $HCO_3^--A^-$) allow the movement of the anionic form across the apical membrane.

In the human colon it has been proposed that approximately 40% of SCFA absorption can be accounted for by the Na^+-H^+ exchange. As SCFA absorption is also associated with a rise in luminal HCO_3^-, the SCFA–HCO_3^- exchange mechanism is suggested to occur. In theory, changes in luminal pH should affect SCFA movements and alterations in acid–base balance should affect their absorption. However, the mucus and unstirred layers at the apical pole of the colonocytes act as a buffer and maintain the surface acid microclimate in the face of considerable changes in the luminal pH.

SCFAs increase the absorption of NaCl partly through the fatty acids acting as metabolic substrates for the colonocytes and partly as a result of the SCFAs directly influencing the transport mechanisms of the apical membranes (see above). Paradoxical results have also been found in animal colons used *in vitro*, such as SCFAs inhibiting Cl^- absorption and in other cases actual secretion of SCFAs by colonocytes. Other studies have shown that SCFAs also cause electrogenic secretion of Cl^- by colonocytes which can be recorded both *in vivo* and *in vitro*. As the SCFAs have been claimed to be a fundamentally important metabolic fuel for the colonocytes, their reduction or near absence in human conditions such as famine (starvation) and malnourishment (marasmus and kwashiorkor) has been suggested as a major cause of colonic dysfunction and – its consequence – diarrhoea. Other studies have shown that colonic and rectal secretory function in starved or malnourished rats can be enhanced, which would again predispose to diarrhoea. There are many unanswered questions and unsolved problems in relation to SCFA and colonic ion and fluid transfer. *See* Kwashiorkor; Marasmus

Bacterial Fermentation

Composition of Colonic Microflora

The bacteria of the human gastrointestinal tract form a complex ecosystem; over 400 species have been identified in the faeces of a single subject. In healthy humans, the upper gastrointestinal tract is sparsely populated by bacteria as most are killed by gastric acidity (except acid-loving forms such as streptococcus, staphylococcus and lactobacillus) and the passage of intestinal contents is rapid. The bacterial flora of the small intestine is between 10^3 and 10^4 colony-forming units (CFU) per ml of content (mainly Gram-positive anaerobes); this increases to 10^6-10^7 CFU per ml in the distal ileum and Gram-negative bacteria now become dominant. After the ileocaecal sphincter, the bacterial concentrations increase enormously, reaching between 10^{11} and 10^{12} CFU per ml of faecal material, which can amount to approximately 1·5 kg wet weight of bacteria. Viable bacteria are said to make up one third of the faecal dry weight. The major species are *Bacteroides*, *Clostridium*, *Eubacterium*, *Peptococcus*, *Bifidobacterium*, *Streptococcus* and *Fusobacterium*. *See* Clostridium, Occurrence of Clostridium perfringens; Clostridium, Occurrence of Clostridium botulinum; Microflora of the Intestine, Role and Effects; *Staphylococcus*, Properties and Occurrence

Metabolic Capacity of Colonic Bacteria

The metabolic capacity of the colonic bacteria is diverse. Luminal contents are potential substrates for bacterial enzymic transformation by hydrolysis (examples are oestradiol glucuronide, cyclamate), dehydroxylation (bile acids, amino acids) or reduction (unsaturated fatty acids, food dyes, benzaldehydes). The bacteria can also synthesize vitamins such as vitamin K, biotin and vitamin B_{12}. Antibiotic treatment of humans is known to lower the plasma levels of the first two, suggesting that the bacteria may play a role in supplying some of the daily requirements for these vitamins. *See* Biotin, Physiology; Cobalamins, Physiology

Carbohydrates are fermented by the bacterial enzymes to SCFA. The major carbohydrate sources are plant cell wall polysaccharides (cellulose, pectins, hemicellulose), starch, intestinal mucus, and mono- and disaccharides. Depending on the amount of fibre in the diet, between 20 and 70 g of carbohydrate are estimated to be fermented per day in the human colon. The SCFAs produced by the fermentation process are absorbed by the colonocytes, for which they represent an important metabolic source and act as a promoter of NaCl and thus fluid absorption (see *Absorption* and *Secretion*). *See* Carbohydrates, Digestion, Absorption and Metabolism; Dietary Fibre, Physiological Effects

Another important feature of the metabolic capacity of the colonic bacteria is the potential for creating candidate carcinogens and mutagens (e.g. nitrosamines) that may play a role in carcinogenesis, especially of the colon. In the USA this is the most frequently diagnosed cancer of internal organs. There is some evidence that the 'Western diet' (high in beef, fat and protein, and low in fibre) is a possible cause of the much higher incidence of colon cancer than is found among Africans, Asians and South Americans. *See* Cancer, Diet in Cancer Prevention; Nitrosamines

Migrants show a cancer incidence that approximates the prevailing rate of their residence rather than their birthplace. There is, however, another side to the bacterial coin of the colon – the inactivation of carcinogenic compounds by bacteria such as *Escherichia coli*, *Lactobacillus* spp. and *Bacteroides* spp.

Urea, Ammonia and Nitrogen

Some 6–9 g of urea (approximately 20% of the daily urea synthesis) is broken down in the human intestine, mainly by the urease of the colonic bacteria. As only 0.4 g of this urea enters the colon from the ileum, and there is no urea and hardly any of its breakdown metabolite ammonia in the faeces, most of the urea apparently has to enter the colon by another pathway in order to be metabolized. Unfortunately, the urea permeability of the cleansed human colon appears to be very low and excludes its transmucosal diffusion as a major route. There is evidence that the low permeability is caused by removal of the colon contents which normally increase the permeability of the mucosa to urea; thus the entry path of urea into the untouched colon is probably transmucosal. The catabolism of the urea load produces 200–300 mmol of ammonia and 100–150 mmol of bicarbonate per day. Practically all the ammonia (99%) is absorbed across the mucosa by nonionic diffusion for at colonic pH (6–7) ammonia is largely present as the ammonium ion (NH_4^+). The absorbed ammonium is transported by the portal system to the liver, where it enters the nitrogen pool and is synthesized to urea or amino acids. This metabolism of urea is of little importance to human nutrition but the enterohepatic circulation of ammonia is important in the genesis of hepatic encephalopathy. In hepatic disease, the liver can fail to detoxify the ammonia and it then enters the general circulation to produce neuropsychiatric disturbances and even coma due to its cerebrotoxic action on the brain. *See* Liver, Nutritional Management of Liver and Biliary Disorders

The origin of ammonia in the large intestine is mainly from the breakdown of urea, as described above, but it can also be produced by the bacteria from non-urea sources such as amine and amide nitrogen of proteins, peptides and amino acids and from plasma glutamine. The colonic bacteria not only produce ammonia but can also utilize it as a nitrogen source for their own synthesis of amino acids and proteins. The oral administration of poorly digested carbohydrates is known to increase the faecal loss of nitrogen. The probable explanation for this is that the nondigestible carbohydrates are metabolized by the bacteria in the colon as a preferential energy source and stimulate the production of new bacteria which are then lost in the faeces.

Effect of Diet on Microflora

While there have been numerous studies both in animals and in humans on the effects of diet on the balance of the colonic microflora, the data are conflicting with regard to the ability of the diet to alter specific components of the adult bacterial population. For example, different studies on individuals fed on omnivorous and then herbivorous diets have reported no change, small increases or decreases in faecal counts of bacteroides. Subjects in Britain and the USA eating the Western diet had more bacteroides and fewer enterococci and other aerobics than subjects eating a vegetarian diet in Uganda, India and Japan. Overall, it appears that the eating of a meat-poor, high-carbohydrate diet increases the faecal counts of aerobic bacteria, and decreases a number of anaerobic bacteria. *See* Vegetarian Diets

Effect of Dietary Intake on Colon Contents

Since the production of colonic gas (see below) and SCFA is so dependent upon the bacterial fermentation of unabsorbed carbohydrate, much attention has been paid to the proportion of dietary carbohydrate that remains undigested, enters the large intestine and is then broken down and 'salvaged'. Starch, rather than dietary fibre, is the major substrate. In healthy adults it is estimated that usually less than 5% of ingested starch is unabsorbed and enters the colon although this may be increased to 12% by food processing.

Colon Gas Production

The major components of intestinal gas are nitrogen, oxygen, carbon dioxide, hydrogen and methane. Gases such as hydrogen sulphide, volatile amines, organic acids, mercaptans, indoles, etc., collectively amount to less than 1% of the total but as they account for the characteristic unpleasant smell of the flatus they are socially important. The colon is the only source for the production of hydrogen, which is either used by the bacteria, expelled in the flatus or absorbed and excreted in the breath. Dietary substrates are the major source for its production as it is low in the fasting subject. Fermentable carbohydrates such as raffinose and stachyose (oligosaccharides found in beans), lactulose and lactose (in subjects with hypolactasia) all increase the production of hydrogen. Measures of breath hydrogen can be used as an index of its colonic production and also as an indication of when food reaches the colon.

Colonic Function and Diarrhoea

It is clear from the various accounts of colonic function that if its absorptive function is impaired or its secretory activity enhanced or both occur, then diarrhoea results. A large number of factors can alter the basic net absorptive 'tone' of the colon to a net secretory one and thus induce diarrhoea. Examples include bacterial toxins (cholera, *Escherichia coli* STa (heat-stable enterotoxin) and LT (heat-labile enterotoxin)), mediators of inflammatory processes (eicosanoids, histamine, kinins, substance P), neurotransmitters (acetylcholine, VIP (vasoactive intestinal peptide), serotonin), hormones (neurotensin, glucagon, cholecystokinin) and specific endogenous luminal contents such as bile acids. Recently, studies on rats and mice to elucidate the enigma of the terminal diarrhoea suffered by human victims of famine and severe malnutrition have shown that starvation induces hypersecretory responses of the enterocytes and colonocytes to neurotransmitters and agents that activate secretion. The mechanism(s) of the hypersecretion is not yet understood but one locus is

probably at the apical membrane after the release of the second messengers that activate the Cl^- secretion.

Bibliography

Binder HJ and Sandle G (1987) Electrolyte absorption and secretion in the mammalian colon. In: Johnson LR (ed.) *Physiology of the Gastrointestinal Tract* 2nd edn, pp 1389–1418. New York: Raven Press.

Goldin BR, Lichtenstein AH and Gorbach SL (1988) The roles of the intestinal flora. In: Shils ME and Young VR (eds) *Modern Nutrition in Health and Disease*, pp 500–515. Philadelphia: Lea and Febiger.

Kasper H and Goebell H (eds) (1982) *Colon and Nutrition*. (Falk Symposium No 32). Lancaster: MTP Press.

Lebenthal E and Duffey ME (eds) (1990) *Textbook of Secretory Diarrhea*. New York: Raven Press.

McBurney MI (1991) Passage of starch into colons of humans: quantitation and implications. *Canadian Journal of Physiology and Pharmacology* 69: 130–136.

Roediger WEW (1990) The starved colon – diminished mucosal nutrition, diminished absorption, and colitis. *Diseases of the Colon and Rectum* 33: 858–862.

Wrong OM, Edmonds CJ and Chadwick VS (1981) *The Large Intestine – its role in mammalian nutrition and homeostasis*. Lancaster: MTP Press.

Roy J. Levin
Sheffield University, Sheffield, UK

Diseases and Disorders

Constipation

The bowel habit of healthy individuals is extremely variable, and consequently there are no universally accepted definitions of constipation. Constipation usually suggests infrequent passage of stools, but some people use the term to imply that their stools are very hard, difficult to expel, or that defecation is painful. Most doctors consider an individual constipated if he or she passes stools less than three times per week or passes an average of less than 30 g stool per day. Some people hold the erroneous belief that they should open their bowels at least once a day to maintain good health, and that missing a bowel action implies constipation. Consequently this may lead to unnecessary prolonged straining at stool or laxative misuse, both of which may be potentially harmful.

Constipation may lead to abdominal distension and discomfort. In the elderly, pressure from a loaded colon and rectum can cause disturbances in voiding urine.

Causes of Constipation

Simple Constipation

Simple constipation is the most common type, in which there is no serious underlying cause. It is more likely to affect women than men. The following factors are relevant:

1. *Diet*. Constipation is to be expected when food or fluid intake is diminished. Faeces consist mainly of water, indigestible fibre and bacteria. On a Western low-residue diet containing 10–20 g fibre, stool weight is approximately 100–150 g. A high-fibre diet will decrease colonic transit time, and increase faecal weight, leading to a softer, bulkier stool. Rural Africans eating such a diet may have a stool output of 400–500 g daily. *See* Dietary Fibre, Physiological Effects; Dietary Fibre, Fibre and Disease Prevention

2. *Loss of habit*. Defecation depends on a conditioned reflex arising from the sensation of a loaded rectum – the 'call to stool'. When the call to stool is ignored, the rectum may become chronically distended and no longer signal the usual desire to defecate. This behavioural change may begin when rushing to work in the morning. Similarly, children may dislike lack of privacy or cleanliness at school and suppress the defecation reflex. Suppressing rectal sensation from consciousness will make the individual unaware of the need to defecate.

3. *Immobility*. Patients confined to bed or immobile due to medical conditions are likely to become constipated.

Thus 'simple constipaton' may be multifactorial and not always solely caused by lack of dietary fibre. In some young women there may be severe constipation from both poor colonic propulsion (slow transit) and also outlet obstruction owing to inappropriate pelvic muscle contractions during defecation.

Irritable Bowel Syndrome

Constipation, often in association with abdominal pain, is a common complaint in patients with the irritable bowel syndrome (see below).

Other Colonic Disease

Diverticular disease and colonic obstruction owing to a benign stricture or a carcinoma may cause constipation.

Pain

Painful defecation resulting from an anal fissure or haemorrhoids will lead to a conscious suppression of the urge to defecate.

Metabolic

Hypothyroidism, hypercalcaemia, and diabetes may all cause constipation.

Neurological

An intact nervous supply to the bowel is required for normal colonic transit and defecation. When disrupted, in conditions such as multiple sclerosis or spinal cord injury, constipation may develop. Aganglionosis (Hirschsprung's disease) is a rare congenital condition in which the nerves within the bowel wall itself are deficient, resulting in constipation. Although usually apparent in infancy, it may not present until adulthood.

Chronic intestinal pseudo-obstruction refers to a rare group of motility disorders causing constipation and episodes of vomiting, abdominal pain and distension. Chronic intestinal pseudo-obstruction may be caused by a primary defect of intestinal neurons or smooth muscle, or may be secondary to other neurological or systemic illness.

Psychological

Depression may be associated with constipation. In children, constipation may be an expression of psychological disturbance.

Drugs

Numerous drugs prescribed for unrelated conditions have constipation as a side-effect. Examples include iron tablets, antacids containing calcium or aluminium, opiates, calcium-channel blockers, anticholinergic agents and tricyclic antidepressants.

Treatment of Constipation

Any underlying causes of constipation should be sought and treated, but the situation is more commonly one of 'simple' constipation. Initial measures include increasing fluid intake, increasing the amount of high-fibre foods in the diet and, if necessary, adding bran supplements. Within the colon, fibre increases stool bulk, retains water and acts as a substrate for bacteria which multiply and augment the bulking effect. The consequent softer, bulkier stool provides a better stimulus to the colon and rectum. In addition, bacterial flora acting on celluloses and hemicelluloses will release volatile fatty acids which have a stimulant effect on the colon. Increasing physical activity where possible may help.

Laxatives

If bran is not tolerated or not taken in sufficient quantity, then a bulking agent (see Table 1) may be added. If ineffective, stool softeners, osmotic laxatives or stimulant laxatives may be necessary. Prolonged use of these latter three types of laxatives is undesirable. Continued purgation may lead to excessive loss of

Table 1. Classification of laxatives on their mode of action

Laxative	Mechanism of action

Bulking agents
  Wheat bran
  Ispaghula husk
  Sterculia
  Methylcellulose
	Increased stool volume (fibre, bacteria, and water retention)

Faecal softeners Dioctyl sodium sulphosuccinate	Facilitate mixing of aqueous and fatty substances in faecal mass to soften it

Osmotic laxatives
  Lactulose
  Magnesium sulphate
	Water retention within bowel increasing stool volume

Stimulant laxatives
  Bisacodyl
  Senna
  Cascara
  Phenolphthalein
  Rhubarb
	Increased colonic motility

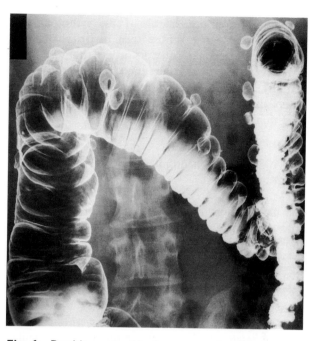

Fig. 1 Double-contrast barium enema showing numerous colonic diverticula.

potassium salts. In the case of stimulant laxatives, prolonged usage can lead to an atonic, poorly propulsive colon, which becomes less and less responsive to laxatives. Unfortunately, misconceptions about bowel habit have led to excessive laxative use. Rectal preparations in the form of suppositories (e.g. glycerol suppositories) or enemas (water, phosphate, arachis oil) are also useful in the management of constipation, particularly in the elderly or those confined to bed.

Diverticular Disease of the Colon

Diverticular disease (or diverticulosis) is a common condition in Western countries describing the presence of diverticula (pouches) arising from the colon. Each diverticulum represents an outpouching of mucosa which has protruded through the muscle layer at an area of weakness – usually the site of entry of blood vessels piercing the muscle wall (see Fig. 1). There is associated thickening (hypertrophy) of the colonic muscle, suggesting that excessive intraluminal pressures have led to the diverticula formation. The thickened muscle results in a narrowing of the colonic lumen. Diverticula are most often seen in the sigmoid colon, although the whole colon may be affected. There may be a few or several hundred diverticula. *See* Inflammatory Bowel Disease

Diverticular disease is rare in people under 30 years of age, but in Western societies about one third of the population over 60 years old will have acquired diverticula. The association with increasing age suggests a decline in the mechanical integrity of the wall of the colon, but colonic diverticulosis is rare in rural Africans when compared to individuals of a similar age in industrialized countries. Diverticular disease seems to be related to the low-fibre diet eaten in Western societies. On a refined diet, colonic muscle contracts more strongly in order to expel the smaller stool mass. Over a period of years, the increased pressure within the colon leads to herniation of the colonic mucosa and formation of diverticula. Africans passing a bulkier stool do not generate such high squeezing pressures in the sigmoid colon and are not prone to diverticula formation. Thus diverticular disease results from a diet low in fibre in an ageing population. Further evidence that dietary fibre (rather than any other Western environmental factor) is causal comes from a study showing that vegetarians, consuming larger amounts of cereal fibre, are less prone to diverticulosis than non-vegetarians within the same community.

Symptoms from Diverticular Disease

Diverticular disease is in the main an incidental finding when a patient undergoes radiological investigation (barium enema), often for unrelated symptoms. Diverticular disease produces no symptoms in 80% of cases. However in some patients there may be left-sided lower abdominal pain thought to be caused by the increased pressure generated by the sigmoid colon musculature. Such pains may be worse after eating. There may be a change in bowel habit, with features of constipation alternating with loose stools. These symptoms are indistinguishable from those seen in irritable bowel syndrome. Indeed many doctors believe that uncomplicated diverticular disease never produces symptoms and that any of the afore-mentioned symptoms are caused by coexistent irritable bowel syndrome in the same individual.

Management of Uncomplicated Diverticular Disease

The fibre content of the diet should be increased, in order to increase stool bulk. This is best achieved using unprocessed coarse wheat bran (20–30 g per day). Bran which is further milled or cooked (as in wholemeal bread) and fermentable fibre (as in fruit and vegetables) are less effective at increasing stool mass and need to be taken in larger amounts to produce the same effect. Increasing stool bulk will lead to a lowering of intra-colonic pressure. Patients with symptomatic diverticular disease will often become pain-free on a high-fibre diet. Fibre supplementation (e.g. ispaghula husk) may be used in those finding bran unpalatable. Antispasmodics such as mebeverine may relax the hypermotile sigmoid colon in diverticular disease, and give symptomatic relief. Simple analgesics (e.g. paracetamol) may be required.

Complicated Diverticular Disease

It must be stressed that diverticular disease is in general a benign condition without symptoms. The following complications are uncommon.

1. Diverticulitis refers to inflammation within a diverticulum and is thought to develop in response to the irritating presence of inspissated faecal material. There is left-sided lower abdominal pain and tenderness, which may be associated with fever, constipation, and vomiting. Hospital admission is necessary and most patients will respond to intravenous fluids and antibiotics without the need for surgery. Diverticulitis can lead to abscess formation outside the colon wall (pericolic abscess), and the ensuing inflammation may occasionally lead to fistula formation. A fistula is an abnormal connection, and may, for example, link the colon to the bladder.
2. Perforation of a diverticulum is a rare but very serious complication. The perforation will allow passage of colonic contents into the abdominal cavity with consequent peritonitis. Surgical intervention is necessary.
3. Haemorrhage from blood vessels present at the neck of a diverticulum can lead to severe rectal bleeding which may settle spontaneously, or occasionally require surgery. Nevertheless, patients who develop rectal bleeding and are known to have diverticular disease should be investigated for concomitant pathology.

Irritable Bowel Syndrome

Irritable bowel syndrome (IBS) is a very common disorder characterized by abdominal pain, disturbance of bowel habit and other gastrointestinal symptoms, without an identifiable cause. There is no strict definition of IBS, and no diagnostic marker, all tests proving normal. In the past the diagnosis has often been one of exclusion, after investigations have ruled out organic gastrointestinal disease. However the following symptoms are more likely to occur in IBS than in organic disease: abdominal distension, abdominal pain relieved by defecation, more frequent and looser stools at the onset of pain, a sensation of incomplete rectal evacuation, and passage of mucus per rectum. Although occurring in all age groups, most patients who report IBS are likely to be young adults (with a female preponderance). Physical examination is usually normal, though some patients complain of abdominal tenderness. Once the diagnosis is made, the patient can be reassured that IBS is a benign condition and not a sinister or life-threatening illness, although it can be troublesome, and at times disabling.

Pathophysiology

It is difficult to imagine how a single mechanism can account for symptoms of pain and constipation in one patient, and bowel frequency in another. It has been suggested that pain in IBS is caused by abnormally increased visceral sensitivity to normal gut events such as intestinal distension. Disturbances of motility patterns throughout the gut (and not just the colon) have been reported in IBS. Psychological factors are also important, many patients recognizing that their symptoms may be worsened by anxiety or depression. In some patients, their abdominal symptoms may represent somatization of underlying psychological problems and indeed these patients may also report many non-gastrointestinal symptoms. Foods do not cause IBS, and there is no evidence to incriminate a faulty or low-residue diet in its aetiology. However, a dietary assessment may on occasion detect hypolactasia, a deficiency of lactase in the small intestinal mucosa; this condition is characterized by abdominal pain, diarrhoea and flatulence after ingesting lactose-containing foods. Such symptoms may be indistinguishable from those of IBS.

Drug Treatment in Irritable Bowel Syndrome

The use of drugs in IBS is often unnecessary, but some patients undoubtedly benefit from drug treatment. The efficacy of drug treatments in IBS has yet to be satisfactorily demonstrated in double-blind placebo-controlled trials. Problems with such trials include definition of IBS, absence of objective markers of improvement and a large (30–60%) placebo response. If used, drug treatments should be tailored to the patient's symptoms.

Constipation

Constipation may be improved by increasing the patient's intake of dietary fibre. If additional coarse wheat bran is unpalatable then proprietary stool bulking agents such as ispaghula husk, sterculia or methylcellulose may be prescribed. These agents increase faecal mass and produce a softer stool. With such treatment, symptoms of abdominal distension, borborygmi or excessive flatus may worsen initially. These will be more tolerable if the amount of fibre or bulking agent is increased gradually.

Diarrhoea

Patients with IBS who complain of diarrhoea do not actually have increased stool output; they defecate more frequently and may have associated urgency. Such patients may benefit from antidiarrhoeal agents such as loperamide, codeine phosphate or diphenoxylate. These drugs delay small and large intestinal transit by stimulation of opioid receptors on intestinal smooth muscle, intrinsic nerves of the enteric nervous system, spinal cord and brain.

Abdominal Pain

Abdominal pain in IBS may result from gastrointestinal smooth muscle contraction, or from gut distension by gas or stool. Antispasmodics are widely used in IBS to relieve abdominal pain, and may be combined with bulking agents. Many antispasmodic drugs are antimuscarinic in action. They antagonize acetylcholine at muscarinic receptors of intestinal smooth muscle, thereby reducing intestinal smooth muscle contraction. Such drugs include dicyclomine and propantheline bromide. Other antispasmodics directly relax intestinal smooth muscle without acting through muscarinic cholinergic receptors. Examples include mebeverine, alverine citrate and enteric-coated peppermint oil.

Associated Affective Disorders

The brain does influence gastrointestinal motility, and, together with the observation that many patients with IBS also have anxiety or depression, this suggests that IBS may represent a disturbance of the 'brain–gut axis'. Drugs modifying central neurotransmitter action might also be expected to modify neurotransmitter action in the enteric nervous system. Some trials have reported symptomatic improvement using tricyclic antidepressants, but the overall improvement reported by patients may be due to treatment of associated depression rather than the IBS itself; in many patients these two conditions are inseparable. Anticholinergic side-effects of such drugs might be expected to improve abdominal pain.

Dietary Manipulation

Many patients not unreasonably expect their diet to be in some way responsible for their symptoms. There have been a few reports suggesting some symptomatic benefit from exclusion diets, leading to the assumption that food intolerances may be relevant in some IBS sufferers. Such dietary studies are difficult to perform in a controlled fashion and at present there is no clear-cut evidence to suggest that food intolerance is a cause of IBS. Nevertheless, some patients (particularly those in whom diarrhoea predominates) will identify certain foodstuffs as precipitating factors. These patients may benefit by avoiding those foods, although this may be a placebo response. In a poorly understood condition, it would seem unwise to totally disregard a possible aetiological role of dietary components.

Increasing dietary fibre is often recommended to IBS sufferers and will help those with constipation. However the efficacy of a high-fibre diet in improving other symptoms of IBS remains doubtful; placebo-controlled studies on the use of added dietary fibre have yielded conflicting results.

Stomas

The term stoma is used to describe the opening created surgically when part of the gastrointestinal tract has been brought to the skin surface. In this article, we discuss the two types of intestinal output stoma – colostomy and ileostomy. A colostomy is constructed when a part of the colon is brought to the skin surface. The actual site of opening on the abdominal wall depends on the nature and site of the underlying disease. With an ileostomy, it is the terminal small intestine which is brought to the exterior as an opening on the lower right quadrant of the abdomen. The effluent from such stomas collects into an appliance incorporating a bag. In the UK there are 100 000 people with a colostomy and 10 000 with an ileostomy. Reasons for such stoma formation are given in Table 2.

Before a stoma is sited, patients should ideally have been prepared regarding what to expect following the operation. Despite prior discussions with the surgeon, a

Table 2. Indications for stoma formation

Type of stoma	Indications
Colostomy	Anal or rectal carcinoma Crohn's disease Complications of diverticular disease Trauma Neurological or anatomical abnormalities impairing normal defecation
Ileostomy	Ulcerative colitis Colorectal Crohn's disease Ischaemic colitis Familial adenomatous polyposis

stoma care nurse, and meeting other patients with stomas, patients often take months to adjust psychologically to having a stoma. Moreover, the decision to fashion a stoma may be made at an emergency operation without adequate time for preoperative psychological preparation. In some cases the stoma may be temporary, and a future operation will restore intestinal continuity.

Colostomy

A distally sited colostomy will produce solid faecal matter and evacuation will be intermittent. Most UK patients manage their colostomy by natural evacuation. The colostomy acts once or twice each day, often at predictable times, allowing some patients to wear the appliance only at those times. Other patients practise irrigation, pouring about 1 litre of warm water slowly into the colon and allowing it to run out through a drainage sleeve into the toilet. Such irrigation is performed on alternate days.

Ileostomy

Most ileostomies are fashioned in association with colectomy (removal of the colon). In health about 1·5 l of fluid passes from the small intestine into the colon daily, and, after absorption by the colon, faecal output is about 100–150 ml. Once established, fluid output from an ileostomy amounts to 400–800 ml daily. The effluent is odourless. As well as the more voluminous and liquid nature of effluent compared to a colostomy, an ileostomy tends to function throughout the day, although output generally increases after meals. Therefore the patient needs to wear the appliance continuously unless an ileal reservoir (Koch continent ileostomy) has been fashioned. Ileostomy patients produce less urine because of their increased intestinal fluid losses, and are prone to developing renal stones. They are also at risk of significant salt and water depletion at times of excessive

sweating in hot climates, and when ileostomy output increases further, e.g. as a result of gastroenteritis. If a significant length of terminal ileum has also been resected, vitamin B_{12} absorption and bile salt reabsorption will be impaired leading to vitamin B_{12} deficiency and a predisposition to cholesterol gall stones.

Stomas and Diet

The nutritional requirements of the individual with a colostomy or ileostomy are not different from those of a normal person. The only exception is the ileostomy (or jejunostomy) patient with a short residual length of intestine who has associated high stomal output and malabsorption necessitating nutritional supplementation. Nevertheless, many stoma patients, discovering a relationship between their diet and stoma output, will restrict their diet in order to control flatus, consistency and odour of the effluent. The patient with a colostomy may notice that eating green vegetables and fruit or drinking beer may lead to a more liquid stool output. Odour from a colostomy is more likely to be troublesome after eating eggs or fish. Aspirin added to the colostomy bag may reduce odour by decreasing bacterial fermentation. Although bacteria tend to colonize the terminal ileum of ileostomy patients, odour is less often a problem. Excessive flatus can occur with either type of stoma, but can be reduced by limiting the intake of cauliflower, green vegetables and onions.

Psychosocial Aspects

Many patients with a stoma have psychological problems in coming to terms with their altered body image. Many will decrease their social activities and there is a high incidence of depression. Following stoma formation, patients of working age are encouraged to resume their previous occupation. In fact, some patients with previously debilitating colitis may find that they can enjoy permanent employment for the first time now that their diseased colon has been removed and an ileostomy created. Re-employment for both types of stoma patients may be limited by inadequate washing and sanitary conditions at work. Younger patients (usually ileostomy patients) tend to readapt more easily than older patients (usually colostomy patients), and may resume their previous social activities, sport and work, but many will have psychological problems in developing personal and sexual relationships.

Bibliography

Almy TP and Howell DA (1980) Diverticular disease of the colon. *New England Journal of Medicine* 302: 324–331.

Devlin HB (1990) Stomas. *Medicine International* (79): 3286–3291.

Devroede G (1989) Constipation. In: Sleisenger MH and Fordtran JS (eds) *Gastrointestinal Disease* 4th edn, pp 331–368. Philadelphia: WB Saunders.

Heaton KW (1988) Functional bowel disease. In: Pounder RE (ed.) *Recent Advances in Gastroenterology 7*, pp 291–312. Edinburgh: Churchill Livingstone.

Painter NS and Burkitt DP (1971) Diverticular disease of the colon: a deficiency disease of Western civilisation. *British Medical Journal* 2: 450–454.

Read NW (ed.) (1985) *Irritable Bowel Syndrome*. London: Grune and Stratton.

D. A. Gorard and M. J. G. Farthing
St Bartholomew's Hospital, London, UK

Cancer of the Colon

Colorectal cancer is the second most common cancer in Western societies, affecting up to 6% of men and women by the age of 75. The cancer is presently thought to develop by a stepwise accumulation of several mutations, the first of which is the loss of a tumour-suppressing gene located on chromosome 5. No direct evidence of the involvement of diet in these changes has so far been shown, but there is a wealth of epidemiological and experimental evidence to suggest that colorectal cancer risk is affected by diet. *See* Cancer, Epidemiology

Epidemiology

Risks of colorectal cancer increase markedly with age, but there remains at least a 15-fold range in age-standardized levels in different parts of the world. Incidence is highest in Australia, New Zealand, and parts of Europe such as northern Italy, Denmark and FRG. Low rates are seen in parts of South America, rural Africa, China and India. Both migrant studies and secular changes in incidence rates show that environmental factors are mainly responsible for these geographical differences. Migrants from low-risk areas (e.g. Japan) adopt the incidence rates of a high-risk population (e.g. in Hawaii) within a single generation. In Japan itself, there have been striking changes: whereas rates were low before Westernization, age-specific colon cancer rates have increased fivefold since 1960, and are fast approaching those recorded in the UK.

Of the many possible environmental risk factors, diet is most strongly associated with colorectal cancer incidence rates, and there are many potential specific dietary factors involved. The majority of investigations have centred around meat, fat, alcohol, and nonstarch polysaccharides (dietary fibre). *See* Microflora of the Intestine, Role and Effects

Meat

The supposition that cancer initiators are formed in the lumen of the large gut has prompted the search for faecal mutagens and carcinogens, of which there are a number of candidates, including polycyclic hydrocarbons, phenols, and *N*-nitroso compounds. Recent attention has focused on the mutagenic heterocyclic amines which are formed in meat cooked at relatively low temperatures. The quinoline derivatives such as IQ (2-amino-3-methylimidazo(4,5-f)quinoline), MeIQx (2-amino-3,8-dimethylimidazo(4,5-f)quinoxaline) and MeIQ (2-amino-3,4-dimethylimidazo(4,5-f)quinoline), probably result from Maillard reactions between a hexose, such as glucose, and an amino acid, with linkage of the resulting Strecker aldehyde to creatinine. MeIQx forms covalent links with mouse DNA (deoxyribonucleic acid) obtained from tissues including the large intestine. MeIQ and IQ are damaging to mouse cells *in vivo*, and IQ induces large bowel tumours in mice. Less than one part per billion of these mutagens are found in food, although the more recently isolated PhIP (2-amino-1-methyl-6-phenylimidazo(4,5-f)pyridine is found in concentrations of 15 mg per kg in fried beef. PhIP is mutagenic, an inducer of sister chromatid exchanges in bone marrow, and a carcinogen causing lymphoma in mice. Other mutagens, the fecapentaenes, are not associated with increased risk of colon cancer in case control studies. However, non-fecapentaene mutagenicity, possibly from heterocyclic amines, has been associated with increased risk. *See* Amines; Mutagens; Nitrosamines; Phenolic Compounds; Polycyclic Aromatic Hydrocarbons

The presence of mutagens in cooked meat would offer a direct link with the epidemiological association of meat consumption and large bowel cancer. Vegetarians are generally at lower risk of colorectal cancer, and both meat and fat consumption are high in high-risk areas. The recent increases in bowel cancer rates in countries such as Japan and Greece have been accompanied by rapidly increasing consumption of meat. To examine risk on an individual basis, 19 case control studies in various geographical locations have reported the risk of colorectal cancer with respect to meat. The majority (12) of these studies yielded non-significant results, but positive associations were found in seven studies, the relative risk increasing with increasing meat consumption. No study yielded inverse associations. These findings have received support from a recent prospective study of 89 000 US nurses in which risk of developing colon cancer was significantly elevated in those who ate beef, pork or lamb as a main dish each day. *See* Vegetarian Diets

Fat

One of the most extensively investigated hypotheses is that secondary bile acids are involved in bowel cancer. Originally, bile acids were thought to be initiators via desaturation to 20-methyl cholanthrene, a polycyclic hydrocarbon. More recently, they have been proposed as promoters, via their damaging and cell-proliferative effects on the colonic mucosa. Deoxycholic acid, in particular, seems to enhance the production of diacylglycerol (DAG) from phosphatidylcholine incubated with bacteria from human faeces. DAG is an activator of protein kinase C, an enzyme which plays a key role in signal transduction and growth control. *See* Bile

Bile acids alone, however, are unlikely to affect the risk of developing colorectal cancer because there is no difference in faecal bile acid output either between cases and healthy matched controls, or between individuals living in a high-risk area and those living in a low-risk area. Nevertheless, it is possible that other factors, such as calcium and pH, may be involved, reducing the solubility of free bile acids, at least in faecal water.

An increased output of bile acids, resulting from a high-fat diet, was a suggested explanation for the epidemiological association between high fat intake and high rates of bowel cancer. The increase in colon cancer in Japan has been associated with an increase in total fat consumption, although not in Greece where the traditional diet is high in fat, from olive oil. Experimental and epidemiological studies offer limited support for a role for fat in bowel cancer, the majority of case control studies of diet and cancer (6 out of 25) having shown no significant associations. In seven, risk was elevated with increased fat consumption, and, in two, an inverse association was found.

Prospective and intervention studies of fat in bowel cancer or in studies of precursor adenoma have also yielded conflicting results. American nurses show mildly increased risk with higher fat intake, less significant than that from meat. Risk of developing adenomas was found to be reduced by a low-fat diet in a prospective study of 45 000 US health professionals, but not in an intervention study of 400 adenoma patients in Australia. Support for a role for saturated fat in bowel cancer could come from large prospective studies if they showed positive associations between risk and blood cholesterol levels. However, in the largest studies of more than 92 000 individuals in Sweden and California, blood cholesterol was positively related to large bowel cancer in one study, with no relation in the other.

In animal studies of large bowel carcinogenesis, induced with chemical carcinogens, recent work shows no overall effect of fat, nor saturated fat when standardized for total energy and for linoleic acid intake. There is increasing evidence that fewer tumours develop in animals fed high levels of n3 fatty acids, whereas there is a tumour requirement for n6 fatty acids. The n refers to the position of the first double bond relative to the methyl carbon atom. In humans, there is no established difference between type of fat and risk of colorectal cancer.

Alcohol

Alcohol, particularly beer consumption, has been linked for some time with large bowel cancer, especially rectal cancer. Time trends in cancer mortality related to changes in food supplies and alcohol consumption, show a positive association between beer consumption and rectal cancer. Alcohol is not a direct acting carcinogen, but beer, wines and spirits contain at least 1200 different compounds, such as aldehydes, higher alcohols, phenols and amines. Acetaldyhyde and urethane are known carcinogens, and acetaldehyde is a metabolic intermediate from alcohol in humans, particularly chronic consumers. A recent report found sufficient evidence to classify alcoholic beverages as carcinogenic to humans, but epidemiological studies were inconsistent for colon cancer, and only indicative for beer consumption in rectal cancer.

Nonstarch Polysaccharides and Starch

The hypothesis that large bowel cancer was caused by prolonged transit time, and concentration of carcinogens in the faecal stream from diminished stool bulk, resulting from lack of dietary fibre (non-starch polysaccharides; NSPs) was first publicized by Burkitt in 1969. Since that time, a number of studies have shown a reduction in faecal mutagenicity, probably by dilution, with bran in humans. Bran, together with cellulose, also appears to have a consistently protective effect against chemical carcinogenesis induced in experimental animals.

There are, however, other aspects to the protective action of dietary fibre, in addition to its effect on stool bulk and transit time. First, NSPs are substrates for anaerobic fermentation by the flora of the large bowel. Second, recent research has shown that as much starch as NSPs may reach the large gut and be fermented by the flora. The amount of 'resistant' starch that reaches the large bowel depends on cooking, processing, and ripeness of food, but in areas where starch is the major contributor to energy supplies in human diets, and where fat intakes are low, substantial amounts of 'resistant' starch may reach the large gut. *See* Dietary Fibre, Physiological Effects; Starch, Resistant Starch

During fermentation, bacterial cell mass and faecal weight are increased and the production of ammonia, amines and other precursor *N*-nitroso compounds is altered. Production of short-chain fatty acids, butyrate, acetate and propionate, is also increased. Butyrate is a well-recognized differentiating and antiproliferative agent in cell culture lines, acting directly as an inhibitor of DNA synthesis and cell growth, mainly via inhibition of histone deacetylase. This may be a general mechanism for allowing access for DNA repair enzymes. Acetate and propionate are much less active than butyrate in this respect. Interestingly, butyrate levels, both *in vitro* and *in vivo*, are enhanced when starch, rather than NSP, is the substrate for fermentation. Starch from different dietary sources also reduces cell proliferation in the colon of mice, particularly in the distal colon. *See* Dietary Fibre, Fibre and Disease Prevention

So far, there has been little testing of the protective effects of butyrate and resistant starch, although two small studies have shown lowered faecal butyrate in cases versus controls. In animal studies, tumour incidence from chemical carcinogens was enhanced in one study, reduced in another, and unchanged in a further study in which butyrate levels were increased either directly or from diet.

Intakes of resistant starch and NSP have not been measured in most dietary studies, but when all case control studies which have measured various indices of 'fibre' consumption are summarized, fibre is associated with a reduction in risk in 11 out of 22 studies, mainly as a result of lower vegetable consumption reported by cases than by controls. In the largest study of 818 cases in Belgium, starch, fibre, cooked vegetables and raw vegetables were all protective factors, with relative risks reduced to 0·82, 0·67, 0·71 and 0·37, respectively. So far, no protective effect of fibre (measured as crude fibre) has been documented in the prospective study of American nurses. Dietary fibre, from both vegetables and cereals, was protective against colorectal adenoma in a prospective study of American males. The recurrence of adenomas has not been reduced on intervention with bran in Australia. More large prospective and intervention trials are required to establish a definite role for NSPs in cancer protection.

Other Dietary Factors

The apparent reduction in colorectal cancer risk from increased vegetable consumption may result from the fact that they are the major sources of NSPs in Western diets, or that they contain micronutrients and pharmacologically active substances for which a general protective role in cancer has been described. A number of intervention trials with β-carotene are presently in progress, although first reports indicate from an Australian study that the incidence of adenomas was actually increased in those subjects receiving β-carotene. In a small trial of colectomized patients with the rare condition, familial adenomatous polyposis, intervention with fibre (as bran) rather than megadoses of vitamins C and E was more effective in reducing recurrence of polyps in the remaining rectal stump. *See* Carotenoids, Physiology

Calcium has been implicated in protection against cancer of the large bowel, following the suggestion that its presence in the large bowel would counteract the irritating effects of free fatty acids or bile acids arising from a high-fat diet. Supplements of calcium carbonate have been shown to reduce cell proliferation in the large bowel in both animals and humans at high risk of colon cancer, although calcium has been viewed in general as an enhancer rather than an inhibitor in various test systems of chemical carcinogens. *See* Calcium, Physiology

Calcium intakes tend to be elevated in areas at high risk of colon cancer, such as the UK and New Zealand, although in some prospective studies and a number of case control studies within populations, the majority suggest that calcium may be protective. The results of further prospective studies are awaited.

Related to the effect of calcium, epidemiological evidence suggests that sunlight exposure and dietary vitamin D may also reduce risk of colorectal cancer. Vitamin D is classically associated with calcium homeostasis, but a more fundamental role in controlling cell growth and differentiation has recently emerged. Nearly all tissues so far examined have been found to have vitamin D receptors, as do most malignant tissues, including breast, colon, cervix and pancreas. Some, but not all, animal studies suggest that the active form of vitamin D (1,25-dihydroxycholecalciferol) may inhibit tumour growth, and there has been one report of an antitumour effect in lymphoma. *See* Cholecalciferol, Physiology

Iron is one of several minerals thought to protect against cancer, particularly at levels sufficient to prevent deficiency, but free iron in the colonic lumen has been suggested to initiate oxygen-centred free radicals which would play a role in carcinogenesis. One study has shown that chemically induced tumour incidence is increased in animals fed high levels of iron, and that this effect is lessened by the addition of phytic acid, known to chelate iron. However, any effect of oxygen-derived free radicals is difficult to reconcile with the highly anaerobic conditions within the gut lumen. *See* Iron, Physiology

Dietary Recommendations

There is accumulating evidence that diet is important in preventing colorectal cancer. Definitive assessments of risk must await the findings of large, well-controlled and validated prospective and intervention trials of diet and

Cancer of the Colon

cancer, coupled with specific testing of hypotheses in relation to molecular genetics. Meanwhile, general dietary advice to restrict alcohol, meat and fat consumption, and to increase the amounts of vegetables, starch and NSPs in the diet will not increase risk of large bowel cancer and is of benefit in the prevention of other diseases common in Western societies. *See* Cancer, Diet in Cancer Prevention

Bibliography

Armstrong B and Doll R (1975) Environmental factors and cancer incidence in different countries with special reference to dietary practices. *International Journal of Cancer* 15: 617–631.

Bingham S (1990) Evidence relating dietary fibre (NSP) and starch to protection against large bowel cancer. *Proceedings of the Nutrition Society* 49: 153–171.

Coleman M and Wahrendorf J (eds) (1988) Directory of ongoing research in cancer epidemiology. International Agency for Research on Cancer, Scientific Publication No. 93. Lyon, France.

Muir C, Waterhouse J, Mack T, Powell J, Whelan F (eds) (1987) Cancer incidence in five continents, 5. International Agency for Research on Cancer, Scientific Publication No. 88. Lyon, France.

National Research Council (1982) *Diet, Nutrition and Cancer.* Washington, DC: National Academic Press.

Poirier LA, Newberne PM and Pariza MA (eds) (1986) Essential nutrients in carcinogenesis. *Advances in Experimental Medicine and Biology* 206.

US DHHS (1988) *The Surgeon-General's Report on Nutrition and Health.* DHHS Publication No. 88, pp 502–510. Washington, DC: US Department of Health and Human Services.

Willett WC, Stampfer MJ, Colditz GA, Rosner BA and Spetzer FE (1990) Relation of meat, fat and fibre intake to the risk of colon cancer in a prospective study among women. *New England Journal of Medicine* 323: 1664–1672.

S. A. Bingham
MRC Dunn Nutrition Unit, Cambridge, UK

COLORIMETRY

See Spectroscopy

COLOURS

Contents

Properties and Determination of Natural Pigments

Natural colours in foodstuffs may arise in basically three ways. They may be present originally in the plant or animal tissue from which the food is derived (e.g. chlorophyll in green vegetables), they may be generated during processing (e.g. brown Maillard products in fried onions), or they may be added deliberately (e.g. β-carotene in orange squash). This article considers the major pigments in these three groups. *See* Browning, Nonenzymatic; Carotenoids, Properties and Determination; Chlorophyll

Naturally Occurring Pigments

The range of compounds responsible for the natural colours of foodstuffs is surprisingly limited. Plants are the primary sources, yielding anthocyanins, carotenoids and chlorophylls as the major groupings, with limited contributions from compounds such as betanins and curcumin.

Properties and Determination of Natural Pigments

Anthocyanins

The anthocyanins are responsible for most of the red, purple and blue colours in plant foodstuffs. The skins of red apples, plums and grapes are rich in anthocyanins, as are strawberries, rhubarb stalks and red cabbage leaves. Chemically, most anthocyanins are based on the six common benzopyrilium aglycones (anthocyanidins) shown in Fig. 1. These aglycones are not stable, and the 250 or so anthocyanins which are known in nature reflect the fact that the aglycone is stabilized by substitution with different sugars at different positions. Substitution at the 3 position is most widespread, but 5 and 7 substitution is also common. The substituent sugars may be simple (e.g. glucose, galactose) or complex and unusual (e.g. rutinose, sambubiose). The sugars themselves are sometimes acylated with other complex organic acids—grapes, for instance, contain significant quantities of the caffeic and p-coumaric acid conjugates of malvidin 3-glucoside. The polar nature of anthocyanins means that they are soluble only in water or polar organic solvents—they are not associated with lipid in the plant cells and they are not soluble in oils nor in organic solvents such as chloroform or hexane.

The colour chemistry of anthocyanins is complex. The benzopyrilium structure can exist in four major equilibrium forms depending upon pH (Fig. 2). The flavylium salt is the most stable and intensely coloured, predominating at low pH. Hence the well-known obser-

vation that red cabbage pigment is intense and stable when cooked in the presence of acid, but rapidly turns blue and degrades at a pH near or above neutrality. The blue colour is due to the generation of the quinoidal base (which is stable under nitrogen, even at pH 10), which rapidly degrades in the presence of oxygen.

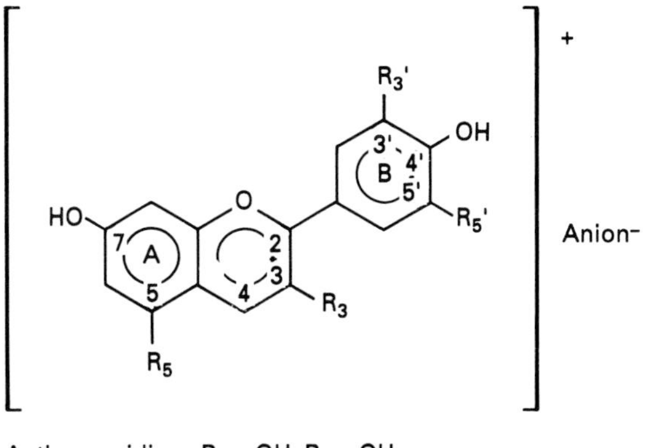

The perceived colour of anthocyanins is also highly dependent on copigmentation effects. In the concentrated environment of intact plant cells, the proximity of pectin, metal ions, organic acids and other polyphenols act to stabilize and to augment anthocyanin colour to a remarkable degree. Hence the skins of red grapes seem intensely dark blue or black but, when the pigment is extracted by ethanol during wine-making, the native anthocyanin is revealed as bright red. The visible absorbance maximum of isolated anthocyanins is somewhat dependent on structure, moving from 506 nm (orange) for pelargonidin derivatives to 534 nm (purple-red) for malvidin, delphinidin and petunidin. A very few anthocyanins are naturally blue, even in the extracted state, due to internal copigmentation with their own sugar acylating groups.

Even at low pH, the anthocyanins are not stable indefinitely, and they tend to polymerize with other polyphenols or reactive carbonyls. After only a few months ageing, therefore, very little monomeric anthocyanin remains in most red wines and the specific E_{520} drops dramatically. The overall visual chromophore is only slightly affected by polymerization, however, giving a colour shift from purple to red. In these circumstances, tristimulus colorimetry is a far more accurate measure of perceived colour than is a spot measurement at 520 nm.

Carotenoids

The carotenoids are a range of lipid-associated pigments widely present in higher plants and algae. They are responsible for many of the orange-yellow colours of fruits and vegetables such as red peppers, tomatoes, carrots and bananas. They are also responsible for the yellow skin ground colour of apples such as 'Golden Delicious'. The structure of carotenoids is more diverse than that of anthocyanins and does not fall into such well-defined groups. The basic unit is a C_{40} hydrocarbon chain (e.g. lycopene), to which additional substituents may be added. In the carotenes, the terminal carbons at each end are cyclized into ring structures. The so-called xanthophyll pigments are carotenoids which contain polar alcoholic or aldehydic end groups derived from oxidative pathways during their biosynthesis. A few carotenoids appear in animal flesh, such as salmon and shrimp, which acquire them via their diet. The dark blue of the live lobster is a carotenoid–protein complex which is destroyed when the animal is boiled and only the pink

Anthocyanidins: R_3 = OH, R_5 = OH

		R_3'	R_5'
Pelargonidin	(Pg)	H	H
Cyanidin	(Cy)	OH	H
Peonidin	(Pn)	OCH$_3$	H
Delphinidin	(Dp)	OH	OH
Petunidin	(Pt)	OCH$_3$	OH
Malvidin	(Mv)	OCH$_3$	OCH$_3$

Anthocyanins: Pg. Cy. Pn. Dp. Pt. Mv with
R_3 = O-sugar or O-acylated sugar
R_5 = OH or O-glucose

Fig. 1 The common anthocyanins and anthocyanidins.

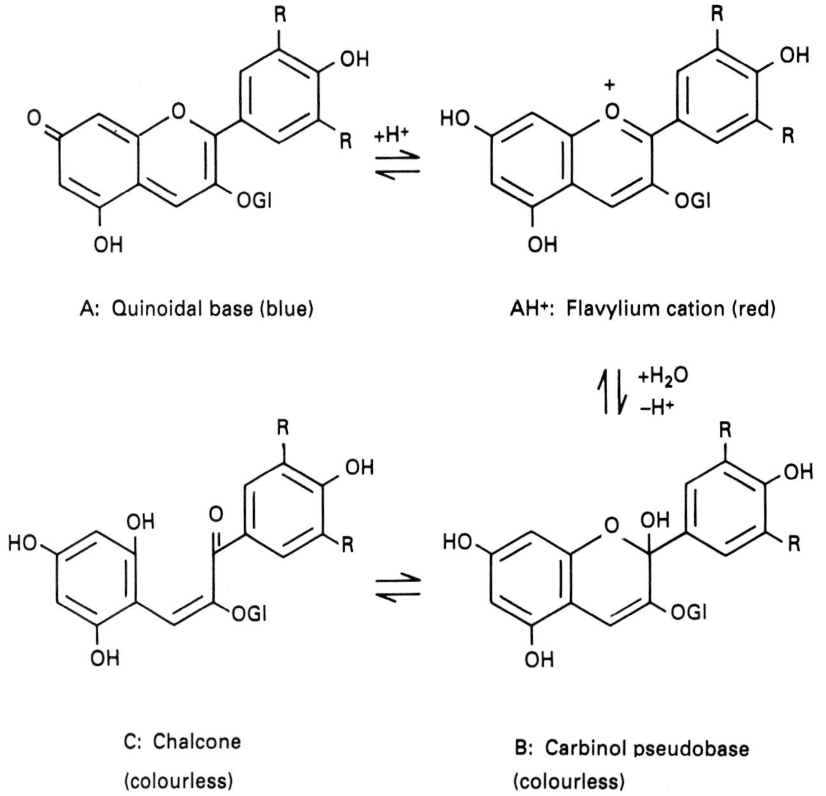

Fig. 2 Equilibrium forms of anthocyanins.

carotenoid then remains. Butter, cheese and egg yolks contain carotenoids which derive ultimately from the vegetable diet of the animals producing them. In animals, many carotenoids act as vitamin A precursors, so have additional value in addition to their properties as pigments. *See* Retinol, Physiology

Although some 500 or so carotenoids are known in nature, very few of them are water-soluble—those that are have achieved a disproportionate importance as food colours as described later. Their general water insolubility means that they tend to be more stable in processed foods than do anthocyanins, since they remain attached to cellular fragments. Thus, the carotenoid pigments of canned tomatoes are more stable than the anthocyanins of canned strawberries. Nevertheless, carotenoids are still prone to degradation once freed from their cellular matrix, and are particularly susceptible to light and oxygen.

Chlorophylls and Haem Pigments

Chlorophylls are amongst the most noticeable of all plant pigments due to their central photosynthetic role. Like carotenoids, they are water-insoluble and are associated with the lipid portion of plant cells in specialized organelles (the chloroplasts). The bright green of native chlorophyll in plants is determined by the presence of a central magnesium atom in a large porphyrin ring. When green leaf vegetables are cooked under normal (slightly acid) conditions, this magnesium is easily lost to form the dull green pheophytins. Although this process can be prevented by the use of alkali during cooking and the green colour thereby retained, this is no longer a common practice since it leads to oxidation and loss of vitamin C. The green colour can also be retained and stabilized if the central magnesium atom is replaced by copper. *See* Chlorophyll

The bright red haem pigments, characteristic of animal blood and therefore of fresh meat, contain similar porphyrin ring structures, but the central atom is iron which shifts the chromophore into the red region. Like chlorophyll, the haem pigments are soon degraded when meat is cooked in the normal way. If preserved in the presence of nitrite, however, as in traditional 'curing', the nitrosohaemoglobin stabilizes the pigment and a red colour is retained. *See* Curing

Other Plant Pigments

Although most orders of higher plants can synthesize anthocyanins to provide red and purple shades, the *Centrospermae* lack this ability and synthesize instead a group of nitrogenous pigments known as the betalains. These occur in both red forms (betanins) and yellow

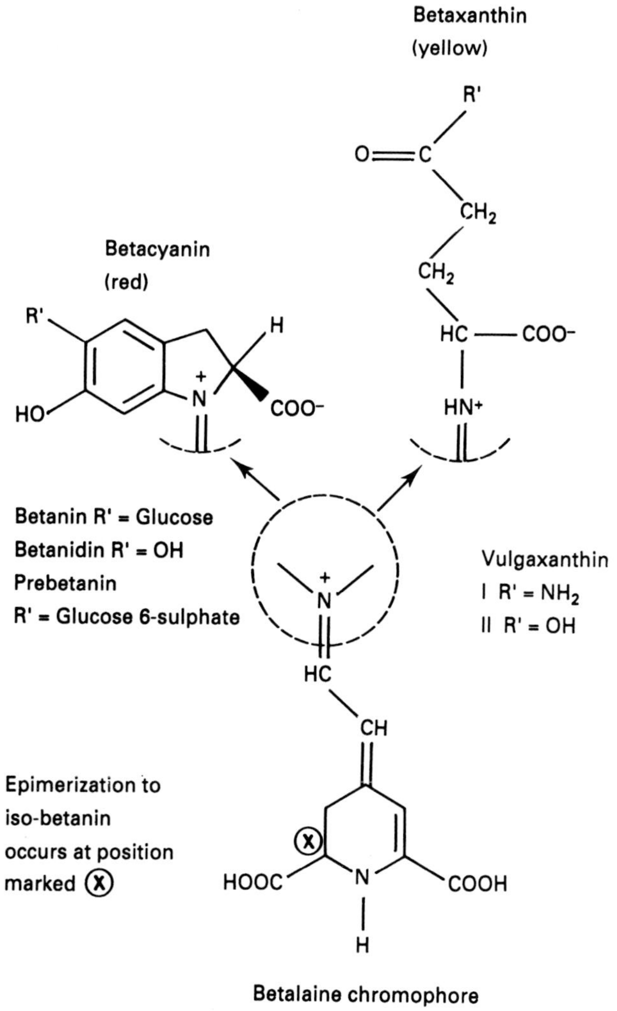

Betaxanthin
(yellow)

Betacyanin
(red)

Betanin R' = Glucose
Betanidin R' = OH
Prebetanin
R' = Glucose 6-sulphate

Vulgaxanthin
I R' = NH₂
II R' = OH

Epimerization to
iso-betanin
occurs at position
marked ⊗

Betalaine chromophore

Fig. 3 The structure of betalains.

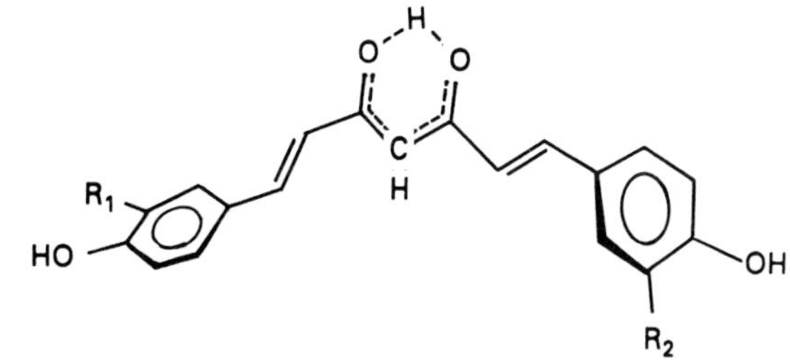

Fig. 4 The structure of curcumin. R=H or OCH₃

structure. They fall into two broad groups—those produced by enzymatic browning (principally from natural phenolics and polyphenoloxidase) and those produced by (nonenzymatic) Maillard reactions between reducing sugars and amino compounds.

Enzymatic Browning

Colours of this sort are generated by the action of polyphenoloxidase or peroxidase enzymes on natural phenolic substrates. The development of colour in a freshly cut apple is a typical example. The principal substrates involved are the catechins or procyanidins, although in older literature the phenolic acids are often mentioned. It is now known that phenolic acids do not themselves brown although they may play a part in coupled oxidation systems which allow the procyanidins to generate the colour. The pigments derived from procyanidins have no specific λ_{max} in the visible region of the spectrum, although those derived from simpler phenolics such as catechins may initially display yellow-orange chromophores about 400 nm before further polymerization occurs.

In some food systems, such as apple juice or white wine, only a limited amount of colour development is desirable before the product becomes unacceptably dark. In these cases, colour formation may be inhibited by antioxidants such as sulphite or by a drop in pH which reduces enzyme activity. In other foods, such as black tea or cocoa, the development of colour during processing is critical to the product and is also associated with flavour development processes. The tea system has been well studied and is known to generate two types of phenolic pigment from catechins. These are the theaflavins, which are bright orange-red, and the thearubigins, which are dull brown. Most oxidized phenolic pigments tend to become browner and duller with time, particularly if further nonspecific oxidation takes place. *See* Antioxidants, Synthetic Antioxidants

forms (vulgaxanthins) (Fig. 3). The betalains are water-soluble and are generally stable at moderately acid pH, although heat, light and oxygen will hasten their decomposition. Although of restricted natural distribution, the importance of betalains, particularly the red betanins, is enhanced by their presence in a number of important food crops such as amaranth, chard and beetroot.

The yellow tubers of turmeric (*Curcuma longa*) are well known as both a spice and a colouring material for food when dried and ground into a powder. The pigment, known as curcumin, has the extended conjugated structure shown in Fig. 4. This is subject to keto/enol equilibrium and the pigment converts to an unstable orange form above pH 7.

Pigments Generated During Processing

Pigments generated during processing or cooking are amongst the least well defined in terms of chemical

Nonenzymatic (Maillard) Browning

This form of colour development is usually associated with heat and is a type of caramelization, in which the

Properties and Determination of Natural Pigments

temperature for degradation of a reducing sugar is lowered by the presence of catalytic amino groups. The sugar degrades to give aldehydic functions which polymerize to give visible chromophores, intensifying after further complex formation with amino groups. Typical desirable examples include the browning of fried onions, the roasting of meat or the manufacture of toffee confectionery.

Almost inevitably, Maillard browning is associated with flavour development. The pigments generated are even less well defined than those from the phenolic browning reaction. Although temperatures above 80°C will generate Maillard pigments rapidly in suitable systems, the reactions will also proceed slowly at room temperature if the water activity is low enough. Thus, apple juice concentrate held at 20°C for several weeks shows discernible colour development from Maillard reactions between fructose and amino acids (in addition to any enzymatic browning which may have taken place earlier). Similarly, tinned condensed milk or dried milk powder develops colour in storage due to reaction between lactose and the lysine ε-amino groups in milk protein. Such slow Maillard reactions are generally considered undesirable, in contrast to the fast reactions under control during cooking.

Natural Pigments Deliberately Added to Foodstuffs

Most of the natural pigments added to food are derived from one of the categories described above. A list of those permitted in the European Economic Community is given in Table 1.

Blues and Reds

Most anthocyanin extracts are derived from grape skins as a by-product of wine or grape juice manufacture. Some extracts are also available from blackcurrant, elderberry or red cabbage. A particularly interesting extract is that from hibiscus, which contains a highly copigmented anthocyanin of much bluer shade than most anthocyanins. The extracts are generally made using acidified water or alcohol, sometimes in the presence of sulphite as an antioxidant (which must be later removed). The extracts are then concentrated to a liquid or dried to a powder. None of the extracts are pure compounds but consist of a variety of anthocyanin structures complete with polymeric degradation products.

Anthocyanin extracts are well suited to aqueous systems but they cannot be used with fatty foods, nor with those of pH much greater than 4. They are susceptible to copigmentation and complexation

Table 1. Natural colours and pigments covered by European Economic Community regulations

Colour	E number
Reds	
Alkannet	
Carmine (cochineal)	E120
Orchil	E121
Red to yellow shades	
Carotenoids	E160
Annatto	E160(b)
β-Carotene	E160(a)
β-Apo-8′-carotenal	E160(e)
Ethyl ester of β-apo-8′-carotenoic acid	E160(f)
Canthaxanthin	E161(g)
Xanthophylls, other	E161
Red to purple shades	
Anthocyanins	E163
Beetroot Red	E162
Yellows	
Curcumin	E100
Lactoflavin (riboflavin)	E101
Riboflavin-5′-phosphate	
Greens	
Chlorophyll	E140
Cu–Chlorophyll	E141
Brown	
Caramel	E150
Blacks	
Carbon black, vegetable	E153
Inorganic colourings	
Calcium carbonate	E170
Iron oxides and hydroxides	E172
Titanium dioxide	E171
Gold	E175
Silver	E174
Aluminium	E173

Source: Lea AGH (1988).

effects – for instance the presence of tin, iron or aluminium (as in canned fruits) can cause noticeable blueing. They are reversibly bleached by sulphite, but tend to be irreversibly degraded by ascorbic acid. Other phenolic compounds such as procyanidin 'tannins' will tend to cause coprecipitation or haze formation. The crude extracts may also react with food proteins such as

Properties and Determination of Natural Pigments

gelatin. Anthocyanins have found considerable application in providing a natural colouring for soft drinks, where they are stable at low pH and moderately resistant to pasteurization temperatures.

Betanin extracts are prepared from beetroot juice, which is fermented to remove the sugar and then dried to a powder. Although generally stable between pH 3 and 7, they are affected by heat, light, oxygen and sulphite. However, they have found considerable application in dairy products such as ice cream, yoghurt and 'instant desserts', where heat is not involved and anthocyanins would be badly affected by the high pH.

The traditional red colour cochineal is derived from the dried bodies of a South American insect (*Coccus cacti*) and consists of a polyhydroxy anthroquinone pigment known as carminic acid. Its aluminium lake is known as carmine, and is water-soluble at pH 3 or above. It is also very stable to heat, light and oxygen. Its principal applications are in soft drinks, sugar confectionery and dairy products.

Orange and Yellow

The carotenoids are generally oil-soluble and therefore well suited for colouring fatty foods such as margarine and cheese. Organic solvent extracts used for this purpose include capsanthin obtained from paprika, lutein from *Tagetes erecta* (Aztec marigold), β-carotene from carrots, and lycopene from tomato. A commonly used extract is annatto, which is obtained from the seeds of a Mediterranean shrub, *Bixa orellana*. This consists mainly of bixin, the fat-soluble methyl ester of a carotenoid carboxylic acid known as norbixin. The free acid itself is water-soluble and thus available for colouring aqueous foods, although it may precipitate out at low pH, and tends to complex with divalent metals at high pH. Annatto can be rendered completely water-soluble by alkaline hydrolysis to yield the salts.

Another traditional water-soluble carotenoid is crocin, an ester of the dicarboxylic acid crocetin, which is the pigment from saffron (the stigmas of *Crocus sativus*). This pigment is also extracted from the seeds of certain oriental *Gardenia* spp. Both annatto and crocin are subject to colour shifts which occur through interaction with food proteins. Crocin is also susceptible to sulphite bleaching and to interaction with heavy metals.

Synthetic but 'nature-identical' carotenoids are also available as food colourants, principally β-carotene, β-apocarotenal and canthaxanthin. These are generally used in oil-based systems but may also be made water-dispersible by physical means (emulsification and encapsulation) and thus are used for colouring cloudy soft drinks. Canthaxanthin is also incorporated into the diet of farmed salmon to replace the carotenoids which wild fish would naturally consume, thereby ensuring a pink flesh. Synthetic carotenoids have also been used in battery chicken feed to ensure that egg yolks give sufficient colour, since the birds have no access to natural carotenoids from greenstuffs.

Curcumin, a deodorized turmeric extract, also provides a useful yellow pigment, although its application is limited by its sensitivity to light and its pH dependency. It has found considerable application, together with annatto, in providing the yellow shade required for vanilla ice cream, as well as in sugar confectionery, soups and sauces.

Greens

Chlorophyll extracts are prepared using organic solvents from sources such as grass and lucerne leaves. The green extracts may be used to colour fatty foods directly, but are more usually converted into their copper complexes to give a brighter green, followed by preparation of water-soluble sodium or potassium salts. In this form they are used to colour sugar confectionery, frozen desserts and dairy products.

Browns and Blacks

These colours are principally obtained by the use of synthetic caramels and carbon blacks. Four types of synthetic caramel are recognized, which differ in their solubilities and isoelectric points. This affects their stability towards such factors as protein binding (in beers) and alcohol solubility (in spirits). The appropriate caramel must therefore be chosen for the product in hand. Synthetic caramels are used at high levels to colour cola beverages. Recently, 'natural' caramels based on malt extracts have also become available. All these colours are based on Maillard browning reactions. Brown pigments based on enzymatic oxidation have not generally been used for addition to food systems, principally on account of their low tinctorial power and instability to further oxidation. *See* Caramel, Properties and Analysis

Analysis of Natural Colours

Analysis of natural colours as individual pigments is really only possible using chromatographic techniques, although the use of tristimulus colorimetry is valuable in defining and maintaining the exact visual specification of a colour in a foodstuff. Extraction of pigments requires specific techniques, e.g. acidified alcohol/water mixtures for anthocyanins, ethyl acetate or dichloromethane for carotenoids. Most analyses are nowadays carried out by high-performance liquid chromato-

Properties and Determination of Natural Pigments

graphy (HPLC) on reverse-phase columns. For anthocyanins, water/alcohol gradients at pH 1·5 are suitable. For carotenoids and chlorophylls, mixtures of dichloromethane, acetonitrile and tetrahydrofuran are often used. Detection must be in the visible spectrum—diode array detectors can be helpful in confirming peak identity. Isolation of standards is often a major difficulty since few are commercially available. Foods which have been subject to processing or maturation, or to which crude pigment mixtures have been added, are not necessarily amenable to HPLC analysis, due to degradation and polymerization of monomeric pigments. Caramels and phenolic oxidation products cannot be analysed as single chemical entities due to their heterogeneous nature, although the presence of by-products such as hydroxymethylfurfural may be useful in indirect assessment of caramel addition. *See* Chromatography, High-performance Liquid Chromatography

Bibliography

Blake CJ (1982) *Determination of Natural Colours in Foods. Scientific and Technical Survey*, No. 130. Leatherhead: Leatherhead Food Research Association.

Coulson J (1980) Naturally occurring colouring matters for foods. In: Walford J (ed.) *Developments in Food Colours*, vol. 1, pp 189–218. London: Elsevier.

Knewstubb CJ and Henry BS (1988) *Natural Colours—a Challenge and an Opportunity*, pp 179–186. London: Institute of Food Science and Technology.

Lea AGH (1988) HPLC of natural pigments in foodstuffs. In: Macrae R (ed.) *HPLC in Food Analysis*, 2nd edn, pp 277–333. London: Academic Press.

Markakis P (1982) *Anthocyanins as Food Colours*. London: Academic Press.

Taylor AJ (1984) Natural colours in food. In: Walford J (ed.) *Developments in Food Colours*, vol. 2, pp 159–206. London: Elsevier.

Timberlake CF and Henry BS (1986) Plant pigments as natural food colours. *Endeavour* 10: 31–36.

A. Lea
Reading Scientific Services Ltd, Reading, UK

Properties and Determination of Synthetic Pigments

This article reviews the use of synthetic colouring materials in foodstuffs, their structural classification, chemical stability, interactions with other food additives, usage in foods, and qualitative and quantitative analysis.

Classification

Food colours classification can be simplified by grouping into the following chemical classes:

- Azo (monoazo, disazo and trisazo);
- Azo-pyrazolone;
- Triarylmethane;
- Xanthene;
- Quinoline;
- Indigoid.

Table 1 lists the food colours currently permitted in the UK, EEC and USA and gives their structural classes.

Azo Food Colours

Azo dyes contain one or more chromophoric azo groups which are usually associated with aromatic systems containing salt-forming substituents generally in the *meta* or *para* position to the azo group. Azo dyes span a wide range of colours, one example is sunset yellow FCF (Fig. 1(a)).

Azopyrazolone Colours

Azo dyes which also contain a pyrazolone group exist essentially as ketohydrazine tautomeric systems. A well-known example of an azopyrazolone dye is tartrazine (Fig. 1(b)).

Triarylmethane Food Colours

Triarylmethane colours are characterized by the presence of a chromophoric system containing a central carbon atom attached to three aromatic moieties with amino, substituted amino and hydroxyl groups in the *para* position, which act as auxochromes. One example of a triarylmethane food dye is green S (Fig. 1(c)).

Xanthene Food Colours

Xanthene dyes are characterized by a chromophoric system comprising essentially of a dibenzo-1,4-pyran heterocyclic ring system with amino or hydroxyl groups in the *meta* position with respect to the oxygen bridge. Erythrosine is the only example of a xanthene dye currently permitted for food use in the UK and USA (Fig. 1(d)).

Quinoline Food Colours

Quinoline yellow (Fig. 1(e)) is the only example of a quinoline dye currently permitted for food use in the EEC. The chromophoric system is based on the 2-(2-quinolyl)-1,3-indandione (or quinophthalone) heterocyclic ring system.

Indigoid Food Colours

The only example of an indigoid dye currently permitted for food use in the UK and USA is indigo carmine (Fig. 1(f)), a blue-violet sulphonated analogue of indigo, a naturally occurring dye which exists as a resonance equilibrium between two hybrid structures.

Pigments and Lakes

Pigments are dyestuffs which are generally insoluble in aqueous and organic solvents and have to be dispersed into foodstuffs to effect coloration. Precipitation of water-soluble dyes onto an inert substrate such as alumina forms water-insoluble pigments known as lakes (see eqn [1]).

$$3(\text{Dyestuff-SO}_3^-) + Al^{3+} \xrightarrow[\text{onto } Al_2O_3 \cdot 3H_2O]{\text{Precipitated and extended}} (\text{Dyestuff-SO}_3^-)_3 Al^{3+} \tag{1}$$

Chemistry and Stability

All of the synthetic colouring materials permitted for food use in the EEC and USA (except lithol rubine BK and citrus red, which have restricted use), apart from the lake colours, are soluble in water to a greater or lesser extent and insoluble in oils and fats. The degree of water solubility is determined by the number and relative position of salt-forming groups present in the dye molecule. The most common of these is the sulphonic acid group ($-SO_3H$) and the less common carboxylic acid group ($-CO_2H$), which form water-soluble anionic dyes. Cationic dyes contain basic groups such as amino ($-NH_2$) or substituted amino ($-NH \cdot CH_3$, $-N(CH_3)_2$, etc.)

Most food dyes are soluble in certain nonaqueous hydrophilic solvents such as glycerine, propylene glycol and sorbitol and this allows the preparation of solutions and pastes for use in certain food products. The triarylmethanes and erythrosine are appreciably soluble in the lower alcohols ethanol and 2-propanol. Turbidity or precipitation of colour may be experienced upon interaction with hard water.

Colouring materials exhibit excellent stability when stored under cool, dry and dark conditions. Many factors can and do contribute to colorant stability such as heat, light, pH, redox systems, other food ingredients (especially preservatives) and trace metals.

Photodegradation

Light is capable of inducing photochemical changes in all dyestuffs, eventually leading to total decolourization.

Table 1. Food colours currently permitted in the UK, EEC and USA

Name	E Number[a]	FD & C[b] classification	Colour index No.[c]	Structure type	Colour shade
Tartrazine	E 102	Yellow No. 5	19140	Azopyrazolone	Yellow
Quinolone yellow	E 104	None	47005	Quinoline	Greenish yellow
Yellow 2G	107	None	18965	Azopyrazolone	Yellow
Sunset yellow FCF	E 110	Yellow No. 6	15985	Monoazo	Orange yellow
Carmoisine	E 122	None	14720	Monoazo	Bluish red
Amaranth	E 123	None	16185	Monoazo	Red
Ponceau 4R	E 124	None	16255	Monoazo	Orange red
Erythrosine	E 127	Red No. 3	45430	Xanthene	Bluish pink
Red 2G	128	None	18050	Monoazo	Bluish red
Patent blue V	E 131	None	42051	Triarylmethane	Violet blue
Indigo carmine	E 132	Blue No. 2	73015	Ingidoid	Deep blue
Brilliant blue FCF	E 133	Blue No. 1	42090	Triarylmethane	Greenish blue
Green S	E 142	None	44090	Triarylmethane	Bluish green
Black PN	E 151	None	28440	Disazo	Bluish black
Brown FK	154	None	—	Azo[e]	Orange brown
Brown HT	155	None	20285	Disazo	Dark brown
Lithol rubine BK[d]	E 180	None	15850	Monoazo	Bluish red
Allura red AC	—	Red No. 40	16035	Monoazo	Yellowish red
Citrus red[f]	—	Red No. 2	12156	Monoazo	Scarlet red
Fast green FCF	—	Green No. 3	42053	Triarylmethane	Bluish green

[a] Numbers without 'E' prefix have provisional listing.
[b] As published by the US Food and Drug Administration.
[c] As published by The Colour Index, Society of Colourists and Dyers, UK.
[d] For colouring of cheese rind only.
[e] Mixture of six main components, for colouring kippers.
[f] For colouring of orange skins only.

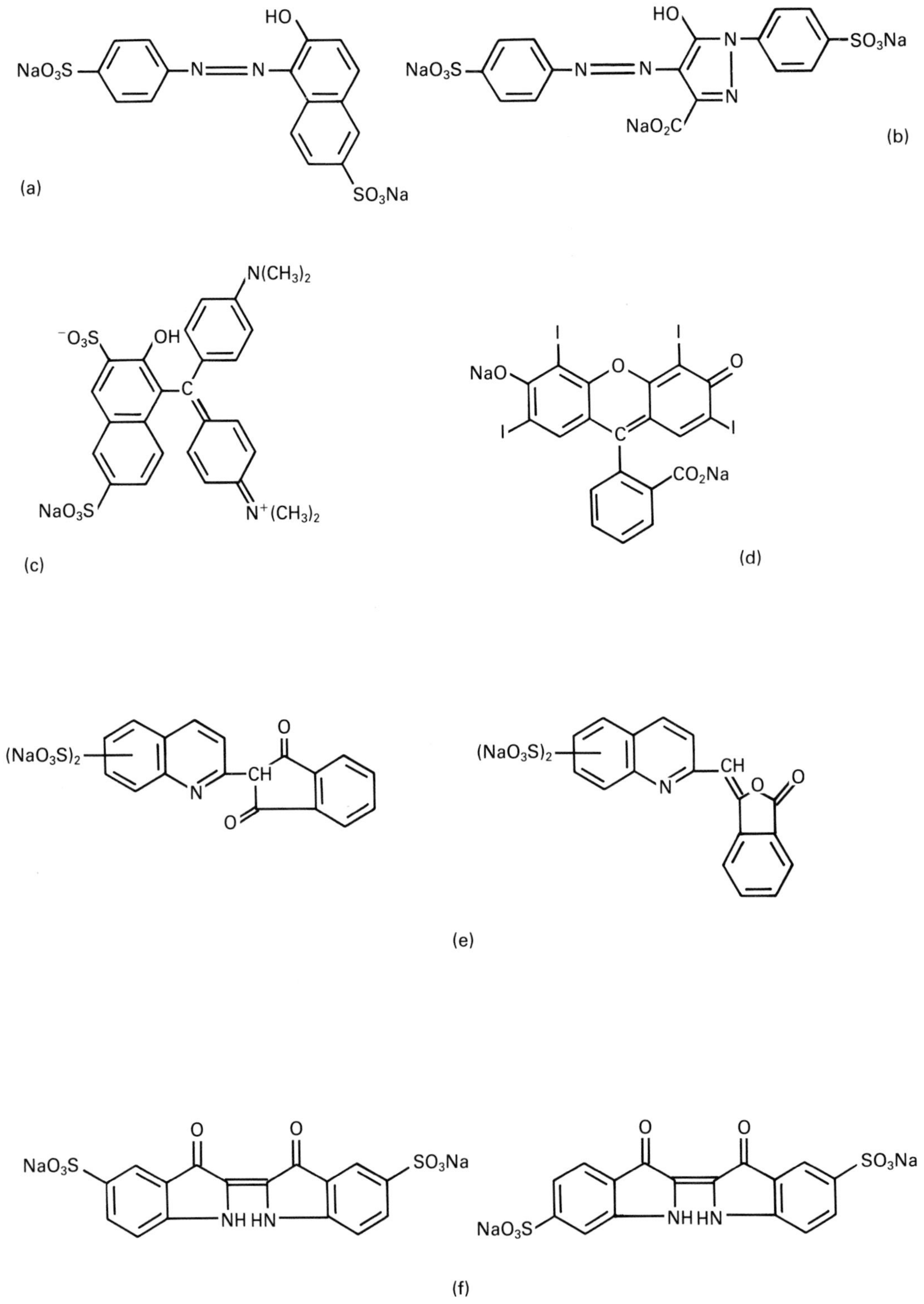

Fig. 1 (a) Chemical structure of the azo dye sunset yellow FCF. (b) Chemical structure of the azopyrazolone dye tartrazine. (c) Chemical structure of the triarylmethane dye green S. (d) Chemical structure of the xanthene dye erythrosine. (e) Chemical structure of the quinoline dye quinoline yellow, showing the two main colouring components. (f) Chemical structure of the indigoid dye indigo carmine, showing the two main colouring components.

Properties and Determination of Synthetic Pigments

Resistance to photochemical degradation is termed 'light fastness'. Heat, other various agents and food ingredients are known to accelerate the photodegradation of dyestuffs, whereas others prove to have a stabilizing effect. True azo dyes can undergo three principal types of photochemical reaction, namely *cis-trans* photoisomerism, photoreduction and photo-oxidation.

Thermal Degradation

Heat can cause losses of colour during food processing and cooking. Colouring materials are added to products at the latter stages of and at the lowest possible temperatures during food processing when further heating is unlikely to take place. For all dyes, processing at very high temperatures will lead to an inevitable loss of colour or change in shade due to carbonization.

Acids, Alkalis and Redox Systems

Not all colours can be used over all pH values and some colouring materials such as erythrosine may precipitate from solution at acid pH whereas others such as indigo carmine will fade rapidly. Colour lakes often exhibit amphoteric properties, with both acids and alkalis tending to solubilize the inorganic substrate, thus releasing the free colorant (i.e. colour 'bleed').

The majority of permitted food colours exhibit instability when used in combination with oxidizing and reducing agents. Since colour depends on the existence of a conjugated unsaturated system within the dye molecule, any substance which modifies this system (e.g. oxidizing or reducing agents such as hydrogen, sugars, acids and salts) will affect the colour.

Metals

All dyes, those with the azo group in particular, will exhibit accelerated fading under both acid and alkaline conditions in the presence of metals, including zinc, tin, aluminium, iron and copper, especially at higher temperatures. This is mostly due to the reducing effect of liberated hydrogen. Dyes will often react with the metal in food cans at a rate proportional to their concentration.

Interaction with Other Food Additives

Preservatives

Canned products containing added colour may degrade in the presence of tartaric and citric acids, which may react with the metal of the container to liberate hydrogen. The stability of nine red colours in comminuted meat products in the absence and presence of nitrite has shown that most of the dyes are destroyed to some extent, but with nitrite more of the colour survives. Subsidiary dye components and colourless fluorescent products are formed as a result of heat processing and, in certain cases, additional products are observed in the presence of nitrite. Nitrite can also cause rapid detinning to produce Sn^{2+}, a strong reducing agent. Sulphur dioxide is known to cause rapid decolorization of dye solutions. The interaction between sulphite and carmoisine results in the formation of a hydrazo compound via hydrolysis. *See* Preservation of Food

Ascorbic Acid

Azo dyes are known to degrade under accelerated conditions in the presence of ascorbic acid at pH 7 but are more resistant to degradation at pH 3. However, ascorbic acid at a concentration of 50 mg l^{-1} can affect all synthetic colouring materials at pH 3 after 3 days of storage at 20°C. *See* Ascorbic Acid, Properties and Determination

Sugars

Reducing sugars such as glucose and fructose can reduce azo dyes in aqueous solution. Amaranth in particular may degrade when incorporated into reducing sugar-containing foods which are baked. The presence of baking soda can promote the degradation of the dye markedly in the presence of glucose. *See* Fructose

Model Food Systems

During accelerated storage in model soft drink systems, tartrazine degrades very little. Amaranth and sunset yellow FCF are also stable to most additives, with the exception of ascorbic acid and sodium metabisulphite. In the latter case the degradation products appear to be higher-sulphonated analogues of the parent dyes. Prolonged storage under these conditions can therefore cause irreversible degradation leading to colourless products. The formation of specific amines from the degradation of amaranth has been used to estimate the amounts of dye added to soft drinks. Red dyes have been shown to degrade both before and after storage in fish paste products. Ponceau 4R may be reduced to a yellow substance by hydrogen sulphide or sulphur compounds liberated during processing and storage of certain foodstuffs, and erythrosine may lose iodine to produce fluorescein when incorporated in canned cherries and stored in unlacquered cans.

Properties and Determination of Synthetic Pigments

Colour Usage in Processed Foods

Certain food processes have been associated with the use of food colouring matter for some time, principally to:

- reinforce colours already present in foods to meet consumer expectations;
- ensure uniformity of colour in batch productions;
- restore the original appearance of certain foods when colour has been, or will be, diminished during processing or storage;
- give colour to otherwise colourless foods such as sweets, instant desserts and ice lollies.

Table 2 gives a brief summary of colour usage in foods in the UK in 1987.

Dye Purity

Most of the dyes used for colouring foods comprise several coloured components as well as the main dye. These are collectively known as 'subsidiary colours'. The manufacture of a dye from its starting materials usually involves a number of synthetic stages and transformations such as reduction, amination, sulphonation, diazotization, condensation and oxidation. The side-reaction products and the precursors of the dyes themselves are collectively known as 'intermediates' and in food dyes these are often sulphonated compounds. Table 3 lists those most commonly found in food colours. Colouring material specifications in general therefore contain criteria for limitations on subsidiary dyes and intermediates as well as certain unsulphonated or free aromatic amines. Separate criteria are prescribed for inorganic impurities such as transition metals, heavy metals and certain salts.

Inorganic Impurities

The most commonly found inorganic impurities in food colours are sodium chloride and sodium sulphate. Small amounts of phosphate, acetate, carbonate and iodide may also be present. The criteria for purity with respect to inorganic matter are somewhat different for lake colours.

Organic Impurities

The most common organic impurities present in synthetic colouring materials are small amounts of reaction intermediates. There may be various unsulphonated aromatic compounds as well as the sulphonated analogues present in the finished colorants owing to impurities in the starting materials. Triarylmethane dyes are prepared by condensation reactions during which an uncoloured leuco base is formed as an intermediate. The leuco base is then oxidized to the fully conjugated coloured dyestuff using oxidizing agents such as lead dioxide, manganese dioxide or dichromate, which might then be present as low-level inorganic contaminants in the finished dye.

Analysis of Synthetic Food Colours

The major components of synthetic water-soluble-food colour formulations are active dye (including subsidiary dyes), inorganic salts and moisture. Other constituents may be permitted diluents or extenders which may be added for standardization purposes or to facilitate the incorporation of the colorant for certain applications.

Dye Content

Azo, triarylmethane and indigoid dyes are readily reducible by tin(II) chloride, which forms the basis of the titrimetric assay method for dye content. Erythrosine (xanthene type) and quinoline yellow (quinophthalone type) are not reducible and have to be assayed by other means. However, erythrosine is the only commonly used food dye which is insoluble in dilute acid and which can consequently be assayed gravimetrically.

Simple spectrophotometric methods are commonly used for the assay of food dyes. Measurement in the ultraviolet/visible range on instruments with scanning and recording facilities is common.

Inorganic Salts

The classical method for the determination of chloride is by the precipitation of chloride as its silver salt. Sulphate may also be determined gravimetrically as the barium salt. Electrometric procedures may be used for specific ion determination. Chloride, sulphate and other ionic species may be determined simultaneously using ion chromatography.

Moisture

Standard procedures for moisture determination are loss on drying, or by nonaqueous titrimetric techniques such as the Karl–Fischer procedure.

Lakes

Alumina is one of the major components of food lakes, but it is rarely determined. Food lakes are generally

Properties and Determination of Synthetic Pigments

soluble in hot dilute ammonia solution, and all alumina lakes, with the exception of erythrosine, dissolve readily in hot dilute hydrochloric acid. The resultant solutions give the identifiable reactions of aluminium with a base and with alizarin. Qualitative identification of the parent dyes and quantitative analysis of the major and minor components of lakes can be carried out using similarly prescribed procedures as for the water-soluble analogues. Certain lake colours such as erythrosine may prove difficult to analyse and may require special procedures for analysis.

Minor Components

Water-insoluble matter is calculated on the basis of 100% dye content and is usually determined by gravimetric procedures. Atomic absorption spectrophotometry has largely superseded the use of wet methods for trace heavy metals, mainly because of the speed with which analyses can be carried out and the high levels of accuracy and precision which can be attained. Other emergent techniques which have been used with limited application because of their high costs are inductively coupled plasma spectroscopy (ICPS), X ray fluorescence (XRF, for mercury) and neutron activation analysis (NAA).

Organic Impurities

Ether-extractable matter content is determined by Soxhlet extraction and is applicable to all dyes except erythrosine.

Primary aromatic amines are usually determined by diazotization and coupling (to N^1-naphthylethylenediamine, NED) of an appropriate extract, followed by spectrophotometric measurement or high-performance liquid chromatography (HPLC). HPLC has superseded classical column chromatographic procedures as the most widely used technique for the separation and quantification of intermediate species. Both gas chromatography (GC) and thin-layer chromatography (TLC) have also been used for the determination of certain intermediate compounds. The leuco base content of triarylmethane dyes is determined by carrying out further oxidation of the parent dyestuff and measuring the subsequent increase in absorbance. *See* Chromatography, Thin-layer Chromatography; Chromatography, High-performance Liquid Chromatography; Chromatography, Gas Chromatography

Analysis of Foodstuffs for Synthetic Colouring Materials

Food colours must first be extracted from the food matrix, purified to remove potentially interfering coex-tractives and concentrated prior to identification and quantification. Some form of sample pretreatment is often required such as defatting of meat products or dilution of sugars and gums in confectionery products before the extraction can proceed.

Leaching

Leaching may be used to remove colorants from the surface of foodstuffs such as sausages, and also from food packaging materials. In the simplest application, the sample is soaked in an appropriate (usually alkaline) solvent which is then filtered or centrifuged to clarify the colorant solution. Further clean-up is performed as necessary. Newer techniques such as supercritical fluid extraction (SFE) may prove to be useful for the extraction of colorants, intermediates and interaction products from foods.

Solvent–Solvent Extraction and Ion Pair Techniques

These are widely used and effective methods of colorant isolation. Simple immiscible solvent pairs may be used where one solvent acts as a carrier for a dye-complexing reagent or soluble ion exchange resin. The higher alcohols, particularly 1- and 2-butanol, are the most useful solvents for this technique. Amberlite LA-2, a liquid anion exchange resin dissolved in butanol (or hexane), has been widely used as a dye extraction medium for foodstuffs.

Quaternary ammonium compounds such as cetylcyclohexyldimethylammonium bromide (biocidan) and cetyltrimethylammonium bromide (cetrimide) have been used for the extraction of synthetic dyes from food. More recently, reagents such as tetra-*n*-alkylammonium halides and cetylpyridinium chloride have also been employed for the rapid extraction of anionic dyes, as hydrophobic ion pair complexes, from food using organic solvents.

Enzymatic Digestion

Pretreatment of a food sample by enzymatic digestion may be used prior to extraction of the colorants in order to release those colorants which may be highly bound or associated with the food matrix. Enzyme–substrate combinations that may be selected include papain (for protein digestion), lipase (lipids), phospholipase (phospholipid), amyloglucosidase (starch), pectinase (pectin) and cellulase (cellulose). Optimization of the pH and temperature conditions are necessary in each case. *See* Enzymes, Use in Analysis

Properties and Determination of Synthetic Pigments

Table 2.   Food colour usage in the UK[a]

Commodity class	Food types	Stability requirements[b]	Additional comments	Main colours used[c]	Typical levels of application (mg kg^{-1} or mg l^{-1})
Soft drinks and other nonalcoholic beverages	Ready to drink, cordials, vending machine concentrates, instant teas	LF, AC, PR, FL	Must not accelerate corrosion of metal containers	TZ, SY, P4R, AM, CA, BB, GS, BHT, QY	10–200 (proportionally higher in concentrates)
Alcoholic beverages	Beers, ciders, fortified wines	—	Limited use	SY, CA, AM, P4R, IC, BPN	Up to 500
Sugar confectionery	Boiled sweets, toffees, caramels, gums, jellies, pastilles, liquorice, chewing gum	TM, SD, FL	Added as late as possible during production	TZ, SY, CA, AM, P4R, ERY, IC	50–300 (some up to 1000)
Dry mixes, edible ices and frozen confectionery	Blancmanges, custards, mousses, coatings, toppings, decorations, ice cream, frozen lollies, ripples, sauces, sorbets, dry mixes, soups	LF, FL, GE	Lakes often used but must not show speckiness in product	TZ, SY, CA, AM, P4R	50–150
Flour confectionery	Biscuits (fillings, coatings, crumb), wafers, cakes, breakfast cereals, home baking ingredients	TM	Raising agents present	TZ, SY, CA, AM, P4R, BHT	50–150 crumb, 50–30 toppings, etc.
Canned fruit, vegetables and soups	Natural, in syrup or brine, pie fillings, purees, fruit for yoghurt, soups	TM, AC	Requires consistent staining of product relative to carrying liquors	SY, CA, AM, P4R, IC, ERY (fruit); TZ, SY, GS, Y2G, (mixtures for vegetables); SY, GS, CA (soups)	10–200
Meat and fish Products	Comminutes, minces, glazes, gravies, fillings, pastries, sausages, sauces, coatings, spreads, patés, pastes, prepared meals	TM, PR	Must show stability in brine (fish) and affinity for protein; sauces, coatings, etc., have other requirements	R2G, ERY (meat) BFK (kippers) TZ (haddock)	Up to 50 in meat products; 200 in fish; may be higher in sauces, coatings, etc.
Milk products	Dairy desserts, mousses, milk shakes, yoghurts, cheese spreads, nondairy creamers	TM, LF	Must have stability to temperatures of pasteurization	TZ, SY, CA, AM, P4R, IC, GS, ERY	20–200

continued

Properties and Determination of Synthetic Pigments

Table 2. *continued*

Commodity class	Food types	Stability requirements[b]	Additional comments	Main colours used[c]	Typical levels of application (mg kg^{-1} or mg l^{-1})
Snack foods	Packet foods, potato crisps, extruded cereals, pizza-type, savoury coatings, hot-instant foods	LF, TM	Products often surface treated	TZ, SY, ERY, GS, BB, IC, P4R	50–300; may be higher in some packet foods
Pickles and relishes	Sauces, ketchups, chutneys, mayonnaises	TM, AC, LF	Dyes often used as mixtures	TZ, GS, Y2G (mayon.); P4R, TZ, SY, (ketchups); SY, AM, Gs, TZ (other mixtures)	50–300; may be higher in mixes (total dye content)
Chocolate confectionery	Solid milk, blended, wafer bars, filled assortments, liqueurs, novelties	TM	Chocolate is not coloured but fillings and coatings are	TZ, SY, CA, AM, ERY, IC	Usually below 200

[a] Based on MAFF (1980) *UK Survey of Colour Usage in Food, Ministry of Agriculture, Fisheries and Food. Food Surveillance Paper* No. 19. London: HMSO.
[b] LF, Light fastness; AC, acids; PR, preservatives; FL, flavourings; SD, sulphur dioxide; GE, gelling agents and emulsifiers; TM, temperature.
[c] TZ, tartarzine; SY, sunset yellow FCF; P4R, ponceau 4R; AM, amaranth; CA, caromoisine; BB, brilliant blue FCF; GS, green S; BHT, brown HT; IC, indigo carmine; BPN, black PN; ERY, erythrosine; Y2G, yellow 2G; R2G, red 2G; BFK, brown FK; QY, quinoline yellow.

Adsorption Techniques

Adsorption techniques have been developed for the isolation of food colorants utilizing a variety of adsorption materials such as wool, powdered leather, cellulose and alumina. More recently, polyamide powder and semimicro adsorption cartridges containing reversed-phase bonded silica materials have found widespread use. Adsorption is achieved by either adding adsorbent directly to a pH-adjusted sample solution or by passage of the sample solution through a column packed with adsorbent. The adsorbent is freed of other sample matrix components by washing with appropriate solvents and the colorants selectively desorbed using a different solvent.

Qualitative and Quantitative Analysis of Food Extracts

Spectroscopy

Numerous techniques are available for the spectroscopic analysis of colorants; measurements at ultraviolet and visible wavelengths are the easiest to perform. Beer's law can simply be applied to extracts containing single colours, whereas extracts containing two or more colours can be problematic. If the identities of the colouring components are known, their concentrations can be determined providing there is no interaction between them. The distinguishing features of the spectra obtained for single colours may be significantly affected by careful adjustment of the pH of the solution with acid or alkali, characterized by shifts in absorption wavelength maxima and intensities.

Other spectroscopic techniques such as infrared, Raman and nuclear magnetic resonance have been used for the analysis of food colours, but do not lend themselves to routine application. *See* Spectroscopy, Overview; Spectroscopy, Infrared and Raman; Spectroscopy, Nuclear Magnetic Resonance

Mass Spectrometry

Because of their inherent lack of volatility, direct analysis of sulphonated azo (and other) food dyes by mass spectrometry (MS) is very difficult. Several reaction schemes may be used to obtain volatile neutral derivatives to facilitate analysis. Alternative ionization techniques other than electron impact (EI) and chemical ionization (CI) may be used for the analysis of food dyes, but have limited application. The most useful of these are fast-atom bombardment (FAB), field desorp-

Properties and Determination of Synthetic Pigments

Table 3. Intermediate compounds commonly found in synthetic food colours

Intermediate name	Trivial name	Occurrence[a]
Aminobenzene	Aniline	R2G
1-Aminobenzenesulphonic acid	Sulphanilic acid	BPN, SY, TZ, Y2G, BFK
4-Aminonaphthalene-1-sulphonic acid	Naphthionic acid	AM, CA, P4R, BHT
6-Hydroxynaphthalene-2-sulphonic acid	Schaeffers acid	AM, P4R, Sy, AR, GS
3-Hydroxynaphthalene-2,7-disulphonic acid	R-acid	AM, GS, P4R, SY
7-Hydroxynaphthalene-1,3-disulphonic acid	G-acid	AM, P4R
7-Hydroxynaphthalene-1,3,6-trisulphonic acid		AM, P4R
4-Acetamido-5-hydroxynaphthalene-1,7-disulphonic acid	Acetyl K-acid	BPN
8-Aminonaphthalene-2-sulphonic acid	1,7 Cleves acid	BPN
4-Amino-5-hydroxynaphthalene-1,7-disulphonic acid	K-acid	BPN
4-Hydroxynaphthalene-1-sulphonic acid	N & W acid	CA
5-Amino-4-hydroxynaphthalene-2,7-disulphonic acid	H-acid	R2G
5-Acetamido-4-hydroxynaphthalene-2,7-disulphonic acid	Acetyl H-acid	R2G
4,4′-Diazoaminodi(benzenesulphonic acid)	Triazene	SY, TZ, Y2G
6,6′-Oxydi(naphthalene-2-sulphonic acid)	DONS	SY
Tetrahydrosuccinic acid	Dioxytartaric acid	TZ
4-Hydrazinobenzenesulphonic acid		TZ
5-Oxo-1-(4-sulphophenyl)-2-pyrazoline-3-carboxylic acid	SPCZ	TZ
2,5-dichloro-4-(3-methyl-5-oxo-2-pyrazolin-1-yl)benzenesulphonic acid	CSPMZ	Y2G
Fluorescein		ERY
2,4,6-Tri-iodoresorcinol		ERY
2-(2,4-dihydroxy-3,5-di-iodobenzoyl)benzoic acid		ERY
1-H-Indole-2,3-dione (and analagous sulphonic acids)	Isatin	IC
5-Sulphoanthranilic acid		IC
1-H-Indole-2,3-dioxo-1-H-indole-5-sulphonic acid	Monosulphonated Indigo	IC
2-, 3- and 4-Formylbenzenesulphonic acids		BB
N-Ethyl-N-(3-sulphobenzyl)sulphanilic acid	ESBSA	BB
m-Phenylenediamine		BFK
4-Methyl-m-phenylenediamine		BFK
4,4′-Bis(dimethylamino)benzhydrol alcohol		GS
4,4′-Bis(dimethylamino)benzophenone		GS
N,N′-Diethylaniline		PBV
m-Hydroxybenzaldehyde		PBV
2,4-Dihydroxybenzylalcohol		BHT
5-Amino-4-methoxy-2-toluenesulphonic acid		AR
p-Hydroxybenzaldehyde-o-sulphonic acid		FG
o-(N-ethylanilino)-m-toluenesulphonic acid		FG

[a] BPN, black PN; SY, sunset yellow FCF; TZ, tartrazine; Y2G, yellow 2G; BFK, brown FK; AM, amaranth; CA, carmoisine; P4R, ponceau 4R; BHT, brown HT; R2G, red 2G; ERY, erythrosine; IC, indigo carmine; BB, brilliant blue FCF; GS, Green S; PVB, patent blue V; AR, allura red AC; FG, fast green FCF.

tion (FD) and secondary-ion MS (SIMS). The potentially very powerful techniques such as liquid chromatography–mass spectroscopy (thermospray LCMS) have as yet found limited use in the analysis of food dyes. *See* Mass Spectrometry, Principles and Instrumentation

Polarography

Differential pulsed polarography and differential pulse adsorptive stripping voltammetry may be used to estimate dye concentrations in food matrices. The addition of gelatin has been found to be advantageous in the partial identification and determination of food colours due to its pronounced affects on measured peak currents.

Electrophoresis

Of the various electrophoretic techniques available, paper electrophoresis has been the most widely used for the analysis of food colours, utilizing a range of different buffer systems and applied potentials. Cellulose acetate and polyacrylamide gel have been used for the electrophoretic separation of azo and triarylmethane dyes.

Capillary zone electrophoresis (CZE) is an emergent technique which may prove to be applicable to the analysis of food dyes. *See* Electrophoresis

Gas Chromatography

GC cannot be used for the direct analysis of food dyes owing to their inherent lack of volatility. It is, however, a useful technique for the analysis of volatile derivatives and certain intermediate compounds.

Paper Chromatography

Paper chromatography (PC) techniques have been widely used in the past for the identification of food colours, but have nowadays been largely superseded by TLC, column chromatography and HPLC techniques. PC maintains popularity in some laboratories because of its relatively low cost and ease of use, and many suitable solvent systems are available.

Thin-layer Chromatography

The use of TLC systems for the separation of food dyes is fairly widespread, but is gradually being superseded by HPLC. Silica gel is the most commonly reported adsorbent used, though alumina, microcrystalline cellulose and high-performance reversed-phase bonded silicas have widespread use.

High-performance Liquid Chromatography

HPLC has become the major analytical technique for the determination of synthetic colouring materials in foodstuffs. The most widely used separation modes are ion exchange and reversed phase. Spectrophotometric detection is applied in the visible wavelength range for dyes and subsidary colours or in the ultraviolet range for intermediates and other organic impurities.

Ion Exchange (IE) HPLC

Dyes, subsidiary colours, intermediates and impurities have all been characterized using IE, mostly on strong anion exchange (SAX) columns using buffered mobile phases such as borate and perchlorate mixtures with gradient elution. Azo dyes and sulphonated intermediates can be separated using weak anion exchange (WAX) columns with a citric acid mobile phase at pH 2·8. Because of poor reproducibility (notably with the use of gradient elution), the requirement for aggressive buffer systems and its consequently relatively short column life, IE has been largely superseded by reversed-

phase HPLC for the analysis of synthetic water-soluble dyestuffs.

Reversed-phase (RP) HPLC

Synthetic dyes require buffered eluents to achieve desired separations on RP HPLC, usually with the organic mobile phase modifiers methanol or acetonitrile. The column materials used are short-chain (C_2), octyl (C_8) and octadecyl (C_{18}) alkyl-bonded silicas, though other bonded phases such as amino (NH_2) and cyano (CN) have also been employed. There has been considerable interest shown in the use of macroporous and highly cross-linked polystyrene–divinylbenzene (PSDVB) copolymer column packing materials. The mobile phase may alter the affinity of ionic species for the stationary phase by both ion suppression and ion pairing mechanisms.

RP HPLC with ion suppression has been used to separate and identify various dyes, eluting with phosphate buffers at various pH values and methanol. Ammonium acetate has recently been successfully used in this mode of RP HPLC.

Ion pair (IP) HPLC is perhaps the most widely used chromatographic technique for the analysis of dyes, subsidiary colours and uncombined intermediates in foodstuffs. Many published methods are available. Most favoured are ion pair reagents derived from quaternary ammonium compounds such as cetyltrimethylammonium bromide (cetrimide) and tetrabutylammonium phosphate.

Both isocratic and gradient systems can be employed to separate dye mixtures, the latter often being preferred for the separation of complex mixtures.

Modern high-performance and computer-aided instrumentation permits the use of many powerful techniques which may be readily applied to aid in the analysis of dyestuffs. These include:

- automated sample handling and processing;
- automated chromatographic methods development;
- High-sensitivity multiple wavelength and rapid-scanning (diode-array) detectors;
- post-run qualitative and quantitative analysis;
- LCMS interfacing.

Figure 2 shows a typical chromatogram of the separation of red food colours by gradient ion-pair HPLC. It is possible to separate many of the UK permitted and several nonpermitted dyes on a single column system by employing a combination of ionpair gradient elution and selective wavelength detection.

Diode Array Detection

Diode array detectors (DADs) have the ability to record the entire spectral range of an eluting dye component

Properties and Determination of Synthetic Pigments

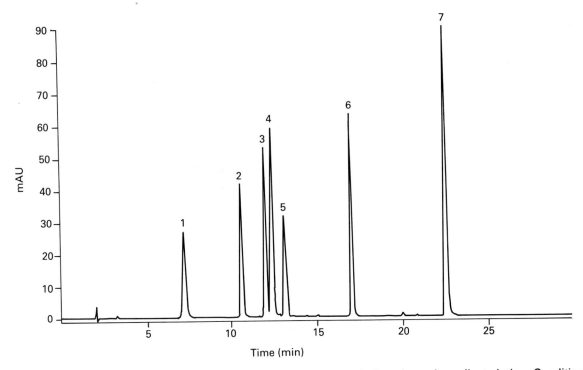

Fig. 2 HPLC chromatogram of a red dye mixture separated by reversed-phase ion pair gradient elution. Conditions: solvent A=0·005 M TBAB in methanol, solvent B=0·005 M TBAB in 0·01 M KH₂PO₄; gradient elution profile 50:50 to 100:0 (A:B) over 30 min linear, 10 min hold; solvent flow rate 0·4 ml min⁻¹; column ODS 20 cm; detection wavelength 520 nm. Peak identification: (1) amaranth (2) allura red AC; (3) red 10B – nonpermitted analogue of (4) red 2G; (5) ponceau 4R; (6) carmoisine; (7) erythrosine. (TBAB, tetrabutylammonium bromide).

during an analysis. Absorbance data may be collected simultaneously from 190 nm to as high as 800 nm and is achieved in real time. The DAD allows the precise determination of absorption maxima of adequately separated solutes and facilitates positive peak identification and peak purity analysis by rapid spectral scanning. Chromatographic peaks may be identified by reference to spectral libraries of previously run reference compounds. Multiple-wavelength monitoring with absorbance ratioing may be used to characterize and identity multicomponent dye mixtures in single chromatographic runs.

Bibliography

Damant A, Reynolds S and Macrae R (1989) The structural identification of a secondary dye produced from the reaction between sunset yellow and sodium metabisulphite. *Food Additives and Contaminants* (3): 273–282.

Dickinson D and Raven TW (1962) *Journal of the Science of Food and Agriculture* 13: 650.

King RD (ed.) (1980) The Determination of Food Colours. In: *Developments in Food Analysis Techniques*, vol. 2, Barking: Applied Science.

Knowles ME, Gilbert J and McWeeny DJ (1974) Stability of red food colours in the presence of nitrite in canned pork luncheon meat. *Journal of the Science of Food and Agriculture* 25: 1239–1248.

Marovatsanga L and Macrae R (1987) The determination of added azo dye in soft drinks via its reduction products. *Food Chemistry* 24: 83–98.

Marmion DM (1984) *Handbook of U.S Colorants for Foods, Drugs, and Cosmetics*, 2nd edn. New York: Wiley.

Reynolds SL, Scotter MJ and Wood R (1988) Determination of synthetic colouring matter in foodstuffs – collaborative trial. *Journal of the Association of Public Analysts* 26: 7–25.

Trace Materials (Colours) Committee (1963) The extraction and identification of permitted food colouring matters with special reference to the changes undergone during processing and subsequent storage. *Analyst* 88: 864.

Venkataraman K (ed.) (1977) *The Analytical Chemistry of Synthetic Dyes*. New York: Wiley.

Walford J (ed.) (1980) *Developments in Food Colours*, vol. 1. Barking: Applied Science.

Walford J (ed.) (1984) *Developments in Food Colours*, vol. 2. Barking: Elsevier Applied Science.

Michael J. Scotter
Ministry of Agriculture, Fisheries and Food, Norwich, UK

COMMINUTION OF FOODS

Determination

The essential requirement for today's high-speed processing factories is the size reduction machine, which not only offers regular sizes of cut, but also operates at large capacities. Development of any machine will need considerable scientific investigation to meet all the required parameters. Past experiences, along with current state of art, relative to the range of materials available, will provide a considerable wealth of knowledge to be evaluated.

Without modern food cutting equipment it would be impossible to produce the uniform and regular sizes essential to the attainment of ideal processing conditions. Production of accurate weight and fill requirements can only be secured where this size control can be achieved.

Techniques are constantly being developed, and now offer many different shapes and sizes. This not only provides products with far greater eye appeal, but also enhances consumer enjoyment.

Extensive consideration must be given to the condition of the product being processed. This is particularly important where food crops or vegetables are being processed. Raw materials can vary greatly, not only throughout the growing season but also because of harvesting from many different areas. Badly stored or overripe items will usually offer very poor finished cuts as well as being very difficult to handle.

The processing temperature of the product along with its heat sensitivity will certainly influence the method of cutting, also the result that can be finally achieved. Choice of machine may be governed not only by the material being processed, but also the size reduction step required. It is not uncommon to have at least one intermediate reduction stage, where initial size, relative to finished requirement, is a relatively large step.

Historical

The initial development was from slicing or cutting by hand, with a knife, to a set of equally spaced, straight knives, mounted in a rigid frame. Product was pushed through these knives, using a ram unit with a suitably profiled face. This system required a great deal of pressure to push product through a large number of knives. The effect was heightened by the product being squeezed through adjacent knives.

Development of this idea resulted in the production of a grid of knives, achieved by placing two frames of straight knives at right angles to each other. Product slices were then pushed through this grid by a similar ram. The great force developed as each dice compressed in two different directions, resulted in serious crushing and cell damage. With fragile products, considerable breakage could occur. This process was also very slow, as the ram had to be returned to its starting point every time, to enable further product to be loaded. An updated method of this dicing unit is still manufactured; it uses the slicing knife directly after the grid to control the length of pieces being cut. The majority of these applications are in the meat industry, but the original design constraints still offer the same problems both for application and product finish.

Development

The greatest breakthrough in three-dimensional cutting was made possible by the invention of a high-speed slicing unit, by Joe R Urschel, President of Urschel Laboratories Inc., USA. Urschel now holds more than 70 patents for food processing equipment.

This new technique subjected the product to a centrifugal force, by rotation in a cylinder. A suitable open-ended impeller driving the product produces this centrifugal force, which holds the product securely in place as it rotates. With controlled feeding of product, the slices will normally generate from the largest face. The prevention of random product movement permits slice thickness of great regularity to be secured.

Another useful feature of centrifugal placement of the largest product face, relative to the slicing knife, is of particular significance where the longest strips are required from product which is not normally round. Now it was possible to produce slices singly, which moved away from the cutting area at high speed, with great capacity. This permitted the addition of linked cutting units, enabling production of three dimensional cuts in many size permutations.

Today most foods are diced in one machine, where slices are first generated, then cut into strips, and finally cut into individual dices.

Immediate exchange and installation of cutting assemblies, without the need for further adjustment, will permit the dicer to be run just for slicing, or strip cutting; many cutting assembly permutations are readily installed or removed.

When dicing fruits and vegetables, the individual slices generated are next cut into strips, one at a time, with no compression of the product. These strips can

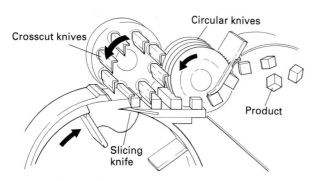

Fig. 1   Model G Dicer.

then be cut into cubes by progressing through a rotating spindle of uniformly spaced circular knives (Fig. 1).

Once the cutting action has started, all three cuts are completed, by moving the product in a straight line. The progressive action of the crosscut spindle knives, as they retain the same operational plane, offers not only square dices, but also a very gentle and clean cut.

Products need to be fed into the centrifugal slicer at a regular rate, to ensure maximum machine capacity. There is no compaction against any machine surface, which is of particular significance where soft or easily bruised products are processed.

The centrifugal action ensures that the product stays securely in place and eliminates any random movement. The uniformity and general quality are greatly improved by this system, and high capacity is attained.

Cutting Assemblies

However well a machine is designed, manufactured and operated, one of the prime considerations will always be the knives used in the cutting assemblies. A critical requirement for knives is similar, well-designed and executed blades, honed to maximum sharpness which is sustainable over considerable periods of operation. It is also essential to have special user equipment, enabling blunt knives to be readily honed very close to the original sharpness. Honing machines must be designed for ease of use by the machine operator.

Even the sharpest knife will cause a small amount of cell rupture in food products; dull or badly designed knives will cause a considerable amount of cell damage, resulting in a reduction in quality and yield.

Clean cutting not only improves product appearance but also enables juices, and thus nutrients, to be retained. For a dehydrator of products this is an essential requirement, but also of considerable importance to any food processor.

Very careful selection of steel alloys, along with specific and closely controlled heat treatment, is essential to ensure maximum knife performance. Great care must also be taken with heat treatment to ensure that, under normal operating conditions, no breakage or

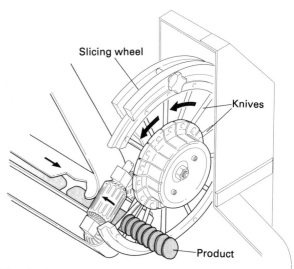

Fig. 2   Model OV Slicer.

fragmentation of the knife takes place. Damage caused by small, hard, foreign materials striking the cutting knife edge should only normally result in turning over of the cutting edge.

To enable harder or tougher abrasive materials to be cut, it is often possible to use special steel alloys and hardening techniques.

Slicing Machines

Many dicing machines will provide slices, strip cuts and dices, depending on the cutting assemblies used and the type of product being processed. Where unusually shaped products or difficult, possibly fibrous materials require to be sliced, a specific choice of machine may be required.

For an elongated product, such as carrot or celery, requiring slices to be made transversely, and at high capacity, there is an obvious choice, shown in Fig. 2. Regularly fed product, entering the machine feed hopper, drops onto two high-speed conveyor belts, arranged to form a 'V' trough cross-section. A third, nonpowered but moving belt, above the 'V' conveyor, completes the product enclosure, ensuring positive feed to the slicing wheel. Knives that are under several thousand N m tension serve as spokes and support the rim of the slicing wheel. The knife mountings are angled, to make a uniform pitch from the hub to the rim. Both the pitch and number of knives determine the thickness of the slice and maintain the feeding speed of the product whilst being sliced. Knives pass through the product at $29 \, \text{m s}^{-1}$. Using a similar principle, slices are available to produce bias cuts of either 30° to the long axis, or an alternative 45°. Slice thicknesses ranging as low as 0·8 mm and a maximum of 54 mm are available. Several options of plain knives are available, plus further alternatives of two patterns of crinkle knife.

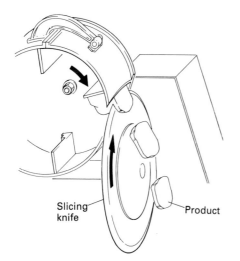

Fig. 3   Model S-A Slicer.

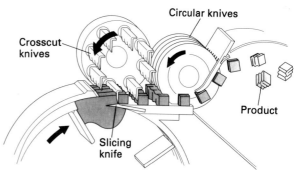

Fig. 5   Model GK Dicer.

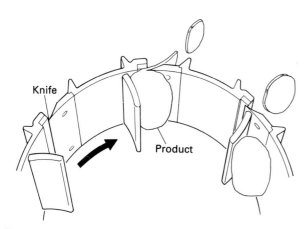

Fig. 4   Model CC Slicer.

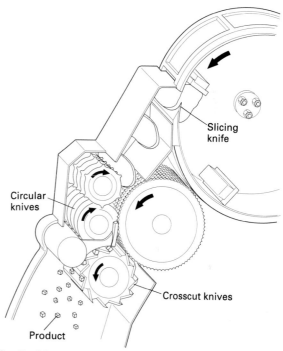

Fig. 6   Model RA Dicer.

Many meat and fibrous vegetable products cannot be effectively cut using a stationary knife edge. A good option in this case is a rotating knife, linked to the simplicity of the centrifugal slicing principle (Fig. 3).

One special slicing requirement is the production of very thin slices for the manufacture of potato crisps (known as potato chips in the USA). The specification is for accurate slice thickness, to restrict under- or over-cooking, and slices generated with the minimum of starch cell damage. For this reason very thin, sharp knives, similar to a safety razor blade, are of the inexpensive throw-away type. Correctly set machines with sharp knives, using average potatoes, will offer 80% of the slices varying less than 0·1 mm. Machine capacity in this case is achieved by having eight cutting stations equally spaced around the periphery (Fig. 4). *See* Potatoes and Related Crops, Processing Potato Tubers

Subsequent development enables crisps with several types of crinkle slices, as well as potato sticks, to be produced. With a small adaption these heads could be

modified to produce shreds from other vegetables and fruits, cheese and similar products.

Dicing Machines

The Model GK Dicer (Fig. 5) will cut uniform crinkle slices and strips, three-dimensional cuts, with four crinkle and two plain cuts, or all plain cuts. The dicer will handle a range of soft ripe fruits and brittle root vegetables, producing well-defined cuts. Slices are generated by the centrifugal principle, but the crosscut knife spindle progresses the slices forward by knives entering at a constant 90°. This progressive cutting action enables clean, square cuts to be produced, with the least possible product loading. The final cut to produce dices is completed by circular knives.

Figure 6 shows a further variant of a three-dimensional dicing machine. One limit in design here, as it is impractical to use a circular knife spacing that is less than 3 mm. The different cutting action developed by a crosscut knife assembly will permit a small dimension of 1·6 mm to be achieved. One special feature of this type of dicer is the ability to by-pass the slicing knife station. This is particularly useful in the reduction of dried fruit, or any suitable material where thickness is already predetermined. Where small products are fed into the machine and these require the minimum of cutting, it is possible to use the impeller as a feeding unit, provided that the slicing knife has been removed.

Material Considerations

The moisture content in most vegetables will lubricate knife surfaces, reducing the pressure required to push the knife through the product. With sticky products, such as glazed fruits or dates, these can readily cause a problem and a rapid build-up of product in the machine. The use of a food-grade lubricant, or even water lightly sprayed over the cutting assemblies at regular intervals, may overcome the problem. Another very good method to lessen the sticky surface effect is the reduction of product temperature.

Fine Controlled Comminution

Machines for the controlled size reduction of products have made several advances in recent years. New concepts have been developed which produce regular-sized pieces in a narrow band, usually with little oversize material. Dependent on the friability of the product being processed, the level of fines secured can also be extremely small. This can very often eliminate a lengthy and expensive sieving operation, and save the consider-able cost of reprocessing fine material.

These concepts are embodied in a machine called the Comitrol® Processor (Fig. 7). Basically, this consists of a cylinder with an internal diameter of 152 mm, com-posed entirely of knives. The dimension used has proved critical where the relationship of centrifugal force, friction and the control of incremental cutting is required.

An extensive number of knife configurations are available in these cylinders, which enable comminution to microfine powders, and even the production of frozen meat chunks. A precision-balanced impeller rotates at high speed within the cutting area, developing a centri-fugal force which pushes the product against, and then through, the knives.

Stepped impeller speeds are available usually ranging from 2000 rpm to a normal maximum of 9000 rpm. Power requirements will be dependent on the machine type and the machine application, starting with a minimum of 7·46 kW and running up to a maximum of 149·2 kW.

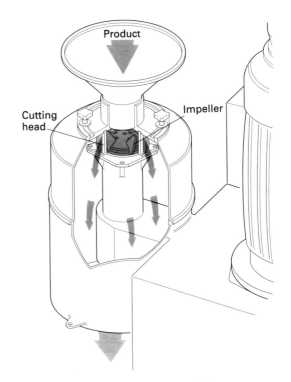

Fig. 7 Comitrol Processor Model 1700.

The use of small-diameter cutting heads employing the incremental shearing principle can still offer impres-sive production rates. It is possible, for example, to flake-cut meat products up to 9000 kg h^{-1} and meat emulsions up to 13 600 kg h^{-1}.

A considerable number of food products can now be cut to size instead of ground, dramatically reducing the frictional heat generated by products rubbing over stationary surfaces. Foods can be sized-reduced in many situations, dependent on the material and the size reduction step required. Thus it is possible to run dry or low-moisture products, material in water or other suspensions, viscous grease and fats, often in the same machines. With ultra-heat-sensitive or tougher mater-ials, the application of cryogenics is extremely useful. With products which deform or compress easily, this step is very often essential.

Design Considerations

The most important criterion is to ensure that there should be no metal-to-metal contact between any part of the cutting assemblies. It is therefore possible to run the machine completely void of product, and no priming or starting media is required. No adjustment is possible on any cutting assembly, thus removing any possible 'art' situation being developed by an operator, if variations were possible.

The clearance between the cutting head and impeller can vary, depending on the type of Comitrol® processor

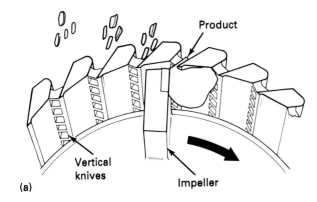

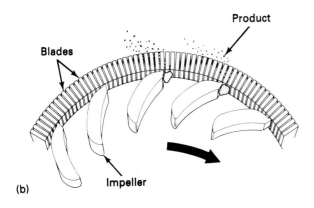

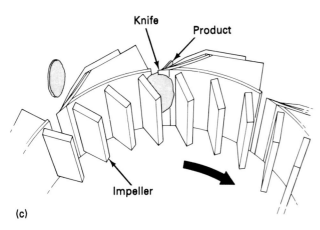

Fig. 8 Three types of reduction heads: (a) cutting head; (b) 'microcut' head; (c) slicing head.

linked to a spindle design. Cutting heads (Fig. 8a) are always made to a standard internal bore, but where precision spindles are used this permits a larger diameter impeller to be fitted, offering less clearance. Several impeller options are available with varying number of arms and approach angles to meet specific requirements.

In 'microcut' head (Fig. 8b) assemblies it is possible to alter the depth of cut, not only by the number of blades fitted but also by the angle at which they are installed in the blade-holding rings. A comprehensive range of 'microcut' heads are available for both standard and degree heads. As the depth of cut is controlled by the

'microcut' blades, all impellers are produced to a standard diameter. In this case, the number of impeller tips and the cutting angle tangent, coupled with speed variations, offer many alternatives.

Completing the trio of cutting assemblies is the slicing head unit (Fig. 8c), which is a precise, miniature version of other Urschel® centrifugal slicers. It consists of a ring of eleven adjustable knife holders, complete with inexpensive throw-away knives. The centrifugal force created by the rotating impeller causes product to press firmly against the inner surface of the knife holders, to produce uniform slices. A specially designed impeller directs product uniformly into all knives, giving the possibility of several thousand kg per hour of uniform slices.

All the foregoing Comitrol® processors and assemblies are intended to be used continuously, enabling maximum hourly product rates to be achieved. If required, all machines and assemblies can be operated on a batch basis, usually with a similar size reduction result.

Current developments now offer a machine with large power and capacity, giving a two-stage size reduction machine. In the first stage, product to be processed enters a rotating impeller, where it contacts the inner ends of the arms that will cause the product to rotate. The ends of these arms are moving at 105 m s^{-1} and strike the product 2480 times per second. As the product being processed begins to rotate within the impeller, centrifugal force attempts to push the product between the arms. The product continues to strike the ends of the arms and this tends to force the product towards the centre. By the time the product reaches sufficient rotational speed to slip between the impeller arms, it has broken into many random size particles.

In the second stage, when the product reaches full rotational speed of the impeller, it moves out towards the periphery of the processing chamber. The product is directed generally in a tangential direction, against a ring of closely spaced knives. The tips of the arms move the product over the knives at a speed of 148 m s^{-1} and, owing to the high centrifugal force produced at this speed, the product is forced against the knife edges by the weight of the product multiplied by 14 746. Pieces of product are sheared off and discharged between the knives. The knives are made either of tungsten carbide or zirconium oxide. Both of these materials are so hard that their shape can only be formed by diamond-faced grinding wheels.

This method of size reduction is so efficient that a single machine has replaced six mills in the manufacturing of peanut butter.

Microbiological and Sanitation Considerations

The extensive use of stainless steel and noncorrodable materials, including castings free from blowholes and blemishes, also food-quality conveyor belts, offers the best possible range of options to reduce bacteriological problems.

By their very design, size reduction machines using a shearing cutting action invariably have dead spots, where product does not self-clean. This is a greater problem where fresh or cooked product is processed immediately ahead of packaging. Control of operational temperatures and regular sanitation programmes are essential to prevent development of a 'snowball effect'.

Many excellent proprietary cleaning agents are available, including solvents for food varnish. Manufacturers' instructions regarding correct usage must be followed with great care; otherwise, irreversible damage to surfaces may occur. *See* Cleaning Procedures in the Factory, Types of Detergent; Cleaning Procedures in the Factory, Types of Disinfectant

The passive state of stainless steel will only be sustained in an air and water situation. Food residues allowed to dry and harden on contact faces will break the passive shield and quickly develop 'mouse holes', which grow at an alarming rate. Great care must be exercised to ensure that certain metals are not exposed to acidic materials, which will cause them to absorb hydrogen and become brittle, resulting in early failure; this is particularly significant where knives are concerned.

Bibliography

Anonymous (1977) *How to Cut Food Products*. Food Product Index and machine specifications. Valparaiso, Indiana: Urschel Laboratories Inc.

Anonymous (1985) *Comitrol Comminuting Machines*. System Bulletin. Valparaiso, Indiana: Urschel Laboratories Inc.

Binsted R and Devy JD (1970) *Soup Manufacture, Canning, Dehydration and Quick Freezing*. London: London Food Trade Press.

Lock A (1969) *Practical Canning*. London: London Food Trade Press.

Maxwell P (1982) *Practical Management of Food Processing Operations*, pp 192–193. Management Publications. Glasgow: WJ Ross Repro Service.

R. A. W. Dickson
Urschel International Ltd, Leicester, UK

COMMON AGRICULTURAL POLICY

See European Economic Community

COMMUNITY NUTRITION

Community nutrition requires a *population approach*. The community rather than the individual is the focus of interest. Community nutrition includes nutritional surveillance, epidemiological studies of diet, and also the development, implementation and evaluation of dietary recommendations and goals. A community may be any group of individuals, e.g. the population of a town or country, or the residents of an old people's home.

Advice to the Community

Dietary advice to the community has changed over the years, depending on the nutrition-related diseases of importance at the time and our understanding of how they are caused. In the 1930s, for example, the primary concern in Europe and North America was the elimination of deficiency diseases. The concept of a 'balanced diet' was developed to try to provide the minimum requirements of protein, vitamins and minerals. By the late 1950s, research suggested that some chronic diseases could be related to overnutrition, and dieting to lose weight became popular. For example, it was recommended that bread and potato intake should be restricted to help avoid becoming overweight. However, by the 1980s, it was recognized that Western diets were short of fibre and wholemeal bread and jacket potatoes were being promoted as good sources of dietary fibre.

Recommended dietary allowances (RDAs) for nutrients were first set in the 1930s and have been revised

Table 1. Comparison of dietary goals from WHO, COMA and NACNE

| | WHO | | COMA | | |
	Lower	Upper	1991 (DRVs)[a]	1984[b]	NACNE[a]
Total energy (MJ)	[c]			Avoid obesity	[d]
Males			10·6[e]		
Females			8·1		
Total fat	15	30	33 (35)[f]	35[g]	30
Saturated	0	10	10 (11)[f]	15[g]	10
Polyunsaturated	3	7	6 (6·5)[f]	6·8[g]	—
Cholesterol (mg per day)	0	300	—	—	—
Total carbohydrate	55	75	47 (50)[f]	—	55
Complex carbohydrate	50	70	37 (39)[fh]	—	—
Dietary fibre (g per day)	27	40	18[k]	—	30
Free sugars	0	10	10[m] (11)[f]	No increase	—
Protein	10	15	—	—	[n]
Salt (g per day)	—	6	1·6	No increase	Down by 3
Alcohol	—	—		Avoid excessive intake[p]	Down to 4

Units are percentage of total energy, unless otherwise stated.
[a] Values are population averages. DRVs, dietary reference values.
[b] Values are upper limits.
[c] Energy intake for normal growth, work, etc., and to maintain appropriate body reserves. Body mass index (kg m^{-2}) in adults 20–22.
[d] Maintain optimal bodyweight and adequate exercise.
[e] Estimated average requirement for men and women, aged 19–49 years, physical activity level 1·4.
[f] Figures in parentheses represent percentage of food energy.
[g] Percentage of food energy.
[h] Intrinsic and milk sugars, and starch.
[k] Nonstarch polysaccharides.
[m] Nonmilk extrinsic sugars.
[n] No change; increase proportion of vegetable protein.
[p] Excessive intake is defined in COMA (1984) as >80 g of alcohol per day for men and >52 g per day for women.

at regular intervals. The RDAs are intended to give the average amounts of essential nutrients considered to be adequate to meet the known nutritional needs of practically all healthy persons in the population, or in a population group. They must be interpreted carefully when used in nutrition education and are not intended to be used by individual members of the public as a guide. In 1991, dietary reference values (DRVs) for the UK were defined for approximately 40 nutrients. The DRVs include a range of intakes covering the distribution of requirements for each nutrient. *See* Dietary Reference Values

Dietary goals or guidelines aim to reduce the chances of developing chronic degenerative diseases and are based on data from animal experiments, metabolic studies, clinical trials and epidemiological research. They provide targets for the population to aim at for some future time. The first set of dietary goals was published in Sweden in 1968. The UK has published its own goals. These are the Health Education Council's publication in 1983 from the National Advisory Committee on Nutrition Education (NACNE) and the Department of Health and Social Security's reports from the Committee on

Medical Aspects of Food Policy (COMA). In 1984 COMA reported on diet and cardiovascular disease, and in 1991 on DRVs for food energy and nutrients for the UK. The World Health Organization (WHO) has also published population nutrient goals in 1990. These are recommended for use in all parts of the world and have been expressed in absolute terms rather than increases or decreases in existing nutrient intake. The desirable change will then vary with the population. For example, in some developing countries the goal for fat intake (lower limit) suggests the need to increase average intakes slightly. Conversely, for most industrialized countries a reduced fat intake is desirable. Table 1 summarizes the COMA, NACNE and WHO nutrient goals. *See* National Nutrition Policies

Nutrient goals and RDAs complement each other. All the reports on goals are concerned with the energy-supplying macronutrients. The RDAs give detail on energy and micronutrient intakes. Both recommendations are based on the best available evidence and may need to be changed in future. The 1991 COMA report on DRVs aims to bring together nutrient requirements and dietary recommendations for health.

Assessing Adequate Nutritional Status

In order to advise the community we need to know what the community is already eating. The nutritional status of the community can be defined as the presence or absence of diet-related diseases and is related to the health and wellbeing of the community. There is no simple or single way to measure it, so that information has to be gathered from many sources. *See* Nutritional Surveillance, In Industrialized Countries

Food and Nutrient Supply

National Level

Information on national food availability is collected annually by many governments in the form of food balance sheets. The Food and Agriculture Organization (FAO) collects and publishes these statistics. They list the total quantity of different foods available for consumption in a country during a specified time (usually one year). Data are limited, since there is no information available about subgroups of the population by region, ethnicity, age, or socioeconomic level, and accuracy is variable, especially for areas with subsistence farming.

Food balance sheets can be used to assess available energy and nutrient intakes per capita. When used repeatedly they can indicate trends towards or away from national food security. *See* Dietary Surveys, Measurement of Food Intake; Dietary Surveys, Surveys of National Food Intake

Household Level

The National Food Survey carried out in the UK by the Ministry of Agriculture, Fisheries and Food (MAFF) assesses trends in food supplies to the home and, by inference, the food eaten. Nutrient intake can be calculated from these data. It records food purchased rather than food eaten and does not distinguish between the intakes of men, women and children, nor does it include alcohol, sweets, soft drinks, or foods eaten away from the home.

As shown in Table 2, the National Food Survey is particularly useful for assessing trends in food and nutrient intake. In general, the food supply was consistent with the amounts recommended to cover the needs of most of the population.

Individual Level

Diet at the individual level is usually assessed by survey, using one of several different methods, such as a weighed intake, dietary recall or record, or a food frequency questionnaire. Attempts have been made to validate the

Table 2. Nutrient intake from the UK National Food Survey, expressed as a percentage of recommended intakes current at the time of the survey

	1958[a]	1968[b]	1978[b]	1988[c]
Energy (kJ)	104	108	94	91
Protein (g)	100	127	121	123
Calcium (mg)	107	191	181	159
Iron (mg)	115	122	100	102
Thiamin (mg)	126	133	125	153
Riboflavin (mg)	108	129	138	123
Vitamin C (mg)	222	181	188	213

Recommended intakes:
[a] BMA (1950) *Report of the Committee on Nutrition.* London: British Medical Association.
[b] DHSS (1969) *Recommended Intakes of Nutrients for the United Kingdom.* London: HMSO.
[c] DHSS (1979) *Recommended Intakes of Nutrients for the United Kingdom.* London: HMSO.
(Nutrient values from MAFF National Food Survey for years stated.)

resulting nutrient levels by measuring biological markers. Surveys may look at a representative sample of the population or a particular 'at-risk' group. A recent survey carried out in the UK by the Office of Population Censuses and Surveys in 1990 studied the current dietary behaviour and nutritional status of adults living in private households in the UK. It aimed to identify characteristics of individuals at risk of coronary heart disease in order to aid implementation of the COMA report and to assist future revisions of DRVs.

Anthropometric Measurements

Weight and height can be used to assess the level of malnutrition or obesity by comparison with reference data. Height can give evidence of past chronic malnutrition, whereas weight is more useful in assessing recent nutritional experience. Overweight or obesity is most practically assessed using the body mass index (weight, in kg, divided by the square of the height, in m^2). *See* Nutritional Status, Anthropometry and Clinical Examination

Health Statistics

Birth statistics such as neonatal, perinatal or infant mortality rates provide indirect information about the nutritional status of a community, particularly its disadvantaged groups. Death rates for diseases which have a nutritional cause can also indicate nutritional status in the community. *See* Epidemiology

Success Level of General Advice

In order to change a population's diet, RDAs and dietary goals must have scientific credibility, political and techni-

Table 3. Percentage of population meeting dietary goals (COMA, NACNE)

Dietary goal	Diet survey of UK adults (1986–1987)[a]		Three Towns Study (1984–1985)[b]		Scotsmen (1980–1982)[c]
	Men	Women	Men	Women	
Total fat <35% food energy	12	15	25	26	28
Saturated fat <15% food energy	45	31	41	39	31
P/S ratio >0·45	40[d]	36[d]	27	26	—
Total carbohydrate > 50% energy	9	12	31	31	—
Refined sugars <12% energy	—	—	19	22	—
Fibre > 25 g per day	45	16	25	10	17

[a] Gregory J et al. (1990).
[b] Cade J and Booth S (1990) What can people eat to meet the dietary goals: and how much does it cost? *Journal of Human Nutrition and Dietetics* 3: 199–207.
[c] Thomson M, Fulton M, Wood DA et al. (1985) A comparison of the nutrient intake of some Scotsmen with dietary recommendations. *Human Nutrition Applied Nutrition* 39A: 443–455.
[d] Percentage consuming P/S ratio 70·4.

cal support, and be recognized as being necessary and acceptable to the consumer. It may take years to achieve the desirable change.

How close to meeting the dietary goals is the UK population? The results of three studies in British adults, showing the percentage who met the UK dietary goals, are presented in Table 3. Most subjects ate more total fat, saturated fat and refined sugars and less carbohydrate and fibre than recommended. Most had a P/S (polyunsaturated fat/saturated fat) ratio lower than recommended.

People who consumed diets that met the nutrient goals were more likely to eat cereals, wholemeal and brown bread, skimmed or semiskimmed milk, polyunsaturated margarine, fruit, vegetables including potatoes, low-fat meat and nonfried fish. They also ate less white bread, butter, margarine, whole milk, high-fat cheese, eggs, fatty meat and fried fish than those who did not meet the goals. Some foods, such as wholemeal bread, low-fat products, polyunsaturated margarine, and fresh fruit and vegetables, were more expensive than the alternatives eaten by people who did not meet the dietary goals. These extra costs may make the cost of a diet which meets the dietary goals too expensive for the elderly, unemployed and low paid. It is worth noting, however, that it is possible to consume a diet which meets the dietary goals *and* is substantially cheaper than the average cost of a diet which does not meet the goals.

The National Food Survey can monitor progress made by a population towards meeting goals. For example, during the 1980s, the amount of fat in household food supplies per person decreased by 13%. This paralleled a similar reduction in the total amount of energy in the national diet, resulting in no real change in the proportion of energy coming into the household as fat (42%) over the decade. There was, however, a marked (26%) increase in polyunsaturated fatty acids in the national diet. Types of food coming into the home have also changed. Less whole milk and more low-fat milk is now consumed. Less white bread and potatoes are eaten but more wholemeal bread is eaten, although the consumption of this is now levelling off.

Community versus Individual Advice

Public health researchers examine risk factors for disease in the population as a whole and then design prevention strategies to reduce them. Meanwhile, the clinician does the same for the individual patient.

Dietary goals for the population are based on identifying population intakes to maintain health, health being defined as a low rate of diet-related diseases. In assessing whether a population is meeting the dietary goal it is the entire range of nutrient intakes which matters. If the intake is normally distributed within the population, then it can be summarized by the average intake of the population and its standard error.

Dietary goals require a population approach to dietary change, leading to a change in the *average* intake. This will result in some individuals consuming more and some less than the stated goal. If the goals were misinterpreted to relate to individuals then the aggregate changes would be greater than intended (Fig. 1).

Methods of Giving Advice to the Community

Much can be done to change a population's diet. Diets are chosen by individuals; government should not enforce recommendations concerning diet and health by restrictive legislation. However legislation concerning the production and sale of food does affect a nation's diet. An alternative approach to change is to increase people's knowledge and awareness of food and its relationship to health.

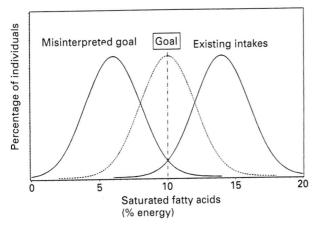

Fig. 1 Distinction between a population nutrient goal and an individual nutrient goal. This figure depicts the distribution of intakes of saturated fatty acids for three hypothetical populations: (Right) an existing population whose intake is higher than recommended by the WHO Study Group; (Centre) a population which has achieved the *population goal* of a maximum intake of 10% of energy as saturated fatty acids; (Left) a population in which nearly all individuals have an intake of less than 10%, a situation which represents the result of misinterpretation of the population goal as an *individual goal*. The figure was prepared by G Beaton and reproduced with permission from the World Health Organization (1990).

Health Promotion

Traditionally, nutrition education campaigns have involved only one or two sections of the community, such as schools or the media. Success, if it was measured at all, was limited. The modern approach is to involve as many groups of the community as possible and to use a variety of educational approaches. For example, in the UK, 'Heart-Beat Wales' is a health promotion programme which involves public education, lay groups, schools, factories, retailers and others. 'Look After Your Heart' is a multidisciplinary campaign, backed by the UK government, to reduce risk factors for coronary heart disease. Evaluating the success of these campaigns in terms of reduction of deaths from heart disease is difficult. *See* Nutrition Education

Knowledge of the health risks associated with consumption of particular dietary components does not inevitably lead to dietary change. The choice of a particular diet is determined by a number of factors. The health effects of particular types of foods may exert only a minor influence. Individual compliance to dietary advice partly depends on the quality of the counselling given. Leaflets are often used, but are ineffective with mass distribution. Health education can change consumers' purchasing and eating habits. For example, the national promotion of low-fat milk immediately increased its consumption by 20%.

Medical Practitioners

In the UK, general practitioners (GPs) are being encouraged to provide health promotion, but they receive little training in nutrition. Patients are rarely referred to a dietitian and the practice nurse often provides most of the advice. Dietary advice provided by members of the primary health care team can be misleading. *See* Dietetics

Most district health authorities in the UK have their own food and health policies which are often limited to measures within their own services. Potential contributors to these policies are groups within the community such as local shopkeepers, industry, and trade unions.

Reaching Vulnerable Groups

Nutrition advice should take account of the special needs of particular subgroups, who may be vulnerable to malnutrition owing to their physiological requirements, their cultural traditions or their economic problems.

Babies and Young Children

The health professions have a role in promoting breast-feeding and the preparation of culturally acceptable and appropriate weaning foods. In the UK, in order to meet the current dietary goals the diet is likely to increase in bulk and so reduce energy density. It is important to maintain adequate energy intakes by not changing babies onto low-fat milks too early. Growth monitoring, particularly in developing countries, can be used to detect growth faltering. Remedial action can then be taken. *See* Children, Nutritional Requirements; Infants, Nutritional Requirements; Infants, Breast- and Bottle-feeding; Infants, Weaning

Adolescents

On the whole, this group is adequately nourished in the UK. There is some concern, however, at the low levels of iron intake in British teenage girls. Adolescents on slimming diets may be at risk of low intakes of some micronutrients. Appropriate nutrition education at school, backed up with the provision of healthy school meals, may help to encourage suitable nutritional habits in this group. *See* Adolescents, Nutritional Problems

Pregnancy and Lactation

Most pregnant and lactating women in the UK consume an adequate diet, but this is a time when women come into contact with health care services and may be open to nutrition education. Particular attention should be paid to the dietary intake of young girls and other women at risk of bearing low birthweight babies. *See* Lactation

Elderly

The current dietary goals are appropriate for the elderly. Energy intakes tend to decrease with increasing age and there is a need for the elderly to consume diets with an increased nutrient density. Health professionals and other carers should be aware of the potential inadequacies of elderly people's diets. *See* Elderly, Nutritionally Related Problems

Low Income Groups

Families on a low income and those living in temporary accommodation may find it difficult to feed themselves properly. Reaching them is not easy. They may not be registered with a GP. Local community groups may provide a forum for education and support of women trying to feed a family in difficult circumstances.

Ethnic Groups

Some ethnic groups consume diets which are characterized by a high fat intake. Women and children in certain communities may be at risk of vitamin D deficiency. Culturally acceptable nutrition education needs to be in a form that can be understood by the whole community. Videos and personal intervention by a trained member of the local community may give the best results in groups that are hard to reach.

Bibliography

COMA (1984) *Diet and Cardiovascular Disease*. Report on Health and Social Subjects 28. London: Her Majesty's Stationery Office (HMSO).

COMA (1991) *Dietary Reference Values for Food Energy and Nutrients for the United Kingdom*. Report on Health and Social Subjects 41. London: HMSO.

DHSS (1979) *Recommended Daily Amounts of Food Energy and Nutrients for Groups of People in the United Kingdom*. Report on Health and Social Subjects 15. London: HMSO.

Gregory J, Foster K, Tyler H and Wiseman M (1990) *The Dietary and Nutritional Survey of British Adults*. London: HMSO.

NACNE (National Advisory Committee on Nutrition Education) (1983) *Proposals for Nutritional Guidelines for Health Education in Britain*. London: Health Education Council.

WHO (1990) *Diet, Nutrition and the Prevention of Chronic Diseases*. WHO Technical Report Series 797. Geneva: World Health Organization.

Janet Cade
University of Leeds, Leeds, UK

COMPUTERS – USE IN FOOD PROCESSING

One of the most rapidly developing fields is that of computer technology and the dramatic evolution of software and hardware systems has affected the whole management of the food chain. Every aspect of farming, processing, storage, product development, marketing and consumption can be monitored, controlled and has been made more efficient with the aid of computers.

Modern Systems

Scientific advances in microchip technology have made systems that are faster, cheaper, smaller and at the same time able to hold vast amounts of information on magnetic or optic disks. Modern systems in the food industry are used for:

- data storage and retrieval;
- process control in factories or analytical instruments;
- robotics;
- quality control;
- computer-aided design;
- artificial intelligence or export systems;
- accounting (spreadsheets);
- modelling and simulation;
- safety management with hazard auditing;
- graphic displays including trend and surface response analysis;
- statistics;
- least cost formulations;
- report writing and presentations (in-house, conferences, sales) and desktop publishing;
- networking and sharing data and software.

Data Storage and Retrieval

Database programs have been developed that allow details of raw material and product quantity and quality to be stored on magnetic or optic discs. The information is accessible from anywhere on earth and allows checks to be made on quality deviations from in-house or government standards. This data can be analysed readily for trends, cross-correlations with other parameters and graphically summarized for reports. Data can be acquired by data loggers in transport, processing and storage areas, and temperature, pH and oxygen sensors can be placed in cans and bottles under high temperatures and pressures. Literature searches can be guided by database sorting and reveal patents or scientific publications within the country or overseas by satellite networking.

Process Control

Process control is the technology used to regulate the control variables of a process to achieve an acceptable result. In the past, manual control meant increased labour cost and the possibility of errors; however, with feedback control of pressure valves, heat and mass transfer and controlled atmospheric equipment, processes can be fine tuned to achieve standards of manufacture. *See* Instrumentation and Process Control

Automation has meant:

- field improvement;
- waste reduction;
- labour savings;
- fuel efficiency;
- optimization with programs that adjust all of the important variables to produce an optimum result for product quality, energy usage or throughput.

Control of Different Food Processes

Biochemical Processing

Control of the activity inside cells or immobilized enzymes is important. Variables such as substrate and product concentration, pH, oxygen tension and temperature must be controlled to optimize the system. Examples are brewing, wine-making, cheesemaking, fruit juice clarification and starch hydrolysis.

Heat Processing

Processes such as blanching, pasteurization, sterilization, baking, frying, extrusion and cooking need to be optimized to maintain quality and save energy. Control of moisture, water activity or colour by time/temperature relationships is critical in heat processing.

Product Formulation and Dispensing

Optimum dispensing and mixing of various ingredients which may be emulsions, liquids, gases and solids are important to maintain quality and consistency.

Process control involves sensors for measurement of parameters, central processing units for computing values and using algorithms to decide the best feedback and hardware actuators that operate a value, motor or switch. Figure 1 indicates diagrammatically a scheme for using computer-based systems for control of food processing.

Robotics

Many food-processing operations make use of robotics that take the place of several humans but have the advantage of working continuously, greater strength, speed and precision of movement. All operations can be controlled and monitored by computers.

However, there have been cases where robots have actually been replaced by humans and this has been due to the greater adaptation to changes in processing line conditions by humans. Large amounts of programming effort need to go into each separate application and changes to production lines or hold-ups often lead to robotic mistiming. An example of this is in a large biscuit factory where 25 varieties of biscuits were made. Variation in production schedules were best suited to human adaptability and tests indicated that robotics at the present stage of development would be less efficient than humans.

Quality Control

Computers can receive data from sensors at production lines, during transport and from analytical instruments such as weighing balances, pH, texture and temperature meters, gas and liquid chromatographs and nuclear magnetic resonance analysers. *See* Quality Assurance and Quality Control

The results can be compared to previous events, standards and government regulations so that a tight check can be kept on all aspects of production and transport of food.

Computer-aided Design

Computer-aided design (CAD) software packages have been available to design food production halls, product flow charts, packaging shapes and labels, equipment

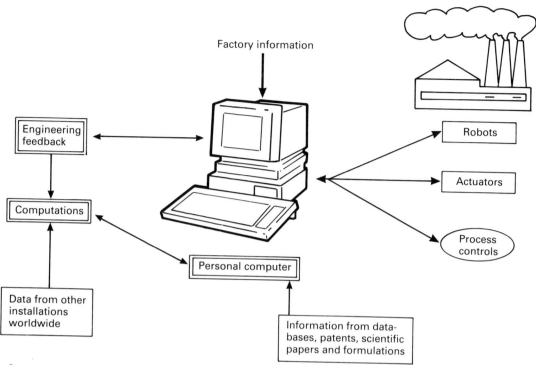

Fig. 1. Computer-based system for control of food processing.

and printed circuits for process control. CAD allows more efficient use of space in equipment design and allows modelling of food processes in conjunction with expert systems. *See* Plant Design, Basic Principles

Artificial Intelligence or Expert Systems

The greatest demand for expert systems (ESs) is in plant automation and process control with increase in productivity, reduction in costs (less machine downtime), shortened design cycles and improved product quality. Captured expert systems contain elements of previous problems encountered in food processing along with procedures of production and hazard analysis. Graphics and databases may be included in the ES. There are many ES packages from Texas Instruments that are 'shell programs' which guide the user through the program, indicating when to set rules, goals, graphics and databases to look up values. There are also rugged versions of computers available that are capable of running ESs on the plant floor, sustaining physical vibrations and extremes of moisture and temperature.

The cost savings of ESs can be large. For example, in 1991 the vice-president of Campbell's in the USA has stated that the $US65 000 cost of an ES package was defrayed by the initial use when 68 000 cans were saved, downtime was eliminated and the cost of bringing in an expert was unnecessary. Other benefits are the use of ESs at many different sites around the world, rapid training of plant personnel and a reduction in anxiety by workers.

Accounting

The revolution in accounting since 1980 has been brought about by electronic spreadsheets such as Excel and Lotus 123. Accountants, food scientists and engineers have not only been kept up to date with costings but also spreadsheets allow people to model 'what if?' situations in regard to food production and marketing. Data can enter spreadsheets from incoming raw material weights to production volume right up to supermarket sales and market surveys. Data may be exported from spreadsheets to graphics, statistics, report writing and desktop publishing programs.

Safety Management and Hazard Auditing

It is imperative that food products are safe and wholesome. There are many stages of farming, transport, processing and point of sale where safety can become an issue. Hazard analysis allows critical points to be monitored and the appropriate remedy to be promulgated. Chemical, physical and microbial contamination as well as loss of nutrients can therefore be minimized. Computers are an essential key in this type of monitoring food safety.

Graphic Displays

High-definition videographic displays allow computers to interact with videotape, optic laser disks or computer graphics, so that decisions can be made on production, equipment of packaging design or marketing.

Surface response or multidimensional scaling grids allow a three-dimensional picture of a food profile such as taste, colour and preference so that interactions between the parameters can be studied; this method is particularly useful in matching the profile of competitor's products. On a geographical basis, surface response grids allow market surveys to be carried out and cross-correlations to be made with socioeconomic factors.

Least Cost Formulations

Food product development requires the food technologist to develop formulations based on several raw materials. Using constraints such as appeal, taste, colour, flavour and texture, least cost formulation with linear programs can determine the relative quantities of ingredients needed to produce a food product at the lowest price. The computer can rapidly optimize the ingredients and formulation can be done daily or whenever there is a change in the availability or cost of the raw materials. Least cost formulation is of particular benefit to producers of pet foods where nutrient composition is the major constraint.

Report Writing and Presentations

The ability to process words, draw colour graphs and project images onto screens for meetings has been vastly improved by computers. High-quality laser or coloured ink jet printers together with the capturing of screen images on slides and video have been developed for desktop and portable computers.

These facilities have been enhanced using scanners with image capturing and editing facilities and optical character recognition (OCR). OCR has allowed words to be reproduced into word-processing programs as well as numbers directly into spreadsheets or graphs. The addition of a spell checker, a thesaurus, language translators and voice recognition have been a revolution to technologists and scientists in the food industry.

Bibliography

Barroclough M (1991) Automation and controls. *Food Manufacturing News* 19: 25–41.
Dziezak JD (1990) Taking the gamble out of product development. *Food Technology* 44: 110–117.
Newell GJ, Skurray GR and Hourigan JA (1986) Use of computers in the Australian food industry. *Food Technology Australia* 38: 456–459.
Pinto JJ (1989) Application of PC-based expert systems in the processing plant. *Food Technology* 43: 145–158.
Shinskey GH (1989) Expert systems in process control. *Food Technology* 43: 139–144.

G. R. Skurray
University of Western Sydney (Hawkesbury), Richmond, Australia

CONDENSED MILK

Some Historical Background

Industrial production for both sweetened and unsweetened condensed milk started around the middle of the last century. However at the beginning of the 19th century, food scientists in Europe, mainly in France, England and the USA had been working on the possibility of preserving milk as a concentrated liquid. Both products have their industrial roots in the USA.

The first sweetened condensed milk in hermetically sealed cans was manufactured and sold in 1856 by Gail Borden in the USA. The business grew rapidly and spread into Europe by 1866 where a sweetened condensed milk factory was set up in Cham, Switzerland, by Charles A. Page, a US consul assigned to the country. The rapid success of this Swiss-based company within Europe led eventually to an expansion of its manufacturing facilities in the USA. This organization, registered as the Anglo-Swiss Condensed Milk Company, sold its US interest in 1902 to a company established and registered at the end of the 19th century as the Borden's Condensed Milk Company. In 1904, the remaining European interests of the Anglo-Swiss Company merged with Henry Nestlé, of Vevey, Switzerland, who also manufactured this product. The new company was called the Nestlé-Anglo-Swiss Condensed Milk Company.

Unsweetened condensed milk until the early 1880s was also produced and was sold open in the market due to the lack of knowledge and success of long-life preservation at that time.

The basic process for preservation of unsweetened condensed milk by heat sterilization was conceived by

John B. Meyenberg in 1882, a Swiss citizen, and an employee of the Anglo-Swiss Condensed Milk Company. The idea to preserve milk without the addition of sugar was crowned by his invention of a revolving sterilizer working with steam under pressure. Lacking sufficient support from his company to continue his work, he migrated in 1884 to the USA and also obtained a patent for his invention in that country. In 1885, Mr Meyenberg was co-founder of the Helvetia Milk Condensing Company in the State of Illinois and, during the same year, he achieved the first successful manufacture of unsweetened condensed milk. The name of this product was changed to evaporated milk for a clearer distinction from sweetened condensed milk which prevails today.

The initial phase of commercial production of both products was hampered by various problems and quality defects. Only at the turn of the century were constant quality standards reached.

Definition of Products

Sweetened Condensed Milk

Sweetened condensed milk is made by the addition of sugar to whole milk, the removal of water from the milk to about one-half of its original volume. The product is canned or packaged in other containers without sterilization, with the sugar acting as a preservative. International standards prescribe:

- a minimum milk fat content of 8%;
- a minimum milk solids content of 28%.

The minimum sugar content is often not precisely specified, but should be sufficient to avoid spoilage.

Permitted stabilizers are usually specified as sodium, potassium and calcium salts of:

- hydrochloric acid;
- citric acid;
- carbonic acid;
- orthophosphoric acid;
- polyphosphoric acid.

The name of the product may either be:

- sweetened condensed milk;
- sweetened condensed whole milk; or
- sweetened full-cream condensed milk.

Legislation in some countries requires a somewhat higher milk solids and fat content; usually 9% milk fat and 31% total milk solids. However, there are also provisions for skimmed sweetened condensed milk with milk solids content up to 24% and low-fat compositions, in principle, of 4% fat and 24% total milk solids.

Frequently this product is fortified by the addition of vitamins, mainly A, D_3 and B_1. *See* Food Fortification

Evaporated Milk

Evaporated milk is made by removal or evaporation of water from milk but without the addition of sugar or any other preservative material. The canned product is heat sterilized at temperatures between 118 and 122°C for several minutes. The product may also be packed in any other sterilizable container.

International standards prescribe:

- a minimum milk fat content of 7·5%;
- a minimum milk solids content of 25·0%.

Permitted stabilizers are usually specified as sodium, potassium and calcium salts of:

- hydrochloric acid;
- citric acid;
- carbonic acid;
- orthophosphoric acid;
- polyphosphoric acid.

In addition, some legislation permits the addition of carrageenan up to 150 ppm.

The main name of the product is:

- evaporated milk;
- evaporated full cream milk; or
- unsweetened condensed full cream milk.

Legislation in some countries requires a somewhat higher fat and milk solids content, up to 9% and 31%, respectively. However, there are also provisions for either skimmed or low-fat milks:

- skimmed evaporated milk with a minimum of 20% milk solids;
- low-fat evaporated milks, 4 or even 2% milk fat and milk solids contents of 20–24%.

Fortification with vitamins of either or both A or D_3 is common practice.

Recombined Milk Products

Sweetened condensed milk and evaporated milk are often recombined in countries outside the traditional dairy belt. *See* Recombined and Filled Milks

For recombining, imported skim milk powder and anhydrous milk fat are used to make up the milk components. In recent years the production of filled milks has gained more and more importance. In this case the milk fat is replaced by locally available and cheaper vegetable fats.

Storage and Packing

An adequate keeping quality of up to 12 months can be achieved for both sweetened condensed milk and

Table 1. Typical comparative figures for standard concentrated products and milk. All values are in grams per 100 g

Product	Protein	Fat	Carbohydrates	Minerals (ash)	Calcium	Phosphorus
Sweetened condensed milk	7·8	8·0	55·2	1·8	0·28	0·23
Evaporated milk	6·5	7·5	9·8	1·4	0·24	0·19
Milk	3·2	3·5	4·6	0·7	0·12	0·09

evaporated milk, but this largely depends on the storage conditions. At storage temperatures above 25°C the ageing process and related physical as well as organoleptical defects appear more rapidly. For recombined products the normal shelf life stability, without major deviations from the original aspect, is reduced by about half of a fresh-milk product. *See* Storage Stability, Parameters Affecting Storage Stability

The most commonly used packing is the tin plate can, which offers absolute protection against light, is basically crash proof and has advantages for handling and storage. Recycling is also an important factor. As alternative packing, glass containers or paper/plastic laminates can be used; however, depending on the packing material, a considerable shelf life reduction should be taken into account. For paper/plastic laminates aseptic filling techniques are used, especially for evaporated milk. *See* Canning, Principles

Nutritional Considerations

Due to the concentrated form, both sweetened condensed milk and evaporated milk have an increased compositional analysis as compared to milk (see Table 1). For sweetened condensed milk the figure for carbohydrate includes the sucrose content necessary for product conservation; the carbohydrates for evaporated milk and nonconcentrated milk are composed of lactose only. The rather high energy value of sweetened condensed milk is mainly due to the amount of carbohydrates present, whereas the protein and fat content compares more or less with evaporated milk. *See* Milk, Dietary Importance

Production and Usage

World production amounts to over 4·5 million tonnes. About one-third is produced as sweetened condensed milk and two-thirds as evaporated milk. As recently as 25–30 years ago, infant feeding was still a major application for either sweetened or unsweetened concentrated milk. Due to the nature of the products, somewhat distinct usages are common practice.

Sweetened Condensed Milk

Due to the high sucrose content of above 40% and its viscous consistency, this product is frequently used as a jam-like bread spread.

An early, but no longer popular, use of sweetened condensed milk was to dilute it with water and consume it as a drink. Presently, coffee or tea whitening and sweetening is the major use of sweetened condensed milk. In many countries, it is also used in combination with cocoa or other milk modifiers in the preparation of homemade drinks.

A growing application is in sweet dessert preparations like ice creams, cakes, cookies, etc. Specific to the Latin American continent is its use for Dulce de Leche, basically a caramelized sweetened condensed milk obtained by boiling the can in water for 2–3 h. Different applications vary from country to country and from one geographical region to another, according to traditional consumption habits.

Evaporated Milk

A large area of application is coffee and tea whitening and for the preparation of milk-based beverages. The other main field for general usage is in the culinary sector to enhance the taste and texture of mashed potatoes, pasta, quiches, soups and a wide variety of savoury and sweet recipes. The main utilization can also vary specifically from one country to another.

Manufacturing Principles

The raw material used for both products is usually cow's milk although in certain regions it may be a mixture of cow's and buffalo's milk. *See* Buffalo, Milk

Sweetened Condensed Milk

A flow diagram for the manufacture of sweetened condensed milk is shown in Fig. 1.

Raw milk is collected and selected according to usual quality criteria. The milk is analysed for fat and solids

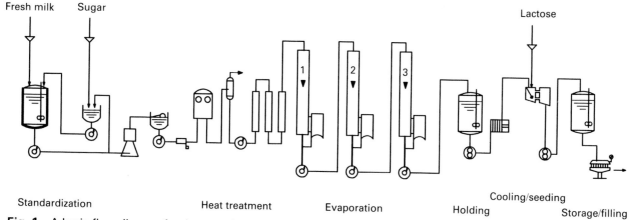

Fig. 1 A basic flow diagram for the manufacture of sweetened condensed milk (continuous process).

Table 2. An example adjustment of the fat and SNF content of raw milk to achieve a final product composition of 8·0% fat and 21% SNF

	Final product	Ratio	Standardized milk	Ratio
Fat (%)	8·0	0·381	3·25	0·381
SNF (%)	21·0		8·52	

not fat (SNF) content and the ratio between both components is adjusted according to fat/SNF ratios of the final product to be manufactured by the addition of either cream or skim milk.

If the final product should have a composition of 8·0% fat and 21% SNF then the raw milk should be adjusted to the same fat/SNF ratio (see Table 2).

Sugar is dissolved in the cold milk, in principle by recirculation through a dissolving vat. The amount of sugar is determined by the quantity of milk prepared for a batch standardization, its fat content, and the compositional requirement of the sucrose content of the final product, e.g.

$$\frac{10\,000\ \text{kg of milk} \times 3{\cdot}25\%\ \text{fat}}{100}$$
$$\times\ \text{Sugar factor}\left(\frac{\text{Sugar content of finished product}}{\text{Fat}}\right).$$

After standardization the milk/sugar mixture undergoes a heat treatment which consists of a temperature/time combination usually above 110°C and holding for seconds or minutes. This heat treatment eliminates nearly all the bacteriological flora of the milk but the choice of temperature/time combinations greatly influences final product characteristics such as the consistency and shelf life stability. *See* Heat Treatment, Chemical and Microbiological Changes

The viscosity of the product is an important factor. It is rather difficult to indicate precise heat treatment conditions since they depend on the equipment used and the characteristics of the raw material milk which can produce different behaviours through regional, climatic and seasonal influences. Constant observations of viscosity and age thickening are necessary to counteract any negative effect. In general lower heat treatments favour increased viscosities and higher, intensive heating tends to give lower viscosities. The viscosity should be sufficient to avoid separation during storage and age thickening should be moderate in order to keep the product pourable during its storage life.

Concentration after heat treatment takes place under vacuum and usually in multiple-effect evaporators.

Sweetened condensed milk is not a sterilized or sterile product; its conservation is assured by the bacteriostatic effect of the high sucrose concentration. The sugar-in-water ratio in the concentrated product must be above 61%. Osmophilic organisms can, however, develop in this medium. Therefore, it is of great importance that the equipment after heat treatment and up to filling is of hygienic design and is operated under the best hygienic conditions to avoid reinfection. Strict controls for equipment cleaning and sterilization are essential.

After evaporation the concentration must be as close as possible to the final product's total solids content; an adjustment by, for example, water has to be omitted due to the risk of contamination.

After evaporation the product is cooled to normally 20–25°C and, at the final concentration, part of the lactose contained in the product is over-saturated. To avoid autocrystallization, fine milled and pasteurized dry lactose crystals are added to the concentrate to provoke instant and controlled crystallization. During storage, product stirring should be maintained for several hours to finalize the crystallization process.

Filling, usually into metallic tin plate cans, is the last delicate operation. Cans and lids must be sterilized, which is often achieved by passing them through a flaming installation. Air in the filling area must be

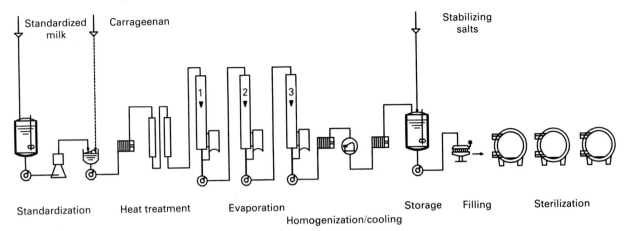

Fig. 2 A basic flow diagram for the manufacture of evaporated milk.

filtered and of an excellent bacteriological quality; the air space in the can must be as low as possible to restrict mould growth. It is not necessary to perform an aseptic operation, but excellent hygienic conditions must prevail.

Evaporated Milk

A flow diagram for the manufacture of evaporated milk is given in Fig. 2.

In principle this product is post-sterilized, which is a conventional process, whereby after filling and closing operations the product is sterilized in the final container (e.g. tin plate cans, glass bottles, etc.).

For stability reasons, the product contains a small percentage of stabilizing salts (either one or a combination of the earlier mentioned salts). Where legislation allows, the hydrocolloid carrageenan may be added. Stabilizing salts are indispensable as manufacturing and technological aids for adjusting or regulating the heat stability of the product during the post-sterilization process. Carrageenan influences phase stability (creaming up and protein sedimentation) during the product storage life.

During the last 10 years, aseptically filled evaporated milks in mainly soft packs have been developed and commercialized. To realise aseptic filling, the product has to be heat treated in-line for final sterilization. Ultra-high temperature (UHT)-type installations are used for this purpose. *See* Heat Treatment, Ultra-high Temperature (UHT) Treatments

The processing steps for milk standardization, heat treatment and concentration/evaporation are similar or identical to those described for sweetened condensed milk, with the exception of the addition of sugar.

After concentration, evaporated milk is homogenized, cooled for intermediate storage and sterilized after filling.

Heat Treatment/Heat Stability

The ability of concentrated milk to withstand high-temperature sterilization is essential. This is commonly described as heat stability and refers to the resistance of milk concentrate to coagulation during sterilization in containers.

Milk has a natural heat stability which is influenced mainly by compositional factors like mineral salt content, protein content, degree of acidity, etc. The natural heat stability also varies according to season and lactation periods. In order to obtain milk sterilizable at different levels of concentrations, this natural heat stability must be improved and adapted. In practice this is achieved by temperature/time combination of preliminary heat treatments on the milk before concentration and the addition of certain mineral salts. Precise indications are rather difficult due to the various influencing factors. The optimal heat stability has to be found by an empirical approach. In principle, more intensive heat treatments increase the heat stability, but above optimum conditions a reverse effect is quickly attained.

It must also be understood that processing operations, such as concentration and homogenization, have a destabilizing effect on the concentrate. The various operations must be balanced so as to ensure a product of optimum quality.

Concentration

After preheating, the milk is evaporated under vacuum. It is of utmost importance that the evaporator works under optimal hygienic conditions despite the fact that the product is sterilized afterwards. In general, falling film evaporators are commonly used today.

Homogenizing

In order to obtain a satisfactory homogenization effect, the homogenizer and, in particular, the homogenizing valves must be kept constantly in the best mechanical conditions.

The homogenizing temperature should preferably be around 65°C.

A homogenizing pressure of 200–250 bar is usually applied and best results are obtained by a two-valve system in series. In principle, the second valve is adjusted to 20–25% of the total pressure. Excessive pressure has a destabilizing effect which is irreversible. Following homogenization, the product is cooled for intermediate storage.

Pilot Sterilization

It is of advantage to fill some cans and to sterilize them at given conditions in order to verify the heat stability of the concentrate. Corrective actions are further possible by addition of stabilizing salt and adaptation of the sterilizing conditions.

Sterilization

After filling into containers (cans), the product is sterilized. The purpose of sterilization is to obtain physical and bacteriological stability. According to practical application, one speaks of a commercial sterility.

The effect of sterility is expressed by the F value as an integral function of the lethality of the microorganisms present, related to *C. botulinum* at the specific destruction temperature of 121°C. Usually, an F value of 4 is considered satisfactory.

Today, modern instruments are available for the measurement of the time/temperature profile within any type of sterilizer.

Usually, rotary and continuous sterilizers are used.

Major Product Defects

Bacteriological Problems

For evaporated milk, the usually applied sterilization processes are proven and sufficiently safe to guarantee product safety and commercial sterility. If problems arise they are mainly traced back to an insufficient can integrity. Faulty soldering, welding of can bodies or closure seams are the weakest points. However, the presence of excessive amounts of thermophilic spores can cause severe spoilage. Appropriate line and finished product controls must be put in place. *See* Spoilage, Bacterial Spoilage

Sweetened condensed milk is less vulnerable to spoilage due to its high sugar content, but it is not protected against osmophilic organisms. Plant and manufacturing hygiene are the keys to success.

Physical Instability

Instability may be of various individual defects, some of which may be interrelated. Separation problems can, and mainly are, a result of inadequate product viscosities. Certain texture problems may be related to nonoptimal heat treatments, but for sweetened condensed milk it may also be a result of coarse lactose crystallization.

Age thickening is a constant problem for sweetened condensed milk. The increase of viscosity over the storage time is basically always present and, from a manufacturing point of view, can only be corrected by an optimal heat treatment of the milk prior to concentration. One needs much practical experience to keep this phenomenon under control.

Age gelation for evaporated milk is a similar phenomenon to age thickening for sweetened condensed milk, but often appears only and suddenly after long storage times. The product can remain with normal physical properties up to 10 or more months and can thicken within a few weeks. This gelation is strictly a storage defect, and should not be confused with thickening or coagulation during the sterilization process nor with coagulation resulting from microbiological activity. The main factors influencing age gelation are, as above, insufficient and nonoptimal preheating conditions of the milk before evaporation, marginal sterilization conditions and an insufficient stabilizing salt level.

Inferior raw milk quality and final product storage conditions can also play an important role within the complex context of age gelation or thickening for either evaporated or sweetened condensed milk.

Products Manufactured by Recombining

As already mentioned, traditional dairy products like sweetened and unsweetened condensed milk are made by recombination using skim milk powder and anhydrous milk fat for the dairy components. The following is a brief description of these processes. *See* Recombined and Filled Milks

When recombining sweetened condensed milk (see Fig. 3), according to a process using only flash cooling evaporation, the skim milk solids have to be dissolved at a concentration of 40%, where some formation of lumps is practically unavoidable. However, these lumps are easily dispersible by mechanical force, as obtained through a colloid mill. A recirculation system has a beneficial effect on skim milk powder hydration.

In principle, sugar dissolving in a low-temperature medium does not pose a major problem but is somewhat time consuming. Therefore, the circulated solution is heated after powder dosage, in order to make the sugar dissolve rapidly.

A slightly simplified process for recombining can be used for evaporated milk (see Fig. 4).

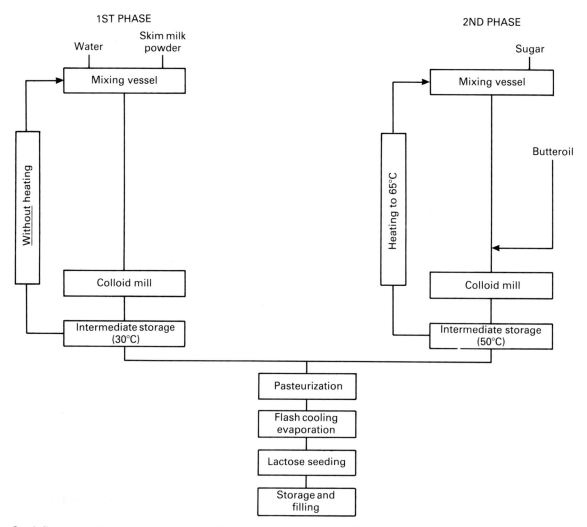

Fig. 3 A flow chart for the recombination of sweetened condensed milk.

Dissolving skim milk powder at low concentration generally poses less problems. Skim milk powder is certainly the most critical raw material and, depending on its characteristics, directly affects the physical properties of the final recombined product. This influence depends to a large extent on the heat treatment given to the liquid skim milk before drying. Seasonal and regional influences may also play a role.

Since milk proteins are sensitive to heat, the extent of their denaturation reflects the heat treatment applied and is used for classifying skim milk powders. The latter have been classified by the American Dairy Products Institute (ADPI) into three groups according to the level of undenatured whey protein nitrogen present in the powder after manufacture. In general terms, this is expressed as the whey protein nitrogen index (WPN index) (see Table 3). Whereas the high-heat-type powders are, in principle, the most appropriate for sterilized products, the low-heat range powders are usually more suitable for nonsterilized recombined products such as sweetened condensed milk.

Anhydrous milk fat is the principal source of fat used in recombined dairy products. It contributes significantly to the taste and milky character of the product. This is a clear indication for the quality requirements for this raw material. In certain cases, vegetable oils are used as butterfat substitutes, primarily for economic reasons. Such products are internationally recognized as 'filled milks'. The vegetable oils used in filled milks should be double refined and deodorized and have a low peroxide value.

Water is a basic ingredient of all recombined dairy products. In general, a good drinking water quality is sufficient and acceptable. However, as water taste, odour and possibly also colour may influence the final product, special monitoring of water quality is important.

Buttermilk powder can be and is used in recombined products. From the technological point of view, buttermilk powder is an emulsifying aid for the fat, since it contains a relatively large amount of the phospholipids which are lost in the separation process of skim milk and

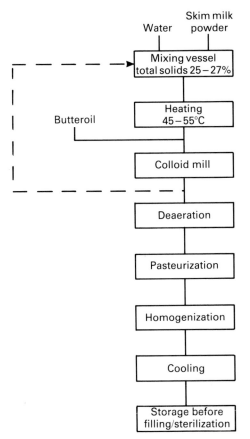

Fig. 4 A flow chart for the recombination of evaporated milk.

Table 3. WPN index (values are in milligrams of nitrogen per gram of powder)

Classification	WPN index
High heat	$\leqslant 1 \cdot 5$
Medium heat	$1 \cdot 51 – 5 \cdot 99$
Low heat	$\geqslant 6 \cdot 0$

For filled milks further addition of vitamin E is carried out and is recommended for nutritional purposes.

Various processing aids, mainly phosphates, but also other emulsifiers or stabilizers are added to achieve specific product characteristics and consistencies.

All additives must be in accordance with legal prescriptions or comply with the Food and Agriculture Organization/World Health Organization standard (Code of Principles). *See* Legislation, Additives

anhydrous milk fat. For most applications only sweet buttermilk is suitable; buttermilk powder obtained from acidified cream for butter production is not suitable. *See* Emulsifiers, Uses in Processed Foods

As the natural vitamin content of fresh milk is usually slightly reduced during processing of the raw materials for recombining, vitamins A, D and B are usually added.

Bibliography

Codex Alimentarium (1984) Rome: Food and Agriculture Organization of the United Nations/World Health Organization.

Hunziker OF (1935) *Condensed milk and milk*, 5th edn. La Grange, Illinois: Hunziker.

Webb BH, Johnson AH, and Alford JA (1974) *Fundamentals of Dairy Chemistry*. Westport, Connecticut: AVI Publishing Company.

H. J. Hess
Nestec Ltd, Vevey, Switzerland

CONFECTIONERY

See Sweets and Candies

CONSUMER PROTECTION LEGISLATION

Development of Consumer Protection in Food

Consumer protection is a relatively recent term and concept, yet protection of the food purchaser's interests has been a primary objective of food legislation throughout history. In each country, measures have been introduced which have sought to provide this basic right whilst simultaneously protecting the honest trader from the excesses of less scrupulous competitors.

This article illustrates the development of consumer protection in matters relating to food, with special reference to British control measures. It is recognized that alternative control systems have been established elsewhere, but whilst differences do occur in the detail of application, the underlying principles and concerns show a similarity of objectives.

British food law has been traced back in history to the Assize of Bread and Ale of 1266, in which the objective was to protect the consumer against short measure. The concern was with quantity rather than with quality. The food purchaser in the Middle Ages received little protection – the weight of food supplied could be checked but there was no possibility of checking a food's quality. Not surprisingly, the opportunities to adulterate foods were substantial and the profits could be significant. The scarcer, more expensive items were particularly susceptible and, for instance, ground pepper commonly contained ground twigs and leaves.

Everyday foods were not immune from adulteration and bread which was supposedly made solely from wheat flour usually also included flour ground from a variety of other grains and seeds. During the eighteenth and nineteenth centuries a variety of product-specific measures attempted to outlaw adulteration of products. Examples include acts referring to the adulteration of coffee, passed in 1718 and 1724 (the second of which also dealt with the adulteration of tea), and a series of acts dealing with bread which were passed in 1709, 1757, 1822 and 1836. *See* Legislation, History

Although well intended, these measures did little to provide the consumer with a general protection against those who set out to cheat. The tide did not begin to turn in the consumer's favour until the mid-nineteenth century, when a combination of circumstances led to the establishment of effective national controls. The key elements were as follows:

1. The development of scientific analysis, in particular analytical chemistry and the increasingly widespread usage of the microscope, allowed for the accurate identification of adulterants.
2. The very rapid shift to urban living transformed the UK from a nation of food producers to a nation of food purchasers. Opportunities for fraudulent practice were considerable and adulteration was rife.
3. Paternalistic social consciousness amongst influential members of society was combined with an interest in scientific developments and provided an environment within which consumer protection measures could be debated.

The work of a number of early food analysts provided the detailed evidence necessary for action. In 1820 Frederick Accum published the first major work, *Treatise on the Adulteration of Food, and Culinary Poisons*. Thirty years later, the *Lancet* took up the issue and established an Analytic and Sanitary Commission. The journal published the results of analyses conducted by Dr Arthur Hill Hassall and Dr Henry Lethaby between 1851 and 1854. In his later book, *Food and its Adulterants* (1855), Hassall summarized adulteration in three categories:

1. Fraudulent but harmless, e.g. chicory in coffee, flour in mustard, water in milk.
2. Indigestible but not toxic, e.g. sawdust, seed husks, brick dust, bone ash.
3. Toxic materials, e.g. mineral pigments derived from lead, arsenic or mercury, or acids included within, for instance, vinegar.

The *Lancet* reports were followed up by the more popular media of the day and parliament was forced to act. Select committees substantiated the *Lancet* claims and called for legislation in reports published in the 1850s.

The select committees' reports stressed and established the principle that the legislation should seek to prevent adulteration rather than merely punish offenders, which would only result in a disruption to trade. The concept of using education to overcome ignorance amongst members of the food trade is one which has direct parallels in food legislation of the 1990s. The subsequent legislation, the Adulteration of Food and Drink Act 1860, was somewhat ineffectual but did serve to establish for the first time that consumer protection measures were the general responsibility of the state. The 1860 act made it an offence knowingly to sell adulterated foods and gave counties the power to appoint public analysts.

Consumer protection was strengthened in 1872 when

the Adulteration of Food and Drugs Act required the appointment of public analysts and provided market inspectors with powers to take samples of food from suspect traders.

A further strengthening of the law came in 1875 when the Sale of Food and Drugs Act clarified a number of legislative difficulties. (For example, the courts had had difficulties in defining what was and what was not an adulterant.) The 1875 act is recognized as being the direct ancestor of current UK primary food legislation.

The 1875 Act introduced the provision that 'No person shall sell to the prejudice of the purchaser anything which is not of the nature, substance or quality demanded by such purchaser'. The term 'to the prejudice of the purchaser' illustrates clearly that the aim was to protect food purchasers (consumers) from malpractice.

The above provision has passed through time and has recently been incorporated into the UK Food Safety Act 1990. The only significant change occurred in 1938 when disjunctive phrasing was introduced to confirm that three separate offences existed. (The wording was changed to '. . . not of the nature, or not of the substance, or not of the quality'). Nature offences apply when the wrong variety of a natural food, such as fish, is supplied. 'Substance' refers to adulterated foods or those containing contaminants, whilst 'quality' offences refer to the commercial quality of the offending food.

The 1875 law (and its antecedents) were primarily concerned with the prevention of adulteration. This legislation was particularly successful at eliminating the addition of harmful adulterants, a fact which reflects its educative role as much as its powers of conviction.

Control of adulteration and gross contamination is only one of a number of concerns relating to consumer protection in the specific context of foods. There are three others of importance in this context:

- Control of food which is microbiologically unsound.
- Control of food standards.
- Provision of consumer information.

Microbiologically unsound food was controlled at the end of the nineteenth century through the Public Health Act 1875. The legislative control, however, was limited by the scientific knowledge of the day. Microbiology was still in its infancy and the principles of food poisoning were not understood. It was only in those instances where gross decomposition could be demonstrated that control was applied. Since 1875 the science of microbiology has developed substantially and this has been followed by progressive improvements in food controls. From 1938 the general control of matters relating to consumer protection from foodborne hazards of microbiological origin has been combined with other food controls within a single enactment. This is currently the Food Safety Act 1990.

Control of food standards, i.e. the establishment of specific compositional requirements for individual foods, was initially achieved by means of individual acts of parliament (e.g. Butter and Margarine Act 1907), Artificial Cream Act 1929) but since 1938 ministers have been given powers to make regulations to control the composition of specific foodstuffs. Control has sought to establish and maintain a standard product and prevent debasement.

The Food and Drugs Act 1938 was also significant since it tackled the general problems of false labelling of foods, and misleading advertisements. Ministerial powers were also given to allow for the establishment of specific labelling requirements.

The 1938 act created the two-tier system of food control which remains in force today. An act of parliament sets out the general principles and provides enabling powers whilst subsequent and subordinate legislation, in the form of regulations, provides the details. The system provides both stability and flexibility. The primary legislation (the act) is designed to be used over a long period of time and is phrased to allow account to be taken of developments without the need for repeated recourse to parliament. The responsibility for secondary legislation (regulations) is delegated to ministers who may rapidly introduce new controls as these become necessary.

Current Situation

The previous paragraphs have established that consumer protection has been an underlying theme of food legislation from the earliest statutes. This section discusses the current situation and considers the major influences on the system as it operates today.

The legislative framework for consumer protection in the area of food remains two-tiered. Primary legislation sets out the general provisions, defines the key terms, and provides ministers with powers that enable them to create regulations providing detailed controls.

The current primary legislation in the UK is the Food Safety Act 1990. This act revises and updates the controls whilst retaining many features which have long been familiar. The act, which came into force on 1 January 1991, includes specific reference to consumer protection in its dealings with matters relating to nature, substance and quality, and to food labelling, presentation and advertising. However, in practice the entire act is concerned with matters relating to the protection of the consumers' interests. The act sets out the broad principles of food-related offences, including the new offence of selling food that does not meet food safety requirements. The act also outlines in some detail the responsibilities of those authorities charged with ensuring compliance, and sets out their powers. *See* Legislation, International Standards; Legislation, Additives; Legislation, Contaminants and Adulterants; Legislation, Packaging Legislation; Legislation, Labelling Legislation

The bulk of the detailed measures which protect the consumer are contained within regulations and the 1990 act continues the established principle of delegating the responsibility for regulations to ministers, rather than requiring that the detail be considered by parliament. The regulations cover the following broad categories:

1. *Compositional standards* require, prohibit or regulate the presence in food or food sources of specified components or ingredients, or, more generally, they regulate the composition of specified foods.
2. *Microbiological standards* exist to ensure that food is fit for human consumption and may set specific microbiological standards either for specific foods or more generally.
3. *Controlling processes* require, prohibit or regulate the use of specific processes and treatments used in food production, processing or manufacture. Controls on food irradiation fall into this category.
4. *Hygiene controls* set out the steps to be followed to ensure that hygienic conditions and practices are used in the production and distribution of foods or food sources. Examples include the setting of specific temperature requirements in the Food Hygiene (Amendment) Regulations 1990 and the forthcoming requirements for the training of food handlers.
5. *Labelling controls* impose particular requirements (for specified foods or more generally) or prohibitions, or regulate in some other way the labelling of food. Such controls also extend to marking, presenting or advertising of foods and may specify particular descriptions which may be used.
6. *Other controls*: the act provides a general provision allowing ministers to regulate or prohibit any commercial operation which is deemed to be hazardous to health or otherwise against the consumer's interest.

Each of the above conditions is directly concerned with consumer protection. Similar provisions allow food contact materials (packaging materials in particular) to be controlled. In addition to the general list, the act permits specific control to be applied to novel foods or foods produced from genetically modified sources as these are developed in the future.

In the past, the UK was solely responsible for its food-related legislation which developed in line with national concerns and national dietary practice. Today, however, a substantial proportion of new measures are introduced as an outcome of membership of the EEC. The community initially attempted to develop a Europewide set of compositional standards but, in time, it was recognized that this programme failed to serve the consumer interest since it was not feasible to submerge the entire culinary history of some 12 nations into codified controls. There was no benefit in specifying the 'Eurosausage' or 'Euroloaf' and the programme was abandoned. *See* European Economic Community, International Developments in Food Law

The present-day European programme focuses on controls that bring real benefits to the consumer:

- Product labelling, including nutritional labelling.
- Controls on additives.
- Controls on materials permitted to come into contact with foods.
- Dietetic foods, i.e. food for particular nutritional purposes.
- Official inspection procedures and standards.

In all matters, UK ministers are required to take advice from appropriate advisory committees. Such bodies are constituted to provide information to specific terms of reference. The principal committee with respect to the safety in use of food components in the UK is the Committee on Toxicity of Chemicals in Food, Consumer Products and the Environment (COT). It is this expert committee which evaluates the scientific questions relating to the possible or continued use of, for example, specific food additives. Questions relating to the use of novel foods or novel processes (e.g. food irradiation) are covered by the Advisory Committee on Novel Foods and Processes. Nutritional matters are examined by the Committee on Medical Aspects of Food Policy. All of the above mentioned committees (cited as examples since there are others) are constituted as expert committees from the nation's scientific community. A more broadly based advisory body is the Food Advisory Committee which includes members from food industry, food law enforcement, medical and research professions, and consumer organizations. This committee advises ministers on matters relating to food labelling and advertising, claims made in food marketing, compositional standards for foods, the need for (rather than safety of) food additives and similar products. *See* Ministry of Agriculture, Fisheries and Food

Matters relating to food labelling and food advertising are of particular concern to consumers who wish to know the exact nature of the products that they are offered. In recent years the food marketing industries have sought to make claims for their products. Claims have covered such matters as nutritional properties (e.g. low in fat, high in fibre), production methods (e.g. free-range), the nature of the product (particularly with respect to the use of the word 'natural') and the presence or absence of particular constituents (e.g. additive-free). Each of these claims has been a matter for public concern in the UK and elsewhere, and advice has been prepared for ministers on each matter. Nutritional claims and the use of the word 'natural' are matters subject to official guidelines, which set out in detail the criteria under which terms may be used. It may be postulated that without such guidance the proliferation of claims would have led to the introduction of legislative control (although it should be noted that the EEC is likely to act in this area). In today's sophisticated market-led environment it is only through very close attention to labelling and to manufacturers' claims that the consumer interest may be addressed. It is no longer possible for the individual consumer to possess a detailed knowledge of each of the products on the market. The shift to prepacked foods sold through major multiple supermarkets has rendered the consumer much more remote from the food producer than ever before, and it is essential to consumer protection that products are adequately and correctly labelled.

Concluding Comment

The protection of the consumer's interests has been central to food controls through the ages. The earliest controls were limited to weights and measures and these have continued to be of importance. Attention then focused on the adulteration of foods and subsequently on the microbiological status of food products. More recently, the consumer voice has called for more information on the foods on sale. This theme will continue to develop, with ever more detail being provided to ensure that foods are properly described, claims substantiated and misleading comments outlawed.

Bibliography

Fallows SJ (1988) *Food Legislative System of the UK*. Oxford: Butterworth Heinemann.
Fallows SJ (1989) *The Food Sector*. Spicers European Policy Reports. London: Routledge.

Stephen J. Fallows
University of Bradford, Bradford, UK

CONTACT PLATE FREEZING

See Freezing

CONTAMINATION

Contents

Types and Causes

The Association of Official Analytical Chemists defines extraneous matter as foreign matter in a product that is associated with objectionable conditions or practices in production, storage, or distribution; included are filth, which is any objectionable matter contributed by animals such as rodents, insects or birds, or any other objectionable matter contributed by insanitary conditions. Bacteria are not included in this definition. Extraneous material is found in all types of foods.

Although proper sanitation and good manufacturing practices reduce contamination, extraneous material cannot be completely eliminated. Methods for detection and identification of extraneous material are designed to differentiate between acceptable and excessive levels of contamination which would reflect poor manufacturing practices and gross insanitation.

Types of Contamination

There are thousands of consumer complaints lodged every year with food industries and government agencies concerning foreign matter in food. Most of these are easily visible, but microscopic contamination such as insect fragments and rodent hairs require specialized laboratory techniques for their detection. Although substantial investment has been made in research into food sanitation, absolute purity has not been achieved. Most contaminants in food are not of concern from a health and safety standpoint although there are exceptions, e.g. glass or large, sharp pieces of material in food or bottled beverages. Infants are at particular risk from these.

The main types of extraneous material that can be found in food are as follows:

1. *Insects*, which are usually grouped into two types – field insects and stored product insects. Field insects are associated with food during growth and harvesting. They do not normally survive during storage. Stored-product insects are able to complete their life cycle entirely in a food in a warehouse. The two groups are not mutually exclusive because some insects which are only classified as stored-product insects in temperate regions are regarded as field insects in tropical regions. Stored-product insects can be found in any of the major groups but most belong to the order Coleoptera (beetles). *See* Insect Pests, Insects and Related Pests; Insect Pests, Problems Caused by Insects and Mites

2. *Excreta*, insect, rodent and mammalian faeces can contaminate foods and therefore have the potential to transmit pathogens. Insect excreta can be detected indirectly by analysing for uric acid (also present in birds) using spectrophotometric tests or by the presence of chitin. Rodent excreta or other animal excreta may be identified by the size and shape of the pellets and the predominant type of hairs in the pellets, as these animals often lick themselves and swallow their hairs. Detection of mammalian faeces involves a chemical assay for the presence of alkaline phosphatase.

3. *Mites*, which can contaminate foodstuffs in large numbers if conditions are favourable. One female can lay 100–400 eggs, and it can take 1–4 months to complete one life cycle under warehouse conditions. Mites need a high relative humidity and so are often found in conjunction with mould growth. As mites feed and reproduce, exuviae, eggs, excreta and bits of food accumulate and appear as a fine brown dust on the food. If it is examined with a magnifying lens, the mites can be seen moving. One way of testing for the presence of mites in the warehouse is to form the dust into a hill and watch it for several minutes. If it begins to flatten on its own it is generally composed of live mites.

4. *Nematodes*, which can be found in foods such as mushrooms, meat, fish and their products. They are, however, destroyed by adequate cooking or processing. *See* Parasites, Occurrence and Detection; Parasites, Illness and Treatment

5. *Hairs*, from many different sources. Common hairs found in foods include human, rat or mouse, and sometimes sheep hairs (found in cheese). Cat, dog, bat and squirrel hairs, and feathers or feather barbules can be present but these are usually accidental contaminants.

6. *Mould*, which can grow on a food as a result of improper storage and also as a result of processing contamination. Mould contamination usually appears as a fine, feathery area which may be white, black or various other colours. Machinery mould (*Geotrichum candidum*) can grow on uncleaned machinery that is used to process foods with a high moisture content, and can therefore accidentally fall into and contaminate food. Often, where insect tunnels are present in a food, mould can be seen along the inside walls of the tunnel. *See* Spoilage, Moulds in Food Spoilage

7. *Heavy filth elements*, including glass, rubber, stones, sticks, plastics, metal, string, and pits from fruits. Depending on the size and hardness, some of these contaminants can cause serious injury, especially to infants.

The food industry aims at minimizing extraneous material in foods because some types can have adverse effects. For example, moulds can produce toxins which can be mutagenic or carcinogenic and can impart a bitter flavour to foods; mites are capable of producing allergic responses in susceptible individuals; pathogens can be transmitted by insect, rodent or mammalian faeces; (cockroaches have been implicated in the transmission of *Salmonella* and the protozoa *Toxoplasma*); some insects (*Tribolium* spp.) produce quinones which may be carcinogenic; some insects (*Dermestes* spp.) have setae (hairs) that can cause nausea and/or diarrhoea. In addition to adverse effects of extraneous material in food, there are aesthetic reasons for concern among manufacturers and consumers. Hence manufacturers generally have in-house quality control programmes aimed at minimizing such contaminants.

Sources of Contamination

Foods can become contaminated by many types of contamination at any of six different stages from the raw material step through to the final product:

1. *Field contamination during growth.* Crops are subject to contamination from field insects or mites, bird feathers, rodent hairs or excreta, mould, parasites, and sand or soil. Sand or soil can be splashed onto fruits and vegetables during heavy rainstorms, cultivating or picking. Large stones or sand that are not removed in processing can pose a hazard to the consumer. The fig wasp, *Blastophaga*, completes its life cycle in the male fig

fruit. The field insect is often seen in figs or fig paste and is unavoidable in the final product. Scale insects are another example of unavoidable field insects found in food. They attach themselves to many types of plants and are difficult to remove during cleaning or processing of the foods. The presence of these insects in high numbers, however, reflects poor agricultural practices and they should be classed as avoidable filth.

2. *Transportation or storage prior to processing*. Stored product insects, mites, moulds and rodents can contaminate food further if present in the transport vehicles or warehouse. Most stored-product insects and mites need temperatures above freezing to reproduce. Warehouses in the temperate zones provide this needed protection. The merchant grain beetle (*Oryzaephilus mercator*) is able to produce four to six generations per year when there is abundant food and the temperature is above freezing. The fungus *Aspergillus flavus*, growing on damp stored grain and peanuts, may produce aflatoxins sufficient to poison animals and has, through chronic exposure, been implicated in human liver damage and carcinogenic effects. Other moulds affecting stored grains are *Penicillium* and *Absidia* species.

3. *Processing*. All the different techniques used to process food have the potential to allow the introduction of contamination. Contaminants include metal fragments from grinding cocoa beans or boning meat, charred particles from the manufacture of skim-milk powder, glass fragments in glass-packaged commodities, various types of packaging material, machinery mould, human hair, and textile fibres from clothes of employees or sacks of ingredients. Animal sources include feathers accidentally introduced, stored-product insects, mites, and rodent hairs. All of these are avoidable, and good manufacturing practices can eliminate or reduce these to numbers that are acceptable.

4. *Storage after processing*. Foods are subject here to the same type of contamination as that which can occur before processing, namely from insects, mites, mould, rodents, birds, and packaging material. The presence of rodents in a warehouse is indicated by faecal droppings (black or brown, rod-shaped pellets, 8–20 mm by 4–8 mm for rats, and 1–4 mm long for mice), runways along floors, walls and ceilings that are dirty, footprints, holes, and gnaw and tear marks on packaging. Rodents can gnaw their way into buildings through wooden doors and windows, or squeeze through pipes. Mites can affect cheese during storage. People who work with mite-contaminated food have been known to break out in rashes or develop asthma. Natural constituents of some food products can form crystals upon storage which look like glass and can be almost as sharp. Examples are magnesium ammonium phosphate (struvite) in canned fish, calcium carbonate in crab paste, calcium phosphate in cheese and naringin in underripe grapefruit. *See* Storage Stability, Mechanisms of Degra-

dation; Storage Stability, Parameters Affecting Storage Stability

5. *Storage at the wholesale or retail level*. Foods that are infested with live organisms can spread the contamination to other sound foods. Cockroaches are often a problem in storage areas. Their presence is revealed by collections of blunt excreta pellets in and around food.

6. *Handling or storage by the consumer*. Common contaminants are mould from other infected products, hairs from pets or humans, metal fragments from opening cans, wood pieces from cutting boards, textile fibres and accidental insect introduction from other infested food.

Illness arising from Contamination

Claims of illness, mostly mild, have arisen from a variety of different kinds of extraneous material. Claims can be placed in four main groups:

1. *Objects that injure through mechanical means*. The most important of these is glass, usually from bottles broken during manufacturing, although it can also derive from a raw product; for example, glass found in canned tomatoes probably comes from bottles that have been thrown on tomato fields and are broken during harvesting. Glass can be present as microscopic fragments or large pieces (up to many millimetres in length); the former are more likely to be ingested, the latter to cut the mouth and be spat out. Other sharp objects are wood splinters, plastic or bone fragments, sharp crystals, e.g. struvites, and stones. These can cut mouths and intestinal linings, as well as break teeth. Metal objects, such as screws, washers, needles and filings, are, after glass, the most frequent forms of extraneous matter causing injury. String, fibrous material, cigarette butts and paper or cardboard material have been responsible for choking and less well-defined gastrointestinal illnesses.

2. *Indigestible objects*. These include hard food particles, e.g. burnt food, rice kernels and unproperly cooked squash, as well as sand. Some of these only affect infants, but burnt food particles have been reported several times as being responsible for gastrointestinal illnesses in adults.

3. *Hydrocarbon-type material*. Material such as oil, grease, paint fragments and asphalt is frequently found around processing areas and can easily come into contact with food on a production line unless it is protected in some way. However, the mode of action in causing illness is not known, although any solvent present could act as an intestinal irritant.

4. *Disgusting objects*. It can be readily understood that the shock of seeing partially digested mice, worms, parasites, slugs, insects or rodent droppings, or tasting slimy, mould-like materials or soap, would cause an immediate vomiting response, but persons eating some

of these have also developed mild gastrointestinal symptoms after incubation periods of several hours. Moulds may produce toxin, and hairs of insect larvae may irritate the gut lining sufficiently to develop diarrhoea.

All of the above examples of extraneous material have been documented as aetiological agents in Canadian national reports over 10 years. It is not always possible to verify each report but over the years repeat complaints indicate that illnesses from a variety of types of extraneous matter should be taken seriously. Health control agencies in other countries may collect this type of data, but it is not published and little work has been done to determine what specific compounds cause the nausea or vomiting and abdominal cramps or diarrhoea which are reported. Since these complaints are frequent, food company representatives have to be able to distinguish genuine illnesses from fraudulent claims, especially if compensation is being sought. Some successful legal settlements have been awarded not only to persons having physical injury (e.g. teeth broken by stones) but also to psychosomatic illnesses brought on by the sight of disgusting objects, especially if the claimant satisfied the judge that the effects were long-lasting or permanent. The impact of extraneous matter being found by consumers in food must therefore be taken seriously by manufacturers.

Techniques and Methods of Detection

The procedures for detecting extraneous material depend largely upon the type of food and the nature of contamination that may be found. The types of detection methods are as follows.

Macroscopic Detection

Direct visual observation is used most often by inspectors and quality control personnel who examine all foods on arrival at the processing plant or warehouse. Seeds, beans and fruit are examples of foods that would be examined in this way in a laboratory. With the aid of a 3–5 × magnifying lens, insects, mites and their damage can be detected. Mould can also be detected this way, although confirmation must be at a higher magnification (100 ×). When foods consist of a variety of particle sizes, as do some of the ground leafy spices, for example, separation by nested sieves makes it easier to detect large and small pieces of extraneous material. X-Ray examination is one nondestructive method of detecting areas of contamination. Insect infestation in grains, and bone fragments in mechanically separated meat are specific applications of this technology. Long-wave ultraviolet light can be used to inspect packaging material or foods

for urine, but positives must be confirmed by chemical analysis. Candling, another nondestructive method, is the technique of gently tilting a bottle of liquid in front of a light source and observing the presence of falling glass.

Microscopic Detection

Extraneous material particles are separated from the food and examined microscopically. In general, microscopic detection involves three steps:

1. Pretreatment. This involves preparation of the food for extraction of light and heavy filth elements by either defatting, dry or wet sieving, digestion by hydrochloric acid or an enzyme, or deaeration to prevent flotation of excessive food particles. This step disperses the food so that the light or heavy filth elements can be released.
2. Extraction. After the food has been dispersed in an aqueous medium the light filth elements are concentrated and filtered. Light filth particles (insects and their fragments, hairs, mites, etc.) are lipophilic and addition of oil to the dispersed food attracts these particles; the oil layer is then separated by means of a trap flask or percolator. The separated oil layer is filtered through a filter paper, where the light filth elements can be identified, measured and counted. For heavy filth the food is dispersed in an aqueous medium with a specific gravity that allows the food to float and the heavy filth elements, such as sand, glass and excreta pellets, to sink to the bottom. These are also filtered onto filter paper.
3. Recovery. In general, extraneous material particles are identified and counted by using a stereoscopic microscope at 30 × magnification. The approximate sizes of the largest and smallest particles are measured by using a micrometer disc. Questionable particles and identification to genus level of insects, mites and hairs is done using a compound microscope.

The majority of foods examined in this way are processed or ground foods. Since it is particulate matter that is sought, separation techniques are based on physical rather than chemical properties.

Methodology

The following organizations have published extraneous material methodology:

1. Association of Official Analytical Chemists, Suite 400, 2200 Wilson Blvd, Arlington, Virginia 22201-3301, USA.
2. Department of Health, Education and Welfare, Public Health Service, Food and Drug Administration (FDA), Washington, DC 20204, USA.
3. Health and Welfare Canada, Health Protection

Branch, Tunney's Pasture, Ottawa K1A 0L2, Ontario, Canada.

4. American Association of Cereal Chemists (AACC), 3340 Pilot Kost Rd, St Pauls, Minnesota, USA.

5. American Spice Trade Association (ASTA), Englewood Cliffs, New Jersey, USA.

6. Leatherhead Food Research Association, Randall's Road, Leatherhead, Surrey, UK.

7. Codex Alimentarius Commission. Joint FAO/WHO (Food and Agriculture Organization, World Health Organization) Food Standards Programme, Rome, Italy.

8. International Organization for Standardization (ISO), PO Box 5059, 2600 GB Delft, The Netherlands.

Good Manufacturing Practices

Good manufacturing practices (GMPs) are the measures used in the manufacturing, processing, packaging and storage of foods to ensure a sanitary product. These measures also reduce extraneous material contamination of food. Good manufacturing practices involve the following:

1. Hygiene in the production and harvesting areas.
2. Good design and hygiene of the establishment.
3. Hygienic and health requirements for personnel.
4. Hygiene in processing and storage.

Specific guidelines for good manufacturing practices are available from various industries, food associations and levels of government. Codex Alimentarius Commission (FAO/WHO) has prepared the *Code of Practice on General Principles of Food Hygiene*.

Actions by Regulatory Agencies

Almost every country and level of government has set standards or guidelines that define limits for extraneous materials in foods. Below are a few examples:

1. International regulations: The Codex Alimentarius Commission has set international standards for various foods that are traded internationally, e.g. coffee beans, dates. *See* Legislation, Contaminants and Adulterants

2. The USA: the FDA has set a number of Defect Action Levels (DALs) that should not be exceeded if the food has been properly handled.

3. Canada: Health and Welfare Canada and Agriculture Canada set standards on processed foods and meat. The Food and Drug Act, administered by Health and Welfare Canada, has two sections that pertain to extraneous material. The Health Protection Branch of Health and Welfare Canada has set regulations and guidelines that pertain to specific foods and contaminants. Agriculture Canada monitors meat under the Meat Hygiene Act.

Each of these regulatory agencies has set tolerances for types of extraneous material in different food commodities. The values assigned are based on data generated from the monitoring of domestic and imported foods. When adhering to GMPs, industry should be able to manufacture a product well within these tolerances. The standards or guidelines also take into consideration the injury hazard associated with certain types of extraneous material, e.g. glass in baby food or bottled beverages. When a product is in violation of a standard or guideline, the manufacturer is notified. Usually this leads to a voluntary recall of the product to the retail level. Sometimes a health alert goes out to the public and this may depend on factors such as the severity of the hazard in relation to the population at risk, and the amount of product still available to the consumer. If the health hazard is very low, the manufacturing practices may be investigated by a regulatory agency to ensure that further contamination can be minimized. In many cases more than one type of filth is found in the same product. In these situations, experience and judgement are used to evaluate the overall cleanliness and acceptability to the consumer.

Bibliography

Codex Alimentarius Commission (1981) *Code of Practice on General Principles of Food Hygiene*. Rome: Food and Agriculture Organization.

McClymont-Peace D and Gardiner MA (1990) *Extraneous Matters in Foods, Detection, Identification and Evaluation*. Quebec: Polyscience Publications.

Smith PR (1983) *Scheme for the Examination of Foreign Material Contaminants in Foods*. Leatherhead, Surrey: Leatherhead Food Research Association.

Todd ECD (1987) Legal liability and its economic impact on the food industry. *Journal of Food Protection* 50: 1048–1057.

Todd ECD (1991) *Foodborne Disease in Canada: A 10-Year Summary, 1975–1984*. Ottawa: Health Protection Branch, Health and Welfare Canada.

Mary-Ann Gardiner and Ewen Todd
Health Protection Branch, Health and Welfare Canada, Ottawa, Canada

Detection

Contaminants in foods can be grouped separately according to their origin and nature. Essentially these are microbiological (bacteria, viruses, parasites), extraneous matter (biological, chemical, physical), seafood toxins, mycotoxins, chemical compounds (pesticides, toxic metals, lubricants, fermentation products, radionuclides), packaging materials, and poisons introduced through tampering. Most of the agents found in food are accidental contaminants from environmental or industrial sources, but some are deliberate additives, including those used for tampering.

Microorganisms

Bacteria that cause foodborne disease occur worldwide, the most common being *Salmonella, Staphylococcus aureus, Clostridium perfringens* and *Bacillus cereus*. These bacteria can multiply rapidly in moist, warm protein-rich foods, such as meat, poultry, fish, shellfish, milk and eggs, and most processed food. Infectious organisms such as *Salmonella* and *C. perfringens* can multiply in the digestive tract and cause illness by invasion of the cell lining, toxin production, or both. Other organisms produce enterotoxins, e.g. *Staph. aureus* and *B. cereus*, or neurotoxins, e.g. *C. botulinum*, in the food during their growth. The staphylococcal and *Bacillus* enterotoxins are heat-resistant, as are spores of *Clostridium* and *Bacillus* species. Two new pathogens, *Listeria monocytogenes* and *Escherichia coli* 0157:H7, have caused several outbreaks of food poisoning and deaths in the last decade. *Listeria*, widespread in the environment, is present in meat, poultry, shellfish, vegetable and dairy products. Most illnesses have resulted from consumption of contaminated soft cheese. *Escherichia coli* 0157:H7 has been responsible for meat (mainly hamburger)-associated outbreaks causing haemorrhagic colitis and haemolytic uraemic syndrome. Cattle seem to be a major source of this organism and other verotoxigenic *E. coli*. Recently, *Salmonella enteritidis* has been the source of many outbreaks involving egg products in the UK and in the USA. Although many of these have occurred as a result of poor preparation and storage practices, transovarian infection from hen to egg has been identified in several studies, and thorough cooking of fresh eggs is recommended. More foodborne illnesses are caused by bacteria than any other group of agents. *See* individual organisms. *See* Food Poisoning, Tracing Origins and Testing; Food Poisoning, Statistics

In addition, some viruses are foodborne, but incidents caused by them are not well documented because of difficulties in their detection. Hepatitis A, Norwalk agent and rotavirus have been implicated, usually in sewage-contaminated shellfish. *See* Viruses

A limited number of parasites are foodborne (water-borne or person-to-person spread is more frequent) and illnesses are usually mild. *Trichinella* is found in garbage-fed pork and wild carnivores, including bears and walruses which are eaten by hunters. *Taenia saginata* and *T. solium* are widespread in beef or pigs, respectively, and up to one third of human infections of *Toxoplasma gondii* arise from contaminated meat. Parasites such as *Anisakis, Pseudoterranova* and *Diphyllo-*

bothrium, are relatively frequent in fish but rarely cause human illness. All parasites can be destroyed by thorough cooking of raw meat or fish, or frozen storage for several weeks. *See* Parasites, Occurrence and Detection; Parasites, Illness and Treatment

Extraneous Matter

Extraneous matter is foreign material entering a food during its production, storage or distribution, and can be (1) biological matter, such as insect parts, rodent excreta, animal hair, mites, nematodes and mould, (2) chemical compounds, such as oil or tar, or (3) physical materials, such as glass, metal objects, stones and string. Most of these are undesirable from an aesthetic point of view, but injuries and gastroenteritis after their consumption have also been reported. In addition, psychosomatic illnesses have been documented from people observing disgusting objects in their food. Manufacturers receive more complaints about extraneous matter than all other food-related problems.

Seafood Toxins

Some seafood toxins have been known for centuries, whereas others have been recently identified. Those of main concern are paralytic shellfish poison (saxitoxins), diarrhoeic shellfish poison (okadaic acid and related compounds), neurotoxic shellfish poison (brevetoxin), amnesic shellfish poison (domoic acid), puffer fish poison (tetrodotoxin), ciguatera poison (ciguatoxin) and scombroid poison (histamine). All but the last are accumulated in fish or shellfish through the food chain from dinoflagellates, diatoms or bacteria. All these organisms are phytoplanktonic or benthic forms of life, naturally occurring in specific areas of the marine environment. Scombroid poison is produced through the decarboxylation of histidine to histamine in certain fish through bacterial spoilage. All these toxins are resistant to normal cooking practices and are not detectable by organoleptic means. Shellfish in potentially toxic areas can be controlled by preventing harvesting until the causative dinoflagellate and diatom blooms have diminished. However, because of their sporadic occurrence and difficulty in detection, it is more difficult to prevent toxic fish from reaching the consumer. *See* Shellfish, Contamination and Spoilage of Molluscs and Crustacea

Mycotoxins

Mycotoxins are widely produced on moist crops by a variety of fungi. Poultry and livestock have been poisoned, with both acute and chronic toxic effects. However, acute poisonings, including deaths, have rarely been documented for human beings; examples of potential problems include ergotism from *Claviceps* growth on rye, alimentary toxic aleukia from *Fusarium* on cereal grains, and aflatoxicosis from *Aspergillus* contamination of maize and other grains. Since food prepared from these usually tastes bad, it is only eaten under starvation conditions. Less conclusive are links to chronic illness from aflatoxins in peanuts, other nuts and grain crops, citreoviridin in mouldy rice, and ochratoxin and zearalenone in grain, trichothecenes (vomitoxin) from winter wheat and patulin from apple juice. However, these crops are monitored and tolerance levels set because milk and meat from animals feeding on mouldy crops are potential sources of carcinogens and teratogens. There is also an indication that mild gastroenteritis can arise from beer and soft drinks in containers contaminated with adventitious moulds penetrating through small holes, e.g. punctured cans and faulty bottle tops. *See* Mycotoxins, Occurrence and Determination

Chemical Compounds

Pesticides

Pesticides are essential for obtaining good crop harvests and also for reducing certain diseases spread by insect or rodent vectors. The definition of a pesticide is a chemical agent which selectively kills target organisms or pests and is nonlethal to nontarget organisms. Pesticides include insecticides, herbicides and fungicides, in solid, liquid, aerosol or gaseous form. More recently, selective biological pesticides have been developed, e.g. spores of *Bacillus thuringiensis* (BT); these are not known to have any adverse affects against humans or domestic animals. *See* Pesticides and Herbicides, Toxicology

For approved use (registration), residue data from field trials, toxicology studies and determination of Acceptable Daily Intake (ADI) must accompany the application. The significance of pesticide residues on plant crops depends on the type and concentration used, number of applications and time from last application to crop harvest, migration in soil away from the plants, environmental degradation, plant and microbial metabolism, harvesting and storage. Lipophilic pesticides tend to be accumulated in fat deposits and this can lead to biomagnification in animals higher up the food chain, e.g. predators and humans. Animals are rarely given pesticides directly (except for control of flies on cattle, for example) but usually obtain these from drift of spray used on adjacent fields or from feed made as by-products of industrial processes.

Organochlorine Pesticides

Organochlorine pesticides were primarily designed against insects and persist in the environment. Dichlorodiphenyltrichloroethane (DDT), and hexachlorocyclohexane (HCH) have been used worldwide for over four decades against mosquitoes and other insects of public health and veterinary health significance. Because of their stability, metabolites of these and other organochloro compounds have now reached all parts of the world's surface. Fungicides such as endrin (hexachlorobenzene) have caused acute human illness and deaths from consumption of treated grain under starvation conditions. *See* Fungicides

Although many countries have banned the use of DDT, it is still of value in controlling diseases such as malaria and cotton infestation. Milk from cattle reared in these areas can be heavily contaminated, over 500 ppm. High levels can also be found in milk products, e.g. ghee, butter, cheese, and infant formula. Hexachlorocyclohexane has also been identified in milk after feed prepared from sprayed crops had been given to cattle, or insecticidal ointment had been applied directly to their skin. Some organochlorine compounds originally unconnected to agricultural use have accumulated in foods because of their long-term persistence, e.g. fish containing mirex, an ant poison and also a fire retardant in household materials.

The long-term effects of organochlorine compounds on human beings are not yet known.

Organophosphates

The next generation of pesticides were the organophosphates, e.g. parathion, malathion and diazanon. Although these are extremely toxic to animals and insects, they do not persist in the environment. They are the most widely used insecticides today. Malathion, for example, is sprayed against malaria and dengue vectors in Mexico, and residues may be found in both domestic and imported fruits and vegetables. Such food consumed raw over a long time may pose a health risk.

Carbamates

In the 1950s, the carbamate group of insecticides was developed with compounds such as carbaryl, aldicarb, baygon and zectran. Dithiocarbamates are fungicides, (e.g. ziram), nematocides (e.g. metham-sodium) and herbicides (e.g. propham). These act in a similar manner to the organophosphates, by inhibiting choline esterase, except that the action is reversible. The toxicity is generally low, with the exception of aldicarb. This last compound is absorbed from the soil systemically, with leaves and fruit accumulating the chemical. Watermelons grown on previously contaminated soil, and hydroponically grown cucumbers treated with aldicarb caused anticholinesterone symptoms in several hundred persons in several recent outbreaks in North America.

Other Pesticides

Arsenic compounds were used as pesticides in pre-World War II years and were considered toxic, but acceptable levels were not properly developed. The need for these largely disappeared with the organochlorine and organophosphate pesticides. Alkyl mercury salts, used as fungicides on seed grain, have caused human illness either through direct consumption of the grain or through meat from pigs eating the contaminated grain. Thallium salts have been used as rodenticides, but are now considered too dangerous for this purpose and are banned in many countries. Compounds derived from certain plants, e.g. rotenone and pyrethrum, are considered to have low toxicity, but have limited use against insects. Bromide fumigants, such as methylbromide, are used against insects, nematodes, viruses, weeds and fungi, and are applied directly to the soil. Crops planted on these soils, particularly lettuce, celery, tomatoes, cucumbers and strawberries, may accumulate bromine, but not enough to be a health hazard. However, when dibromoethane was found in flour and cake mixes arising from fumigation of wheat during storage, its use was banned because of its mutagenic, carcinogenic and teratogenic properties. *See* Fumigants

Pesticide Contaminants

In addition to pesticides themselves, certain impurities in formulations can be toxic; for example, acute delayed toxic effects including weight loss, red staining of mouth and nose, and pneumonia have developed from exposure to trimethylphosphorothioate (TMR) present in malathion sprays.

Nitrosamines have long been known for their carcinogenic properties in animal studies, although there have been no documented human cases. These compounds, in particular nitrosodimethylamine (NDMA), have been found as contaminants in certain pesticides, notably dinitroaniline and acidic herbicides. These nitrosamines have arisen by nitrosation of amines or amides, or during synthesis with dinitroaniline. Improved pesticide production practices have since reduced the level of these. In addition, plants do not take up these compounds readily, and the risks from contaminated food, as compared to smoking, for these carcinogens is very low. *See* Nitrosamines

Summary

Several pesticides are potentially carcinogenic or teratogenic; this statement is based on various tests including animal studies. However, human data are limited

(except perhaps for the use of the defoliant Agent Orange in Vietnam), and there is no epidemiological evidence that any pesticide is a human mutagen, carcinogen, or teratogen at normal exposure levels. Future work needs to concentrate on mechanisms of pesticide toxicity and metabolism, re-evaluation of acceptable limits, and their control in the environment. The use of pesticides will not be eliminated in the future but may be reduced; DDT and other organochlorines will remain in the environment for many years, despite the fact that their use is decreasing, and the demand for organophosphates and carbamates is increasing.

Toxic Metals

Cadmium

Cadmium is naturally present at a very low level in the environment, but large concentrations are produced as waste by-products of electroplating, rust proofing, colour tints for paint, plastic stabilizers and batteries. Effluents also arise from textile, porcelain and enamel manufacturing. When cadmium salts are released into an aquatic environment, crustaceans and fish accumulate quantities large enough to be hazardous if they are a part of the regular diet, but these are usually found in limited areas. *See* Cadmium, Toxicology

Lead

Lead is present in rocks and soil and may be accumulated in plants and transmitted to humans through the food chain, but most lead comes from atmospheric aerosols and dust particles through industrial processes and automobile emissions. Urban areas therefore contain more lead particles than rural regions. These fall on soil and are absorbed by crops. Fields near highways can have concentrations as high as 950 μg per g of soil. From there lead can reach a food source directly. Another source is lead solder in unlacquered cans; sealed cans opened for 5 days can accumulate two to eight times the original level, depending on the pH of the canned product. The demise of the Franklin expedition to the Arctic in 1845 has been at least partially attributed to the lead poisoning of the sailors fed exclusively from food in cans sealed with lead solder. Today, the use of lacquer, side-seam welds and seamless two-piece cans avoids the possibility of lead leaching from the container. Lead in glazed vessels has also contributed to human illness from prehistoric times to the present. In addition, the alimentary tract can receive lead from potable water transported by lead piping or stored in lead-lined tanks, and through the compulsive nibbling by children of paint chips containing lead, with up to 550 μg per day being accumulated. High concentrations may cause acute illness, but are more likely to be responsible for chronic damage to the central nervous system (CNS), reproductive, renal and immune systems. *See* Lead, Toxicology

Arsenic

Arsenic reaches food sources through industrial processes (atmospheric fallout and discharge into water). Most of these sources are seafood and certain crops. Several hundred micrograms are ingested every day in certain areas of the world, but now that few arsenic-based pesticides are used, chronic poisoning from arsenic is unusual.

Mercury

As previously mentioned, organomercury compounds have been used as fungicides. In the environment the most toxic form is methyl mercury, found in fish and shellfish living in water contaminated from industrial wastes and in large lakes artificially created for hydro-electric power from drowned, decaying vegetation. Acid rain also helps to mobilize industrial aerosols into water supplies. People with a regular diet of fish containing high levels of organic mercury, or shellfish with inorganic mercury, are at the greatest risk. *See* Mercury, Toxicology

Tin

Although tin can reach aquatic environments through natural sources, industrial pollution and antifouling paint on boat hulls, there is little evidence that it can cause chronic human illness. However, acid foods in tin-lined cans can dissolve enough metal to cause acute gastroenteritis. For example, several hundred parts per million can accumulate either gradually over several years of storage, or rapidly if the lid is opened and oxidation accelerates the leaching process.

Copper and Antimony

In common with tin, both copper and antimony cause problems only when acidic liquids are in contact with them. Copper pipes used in soft-drink vending machines, and antimony-lined bowls or cups have been implicated in acute illness. The speed of metal solubilization depends on the acidity of the liquids, temperature and time of exposure.

Cobalt

Only once has there been a problem with cobalt. This was when a cobalt-based antifoaming agent was added to beer in the 1960s. Some heavy drinkers in Quebec (Canada), Minnesota (USA) and Belgium received enough cobalt to develop severe heart disease (cardiomyopathy) with a high mortality rate. *See* Heavy Metal Toxicology

Lubricants

Tricresyl phosphate was developed as a hydraulic fluid and lubricant because of its stability at high temperatures. Delayed paralysis affecting the hands and feet occurred when an alcohol substitute, ginger extract, and cooking oils were adulterated in the 1930s with this compound. This was replaced by other lubricants, e.g. polychlorinated biphenyls (PCBs) and polychlorinated naphthalenes (PCNs). However, problems were also associated with these compounds. They reached cattle as a result of lubricating oils on farm machinery being licked directly by the animals or through leaks onto animal feed; the animals developed a debilitating condition, and human ingestion of milk was considered hazardous. Because of their extreme persistence in the environment, PCBs are not only banned from future use but are being removed from ageing equipment, e.g. transformers, and destroyed by incineration. Polybrominated biphenyls (PBBs) have also been accidently fed to livestock with resultant human exposure through milk and meat.

Fermentation Products

The carcinogen ethyl carbamate is a natural fermentation product in the production of wine, either through reaction of ammonia with the antimicrobial agent diethyl pyrocarbonate, or through ethanol with carbamyl phosphate. Limits of 30 μg per kg of wine and 400 μg per kg of brandy have been set to reduce the level of carbamates for human exposure. Recently, there have been over 1500 cases and 20 deaths owing to eosinophilic myalgia syndrome in the USA from tryptophan dietary supplements contaminated with derivatives of L-tryptophan. These contaminants probably arose during the fermentation process when a genetically modified strain of *Bacillus amyloliquefaciens* was used to produce the tryptophan.

Radionuclides

Radionuclides are normally present in the environment at low levels from naturally radioactive rock, but can also arise from atmospheric fallout from nuclear tests and gaseous emissions and spills from accidents at nuclear reactors. Food is one possible means of transmitting radionuclides to the human body, with a danger

Detection

for long-term carcinogenic, teratogenic, or mutagenic effects. Higher doses may also affect reproductive capability and shorten the lifespan. Radium-226 and uranium-238 are naturally occurring radioactive elements that may be at high levels in certain locations because of the underlying rock structure. Cereals are the food items that contribute the most radium-226 to our diet. Fallout from tests or accidents persists longer in arctic zones, and persons eating an exclusive meat diet, such as Lapps and Eskimos, are at highest risk from lead-210 and polonium-210. Milk and meat supply most of radionuclides, such as strontium-89, strontium-90, iodine-131 and caesium-137 to our bodies. The effect of the Chernobyl nuclear reactor explosion in the Commonwealth of Independent States is still being evaluated, but the effect of the contamination worldwide was not as high as was originally feared, although the damage to life in the immediate area of the reactor was extreme. *See* Radioactivity in Food

Packaging and Storage

Packaging can exist in various forms, from crates to wraps. Wood preservatives, such as phenols or copper arsenates and insecticides against termites, used in crates, can contaminate food during shipping through direct contact or vapours. For example, dieldrin has been found at 0·08 mg kg^{-1} on cocoa beans. Wood shavings used for packing can also transfer these chemicals to foods, or to animals if the shavings are used for bedding. In addition, food stored in rooms with walls covered with insecticidal paint, or containing pest strips from which pesticides evaporate over a long period of time, may become exposed to the chemical. Experiments have shown that strips containing dichlorovos can contaminate most home-made meals with up to 0·09 mg kg^{-1}, but lipid-type food had even higher levels, e.g. up to 0·3 mg kg^{-1} in wax-covered apples. Even pesticide-treated shelf paper can produce enough residues to penetrate packages of flour over a period of time.

Paper, cardboard, plastic wrap or aluminium foil do not keep out lindane vapours. Phosphoric acid esters as flame retardants in paper, adhesives and plastic wrappers, e.g. bread bags, margarine or butter wraps can reach food. Diffusion through these is dependent on time of contact and type of food wrapped (lipid-rich or moist foods absorb better than other foods). These retardants have a similar toxicity to organophosphorous insecticides. Exhaust from tractors in warehouses in the Arctic, where food is stored for long periods of time, has penetrated packages to cause undesirable tastes and complaints of mild illness after their consumption. Hermetically sealed containers protect food from all chemical and microbial contaminants if the process is carried out correctly.

Tampering Problems

Food has for centuries been adulterated for purposes of fraud, or poisoned for injuring or killing specified persons. More recently, commercially produced food has been tampered with for a variety of reasons, some of which are not clearly understood. The more obvious of these are product extortion to obtain money from a company or life insurance firm, attempts to ruin a company by a dissatisfied customer or disgruntled employee, attention in the media for a political cause, or as a joke to observe the reaction of those affected. Tamper-resistant and tamper-evident packaging has reduced but not eliminated these problems. *See* Adulteration of Foods, History and Occurrence; Adulteration of Foods, Detection

Bibliography

Concon JM (1988) *Food Toxicology*, parts A and B. New York: Marcel Dekker.
Doyle MP (ed.) (1989) *Foodborne Bacterial Pathogens*. New York: Marcel Dekker.
Nriagu JO and Simmons MS (eds) (1990) *Food Contamination from Environmental Sources*. New York: John Wiley.

Ewen Todd
Health Protection Branch, Health and Welfare Canada, Ottawa, Canada

Detection

CONTROLLED ATMOSPHERE STORAGE

Contents

Applications for Bulk Storage of Foodstuffs

Planting and harvesting of fruits and vegetables is controlled by season and climatological conditions in many growing areas. In addition, since the majority of the consumers of fruits and vegetables are often located far from growing areas, most crops must be stored then transported to marketplaces if demand for them is to be satisfied throughout the year and the world. Storage, because it acts to allow for the development of a consistent supply of fruits and vegetables in the marketplace year-round, results in stable marketing and financial benefits to the producers. Although the primary goal of storage is to lengthen the shelf life of crops by controlling their level of transpiration, respiration and disease/microbial infection, storage, in some cases, also improves crop quality. *See* Storage Stability, Mechanisms of Degradation

Control of Undesirable Plant Processes

Since fruits and vegetables are living tissues, their physiological processes continue after harvest and, in general, shorten the storage life of the crop. Under inadequate storage conditions, sprouting, elongation of existing structures, rooting, seed germination, greening and toughening responses have been observed. These processes can be minimized by using storage conditions which are capable of minimizing physiological processes, i.e. transpiration and respiration.

Control of Transpiration

A 5% transpiration weight loss from fruits and vegetables is sufficient to produce shrivelling, shrinkage and product loss. Reducing the rate of transpiration in these foods can be achieved by maintaining low temperatures, high relative humidities and small vapour pressure differences during storage.

Control of Respiration

Respiration is a catabolic process which can indirectly affect the transpiration rate. Respiration, if allowed to occur to any extent, produces heat, thus affecting the temperature of the product. The control of respiration can be achieved, to a limited degree, by controlling temperature through refrigeration. However, many fruits, such as melons, peppers, cucumbers, etc., cannot be stored for long periods of time under refrigeration because of their susceptibility to chill injury. Respiration can also be controlled by altering the gaseous environment during storage.

Pioneering work by Kidd and West (1927) led to the development of controlled atmosphere (CA) storage, a sophisticated technique that can extend the life of some produce by controlling the gases within the storage environment. In present-day postharvest handling of fruits and vegetables, CA storage is usually used in conjunction with refrigeration. The first studies regarding fruit preservation in a gaseous medium were carried out in an atmosphere consisting of more carbon dioxide and less oxygen than is normally present in the air. Carbon dioxide played the dominant role, and that is why the method is also called the carbon dioxide preservation method. Increased carbon dioxide in the atmosphere helps to slow down the respiration rate of living tissues of fruits and vegetables and extends the length of time of their usability.

CA storage has been proven to be good for vegetables such as cauliflower, asparagus and broccoli. Among vegetables, artichokes may be held in 3% carbon dioxide and 3% oxygen, asparagus in 7 ± 2% carbon dioxide, broccoli in 5–20% carbon dioxide, cabbage in 1–2·5% oxygen and 5·5% carbon dioxide, carrots in 1–2% oxygen at 2°C, okra in 10–12% carbon dioxide at 7·2°C, radish in 1–2% oxygen level at 5 or 10°C, tomatoes in 3% oxygen without carbon dioxide at 12·8°C, and lima beans can be stored at high levels of carbon dioxide.

One of the principal commercial fruits with which CA storage has been used successfully is apples. Because many varieties may be injured by long-term storage at −1·1 to 0°C, a combination of low oxygen (2–3%) and high carbon dioxide (1–8%), depending on variety, combined with temperatures of 2·2–4·4°C permits extended storage of cold-sensitive apple varieties.

It has been reported that equal amounts of oxygen and carbon dioxide (5%) at 11·7°C were suitable for Gros Michel bananas held for 20 days. Lacatan and

Dwarf Cavendish bananas were effectively stored for 3 weeks using CA storage conditions of 6–8% carbon dioxide and 2% oxygen at 15–15·5°C. A mixture of 8% oxygen and 12% carbon dioxide was reported to be effective for oranges, 5% oxygen and 7% carbon dioxide for lemons, 2–3 to 18% carbon dioxide and 10·0–19·0% oxygen for lychee nuts, 5% oxygen and carbon dioxide at 12·7–14·4°C for mango, and 10% carbon dioxide at 18·3°C for papayas. However, different studies have shown great variation in the effective combinations and ranges of gases used in CA storage of both fruits and vegetables.

Control of Ripening

Fruits can be divided into two categories based on their ripening physiology. Some fruits, such as apples, tomatoes and bananas, are referred to as climacteric; while other fruits, such as oranges, grapes and pineapples, are nonclimacteric. One way these two types of fruits are distinguished is by their response to the gas ethylene. Climacteric fruits when exposed to ethylene exhibit a respiration surge/climax which is coincident with their ripening, while nonclimacteric fruits do not have a respiration climax and show no ripening changes. Also, during ripening, climacteric fruits produce and release ethylene into the atmosphere. Ripening in climacteric fruits hastens their transition into senescence and, therefore, shortens their storage life. Therefore, in order to prolong the storage life of climacteric fruits, it is important to control the level of ethylene in the environment. *See* Ripening of Fruit

Present knowledge of the role of ethylene in CA storage is still incomplete. However, there is evidence that ethylene synthesis may be inhibited at low oxygen concentrations and ethylene action may be blocked or modified by high carbon dioxide and/or low oxygen concentrations. Maintenance of ethylene concentrations of <1 μl per litre in CA storage delays fruit softening and other ripening changes, including the development of disorders, such as superficial scald and bitter pit in apples, both of which are also markedly influenced by preharvest factors and maturity. It is clear that the potential for disorder development, which would be readily manifest in air or refrigerated storage, can be modified significantly by storage in conditions that induce markedly reduced ethylene production rates and/or prevent build up of ethylene in the storage atmosphere.

Carbon monoxide has also been used in CA storage. Carbon monoxide is an air pollutant that is hazardous to humans and can detrimentally affect vegetable crops before and after harvest because of its ethylene-mimicking capabilities. In a study, carbon monoxide added to air, or 2% oxygen, reduced the respiration rate of head

lettuce during storage at 2–5°C. Carbon monoxide can stimulate carbon dioxide and ethylene production by climacteric fruits, but has little effect on respiration rates of nonclimacteric fruits, such as strawberries. However, it has been reported that a combination of 4% oxygen, 2% carbon dioxide and 5% carbon monoxide may be optimal for delaying maturation and ripening, maintaining good quality and retarding decay during storage of mature green tomatoes at 12·7°C. It has also been found that packaging precut vegetables, i.e. lettuce, cabbage, celery, broccoli, cauliflower, parsley and green onions, in 1·5 mil (a mil is a full unit used for thickness), polyethylene bags and modifying the atmosphere within these packages to include 25–50% oxygen and 3–10% carbon monoxide retarded brown discoloration. Carbon monoxide has also been shown to prevent browning of mushrooms by inhibiting polyphenol oxidase activity.

Many investigations have shown that the basic advantages of preserving produce with CA storage are as follows:

(1) Reduction of low-temperature diseases, such as chill injury, encountered in certain varieties of apples and other fruits during refrigeration.
(2) Reduction of microbial infection and pest infestation of fruits and vegetables which are frequently encountered when stored in conventional storage.
(3) Taste and aroma are preserved better.
(4) Consistency (texture) of fruits are preserved better.
(5) Losses under CA storage are half to one-third, while the period of preservation is significantly longer than when kept in an uncontrolled atmosphere.

However, each fruit or vegetable, and even each variety, may differ in their reaction to changes in the composition of the atmosphere. Therefore, different gaseous regimes may be required for different commodities, depending on their physiological processes.

Control of Microorganisms

Fruits and vegetables contain water and other solutes which are utilized by microorganisms deposited on their surfaces during the growing season. Most of the microorganisms are opportunist, invading the tissue as it matures, particularly if the crops are stored under conditions of high temperature and humidity. Although fungi and bacteria cause substantial losses in vegetables and soft fruits, most losses are caused by moulds since the inherent acid conditions of the product retard bacterial growth. *See* Spoilage, Bacterial Spoilage; Spoilage, Moulds in Food Spoilage

It is difficult to determine the full extent of postharvest losses due to microorganisms; however, conservative estimates place US losses at around 24% of the harvested crop of fruits and vegetables. Worldwide, post-harvest losses have been estimated to be 50% of the harvested crop, and much of this is due to rot caused by microbes.

Fruits and vegetables, are frequently washed with recirculating water after harvest. This water is often contaminated with soft rot bacteria and fungi due to the recirculation and will contaminate fresh commodities. Therefore, an effective concentration of a broad-spectrum antimicrobial agent should be maintained in water used for handling fruits and vegetables in order to kill introduced pathogens. Chlorine and sodium orthophenylphenol (SOPP) have been used for this purpose. Bananas are generally surface contaminated with several fungi, i.e. *Cephalosporium*, *Gloeosporium*, *Fusarium* and *Verticillium* species, which may cause crown rot during marketing. These fungi can be killed by an exposure of 1 min to 2 ppm chlorine in water.

Care must also be taken in properly maintaining the storage environment of fruits as a means of controlling microbial losses. Rooms used for ripening bananas, degreening citrus fruits, and refrigerated storage can become heavily infested with spores of pathogenic fungi. These rooms may be disinfected easily and economically by atomizing a water solution containing 1% formaldehyde or 5% sodium hypochlorite into the atmosphere and closing the room for a few hours. Gaseous nitrogen trichloride and sulphur dioxide have also been used to disinfect lemon and grape storage rooms, respectively.

Brief heat treatments have been most successful in eradicating latent or incipient fungal infections in several fruits. Hot water is the best heat transfer medium because of availability, heat capacity and lack of residue on the fruit. Hot water has been advocated for control of *Penicillium* and *Diplodia* species on oranges, *Colletotrichum* species on papaya and mango, and crown rot of banana. Gamma-irradiation is the only treatment that has shown promising results for true therapy of established infections, but its use is limited due to low consumer acceptance of the technology. Overall, low-temperature storage is the most effective and useful method for delaying the development of postharvest decay in fruit and vegetables with deep-seated infections.

Infection may also be prevented by the use of fungicides before harvest or before storage. Many weak acids, such as benzoic, sorbic, propionic, acetic, nitrous or sulphurous acid, are used to control moulds in foods and stored products. *See* Fungicides

Biological control of postharvest diseases is a newly emerging area of research. *Trichoderma viride* applied to strawberry plants partially controlled grey mould caused by *Botrytis cinerea* on strawberry fruits after harvest. Brown rot of peach has been controlled by *Bacillus subtilis*.

A storage atmosphere that has been modified by reducing the oxygen level and increasing the carbon dioxide level can influence the development of postharvest diseases either by direct inhibition of the pathogen or by altering the resistance of the host. It has been found that 30–40% carbon dioxide in the storage atmosphere inhibited the development of several pathogenic fungi on temperate zone fruits. Tropical fruits may be less tolerant to high levels of carbon dioxide; it has been reported that the Alphonso mango is injured by storage for several days in 10% carbon dioxide. Papayas and pineapples have benefitted slightly from storage in low-oxygen atmospheres. While an atmosphere of 1% oxygen and 99% nitrogen inhibited ripening in peaches, green bananas and tomatoes and less decay was observed. It must be emphasized that fungicide-impregnated wrappers usually do not prevent decay of infected fruit, but may prevent the spread of disease to adjacent sound fruits.

The most commonly used gas combination is 5% carbon dioxide and 3% oxygen, a mixture which provides good storage conditions, along with low temperatures (0–4·4°C). Dry ice can be used to increase the carbon dioxide content to 10%–45% during transit or short-time storage. Such treatment is beneficial for sweet cherries, strawberries, raspberries and some other products, the carbon dioxide has strong antiseptic properties, retards decay and helps to maintain a fresh appearance.

Among vapour treatments, sulphite fumigation is a standard practice for control of decay of grapes in storage, but it is injurious to most other fruits and vegetables. Biphenyl pads have been used to control decay in packages of some citrus fruits. *See* Fumigants

Ozone in low concentrations is sometimes used as a deodorizing agent but extreme caution must be taken as it is harmful to humans. Sodium orthophenylphenate is frequently used as an antiseptic wash or in a wax on several crops including citrus fruits, pears, sweet cherries and sweet potatoes.

Control of Insect Pests

Insect pests along with fungal and bacterial diseases and spoilage are responsible for much storage loss that causes extensive economic losses. Many insects are found associated with fruits and vegetables. Various control methods are available for these pests, such as hygiene and cultural control, physical control, physical barrier, chemical control and biological control. *See* Insect Pests, Insects and Related Pests; Insect Pests, Problems Caused by Insects and Mites

Use of Fumigants

Typical fumigation procedures expose the fruit, at ambient or near ambient temperatures, for several hours to methyl bromide or ethylene dibromide at concentrations of 45 g to a few kilograms per 1000 m³ of air space in air-tight chambers. The fumigants are highly toxic and their residues can pose an additional problem in the use of chemical fumigants.

Use of Gas Control

The observed increased mortality of San Jose scale on apples in CA storage was thought to be a consequence of either the higher carbon dioxide or lower oxygen in the atmosphere. Similar biocidal effects with mites on apples under CA storage have been observed. Treatment of European red mite on Delicious and Spartan apples with close to 100% carbon dioxide or nitrogen at 21–24°C provided a 100% kill in 2 days. A mixture of 60% carbon dioxide with nitrogen was equally effective, but 60% carbon dioxide with air provided no mite mortality even after 7 days of exposure. This indicated that the biocidal effect resulted from low oxygen. The effects of carbon dioxide were also more or less the same on a number of other insects of economic importance.

The codling moth is also sensitive to high carbon dioxide and low oxygen. The possible phytotoxicity caused by such an atmosphere indicated a potential for using high levels of carbon dioxide on some apple cultivars. Laboratory tests have shown the effects of high carbon dioxide (60%) and low oxygen (0·5%) atmospheres, applied at 25°C and at relative humidities of 60 and 95%, as reducing the amount of time required for codling moth mortality.

Design of Storage Areas

Fruits and vegetables can be stored in a CA most effectively in special chambers. These chambers are equipped with a cooling system, devices for creating the necessary gas composition, and devices for controlling and regulating relative humidity. In addition, they generally also have a system which monitors and records the conditions in the chamber over time.

Volume Planning Decisions

The requirements which should be kept in mind before planning of storage chambers are the level of produce loading which can be expected, the distribution of temperature and gases in the mass of produce, and the geometry and parameters of the chambers. If the chambers have very high loads, then it will be difficult to obtain a gas mixture of the required composition to maintain CA. It has been shown that produce must be loaded in a continuous stack with a minimum gap

between them and the walls. For instance, in the UK the standard distance between boxes in the stack is 0·5 cm. When loading containers in the chambers, the gap between them is 2·5 cm; in the case of boxes on racks, the gap between them is 5 cm. In all cases, the gap between the stack of produce and the enclosure wall is 2·5 cm. At the same time, it must be considered that these chambers should be economical. Studies in the USSR have shown that, from the viewpoint of minimum cost of enclosures, chambers with a height up to 5·4 m are considered to be economical. In other countries this value is 4·0–4·8 m (UK), and 5·6–6·6 m (USA, Italy, France).

Modern CA fruit storage areas consists of individual chambers having load capacities of 50–150 tonnes, or more. Volume planning designs regarding these chambers are generally made on the basis of following considerations:

(1) the specific volume of the chamber must be 4–5 m³ tonne⁻¹;
(2) the size of chambers must correspond to the size of boxes;
(3) the chamber net height must be in the range 4·8–5·4 m;
(4) when arranging the produce in chambers, a gap of 1–2 cm for boxes and 5–10 cm for trays should be maintained;
(5) the minimum capacity of chambers should be about 30–50 tonnes;
(6) the arrangement of internal engineering equipment in the chamber must ensure its optimum specific volume; and
(7) the most rational plans will be chambers measuring 6 × 6 m, 6 × 12 m and 12 × 12 m with a net height of 4·8–5·4 m.

Hermetic Sealing and Gas Insulation

To maintain the desired gas mixtures it is necessary that chambers be airtight, and because of the cost of airtight insulation of partition walls, these chambers should not be very high. Another important factor is the selection of the gas-impermeable material used for construction of the chambers. The most reliable gas insulation materials are galvanized iron sheets, aluminum foil covered with asphalt on one or both sides, vinyl-based resins, polyester and epoxy resins, reinforced fibre glass, and asphalt matriced with rubber. Besides these, plastic sheets, gas-impermeable varnish, paints, etc., have also been used. Galvanized iron sheets and aluminum foil covered with asphalt are the materials which are used most widely in Italy, the USA and the UK.

The most difficult places to design in chambers with a CA are the joints between walls, ceiling and floors and inlets and outlets of pipelines in the building. Doors lined with galvanized iron sheet on both the inner and outer sides have been used. The cost of these insulated doors comes to about 11–14% of the total cost of construction of the storage facility.

At present, there is no unanimous opinion on how to make cold storages airtight for storing fruits and vegetables under CA conditions. Research is in progress studying the hermetic sealing of the chambers in order to find more economical and reliable gas insulation materials and methods for sealing the walls of chambers.

Bibliography

Eckert JW (1975) Postharvest physiology. Part 1. General principles. In: Pantastico EB (ed.) *Postharvest Physiology, Handling and Utilization of Tropical and Subtropical Fruits and Vegetables*, pp 393–394. Westport: AVI.

Eckert JW (1978) Pathological diseases of fresh fruits and vegetables. In Hutlin HO and Milner M (eds) *Postharvest Biology and Biotechnology*, pp 161–209. Westport: Food and Nutrition Press.

Kader AA (1987) Effects of adding CO to controlled atmospheres. In: Weichman J (ed.) *Vegetables and Postharvest Physiology* pp 277–284. New York: Marcel Dekker.

Metlitskii EG, Sal'kova EG, Volkind NL, Bondarev VI and Yanyuk VYa (1972) *Controlled Atmosphere Storage of Fruits*, pp 150. Moscow: E'konomika.

Soderstrom EL and Brandl DG (1985) Controlled atmospheres to reduce post harvest insect damage to horticultural crops. *Proceedings of the 4th National Controlled Atmosphere Research Council*, pp 207–212.

Jyoti Saxena, S.L. Cuppett and L.B. Bullerman
University of Nebraska-Lincoln, Lincoln, USA

Effect on Fruit and Vegetables

The composition of gases in the storage atmosphere of fruit and vegetables can affect their storage life. Controlled-atmosphere storage (CAS) usually refers to the reduction of oxygen (O_2) and the elevation of carbon dioxide (CO_2), in comparison with the ambient atmosphere, and sometimes includes the removal of ethylene (C_2H_4) or the addition of carbon monoxide (CO). Controlled-atmosphere storage implies continuous and precise control of these gases, whereas the term 'modified-atmosphere storage' (MAS) is used when the composition of the storage atmosphere is not actively controlled, e.g. in plastic film packaging. *See* Chilled Storage, Use of Modified Atmosphere Packaging

The scientific basis of CAS was originally established in England by F Kidd and C West in the early twentieth century. It is the most advanced method for the storage of fruit and vegetables. If CAS is carried out appropriately, the product so stored will maintain its freshness and eating quality for a significantly longer time (usually at least twice as long) than it would if stored at the same temperature in the air.

This article will review the physiological changes that occur in stored produce under high CO_2 and low O_2 conditions.

Gaseous Atmosphere in Commercial Use

Recommended CA conditions during storage and transport are summarized in Table 1, which also shows an estimate of the potential benefits and extent of current commercial use. Originally, it was hoped that CAS could replace refrigeration, but it is now generally used as an adjunct to low temperatures to obtain additional benefits. Generally speaking, CA has its most beneficial effects on climacteric fruits at the preclimacteric stage by prolonging this period. The effects are less marked in climacteric fruits at the ripening stage, and in nonclimacteric fruits. For example, in green bananas, the storage life can be increased 12-fold in an atmosphere of 5% CO_2, 3% O_2, and 92% nitrogen (N_2) in the absence of C_2H_4, compared with air storage. Climacteric fruits are sensitive to C_2H_4, so that its removal is recommended for long-term CAS. *See* individual fruits and vegetables *See* Ripening of Fruit

The commercial adoption of CA or MA storage for a given kind of produce depends on the balance between cost and benefits, because control of the gas composition is expensive. The major commercial application of CA has been confined to some apple and pear cultivars; MA has been used successfully for the storage and transport of some fruits and vegetables.

In general, the lower the O_2 level and the higher the CO_2 level, the more CA effects such as retardation of ripening and senescence can be anticipated. However, the reduction of the O_2 level and the elevation of the CO_2 level are limited by shift from aerobic to anaerobic metabolism, which results in off-flavours or odours. Excess CO_2 induces and aggravates specific physiological disorders such as black heart in potatoes, brown stain on lettuce, and brown heart in apples and pears. The optimum CA conditions depend on the kind of produce, cultivar, maturity, season of harvest, and temperature and duration of storage. About 2% O_2 is the lower limit tolerated by most fruit and vegetables, and CO_2 build-up to concentrations above about 5–10% should be avoided in long-term storage. When exposure time is short, some horticultural crops might be tolerant of more extreme CA conditions ($<1\%$ O_2, $>20\%$ CO_2) than are normally used. Some recent tests have shown such extreme conditions to be a possible method for the control of pest and fungi for some produce. Short-term treatment with high CO_2 (10–20%) before CAS has beneficial effects on the storage life of a few kinds of fruits. *See* Storage Stability, Parameters Affecting Storage Stability

Table 1. Summary of recommended CA or MA conditions during storage and transport of selected fruit and vegetables

Produce	Temperature (°C)	CA O$_2$ (%)	CO$_2$ (%)	Potential for benefit[a]	Remarks[b]
Climacteric fruits					
Apple	0–5	2–3	1–2	A	About 40% of production is stored under CA in USA
Banana	12–15	2–5	2–5	A	Some commercial use
Kiwifruit	0–5	2	5	A	Some commercial use
Pear	0–5	2–3	0–1	A	Some commercial use
Persimmon	0–5	5	5–8	A	Some commercial use in Japan
Avocado	5–13	2–5	3–10	B	Limited commercial use
Peach	0–5	1–2	5	B	Limited commercial use
Plum and prune	0–5	1–2	0–5	B	No commercial use
Tomato	8–12	3–5	0	B	Limited commercial use
Nonclimacteric fruits					
Lemon	10–15	5	0–5	B	No commercial use
Orange	5–10	10	5	C	No commercial use
Grapefruit	10–15	3–10	5–10	C	No commercial use
Grape	0–5	None	None	D	Incompatible with sulphur dioxide fumigation
Strawberry	0–5	10	15–20	A	Increasing use during transit
Nuts and dried fruits	0–25	0–1	0–100	A	Effective for insect control method
Vegetables					
Asparagus	0–5	Air	5–10	B	Limited commercial use
Broccoli	0–5	1–2	5–10	B	Limited commercial use
Cabbage	0–5	3–5	5–7	B	Some commercial use
Lettuce	0–5	2–5	0	B	Some commercial use with 2–3% CO added
Cauliflower	0–5	2–5	2–5	C	No commercial use
Cucumber	8–12	3–5	0	C	No commercial use
Onion, green	0–5	1–2	10–20	C	Limited commercial use
Spinach	0–5	Air	10–20	C	No commercial use
Potato	4–12	None	None	D	No commercial use
Carrot	0–5	None	None	D	Relative humidity of 98–100% is best

Source: Kader AA (1985).
[a] A, excellent; B, good; C, fair; D, slight or none.
[b] A relative humidity of 90–95% is recommended unless otherwise indicated.

Influences of Storage Gases on the Respiratory and Other Metabolic Activities in Plant Tissues

Effects of Low O$_2$

The effects of the O$_2$ concentration on the respiration rate of plant tissues are shown in Fig. 1. If the O$_2$ concentration of the storage atmosphere is reduced, below 8% in particular, the respiration rate decreases as a function of the O$_2$ concentration. When the O$_2$ concentration drops to the extinction point, anaerobic respiration begins. As the concentration of O$_2$ further decreases, anaerobic respiration becomes predominant, and the CO$_2$ output starts to increase after it reaches its lowest value at the critical O$_2$ concentration. At O$_2$ concentrations below the critical point, the glycolytic pathway replaces the Krebs cycle as the main source of

the energy needed by the plant tissues. Pyruvic acid is no longer oxidized but is decarboxylated to form acetaldehyde, CO$_2$ and, ultimately, ethanol; this results in the development of off-flavours and tissue breakdown. Thus the minimum O$_2$ level needed to ensure aerobic metabolism and help to prevent fermentation is optimum for the storage atmosphere. This concentration depends on the kind of produce, temperature and duration of storage, etc., but it is usually 2–5%.

The decrease in O$_2$ uptake in response to reduced O$_2$ levels when not less than about 2% is not the result of suppression of the basal metabolism mediated by cytochrome oxidase, for which the K_m is 10^{-8}–10^{-7} M O$_2$. That is, the storage atmosphere must contain less than 2% O$_2$ for the activity of cytochrome oxidase to be affected. The decrease in the O$_2$ uptake stems from the decrease in the activity of other oxidases, e.g. polyphenol oxidase, ascorbic acid oxidase, and glycolic acid

Effect on Fruit and Vegetables

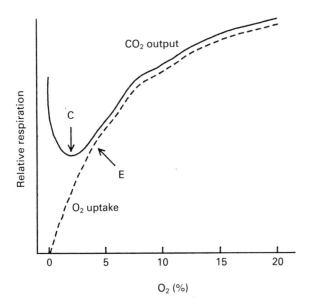

Fig. 1 Schematic diagram of the effects of the O_2 concentration in O_2 uptake and CO_2 evolution by harvested crops. E, extinction point: the lowest concentraton of O_2 at which all aerobic respiration ceases. C, critical O_2 concentration: the O_2 concentration at which CO_2 production is lowest.

oxidase; their affinity for O_2 may be about 20% of that of cytochrome oxidase. The development of fermentation under lower O_2 levels does not depend on the increase in the activities of pyruvate decarboxylase and alcohol dehydrogenase, because these enzymes are often active before exposure to low O_2 levels.

Beneficial aspects of a low-O_2 atmosphere also depend on the effects of the atmosphere on the biosynthesis and action of C_2H_4, which is closely related to the ripening and senescence of harvested crops. The final step of C_2H_4 biosynthesis, catalysed by an ethylene-forming enzyme, is shown in eqn [1].

$$1\text{-aminocyclopropane-1-carboxylic acid} + \tfrac{1}{2}O_2 \rightarrow \quad (1)$$
$$C_2H_4 + CO_2 + HCN + H_2O$$

The concentration of O_2 that gives half the maximum C_2H_4 production rate ranges between 5% and 7% in various tissues, so that the 2–5% atmosphere usually used in CAS directly interferes with C_2H_4 synthesis. The action of C_2H_4 on plant tissues at 3% O_2 is about 50% of that in the air.

Effects of High CO_2

Most researchers have believed that the respiration rate would decrease as the CO_2 concentration in the atmosphere increases, because CO_2 is a product of respiration. However, recent studies raise doubts about this assumption.

Studies of the effects of a high-CO_2 atmosphere on glycolytic intermediates and enzymes in pears have shown that fructose 6-phosphate accumulates and fructose 1,6-diphosphate decreases because the activity of phosphofructokinase, one of the key enzymes of glycolysis, is inhibited. In the Krebs cycle, exposure to high CO_2 levels causes the accumulation of succinic acid in several crops, including apples, pears, lettuce, and podded pea, and reduces succinic dehydrogenase activity in pears. In studies of mitochondria isolated from apples, treatment with high levels of CO_2 suppresses the oxidation of several intermediates of the Krebs cycle. With a high-CO_2 atmosphere, even if there is sufficient O_2, several crops form aldehyde and ethanol; this phenomenon is called 'CO_2 zymasis'. These findings are indirect evidence of a shift from aerobic to anaerobic metabolism with a high-CO_2 atmosphere, as also occurs with low O_2 levels.

The results of measurement of O_2 uptake in climacteric fruits, such as bananas and avocados, show that without affecting the respiratory activity before the climacteric, a high-CO_2 atmosphere delays the onset of the climacteric rise (Fig. 2), triggered by endogenous C_2H_4. These results suggest that a high-CO_2 atmosphere delays the burst of C_2H_4. Depression of O_2 uptake by high CO_2 has not been found in nonclimacteric fruits, such as citrus, grapes and Japanese pears, or in most vegetables; it occurs only in ripening climacteric fruits and broccoli, accompanied by inhibition of C_2H_4 synthesis. Furthermore, in some crops susceptible to high CO_2 levels, e.g. lettuce, cucumber and lemons, the opposite effect has been reported, that of elevation of O_2 uptake with induction of C_2H_4 synthesis by exposure to CO_2 at levels of 10% CO_2 or more. These observations indicate that the respiratory response of crops to high CO_2 levels might be mediated mainly by the effect of CO_2 on the synthesis or action, or both, of C_2H_4. In other words, retardation of ripening or senescence and associated biochemical and physiological changes caused by high CO_2 levels depend on the effect of the CO_2 concentrations on the action or synthesis of C_2H_4 rather than on any direct effect on the respiratory metabolism.

Dark fixation of CO_2, which might be mediated by phospho(enol) pyruvate carboxylase or $NADP^+$ (the oxidized form of nicotinamide adenine dinucleotide phosphate) malic enzyme, has been found in studies of $^{14}CO_2$ in lemons, stored in a CO_2-enriched atmosphere. This phenomenon is also observed in apples, pears and persimmons. The incorporated $^{14}CO_2$ is mostly taken up into malate, with a lesser amount being taken up into other carboxylic acids and amino acids. This incorporation of CO_2 by harvested crops might be involved in a disturbed metabolism of organic acids, resulting in the accumulation of succinic acid, development of fermentation, and increased retention of acidity, discussed above.

Effect on Fruit and Vegetables

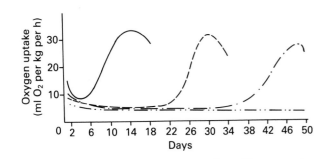

Fig. 2 Effects of CO_2 on the respiration of bananas at a constant O_2 tension. —— Air; – – – 10% O_2; – · – · – 10% O_2 plus 5% CO_2; – ·· – ·· – 10% O_2 plus 10% CO_2. Data from Biale (1960).

A high-CO_2 atmosphere prevents or delays many responses of crops to C_2H_4, such as fruit ripening, abscission, growth inhibition, floral senescence, and the induction of some enzymes. A comprehensive study of the effect of CO_2 in reversing the action of C_2H_4 in growth of pea segments has suggested that CO_2 competes with C_2H_4 for binding sites, and that the relative affinity of the site for 15% CO_2 is equivalent to that for 1 ppm C_2H_4. However, the calculation of the binding of the site with radioactive C_2H_4 suggests that the inhibition of C_2H_4 binding is indirect or due to secondary effects such as pH changes.

Carbon dioxide is dissolved easily in plant tissues by the dissociation of carbonic acid into bicarbonate and hydrogen ion; it has therefore been generally assumed that exposure to high CO_2 levels would lower the pH in the tissue. However, reported measurements of pH changes in several plant tissues stored in a high-CO_2 atmosphere have been contradictory. A nuclear magnetic resonance (NMR) study of intact lettuce tissue exposed to 15% CO_2 for 6 days showed a drop of about 0·4 and 0·1 pH unit in the cytoplasm and vacuoles, respectively. Assays of a tissue homogenate or juice extracted from a crop exposed to high CO_2 levels have shown increased pH. As any change in the pH in plant cells might affect most metabolic activities, the effect of CO_2 on the pH could be included in both the beneficial and harmful aspects of high CO_2 conditions for harvested crops. The significance of pH changes under CA conditions is not yet fully understood. *See* pH – Principles and Measurement

Effects of CAS on Quality for the Consumer

Texture

In general, CAS effectively helps to maintain the desirable texture of apples, because of the delay in ripening described earlier. Retention of firmness is one

of the most important advantages of the commercial CAS of apples. This advantage has been obtained with other climacteric fruits, including pears, peaches, apricots and tomatoes. High CO_2 and low O_2 conditions both contribute to the retention of flesh firmness in these fruits. The effect of high CO_2 levels is more prominent than that of low O_2 levels and sometimes becomes noticeable after the transfer of those fruits to air. The induction of polygalacturonase, a key enzyme in the degradation of pectic substances, is prevented by the storage of mature green tomatoes in 5% O_2 and 5% CO_2 for up to 8 weeks at 12·5°C. On removal of the tomatoes to the air, polygalacturonase is synthesized, and fruit softening resumes. In kiwi fruit, retention of fruit firmness is better in CAS, but contaminating C_2H_4, even if at a very low level, counteracts this positive effect.

The textures of most other fruits and vegetables are influenced little, if at all, by low O_2 conditions. Some positive effects have been reported for high CO_2 conditions, such as a delay in the softening rate of strawberries and bush-type berries and the retardation of the toughening of asparagus spears, cauliflower, and snap beans.

Flavour

Changes in organic acids, carbohydrates, volatile compounds and other components can affect the flavour of harvested crops. Most reports agree that CAS delays normal losses of acidity and the decomposition of starch to sugar during apple storage, provided that the concentrations of CO_2 and O_2 are suitable. Similar effects have been obtained in other climacteric fruits, including pears, tomatoes, and kiwi fruit. The organic acids, especially malic acid, of apples are retained better, if favourable CA conditions are reached quickly. However, if the CO_2 level reaches 3%, loss of acidity is sometimes stimulated in these fruits. Leafy vegetables, such as lettuce, spinach and broccoli, always contain higher amounts of titratable acid after storage in the air than after storage in a CA. *See* Flavour Compounds, Structures and Characteristics

In some nonclimacteric fruits and vegetables, undesirable changes in carbohydrates such as starch-to-sugar conversion in potatoes, sugar-to-starch conversion in peas and sweet corn, and acidity losses in sweet cherries are delayed by CAS.

Controlled-atmosphere storage can decrease the production rate of volatile compounds such as alcohols, aldehydes and esters; sometimes, as a result, the characteristic desirable aroma of the produce is reduced. Off-flavours and off-tastes can develop in any produce if it is exposed to unfavourable O_2 or CO_2 concentrations, especially for a long time. For example, more than 15% CO_2 easily induces odours in broccoli and cauliflower.

Ascorbic Acid

The nutritional significance of ascorbic acid makes the effect of CAS upon its retention in produce of special interest. In general, a low-O_2 atmosphere is favourble to the retention of ascorbic acid because of the low affinity of ascorbic acid oxidase to O_2. On the other hand, the effects of high CO_2 are not clear-cut; they are sometimes dual, depending on the kind of produce, storage temperature, and concentration of CO_2. For example, the degradation of ascorbic acid in parsley leaves is retarded with storage in 4·2% O_2 and 1% CO_2 compared with storage in the air, but it is accelerated with storage in 4·2% O_2 and 6% CO_2. Slightly elevated CO_2 (<3%) sometimes retards the loss of ascorbic acid, but higher CO_2 (>5%) greatly stimulates it. *See* Ascorbic Acid, Physiology

Colour

Improved retention of their green colour, mainly because of reduced breakdown of chlorophyll, is one characteristic of plants stored under CA conditions. High CO_2 concentrations in particular preserve the chlorophyll content. The effect is obvious in green vegetables such as spinach, asparagus spears, broccoli and snap beans, and in green citrus fruit such as limes. Pigment biosynthesis that accompanies fruit ripening, such as lycopene in tomatoes and anthocyanin in plums, is slowed down by CA conditions. *See* Chlorophyll; Colours, Properties and Determination of Natural Pigments

Growth and Development

Controlled-atmosphere conditions help to prevent undesirable sprouting and rooting in onions, garlic, and other root crops. The sprouting of potatoes is inhibited by 15% CO_2 at 10°C, but is encouraged by 2–5% CO_2 or 2–4% O_2. Concentrations of CO_2 greater than 5% inhibit the elongation of asparagus spears, and the growth and cap opening of mushrooms.

Pathological Breakdown

The onset of ripening in climacteric fruit, and senescence in all produce, render them susceptible to infection by pathogens. Controlled-atmosphere conditions delay the ripening of climacteric fruits and the senescence of some vegetables; consequently, such produce retain greater resistance to post-harvest diseases.

Oxygen levels below 1% or CO_2 levels above 20% directly suppress fungus growth and spore germination. These extreme conditions can induce physiological breakdown in most produce, but some crops may tolerate these conditions for a short time. Carbon dioxide at a concentration of 10–20% has been used successfully with strawberries to suppress *Botrytis cinerea*, and with sweet cherries to suppress *Monilinia fructicola* and *B. cinerea* during transit periods of up to 8–10 days. Similar effects have been obtained in fresh figs. *See* Spoilage, Bacterial Spoilage; Spoilage, Moulds in Food Spoilage

Bibliography

Biale JB (1960) The postharvest biochemistry of tropical and subtropical fruits. *Advances in Food Research* 10: 293–354.

El-Goorani MA and Sommer NF (1981) Effects of modified atmospheres on postharvest pathogens of fruits and vegetables. *Horticultural Review* 3: 412–461.

Isenberg FMR (1979) Controlled atmosphere storage of vegetables. *Horticultural Review* 1: 337–394.

Kader AA (ed.) (1985) *Postharvest Technology of Horticultural Crops.* pp 58–64. University of California, Oakland: Division of Agriculture and Natural Resources Publications.

Kader AA (1986) Biochemical and physiological basis for effects of controlled and modified atmospheres on fruits and vegetables. *Food Technology* 40: 99–104.

Smith WH (1963) The use of carbon dioxide in the transport and storage of fruits and vegetables. *Advances in Food Research* 12: 95–146.

Smock RM (1979) Controlled atmosphere storage of fruits. *Horticultural Review* 1: 301–336.

Weichmann J (1986) The effect of controlled-atmosphere storage on the sensory and nutritional quality of fruits and vegetables. *Horticultural Review* 8: 101–127.

Wills RBH, Lee TH, Graham D, McGlasson WB and Hall EG (1981) *Postharvest: An Introduction to the Physiology and Handling of Fruit and Vegetables.* Kensington, Australia: New South Wales University Press.

Y. Kubo
Okayama University, Okayama, Japan

CONVENIENCE FOODS

Convenience foods may be broadly defined as foods that have undergone major processing by the manufacturer such that they require little or no secondary processing or cooking before consumption. This means that apart from heating, regeneration or rehydration the food is 'ready to eat'. A food may be classified as convenience food if it meets the following criteria:

1. The food must have undergone a considerable amount of food preparation by the manufacturer before it reaches the retailer.
2. The food produced must require minimal cooking or processing by the consumer before consumption.
3. The preparation time required before consumption by the consumer must be minimal.

Earliest examples of convenience foods include bread, dried fruits, dried meat, fish and vegetables. Today the term 'convenience foods' encompasses a variety of processed foods, including canned foods, frozen or chilled foods, breakfast cereals, microwave ready meals, boil-in-the-bag, cook-in-the-pot, baking mixes, soup and gravy mixes. Table 1 shows a simple classification of convenience foods based on the degree of secondary processing required of the consumer before consumption. Convenience foods have evolved into their current position in the food industry simply because they meet the demands of our modern society.

Table 1. Classification of convenience foods

Product	Food examples	Secondary processing required
Baked goods	Bread, rolls, pizza, sausage rolls	Nil or mild heating
Breakfast cereals	Cornflakes, Rice Krispies	Nil
Canned foods	Canned fruits, vegetables, soups, gravy, meat	Nil or mild heating
Cook/chill foods and frozen foods	Vegetables, prepared meals	Reheat
Cook-in-the-pot	Pot Noodles, Pot Rice, Pot Spaghetti, etc.	Add boiling water
Boil-in-the-bag	Fish-in-sauce, chicken-in-sauce, etc.	Boil in water for a few minutes
Baking mixes	Cakes, pastries	Add water and bake

Historical Perspective

Since antiquity, humans have preserved and extended the shelf life of foods. For example, early humans dried meat and fish by the fire and ground it to a powder. This was either used by itself as a relish or made into a paste with the addition of fat. The resultant product could be used at any time without adhering to the old practice of 'feast or famine', depending on the availability of food. This perhaps represents the first examples of a 'convenience food'.

The earliest documented large-scale preservation of food was practised by the Egyptians (4000 BC) who, in addition to drying fruits and vegetables, were also expert bread makers. The natives of Andes dried potatoes known as 'chuños' over 3000 years ago. In Roman times, fruits were preserved in honey. By the Middle Ages, several methods of food preservation were in practice, including smoking, salting and pickling. In countries with warm climates fermentation was also used as a method of preservation. Although food preservation has existed for thousands of years, only in the last two centuries have many new food-processing techniques developed. Previously, the consumer had to perform a series of processes to transform a food item into an edible commodity. This is well illustrated by the transformation of wheat to bread. Today, large industrial bakeries produce millions of loaves of bread for the consumer. Similarly, other food factories produce a whole selection of foods for the consumer. In fact, new developments in food technology have paralleled the evolution of convenience foods.

Evolution of Modern Convenience Foods

Most populations in the developed world live in urban centres far removed from the source of food production. In order to sustain such populations it was clearly necessary to evolve convenience foods.

Canning

The single most important development in the evolution of convenience foods happened a little under 200 years ago. In 1795 Nicholas Appert showed that when foods were placed in bottles (cans were not available at that time) and the bottles heated in hot water and then sealed, they stored well for a long period of time. This was the beginning of the 'canning' process as we now know it. By 1805 Appert had established a small factory in France. Canned foods played a significant role in feeding the armies of the Napoleonic War of 1810. In the years that followed, canneries opened in both Europe and North America. Seafarers found canned foods a very convenient and reliable method of transporting food. Captain Parry, for example, took large supplies of canned foods when in 1818 he sailed from England in the hope of finding a passage to the Pacific Ocean. Within a few years canned foods became an integral part of sea voyages and expeditions. By 1820 the first canning plant opened in the USA. With the introduction of canning, the consumers had a variety of foods, such as fruits, vegetables, meats, fish and soups, all year round and at a reasonable price. Canned foods also played an important role in feeding the armies of World Wars I and II. Since 1920, commercial canning processes have produced over a trillion (10^{18}) cans. Canned foods can truly be called the first mass-produced convenience foods. More recently, canned foods played a significant role in feeding troops in the Gulf war (1991). A recent extension of the canning process is the 'self-heating can', which is able to heat the food inside it. The Japanese and the US army have several products that are manufactured and sold in self-heating cans. Whilst costs preclude their extensive use today, in the future it is likely that they will become as common as canned foods. In the UK, canned vegetables, including baked beans, have the largest market, followed by soups and sauces, fruits, meat and fish. Production of canned food in the UK (for 1988) was approximately 5.5×10^6 cans. Despite new technological innovations, canned foods will remain an important part of our repertoire of convenience foods. *See* Freezing, Principles

Freezing

The Chinese (in the eighteenth century BC) were perhaps the first to use freezing as a method of preservation. Early man used blocks of ice to preserve and extend the shelf life of meat and fish, but it was only 100 years ago that commercial refrigeration became a reality. By the late 1880s refrigeration was used to transport meat by rail and ship over long distances. This was possible due to the invention of an ammonia compressing machine which resulted in the manufacture of the first refrigerator. It was, however, Clarence Birdseye who realized the full market potential of frozen foods. By 1930 Birdseye commercialized the marketing of frozen fruits, vegetables, meat and fish. Despite the great depression (1930) and the slow progress in the construction of storage and distribution facilities, frozen foods rapidly became a popular and expanding industry. One of the first frozen prepared foods for large-scale distribution

was 'Chicken à la King'. The product quickly gained popularity because it retained all the characteristics of a 'home-made' product. Commercial freezing of small fruits commenced in the USA by 1905, and the freezing of vegetables by 1917. The earliest expansion in the purchase of frozen food was noted in frozen potatoes (french fries). Today, we would not think of frozen peas as a 'convenience food' yet they are considered as such because they fulfil the three main criteria outlined earlier. It is currently more popular to find 'ready-to-eat' frozen meals, such as chilli con carne with rice, spaghetti bolognese, lasagne, and Chinese fried rice with prawns. This is a shift away from single 'commodity' products (frozen peas, carrots, etc.) to complex commodity products. 'Frozen foods' are the largest growing convenience food market and represent approximtely 5% of the total food expenditure in the UK. *See* Freezing, Principles

Cook/Chill Foods

Cook/chill is a process whereby the food is cooked in a central location, placed in suitable containers and chilled immediately to 3°C within 90 min. It is then stored at 0–5°C for subsequent consumption. Before consumption the food is heated to at least 70°C. Cook/chill foods can clearly be classified as convenience foods. They are widely used by industrial canteens, district health authorities, social services departments, hotels and airlines.

Demand for Convenience Foods

The increasing demand for convenience foods may be traced to the following developments:

1. Changes in demographic, social and economic patterns.
2. Increasing participation of women in the workforce.
3. Changes in meal patterns and existing food habits.
4. Altered attitudes to leisure activities and time spent in conventional 'cooking'.
5. Increased foreign travel and integration of 'ethnic foods' into local food habits.
6. Rising real income and disposable income.
7. Increasing demand for home entertainment (TV).
8. New advances in food technology and packaging.
9. Increased interest in 'healthy eating' and low-calorie foods.

Many of these factors are clearly interrelated. For example, with the increasing participation of women in the workforce, less time is available to plan and cook meals. At the same time, women's earning capacity enables them to purchase convenience food at an affordable price. Two-career couples and single parents prefer to eat high-quality convenience foods without the drudgery of spending long hours in the kitchen. Our eating habits have also undergone remarkable changes. The conventional three meals a day has been replaced by 'grazing', in which snack-type meals are eaten several times a day. Convenience foods have filled in a real demand for such changes in food habits. Overseas travel, coupled with the introduction of Indian, Chinese, Mexican, and West Indian foods to the Western palate, has created a demand for 'ethnic' meals. This has given rise to the production of such foods in the form of frozen or chilled ready meals.

The Home Appliance Revolution – Interaction with Convenience Foods

Several kitchen appliances now taken for granted have only recently become widely available at an affordable price. The percentage UK ownership of deep freezers in 1985, 1986 and 1988 was 66%, 72% and 77%, respectively; the ownership of microwaves rose from 23% in 1986 to 39% in 1988. Forward projections suggest that by 1995, 95% of the UK population will have deep freezers and 75% microwaves. The food industry has taken advantage of this booming trend in kitchen appliances and formulated food products – notably convenience foods. The combination of freezer and microwave ownership has led to the manufacture of foods that are not only convenient but appealing, nutritious and appetizing. *See* Cooking, Domestic Use of Microwave Ovens

The appliance which has offered the greatest opportunity and innovation for the development of a range of convenience foods is the microwave. The UK market for microwaves really only developed in the 1980s. Microwave oven owners have demanded that convenience foods have the following attributes:

1. The product must be packaged in such a way that it goes into the microwave directly.
2. The product must have easy-to-follow cooking instructions.
3. The product must have comparable taste to conventionally cooked food.

The food industry has risen to the challenge and produced a range of convenience foods suitable for the microwave. Foods stored at low temperatures (frozen foods) can be effectively and safely heated within a few minutes in the microwave. Microwave foods have now become the largest sector of the 'frozen meal' market.

Mention must also be made of that other valuable kitchen appliance, the refrigerator. The ownership of refrigerators meant that in addition to being able to

store 'conventional' foods such as milk, cheese and other dairy products, prepared meals and ready-to-eat meals could also be stored.

Healthy Eating – Impact on Convenience Foods

Since the mid-1980s, interest in healthy eating and low-calorie diets has dramatically increased. The demand for such foods has encouraged food manufacturers to produce products specifically tailored for this market. For example, in the case of 'frozen meals', a range of products which are low in calories, high in fibre but rich in flavour and appeal are now widely available.

Advantages and Disadvantages of Convenience Foods

The salient advantages of convenience foods may be summarized as follows:

1. The products are reliable and consistent in quality.
2. A greater variety of composite foods are available at all seasons.
3. Productivity is higher and unit costs are lower (due to bulk buying).
4. 'Ethnic' food and 'exotic' meals are more readily available.
5. There are savings in space and labour.
6. There is less reliance on skilled chefs for meal preparation.

The disadvantages of convenience foods are twofold:

1. Improper handling or reheating of convenience foods such as cook/chill can lead to food spoilage or poisoning.
2. High initial investment is required to produce convenience foods.

Importance of Convenience Foods in the Diet of Various Groups

Whilst it is impossible to be precise and detailed about the role convenience foods play in all sectors of our society, the following examples illustrate their importance in certain groups.

Airlines

A *single* commercial airline operating international routes serves approximately 30 million meal units per year. This implies that foods of high volume and quality need to be supplied to this industry. Cook/chill foods have formed the basis of several airlines' catering practice. They provide versatility, convenience and variety to its passengers. It is hard to think of how the expanding airline industry would feed its passengers if not for the evolution of convenience foods.

Hospital Patients and the Elderly

Convenience foods (cook/chill) have come to play an important part in the varying dietary needs of patients. Emerging trends suggest greater use of convenience foods in this sector.

By the year 2000 roughly 20% of the Western population will include people over the age of 65. This significantly increasing population group will find the availability of convenience foods a real bonus. It allows those who have difficulty in preparing foods for themselves the convenience of the 'ready meals' that are both nutritious and appetizing.

Conclusion

Marked changes in the lifestyle, age structure of the population and the impact of 'ethnic foods' in our diet has significantly influenced the growth of convenience foods. Convenience foods offer a range of highly palatable, nutritious foods, without the drudgery of a long preparation time. Convenience foods are here to stay and in future will play an even more significant role in the marketplace.

Bibliography

Arthey D and Dennis C (1991) *Vegetable Processing*. Glasgow: Blackie.
Kroger M and Shapiro R (1987) *Changing Food Technology*. Pennsylvania: Technome Publications.
Thorne S (1989) *Development in Food Preservation*, vol. 5. London: Elsevier Applied Science.

C. J. K. Henry
Oxford Polytechnic, Oxford, UK

COOKIES

See Biscuits, Cookies and Crackers

COOKING

Contents

Domestic Techniques

As with all forms of cooking, domestic cooking is intended to improve the palatability of the food, making it more appetizing. Unlike industrial food preparation and catering or food service, domestic cooking is carried out in the end user's home, by people who may not have any technical knowledge of what is happening from an engineering or biochemical point of view. By definition cooking raises the temperature of the food. This results in a number of simultaneous and interrelated processes which influence the flavour, texture, appearance, nutrient content and safety of the food.

The different techniques of domestic cooking reflect the way in which the temperature of the food is raised (Fig. 1). Clearly, there are two basic ways in which energy can be applied to a food stuff, resulting in a rise in temperature. The traditional route is by contact with a heated medium which causes heat to flow to the surface

Energy transferred by contact with a heated:							Energy transferred by electromagnetic radiation	
Solid	Liquid		Gas or vapour				Typical wavelength	
	Oil	Water	Steam		Air convection		0·03mm	300mm
			Atmospheric	Pressure	Natural	Forced		
All these techniques achieve surface heating, heat flow to centre by conduction							Heat generated throughout	
Griddling	Frying	Boiling Simmering	Steaming	Pressure cooking	Roasting Baking		Grilling	Microwave

Fig. 1 Classification of domestic cooking techniques.

of the food and then on to the centre by conduction. An alternative route is to apply electromagnetic radiation. Of the two types of electromagnetic radiation commonly used in domestic cooking, infrared, radiant heating (grilling) employs short-wavelength radiation which is only able to penetrate a couple of millimetres below the surface of the food. The inner regions of the food heat by conduction. Microwaves have longer wavelengths which are able to penetrate deep into foods, generating heat *in situ*.

In many cases energy transfer during cooking is not by a single mechanism. For example, ovens absorb and emit infrared energy and baked food heat by a combination of convection and radiation. Similarly, barbecues emit infrared radiation as well as generating hot combustion gases which flow around the food, heating it by convection.

Some of the mechanisms by which foods heat up are illustrated in Fig. 2.

Cooking by Direct Contact with a Heated Medium

Surface Heat Transfer

The crucial difference between the different techniques of heating by contact with a heated material is what happens at the surface of the food.

When a solid food is placed in a hot fluid, there is a stagnant layer of fluid around the food. This boundary layer acts as an insulating barrier which slows the flow of heat from the fluid to the food.

Air is a good insulator (thermal conductivity, $0·024$ W m^{-1} K^{-1}); therefore a boundary layer consisting of air greatly slows the flow of heat from an oven to the food (Fig. 2a). One way of reducing the thickness of this boundary layer is to agitate the heating medium. In

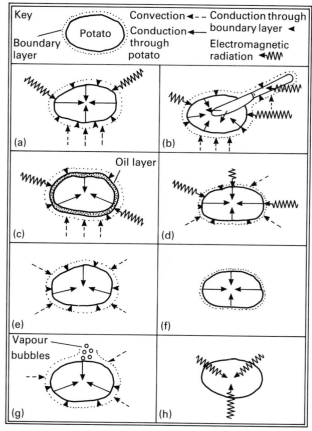

Fig. 2 Eight ways to cook a potato: (a) bake; (b) bake with a good conductor (e.g. knife) inserted; (c) roast; (d) forced convection (fan-assisted oven); (e) boil; (f) steam or pressure-cook; (g) fry (chipped); (h) microwave.

the case of fan-assisted ovens, the air is forced to circulate, thereby impinging on the surface of the food and physically reducing the thickness of the boundary layer (Fig. 2d). The surface heat transfer coefficient in a fan-assisted oven is about 10 times greater than in a conventional oven.

Heat travels by conduction through static boundary layers. Heating media which are better conductors of heat than air will increase the rate of heat flow to the surface of the food. Water has a thermal conductivity of 0.573 W m^{-1} K^{-1}, and the rates of convective heat transfer during boiling and simmering are therefore considerably faster than in ovens at the same temperature (Fig. 2e). However, the maximum temperature attainable with water is limited by its boiling point. Alternative liquid heating media, such as oil, have thermal conductivities in the same region and can operate at temperatures around 180°C. Hence rates of heat flow to the surface in frying are considerably greater than in boiling. This is also partly attributable to physical agitation of the boundary layer caused by the generation of water vapour at the surface of the food in contact with the hot oil (Fig. 2g).

When saturated steam is used as the heating medium, heat flow to the surface of the food is accompanied by a simultaneous condensing of the steam. The dramatic volume change during condensation results in fresh steam flowing to occupy the void, thereby maintaining a virtually negligible boundary layer (Fig. 2f). However, if the steam is not saturated, then the noncondensing air accumulates at the surface of the food, forming an insulating layer. In fact, as little as 6% air in steam reduces the surface heat transfer by 90%.

Heat Flow from the Surface to the Centre of the Food

As heat flows through the boundary layer, the surface temperature of the food begins to rise. The rate at which the heat is carried from the heated surface to the rest of the food is governed by the physical properties of the food and the difference in temperature between the surface and the bulk. This temperature difference is the driving force; obviously, as the bulk of the food heats up the temperature difference becomes less and the rate of heat transfer diminishes with time.

The rate of heat flow is directly related to the thermal conductivity, and inversely to the specific heat and the density. In general, foods tend to be poor conductors of heat, with the consequence that the surface gets hot while the centre remains relatively cool. It is only with extended heating times that the centre temperature approaches that of the heating medium.

The final factor which influences the rate of heat flow from the surface to the centre is the geometry of the food (the shape, size and surface area being exposed to the heating medium). The critical length is the shortest distance from the surface to the centre of the food. The shape dictates the surface:volume ratio; obviously, the greater the ratio of heated surface to volume, the more rapidly the food heats at its centre. This is exemplified by

deep and shallow frying, the only real distinction between the two being the surface area exposed to the hot oil.

Cooking by Electromagnetic Radiation

Infrared

As with the other *traditional* forms of cooking, grilling (broiling) causes the surface of the food to heat, and the centre then heats by conduction. Absorption of infrared radiation at the surface is proportional to the difference of the fourth power of the temperature of the radiation source and the surface of the food. However, various foods absorb infrared radiation to differing extents depending on their absorbtivity (e.g. black body, 1; perfect reflector, 0; water, 0.96).

Conventional grilling and barbecuing are restricted by the fact that radiant energy is supplied from one direction; cooking of all sides is only achieved by frequently turning the food, e.g. on a spit.

In practice, infrared heating is involved in many cooking techniques, such as baking and roasting. In these cases the oven walls heat up by convective heat transfer and then emit infrared radiation.

Microwaves

Microwaves penetrate deep into most foods; their sinusoidal electromagnetic waveform causes dipoles (e.g. water) to oscillate, which in turn causes heat (Fig. 2h). As microwaves pass through a food material their energy is lost; although heating does occur within the food, it is greatest at the surface. The actual temperature achieved within the food depends on several factors, including the frequency of the radiation, the strength of the field, the dielectric loss factor of the food, the free moisture present, and the shape of the food.

Quality Changes during Cooking

General Considerations

Mrs Beeton tells us that there are only two basic cooking methods: wet and dry. Wet cooking includes boiling, simmering, steaming, pressure cooking, stewing, and poaching. During wet cooking the surface temperature of the food does not exceed the boiling point of water (usually 100°C, but up to about 120°C in domestic pressure cookers); consequently, the surface remains moist. Dry cooking includes frying (deep and shallow), baking, roasting (in an oven with natural or added fat), grilling (broiling), barbecuing, and griddling. The surface temperature during dry cooking may well exceed 100°C, leading to evaporation of moisture and a dry or crisp surface.

Whatever is being cooked it is worth bearing in mind that most foods are biological in origin and many are still respiring up to the time of cooking. The rise in temperature during cooking can result in a severe disruption of structural integrity and the termination of normal metabolic activity.

We eat a diverse range of foods, each with its own criteria of quality. Since the changes that occur during cooking are dependent on both the temperature achieved in the product and the time at which the food is held at each temperature, the quality of the product is constantly changing. Most of the quality changes that take place during domestic cooking can be described by first-order Arrhenius kinetics (i.e. after a finite activation energy is reached, the rate of change is proportional to a rate constant, which is itself exponentially affected by temperature). The activation energy and rate constant vary for different quality factors; moreover, any particular factor may behave differently in each food (e.g. thiamin is destroyed more rapidly during cooking of rainbow trout than in a buffered solution with the same temperature–time profile). This means that if a food is cooked on the basis of one quality characteristic (e.g. colour in meat, or texture in cakes) and if the time–temperature treatment is varied from an established procedure, then the other quality parameters may be suboptimal. For example, microwaved meat may not develop the same flavour as conventionally roasted meats.

Textural Changes

No single mechanism is responsible for the texture of foods, yet changes in protein structure and solubilization of polysaccharides (and some proteins) are the two primary phenomena involved.

Heat causes proteins to unwind their tertiary structure. Heating for long periods or high temperatures frequently results in irreversible changes in tertiary structure, termed denaturation, which causes changes in functional properties. If the protein is highly charged, the uncoiled amino acid chains tend to repel each other and the protein increases its affinity for water, leading to an enhanced solubility. *See* Protein, Interactions and Reactions Involved in Food Processing; Protein, Functional Properties

If the protein molecules are reasonably close to their isoelectric point, the amino acid chains tend to attract each other with hydrophobic interactions and hydrogen bonds, forming a network of chains. This association of molecules results in a reduction in the amount of water which is associated with protein, and hence the following consequences: a loss of protein solubility; precipitation of the protein from solution, giving rise to a solid structure (such a change is responsible for the thermal setting or gelation); loss of water-holding capacity accompanied by an aqueous exudate from the product (often observed when cooking meats); shrinkage of the product as both the above occur; and increase in the opacity of the food (e.g. egg white).

Some proteins undergo reversible thermal transitions when heated. For example, collagen (and its partially hydrolysed derivative, gelatin) is solubilized when heated. Owing to its prevalence in connective tissue, this has important implications in tenderness of cooked meat and is partly responsible for the softening action of long-duration stewing.

Solubilization is also a process which affects polysaccharide material between the cell walls of plants. Dissolution of these pectins results in softening of the plant tissues. Addition of sodium bicarbonate enhances solubilization of pectin by producing the sodium salt and displacing the calcium ions which are naturally chelated in the structure. *See* Carbohydrates, Interactions with Other Food Components

Another mechanism commonly involved in providing rigidity in plant tissues is turgor. Denaturation of the proteins present in the cell membranes causes a termination of osmoregulation and a subsequent softening of the tissues. Deliberate protein denaturation is the aim of blanching, a brief exposure to temperatures around 85°C, with the intention of destroying flavour-modifying enzymes prior to home freezing.

Starch is present in many plant foods. Heating starch with an ample supply of water leads to gelatinization. The granules swell as they absorb water and the crystalline regions are disrupted. This has both a softening and a thickening effect, which is why gelatinized starch provides the viscosity of many sauces. *See* Starch, Structure, Properties and Determination

The light, open texture of baked flour products is due to the presence of gas or air cells in the prebaked dough or batter. During heating the gases expand; this expansion is aided by the generation of additional gas from chemical leavening agents (e.g. sodium bicarbonate) and from an increase in the vapour pressure of the water present. Finally, the liquid matrix is heat-set by denaturation of proteins and starch gelatinization. In the case of popcorn the impervious grain coat acts as the wall of pressure vessel. As the grain is heated the water vapour pressure increases until the wall ruptures. The vapour then flashes off, opening out the endosperm which then heat-sets.

A crisp outer surface is often associated with dry cooking. The temperature in excess of 100°C results in moisture being lost from the surface.

Domestic Techniques

Colour and Flavour Changes

With the exception of added colours sometimes used in domestic cooking (e.g. saffron or cochineal), two types of colour change result from domestic cooking: modification of natural pigments present in the raw materials, and browning reactions. Most natural colours tend to be relatively unstable when cooked. In addition to these chemical reactions, in wet cooking loss of natural colour may result from leaching of water-soluble pigments into the cooking medium.

Metalloporphyrin colours are found in foods of both animal and plant origin. Myoglobin, the pigment found in muscle, undergoes colour change from red-purple to brown when heated; this is a result of certain amino acids in the globin protein constituent of the molecule becoming coordinated with the central iron atom. Chlorophylls are also prone to lose their colour when heated in acid conditions. The change from bright green to a greyish green is the result of demineralization of the central magnesium atom from the molecule. *See* Colours, Properties and Determination of Natural Pigments

Sensitivity to pH is exhibited by other natural pigments. Anthocyanins, for example, change from red (in acid conditions), through colourless (when neutral) to blue (when alkaline). This can result in colour changes when heat disrupts cells and allows these water-soluble pigments to mix with the cooking water.

Browning reactions tend to occur at low levels of available water. They are therefore common in dry cooking where the surface layers may dry out. Caramelization occurs when concentrated sugars are heated, particularly in the presence of acids or alkalis. Caramelization is of importance in both sugar and flour confectionery. The most famous of these reactions is Maillard browning, which involves the reaction between carbonyl groups (as found in reducing sugars) and amino groups. The reaction gives rise to a variety of brown compounds and characteristic aromas. Simple mixtures of one amino acid and one reducing sugar have been shown to produce distinctive aromas, reminiscent of particular foods (e.g. glucose and cysteine heated at 180°C for 30 s smells of puffed wheat, yet after 3 min it smells of over-roasted meat). *See* Browning, Nonenzymatic

Generally speaking, volatile components are lost during cooking, and this can result in a loss of the uncooked flavour. Since domestic cooking is carried out by the end user, loss of volatiles is not completely wasted and may act as an appetizer.

Sustained heating of dry surfaces can result in carbonization, usually accompanied by the generation of smoke. In such circumstances the surface browns, then blackens as it burns; such products are usually regarded as spoiled.

Nutritional Changes

Although the act of cooking involves raising the temperature of the food, the term is frequently undifferentiated from other food preparation procedures, many of which commonly precede cooking. Peeling and trimming are two such operations which can lead to substantial loss of available nutrients, by cutting unsightly portions off the food and throwing them away!

Nutrient loss during cooking is attributable to two basic routes: thermally induced chemical reactions, and leaching of nutrients into the cooking medium.

Many nutrients are thermally unstable and when heated their concentration falls exponentially with time. Obviously, different nutrients have their own rates of destruction. The most sensitive vitamins are ascorbic acid (vitamin C) and folic acid, both of which can be completely destroyed by domestic cooking. Of the essential amino acids, lysine is the least stable to heat and up to 40% may be lost by domestic cooking practices. In general, rapid cooking methods, using high temperature for short times, or microwaves cause less nutrient destruction than long-duration, low-temperature cooking methods such as stewing. *See* Amino Acids, Properties and Occurrence; Ascorbic Acid, Properties and Determination; Folic Acid, Properties and Determination

In addition to thermal decomposition, nutrients can be lost by reacting with each other. For example, proteins will participate in Maillard reactions, particularly when ε-amino groups are present.

Sodium bicarbonate is sometimes added to vegetables for its softening effect. Unfortunately its addition leads to the destruction of vitamin C, as well as chemically modifying proteins, lowering their biological value.

Safety Aspects

A common misconception is that domestic cooking is performed purely to improve the gastronomic experience at the detriment of the food's biological value. In fact, domestic cooking can make safe products which would otherwise contain harmful or toxic components.

Harmful components in food arise in the form of naturally present toxins (e.g. cyanides in kidney beans and cassava), or compounds that interfere with digestion effectively making the food less nutritious (e.g. trypsin inhibitors found in many legumes). The presence of pathogenic microorganisms may lead to infections, while other microorganisms produce toxins, both of which result in food poisoning. *See* Plant Toxins, Trypsin Inhibitors; Plant Toxins, Haemagglutinins; Plant Toxins, Detoxification of Naturally Occurring Toxicants of Plant Origin

Cooking is effective at destroying or removing many of these harmful components. However, some toxins are relatively heat-stable (e.g. the toxin produced by *Staphylococcus aureus*) and may not be destroyed by the temperatures and times incurred during domestic cooking. It is of course likely that untrained domestic cooks will be oblivious to the risks involved in eating particular foods, or to the neutralizing effect of cooking. A further risk arises from cross-contamination of cooked food by raw ingredients, resulting in a potential for fresh growth of pathogenic micro-organisms.

Bibliography

Glew G (1985) *Advances in Catering Technology – 3*. Essex: Elsevier Science Publishers.

Karmas E and Harris RS (1988) *Nutritional Evaluation of Food Processing*. Westport, Connecticut: AVI Publishing.

McGee H (1991) *On Food and Cooking: The Science and Lore of the Kitchen*, 2nd edn. London: Harper Collins.

A. J. Rosenthal
Oxford Polytechnic, Oxford, UK

Domestic Use of Microwave Ovens*

What are Microwaves and how do they Heat Foods?

Microwaves are, by definition, electromagnetic waves in the frequency range of 300 to 300 000 MHz, corresponding to wavelengths of 1 m to 1 mm. For food cooking applications these are, however, limited to the industrial/scientific/medical (ISM) band 2450 ± 50 MHz. In the USA 915 ± 15 MHz is also a much used ISM frequency. In Europe 915 MHz is not a generally available ISM frequency with the exception of the UK.

Heating foods is accomplished both by the absorption of microwave energy by rotation of the water molecules and translation of the ionic components of a food. This energy is converted to heat. Both the water content and the dissolved ion content (often salt) are important factors in the microwave heating of food.

The dielectric heating mechanism relies on the fact that the water molecule is a dipole, i.e. it has a positive and a negative end. When the dipole is subjected to a microwave field that rapidly changes direction, the dipole tries to align itself with the direction of the electrical field. This is achieved with a time lag as the

water molecules overcome the inertia and intermolecular forces in the water. The electrical field provides energy for the water molecule to rotate into alignment. The energy is then lost to the random thermal motion of the water. This energy is equivalent to a temperature increase. *See* Water, Structure, Properties and Determination

The energy transfer mechanism will be efficient only if the time between the changes of direction of the electrical field is so short that the dipolar molecule aggregates barely follow its changes. If the time is long (frequency is low), the alignment will be good and the energy transfer slow. If the time is short (frequency is high), the aggregates will not move much between field polarity reversals and the energy transfer rate will again be slow. The number of water molecules bound together by hydrogen bonds is lower at higher temperatures so the inertia is reduced. As the applied microwave frequency is constant and lower than the energy transfer efficiency optimum, this efficiency will decrease with increasing temperature. Hydrated ions, such as Na^+ and Cl^- from table salt, try to move in the direction of the electrical field. The ions are surrounded by water molecules and in their movement transfer energy randomly to the water molecules. The water molecules are more mobile at higher temperatures and not so tightly bound to the ions. They can move more freely, and absorb and dissipate more energy. Conductive heating due to dissolved ions increases with increasing temperature. *See* Heat Transfer Methods

Microwave Properties of Foods

The macroscopic interactions between a food material and a microwave field are expressed by a complex dimensionless number, the permittivity; ε^*. The real component, the dielectric constant, ε', expresses the ability to store energy in the material. The imaginary component represents the energy losses and is called the dielectric loss factor, ε''. The quotient is also often used, which is expressed as the loss tangent; $\tan \delta = \varepsilon''/\varepsilon'$.

For practical understanding of the meaning of the values of the dielectric properties of foods, a so-called penetration depth is calculated:

$$d = (3{\cdot}38 \times 10^7/f\varepsilon'^{1/2})[(1 + \tan^2 \delta)^{1/2} - 1]^{1/2} \quad \text{(m)}. \quad (1)$$

It represents the depth into the material where 1/e (37%) of the incident surface power remains. An approximation gives sufficient accuracy for most foods. For 2450 MHz it gives

$$d \simeq 0{\cdot}019\,5\sqrt{\varepsilon'}/\varepsilon'' \quad \text{(m)}. \quad (2)$$

Cooking vessel materials can be classified into reflecting, absorbing or transparent according to their interaction with the microwave field. Reflecting materials are

---

* The colour plate section for this article appears between p. 1146 and p. 1147.

mostly metals, where the microwave energy creates surface currents penetrating some few micrometres into the material. Transparent materials, on the other hand, only to a very small extent absorb microwave energy. Glass and most plastics are typical examples. Materials that will absorb microwave energy, according to the heating mechanism explained above, are those containing polar constituents, predominantly water, or which have a relatively low conductivity.

For foods the water content will be important for determining the microwave heating properties. Basically, the higher the water content, the higher the dielectric constant. Many foods also contain salt. Reduction in dielectric losses with increasing temperature, due to the dipole absorption of water at higher temperatures, is more or less balanced by increases in conductive losses, due to the contribution of the dissolved ions of the salt to the dielectric losses.

Dielectric properties for foods are material constants and must be experimentally measured. Data is reasonably available for basic food components, especially for 2450 MHz. However, very little data is available for formulated foods and ready meals. A few prediction models are available with limited applicability.

In addition to the influence of water and salt, density of the food greatly influences the dielectric properties.

Chemical components that affect the possibilities of the water dipoles to freely participate in the heating mechanism can also influence the dielectric properties. These can be components that 'bind' the 'free' water or influence the formation of oil and water emulsions.

Frozen foods show much lower dielectric properties than thawed foods. Most of the water in frozen foods is present as ice crystals inside the food. However, approximately 10% of the water may remain as a strong salt solution in the food. Recent dielectric measurements have shown that the solution can successfully be heated by microwaves. Ice hardly absorbs microwaves at all. The differences in dielectric properties between the frozen and the thawed food are thus large. They lead to the well-known problems of 'run-away' heating during microwave thawing of foods, where the part of the food that is starting to thaw increases its microwave absorption properties and thus tends to absorb more of the available microwave energy. As a result, the thawed parts rapidly increase in temperature at the expense of the frozen parts. This is illustrated in Fig. 1, showing a computer simulation of the temperature profile through a slab of fish during microwave thawing. *See* Freezing, Structural and Flavour Changes

Microwave absorption properties of foods can also be expressed in terms of penetration depth of the microwave energy into the foods. It should be noted that for most foods about 0°C the penetration depth is between 10 and 15 mm, and almost the same over the temperature range 0–100°. For salted foods such as ham the

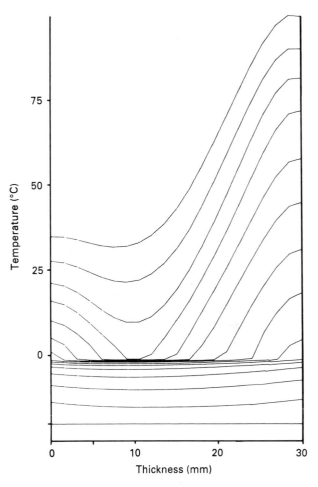

Fig. 1 Temperature profile for microwave thawing of a slab of fish.

penetration depth is only 3–5 mm. The large differences in the microwave properties between frozen and thawed foods are illustrated by the large differences in penetration depth.

Heating Uniformity

The limited penetration ability of microwave energy into compact foods is shown in Fig. 2. Both practical experience and computer simulations have shown that uniform temperature distribution through the full depth of the food can only be achieved if the thickness of the food is less than about 2·5 times the penetration depth. In other situations, the surface part of the food will absorb most of the energy and heat conduction will not be sufficiently rapid to transfer the heat from the surface to the centre. This leads to surface temperature 'run-away' phenomena which can be aggravated in situations where the dielectric loss increases with temperature, e.g. for a food which high salt content.

Microwaves are electromagnetic waves and some of the heating mechanisms can be explained by compari-

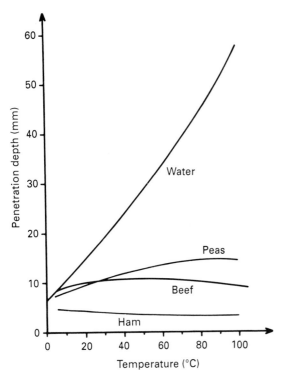

Fig. 2 Penetration depth at 2450 MHz for some foods

son to geometrical optics. Microwaves are reflected at the interfaces between materials of different dielectric properties. This may lead to standing waves developing in layered materials, with different dielectric properties.

When microwaves are transmitted into foods with round or rounded shapes, the propagation direction of the microwave energy inside the food is in many cases directed approximately perpendicular to the surface. This may lead to high concentrations of energy in the centre of round foods if the centre is within a few penetration depths of the food. Overheating at the centre may occur for round food items with diameters between 25 and 55 mm. An example is eggs, which have a tendency to explode.

Sharp edges and corners of foods, including those created by the design of the package, will act as antennae for the microwave field and absorb disproportionally high amounts of microwave energy. This causes quality defects such as drying out or even burning of the food at areas close to the edges of the top open surface in packaged foods. Thus, microwave heating uniformity is effected both by the geometry of the food and the package and by the composition of the food.

Packaging material that is reflecting or transparent has a large influence on the resulting temperature distribution. Another influential factor is the microwave field distribution created by the system for feeding the energy into the microwave oven and by the various means for distributing the energy inside the cavity, typical for each microwave oven.

Both the temperature and moisture distributions in microwave-heated food is different compared to conventionally heated foods. Conventional heating dries out the food surface and moisture is gradually transferred from the interior to the drier surface. Many important flavour components are formed in the dried surface at the elevated temperatures that exist there. With microwave heating the surface temperature of the food is, in contrast, usually slightly lower than temperatures a few millimetres below the food surface, due to evaporative cooling. Evaporation is by no means sufficient to dry out the surfaces. Water migrating from the interior can even condense on the cooler surface of microwave-heated foods. The typical flavour and appearance of roasted foods are therefore not created in microwave-heated foods, as the water content at the surface is too high and the surface temperatures too low. Various means of overcoming this limitation of microwave heating are available, e.g. the use of ingredients that enhance microwave heating at the surface, susceptor packaging that browns or crisps the food surface, and combination heating with hot air.

The Speed of Microwave Heating

The rate of heating of food in a microwave field is often expressed by the power equation

$$P_v = 55 \cdot 6 \times 10^{16}\, f|E|^2\, \varepsilon''\ (\text{W m}^{-3}), \tag{3}$$

where P_v is the power density per unit volume. However the electrical field strength, E, varies greatly in the microwave oven and is complicated to predict, so the power equation is not very useful in practice. A simple energy balance is much more useful for predicting heating time (t) or speed of heating:

$$P_{mw}t = mc_p(T_e - T_i), \tag{4}$$

where m is the mass of the food to be heated, c_p is the specific heat of the food and T_e and T_i are the final and initial average temperatures. P_{mw} is the microwave output power of the oven, usually 600–700 W. An important consequence of the energy balance is the 'rule of thumb': twice the amount of food – twice the heating time. Since P_{mw} is lower for smaller masses of foods, this rule is, however, most relevant for large quantities of food.

Advantages and Limitations of Microwave Heating

The advantages of microwave heating are:

- convenient, clean heating;
- heating of food only;
- in-depth heating;

Domestic Use of Microwave Ovens

- rapid heating;
- energy efficient.

There are of course also limitations, some of which are inherent to the heating method and some that may be overcome. The limitations of microwave heating are:

- lack of control of temperature distribution;
- no surface browning;
- best suited for small food masses.

Microwave Ovens

The microwave oven consists of a number of basic components. The microwaves are generated by a magnetron, which is an electronic vacuum tube with a cathode and an anode. It needs high-voltage direct current and thus a transformer and rectifier. The microwaves are transferred to the heating cavity by various electromechanical devices that are designed to efficiently distribute the energy inside the cavity. This enables foods of many different sizes to be heated as uniformly as possible. Oven cavity dimensions generally allow room for a few wavelengths of microwaves (at 2450 MHz being 12 cm) inside the cavity, creating a pattern of standing waves. This three-dimensional mode pattern has areas of both high and low power density. A few mode patterns normally exist in a well-designed microwave oven. Heating from a number of mode patterns is often desirable, as they will combine to a more uniform distribution. In addition, microwave ovens often contain devices that help to direct the microwaves on to the central area where foods are placed for heating. Most microwave ovens have a combination of direct heating and multimode standing wave pattern heating.

Solid state controls with microprocessors are increasingly included in modern microwave ovens. Turntables, where the food is placed on a slowly rotating shelf, allow the food to pass through areas of high and low power density from the multimode field pattern. Combination ovens where microwave heating functions are built into conventional ovens, or microwave ovens are combined with circulating hot air or grills, are becoming increasingly popular.

Safety requirements for microwave ovens are regulated through international agreements. The microwave oven is by far the most thoroughly tested safety appliance in the home. Statistics from insurance companies show few home accidents due to microwave ovens compared to other risks in the home. Possible hazards caused by leakage of microwave energy from ovens was a concern some years ago and the current stringent testing procedures were developed as a result of these concerns. The most frequent problem of microwave oven safety is the risk of setting fire to foods in the microwave oven by heating food for too long. The food material can dry out and, if the conditions are unfavourable, can catch fire.

Microwaveable Foods

The 1980s have been called the 'decade of the microwaves' in the USA, where an enormous growth of microwaveable foods was seen during these years. The growth of the market has, however, slowed down considerably in the last few years, with decreases in volume for many products. The two major reasons for this are poor quality and high prices. Many consumers have found that cheaper conventional products when heated by microwaves present almost the same quality on the plate as the high priced microwaveable product.

The frozen food category is the largest in volume for microwave foods. Important segments are ready meals, pizzas, snack items such as hamburgers, vegetables and potato products. Light, low-energy meals are becoming an important selling feature among the microwave frozen meals. In the USA special meals for children have also been successful. Shelf-stable microwave foods are another important food product segment, consisting mainly of meals in plastic retortable containers, suited for microwave heating before serving. These products have developed very well both in the USA and in Europe. Some are microwave sterilized in industrial production. *See* Convenience Foods, Definition and Classification

Microwave popcorn has seen phenomenal growth. It is the largest single microwave product in the USA and is rapidly growing in Europe. It is based on susceptor technology to reach the high temperatures needed for 'popping' the kernels. It is a high-technology product compared to many other food products, but there are many microwave popcorn producers that do not deliver good-quality products.

Heating and cooking food in microwave ovens have become important and even preferred methods in the home. Many food products that are not normally associated with microwave heating now have microwave cooking instructions.

The markets in Europe are all at stages where more microwave food products are being introduced. Both internationally well-known and accepted products are found on the market, such as lasagne or French fries/chips, and products that promote more nationally oriented dishes, such as Salisbury steak or 'Schweinbraten mit Sauerkraut'. Although much can be learnt from development of the microwave food market in the USA, it is important to recognize the differences in eating habits and food preferences in Europe compared to the USA.

An important factor in the growth of the microwave

Domestic Use of Microwave Ovens

food market is the percentage of homes having a microwave oven. Penetration of microwave ovens into households is considerably higher in the USA and Japan than in Europe. A number of steps in the development of microwave food products can be identified both by observing the market evolution in the USA and its development in Europe.

In most food companies the chain of development for microwave food products goes through three stages.

In stage 1, the quality of available prepared food products after microwave heating is tested. For products that give an acceptable quality and performance, microwave cooking instructions are added to the package.

In stage 2, the food industry develops food products with a view towards microwave heating at the initial stages of the development process and tries to ensure good food quality after either microwave or conventional heating. This often requires use of packaging able to be used in a microwave oven and heating conventionally and making compromises when selecting ingredients. Many of the recently introduced prepared food products in Europe are at this stage.

In stage 3, foods are developed for microwave heating only, including all the specific considerations that microwave heating requires with regard to the selection of ingredients, product shape and layout. Packaging selection may also be easier as the temperature requirements are lower than in stage 2.

Nutritional Quality of Microwave-heated Foods

In the early days of microwave heating of foods, consumers were concerned about microwaves remaining in the food, or even radioactivity in the microwave heated food. These concerns were easily allayed by the scientific community. Experimental results showing that nutrient retention was often better in microwave heated foods allayed fears about the nutritional value and wholesomeness of microwave-heated foods.

The nutritional value of raw food may be improved or reduced during cooking. Antinutritional components that bind nutrients, making them unavailable for digestion, may be destroyed by cooking, increasing availability of the nutrients to the body. Nutrients may be lost or made unavailable, due to both leaching to the surrounding boiling liquid and to chemical and enzymatic reactions, where the rate depends on factors such as the amount of water, time/temperature, pH, light and oxygen level.

There is much variability in published comparisons of nutritional data. A fair comparison between microwave and conventional cooking, where samples have been cooked to the same final temperature, is essential. Biological variation between samples has often resulted in larger differences in nutritional quality than any differences due to the cooking methods.

The protein quality of meats cooked in microwave ovens has frequently been studied. A slightly higher protein content in microwave-cooked meats has often been found. This is caused by reduced losses of protein in the cooking juices during the shorter duration of microwave cooking.

The amino acids of animal proteins and carbohydrates may react in the so-called Maillard reaction, causing the formation of a brown crust on meats and bread. The components formed give a pleasant and desired aroma to the foods but reduce the protein quality. High surface temperatures and drying out of the food surface do not occur in microwave cooking. This will result in little or no browning and improved nutrient retention. *See* Browning, Nonenzymatic

Some cooking methods may reduce the fat content of food due to the fat melting. With other methods, cooking fats may be absorbed by the food. Literature studies do not give any clear differences for changes in fat content between microwave and conventionally cooked foods. Neither have differences been found in the degree of rancidity due to cooking, as measured by the so-called thiobarbituric acid (TBA) values.

Few investigations have covered the effect of microwave cooking on the mineral composition of foods. As microwave cooking requires little or no added water, losses of minerals due to leaching are small. This has also been shown for potassium in potatoes. *See* Minerals, Dietary Importance

In contrast, water-soluble vitamins such as thiamin (vitamin B₁) and ascorbic acid (vitamin C) have been much investigated. Up to 20% of the thiamin content may be lost during cooking due to thermal degradation. No significant differences between microwave and conventional cooking have been found in the many foods studied. *See* Ascorbic Acid, Properties and Determination; Thiamin, Properties and Determination; Vitamins, Overview

Ascorbic acid, mainly lost due to oxidation and leaching during cooking, has been reported to be better retained with microwave cooking. This has been demonstrated for vegetables by many researchers. The main reason is the smaller amount of cooking liquid used in microwave cooking, which reduces leaching.

Although a large number of investigations on the nutritional values of foods cooked in microwave ovens have been published, sufficient data for many important nutrients are lacking. Also, in many older investigations microwave cooking was poorly controlled, leading to poor results. The conclusions from investigations during the last few decades are that microwave heating *per se* does not have any negative effects on nutrients. As in cooking in general, it is the time/temperature of the cooking operation and the amount of liquid lost from the food, or added to cook the food that determines whether there are positive or negative changes in nutritional quality. In general terms, microwave cooking, compared to conventional cooking, results in the same or in some cases improved nutritional quality of the foods. Smaller losses due to leaching of water-soluble nutrients and the lack of surface browning account for most of the often slight improvements. Nutritionists often recommend microwave cooking as a healthy alternative to conventional roasting and frying.

Safety of Microwave-heated Foods

In the last few years questions about the microbiological safety of microwave-heated foods have been raised. It was pointed out some 10 years ago that with microwave heating an end temperature above 70°C in foods is needed to inactivate food poisoning microorganisms. Studies on the temperature distribution in rectangular samples of mashed potatoes, in a large number of microwave ovens, showed that for a number of ovens the centre of the mashed potato sample did not reach 70°C after microwave heating according to the cooking instructions on the package. There is some concern by consumers about the safety of microwave ovens and microwave heated foods, often associated with poor knowledge about the microwave heating method. Further investigations into the safety and nutritional quality of microwave-heated foods are necessary, but all scientific evidence to date shows that microwave heating is a convenient and safe method for preparing and cooking foods, if care is taken as with conventional cooking methods.

Bibliography

Bengtsson NE and Risman PO (1971) Dielectric properties of foods at 3 GHz as determined by a cavity perturbation technique. II. Measurements on food materials. *Journal of Microwave Power* 6: 107–123.

Cross GA and Fung DYC (1982) The effect of microwaves on nutrient value of foods. *CRC Critical Review* 16: 355–381.

Kent M (1987) *Electrical and Dielectric Properties of Food Materials – COST 90/bis*. Hornchurch, Essex: Science and Technology Publishers.

Ohlsson T (1983) Fundamentals of microwave cooking. *Microwave World* 4(2): 4–9.

Ohlsson T (1989) Dielectric properties and microwave processing. In: Singh RP and Medina AG (eds) *Food Properties and Computer Aided Engineering of Food Processing Systems*, pp 73–92. Dordrecht: Klüwer.

Ohlsson T and Åström A (1982) Sensory and nutritional quality in microwave cooking. *Microwave World* Nov.–Dec.: 15–16.

Ohlsson T and Bengtsson NE (1971) Microwave heating profiles in foods. A comparison between heating experiments and computer simulation. A research note. *Microwave Energy Applications Newsletter* 4(6): 3–8.

Ohlsson T and Risman PO (1978) Temperature distribution of microwave heating. Spheres and cylinders. *Journal of Microwave Power* 13(4): 303–310.

Ohlsson T, Bengtsson NE and Risman PO (1974) The frequency and temperature dependence of dielectric food data as determined by a cavity perturbation technique. *Journal of Microwave Power* 9: 129–146.

Risman PO (1988) Microwave properties of water in the temperature range +3 to 140°C. *Electromagnetic Energy Reviews* 1: 3–6.

Risman PO, Ohlsson T and Wass B (1987) Principles and models of power density distribution in microwave oven loads. *Journal of Microwave Power* 22(4): 193–198.

Walker J (1987) The secret of a microwave oven's rapid cooking action is disclosed. *Scientific American* Feb. 98–102.

Thomas Ohlsson
Swedish Institute for Food Research, Göteborg, Sweden

COPPER

Contents

Properties and Determination

Copper occurs in nature as ores and, less commonly, as metal deposits. The most common ores of copper are sulphide, oxide and carbonate salts. All soils, and plant and animal tissues contain at least trace amounts of copper.

The earliest use of copper was to make tools and other utensils thousands of years ago. Today, copper and its alloys are second in use only to iron. Major copper alloys are brass (copper–zinc), bronze (copper–zinc–

tin), sterling silver (copper–silver), aluminum bronze (copper–aluminum) and German silver (copper–zinc–nickel). Copper is widely used for plumbing, electrical wire, coins, cooking utensils, decorative objects and jewellery.

Speciation and Chemical Properties

Copper is a reddish metal that is an excellent conductor of heat and electricity. The aqueous solubility of copper salts depends on the accompanying anion, and many highly soluble salts are available. Copper has an atomic weight of 63·546 and a valency of either 1 or 2. This ability of copper to change oxidation states is essential in the electron transport chain of the mitochondria for energy production, and for numerous other biologically important reactions mediated by copper metalloenzymes. However, as is the case with iron, changes in oxidation state can also be hazardous to biological systems. For example, copper enhances lipid peroxidation in foods and animal tissues, and can cause haemolysis of red blood cells. *See* Oxidation of Food Components

Isotopes

The characteristics of copper isotopes present unique challenges and opportunities for studies of copper metabolism. The short half-lives of the radioisotopes are frustrations for metabolic studies in plants and laboratory animals, but are advantages when seeking to limit radiation exposure in humans. The stable isotope, ^{65}Cu, is present in such high abundance that true tracer studies are difficult to perform and the instrumentation must be highly precise and accurate to measure enrichment in tissues.

Radioactive isotopes of copper include ^{64}Cu ($t_{1/2} = 12\cdot7$ h) and ^{67}Cu ($t_{1/2} = 61\cdot9$ h). Because of its relatively long half-life, ^{67}Cu is the most widely used radioactive isotope for tracer studies in plants and animals. ^{67}Cu is prepared by irradiation of zinc followed by electrochemical purification.

Because copper forms stable chelates with numerous chemicals, it has been proposed that radiocopper-labelled compounds may be useful in nuclear medicine to image organs and tumours. ^{67}Cu is suitable for γ camera imaging and ^{64}Cu for positron emission tomography. The short half-lives of these radionuclides limit radiation exposure. Porphyrins are being actively studied because of the strong complexes they form with copper and the unique biodistribution of porphyrin compounds.

Copper exists in nature as the stable isotopes ^{63}Cu (69·174 atom %) and ^{65}Cu (30·826 atom %) at a ratio of 2·24. Enriched ^{65}Cu (99·6%) can be obtained commercially. ^{65}Cu has been used in humans to study the effects of protein level, protein source, phytate, fibre, zinc, vitamin C and copper level on copper absorption from the diet. Mass spectrometry is used to measure these stable isotopes. *See* Bioavailability of Nutrients

Soil

The levels of copper in plants and grazing animals are dependent, in part, on the copper levels of the soil. For example, the low copper levels of pastures in Western Australia has been associated with severe copper deficiency in grazing sheep. Studies of this situation furthered understanding of the manifestations of copper deficiency in animals and of the dietary components that affect copper uptake.

Soil copper levels are usually between 5 and 50 mg kg^{-1} dry weight, but can range from 0·5 to 600 mg kg^{-1}. The copper content depends on geochemical history, adjacent or nearby mineral deposits, agricultural practices, industrial pollution, specific soil characteristics (e.g. pH, organic matter, sand, silt, clay and carbonate levels), and the presence of other mineral salts such as those of manganese and iron.

Human and Animal Foods

The range of copper levels in selected human foods is shown in Table 1. The amount of copper in a typical serving size can be roughly approximated by using portion sizes of 250 g for fluid milk and juices, 120 g for small servings of fish or meat, 100 g for fruits, vegetables and legumes and 30 g for a slice of bread, small bowl of cereal or slice of cheese. Copper contents of foods vary widely and depend on where a given food was produced and how it was processed. Within a single type of food of plant origin, the variation in copper content may be the result of soil conditions, type of fertilizer or other agricultural chemicals, weather, time of harvesting, and processing. Generally, processed grains contain less copper than whole grains because much of the copper is removed with the bran fraction and seed coat. Seeds, nuts and legumes have the highest copper contents of the plant foods. More than 60% of the copper in Western diets is derived from plant foods (Table 2). *See* Food Composition Tables

Among foods of animal origin, the highest levels are found in shellfish and in liver. Copper levels in the liver and kidney vary substantially and depend on age and dietary copper intakes. The very low levels of copper in dairy products contribute to the development of copper deficiency in premature or malnourished infants.

The copper content of animal feeds varies from 1·7 to

Table 1. Copper in selected human foods

Food	Copper content (mg kg⁻¹)

Food	Copper content ($mg\ kg^{-1}$)
Dairy	
Cheese	0·4–0·8
Chocolate milk	0·2–0·3
Cottage cheese	0·1–0·2
Cow's milk (skim, 2%, whole, buttermilk)	0·02–0·08
Human milk	0·02–0·8
Yoghurt	0·01–0·09
Eggs (fried, scrambled or soft boiled)	0·4–0·8
Fish and shellfish (cooked)	
Cod, fish sticks, haddock salmon, sardines, tuna	0·3–0·8
Shrimp	2–3
Oysters	0·3–16
Fruits	
Apples (red, with peel, raw)	0·1–0·4
Apple juice (canned)	0·02–0·2
Banana (raw)	1–2
Grapes (raw, purple or green)	0·4–1·4
Grape juice (canned)	0·01–0·13
Orange (raw, all varieties)	0·1–1
Orange juice	0·1–0·3
Dried fruits (currants, dates, figs, prunes, or raisins)	1–5
Grains and cereals (cooked or processed)	
Barley, pearl	0·4
Bread	
White (loaf, rolls, biscuits)	1–2·6
Whole wheat	2–3
Rye	1·6–2·8
Corn (fresh, frozen, cream style, grits)	0·1–0·4
Flour	
Whole grain	2–8
White	1–3
Macaroni (cooked)	0·6–1
Oatmeal (cooked)	0·3–1·2
Wheat bran	10–20
Wheat cereals (shredded, bran flakes, puffed wheat, raisin bran)	4·5–5·5
Legumes	
Beans (boiled or baked: cowpeas, kidney, lima, navy or pinto)	1–4
Beans (dry: cowpeas, kidney or lima)	5–10
Peanuts (fresh, roasted or butter)	3–10
Meats (cooked: beef, pork and poultry)	
Muscle meat	0·7–1·4
Liver	20–180
Nuts and seeds (almonds, brazil nuts, hazelnuts, pecans, pistachios, sesame seeds, sunflower seeds or walnuts	8–18
Vegetables	
Broccoli (fresh, frozen or boiled)	0·1–0·9
Cabbage (fresh, boiled or cole slaw)	0·1–0·2
Carrots (raw or boiled)	0·5–1
Cauliflower (fresh, frozen or boiled)	0·2–1
Onions (raw or cooked)	0·2–1
Peas (green, canned, cooked)	1–1·5
Potatoes	
Baked (with peel)	0·6–1·8
Boiled (without peel)	0·3–1
Spinach (canned, fresh, frozen or boiled)	0·6–1·2
Sweet potatoes (boiled or baked)	1·6–2·0
Tomatoes (raw, canned or juice)	0·3–1·4

Adapted from Kies C (1989) and Davis GK and Mertz W (1987) with permission.

Properties and Determination

Table 2. Contribution of food groups to copper intakes in Western diets

Food group	Contribution (%)
Meat, poultry, fish	21
Vegetables	20
Grain and cereal products	18
Legumes, nuts and soy	18
Fruits	7
Dairy	4
Sugars and sweeteners	3
Eggs	1
Fats and oils	<0·5
Miscellaneous	8

Adapted from Life Sciences Research Office (1989) and Johnson MA and Kays SE (1990) with permission.

22·3 mg kg^{-1} (Table 3). Additional copper is sometimes added as a mineral salt mixture or provided in salt licks in the pasture.

Human Tissues, Fluids and Excretions

Copper is present in all tissues and bodily excretions (Table 4). Although serum is the most commonly used indicator of copper status, it poorly reflects the body pools of copper and becomes subnormal only when the stores of copper are nearly exhausted. Similarly, there is little correlation between copper in hair and body levels of copper. Sweat is under investigation as an indicator of copper status, but it is difficult to collect sufficient quantities for analysis without contamination, and the relationship between body copper stores and sweat levels has not been established. Losses of copper in the faeces are proportional to intake, while urinary excretion is less than 5% of intake. Except under conditions of profuse sweating, sweat is not considered a major excretory route. Unlike for iron, variations in menstrual losses are not believed to influence body levels of copper.

Although there are some species differences, the concentration of copper in human tissue is similar to other animals. Liver copper is the most variable because it is highly correlated with copper exposure. Sheep, cattle, ducks, frogs and certain fish generally have higher levels in their liver than humans. In most species, liver copper is highest at birth. Abnormally high liver copper occurs in a variety of diseases.

Most tissues are less sensitive than the liver to variations in usual copper intakes. However, the level of copper in the kidney shows some correlation with intakes because, like the liver, it contains an abundant amount of the copper storage protein metallothionein. *See* Kidney, Structure and Function

Properties and Determination

Analytical Methods

Numerous methods exist for determination of copper. Atomic absorption spectrometry is by far the most widely used and available technique for routine analysis; however, inductively coupled plasma emission spectroscopy is becoming more popular because it can analyse up to more than 40 elements simultaneously in a single sample.

General Considerations

General principles of sample preparation are discussed by Evenson (see the Bibliography). Copper is somewhat easier to analyse than other trace elements because sample contamination is readily controlled and predictable. For example, contamination from copper salts used in assays for protein, glucose or other compounds is easily avoided with good laboratory practices and common sense.

A high-quality 'clean room' is usually not necessary; however, samples, reagents and containers must be kept free of laboratory dust. High-purity water that has been distilled and deionized and high-purity reagents must be used.

Teflon is the best material for sample storage and preparation, but is quite expensive. Sample containers with the least impurities at the most economical price are polyethylene or polypropylene. Polypropylene is preferable because it tolerates freezing, mild heating and certain organic solvents better than polyethylene. Quartz and Pyrex glass are also suitable if great care is taken to ensure that they are free of copper contamination. Any metal utensils such as knives, blades and needles must be made of stainless steel.

All sample containers and collection or transfer devices (e.g. syringes and pipette tips) must be routinely checked for trace copper contamination by rinsing or soaking in water (metal) or weak acid (quartz, Pyrex, plastic) and then analysing this fluid for copper. A routine procedure for eliminating copper contamination is to rinse containers thoroughly with acetone, 2 M nitric acid and high-quality water before use. Persistent cases of copper contamination on nonmetal objects can be eliminated by soaking in 1 M nitric acid or 1 M hydrochloric acid for a few hours.

Calibration standards of 1000 mg l^{-1} in dilute acid are available from several chemical companies.

Sample Preparation and Removal of Matrix Effects

Usually only 15–500 mg or μl of biological sample is sufficient for copper determination. Depending on the

Table 3. Copper in some animal feeds

Feed	Copper content (mg kg^{-1} dry matter basis)
Alfalfa (*Medicago sativa*), dehydrated	3·2–9·0
White clover (*Trifolium repens*) hay	12·7–18·4
Soya bean (*Glycine max*) hay	8·0–11·5
Wheat (*Triticum aestivum*) straw	3·0–3·7
Oat (*Avena sativa*) straw	7·2–11·0
Corn (*Zea mays*) stover	1·7–5·0
Cottonseed meal (*Gossypium* spp.), 41% protein	20·2–22·0
Soya meal	9·0–22·3
Bermuda grass (*Cunodon dactylon*)	4·9–9·2
Kentucky bluegrass (*Poa pratensis*)	1·6–12·7
Lespedeza (*Lespedeza striata*)	6·0–10·2
Orchard grass (*Dactylis glomerata*)	2·3–9·8
Ryegrass (*Lolium* spp.)	5·6–15·0
Wheat grain	6·3–13·9
Oat grain	6·3–11·0
Corn grain	3·3–22·3

From Davis GK and Mertz W (1987) with permission.

Table 4. Copper in human fluids, excretions, tissues

Fluids and excretions	Level
Serum	0·5–1·5 mg l^{-1}
Sweat	20–100 μg l^{-1}
Urine	4–66 μg l^{-1}
	5–50 μg day^{-1}
Faeces	0·5–2·5 mg day^{-1}
	20–100 mg kg^{-1} dry weight
Menstruation	0·5 mg per period
Hair	10–50 mg kg^{-1} dry weight

Tissues	Concentration (mg kg^{-1} wet weight)	Estimated % of total body copper
Bone marrow	5–7	15
Liver	5–7	8
Brain	5–7	8
Bone	2–3	19
Skin	2–3	15
Lungs, heart, kidney	2–3	<5
Muscle	<2	25
Blood	<2	5
Spleen	<2	<1

Data from Davis GK and Mertz W (1987) and Johnson MA and Kays SE (1990).

instrumental technique, fluid materials such as serum or urine can be analysed directly after a threefold (or more) dilution or they may require protein precipitation or removal of interfering salts. Matrix effects in fluid samples can sometimes be controlled by the technique of standard additions which involves adding known amounts of copper to the sample. Nonfluid samples such as plant tissue, animal organs or faeces require wet digestion with acid or dry ashing at approximately 450°C for 20–24 h to remove organic material.

Other matrix effects such as interfering salts can be removed by ion exchange chromatography. Removal of copper from a salt matrix or concentration of copper from biological samples is accomplished by complexing copper with various ligands followed by extraction with organic solvents such as methylisobutylketone.

Spectrophotometric Methods

In the 1950s a colorimetric method for determination of copper in biological samples was developed. Copper is liberated from proteins in tissues such as whole blood, red cells or plasma by hydrochloric acid and trichloro-acetic acid. The copper complexing agent sodium diethyldithiocarbamate is added to the supernatant liquid and the copper concentration is determined. Detection limits are around 100 μg l^{-1}. This method has largely been replaced by more sensitive techniques such as atomic absorption spectrometry (AAS). *See* Spectroscopy, Visible Spectroscopy and Colorimetry

Atomic Absorption Spectrometry

AAS is the most well-established technique for copper analysis in the clinical and industrial laboratory. The main advantages are: high accuracy, precision and sensitivity; controllable matrix and chemical effects; relatively inexpensive instrumentation and operating

Properties and Determination

costs compared to other techniques; and ease of use by technical staff.

AAS comprises two types: flame (FAAS) and electrochemical atomization (ETA-AAS). About 10–100 times less sample is needed for ETA-AAS than for FAAS. The detection limit for copper by FAAS is $< 10\ \mu g\ l^{-1}$ in 0·5 ml, and by ETA-AAS it is $< 1\ \mu g\ l^{-1}$ in 0·05 ml. FAAS is by far the most common technique in the clinical and industrial laboratory. For technical and economical reasons, ETA-AAS instrumentation is not as well established for routine copper analysis as FAAS.

Inductively Coupled Plasma Atomic Emission Spectrometry (ICP-AES)

The major advantage of ICP-AES is that simultaneous multielement analyses can be performed and that the standard curves for the elements are linear over several orders of magnitude. As little as 10 mg of sample can be analysed for more than 40 elements in a total volume of 1–3 ml. Detection limits for copper are around $1–5\ \mu g\ l^{-1}$. If copper is one of several elements to be determined, this technique is faster than AAS. Lower detection limits can sometimes be achieved for certain elements with ICP-AES, but this depends on how well the operating conditions for ICP-AES are optimized specifically for copper. ICP-AES is not as routine as AAS in most clinical and industrial laboratories because of the somewhat higher cost of the instrumentation. However, when many samples are to be analysed for several elements it is the method of choice.

Anodic Stripping Voltammetry (ASV)

ASV is less commonly used than AAS for analysis of biological samples because it is more sensitive to matrix effects. Adequate sample preparation with careful selection of extraction techniques and analytical solvents can control these products.

Electrochemical Detection (ED)

ED is also used less frequently than AAS for routine copper determination of plant and animal materials for reasons similar to those discussed for ASV. However, with further refinement, microelectrodes may become useful detectors for chromatographic separation of copper compounds in the complex biological matrices in plant and animal tissues. Detection limits for copper are around $1–5\ \mu g\ l^{-1}$.

Neutron Activation Analysis (NAA)

NAA is accomplished by irradiation of the sample with neutrons and measuring the corresponding radioactive nuclides from the elements of interest. Copper determination is achieved by measuring γ rays from ^{64}Cu. Compared to other elements, NAA is somewhat less reliable for copper because ^{64}Cu can be produced by other elements after neutron bombardment. Detection limits around 0·035 ng have been achieved.

Mass Spectrometry (MS)

MS is used to determine absolute concentrations and ratios of the stable isotopes, ^{63}Cu and ^{65}Cu. Of the various types of mass spectrometry, two commonly used for copper are inductively coupled plasma MS and thermal ionization MS. *See* Mass Spectrometry, Principles and Instrumentation

Bibliography

Davis GK and Mertz W (1987) Copper. In: Mertz W (ed.) *Trace Elements in Human and Animal Nutrition*, 5th edn, vol. 1, pp 301–364. New York: Academic Press.

Delves HT (1987) Atomic absorption spectroscopy in clinical analysis. *Annals of Clinical Biochemistry* 24: 529–551.

Dipietro ES, Bashor MM, Stroud PE, Smarr BJ, Burgess BJ, Turner WE and Neese JW (1988) Comparison of an inductively coupled plasma-atomic emission spectrometry method for the determination of calcium, magnesium, sodium, potassium, copper and zinc with atomic absorption spectroscopy and flame photometry methods. *Science of the Total Environment* 74: 249–262.

Evenson MA (1988) Measurement of copper in biological samples by flame or electrochemical atomic absorption spectrometry. *Methods in Enzymology* 158: 351–357.

Hee SSQ and Boyle JR (1988) Simultaneous multielemental analysis of some environmental and biological samples by inductively coupled plasma atomic emission spectrometry. *Analytical Chemistry* 60: 1033–1042.

Jensen A, Riber E, Persson P and Heydorn K (1983) Determination of manganese, iron, cobalt, nickel, copper and zinc in clinical chemistry. In: Sigel H (ed.) *Metal Ions in Biological Systems, Volume 16, Methods Involving Metal Ions and Complexes in Clinical Chemistry*, pp 167–181. New York: Marcel Dekker.

Johnson MA and Kays SE (1990) Copper: its role in human nutrition. *Nutrition Today* 25: 6–14.

Kies C (1989) Food sources of dietary copper. In: Kies C (ed.) *Copper Bioavailability and Metabolism. Advances in Experimental Medicine and Biology* 258: 1–20.

Life Sciences Research Office, Federation of American Societies for Experimental Biology (1989) Copper. In *Nutrition Monitoring in the United States – An Update Report on Nutrition Monitoring*. Prepared for the US Department of Agriculture and the US Department of Health and Human Services. DHHS Publication No. (PHS) 89-1255, Public Health Service, pp. 70, II176–II178. Washington, DC: US Government Printing Office.

Luscombe DL and Bond AM (1990) Copper determination in urine by flow injection analysis with electrochemical detection in platinum disk microelectrodes of various radii. *Analytical Chemistry* 62: 27–31.

McGrath SP (1986) The range of metal concentrations in topsoils of England and Wales in relation to soil protection guidelines. *Trace Substances in Environmental Health* 20: 242–252.

Singh JP, Karwasra SPS and Singh M (1988) Distribution and forms of copper, iron, manganese, and zinc in calcareous soils in India. *Soil Science* 146: 359–356.

Mary Ann Johnson
University of Georgia, Athens, USA

Physiology

Copper is essential in enzymes required for heart function, bone formation, energy metabolism, nerve transmission, elastin synthesis, pigmentation of the skin, normal hair growth, and red blood cell production. Because copper deficiency is not widely recognized, many patients have been misdiagnosed as having iron deficiency, rickets, scurvy and even cancer.

Infants are more likely than adults to become copper deficient. Adults who take high levels of zinc and possibly other supplements may impair their copper status.

Role in the Body

Signs of severe copper deficiency, such as brain, heart, bone, lung and blood disorders, are explained by decreases in copper metalloenzymes (Table 1). Iron absorption, mobilization from storage, transport, and incorporation into haemoglobin require changes in the oxidation state of iron which are in part mediated by the copper-protein, caeruloplasmin. Iron and copper metabolism are also linked through their joint presence in cytochrome *c* oxidase. *See* Iron, Physiology

Alterations in lipid and carbohydrate metabolism during copper deficiency are not so readily explained by the copper-proteins in Table 1. Thus this is an active area of research. *See* Carbohydrates, Digestion, Absorption and Metabolism

The severe heart dysfunction that occurs during copper deficiency in livestock and experimental animals has led to interest in the role of copper in heart disease. Because of its role in bone formation and protection against free radicals, it has also been proposed that copper may play a role in human bone diseases and cancer. However, little research has been conducted on the relationship between copper and these diseases in humans. *See* Bone

Absorption, Distribution and Storage

Absorption of copper occurs primarily in the proximal small intestine by passive absorption and amino-acid-facilitated active transport. Proposed regulatory factors include metallothionein, hormones and secretions from the pancreas and intestine. Absorption is influenced by dietary composition, chemical form of copper, age and disease.

For portal delivery to the liver copper is loosely bound to albumin or amino acids, and possibly to a newly proposed protein 'transcuprein'. Copper proteins such as caeruloplasmin are synthesized in the liver. The majority of serum copper is bound to caeruloplasmin, which serves as the transport protein from the liver to other organs.

The adult human contains 50–120 mg of copper. The

Table 1. Copper-proteins[a]

Common name	Function	Known or *possible* consequences of deficiency
Cytochrome *c* oxidase	Electron transport	*Muscle weakness; heart and brain disorders*
Superoxide dismutase	Free radical detoxification	*Membrane damage; other free radical damage*
Tyrosinase	Melanin production	Lack of pigmentation
Dopamine β-hydroxylase	Catecholamine production	*Neurological defects*
Lysyl oxidase	Cross-linking of collagen and elastin	Blood vessel, skin, bone and lung disorders
Caeruloplasmin	Ferroxidase, amine oxidase, copper transport	*Anaemia, impaired copper transport*
Metallothionein	Storage of copper	Decreased body stores of copper
Clotting factor V	Blood clotting	*Bleeding tendency*
Enzyme not known	Cross-linking of keratin (disulphide bonds)	Abnormal hair

[a]Adapted from Danks DM (1988), with permission.

Table 2. Blood indicators of severe copper deficiency

Blood indicator	Effect of copper deficiency on levels	Problems with interpretation
Haemoglobin[a]	↓ ⎫	Indicator for numerous abnormalities
Plasma iron	↓ ⎭	including iron deficiency
Plasma caeruloplasmin[a]	↓ ⎫	Increased by cigarette smoking, oral contraceptives,
Plasma copper[a]	↓ ⎭	pregnancy, infection and inflammation
Plasma neutrophils[a]	↓	Altered by infections and other diseases
Red blood cell superoxide dismutase	↓	Method not standardized among laboratories, so range of normal not established

[a] High probability of copper deficiency when three out of four of these indicators are subnormal.
↓ = decrease in levels.

Table 3. US recommended oral and intravenous intakes of copper[a,b]

Route	Population	Amount
Oral	Infants and children	80 μg per kg of bodyweight
	Adults	1·5–3 mg per day
Intravenous, total parenteral nutrition		
	Premature and fullterm infants	20 μg per kg of bodyweight
	Children	20 μg per kg of bodyweight, < 300 μg per day
	Adults	500–1500 μg per kg of bodyweight

[a] Data from National Research Council (1989) and Greene HL (1988).
[b] Table from Johnson MA and Kays SE (1990), with permission.

liver is believed to be the primary storage organ, but brain, bone marrow, skin, bone and muscle are each estimated to contain an equal or greater percentage of body copper compared to the liver. The concentration of copper in various tissues is (mg per kg wet weight): muscle, blood and spleen; < 2; bone, skin lungs, heart and kidney; 2–3; bone marrow, brain and liver; 5–7.

During gestation copper is stored in the liver and at birth the human liver has 5 to 10 times the adult concentration. This gradually decreases during the first year of life, as the stores are used.

Assessment of Nutritional Status

The hallmark biochemical signs of severe copper deficiency in infants and adults are subnormal levels of neutrophils, copper, caeruloplasmin and haemoglobin in the blood (Table 2). Copper deficiency has often been mistaken for iron deficiency because of the low haemoglobin values. However, the anaemia of copper deficiency does not respond to iron supplementation and hence is one form of 'iron refractory' anaemia. *See* Anaemia, Other Nutritional Causes

Marginal copper status is nearly impossible to detect at the present time. Indices of copper status such as plasma copper and plasma caeruloplasmin are elevated by numerous factors and are therefore not useful in the assessment of marginal copper status. Also, in a human study serum copper and caeruloplasmin were not increased when dietary intakes were increased 10-fold from 0·8 to 8 mg per day. Moreover, a marker protein for body stores of copper (like ferritin for iron stores) has not been identified. Although metallothionein contains copper, it also contains zinc and could reflect zinc rather than copper intake. *See* Zinc, Physiology

Dietary Requirements and Intakes in Adults

An 'estimated safe and adequate dietary intake' for the USA was established in 1989 for copper because insufficient data were available to set a 'US recommended dietary allowance' (Table 3). There is some discrepancy between the actual intakes (∼1–1·5 mg per day) and the estimated safe and adequate dietary intake (1·5–3 mg per day) for copper. Whether or not 1 mg of copper would be adequate in the presence of dietary or physiological factors that increase requirements remains to be explored.

Copper Requirements of Total Parenteral Nutrition Patients

As with many nutrients, less copper is needed when the nutrient is acquired intravenously from total parenteral nutrition (TPN) than when acquired orally (Table 3). Copper should be added to parenteral feeds under most circumstances, especially in patients with jejunostomies or exterior biliary drainage. However, additional copper is generally not needed when the parenteral nutrition is supplemental, when TPN is limited to less than four weeks, or when biliary excretion or liver function is impaired.

Nutrient Interactions

High intakes of zinc, ascorbic acid and iron are common in people who take large doses of vitamin and mineral supplements. It is well established that these nutrients interfere with the copper status of animals. In humans, as little as 50 mg of zinc per day impairs copper status and higher intakes result in severe anaemia. Zinc supplements commonly contain 30–60 mg of zinc per tablet. One person suffering from zinc-induced copper deficiency was inappropriately diagnosed with pre-leukaemia. However, the high zinc intakes were discovered before chemotherapy was initiated. The copper status of humans fed 600 mg of ascorbic acid per day show few changes, but 1500 mg of ascorbic acid per day significantly decreases caeruloplasmin. The influence of ascorbic acid in excess of 2000 mg per day on the copper status of humans is unknown. *See* Ascorbic Acid, Physiology; Health Foods, Dietary Supplements

Iron has primarily been studied in infants, so it is not known if iron supplements in the range of adult intakes adversely affect copper status. Although fibre adversely affects zinc status, it has only small and variable effects on copper status. *See* Dietary Fibre, Effects of Fibre on Absorption

Fructose and sucrose adversely affect the copper status of copper-deficient rats, but not pigs, Whether or not this is a practical problem for humans is unclear. For example, in one human study, fructose (20% of calories) depressed copper-zinc-superoxide dismutase in the blood, but unexpectedly improved the absorption of copper. In recent years there has been concern about the partial replacement of sucrose by high fructose corn syrups. However, these syrups contain both glucose and fructose, often in roughly equal amounts, although the fructose content may range from 42% to 90%. Because sucrose is 50% fructose, concern for the postulated effects of simple sugars on copper status must be directed toward both sucrose and fructose. *See* Fructose; Sucrose, Dietary Importance

Copper Deficiency in Infants

Infants are more susceptible to severe copper deficiency than all other population groups. Copper accumulates in the fetal liver during the latter part of gestation. Human milk is low in copper, so the liver stores are needed during the first months after birth. Infants who are malnourished, premature or of low birthweight are at the highest risk for copper deficiency. When these physiological conditions are combined with feeding practices such as cow's milk or TPN, the risk increases. *See* Infants, Breast- and Bottle-feeding; Infants, Nutritional Requirements

Although relatively uncommon (< 11% of cases), infants with copper deficiency may develop an osteoporotic and fractured skeleton that can be mistaken for scurvy, rickets and even child abuse. The symmetrical pattern of abnormalities from bone radiographs accompanied by abnormal copper status in the blood will distinguish copper deficiency from child abuse.

The likelihood of an infant becoming copper deficient is decreasing because infant formulas are supplemented with copper and it is recommended that copper is added to TPN feeds for infants as well as adults. However, in certain parts of the world where malnutrition is prevalent, copper deficiency continues to be a problem and can be more common than zinc deficiency. *See* Infant Foods, Milk Formulas; Infant Foods, Weaning Foods; Malnutrition, Malnutrition in Developing Countries

Genetic Disorders of Copper Utilization

Two genetic disorders of copper utilization are known in humans (Table 4). The combined frequencies of Menkes' disease and Wilson's disease are approximately five times less than phenylketonuria. Techniques for prenatal diagnosis are an active area of research. Several animal models have disturbances in copper metabolism that are remarkably similar to these human disorders.

Menkes' disease is characterized by the unusual 'steely' texture of the hair and by severe developmental delay. The symptoms are similar to dietary copper deficiency, yet oral copper is not effective in relieving the condition. Intestinal cells absorb copper but cannot release it to the general circulation. Injections of copper restore copper levels in the liver and serum but do not increase brain copper or prevent brain damage or premature death.

In contrast, early diagnosis and treatment will reduce

Table 4. Genetic disorders of copper utilization[a,b]

	Menkes' disease	Wilson's disease
General description:	Copper deficiency	Copper excess
Frequency:	~1:100 000 population	~1:100 000 population
Inheritance:	X-linked chromosomal	Autosomal recessive
Age at appearance:	Before three months	Between six years and early adulthood
Survival:	Only three months to three years	Good, if treated
Treatments:	None successful	Pencillamine, zinc, thiomolybdate
Key features:	Abnormal hair	Liver disease
	Developmental delay	Neurological disease
	Cerebral degeneration	Kayser–Fleischer rings
	Hypopigmentation	Haemolytic crises
	Bone changes	Bone and joint problems
	Arterial abnormalities	Renal stones
	Hypothermia	Renal tubular acidosis
Copper metabolism		
Intestinal transport:	Decreased	Normal
Biliary excretion:	—	Decreased
Urine excretion:	—	Increased
Balance[c]:	Negative	Positive
Serum copper or caeruloplasmin:	Very low	Often low
Liver copper:	Low	Elevated
Duodenal copper:	Elevated	—
Radioisotope studies (^{64}Cu or ^{67}Cu):	Excess accumulation in cultured fibroblasts	Not incorporated into caeruloplasmin

[a] Information from Danks DM (1983).
[b] Table adapted from Johnson MA and Kays SE (1990), with permission.
[c] Balance is copper intake minus faecal copper excretion.

morbidity and mortality from Wilson's disease. Liver diseases and/or neurological disorders develop because toxic levels of copper accumulate in these tissues. The genetic defect results in impaired incorporation of copper into caeruloplasmin, and decreased biliary excretion of copper. If copper is elevated in a liver biopsy, the diagnosis can be confirmed by copper deposits in the cornea (Kayser–Fleischer rings), by abnormally high levels of copper in urine and blood, and/or by lack of incorporation of radioactive copper into plasma proteins (i.e. caeruloplasmin). Siblings of Wilson's patients have a 25% chance of having the disease and should be screened. *See* Liver, Nutritional Management of Liver and Biliary Disorders

Toxicity

In experimental animals and livestock, mild to fatal signs of copper poisoning occur with as little as 20 to 40 times the usual intake of copper. In humans, only 10–30 mg of orally ingested copper from various ionic salts or from foods stored in copper vessels may cause intestinal discomfort, dizziness and headaches. Ingestion of copper salts in excess of 500–1000 mg has caused acute poisoning in humans and has been fatal. Acute copper poisoning is very similar to poisoning by other heavy metals and causes vomiting, diarrhoea with bleeding, circulatory collapse, failure of liver and kidneys, and severe haemolysis. Acute poisoning is rare but has occurred from accidental ingestion of copper sulphate by children, soft drinks served from defective equipment, and consumption of foods, alcohol, or other beverages cooked or stored in copper-lined vessels. Copper poisoning is a common method of suicide in India, where it accounts for one third of all poisonings in some hospitals. Industrial exposure to high levels of copper has been associated with breathing and skin problems.

The healthy liver of normal individuals prevents excess accumulation of copper in the body. However, copper accumulation can occur during prolonged liver diseases that disrupt normal biliary excretion of copper. Hepatitis or cirrhosis may result from the excess accumulation of copper in the liver. When the capacity of the liver to store copper is exceeded, a sudden release of copper may occur and result in a haemolytic crisis similar to that seen in acute copper poisoning. *See* Liver, Nutritional Management of Liver and Biliary Disorders

One of the benign but alarming manifestations of copper toxicity is green hair. This occurs when hair is exposed to chlorinated water, copper-based swimming pool algicides, water from corroded copper pipes, or certain industrial agents.

Bibliography

Danks DM (1983) Hereditary disorders of copper metabolism in Wilson's disease and Menkes' disease. In: Stanbury JB, Wyngaarden JB, Fredrickson D S, Goldstein JL and Brown MS (eds) *The Metabolic Basis of Inherited Disease*, 5th edn, pp. 1251–1268. New York: McGraw-Hill.

Danks DM (1988) Copper deficiency in humans. *Annual Review of Nutrition* 8: 235–257.

Davis GK and Mertz W (1987) Copper. In: Mertz W. (ed) *Trace Elements in Humans and Animal Nutrition*, Volume 1, 5th edn, pp. 301–364. New York: Academic Press.

Greene HL, Hambidge KM, Schanler R and Tsang RC (1988) Guidelines for the use of vitamins, trace elements, calcium, magnesium, and phosphorus in infants and children receiving total parenteral nutrition: report of the Subcommittee on Pediatric Parenteral Nutrient Requirements from the Committee on Clinical Practice Issues of the American Society for Clinical Nutrition. *American Journal of Clinical Nutrition* 48: 1324–1342.

Johnson MA and Kays SE (1990) Copper: its role in human nutrition. *Nutrition Today* 25: 6–14.

National Research Council (1989). In: *Recommended Dietary Allowances*, 10th edn, pp. 224–230. Washington DC: National Academy Press.

Reiser S, Smith JC, Mertz W *et al.* (1985) Indices of copper status in humans consuming a typical American diet containing either fructose or starch. *American Journal of Clinical Nutrition* 42: 242–251.

Shaw JCL (1988) Copper deficiency and non-accidental injury. *Archives of Disease in Childhood* 63: 448–455.

Turnlund JR, Keyes WR, Anderson HL and Acord LL (1989) Copper absorption and retention in young men at three levels of dietary copper by use of the stable isotope ^{65}Cu. *American Journal of Clinical Nutrition* 49: 870–878.

Mary Ann Johnson
University of Georgia, Athens, USA

CORONARY HEART DISEASE

Contents

Aetiology and Risk Factors

Coronary heart disease (CHD) is caused by atherosclerosis of the coronary arteries. This pathological process is initiated by the uptake of cholesterol into scavenger macrophages which become transformed into foam cells. Smooth muscle proliferation takes place and the arterial wall becomes thickened within its inner region, with consequent loss of lumen diameter. When the loss of lumen diameter reaches a critical stage the maximum blood flow rate through the artery may be insufficient to meet the demand of the heart muscle supplied. At this stage the patient may suffer from angina (chest pain). This condition may progress or remain stable, or develop further into a coronary thrombosis. Coronary thrombosis occurs when, following a split in the endothelium lining over a patch of atherosclerotic plaque, platelets become adherent, tissue factors are released and blood clot develops. Fibrinolytic processes also come into play and the final outcome in terms of the size of the thrombosis depends on the balance between clotting and fibrinolytic factors. The thrombosis causes further narrowing of the lumen diameter and thus an acute reduction of blood flow which further exacerbates any ischaemia. If blood flow falls to a very low level or is totally obstructed, the heart muscle supplied by that particular coronary artery or branch ceases to function and dies. This death of heart muscle (myocardial infarction; the area of dead tissue is surrounded by living but malfunctioning tissue) causes effects ranging from sudden death, through severe chest pain, irregularities of heart rhythm, acute heart failure to no symptoms at all where the area affected is small. *See* Atherosclerosis

Extensive epidemiological studies have shown that

the risk of developing CHD is high in smokers, hypertensives, hyperlipidaemic patients, diabetics, those who are overweight or obese, and those who are physically inactive and subjected to stress. The risks are also high in women who use some forms of contraceptive pill, in those who have a strong family history of CHD, and in men rather than women (although beyond the age of 50 years the rates for women are very similar to those for men).

Smoking causes atherosclerosis through direct effects of smoke components (notably nicotine) on the arterial wall, but may also have indirect effects. Smokers eat less fruit and vegetables than non-smokers, are thus expected to consume less dietary antioxidant substances (e.g. β-carotene and lycopene, as well as vitamin C), and are thus at greater risk of oxidative damage to lipoprotein particles. Oxidized low-density lipoprotein (LDL)-cholesterol is readily taken up by scavenger macrophages. There is evidence that both the dose of cigarettes smoked and the duration of smoking (smoking years) determine CHD risk. In hypertension, changes in arteries, including smooth muscle hypertrophy, and facilitation of lipid entry serve to accelerate the atherosclerosis process. Risk of CHD is related to the extent of both diastolic and systolic hypertension, and the duration. Although the duration of exposure to hypertension is rarely known precisely, longer exposure increases risk. Risk is also increased at raised blood pressures, even in the lower range, emphasizing that even slightly raised blood pressure should be treated. *See* Hypertension, Hypertension and Diet; Smoking, Diet and Health

High Blood Cholesterol

Many studies have demonstrated the positive relationship between total blood cholesterol and CHD mortality. In most studies, the least risk of CHD corresponds to a total blood cholesterol of $5 \cdot 2$ mmol 1^{-1}. In studies reported more recently high-density lipoprotein (HDL)-cholesterol has been shown to be inversely related to CHD mortality. Some studies of apolipoprotein concentrations have shown that these too can be good markers of risk. Blood cholesterol can be raised in an individual because he or she is at the upper end of the biological distribution for cholesterol in the population, or because the individual is a member of a group with a specific genetic hypolipidaemia. For example familial hypercholesterolaemia has a frequency of about 1 in 500 in Western populations. It is a monogenic dominant condition and is thus expressed in the heterozygote form. Functioning (high affinity) LDL receptors are reduced in number by about 50% in heterozygotes and by about 100% in homozygotes, with consequent high LDL-cholesterol levels (perhaps up to 15 mmol 1^{-1} in

heterozygotes and higher in homozygotes). Atherosclerotic arterial disease is accelerated in these people and they present with CHD and other manifestations of atherosclerosis at a relatively young age compared to the 'normal' population. They account for about 5% of cases of CHD, although their frequency in the population is only 1 in 500. *See* Cholesterol, Role of Cholesterol in Heart Disease; Hyperlipidaemia; Lipoproteins

Diabetes and Obesity

Studies on diabetic patients treated according to standards of care in the 1960s and 1970s show an increased risk of CHD between two and nine times that of nondiabetics, according to age and sex (young male subjects having the highest relative mortality). Factors in diabetics which increase the risk include disordered cholesterol metabolism and increased smooth muscle cell proliferation, both possibly insulin-induced. Lipid oxidation may also be more of a problem in diabetics. There is some evidence that, compared to nonobese people, nondiabetic obese individuals may be at slightly higher risk of CHD, but obesity may not be an independent risk factor; rather, it may be linked via hypertension and diabetes. Seventy per cent of diabetics are overweight or obese, and a high proportion of CHD patients have evidence of insulin resistance and/or glucose intolerance. Thus endogenous overproduction of insulin to meet relatively high demands owing to insulin resistance, or exposure to relatively high exogenous insulin doses for treatment purposes may be factors. Diabetics are particularly predisposed to hypertriglyceridaemia when not well controlled, but there is little evidence that raised triglyceride is an independent risk factor for CHD. *See* Obesity, Aetiology and Assessment

Exercise and Stress

Population studies have shown that a sedentary lifestyle is associated with higher rates for CHD. Early studies clearly showed that the level of physical activity at the workplace was clearly linked to CHD risk. Exercise has been shown to modify blood lipids, raising HDL-cholesterol, to alter platelet adhesiveness and, if sufficiently strenuous on a regular basis, to improve the myocardial circulation. Exercise may also ameliorate some of the effects of stress. In susceptible individuals, stress may raise blood pressure, raise blood lipids and increase vascular tone, all of which, if sustained or repeated frequently, might be expected to accelerate atherosclerosis. Quantification of stress is difficult, and detection of those who respond adversely to it is not part of routine screening, but the response of blood pressure

Coronary Heart Disease 1249

to a standard stress test might become more widely used. *See* Exercise, Metabolic Requirements; Stress and Nutrition

Assessment of Risk

Several large-scale trials, e.g. the PROCAM trial in the FRG and the British Regional Heart Survey, have resulted in the development of formulae designed to quantify risk. The risk is usually defined in terms of the probability of death from CHD within a defined period. Such formulae are of interest because they are based on data from many thousands of individuals and they can be used to predict the change of risk resulting from intervention on risk factors. They then show clearly the relative importance of the different risk factors and show where the effort needs to be placed. All show quite clearly the overriding role of smoking and the clear benefit to most patients of stopping smoking. In some formulae, well-known risk factors do not appear; for example, in the British Regional Heart Survey blood cholesterol seems not to be a major predictor of risk, but is included in the PROCAM formula. In the latter, reductions of blood cholesterol do not seem to be associated with big reductions of risk. It must be remembered, however, that while based on data from thousands of individuals studied for several years, results can only be used to predict risk in similar population groups (usually older individuals). It may be that some risk factor modifications are more effective if undertaken earlier in life.

Bibliography

Committee on Diet and Health, National Research Council (1989) *Diet and Health: Implications for Reducing Chronic Disease Risk*. Washington, DC: National Academy Press.

Committee on Medical Aspects of Food Policy (1984) *Diet and Cardiovascular Disease*. Report of the Panel on Diet in Relation to Cardiovascular Disease. London: DHSS.

Study Group, European Atherosclerosis Society (1987) Strategies for the prevention of coronary heart disease. A policy statement of the European Atherosclerosis Society. *European Heart Journal* 8:77.

The Health of the Nation (1991) Presented to Parliament by the Secretary of State for Health by Command of Her Majesty, June 1991.

WHO Expert Committee (1982) *Prevention of Coronary Heart Disease*. Technical Report Series, 678.

A. R. Leeds
King's College, London, UK

Antioxidant Status

The Rationale for the 'Antioxidant Hypothesis'

The major recognized risk factors for coronary heart disease are smoking, hypertension and blood cholesterol concentration but these account for less than 50% of the variance in the incidence of the disease. The 'antioxidant hypothesis' attempts to account for some of this unexplained variation by introducing a low dietary intake of nutritional antioxidants as an additional risk factor. The associated reduction in the concentrations of antioxidants such as vitamin E, carotenoids and, possibly, ubiquinone in the low-density lipoprotein (LDL) molecule, and a low concentration of vitamin C in the aqueous phase render the LDL-cholesterol more susceptible to oxidative modification by free radicals and thereby increases its atherogenic properties. *See* Atherosclerosis

Free Radicals and Antioxidants

Free radicals are molecules or molecular fragments with an unpaired electron; they can be highly reactive and, by abstracting a hydrogen, can damage many biomolecules, including proteins, thiols, nucleic acids, nucleotides, polyunsaturated fatty acids and others. Free radicals are formed during normal metabolism, and by secondary reactions with protons and transition metals such as copper and iron. For example, the superoxide anion (O_2^-) is produced in many cell redox systems, including those involving xanthine oxidase, aldehyde oxidase, membrane-associated NADPH (nicotinamide adenine dinucleotide phosphate, reduced form) oxidases and the cytochrome P-450 systems. About 1–4% of the total oxygen uptake by mitochondria may be converted to O_2^- and about 20% of this may then be ejected into the cell. In addition, stimulated macrophages and monocytes can release large amounts of O_2^- via the respiratory burst. Although O_2^- is not particularly reactive, having a low second-order rate constant with biomolecules, it can diffuse relatively large distances through the cell before it is converted to the highly reactive hydroxyl radical (OH$^\cdot$) in a Haber–Weiss reaction catalysed by iron or copper ions.

Potentially injurious free radicals are also present in pollutants and halogenated anaesthetics. Moreover, each puff of a cigarette contains approximately 10^4 free radicals in the tar phase and approximately 10^{15} in the gas phase. Long-lived quinone-semiquinone radicals (Q$^\cdot$) associated with the particulate phase are generated by the oxidation of polycyclic hydrocarbons. In aqueous

Antioxidant Status

medium, $Q^{\cdot}$ can reduce oxygen to O_2^- and hydrogen peroxide (H_2O_2) and catalyse the conversion of H_2O_2 to $OH^{\cdot}$. In the smoke phase, reactive carbon- and oxygen-centred radicals ($ROO^{\cdot}$) are continuously generated by a reaction between nitrogen dioxide (NO_2) and aldehydes and olefins. Moreover, NO_2 may react with H_2O_2 to produce $OH^{\cdot}$. Pulmonary macrophages activated by nicotine may provide a source of H_2O_2 which may then be converted to $OH^{\cdot}$ in a Fenton reaction catalysed by free copper or iron ions. *See* Smoking, Diet and Health

A complex antioxidant defence system normally protects our mammalian cells from the injurious effects of free radicals. Antioxidants are substances which, when present at much lower concentrations than an oxidizable substrate, significantly delay or prevent its oxidation. Certain essential antioxidants need to be provided by the diet. Vitamin E is a major lipid-soluble antioxidant which breaks the chain of free-radical-mediated lipid peroxidation of polyunsaturated fatty acids in cell membranes. β-Carotene and other carotenoids may have a similar function, particularly in tissues with a low partial pressure of oxygen. Vitamin C scavenges free radicals in the water-soluble compartment of the cell and may also regenerate vitamin E. In addition, several antioxidant enzymes, such as glutathione peroxidase, catalase and superoxide dismutase, metabolize the toxic intermediates produced on oxidation of biological material. These require micronutrient cofactors, such as selenium, iron, copper, zinc and manganese. *See* Antioxidants, Role of Antioxidant Nutrients in Defence Systems; Ascorbic Acid, Physiology; Carotenoids, Physiology; Tocopherols, Physiology; Trace Elements

The efficiency of this antioxidant defence system depends in part on an adequate intake of foods that are enriched in these antioxidants and trace metal cofactors. Thus the antioxidant status of the body may be influenced by diet. If the antioxidant status of the body is lowered, possibly because of inadequate dietary intake of these micronutrients, then free-radical-mediated modification to the various components of the cell, including the LDL, may occur, with increased risk of the onset of coronary heart disease.

Biochemical Evidence to Support the Antioxidant Hypothesis

Low-density lipoproteins contain a high proportion of polyunsaturated fatty acids (PUFAs) in the phospholipid layer which are susceptible to free-radical-mediated peroxidation. Oxidation of LDLs results in a loss of PUFAs and an increase in lipid hydroperoxides, aldehydic products and lysolecithin. Experiments with cell cultures suggest that such oxidation modifies the chemical and physical properties of the LDL to render it more atherogenic. The consequences of these oxidative changes include the following: *See* Lipoproteins

1. Recognition and preferential uptake of modified LDL by scavenger receptors of macrophages.
2. Enhancement of chemotactic responses with respect to other monocytes or macrophages, leading to accumulation of macrophages at specific sites.
3. Increased production through the action of a platelet-derived growth factor by endothelial cells, with a resultant increase in the tendency for platelet aggregation.
4. Increased release of adhesion molecules by endothelial cells.

An important step in the development of the atherogenic plaque is the formation of foam cells on the wall of the artery. This can be explained by increased oxidation of LDL and a series of related events (Fig. 1). If the intake of nutritional antioxidants is less than that required to cope with the exogenous free radical load incurred by smoking and/or excess dietary intake of PUFAs, there will be an increased burden of lipid hydroperoxides. This cytotoxic by-product of the peroxidation of PUFAs may then cause the initial lesion in the artery wall. Uptake of oxidized LDL by monocytes which are attracted to this site of injury promotes chemotactic attraction by further monocytes. On transformation of monocytes to macrophages, the oxidized LDL appears to limit further macrophage mobility and decreases their ability to migrate away from the artery wall. The enhanced rate of uptake of oxidized LDL may then convert macrophages into foam cells. Since the macrophage can oxidatively modify native LDL via the respiratory burst, autocatalytic progression may lead to the continuous growth of the atheroma. Elevated concentrations of lipid hydroperoxides also appear to promote platelet aggregation, thus eventually contributing to thrombus formation. High intakes of those saturated fatty acids that increase LDL would provide increased substrate for the above reactions.

The susceptibility of LDL to oxidation may also be influenced by its own antioxidant content. When LDL is subjected to a copper-mediated oxidation *in vitro*, ubiquinone and vitamin E disappear first, followed by the carotenoids, e.g. lycopene and β-carotene. However, LDL oxidation can be delayed if vitamin C is present in the external medium, presumably through regeneration of vitamin E. Increasing the vitamin E content of the LDL also inhibits oxidation. If similar reactions occur *in vivo*, then dietary antioxidant intake may influence LDL oxidation.

The mechanisms by which LDL is oxidized *in vivo* have yet to be clearly characterized. Oxidation is unlikely to occur in plasma which has an effective

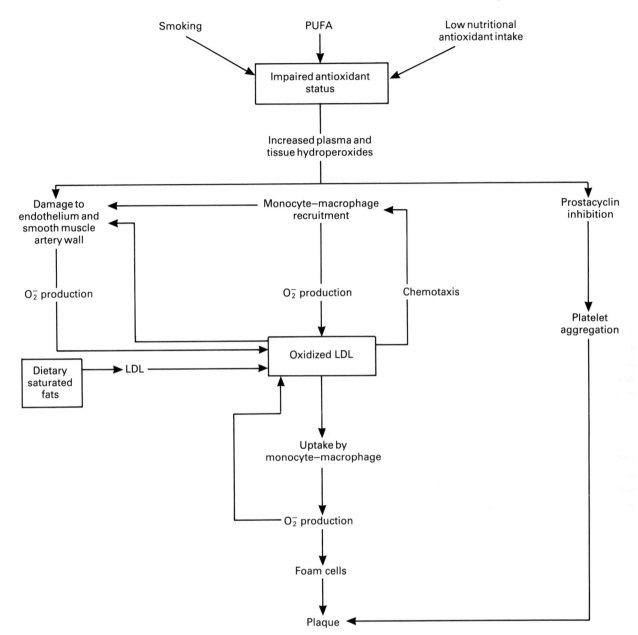

Fig. 1 The possible oxidative interactions which contribute to the development of the atheromatous plaque. PUFA, polyunsaturated fatty acid; LDL, low-density lipoprotein.

antioxidant capacity and may be restricted to regions of the vascular intima. Although LDL can be modified by lipoxygenases and phospholipase A_2, oxygen radical reactions with copper are likely to play a more dominant role. Copper ions effectively promote oxidation of LDL *in vitro*, and release of copper from caeruloplasmin within the atherosclerotic lesion may lead to peroxidation of preformed hydroperoxides. These may themselves be formed within the lesion by initiation with OH· produced by macrophage-derived O_2^- and H_2O_2. The evidence for LDL oxidation *in vivo* is still sparse but LDL extracted from aortic lesions does react with antibodies specific for oxidatively modified LDL.

Epidemiological Evidence to Support the Antioxidant Hypothesis

Support for the premise that a low nutritional antioxidant intake contributes to atherogenesis has been provided by cross-cultural investigations which found that mortality was inversely correlated with a 'cumulative antioxidant index'. This was defined as follows:

$$(\text{vitamin E} \times \text{vitamin C} \times \beta\text{-carotene} \times \text{selenium})/\text{cholesterol}$$

All concentrations are those in plasma. Mortality from coronary heart disease can be strongly correlated with

Antioxidant Status

plasma vitamin E in its own right, and case-control studies indicate that in subjects with angina plasma concentrations of vitamin E and C and β-carotene are decreased, while those of lipid hydroperoxide-related substances are increased. In northern latitudes, smokers – a group at a two- to threefold increased risk of coronary heart disease – are also characterized by their low plasma vitamin C and carotenoid concentrations, and increased plasma indices of oxidative damage.

Summary

The antioxidant hypothesis augments the lipid hypothesis of coronary heart disease by identifying oxidized cholesterol rather than cholesterol *per se* as the risk factor. The recent experimental evidence for free-radical-mediated modification of LDL, and the epidemiological inverse correlations between plasma levels of antioxidants and mortality from coronary heart disease indicate that oxidant stress may provide a mechanistic basis for development of the disease.

Bibliography

Duthie GG, Wahle KWJ and James WPT (1989) Oxidants, antioxidants and cardiovascular disease. *Nutrition Research Reviews* 2: 51–62.
Gey KF (1990) The antioxidant hypothesis of cardiovascular disease: epidemiology and mechanisms. *Biochemical Society Transactions* 18: 1041–1045.

G. G. Duthie
Rowett Research Institute, Aberdeen, UK

Intervention Studies

Definition and Aims

In the section on Epidemiology a number of research strategies are discussed. These fall into two very obvious groups: observation and intervention. In general, observation studies seek to ascertain more about the natural course of a disease process, whereas intervention studies test the effect of a possible therapeutic or prophylactic measure. *See* Epidemiology

In nutrition research, intervention trials can be thought of, first, as those in which a foodstuff or a nutrient is given to subjects, and the effect upon a mechanism, or a metabolic pathway, is observed. Measuring the rise in blood lipids following changes in dietary fat intake, or measuring the blood pressure response to coffee prepared in different ways, illustrates this kind of study. In these, the numbers of subjects can be relatively small, because a measurement of the outcome variable (serum cholesterol, or blood pressure, etc.) is obtained for every subject. The cardinal rules for a randomized controlled trial (RCT) apply here just as much as to the studies which will be described later, though a 'cross-over' design, in which each subject serves as his own control, is efficient and may be appropriate if the effect being tested is relatively short lived.

In the second kind of intervention trial the effect of a dietary change on the incidence of a disease is studied. This is very much more difficult because the outcome is an event, such as death or a nonfatal heart attack, and this occurs in only a very small proportion of subjects. Numbers have therefore to be very large and/or the period of observation long.

Design

The only designs for an intervention study which are now acceptable, are those that fulfil the basic criteria for an RCT. These criteria include the following:

1. Allocation of only a proportion (usually half) of the subjects in the group defined for the trial, to the intervention procedure, the other subjects not receiving the intervention.
2. Identical advice, handling and monitoring of the two subgroups of subjects – those receiving the intervention and those not.
3. Assessment of the outcome, be it the change in a biochemical or other variate, or a disease event, by an observer who is blind as to whether or not the subject had received the intervention.

Unfortunately, it is rarely possible in dietary RCTs to comply with a further criterion which many would regard as cardinal, namely blindness of the participants as to whether they are receiving the intervention measure or not. This is achieved in drug trials by the use of a placebo tablet but in dietary trials the use of a dummy foodstuff is just not possible.

A recent trial by Burr *et al.* of three dietary measures (fat, fish and fibre) in the prevention of coronary heart disease (CHD) has demonstrated the value of a factorial design. In this trial, each of the different interventions are randomized independently to half the subjects. Equal numbers of subjects therefore receive each possible combination of the interventions, with some receiving all and some none. This design is acceptable provided that there is no reason to expect strong interaction between the different interventions. It is highly efficient as the main effects are all tested simultaneously without loss of power.

Compliance of subjects with an intervention is of great importance and should be taken into account in drawing conclusions from a trial. In fact, it is important to monitor both the degree of compliance by those who have been given advice about the dietary factor being tested and the extent to which the control subjects may spontaneously change their consumption of that factor. Ideally, compliance should be monitored in an objective way; for example, the estimation of plasma eicosapentaenoic acid will indicate how much fatty fish has been consumed. If an appropriate objective measure is not available, then at intervals the subjects (both those advised and the controls) can be asked to keep a diary of the food they consume.

Careful attention should always be given to the likely power of a study, i.e. the likelihood that the planned trial will be sensitive enough to detect a statistically significant beneficial effect, should one occur.

A number of things affect power, including the variability of the predictive factor (e.g. fat intake) within different subjects, the number of subjects and the number of outcome events. A further item which is required if numbers are being estimated in a power calculation is the likely effect of the intervention on the outcome variable. This will not be known and an estimate will therefore have to be made. Clearly, this should be a compromise between what might be desired (even a very small beneficial effect is worthwhile) and what is feasible.

Power calculations should always be done with care, but – to give a very rough guide – to have a reasonable chance (say 80–90%) of detecting a reduction in CHD incidence of about 20–25% as statistically significant (at, say, $P < 0.05$), a primary preventive trial will have to yield around 50 000 man-years of evidence and a secondary preventive trial about 5000.

This does not mean that smaller trials should not be undertaken. The play of chance is such that no single trial, however large, can give conclusive evidence, and the value of 'overviews' of a number of trials has been repeatedly demonstrated. To be acceptable for inclusion in an overview, a trial must make no compromise of the cardinal rules of an RCT, and for an overview to be acceptable every trial should be included. This last will be difficult because there is a publication bias, and trials which fail to demonstrate an effect are unlikely to be reported. However, extensive enquiries should be pursued and every attempt made to locate such trials.

Primary and Secondary Trials in CHD

The terms 'primary' and 'secondary' are used to distinguish trials which test a preventive measure in men who have not already had a clinical episode of ischaemic heart disease (IHD) (primary) from those based on patients who have already had a myocardial infarct or other clinical event (secondary).

Ideally, all preventive measures should be tested in a primary RCT, but the numbers required for this are formidable. Further difficulties arise in persuading healthy subjects to comply with the intervention to a sufficient degree and for a sufficient time. On this last, it may be that no trial has yet been realistic in that, if the aim is to prevent or reduce atherosclerosis, the trial should be commenced in childhood or adolescence and continue into late middle life, or beyond. See Atherosclerosis

On the other hand, most subjects who have already had a clinical event of a disease consider themselves to be at high risk and are likely to be more easily persuaded to comply with a dietary change for a very long period, if not indefinitely. At the same time it can be argued that the underlying disease of survivors of a myocardial infarction (MI) is too far advanced to be reversible within the time span of trials of less than, say, 10 or more years. While this may be true of measures aimed to reduce atherosclerosis, the success of Burr et al.'s recent trial of fatty fish in the reduction of mortality indicates that dietary factors are relevant to mechanisms in heart disease other than atherosclerosis. It is perhaps on these other mechanisms that research should now focus. Force is given to this statement by the growing evidence that haemostatic factors are far more highly predictive of CHD than lipid levels, and by the suggestion that one of the main effects of fish oil may be on the electrical stability of the myocardium. See Fish Oils, Dietary Importance

The Main Dietary Trials Conducted

Fatty Fish

The hypothesis that fatty fish, fish oil, or eicosapentaenoic acid (EPA) might reduce the risk of CHD has recently received new impetus by the report by Burr et al. of an RCT in secondary prevention. In this, 2033 men were randomized factorially to three interventions, one of which was fatty fish. The amount of fish recommended was modest – at least two main meals per week, contributing around 2·5 g of EPA per week.

Mortality in the 1015 men advised to eat fatty fish was 9·3% over the next 2 years, and it was 12·8% in the 1018 men who had been given no advice about fatty fish. This represents a reduction in mortality of about 29% and a saving of lives of about 36 per 1000 men advised. Because these last are derived from the results of a single trial they carry a considerable uncertainty.

It is notable, however, that this trial gave no evidence that nonfatal infarctions were reduced by fish-eating. Indeed, there were rather more nonfatal infarctions in the men advised (4·8%) than in the other men (3·2%). It is therefore possible that the effect of fish is to reduce the risk of death after infarction rather than to reduce the incidence of infarction; evidence consistent with this

Table 1. Trials of dietary fat reduction in primary prevention

	Advised	Control	Duration (years)	Total deaths		Nonfatal MI	
				Advised	Control	Advised	Control
WHO[a]	30 489	26 971	6	1325	1186	505	505
Goteborg[b]	10 004	20 018	12	1293	2636	501	978
MRFIT[c]	6428	6438	7	265	260	294	323
Helsinki[d]	612	610	15	67	46	15[f]	8[f]
Oslo[e]	604	628	5	16	24	14	24

[a] WHO European Collaborative Group (1986). European collaborative trial of multifactorial prevention of coronary heart disease: final report on the six-year results *Lancet* i: 869–872.
[b] Wilhelmson L, Berglund G, Elmfeldt D, Tibblin G *et al.* (1986) The multi-factorial primary prevention trial in Goteborg, Sweden. *European Heart Journal* 7: 279–288.
[c] Multiple Risk Factor Intervention Trial Research Group (1982) Multiple risk factor intervention trial. *Journal of the American Medical Association* 248: 1465–1477.
Multiple Risk Factor Intervention Trial Research Group (1986) Coronary heart disease death, non-fatal acute myocardial infarction and other clinical outcomes in the Multiple Risk Factor Intervention Trial. *American Journal of Cardiology* 58: 1–13.
[d] Miettinen TA, Huttunen JK, Naukkarinen Y *et al* (1985) Multifactorial primary prevention of cardiovascular diseases in middle-aged men. *Journal of the American Medical Association* 254: 2097–2102.
Strandberg TE, Salomaa VV, Vanhanen HT, Naukkarinen V, Sarna S and Miettinen TA (1990) 15-year mortality rates for participants in a multifactorial primary prevention trial of cardiovascular diseases. *International Symposium on Multiple Risk Factors in Cardiovascular Disease*, Washington DC.
[e] Hjermann I, Velve Byre K, Holme I and Leren P (1981) Effect of diet and smoking intervention on the incidence of coronary heart disease. *Lancet* ii: 1303–1310.
[f] Five year nonfatal MI incidence, data for 15 years not available.

hypothesis comes from work on the electrical stability of the myocardium in experimentally induced infarction in animals.

Dietary Fat

Undoubtedly, fat reduction has been more investigated in the prevention of CHD than any other potential prophylactic. The early trials focused largely on the reduction of total fat in the diet; more recently interest has focused on the P:S ratio (the ratio of polyunsaturated to saturated fats). Mono-unsaturated fats are also of current interest. The interest in the poly- and monounsaturates arises largely from the fact that they lower cholesterol levels, while saturated fats raise circulating cholesterol. *See* Cholesterol, Role of Cholesterol in Heart Disease; Fats, Requirements

Table 1 summarizes the published trials of primary prevention by dietary fat reduction. The interventions in these trials have differed somewhat but all have included advice to reduce dietary fat consumption and fat of animal origin in particular. In all the trials, advice on smoking cessation was also given, and, in all but one, treatment of raised blood pressure was offered. *See* Smoking, Diet and Health

A number of overviews of these trials have been published. These show that while there is a reduction in CHD events there is no reduction in overall mortality. This last is important and makes it difficult to judge the value of dietary fat reduction. This difficulty is com-

pounded by the finding that noncardiovascular causes of death are increased in the subjects advised to reduce their dietary fat, and this increase is most clearly shown in deaths which have been certified as due to violence, suicide and accidents. This excess has also been shown in trials of cholesterol lowering drugs.

Trials of fat reduction in secondary prevention are summarized in Table 2. Again, there is no convincing evidence of a reduction in mortality, particularly if one only accepts evidence from the randomized trials. At the same time there is evidence of a reduction in nonfatal infarctions.

Dietary Fibre

Unfortunately, again, there has been only one RCT of dietary fibre, reported by Burr *et al.* In this, advice given to 1017 men led to an increase in cereal fibre intake to 19 g per day, compared with 9 g in 1016 controls. After 2 years there was no significant difference in the deaths in those given the advice about fibre (12·1%) compared to those not so advised (9·9%).

Interest in fibre has shifted again, and attention is now being focused on 'soluble' fibre, which is quite a change from the early ideas about 'roughage' and insoluble fibre. Interest in soluble fibre arises primarily because it has been shown in numerous small feeding trials to reduce serum cholesterol if eaten in sufficient quantities. There is also interest in fruit and vegetables, the main source of soluble fibre, because these are also a significant source of

Table 2. Trials of dietary fat reduction in secondary prevention

	Number of patients		Duration (years)	Allocation to diet	Cholesterol reduction (%)	Deaths		Reinfarctions	
	Low fat	Control				Low fat	Control	Low fat	Control
Morrison[a]	50	50	12	Alternate	29	31	50	—	—
Bierenbaum[b]	100	100	10	Later: matched	10	16	28	—	—
MRC[c]	123	129	4	Random	16	20	24	43	44
Rose[d]	28	52	2	Random	17	5	4	6	11
Leren[e]	206	206	10	Random	14	101	108	24	31
MRC[f]	199	194	4	Random	16	28	31	20	26
Woodhill[g]	221	237	2–7	Random	4	39	28	—	—
Burr[h]	1017	1015	2	Random	4	111	113	35	47

[a] Morrison LM (1960) Diet in coronary atherosclerosis. *Journal of the American Medical Association* 173: 884–888.

[b] Bierenbaum ML, Fleischman AI, Raichelson RI, Hayton T and Watson PB (1973) Ten year experience of modified-fat diets on younger men with coronary heart disease. *Lancet* i: 1404–1407.

[c] Medical Research Council, Research Committee (1965) Low fat diet in myocardial infarction; a controlled trial. *Lancet* ii: 501–504.

[d] Rose GA, Thomson WB and Williams RT (1965) Corn oil in treatment of ischaemic heart disease. *British Medical Journal* 1: 1531–1533.

[e] Leren P (1966) The effect of plasma cholesterol lowering diet in male survivors of myocardial infarction. *Acta Medica Scandinavica* Suppl. 466: 1–92.

Leren P (1970) The Oslo Diet-Heart Study. Eleven-year report. *Circulation* 40: 935–943.

[f] Medical Research Council, Research Committee (1968) Controlled trial of soya-bean oil in myocardial infarction. *Lancet* ii: 693–700.

[g] Woodhill JM, Palmer AJ, Leelarthaepin B, McGilchrist C and Blacket RB (1978) Low fat, low cholesterol diet in secondary prevention of coronary heart disease. *Advances in Experimental Medical Biology* 109: 317–330.

[h] Burr ML, Fehily AM, Gilbert JF, Rogers S, Holliday RM, Sweetnam PM, Elwood PC and Deadman NM (1989) Effects of changes in fat, fish, and fibre intakes on death and myocardial reinfarction: Diet and Reinfarction Trial (DART). *Lancet* ii: 757–761.

antioxidant nutrients (vitamin C, β-carotene and E). Whatever the biochemical effects of these various dietary items, the ultimate need is for RCTs and, in the first instance, these trials could well be of secondary prevention. *See* Antioxidants, Natural Antioxidants; Dietary Fibre, Fibre and Disease Prevention

Interpretation of the Results of RCTs

A clear distinction must always be made between the testing of a hypothesis which was defined before a study was set up, and the generation of new hypotheses from detailed analyses of data from subgroups within a trial. This latter, which is often dismissed under the name 'fishing' or 'dredging' is permissible only if it is recognized for what it is and if the associations detected are tested in further *ad hoc* trials.

Firm conclusions should only be based on evidence drawn from a number of trials. The play of chance can never be ruled out, whatever the level of statistical significance, and consistency in a number of studies is likely to be a better guide to truth than the results of a single study. Hence the importance of 'overviews' of studies, or 'meta-analyses' of data from a number of different studies. This approach is particularly appro-priate with RCTs, but it is important that data from every relevant RCT is included. Unfortunately certainty on this last is impossible, as there is always a publication bias, and reports which report an effect are generally more likely to be accepted by a journal than those which show no effect.

There is another aspect of the last point. Not only does one like to see consistency in the results of different studies, one should also look for consistency in the results of studies with different approaches. This is necessary because, for example, in every trial in which the consumption of one nutrient, or one foodstuff, is increased, there may be a consistent compensatory decrease in the consumption of some other nutrient or food item. Confidence is enhanced, however, if prospective studies demonstrate an association between a food item and a disease, if RCTs show a change in the disease incidence, and if these effects are consistent with the results of metabolic studies. Examples of such consistency are rare in dietary research but the benefit of fatty fish is consistently shown in all these approaches.

Bibliography

Burr ML (1983) Epidemiology for nutritionists. 3. The design of studies. *Human Nutrition: Applied Nutrition* 37A: 339–347.

Burr ML, Fehily AM, Gilbert JF, Rogers S, Holliday RM *et al.* (1989) Effects of changes in fat, fish, and fibre intakes on death and myocardial reinfarction: Diet and Reinfarction Trial (DART). *Lancet* ii: 757–761.

Muldoon MF, Manuck SB and Matthews KA (1990) Lowering cholesterol concentrations and mortality: a quantitative review of primary prevention trials. *British Medical Journal* 301: 309–313.

Peto R, Pike MC, Armitage P, Breslow NE, Cox DR *et al.* (1976) Design and analysis of randomized clinical trials requiring prolonged observation of each patient. I. Introduction and design. II. Analysis and examples. *British Journal of Cancer* 34: 585–612 and 35: 1–39.

Peter C. Elwood
Llandough Hospital, Penarth, UK

Prevention

Coronary heart disease (CHD) (atherosclerotic arterial disease of the coronary arteries) accounts for about one in four deaths among men in the countries of western Europe and North America and a slightly smaller proportion of deaths in women. Some of these deaths occur in relatively young men, especially those with high CHD risk factors, but the condition also causes considerable morbidity (reduction of quality of life by cardiac symptoms, such as angina) in middle-aged to older men and women. It must also be remembered that the underlying pathological process also causes damage to other major arteries, with serious consequences for the legs, kidneys, gut and brain. Prevention of CHD should be considered as prevention of atherosclerotic arterial disease. *See* Diseases, Diseases of Affluence

The objective in preventing CHD is to reduce morbidity and mortality and a wide variety of end-points have been used in studies. Correct definition of cases of coronary arterial disease requires use of either noninvasive techniques (clinical history, electrocardiographic assessment) or invasive angiographic techniques, and intervention studies have followed variables derived from these techniques as well as changes in risk factor variables.

Prevention of CHD is either primary (before any clinical event has occurred) or secondary (after nonfatal myocardial infarction, or after diagnosis based on clinical, electrocardiographic and biochemical assessment). Primary prevention requires either that individuals at high risk be identified as such and be required to change those risks, or that whole populations or groups change their group characteristics, e.g. by reducing the proportion who smoke, the numbers with undiagnosed diabetes, the numbers with inadequately treated hypertension, and the numbers with high blood cholesterol and other lipid variables. *See* Cholesterol, Role of Cholesterol in Heart Disease; Hypertension, Physiology; Smoking, Diet and Health

There is still debate about the advantages and disadvantages of attempting to prevent CHD. There is little doubt in the minds of most clinicians that in most cases of established CHD there should be aggressive intervention, but considerable discussion about the benefits in relation to costs and other disadvantages of whole-scale population risk-factor interventions.

Primary Prevention

A number of expert committees, including a group from the European Atherosclerosis Society, have identified strategies for primary prevention. There are two main strategies: the population approach and the high-risk approach. The population approach primarily involves education of a population group about risk factors of CHD: the hazards of smoking, the characteristics of a healthy diet, the benefits of exercise and stress avoidance. It requires the adequate provision of facilities to enable people to make the advised changes: 'stop smoking' clinics, wide availability of suitable foods (e.g. low-fat foods, and a wide variety of carbohydrate foods), sports and exercise facilities. Studies to determine whether or not the population approach is effective have been undertaken in Finland, Norway, the USA and the UK (South Wales), and some evidence for efficacy has been produced. However, it has always been virtually impossible to undertake 'controlled' trials. It has always been difficult to isolate the target province or region from a control region in the same country – information would always 'leak' from the treatment region to the control. When North Karelia, in Finland, was the subject of intervention and CHD rates fell, rates also fell in the 'control' western provinces. Thus, while there is evidence that population interventions are followed by reduced CHD rates, there is no absolute certainty that changes resulted from the interventions. *See* National Nutrition Policies

The high-risk approach involves the identification of individuals who are at high risk of CHD, followed by appropriate treatments. Screening for such individuals can be carried out either systematically, e.g. by deliberately checking all other risk factors in a group known already to have a high risk, such as diabetic and hypertensive individuals, or randomly, e.g. by screening those who attend a GP surgery if they have one or more risk factors including a family history of heart disease. Evidence for the efficacy of the high-risk-factor approach comes from a large literature reporting results on clinical trials of specific risk-factor interventions. Much of the evidence concerns the effects of blood-lipid-lowering regimens applied to those with high initial values. The interventions studied have been either diet only or diet and drug, and the end-points have generally been fatal or nonfatal myocardial infarction reported along with changes of blood lipid variables. Studies of this type, e.g. the Lipid Research Clinics Coronary Prevention Trial, provide evidence that within the study period there can be significant reductions of mortality and morbidity. Multiple-risk-factor intervention trials have also been carried out and have provided evidence for efficacy of intervention.

Secondary Prevention

Patients already diagnosed as having CHD can be treated to slow the progress of the disease or to reverse it. Demonstration of nonprogression or regression of coronary artery stenosis requires serial coronary angiography – an increasing number of reports describe effects of diet or diet and drugs on arterial change. The recent 1992 St Thomas' Arterial Regression Study (STARS) showed that both dietary intervention and diet and drug treatment (cholestyramine) could cause nonprogression and regression of arterial disease. Other studies have used mortality as the end-point, for example the Diet and Re-infarction Trial (DART) examined the effect of three dietary variables (fat – high-fat or low-fat; fibre – high-fibre or normal fibre; and fish – taking fatty fish or no fatty fish) on survival over a 2-year period following an initial myocardial infarction. After 2 years, survival was significantly greater in those who had received fatty fish compared to those who had not. Neither a low-fat diet nor a high-fibre diet had any effect on mortality over 2 years. It has to be remembered, however, that the subjects were individuals in whom the disease was well advanced and it can be presumed that the protective effect of fish was attributable to modification of the clotting and fibrinolytic variables. Thus there is adequate evidence, from these and many other studies, to conclude that dietary and drug interventions in patients with existing arterial disease can reduce mortality (i.e. prolong life) and slow or even reverse the progression of coronary arterial disease. *See* Dietary Fibre, Fibre and Disease Prevention; Fish Oils, Dietary Importance

Secondary prevention of CHD is a medical 'treatment' activity, rather than a public health programme, and requires proper assessment of the factors responsible for the development of the disease. Treatment consists of several stages, starting with a full assessment of risk factors: the family history; the patient's smoking history; proper measurement of blood pressure; assessment of body composition (the degree of adiposity); biochemical assessment of blood lipid variables, including total blood cholesterol, high-density lipoprotein (HDL)-cholesterol, calculated low-density lipoprotein (LDL)-cholesterol, apoprotein concentrations and total triglyceride, measured on a fasting blood sample; tests for diabetes; dietary history including alcohol use; exercise history; and relevant drug usage including the contraceptive pill. Some centres might measure clotting factor VII and fibrinogen. There is a great debate about how aggressive subsequent intervention should be, especially in relation to age (when is an individual too old to benefit from intervention?) and whether intervention should be in terms of diet and life style only, or should include, for example, the use of lipid-lowering drugs. Obviously, treatment of hypertension and diabetes should be effective, but this is probably not so in all cases. Indeed, there is now evidence that the choice of drug in the treatment of hypertension may modify the progress of coronary arterial disease.

Blood lipids should be assessed and diagnosis made of the type of lipid abnormality, if any. Is the hyperlipidaemia primary or secondary? If the latter, have the commonest causes, e.g. hypothyroidism, diabetes, excessive alcohol intake (for raised triglycerides), been excluded? What type of primary hyperlipidaemia is present? All cases are first treated by dietary measures: an isoenergetic, modified-fat diet (e.g. 30% of energy from fat, 10% each from saturated, polyunsaturated and monounsaturated fat) for those of ideal weight, an energy-reduced modified-fat diet for those who are overweight. Those with primary hyperlipidaemias are also initially treated by diet only, even though they may not respond as well as other patients. After an adequate trial of diet, drugs may be introduced to try to achieve the target lipid levels (based on population studies, this might be a total blood cholesterol of $5 \cdot 2$ mmol l^{-1} unless the HLD-cholesterol is known to be high, in which case a higher total cholesterol may be an acceptable target). How much effort is put into achieving the initial dietary compliance, and how much measurement and therapy change is used to achieve an optimal lipid profile depends on the physician's expertise and preferences. *See* Hyperlipidaemia; Lipoproteins

Following the initial assessment and first round of interventions, it is necessary to reassess patients at intervals in order to check that improvements in risk-factor profile have been maintained and to apply further life style changes or drug therapy as necessary. At some stage, other family members, especially children of known cases, might be assessed in terms of their predisposition to CHD.

The Future

Improvements which can be expected in the prevention of CHD over the coming years include improved methods for assessing risk, such as further development of formulae and indexes based on results from major trials. Use of indexes of clotting and fibrinolysis will enter more widespread use. Better methods of achieving long-term compliance with diet and life style changes will be developed. There will be further advances in the drug therapy of hypertension, diabetes and hyperlipidaemia. While there will probably be a degree of success in changing risk-factor profiles in populations, the big changes necessary to achieve big reductions of risk may meet with some resistance. Identification of those at high risk of early development of CHD will probably be the major approach to prevention in the future.

Bibliography

Committee on Diet and Health, National Research Council (1989) *Diet and Health: Implications for Reducing Chronic Disease Risk.* Washington, DC: National Academy Press.
Committee on Medical Aspects of Food Policy (1984) *Diet and Cardiovascular Disease.* Report of the Panel on Diet in Relation to Cardiovascular Disease. London: DHSS.
Study Group, European Atherosclerosis Society (1987) Strategies for the prevention of coronary heart disease. A policy statement of the European Atherosclerosis Society. *European Heart Journal* 8:77.
The Health of the Nation (1991) Presented to Parliament by the Secretary of State for Health by Command of Her Majesty, June 1991.
WHO Expert Committee (1982) *Prevention of Coronary Heart Disease.* Technical Report Series, 678.

A. R. Leeds
King's College, London, UK

CORROSION CHEMISTRY

For most people, the word 'corrosion' carries the image of rust specific to iron-containing metals, surmising that only iron is subject to this phenomenon. In fact, corrosion is the general term for the damage and destruction of all man-made metallic materials. This destructive force of corrosion has always existed but has grown in importance only in the modern era due to the advancement of civilization and technology.

Corrosion may be considered as the deterioration of metals and alloys made by humans, which tend to return to their original state; thus, 'rust' is the natural state of iron, as steel is obtained from iron oxides found in the earth's crust. The same can be applied to many metals (such as aluminium, zinc, copper and so on) which are unstable.

Thus, corrosion is an unavoidable problem and the most important aim is to reduce its occurrence as much as possible. Annual damage due to corrosion in the world is very important. Every domain of industry is affected, including the food industry.

How Corrosion Starts

Prior to corrosion a disparity or a heterogeneity can always be found, either physical or chemical. The most conspicuous physical disparity is obtained by the contact of two different metals (e.g. tinplate, galvanized steel) present in the same solution (e.g. salt water). In this case, an electrochemical cell is formed.

Chemical heterogeneity may be represented by differences of ion concentration near identical electrodes or by the Evans cell which results from differential aeration. The case of a salt water drop on a ferrous material is well known (Fig. 1). The anodic site (i.e. the area of corrosion) is always at the centre of the drop where there is an oxygen deficit relative to the peripheral zone where aeration (and thus oxygen) is more extensive than in the centre of the drop.

Microscopic disparities can also be found; there is no practical industrial process which yields metals with an absolutely homogenous surface, in the strict physical sense: a touch of the metal surface with the hand or simple machining with any tool may be sufficient to damage the surface. A cold-worked zone becomes less 'noble', that is, more easily corroded, than the surrounding zones as the atoms found in stressed cycles tend more easily to leave the metallic crystal lattice. The various chemical treatments sustained by the metallic material are other sources of heterogeneity.

The Electrochemical Basis of Corrosion

A study of corrosion phenomena at a molecular level shows an electron exchange between donating and

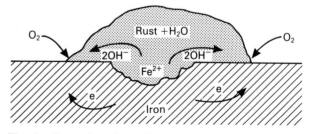

Fig. 1 Formation of rust through the formation of a differential aeration (Evans) cell.

Anode

Excess of electrons

Release of electrons

$\xrightarrow{\ \ e\ \ }$

Oxidation

Destruction of material

(e.g. $Sn \rightarrow Sn^{2+} + 2e$

$Al \rightarrow Al^{3+} + 3e$

$Fe \rightarrow Fe^{2+} + 2e$)

Cathode

Deficit of electrons

Capture of electrons

Reduction

Protection of material

(e.g. $2H^+ + 2e \rightarrow H_2$

$O_2 + 4e + 4H^+ \rightarrow 2H_2O$)

Fig. 2 Corrosion as an electrochemical process.

accepting sites. This is a reduction–oxidation or 'redox' reaction: the oxidizing part (which acts as a cathode) is reduced through electron capture while electrons are donated by the reducing material (which acts as an anode), which becomes oxidized (Fig. 2).

Parameters Driving Electron Transfer

The most important factors governing electron transfer are potential and easiness.

The potential factor is governed by the electron affinity difference between the two transferring elements. The greater the difference, the faster the corrosion may develop. The potential factor is sometimes called the dissolution potential. Consider, for example, a metal M in a solution containing M^+ ions. The potential of the metal is given by the Nernst formula

$$E = E_0 + \frac{RT}{nF} \log_e(a_{M^+}), \qquad (1)$$

where E_0 is a constant factor, independent of the solution concentration, a_{M^+} is the activity of the M^+ ions in the solution, (activity is proportional to concentration) R is the gas constant ($8\cdot31$ J K^{-1} mol^{-1}), n is the number of moles of electrons driven by the cell potential E, F is the Faraday ($96\,500$ coulombs) and T is the absolute temperature. The Nernst formula is commonly used as

$$E = E_0 + \frac{0\cdot06}{n} \log_{10}(a_{M^+}) \qquad (2)$$

for convenience. From measurements of differences in potential between a metal and a reference electrode, a series can be produced of dissolution voltages (Table 1). Elements that have a greater tendency than hydrogen to lose electrons are described as electropositive, while those that gain electrons are called electronegative, e.g. sodium is more electropositive than aluminium. From this series, it can be seen which of two metals, if placed in contact with each other, will become corroded. For example, in this series, zinc has a much greater dissolution voltage than iron; thus if a piece of iron is coated with zinc and placed in water, the iron will not rust if the zinc coating is scratched, because zinc loses electrons in preference to iron. This is the principle behind the galvanizing of steel.

Table 1. The electrochemical series

Metal	Electrode reaction	Standard electrode potential (V)
(Active end)		
Sodium	$Na \rightarrow Na^+ + e$	$-2\cdot712$
Magnesium	$Mg \rightarrow Mg^{2+} + 2e$	$-2\cdot34$
Beryllium	$Be \rightarrow Be^{2+} + 2e$	$-1\cdot70$
Aluminium	$Al \rightarrow Al^{3+} + 3e$	$-1\cdot67$
Manganese	$Mn \rightarrow Mn^{2+} + 2e$	$-1\cdot05$
Zinc	$Zn \rightarrow Zn^{2+} + 2e$	$-0\cdot762$
Chromium	$Cr \rightarrow Cr^{3+} + 3e$	$-0\cdot71$
Iron	$Fe \rightarrow Fe^{3+} + 3e$	$-0\cdot44$
Cadmium	$Cd \rightarrow Cd^{2+} + 2e$	$-0\cdot402$
Cobalt	$Co \rightarrow Co^{2+} + 2e$	$-0\cdot277$
Nickel	$Ni \rightarrow Ni^{2+} + 2e$	$-0\cdot250$
Tin	$Sn \rightarrow Sn^{2+} + 2e$	$-0\cdot136$
Lead	$Pb \rightarrow Pb^{2+} + 2e$	$-0\cdot126$
Hydrogen	$H_2 \rightarrow 2H^+ + 2e$	$0\cdot000$ (reference)
Copper	$Cu \rightarrow Cu^{2+} + 2e$	$+0\cdot345$
	$Cu \rightarrow Cu^+ + e$	$+0\cdot522$
Silver	$Ag \rightarrow Ag^+ + e$	$+0\cdot800$
Platinum	$Pt \rightarrow Pt^{2+} + 2e$	$+1\cdot2$
Gold	$Au \rightarrow Au^{3+} + 3e$	$+1\cdot42$
(Noble end)		

The easiness factor reflects any factors affecting the reaction arising from the conditions of the electrolytic media where the electron transfer takes place. If the electron donor (the anodic site) does not easily let electrons loose, the corrosion is said to be donor controlled and there is an anodic overvoltage. On the other hand, the corrosion is controlled by the electron acceptor if it cannot freely accept the electrons; a cathodic overpotential then exists.

Any corrosion cell can be studied through intensity voltage curves or polarization plots. In the laboratory, special devices quantitatively measure the ease of electron transfer from an anodic site to a cathodic one. Evans diagrams are mostly favoured as they are very simple; three examples are shown in Fig. 3 as illustrative cases.

The ideal situation would be a corrosion battery with the lowest possible activity as a result of strong anodic and cathodic overvoltages.

The role of corrosion inhibitors is to increase the overvoltage either on the anode or on the cathode or on both electrodes simultaneously. They polarize the cell, thus reducing its electron flow, often through the formation of an insoluble compound on the surface of one electrode. The corrosion inhibitor behaviour (especially the anodic inhibitors) is sometimes unpredictable as most of the compounds used, depending on their concentration and other environmental factors, may have a role as either an accelerator or inhibitor of

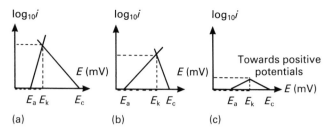

Fig. 3 (a) Low anodic overtension, high cathodic overtension; the galvanic couple is under cathodic control. (b) High anodic overtension, low cathodic overtension; the galvanic couple is under anodic control. (c) High anodic and cathodic overtensions; the galvanic couple is under mixed control. $\log_{10}i$, $\log_{10}$ of the corrosion current (or electrons), E_a, from the equilibrium potential: anodic polarization or overtension on the electrode supplying the electrons; E_k, mixed and common potential of both; E_c, from the equilibrium potential: cathodic polarization or overtension on the electrode capturing the electrons.

corrosion. A corrosion accelerator is the reverse of an inhibitor. Every electroactive compound in the electrolyte which is able either to complex the positive ions coming from the anode or to use the electrons arriving at the cathode, either directly or through nascent hydrogen formation, must be considered as a corrosion accelerator.

Appearance of Corrosion

Macroscopically, corrosion can appear in the following ways (Fig. 4):

- Generalized or uniform corrosion, which appears at the same speed on the whole surface of the metal.
- Pitting corrosion, which appears on localized sites, e.g. at the interface between the metal and an inclusion, on the breaks of a passivation film or coatings. Current density is high in the vicinity of the deficit as the anode is small while the cathode is very large.
- Crevice corrosion, which appears in cracks mainly on stainless steels and under metallic coatings.
- Intergranular corrosion, which appears only on intergranular joints.
- Intragranular corrosion: arborescent corrosion cracks which appear in metallic crystals. Stress often initiates this type of corrosion.

Corrosion Reactions in the Food Industry

Most foodstuffs are in aqueous solution, they are thus conductors, and, to some extent active electrolytes.

Metals used in the food industry are found chiefly in two separate areas:

- metallic cans used for preservation of foodstuffs:
- processing equipment and storage vessels – aluminium alloys and stainless steels are most widely used for this application.

Corrosion of Metal Cans

In the world, over 40 000 million cans are used every year to preserve and protect a very wide range of foods. Preservation of foodstuffs in closed cans by heat was proposed by the Frenchman Nicolas Appert at the beginning of the 19th century. A few years later, the first metallic cans in tinplate were produced in England, a material made from the tin/iron couple used since the Middle Ages for kitchen utensils. The preserved food industry developed most rapidly in the USA.

The shelf life of cans should be several years, that is if the rate of corrosion is kept as low as possible.

The metal canning of foodstuffs makes use of two base materials:

- Steel coated on both sides with a layer of tin of varying but uniform thickness (0·4–1·6 μm). For some 20 years, tin has been replaced, from time to time, by a layer of metallic, oxidized chromium not thicker than 0·015 μm. This composite is usually called 'tin-free steel'.
- Aluminium-based alloys, which have only been used extensively since the World War II.

Tinplate is a very assymetric material; the behaviour of the tin/iron cell is shown schematically in Fig. 5. Tin in the presence of most foodstuffs behaves as a sacrificial anode and steel is thus cathodically protected. The anodic behaviour of tin is due to the formation of many complexes with organic acids and phenolic compounds (tannins) found in fruits and vegetables. The uncomplexed fraction of tin in solution or in the foodstuff is very low. Following the Nernst equation, tin is more electronegative than it appears from the electrochemical series. *See* Tin

Tinplate producers sell about 13 million tonnes per year, two-thirds of which is used for foodstuff canning. Tinplate is not a single product: many types can be manufactured, depending on the quality of the steel and the thickness of the tin coating.

Pure tin exhibits good resistance to the acid medium of foodstuffs without oxidizing agents. This corrosion is considered as normal. It even has a beneficial effect on the retention of some organoleptic qualities of the foodstuffs. The most important corrosion accelerators (that is, electron acceptors) which may be found in foods are oxygen (air), sulphur dioxide (preservative), sulphur (pesticide), nitrates (water, fruit, vegetables) and tri-

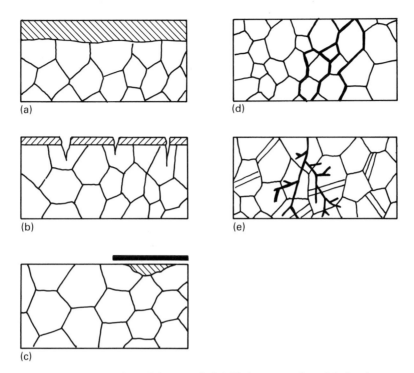

Fig. 4 (a) Generalized or uniform corrosion of the metal. (b) Pitting corrosion. (c) Crevice corrosion. (d) Intergranular corrosion. (e) Intragranular corrosion.

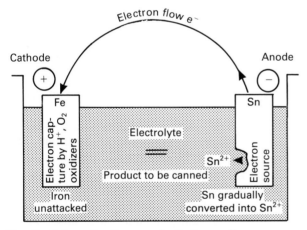

Fig. 5 Schematic diagram of a tin/iron cell.

methylamine oxide (fish). Farming techniques are always changing and have an influence on the chemical composition of foodstuffs. Corrosion problems have multiplied during the last 20 years as a result of, for example, fast detinning by nitrates, which is even faster as the pH is lowered and the preferential dissolution of iron due to the presence of pesticide residues such as dithiocarbamates. Contents of up to 40 mg per kilogram of foodstuff, which have no adverse effect on the consumer's health may, in some cases, lead to significant dissolution of tin through corrosion. Similarly, dithiocarbamate residues (a few milligrams per kilogram) are

sufficient to invert the tin/iron cell and induce corrosion of the steel. When these additional corrosion risks appear, organic coatings inside the can are needed. For this purpose, lacquers (macromolecular compounds or high polymers) are used. They are insoluble and inert in aqueous media. On account of the nature of the foodstuffs and the various mechanical stresses these lacquers have to withstand, several different types are used. These are characterized either by their barrier behaviour, or their degree of flexibility: oleoresinous, organosols, epoxyphenolics, epoxyesters, epoxyurea and so on are commonly used. These organic films are deposited either on the flat sheet or after can making. In both cases, they are cured thermally in an oven, usually at 200°C for 10–15 min. Their thickness ranges between 5 and 15 μm, depending on the requirements for preservation of the can and/or the foodstuff. They must also withstand sterilization temperatures (125–130°C).

Tin-free steels cannot be used alone as they are much more sensitive to acid corrosion, and an organic protective coating is thus essential.

Aluminium is widely used in the food industry, either as canning material or in various equipment for preparation, storage and transport of foodstuffs. For metallic canning, it is used much less than steel-based materials: only 2·5 million tonnes per year. In the USA about 2 million tonnes per year are used due to the large market for beverage cans (beer, soft drinks). In foodstuff cans, aluminium is always used as an alloy (with magnesium or manganese), the exact composition depending on the mechanical properties needed: for aerosol cans 99·5% aluminium is used and for collapsible tubes 99·7%. Aluminium is also used in composite packaging materials associated with polymer films (polyethylene, polypropylene, polyester, etc.). Theoretically, aluminium is a very passive metal as it is easily covered with an alumina film (hydrated aluminium oxide). But being an amphoteric metal, it is still highly sensitive to corrosion in acid media (aluminium salts) or alkaline media (aluminates). Pure aluminium is subject to all the corrosion forms mentioned above (uniform, pitting, stress, inter- and intracrystal, galvanic). For this reason, aluminium is often chemically or electrochemically passivated (anodization through chroming or in sulphuric media). The surface treatments greatly improve the adhesion of organic coatings (or lacquers) always used for internal protection of metallic cans to achieve chemical inertness over several years. Epoxyphenolic, vinyl organosols or polyesters are usually used, in one or two layers, as the situation requires. Corrosion of aluminium cans is very rare with such protection. *See* Aluminium, Properties and Determination; Aluminium, Toxicology

Whether the can is in tinplate or aluminium, beer can only be stored in totally inert cans as it is extremely sensitive to contamination by iron or aluminium, resulting in cloudiness and taints.

Low density, high thermal conductivity and low sensitivity to atmospheric corrosion are the three main specific advantages of aluminium over steel for cans.

Equipment Corrosion

Many aluminium alloys are still used in tanks and containers of all kinds (jars, cans, trolleys, tables and so on). The meat, fish, milk, cheese, pastry and confectionery industries all use such equipment. However, in the modern food industry, stainless steels are now more commonly used on account of their good mechanical properties and robustness to frequent cleaning. Similarly, glass and porcelain are now more commonly being used.

There are two main families of stainless steel which possess ferritic and austenitic structures. The first is mostly chromium and iron while the second contains additional nickel. In both families, some molybdenum may be added to improve corrosion resistance. To prevent corrosion of welded zones, it is necessary to reduce the carbon content of austenitic steels or to stabilize them by adding titanium and/or niobium. Corrosion resistance, and also cost, increase with the amounts of other elements used in alloys. It is thus essential to evaluate, as far as possible, the risks and the corrosion resistance properties of the steels used, to eliminate all technical problems, yet at the same time avoiding high costs of production and maintenance. Stainless steels can with-

stand different types of localized corrosion: intergranular corrosion, pitting and cracking. Chloride solutions at high temperature can be highly aggressive: any cracks in the passive layers may lead to rapid corrosion as they become anodic sites with regard to the remainder of the surface. Depassivation may have a mechanical origin (abrasion, wear), and the metal is then permanently depassivated or 'active'. It must be kept in mind that stainless steels have extensive but not universal corrosion resistance. Every use of stainless steel in corrosive media must be treated as a particular problem. The choice of the material must be made in conjunction with a metallurgist, the equipment builder and user in order to study all aspects of the problem (both economic and technical).

Some food industries experience more corrosion problems than others, such as pork butchers and salt meat producers as a result of chlorine- and salt-containing vapour in plants (from brines).

The dairy industry has used for a long time large quantities of austenitic stainless steel (18% chromium, 10% nickel) for tubes, heat exchangers, tanks, centrifugation bowls, etc. New varieties of ferritic steels, containing 17% chromium, a low percentage of carbon and some titanium, are now being successfully introduced for boilers.

Corrosion by Cleaning and Disinfecting Products

To obtain regular production of good-quality foodstuffs it is necessary to clean, disinfect and descale surfaces in contact with food. The frequency of such treatments varies from one industry to another: two to four times a day in the milk industry to once a year in the sugar industry. These treatments require the use of chemical products which may themselves exert a considerable corrosive action, generating microcavities which will, as the damage increases, be more and more difficult to clean. *See* Cleaning Procedures in the Factory, Types of Detergent; Sanitization

With regard to alkaline cleaning agents, stainless steels withstand corrosion well while aluminium alloys are very sensitive, although corrosion may be reduced by addition of silicates.

Corrosion of stainless steels in acidic media varies with the particular acid, pH and oxidizing potential of the solution. In nitric acid solution, austenitic stainless steels face no generalized corrosion, being naturally autopassive. In some cases, slight pitting of the whole surface can be seen. However, aluminium alloys do not exhibit passivation in nitric acid but, here too, it is possible to reduce corrosion speed by adding organic acids such as malic or citric acids. Cleaning solutions based on sulphuric acid always contain corrosion inhibitors for stainless steels.

Chlorination is frequently used by many food industries, owing to its simultaneous strong and cheap disinfecting and bactericidal actions. Its effect is still not fully understood, but it is known that chlorine is effective between pH 7 and 9. As sodium hypochlorite, its effect would be due to nascent oxygen, which is very effective against microbial germs. The problem with the use of chlorine is to know the level of addition required. Resistance to chlorine varies widely between microbial species which are to be killed. In terms of corrosion, chlorine is a strong oxidizing agent. For metallic cans, chlorination of $0.5–2$ mg l^{-1} of free chlorine is sufficient to prevent their recontamination through suction via seams in the cans due to the increasing vacuum level developing inside. Higher chlorine levels may induce corrosion phenomena (detinning and rust on tinplate, pitting on aluminium cans).

With the very high chlorine concentrations (300 to 1500 mg l^{-1}) needed for thorough disinfection (in dairies, for example) the risk of pitting and crevice formation on stainless steel is higher as the temperature and contact durations increase. The lower the pH value, the higher the risk. Sometimes, corrosion inhibitors are also needed to improve the chemical inertness of stainless steels.

Iodine containing compounds are considered as having no action on stainless steels, but should not be used for cleaning and disinfecting aluminium and aluminium alloys.

Solutions of peracetic acid (300 mg l^{-1}) made from acetic acid, hydrogen peroxide and water, which have very good bactericidal properties, may be used at room temperature, for short durations (about 20 min) on austenitic steels and aluminium alloys.

Bacterial corrosion, although uncommon, may appear in some food industries, e.g. in buried tubing. Every material, even metals may be attacked by microorganisms adhering to surfaces and inducing there, through their bioactivity, accumulation of acids and dissolved gases. For example, we may quote ferrobacteria and sulphate-reducing bacteria. Ferrobacteria, acting on the anodic site, take their energy from the oxidation of ferrous ions to ferric ions, thus producing rapid formation of rust as they continuously modify the equilibrium by simultaneous anodic and cathodic depolarization. Sulphate-reducing bacteria use hydrogen and induce cathodic depolarization: jelly-like vesicles appear, which are living bacterial colonies.

Ways to Prevent Corrosion

Some common ways of preventing corrosion of metals have already been mentioned:

- Organic coatings with inert macromolecular polymers used for cans and for steel-based equipment in food industry plants.
- When using unprotected metals (aluminium alloys and stainless steels), the following must be considered:
  -avoid as far as possible two metals joining;
  -choose the best suitable material;

-modify aggressive media composition with inhibitors;
-use cathodic protection by coupling a sacrificial anode metal to the material to be protected. The use of a metal as a sacrificial anode does not suppress corrosion and theoretically is not to be used for materials in contact with food (unless the corroding metal is specifically authorized for contact with food (e.g. tinplate).

Regulations on Materials in Contact with Foodstuffs

The corrosion of a metallic material induces migration of metallic elements to the foodstuff with which it is in contact. Thus, materials and objects to be used in contact with foods must be inert with regard to foodstuffs. That is, they must not, under their various conditions of use, liberate elements liable to modify the foodstuff composition significantly, i.e. imparting a toxic character or changing its organoleptic qualities (contamination, for example, by iron or tin).

Firm regulations are always based on definite listing: everything which is not precisely authorized is forbidden. Some local regulations stipulate limits for global or specific migration levels. They vary from one country to the other. On a worldwide basis, the *Codex Alimentarius* is the reference. *See* Legislation, Packaging Legislation

Traces of cleaning agents incompletely rinsed may pollute the foodstuff, although this operation is mandatory. The choice of corrosion inhibitors to be added to the cleaning products must always be done with reference to the list of compounds authorized for cleaning.

Bibliography

Bosich JF (1970) *Corrosion Prevention for Practising Engineers.* New York: Barnesand Noble.

Centre Français de la Corrosion (CEFRACOR) (1980) *Corrosion dans les Industries Alimentaires.* Symposium, Rennes (France), 23–25 September 1980. Paris: CEFRACOR.

International Tin Research Institute (1975) *Tin versus Corrosion.* Publication No. 150. Greenford, Middlesex: International Tin Research Institute.

International Tin Research Institute (1980) *Guide to Tinplate.* Publication No. 622. Greenford, Middlesex: International Tin Research Institute.

Marsal P (1965–1985) [Various publications on the subject, particularly on the corrosion of metal packaging including (1981–1982) *On some corrosion factors in canned foods*; (1977) *Matching tinplate cans to their contents*; (1979) *Influence of nitrates upon tinplate corrosion*; (1985–1986) *Practical use of organic coatings in the protection and decoration of metal containers.*] Thionville: French Tinplate Research Centre.

Vargel C (ed.) (1979) *Le Comportement de l'Aluminium et de ses Alliages.* Paris: Dunod Technique.

P. Marsal
Thionville, France

CRAB

See Shellfish

CRACKERS

See Biscuits, Cookies and Crackers

CRANBERRIES

See Fruits of Temperate Climates

CRAYFISH

See Shellfish

CREAM

Contents

Types of Cream
Clotted Cream

Types of Cream*

Cream, a concentration of the natural emulsion of milk, is available to the consumer in many forms. This article will review the range of products, legal standards, composition, production and uses.

* The colour plate section for this article appears between p. 1146 and p. 1147.

Types of Cream

Range of Products, Legal Standards and Compositional Data

A variety of creams, with differing compositions, functions and types of packaging, can be obtained for consumption. Cream consists of emulsified globules of fat (range of diameters approximately 0–10 μm) in a skim milk serum. The fat provides flavour, and the emulsion form gives characteristic textural attributes and functional properties. The fat content is generally used for legal classification of products.

Table 1 gives the standards as recommended by the United Nations Food and Agriculture Organization (FAO) and the World Health Organization (WHO) with the legal standards currently in force in the UK. Each country has its own standards to suit the particular products marketed.

Other regulations cover declarations on the heat treatment applied to the cream – untreated, pasteurized, sterilized or ultrahigh temperature (UHT) treated – as well as limits on allowed additives and normal regulations relating to labelling. Several countries do not allow the sale of unpasteurized cream.

Low-fat creams are used as pouring creams for desserts or for addition to coffee or tea. Creams with higher fat contents may be used as whipping creams. Aerosol cream is a special form of whipping cream, the cream (UHT) is packed in a can with nitrous oxide gas as a propellant. Allowed additives vary from country to country. Typical additives are sugar, emulsifiers, stabilizers and stabilizing salts.

As fat content rises, the viscosity of the cream increases and creams with fat content greater than 60% can be used as spreads. However, fat content is not the only determining factor in consistency, and spreadable creams can be made with lower fat contents by reducing fat globule diameters (homogenization) and adding thickeners.

Although cream is generally defined by its fat content, the suspending serum is also important. This serum consists largely of water (approximately 91%) with lactose (approximately 5%), protein (approximately 2·8% casein and 0·7% whey protein) and other minor constituents such as minerals (0·7%) and vitamins. The fat and the solids-not-fat (SNF) content of milk are influenced by breed, nutrition of the cow and lactational or seasonal factors. *See* Milk, Dietary Importance

Another very important component of cream is the membrane which surrounds the fat globules. The major components of this membrane are protein (41%), phospholipids (27%), neutral glycerides (14%), water (13%), cerobrosides (3%) and cholesterol (2%). Many of the properties of cream are influenced by the membrane and its surface-active components as they affect the stability of the globules and their tendency to agglomerate. Vitamins, minerals and enzymes are important minor components of the fat and the membrane.

Production and Packaging of Cream

Separation and Standardization

Cream is produced from whole milk by 'separation' which relies on the density difference between the fat and the aqueous serum. Fat globules will rise in milk according to Stokes law:

$$v_g = \frac{d^2(\rho_f - \rho_1)g}{18\eta}$$

where v_g = velocity of globule (m s^{-1}); d = diameter of globule (m); ρ_f = density of globule (kg m^{-3}); ρ_1 = density of serum (kg m^{-3}); g = acceleration due to gravity (m s^{-2}); η = viscosity of serum (kg m^{-1} s^{-1}). Note that v_g is negative as the equation represents a velocity of settling: $\rho_f < \rho_1$.

The rate of separation can be increased by applying a centrifugal force field and this forms the basis of the milk separator:

$$v_g = \frac{d^2(\rho_f - \rho_1)r\omega^2}{18\eta}$$

where r = radial distance of globule from axis of rotation (m); and ω = angular velocity (rad s^{-1}).

The continuous separation of fat-rich fraction (cream) and serum (skim milk) is achieved through a stack of rotating discs into which the milk is distributed (Fig. 1). Each gap between the discs acts as a zone of separation. Separation takes place in the gaps between the discs, where the denser aqueous phase moves outwards at greater velocity than the fat globules and is channelled via the underside of the discs to the outside and the skim outlet. The fat globules concentrate toward the axis of the spinning discs and are channelled out via the upper surface of the discs to the cream outlet. The position of the rising channels is important in maximizing separation efficiency, and their position on the discs should be in relation to the flows of the two products.

The rotational energy of the streams can be converted to hydrostatic pressure by paring discs (centripetal pumps), and used to pump the products away. Effi-

Table 1. WHO/FAO-proposed cream standards and UK legal standards for fat content

Authority	Cream type	Required fat content (%)
WHO/FAO	Pasteurized, sterilized or UHT treated	≥ 18
	Double	≥ 45
	Heavy whipping	≥ 35
	Whipping	≥ 28
	Half	10–18
UK	Clotted	≥ 55
	Double	≥ 48
	Whipping and whipped	≥ 35
	Sterilized	≥ 23
	Cream and single cream	≥ 18
	Half	12–18

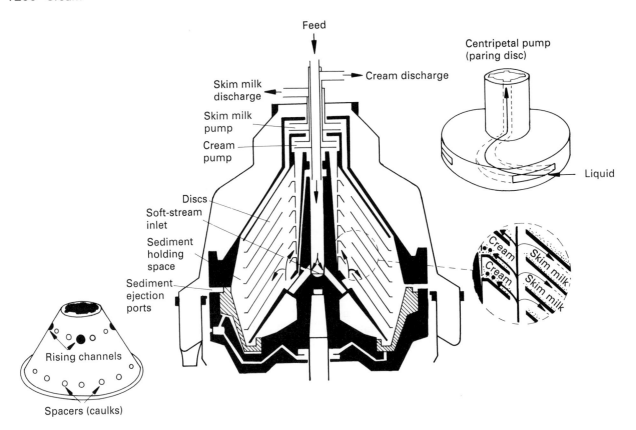

Fig. 1 Elements of a milk separator (from Lehmann and Zettier, 1987). (Courtesy of Westfalia Separator AG, Oelde, Germany.)

ciency of separation is measured by fat content in the skim milk, usually in the form of very small fat globules (less than 1 μm). Separation efficiency is influenced by the number of discs, their distance apart and the bowl rotational speed. However, there are practical limits to these parameters and little improvement is made even with very high rotational speeds. A commercial separator would normally work at around 6000 r.p.m. to give cream with a fat content of approximately 40% and skim milk with a fat content of 0·06%. Air incorporation markedly reduces separation efficiency and hermetic separators use mechanical seals to eliminate air. Hermetic separators are fed under pressure and do not require paring discs to remove the products.

The fat content of the cream is controlled by the relative flows of the outlet streams. If the flow of cream is restricted, the fat content will increase, but separation efficiency will decrease if fat content becomes very high. Separation temperature will also influence separation efficiency due to the effects on cream viscosity and the relative densities of fat and serum. However, higher temperatures may disrupt the membrane, resulting in more free fat in the cream. Phospholipids migrate from the membrane into the serum as temperature increases; this affects functional properties of the cream, notably whipping which may be adversely affected. Milk is

usually separated at optimum temperatures of 40–55°C depending on history of the milk, but some separators are designed to separate milk at around 5°C, the temperature at which it reaches the processing facilities.

Cream is normally standardized continuously by automatic control of the flow of the various streams. The fat content of the cream can be monitored through rapid instrumental analysis or by in-line density measurement and the resultant signals may be used by process logic controllers (PLCs) to adjust back pressures in the product lines automatically, in order to control fat contents.

Pasteurization, Sterilization and Packaging

Cream may be batch-pasteurized with a temperature of 63–65°C and holding time of approximately 30 min. Continuous pasteurization in a plate heat exchanger is more common. Whereas 72°C for 15 s is the legal minimum in most countries and the regime normally used for milk, it has been found advantageous to use a higher temperature of 80°C for cream. Higher temperatures of up to 85°C can shorten shelf life, possibly through the activation of bacterial spores. It is important that the cream is handled with care during any

Types of Cream

processing; positive pumps are recommended to avoid disruption of the fat globule membranes and release of free fat. Pasteurized cream may be packed in glass, cartons or plastic pots. *See* Pasteurization, Principles

Cartons require a watertight barrier between the cardboard and the cream and polyethylene is almost universally used, having replaced wax. Pots can be made of polystyrene or polypropylene, the latter being more popular. Aluminium foil lids are sealed onto the pots and a snap-on plastic cover can be added to provide a method of resealing after opening.

Alternatively, the cream may be in-can sterilized for extended shelf life. The cream, which must be of low bacterial count and low acidity, is standardized to a fat content close to the legal 23% minimum (often called 'reduced cream') then preheated and homogenized. Homogenization breaks large fat globules into smaller ones to reduce the tendency for fat globules to rise (creaming), creating at the same time a more stable fat globule membrane as protein is adsorbed from the serum to cover the new fat–serum interface. To obtain a smooth product without graininess, it may be necessary to add stabilizing salts, such as sodium carbonate, trisodium citrate or a sodium phosphate, which increase the availability of serum casein. The cream is filled into lacquered cans which are sealed and sterilized in a suitable retort or continuous sterilizer. UK regulations specify that the cream must be held at $\geq 108°C$ for ≥ 45 min or at conditions to give the equivalent effect. Temperatures of 115–120°C are normally used, with holding times dependent on size of can and whether agitation is applied during the sterilization process. The volume of a can is restricted (< 300 ml) as the prolonged heat treatment necessary for larger volumes would increase Maillard browning reactions between protein and lactose, and adversely affect colour and flavour. *See* Browning, Nonenzymatic; Sterilization of Foods

Cream may be UHT sterilized ($\geq 140°C$ for ≥ 2 s) and aseptically packed. Aseptic packaging material includes laminated cartons with plastic (e.g. polyethylene) on the inside, an intermediate aluminium foil barrier and cardboard on the outside. The cartons may be preformed, or formed continuously from a roll of laminate. The material must first be sterilized with hydrogen peroxide and the residual sterilant removed by draining and heating before filling. Pack sizes normally range from 100 to 1000 ml. Plastic pots may also be used, thermoformed continuously from a sheet before aseptically filling in a laminar air flow and final sealing with an aluminium foil (form–fill–seal). Pack sizes range from approximately 7·5 ml, for coffee cream, to 1000 ml. Lacquered metal cans are used for UHT aerosol cream. *See* Heat Treatment, Ultra-high Temperature (UHT) Treatments

Cream is packed in bulk with plastic pouches or plastic/foil laminate pouches contained in cartons or returnable plastic crates. UHT cream may be packed in bulk with special aseptic filling systems. Volumes up to 1000 litres can be packaged.

Hygiene and Storage

Cream is very susceptible to deterioration because of microbial, enzymatic and physicochemical changes. Pasteurized cream has a limited shelf life of several days and must be kept chilled ($< 5°C$). Although microbial deterioration is the major hazard, lipases in the cream release fatty acids which cause rancid flavours. The fat globules will tend to rise to the surface and agglomerate unless the cream is homogenized. Homogenization is advantageous for low-fat creams to increase the viscosity and to inhibit creaming. Storage at low temperature retards the 'plugging' of non-homogenized cream as creaming is retarded due to the higher viscosity, and the lower proportion of liquid fat in the globules minimizes agglomeration. Cream in glass bottles should be kept in the dark as light will cause photo-induced oxidative changes in the milk fat, with consequent deterioration in flavour. The shelf life of sterilized cream is limited by chemical and physical changes. Spore-forming organisms may be a problem if not eliminated by preheating. In-can sterilized cream has a long shelf life at ambient temperature, although Maillard reactions, which are initiated in the sterilization process, and serum separation (syneresis) may occur during storage. *See* Storage Stability, Mechanisms of Degradation

The greatest problem with UHT cream is physical separation of fat with subsequent agglomeration, although this can be minimized by homogenization. The addition of stabilizing salts, sodium caseinate or gum stabilizers will also inhibit agglomeration of fat globules. Psychrotrophic bacteria in the milk may release heat-resistant proteolytic enzymes which will result in coagulation and bitter flavours. The shelf life of UHT cream is limited to some extent by the packaging. Plastics are permeable to air and consequent oxidation adversely affects flavour. A layer of aluminium foil in a laminate will prevent oxygen entry, but flavour will still deteriorate due to nonoxidative reactions.

The principal defect of coffee cream is an increased tendency to 'feather' with storage time. This phenomenon is associated with migration of calcium from the serum to the membrane, resulting in reduced stability with consequent precipitation of protein and release of free fat when added to hot coffee. This can be minimized by careful control of homogenization and UHT conditions to produce a small fat globule (around 0.4 μm) and to eliminate globule clusters. The addition of calcium-sequestering agents and additional stabilizing protein, such as sodium caseinate, will also alleviate the problem.

Types of Cream

Freezing of Cream

Freezing cream will provide protection against microbial deterioration. However, unless the freezing is very rapid it will disrupt the emulsion, resulting in separation on thawing. Bulk frozen cream is used for manufacturing processes when the separation is not important. Cream is frozen rapidly by keeping unit volumes small, through film formation or by cryogenic freezing with liquid nitrogen. Frozen cream must be stored at less than −18°C for a long shelf life, and temperature cycling must be avoided as this will result in the formation of ice crystals which will damage the fat globule membranes. *See* Freezing, Cryogenic Freezing

Cultured (Sour) Cream

Cream can be cultured with suitable organisms which metabolize lactose to lactic acid and also provide other flavouring compounds. The reduction of pH coagulates the protein, which thickens the product and gives a somewhat extended shelf life. Pasteurized single cream is normally used as the starting material for culturing. Sour cream is used as an ingredient in many savoury foods (e.g. stroganoff, vegetable dishes, dressings, snack dips, etc.). *See* Lactic Acid Bacteria

Industrial Uses

Whipped Cream

Mechanical agitation of cream will introduce air into the cream as dispersed bubbles. Fat globules concentrate at the air–serum interface, where the surface tension is believed to disrupt the globule membrane. As agitation continues, the air bubbles become smaller and the globules interact to form a stable network. The interaction depends on several factors. The fat content has to be sufficiently high to give the necessary density of the globules at the interface. The membrane round the fat globules must not be too stable as some mechanical breakdown is necessary to develop the interaction and 'welding' of the globules. Homogenization or addition of stabilizing substances, such as protein, have an inhibitory effect on whipping. The temperature and ageing of the cream are important. If the temperature is above 10°C, excessive liquid fat will weaken the structure and act as a foam depressant. Cream should be stored refrigerated for at least 12 h before whipping to optimize fat crystallization and membrane destabilization. The addition of emulsifer can result in increased overrun (percentage increase in volume on whipping) of the whipped cream. Some emulsifiers can increase the interaction of the globules with consequent shorter whip

times and stiffer structures. However, the addition of these is only really of advantage when the cream has to be homogenized for long shelf life products, and their addition is restricted by legislation. *See* Emulsifiers, Uses in Processed Foods

The major industrial use of cream is as whipped cream in baking and confectionary to decorate cakes and desserts. Whipped cream can be produced commercially in large batch mixers or in continuous machines which use a pump to take the cream through a whipping device such as a static mixer. Air is drawn into the mixer, and degree of whipping is controlled by the air:cream ratio.

Control of cream whipping is very important as 'overwhipping' will result in the complete breakdown of the emulsion with 'churning' of the fat and release of free serum. 'Underwhipping' will give a soft foam without adequate structure to hold its shape. Whipped cream has better freeze–thaw stability than the unwhipped product so can be successfully incorporated in frozen confections. Addition of stabilizer, such as carrageenan or sodium alginate, will reduce the tendency of the whipped product to synerese. *See* Stabilizers, Applications

Other Industrial Uses

Cream soups are products which incorporate cream as an essential ingredient. Products may be canned, or sold as dry powders to be reconstituted in water.

Cream can be used industrially as a source of fat for other food products. However, butter or anhydrous milk fat, which are both manufactured from cream, would be more generally used for reasons of storage stability and economy. Cream may be used if flavour is of prime importance; fresh cream makes the best quality ice cream.

Cream can be dried to produce high-fat powders which may be used as ingredients in foods and may be particularly useful for dry blends (e.g. cake mixes, soup mixes or soft-serve ice-cream powders). The spray drying of cream demands formulations to suit the end use and special driers are required to handle the high-fat product. Cream powders are not produced in large quantities because vegetable-fat-based products are much cheaper and easier to produce. Cream-based powders have the advantage of superior flavour, but protection against lipid oxidation is required to give the product adequate shelf life. Cream liqueurs are popular beverages which use the preservative powers of alcohol for long shelf life. *See* Drying, Spray Drying; Oxidation of Food Components

Bibliography

Alfa-Laval (1980) *Dairy Handbook*. Lund, Sweden: Alfa-Laval AB, Dairy and Food Engineering Division.

Buchheim W (1990) Milk and dairy-type emulsions. In: Larsson K and Friberg S (eds) *Food Emulsions* 2nd edn, pp 203–246. New York: Marcel Dekker.

Lehmann HR and Zettier K-H (1987) *Separators for the Dairy Industry*, Technical scientific documentation No. 7, 3rd revised edn. Oelde, Germany: Westfalia Separator AG.

Mulder H and Walstra P (1974) *The Milkfat Globule. Emulsion Science as Applied to Milk Products and Comparable Foods.* UK: CAB International, Wallingford/The Netherlands: PUDOC, Wageningen.

Rothwell J (ed.) (1989) *Cream Processing Manual* 2nd edn. Huntingdon, Cambridgeshire: The Society of Dairy Technology.

Towler C (1986) Developments in cream separation and processing. In: Robinson RK (ed.) *Modern Dairy Technology*, vol. 1, pp 51–92. London: Elsevier Applied Science Publishers.

C. Towler and P. A. E. Cant
New Zealand Dairy Research Institute, Palmerston North, New Zealand

Clotted Cream

Clotted cream, often referred to as 'Cornish cream' or 'Devon cream', is a high-fat cream which has been specially processed so that it acquires a characteristic nutty flavour, a consistency which is a mixture of thick and thin regions and a texture which alternates between granular and smooth. The colour can vary from cream to golden yellow depending on breed of cow and season of year, and the product from each small manufacturing unit has its own typical flavour and physical characteristics. The most popular method of consumption is with scones and jam, ideally strawberry, or with fruit.

Traditionally, clotted cream has always been manufactured in the counties of Devon and Cornwall (UK) – 'the West Country' – where small herds of cows of Channel Islands and South Devon origin produce high-fat milk, especially in the spring and summer.

During this period, some of the warm milk, i.e. straight from the cow, was transferred to shallow pans (150 mm high and 500 mm in diameter) standing on slate shelves in a cool dairy. Overnight, the cream rose to the surface and, next day, the pans were slowly heated (scalded) over a period of 2–3 h until the surface of the cream had a strawlike appearance. The milk was never allowed to boil, for the 'bubbling action' would have disrupted the crust. Once the heating stage was complete, the pans were cooled, either in running water or by standing on the slate shelf until the following day. Either way, the cream had then hardened and could be skimmed off, using a large, flat, perforated spoon, into a dish ready for eating. The skimmed milk was used for drinking, cooking or for feeding calves or pigs.

The Current Position

The most significant change in the manufacture of clotted cream occurred with the introduction of cream separators onto the farm. The separated cream was then scalded in pans using the method described above, but with the difference that, after cooling, the entire contents of the pan could be eaten, i.e. no skim-milk was present. Any surplus clotted cream was made into butter for use during the winter months when milk supplies were reduced.

In addition, the last 10 years has seen a major increase in factory-produced clotted cream, and as much as 30 000 l of whole milk is processed daily to give approximately 2 t of product. This development, along with the improvement in chilled distribution to the supermarkets, has meant that clotted cream is now available to many more customers.

These large factories have their own specially designed processing plants, configured according to systems that they have developed themselves, and employing modern technology to provide the product safety required today. Thus, regardless of volume of manufacture, the scalding of the cream must give a product that is both bacteriologically safe and readily saleable, and control of this stage is critical for success. In particular, the scalding time depends on the following: (1) the butterfat content of the cream, and any heat treatment that the cream may have received prior to scalding; (2) the volume of cream to be processed, and the surface area in contact, directly or indirectly, with the heating medium; (3) the temperature of the heating medium, and its volume in relation to the volume of product.

The minimum time and temperature conditions are 30 min at 65°C to give a bacteriologically safe product, and care must be exercised when choosing where in the system this temperature is measured. However, a further heating time is required to give the product its desired characteristics of flavour and texture, and hence survival of pathogens should not be a problem. An additional consideration is the fact that, with the cream reaching 70–80°C, evaporation can cause a loss in weight of up to 15%, depending on the surface area exposed. Control of the humidity in the scalding chamber or room may help to reduce this loss and give an even heat treatment, but especial care is needed to avoid condensation contaminating the product.

The system of cooling in a factory operation needs careful planning to avoid atmospheric contamination of the product, and expensive air filtration systems are installed to give a positive-pressure airflow in the high-risk areas. Although too rapid cooling can reduce the viscosity of the final product, all cream should be cooled to below 5°C within 12 h of production.

Legal and/or Advisory Standards

The statutory regulations insist that clotted cream must have a minimum butterfat content of 55%, and that the only acceptable preservative is nisin. *See* Preservation of Food

In addition, local authorities expect the product to conform to certain bacteriological standards, and these include a requirement that the total colony count (TCC) 24 h after manufacture should be less than 1000 colony-forming units (cfu) per g (Yeastrel milk agar at 30°C for 72 h); coliform bacteria should be absent in 1 g; yeast and moulds should be less than 100 cfu g^{-1}.

Manufacturing Procedures

In a Small Dairy using up to 2000 l per day (*On Farm*)

Each dairy manufactures clotted cream with certain individual characteristics which their customers accept as normal. The great advantage that these producers enjoy is the availability of a fresh supply of raw milk, which is produced at the required standards for a good product, i.e. low TCC, high fat level and freedom from taints or off-flavours. The milk, at around 35°C, is pumped directly from the receiving jars in the milking parlour to the separator. There are many types of separator in use, and capacities range from 30 to 500 l of whole milk per h. The cream screw is kept in a fixed position on the top plate, and the final cream thickness is regulated by the flow of milk through the separator. Real problems only occur when the milk is too cold owing to ambient conditions, for there is then an increased fat loss into the skim-milk. *See* Milk, Processing of Liquid Milk

Various methods are used to scald the separated cream, and these include the hot plate of a solid fuel cooker, a catering-size *bain-marie*, special hot-water scalders designed specifically for clotted cream (see Fig. 1) and hot-air ovens with forced air circulation. The actual product is scalded in pans made of stainless steel or aluminium; aluminium conducts the heat more efficiently but is not as easily cleaned as stainless steel. The pans vary in size according to the method of scalding.

Cream made in *bains marie* is stirred to ensure even heating, and is then often cooled to 50°C and poured into the retail pots, followed by overnight refrigeration; a very smooth, homogeneous product is obtained by this

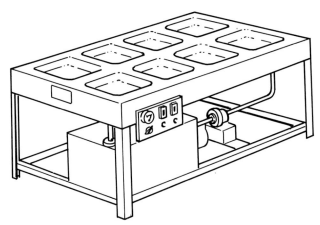

Fig. 1 The Clotted Cream Maker produces the real clotted cream usually associated with Devon and Cornwall, is available in two models (four and eight pans) and is very simple to operate, with automatic temperature control.

Produced in quality stainless steel, the Clotted Cream Maker is extremely durable and cleans easily. Water in the system is heated by three 3-kW heaters and is circulated by a pump around the tray in which the pans are located. The water temperature is thermostatically controlled to ensure that the correct level of heat is maintained. Following the heating process, cold water may be circulated through the system to cool the pans. When the temperature of the cream is sufficiently reduced, the pans are removed from the tray and placed in a refrigerator for final cooling prior to potting.

(By courtesy of MM Services, Truro, UK.)

method. In hot-air ovens, the cream can be scalded in the retail pot.

More traditional scalders are available to produce from 4·5 to 9·0 kg of cream in one batch, and one commercial form is shown in Fig. 1. This type is heated by electricity, and the hot water is circulated in the shallow tank underneath the pans; this ensures even heat distribution. At the end of scalding, the hot water is diverted into the heating section and cold water is circulated under the pans. If required, insulated covers can be placed over the scalder to give more consistent heating by controlling the airflow over the cream; the covers also reduce the risk of atmospheric contamination. The cream is cooked to the desired degree when the surface has a strawlike, even colour, and there are small globules of free fat around edge of the pan. The surface of the cream should not be disturbed during transfer to the cold room. The cream should then be refrigerated overnight to allow the surface fat to crystallize, so giving the granular texture expected in the retail product, and making the cream easier to handle next day, and with less waste.

The room where the bulk cream is packed into retail packs should be separate from the production area, as this will reduce the possibilities of both contamination from the raw materials and yeast or mould infection from the air. The shelf life of properly made clotted cream should be at least 6 days at 5°C.

In general, farm-produced clotted cream varies in fat content between 60% and 65%, and it tends to have more flavour and a more varied texture than factory processed cream.

Factory-produced Clotted Cream

With factory-scale operations, the individual milk supplies are bulked to give a more consistent raw material and, in order to maintain product viscosity, the percentage of fat in the cream has to be adjusted, prior to scalding, to compensate for seasonal variations. Modern process technology and laboratory control are used to monitor the quality of both the raw material and the cream emerging from the separator, and design parameters that minimize the shear on the fat during pumping are important.

The use of milk more than 24 h old should be minimized, and the separated cream must be scalded within 4 h. Modern, automatic desludging separators are designed to minimize fat losses into the skim-milk during the production of cream at 50% butterfat, and at high separating temperatures. However, separation at milk temperatures above 43°C can affect the final viscosity of the retail product. In general, the cream is separated at 54–59% butterfat, depending on the method of scalding that is to follow, and each batch is standardized to a preset figure.

In most factories, the separated cream is then pasteurized through a plate heat exchanger designed to heat the cream to 75°C for 15 s, followed by cooling to 60°C if the cream is to be scalded immediately, or to below 20°C if it is to be stored. Compensation for any loss of viscosity in the final product as a result of handling of raw milk and pasteurization of cream is made by adding a small percentage of homogenized cream to the mix prior to scalding. *See* Pasteurization, Principles

At present, there are two methods of scalding practised in the industry, one using hot water and one using hot air. The hot-air technique is generally employed on a batch system, and all the retail product is scalded in pots ranging from 125 g to 2·25 kg. The accuracy of fill is much easier to achieve with the uncooked cream, and the risk of postpasteurization contamination is reduced as the final product needs only to be lidded. A continuous approach is adopted with hot-water scalding. The pans are taken through the heated water on bars which move at a given speed. Each pan holds 1·5–2·25 kg of cream, and the depth of the cream is approximately 25–30 mm; a scalding time of 1–1·5 h is usually employed. Monitoring of air and/or water temperatures at each process stage is important to ensure even heating.

Alternative sources of heating using infrared and microwave technology will be introduced when they become cost effective, but as the total volume of clotted cream produced annually is comparatively small, it is difficult to justify high capital expenditures.

A separate room, which has a positive-pressure airflow of good bacteriological quality, is required for when the cream comes off the scalder and is placed onto trolleys before entering the refrigerator, the trolleys having been previously washed and sterilized in a tunnel-wash system. The refrigerator, which will operate at 5°C, should have a level floor and be divided into separate sections, each holding the total production for one day.

Packaging

Cream Scalded in the Pot

A number of systems are available for lidding, and these employ either a foil lid that is heat-sealed to the plastic pot, or a plastic snap-on lid. Each pot can be coded as required. Underweight packs have to be rejected, as any manual additions of cream will spoil the visual impact, and hence this fault must be corrected as the prescald cream is filled into the pot.

Packing of Bulk Cream into Retail Packs

Filling machines, rotary or linear, must be designed to give minimum breakdown of the cream during dispensing, and control of the final weights can be difficult owing to texture variations in the product. The cream, after a short cooling period, can be packed into the retail pots at between 20°C and 30°C, and then returned to the refrigerator, where final cooling gives a desirable increase in viscosity. The shelf life of factory-produced cream should be 10–14 days, and supermarkets expect 6 days in store. In general, this type of clotted cream has a smooth, tacky consistency, little trace of the traditional crust, a pale cream colour – as a result of the increased heating – and a bland flavour; the average butterfat content is 60%. Some factory-produced clotted cream is used for the manufacture of luxury ice cream, and this manufacturing cream would be made to a final fat level of 56%; texture is not important as will be further processed in the ice-cream mix. *See* Ice Cream, Methods of Manufacture

Mary Mikalsen
MM Services, Truro, UK

Clotted Cream

CREAM LIQUEURS

See Liqueurs

CRUSTACEA

See Shellfish

CRYOGENS

See Freezing

CRYSTALLIZATION

Basic Principles

Crystallization is one of the basic thermal unit operations and is the process in which solids – crystals (from the Greek word, *krystallos*, meaning ice) – are formed from a previously homogeneous system, with a certain well-defined spatial arrangement of their components (atoms, ions, molecules).

Crystallization serves three main purposes: purification, separation and production of specific crystal forms. The production of well-formed crystals for specific applications (monocrystals for optical or electronic purposes, precious stones) is termed crystal drawing.

As a physical process, crystallization takes place in two stages, whereby crystal growth follows nucleus formation. The conditions necessary for nucleation and crystal growth are that the equilibrium concentration of the solution should be exceeded to a certain extent (supersaturation, supercooling). Usually, crystallization is then induced by addition of 'seed nuclei', e.g.

crystal fragments. Not every substance can be crystallized; the tendency for crystallization decreases with an increase in molecular weight and the number of components (e.g. tar, pitch, resins). Crystallization can take place from solid, liquid (solutions, melts) or gaseous phases.

Technically, crystallization from solid phase is of minor importance, nucleation and crystal growth being usually exceptionally slow. However, in downstream process steps, such as drying and storage, changes in the crystalline state can have a decisive effect on the product quality.

Crystallization from solutions – particularly from aqueous solutions – is of major importance for the recovery of crystalline bulk goods, such as sugar, salt, potassium chloride and some nitrogen fertilizers. Depending on the dissolving characteristics of the solid, crystallization is effected either by removal (evaporation) of the solvent or by cooling, until the solubility limit of the relevant substance is exceeded. Dissolution represents the reverse of crystallization.

Crystallization from solutions can take place at rest or in motion. Crystallization at rest from solutions of low supersaturation to produce large, well-formed, pure crystals requires several days to weeks. However, crystallization in motion, introduced by Wulff at the end of the nineteenth century, is more suitable for industrial-scale recovery of crystalline products, guaranteeing a high throughput per unit volume of crystallizer.

Mechanical separation methods are used to separate the crystals from the mother liquor (e.g. centrifuging, filtration, screening).

The formation of solids from solutions can also take place by precipitation. In contrast to crystallization, precipitation is defined as the operation in which the addition of a further substance to a solution causes the formation of a precipitate, regardless of whether this precipitate is amorphous or crystalline. The fundamental mechanism is either chemical reaction (reaction precipitation) or reduced solubility (displacement precipitation, salting out). If during precipitation crystals are formed directly, the processes of precipitation and crystallization become entwined and one can speak of 'precipitation crystallization'.

In adductive crystallization, an auxiliary substance, e.g. urea, capable of forming a crystalline adduct with the desired substance, is added to the solution; the adduct is recovered by separation from the mother liquor and decomposed to recover the desired substance. An example is the dewaxing of crude oil with aqueous urea solution and methylene chloride.

Crystallization from melts takes place by cooling. Here too a supersaturation may be reached, from which the addition of nuclei causes spontaneous crystallization with the production of heat. In chocolate manufacture, the correct regulation of fat crystallization in the melt obtained from conching is of vital importance for the product quality. Similarly, in metals and alloys the microcrystalline structure determined by the rate of crystallization can have a great effect on the properties of the material. *See* Cocoa, Chemistry of Processing

Solutions or melts often contain several substances. If there are appreciable differences in their solubility, they can be separated from each other by 'fractionated crystallization', i.e. by repeated recrystallization and thus be recovered relatively pure.

Crystallization from the gas phase (solidification, desublimation) is the direct condensation of a vapour into the solid crystalline state. The condensation temperature must be lower than the triple point in the phase diagram. The solidification usually follows the volatilization of a solid. The overall process is called sublimation. It serves mainly for purifying organic and inorganic solids in the chemical industry.

For industrial-scale crystallization a large variety of different batch and continuous crystallizers is available.

In classifying crystallizers the part for creating the supersaturation is separated from the actual crystallization space. This allows maintenance of a definite supersaturation, and crystals which are sufficiently large may be drawn off.

The selection of a crystallizer depends essentially on the following considerations:

1. The physical data of the substances involved, e.g. the difference in density between crystals and mother syrup.
2. The crystallization method to be employed.
3. The quality criteria for the crystalline product (purity, crystal size distribution).

Extensive research on crystallization carried out to date notwithstanding, the design of crystallizers is still largely based on empirical knowledge.

Factors Affecting Crystal Growth

Saturation and Supersaturation

A solution in thermodynamic equilibrium with a solid phase is termed saturated in relation to the solid. However, it is also possible to produce solutions containing a larger proportion of the solute than that contained in a saturated solution. These solutions are called supersaturated.

The degree of supersaturation of a solution is expressed in practice either by the difference in concentration ($\Delta c = c - c^*$) or by the supersaturation number ($S = c/c^*$); c is the actual solution concentration and c^* the equilibrium solubility. The temperature solubility diagram shows the solution equlibria of the solid and is the basis of the crystallization process to be used. The prerequisite for crystallization is a supersaturation number greater than one. The crystals are formed and grow until the supersaturation is removed, but a crystallizing solution reaches its equilibrium value only slowly from the side of supersaturation. Ostwald introduced the term supersolubility for this apparent stability of supersaturated solutions.

The range included by the solubility and supersolubility curves is called the metastable or Ostwald–Miers range (see Fig. 1). This is followed upwards by the so-called labile zone. On closer examination two supersolubility curves can be distinguished. As the first supersolubility curve is exceeded, crystal nuclei are formed in the intermediate range only when crystals are already present in the solution; above the second, spontaneous nuclei formation occurs at high speed, with a measurable heat effect.

In the actual metastable region the probability of nuclei formation is extremely low. Metastable solutions, with a concentration differing only slightly from the equilibrium solution, are almost ideal for crystal growth

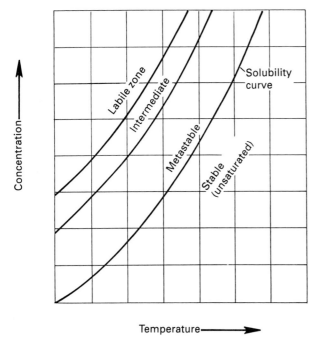

Fig. 1 Solubility–supersolubility diagram.

with the addition of seed crystals. The metastable range therefore has great practical importance for all crystallization processes.

Crystal Nucleation

Depending on the conditions of formation of submicroscopic crystals – 'nuclei' – in supersaturated solutions, two types of nucleation may be distinguished:

1. Primary nucleation – in the absence of crystals.
2. Secondary nucleation – in the presence of identical crystals (homogeneous nucleation) or under the influence of foreign matter (heterogeneous nucleation).

Crystal nuclei which fail to reach a certain critical size are unstable and redissolve. Based on thermodynamic data the critical nucleus size can be calculated. It is smaller with increasing supersaturation. The time after reaching supersaturation until the beginning of nucleation (induction time) also decreases as supersaturation increases.

In industrial-scale processes only secondary (induced) nucleation is of importance, in contrast to the laboratory trials.

Crystal Growth

The formation of stable nuclei is followed by crystal growth where ions or molecules from the supersaturated solution are deposited on the preformed nucleus surfaces.

According to Volmer, the crystals are surrounded by a layer in which the molecules transported there by diffusion, although able to move relatively freely, are already subject to the attractive forces of the crystal surface. These molecules are displaced to energetically favourable positions and finally incorporated into the crystal lattice.

The growth rate of a crystal is thus determined by the mass transfer by diffusion from the supersaturated solution through the Prandtl layer to the Volmer layer on the crystal and the boundary layer reaction (adsorption, surface diffusion, incorporation into the energetically favourable lattice position).

The mathematical description of these complex procedures represents an exceptionally difficult task. Approximate formulae are described in the literature.

The growth rate of the crystals can be principally governed by any of the mentioned steps. In any case it increases, according to the Arrhenius relationship, with the temperature. Furthermore, it increases with supersaturation, often following a first-order reaction.

The overall mass transfer rate is enhanced by increasing stirring efficiency, or the relative velocity between the crystals and solution, as well as by decreasing dynamic viscosity of the solution.

The development of individual crystal surfaces during growth depends on the crystallization conditions (temperature, supersaturation, impurities) and determines the shape and form of the crystals.

Crystallization leads to crystals of different sizes, the crystal size distribution representing an important quality criterion for the final product.

Low-temperature Techniques

When the product is heat-sensitive or there is a favourable position of the thermodynamic equilibrium in the solid–liquid range, crystallization may be performed at low temperatures.

For example *p*-xylol, which is an important intermediate in the production of plastics, is recovered from the mixture of isomers obtained in petroleum distillation by crystallization at a temperature of about $-70°C$. Deparaffining of some crude oil fractions also takes place by crystallizing out the paraffins by cooling to about $-30°C$.

'Freezing out' is a specific type of crystallization in which the solvent is crystallized out instead of the solute. Known examples are seawater desalination and the mild technique of concentrating fruit juices by freezing out ice. Moreover, beer, wine and coffee extracts may also be concentrated by this method. The highest solute concentration achievable is determined by the position of the eutectic point in the solidification diagram. *See* Freezing, Principles

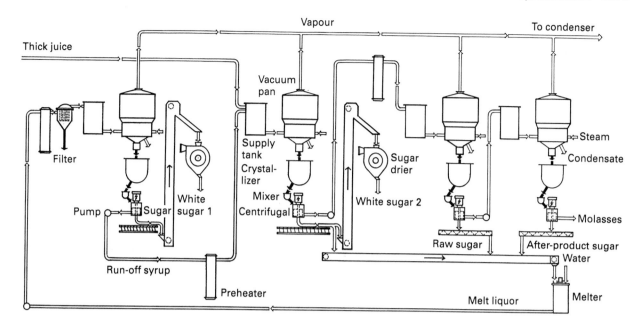

Fig. 2 Flow sheet of industrial sugar crystallization.

The heat removal can be effected through heat exchange surfaces by evaporating a highly volatile solvent, e.g. *n*-butane, or by flash vaporization under vacuum.

Specific Applications

Sugar Refining

Sugar refining is achieved in both the beet and the cane sugar industries by crystallization from concentrated juice (see Fig. 2). The raw juice obtained from sugar beet by extraction with water and/or from sugar cane by pressing with roller mills is concentrated, after purification steps, in a multistage evaporator to a solids content of about 70–75%. Because of the nonsugar materials still present in varying amounts in the thick juice, and their influence on the purity of sugar, the crystallization must be carried out in several steps to obtain a sufficiently pure product. *See* Sugar, Handling of Sugar Beet and Sugar Cane; Sugar, Sugar Cane

From the thick juice 85–90% of the sucrose present can be recovered as a crystalline form by multistage crystallization without using other methods such as ion exchange. The residual sucrose and practically all the nonsugar substances present in thick juice go into molasses, the mother liquor from the last crystallization step.

The evaporative crystallization is carried out in steam-heated vacuum pans under reduced pressure and low temperature (70–75°C).

In batch operation, enough juice (syrup) is initially introduced to keep the heating chamber (calendria) covered during further concentration.

As soon as sufficient supersaturation is reached, a predetermined number of seed crystals of defined size, governed by the grain size of the final product, is added. Subsequently, the pan is filled up by continuous addition of juice, whereby the crystals present grow to their final size. Finally, the crystal magma is concentrated to the proper consistency for the subsequent centrifuging (optimum crystal content).

In continuous crystallizers, which have found increasing acceptance in the sugar industry in recent years, the process steps described are run one after the other in individual chambers of the pan.

Separation of the sugar crystals from the mother liquor takes place in centrifuges. Thus the mother liquor, which still sticks to the crystal surface, is removed with a syrup of higher purity followed by hot water and steam. The white sugar obtained is then dried. The resulting syrups are subjected to two further crystallization steps (raw sugar and after product).

Refined sugar is produced from raw sugar by dissolving, filtering and recrystallization, resulting in a sugar of higher purity.

Oil Fractionation

The crude oils of plant or animal origin obtained by pressing, extraction, melting out, etc., are subjected to an initial refining step in order to remove undesirable impurities, e.g. gums. The aim of fractionation is to obtain components with specific properties or to separate further constituents, which may impair the suitability of the oil for its intended application. *See* Fats, Uses in the Food Industry; Vegetable Oils, Refining

The higher-melting glycerides are crystallized out, e.g. during 'winterization' of the edible oils, by cooling over several hours to 6–10°C, and then removed by filtration. As a result, cloudiness of edible oils at refrigerator temperature is avoided. *See* Triglycerides, Structures and Properties

In addition to liquid–liquid extraction, fractionated crystallization is employed to separate oil components. The molten fat to be fractionated is cooled slowly in agitated vessels, in order to obtain the largest possible and most easily filterable crystals of the higher-melting glycerides, which are then separated, on filter presses or rotary drum filters. This separation can be simplified by selective wetting, e.g. with sodium lauryl sulphate in aqueous solution. The crystal suspension produced in batches or continuously is mixed with the solution of the wetting agent. The wetted fat crystals go into the aqueous phase and can easily be separated by centrifuging.

By using solvents such as acetone or ethyl methyl ketone in the fractionated crystallization, the separation between higher- and low-melting glycerides may be improved.

However, additional equipment for solvent recovery is necessary. Moreover, foodstuff regulations have to be taken into account.

Palm oil is important for the manufacture of margarines, baking, roasting and frying fats. Refined palm oil may be separated into a solid and a liquid fraction. The palm oil stearin (20–25%) is suitable for margarines as the hard component and the palm oil olein (75–80%) is used, for example, as a frying fat. *See* Vegetable Oils, Oil Palms

With a more sophisticated fractionation, e.g. using acetone, palm oil yields not only the stearin and olein fractions, but also a middle fraction very much resembling cocoa butter.

Bibliography

McGinnes RA (ed.) (1982) *Beet-Sugar Technology* 3rd edn. Fort Collins, Colorado: Beet Sugar Development Foundation.

Meyerson AS and Toyokura K (eds) (1990) *Crystallisation as a Separations Process*. ACS symposium series 438. Washington, DC: American Chemists Society.

Mullin JW (1972) *Crystallisation* 2nd edn. London: Butterworth.

Nyvlt J (1971) *Industrial Crystallisation from Solutions*. London: Butterworth.

Thomas A (1987) Fats and fatty oils. In: *Ullmann's Encyclopedia of Industrial Chemistry* (Gerhartz W, ed.), vol. A10, pp 173–243. Weinheim: VCH.

H. Schiweck and G. Witte
Südzucker AG Mannheim/Ochsenfurt, Grünstadt, FRG

CUCURBITS

See Vegetables of Tropical Climates

CULTURED MILK PRODUCTS

See Fermented Milks and Yoghurt

CURING

History of Curing

Curing by salting was originally used for the preservation of meat during times of abundance to be consumed in times of scarcity. Its origin is lost in antiquity. It was discovered that impurities in salt, mainly saltpetre (potassium nitrate), produced a characteristic flavour and colour. However, the scientific knowledge of the role and mode of action of nitrates was not established until the latter half of the 19th century. It was shown by Polenske, in 1891, that nitrate was reduced to nitrite by bacterial action while Lehman, in 1899, indicated that the characteristic colour of cured meat products was due to nitrite. Two years later, Haldane explained the colour formation as a result of the reaction of nitric oxide, one of the degradation products from nitrite, with meat pigments. All these advances led to the direct use of nitrite instead of nitrate because of some important advantages such as lower levels of addition required and less residual nitrite. However, it also became clear that, in long ripening processes for the production of dry-cured or fermented meat products, nitrate was required for slow nitrite generation by bacterial reduction. Today, due to the availability of industrial and domestic refrigerators, curing has lost some of its importance for meat preservation but now has a new dimension as a means for obtaining a great variety of products with characteristic colour and flavour.

The term 'cured' is used for a great number of meat products although the meaning of the word varies slightly depending on the country and kind of product. Cured meat products are generally understood to have been treated with salt, nitrate and/or nitrite, but they also include products that have been subjected to a long ripening or ageing process where complex biochemical reactions, of proteolytic and lipolytic nature, have produced a characteristic flavour.

Curing Ingredients and their Functions

Salt, nitrate and/or nitrite are the main curing ingredients. Salt is basic to all curing mixtures. Its main role is as bacteriostatic agent, but it also affects the flavour and increases protein solubility as well as the water-holding capacity, which is very important in cooked meat products. Salt levels in meat products may be as high as 3% although this is not high enough to exert a complete bacteriostatic action. Therefore, other preservation techniques such as refrigeration, dehydration, acidifica-

tion, cooking or smoking are required. On the other hand, salt may cause undesirable effects in that it may accelerate oxidation of pigments and fats, resulting in brown off-colours and rancid taste. Nitrate and nitrite play an important role in the prevention of these changes. Nitrite is the active agent in the curing mixture and, in fact, all reactions taking place during curing have some kind of relation with nitrite chemistry. Nitrite can be part of the cure formulation, but may also be generated through nitrate reduction by the action of naturally occurring bacteria or added starter cultures. The nitrite ion (NO_2^-) is very reactive and, depending on the conditions, may act as an oxidizing or reducing agent. In biological systems with a slightly acid pH (5·5–6·2), which is generally the case in post-mortem muscle, a small quantity of the added nitrite, as sodium or potassium salt, is transformed into nitrous acid. This metabolite can take part in many chemical reactions with meat components, depending on the pH, temperature, redox potential and presence of other added substances. These chemical reactions have been studied extensively, but the results are not conclusive due to the high reactivity of nitrite, the complexity of the substrate (meat) and the type and method of processing of the product. In meat curing, a major part of the added nitrite disappears as the result of the reaction of nitrous acid with proteins and other meat components. The Van Slyke reaction (eqn [1]),

$$RCHNH_2COOH + HONO \rightarrow RCHOHCOOH + N_2 + H_2O \quad (1)$$

where nitrous acid reacts with α-amino acids (R denotes an organic group), is major mechanism for nitrite disappearance which, depending on processing conditions, represents between 30 and 50% of the amount initially added. Nitrous acid produced from the added nitrite may decompose, in the presence of favourable reducing conditions (eqn [2]).

$$3 HONO \rightleftharpoons HNO_3 + 2NO + H_2O \quad (2)$$

The most important reaction in curing is the formation of nitric oxide (NO), which reacts with the meat pigment myoglobin giving the characteristic colour of cured meat products. *See* Oxidation of Food Components; Preservation of Food; Starter Cultures

Nitrate is added as the sodium or potassium salt, which is transformed to nitrite by bacteria with nitrate reductase activity, naturally occurring in meat or added as starter cultures, usually of the family *Micrococcaceae*.

Other substances can be used as curing adjuncts. Examples are sugars, ascorbic and erythorbic acids or their sodium salts, phosphates, flavouring agents and flavour enhancers. In some countries, sugars, such as sucrose or glucose, at concentrations around 2% are used as additional curing ingredients. They serve to counteract the harsh hardening effects of salt and, at the same time, they constitute an excellent substrate for bacterial growth in some applications such as the dry curing of sausages. Ascorbic and erythorbic acids play an important role in colour development because they facilitate the formation of nitric oxide, take part in the reduction of metmyoglobin to myoglobin, stabilize both colour and flavour as a result of their antioxidant activity and, finally, reduce the rate of formation of nitrosamines in cured meat products. In some countries, legislation dictates the addition of about 500 ppm of ascorbic or erythorbic acid because these substances inhibit the formation of nitrosamines. Phosphates are added to solubilize meat proteins and increase the water-holding capacity. This is very important as the yields of wet-cured products increase. Maximum concentrations are usually around 3000 mg of P_2O_5 per kilogram. All the above-mentioned substances have an antioxidant activity which improves both colour and flavour. Flavouring agents and flavour enhancers, such as spices or protein hydrolysates, are sometimes added to accentuate a specific flavour. *See* Antioxidants, Synthetic Antioxidants; Ascorbic Acid, Properties and Determination; Colours, Properties and Determination of Synthetic Pigments; Meat, Sausages and Comminuted Products; Nitrosamines

Effect of Curing on Meat Properties

Curing plays an important role in the development and fixation of the characteristic cured colour, the prevention of the growth of pathogenic and spoilage microflora and the development and stability of flavour. *See* Spoilage, Bacterial Spoilage

Colour Development

The colour of fresh meat may vary depending on the oxidation state of the iron and the radical attached to the haem group of the myoglobin pigment. When nitrite is added, numerous and complex chemical reactions, take place. Eventually, these lead to the development of the cured pigment nitrosomyoglobin or nitric oxide myoglobin. Figure 1 includes a schematic presentation of these reactions. Although these reactions have been thoroughly studied by numerous research groups, the exact nature of some reactions is still not well understood because meat is such a complex substrate. All evidence suggests the existence of an intermediate step for the formation of metmyoglobin pigment (ferric form of iron, Fe^{3+}) as a consequence of pigment oxidation by

nitrite. Metmyoglobin is then reduced and combined with nitric oxide, which substitutes the molecule of water bound to the iron in the haem group, giving a bright red coloured pigment (ferrous form of iron, Fe^{2+}). This molecule, called nitrosomyoglobin or nitric oxide myoglobin, is the desirable pigment in cured meats. The mechanism of formation of this pigment still remains unclear and several mechanisms, including reducing substances present in meat such as sulphydryl groups (—SH), respiratory coenzymes like nicotinamide adeninedinucleotide (NADH), the mitochondrial enzyme ferricytochrome c or added reducing substances such as ascorbic acid, have been suggested. Under the influence of heat, the pigment nitrosohaemochromogen is formed, which is the desirable and stable pink pigment characteristic of cooked cured meat products. The haem group of the pigments may be degraded by both bacterial action or photochemical oxidation, resulting in the formation of porphyrins (decoloured or green/yellow colours) typical of spoiled meat products.

Bacterial Inhibition

Numerous studies have shown different sensibilities of bacteria to nitrite. Gram-positive bacteria, such as those of the genus *Lactobacillus* and family Micrococcaceae, which play an important role in the fermentation of sausages, are more resistant to nitrite. Thus, in cured sausage manufacture nitrite is very important because it helps the selection of an adequate fermentation flora. However, the most important function of nitrite is to inhibit the outgrowth and toxin formation of *Clostridium botulinum*, a bacterium that produces a highly potent and dangerous toxin. This is the major reason why nitrates and nitrites are considered essential in producing safe cured meat products. The minimum input level required is 120 mg kg^{-1}. The inhibitory process is not yet completely understood, but it is believed that nitrite interacts with components of the cellular metabolism. Other factors such as salt concentration, pH, redox potential, water activity, heat treatment and storage conditions also play important roles in bacterial inhibition. *See* Clostridium, Occurrence of *Clostridium botulinum*; Lactic Acid Bacteria

Flavour Effects

It is well established that nitrite contributes to the development of cured meat flavour although it is characteristic and distinctive for each kind of product. It should be taken into account that many substances, like flavouring agents or enhancers which are added, and treatments, like smoking, may contribute significantly to the flavour. It is generally recognized that 'cured flavour' is the result of multiple components. The most important contribution of nitrite to the curing flavour relies on its delaying the development of oxidative

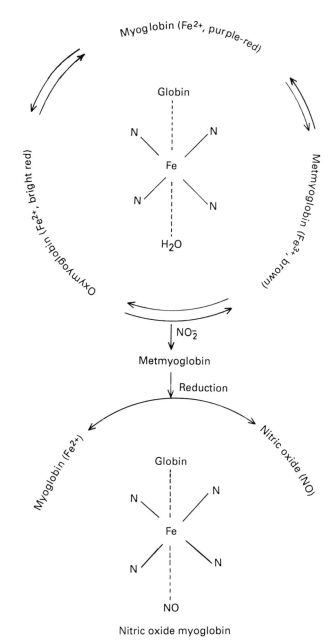

Myoglobin (Fe²⁺, purple-red)

Globin

NO_2^-

Metmyoglobin

Reduction

Myoglobin (Fe²⁺)   Nitric oxide (NO)

Globin

NO

Nitric oxide myoglobin

Fig. 1 The main changes in the pigment haem during meat curing.

rancidity. Nitrite also prevents the development of warmed-over flavour (WOF), which is an undesirable oxidized flavour appearing during the storage of nitrite-free cooked meats. These effects are probably due to the same reaction that is responsible for colour development. The reaction of nitrite with the haem iron avoids the formation of ferric iron, which is considered the most important catalyst in meat for lipid oxidation.

Curing Processes and Applications

There is a wide variety of cured meat products as a consequence of different customs and habits of different countries. These include variations in raw materials, formulations, processes and techniques applied. Meat products made from entire primal cuts (hams, shoulders and bellies) are termed cured. Yet, sausages, although also cured, are usually classified separately, depending on the technology used. However, from a general point of view, two basic curing processes should be distinguished: 'dry curing' and 'wet' or 'pickle curing' (see Fig. 2). Other curing processes are combinations or modifications of these processes mentioned above but, as there is a great variety and many are of minor importance, these will not be discussed in detail.

Dry Curing

This process is the oldest and uses a mixture of curing ingredients (mainly salt, nitrate and/or nitrite and sugars) rubbed into the surface of pieces of meat. The dry cure is applied without any added water. Consequently, the curing agents are solubilized in the original moisture present in the meat and they penetrate by diffusion. The temperature in the curing room during salting is held at 2–4°C for a period of time depending on the characteristics of the pieces, usually 1–1·5 days per kilogram. After curing is completed, the excess cure is washed off and the meat is placed under refrigeration (2–4°C) for 20–40 days for salt equalization. The objective of this post-salting phase is to achieve a complete and homogenous salt distribution throughout the piece of meat. The next step involves time–temperature interactions. The pieces are placed in natural or air-conditioned drying chambers (see Fig. 3) and ripened (aged) for a minimum of 6 months and up to 12 or more months, depending on each country's tradition. The temperature is usually varied between 14 and 20°C at relative humidities between 90 and 70%. Complex biochemical reactions, mainly proteolytic and lipolytic, take place and a characteristic flavour is developed. Some of the most representative products are the Spanish Serrano ham, Italian Parma ham and French Bayonne ham. Other products, such as the American country-style ham, the German Westphalia ham and northern European hams may be smoked after postsalting and subsequently aged over 1–3 months.

The dry curing of minced meats is used for the manufacturing of fermented dry-cured sausages. Curing ingredients and adjuncts are mixed with the minced meat and, subsequently, stuffed into natural pork or veal casings or artificial casings made from reconstituted collagen. Sausages are placed into natural or air-conditioned drying chambers at 20–23°C for about 2 days to promote the development of the microbial flora responsible for ripening. Starter cultures may be added to accelerate this process. Sugars are metabolized to lactic acid and the pH drops to 4·5–5·0, very close to the

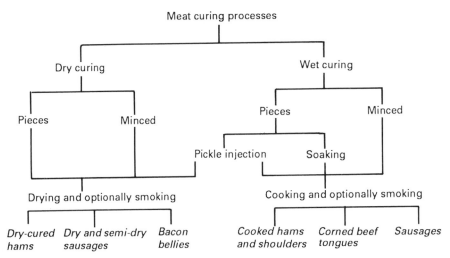

Meat curing processes
Dry curing — Wet curing
Dry curing: Pieces, Minced
Wet curing: Pieces, Minced
Pickle injection — Soaking
Drying and optionally smoking
Cooking and optionally smoking
Dry-cured hams | Dry and semi-dry sausages | Bacon bellies
Cooked hams and shoulders | Corned beef tongues | Sausages

Fig. 2 Schematic diagram of the most important meat curing processes.

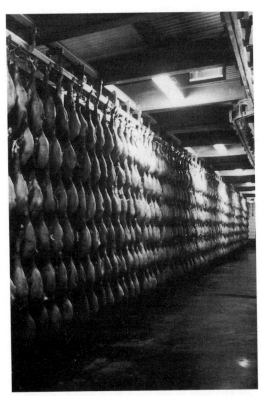

Fig. 3 Controlled temperature and humidity chamber for the dry curing of hams. Courtesy of Navidul, S.A., Torrijos-Toledo, Spain.

isoelectric point of meat proteins. Thus, three objectives are achieved: (1) selection of the microbial flora, eliminating the pathogenic microorganisms, (2) a reduction of the water-holding capacity of proteins, favouring drying and, finally, (3) protein coagulation giving the sausage a characteristic texture. The length of the ripening period, depending on the kind of product and its diameter, usually takes 20 (rapid process) to 90 days (slow process).

Temperatures usually range from 14 to 16°C and relative humidities from 90 to 70%. Typical sausages include the Italian salami, Spanish chorizo and French saucisson sec. Other countries, like Germany, smoke most of their sausages.

Wet Curing

The curing ingredients and adjuncts are essentially the same as those for dry curing, except that they are now dissolved in water to form a pickle or brine which is used as a vehicle for cure penetration into the meat. Phosphates are usually added to aid water retention and increase yields. In essence, two techniques are used for wet curing of meat pieces: brine soaking and pickle injection. In brine soaking, the pieces of meat are immersed in the curing brine until the cure has penetrated the entire piece. This process is slow and if large pieces are used, spoilage can develop. Thus, its primary use is in producing small items such as corned beef, tongues, etc. The other technique, pickle injection, allows a more rapid and uniform cure diffusion throughout the entire piece. It has numerous variants like artery pumping, stitch pumping and multiple needle injection pumping, the latter being widely utilized today.

Figure 4 shows a complete line for producing cooked ham and shoulder. Three important steps can be observed: the multiple needle injection pumping, the mechanical tumblers for massaging to accelerate and improve brine uptake and, finally, the packing section where the pieces are stuffed or moulded before cooking. When producing bacon, one important modification involves deleting massaging and, instead, allowing pieces to dry for a short period and/or smoking.

In the case of wet curing of minced meat, the curing ingredients and adjuncts are directly added to the meat

Curing

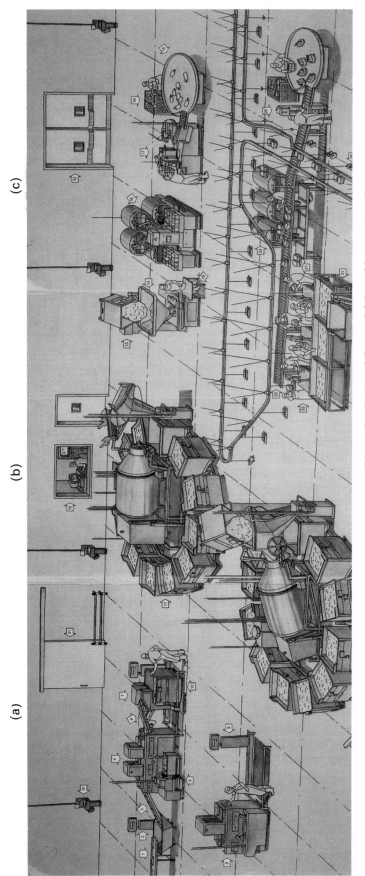

Fig. 4 Cooked ham and shoulder production plant. (a) Pickle injection, (b) mechanical tumbling and (c) packing section. Courtesy of Metalquimia, Gerona, Spain.

and fat and mixed into the products when preparing the paste or emulsion. Ice is also added to the mixture to cool the meat paste to between 5 and 11°C, allowing emulsification of fat and preventing protein denaturation which might break the emulsion. The meat paste is stuffed in cellulose, plastic or reconstituted collagen casings, heat treated and, optionally, smoked. Wet-cured sausages are available in many varieties, but frankfurters, Bologna sausages and mortadella are well known.

Dietary Implications of Cured Products

Cured meat products have an important nutritive value which is mainly due to the high content (up to 30% in dry-cured ham) of protein of high biological value. However, cured products have been implicated in the debate over nitrosamines. Numerous scientific studies have shown the existence of nitroso compounds in foods, especially nitrosamines. Most of them exhibit carcinogenicity. Current research efforts are focused on the development of methods for detecting precursors (nitrate, nitrite and amines), volatile nitrosamines and nonvolatile nitroso compounds. The results of surveys of cured meat products indicated that nitrosamines were only detected in bacon after frying. Nitrosamines found in fried bacon were N-nitrosopyrrolidine and N-nitroso-dimethylamine; however, levels were very low, 1–20 and 1–10 $\mu g\ kg^{-1}$, respectively. In other types of cured meat products, even if fried, no nitrosamines have been detected, probably because none of these products are dried completely as in the case of fried bacon. Other research efforts are focused on substitutes for nitrites but, so far, no effective alternatives for inhibiting the outgrowth of *C. botulinum* have been found.

International Curing Regulations

As a consequence of the nitrosamine issue, regulatory agencies around the world have tried to reduce the residual levels of nitrates and nitrites in foods and, especially, in cured meat products. For instance, in the USA, the maximum levels of sodium nitrite or potassium nitrite permitted in bacon are 120 and 148 ppm, respectively. Incorporation of 550 ppm of sodium ascorbate or erythorbate, as nitrosamine inhibitors is also recommended. Nitrates are not allowed in bacon and are only used in dry-cured meat products. Currently, nitrates and nitrites are under study in Europe because a new European Economic Community (EEC) list of positive additives for foods is being prepared. The trend is to use nitrite in the wet-curing processes only and to rely on nitrate for dry curing. It is likely that the use of a combination of nitrates and nitrites will be exclusively permitted for those products where a slow nitrite production would be required to keep the colour. The estimated maximum input levels in Europe are 150 ppm for sodium nitrite and 300 ppm for potassium nitrate but are not still definitive. Until the official list is approved by the EEC Commission, these estimates might serve as reference values. *See* Legislation, Additives

Bibliography

Cassens RG, Greaser ML, Ito T and Lee M (1979) Reactions of nitrite in meat. *Food Technology* 17: 46–62, 93.

Frentz JC and Zert P (eds) (1990) *L'Encyclopedie de la Charcuterie*, 3rd edn. Paris: Soussana.

Gray JI and Pearson AM (1984) Cured meat flavor. *Advances in Food Research* 29: 1–86.

Haldane J (1901) The red color of salted meat. *Journal of Hygiene, Cambridge* 1: 115.

Institute of Food Technologists (1987) Nitrate, nitrite and nitroso compounds in foods. A scientific status summary by the I.F.T. Expert Panel on Food Safety & Nutrition. *Food Technology* 14: 127–134.

Lawrie RA (ed.) (1985) *Meat Science*, 4th edn, pp 149–158. Oxford: Pergamon Press.

Lehman KB (1899) Uber das Hämoglobin ein neves weitverbreitetes blutfarbstoffderivat. *Sitzungberichte der Physikalisch Medizinischen Gesellschaft* 4: 57.

Pearson AM and Tauber FW (eds.) (1984) Curing. *Processed Meats*, 2nd edn, pp 46–68. Westport, CT: Avi.

Polenske E (1891) Uber den Verlust, welchen das Rindfleisch an Nahrwert durch das Pokeln erleidet, sowie uber die Veranderungen saltpeter-haltiger Pokellaken. *Arbeiten aus dem Kaiserlizhen Gesundheitsamte.* 7: 471.

Potter NN (ed.) (1978) Cheese. *Food Science*, 3rd edn, pp 401–402. Westport, CT: Avi.

Townsend WE and Olson DG (1987) Cured meats and cured meat products processing. In: *The Science of Meat and Meat Products*, Price JF and Schweigert BS (eds) 3rd edn, pp 431–456, Westport, CT: Food and Nutrition Press.

J. Flores and F. Toldrá
I. A. y Tecnologia Alimentos (CSIC), Valencia, Spain

CURRANTS AND GOOSEBERRIES*

The domestication of currants and gooseberries has taken place within the last four or five hundred years. Horticulturally these fruits are not major crops, but they are widely grown in northern European regions. The crop is mainly used in the production of juices, jams and jellies. Blackcurrant has a strong colour and aromatic taste and is an excellent source of ascorbic acid. Long before vitamins were known, people used blackcurrants for medicinal purposes, mostly as a hot drink against the common cold. *See* Ascorbic Acid, Properties and Determination

Global Distribution

The genus *Ribes*, of the *Saxifragaceae* family, consists of about 150 species of currant and gooseberry, mainly distributed in the northern temperate regions of Europe and North America. Of the edible types the main commercially grown species are blackcurrant (*Ribes nigrum* L.), red- and whitecurrants (*R. rubrum* L., *R. sativum* Syme and *R. petraeum* Wulf.) and the gooseberry (*R. grossularia* L.).

Commercial Importance

The majority of currants and gooseberries are produced in Europe (Table 1) with Germany and Poland as the main producers. Blackcurrants account for more than half of the total world production; this species is dominant in the UK and Scandinavia, and gaining in importance in other countries. About one quarter of the *Ribes* production is gooseberry, but the production of this fruit is decreasing in most countries. Germany, UK, Poland, Czechoslovakia and the USSR are the major gooseberry-producing countries. Countries with a high proportion of redcurrants compared to blackcurrants are Germany, Belgium, Netherlands and Austria. Currants and gooseberries are at present of little commercial significance in North America (45 t), as it is an alternative host of white pine blister rust (*Cronartium ribicola* Fisch.), but there is increasing interest in the USA in *Ribes* fruits, and some legislative controls on their cultivation are changing.

Machine harvesting is prevalent in industrial produc-

Table 1. World production of *Ribes* fruit

	1979–1981 ($\times 10^3$ t)	1987–1989 ($\times 10^3$ t)
Austria	25	29
Czechoslovakia	21	35
France	6	8
Germany	139	168
Hungary	17	18
Poland	131	145
Scandinavia	35	30
UK	21	22
Europe	395	455
USSR	83	101
Oceania	2	3
World	480	559

Data from Food and Agriculture Organization (FAO) production yearbooks, corrected for national statistics in Scandinavia.

tion of blackcurrants. The machines are useful for redcurrants as well, but work less satisfactorily for gooseberries.

Besides commercial production, currants and gooseberry are important home garden crops in many countries. They tolerate both low summer and winter temperatures, and may therefore be grown in the far north, where few other fruits can be cultivated.

Blackcurrant Cultivars

The cultivars Baldwin, Booskop Giant, Silvergieters Zwarte, Roodknop and Øjebyn have been dominant in Europe in the past, but in most countries there is a swing toward Ben Lomond and Ben Nevis, two high yielding cultivars with good processing quality. There is also an increasing demand for new cultivars, such as Ben Alder and Ben Tirran from the UK. The USSR has a large range of blackcurrant cultivars adapted to the climatic conditions in different regions. Fertödi 1 is the main cultivar in Hungary, and is gaining popularity in other Eastern European countries. Øjebyn is still dominating in Poland, Finland and Sweden.

Redcurrant and Whitecurrant Cultivars

The major red cultivars grown in Europe are Jonkheer van Tets, Red Dutch, Rondom and Stanza. For fresh

---

* The colour plate section for this article appears between p. 1146 and p. 1147.

fruit and dessert markets, Red Lake and Jonkheer van Tets are the most popular because of their good eating quality. There is a considerable interest in newer cultivars, especially Redstart from the UK, and the Dutch cultivars, Rovada, Rolan and Rotet. White Dutch and White Versailles are most widespread among the whitecurrant cultivars. The whitecurrants lack colouring pigments and are in fact a colour form of redcurrants.

Gooseberry Cultivars

In the nineteenth century gooseberry was a popular fruit in home gardens in Europe, especially in the UK, and amateur breeders raised hundreds of cultivars. Selection was largely for fruit size. However, the appearance of American gooseberry mildew (*Sphaerotheca mors-uvae*) in 1905 soon drastically reduced the acreages of gooseberry, as the large-fruited types all proved more or less susceptible to the pathogen. Mildew-resistant cultivars have been released but they are inferior to the old types, in terms of both fruit size and quality, and none of them have become widespread. One which is gaining popularity is the green-fruited Invicta, bred in the UK. Among the old cultivars, Careless, Keepsake and Whitesmith are most widely grown of the green types, and Whinham's Industry is most popular among the red-fruited cultivars. The hardy and small-fruited red and yellow types of the Finnish cultivar Hinonmäen are widely grown in Scandinavia. New cultivars, such as Greenfinch from the UK, and Rixanta, Reflamba and Rolanda from Germany, are promising.

Other *Ribes* Cultivars

Artificial hybridization between *R. nigrum*, *R. divaricatum* and *R. grossularia* has given rise to the new species *Ribes* x *nidigrolaria*. The fruit quality is somewhere between blackcurrant and gooseberry. Josta, the first cultivar to be released from Germany, is planted to some extent, mostly in home gardens.

Morphology and Anatomy of the Fruit

The fruits of currants are borne in clusters, with every single fruit adjoined to the main strig by a short stem. The fruits ripen in order along the strig, the fruit closest to the branch first and the terminal fruit last. Gooseberry fruits develop singly or in small clusters with two or three fruits.

The berry of currants and gooseberry is a true fruit, with the seeds enclosed in a fleshy pericarp. Table 2 gives a guide to the range of variation concerning fruit

Table 2. Fruit characteristics of currants and gooseberry

	Number of fruits per strig	Fruit weight (g)	Number of seeds per fruit	Weight per seed (mg)
Blackcurrant	5–10	0·6–1·5	30–50	1–2
Redcurrant	6–14	0·4–0·9	5–11	6–8
Gooseberry	1–3	1·6–14·0	3–5	4–6

characteristics. Gooseberry has the largest fruits and redcurrant the smallest. Redcurrants and gooseberries have fewer and larger seeds than blackcurrants. The skin of some gooseberry cultivars is hairy, while the skin of currants is always hairless.

The pigments of the blackcurrant fruit are located in the skin, the flesh remaining green. The pigments of redcurrant and gooseberry, however, are present both in the skin and in the fruit flesh. Unlike currants, the cultivars of gooseberry cover the whole range of fruit colours, from dark to light red, through various shades of green, to yellow and almost white. Blackcurrants have a dark purple colour, while redcurrants are pure red. The white currants are lacking anthocyanins and have a light yellow-greenish colour. *See* Colours, Properties and Determination of Natural Pigments

Chemical and Nutritional Composition

The energy in fruits of currants and gooseberries comes mainly from carbohydrates (Table 3). Only a small part comes from protein and fat. Fructose and glucose are the main sugars, with about equal amounts of each. Sucrose is present, but to a lesser extent. Gooseberries contain small amounts of sorbitol, while only traces of sorbitol are present in currants. A characteristic feature of the fruits is the high content of acids. Citric acid is dominating in currants, while citric and malic acid are present in almost equal quantities in gooseberries. See individual nutrients.

Ascorbic acid (vitamin C) has probably received more attention than any other constituent of blackcurrants. Less than 50 g of the fruits meets the recommended daily requirement of ascorbic acid. However, considerable variation exists between cultivars and years (Table 4). Other vitamins are also present in the fruits, and the content of minerals is worth mentioning, especially the high content of potassium.

Blackcurrants possess a high flavonoid content compared to other soft fruits. The most important group of the flavonoids are the anthocyanins. The anthocyanins are the dominant pigments, and blackcurrants contain from 1250 to 2000 mg per 1000 g of fresh weight. The anthocyanins of blackcurrant are mainly cyanidin and

Table 3. Chemical composition (per 1000 g of fresh fruit) of currants and gooseberry

Nutrient	Black-currant	Red-currant	Goose-berry
Water (g)	815	845	880
Soluble solids (g)	155	105	125
Carbohydrates (g)	128	96	78
Protein (g)	13	12	8
Fat (g)	2	2	2
Fibre (g)	43	39	22
Pectin (g)	8	7	5
Glucose (g)	35	27	26
Fructose (g)	37	26	24
Sucrose (g)	13	4	6
Total sugar (g)	85	57	56
Citric acid (g)	40	25	14
Malic acid (g)	6	4	13
Titratable acid[a] (g)	38	24	23
Energy (J)	2600	2050	1650
Sodium (mg)	17	13	15
Potassium (mg)	3130	2260	1550
Magnesium (mg)	190	142	113
Calcium (mg)	570	380	240
Iron (mg)	13	9	6
Phosphorus (mg)	480	330	250
Ash (mg)	7200	6400	4800
Ascorbic acid (mg)	1600	650	350
Thiamin (mg)	0·5	0·4	0·4
Riboflavin (mg)	0·4	0·3	0·2
Pyridoxine (mg)	1·2	0·5	—
Nicotinic acid (mg)	2·8	2·5	2·5
Pantothenic acid (mg)	4·0	6·0	2·3
β-Carotene (mg)	1·2	0·6	1·5

[a] Acid content measured using equivalent weight of citric acid.

Sources:
Souci SW and Bosch H *Lebensmittel-Tabellen für die Nährwertberechnung* (1978) Stuttgart: Wissenschaftliche Verlagsgesellschaft.
Kuusi T (1970).
Hulme AC (ed) (1971) *The biochemistry of fruits and their products* Vol. 2. London: Academic Press.
Heiberg N and Maage F Unpublished data.

Table 4. Ascorbic acid content (mg per 1000 g of fresh fruit) of four blackcurrant cultivars

Cultivar	1988	1989	1990	Mean
Hedda	640	740	790	720
Ben Nevis	1260	1800	1760	1610
Ben Alder	1220	1950	1490	1550
Ben Tirran	1690	2480	1560	1910
Mean	1200	1740	1400	1447

From Maage F and Heiberg N Unpublished data.

delphinidin 3-glucosides and 3-rutinosides. In redcurrant, six different cyanidins have been isolated. Most red European gooseberry cultivars contain only cyanidin 3-glucoside and 3-rutinoside. Another important group of flavonoids are the flavonols, of which glycosides of kaemferol, quercetin and myricitin are present in blackcurrants and redcurrants.

The characteristic aromatic compounds of blackcurrant are present in the whole plant. Several studies have been carried out to identify the aromatic components of blackcurrants, and a wide range of the volatile compounds have been identified, but the exact chemical nature of the specific aroma in blackcurrants is unknown.

The degree of ripening has great influence on the quality characteristics. The colour intensity, the content of dry matter, soluble solids and sugars increase with ripening, while viscosity and content of ascorbic acid decrease. Content of titratable acids reaches its peak about 2 weeks before harvest and does not change much during ripening. The development of some quality factors is shown in Fig. 1. *See* Ripening of Fruit

The seeds of currants and gooseberry contain about 20% fat, of which 5–20% is γ-linolenic acid, the highest content occurring in blackcurrant. *See* Fatty Acids, Gamma Linolenic Acid

Handling and Storage

The strong flavour and the high acidity of currant fruits makes them less attractive for fresh consumption. However, there is still a fresh market, as berries are bought for home processing. Gooseberries have a milder flavour and a considerable part of the crop is used for dessert purposes. Gooseberries are sold both as unripe, green fruits, and as ripe fruits. For fresh consumption the *Ribes* fruits are still picked by hand, because the harvesting machines reduce the post-harvest quality. The currants are picked on strigs, while gooseberries are sold as single fruits. The berries should be picked when dry, they will quickly spoil if gathered and packed when wet.

Compared to other soft fruits, currants and gooseberries keep reasonably well, but without cooling the fruits degrade rapidly after harvest. The weight loss may reach 2–3% within 24 h without cooling. The fruits are usually cooled to 0–5°C immediately after harvest. Forced-air cooling is recommended. At low temperatures the fruits have a shelf life of 2–6 days, greatly dependent on maturity stage. Unripe gooseberries can be stored for 4 weeks. Picking the berries slightly unripe increases the shelf life. The fruits should be kept cooled during transportation and marketing. To increase shelf life beyond a week the fruits must be stored in controlled atmosphere conditions. *See* Controlled Atmosphere Storage, Applications for Bulk Storage of Foodstuffs; Storage Stability, Parameters Affecting Storage Stability

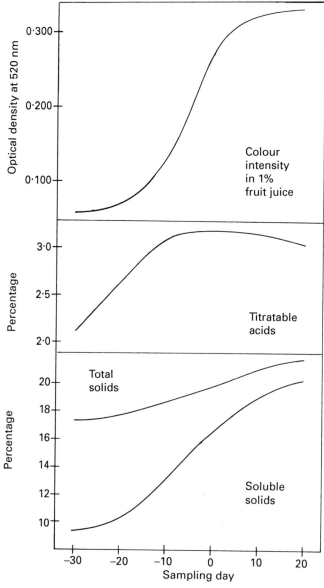

Fig. 1 Changes in fruit quality components in blackcurrants from 30 days before to 20 days after normal harvest time. (Titratable acid expressed in terms of citric acid.) (From Heiberg N, 1986.)

Industrial Uses

The most important products of blackcurrant are different types of juices and syrups. Due to the special aromatic taste, and the high content of ascorbic acid, blackcurrant products are popular in northern Europe, and are commonly regarded as healthy preparations. The fruits are also used for jams and jellies, and are suitable for flavouring other foods, such as yoghurt and other dairy products.

Redcurrants are mainly grown for juice and jelly processing, often mixed with other fruits with lower acidity. Gooseberries are mainly used for jams and canned products. All three fruits find some use in wine and sweet liqueur production, alone or in combination with other fruits.

The γ-linolenic acid produced from blackcurrant seeds is used as a health preparation. Manufacture of the oil is based on press cake from blackcurrant juice processing.

In blackcurrant other parts of the plant are also of commercial interest. Bud extract is used as a flavour component in other foods, and as an ingredient in some fragrances.

Bibliography

Brennan RM (1990) Currants and gooseberries. In: Moore JM and Ballington JR (eds) *Genetic Resources of Temperate Fruit and Nut Crops*, vol. 1, pp 459–488. The Netherlands: International Society for Horticultural Science.

Green A (1971) Soft fruits. In: Hulme AC (ed.) *Biochemistry of Fruits and their Products*, vol 2, pp. 375–410. London: Academic Press.

Heiberg N (1986) Quality components of blackcurrant (*Ribes nigrum* L.) fruits as related to degree of ripeness and cultivar. *Meldinger fra Norges landbrukshøgskole* 65.

Keep E (1975) Currants and gooseberries. In: Janick J and Moore JN (eds) *Advances in Fruit Breeding*, pp 197–268. West Lafayette, Indiana: Purdue University Press.

Keipert K (1981) *Beerenobst*. Stuttgart: Verlag Eugen Ulmer.

Kuusi T (1970) Uber die chemische Zusammensetzung und Kennzahlen einiger finnischer einheimischer Beeren. *Flüssiges Obst.* 37: 188–190, 253–263.

Nina Heiberg
Njøs Research Station, Hermansverk, Norway
Finn Maage
Agricultural University of Norway, Norway

CYCLAMATES

Cyclamate is the term given to the artificial sweetener cyclamic acid (cyclohexylsulphamic acid) and its calcium or sodium salts (see Fig. 1). Cyclamate was discovered in 1937 at the University of Illinois following the accidental contamination of a cigarette with a derivative of cyclohexylamine. In 1940 DuPont obtained a patent for its production and in 1950 it was available to consumers. Consumption of cyclamates increased steadily from that time up to about 1969, when it was banned in the USA by the Food and Drug Administration and also in other countries due to safety concerns related to its potential carcinogenicity. Cyclamate is not metabolized by the human body, thus it contributes no energy to the diet and is considered a nonnutritive sweetener.

Sweetness

In a comparison with other intense sweeteners, cyclamate is perhaps the least sweet, being only 30–80 times as sweet as sucrose in actual food uses, depending upon concentration, pH, flavouring agents and other ingredients which may constitute a part of the food product. Aspartame by comparison is about 200 times sweeter than sucrose while saccharin is about 300 times sweeter. In high concentrations cyclamate has an unpleasant aftertaste. However, at low concentrations it has some bitterness-masking ability that makes it attractive for use in pharmaceutical products. During the 1960s, cyclamate–saccharin combinations became very popular. At ratios of 10:1 (cyclamate:saccharin) on a weight basis, the combination resulted in a pleasant sweetness minimizing the somewhat disagreeable aftertastes of both sweeteners individually. The synergistic effect of saccharin in combination with cyclamate increased the sweetening power of the mixture compared to the individual sweeteners. *See* Saccharin; Sweeteners – Intense

Production, Physical and Chemical Properties

Cyclamate and its calcium or sodium salts are white crystalline powders with intensely sweet tastes. Cyclamate has a melting point of about 169–170°C. It is soluble in water up to a concentration of about 1 g in 7·5 ml, while the calcium and sodium salts are slightly more soluble, to the extent of about 1 g in 4 ml of water. Cyclamate is rather acidic (the pH of a 10% aqueous solution being 0·8–1·6), while similar solutions of the calcium and sodium salts are neutral (pH 5·5–7·5). Cyclamate is relatively heat-stable, microbiologically inert and nonhygroscopic.

Table 1. Cyclamate use levels in diet food products

Diet food	Cyclamate level
Table top sweeteners	25 mg g^{-1}
Milk beverages	0·8 mg ml^{-1}
Beverages and beverage bases	4 mg ml^{-1} prepared drink
Gelatin, puddings, filling	27 mg ml^{-1}
Salad dressings	1·6 mg ml^{-1}
Jellies, jams, preserves	30 mg ml^{-1}
Sweet sauces, toppings, syrups	30 mg ml^{-1}
Chewing gum	20 mg per stick
Hard confectionery	5 mg g^{-1}
Baked goods, baking mixes	2·6 mg g^{-1}

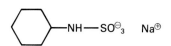

Fig. 1 Structure of cyclamate (sodium salt).

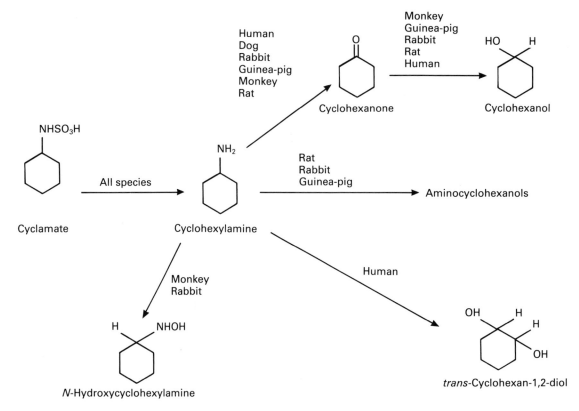

Fig. 2 Schematic of the metabolic routes for cyclamate in several mammalian species.

Cyclamate is synthesized by sulphonation of cyclo-hexylamine with chlorosulphonic acid in chloroform followed by treatment with barium hydroxide and sulphuric acid. Variations of this reaction scheme followed by treatment with sodium or calcium hydroxides yields the salts of cyclamate. Commercial production of cyclamate reached a peak in the USA in 1968 when an estimated 7400 tonnes were produced. Commercial production dropped dramatically after bans on its use in foods went into effect in many countries around 1970.

Food Uses

Cyclamate is no longer permitted as a food additive in most developed countries including Canada, the USA and many European countries. It is, however, available in many countries as a table top sweetener. Prior to 1970, cyclamate was used in a variety of diet food products. In 1969, 70% of the usage of cyclamate was in beverages while 15% was in dietetic foods and 15% in table top products. Table 1 lists some of its past applications and approximate concentration levels. Like saccharin, cyclamate is rather stable to heat and moisture and thus it was suited to sweetening a wide variety of food products. It found wide use as a sweetener in combination with saccharin as mentioned above.

Metabolism and Safety

Fig. 2 shows a schematic of the overall metabolism of cyclamate in a number of mammalian species. In humans, orally administered cyclamate is rapidly excreted via both the urine and faeces. Greater than 98% of the dose is excreted within 1–2 days. Studies with rats and dogs have shown that small amounts of cyclamate can be distributed to all tissues (except the brain) although accumulation is negligible.

Conversion of cyclamate to cyclohexylamine in human subjects was first reported by Japanese researchers in 1966. Very small amounts of cyclohexylamine (0·7% of the administered dose) were found in urine. This finding stimulated a large number of feeding studies in humans and animals. It appears that *Entero-cocci* organisms in the intestine convert cyclamate to cyclohexylamine. Cyclohexylamine may be converted to other metabolites as shown in Fig. 2. The metabolism of cyclamate to cyclohexylamine and other products is dependent upon the individual concerned. In one study involving 1000 human subjects 10–30% of the subjects converted ingested cyclamate to cyclohexylamine mostly in the range of <0·1–8% of the administered dose. However, some individuals converted up to 60% of the cyclamate.

Cyclamate was banned from use in many countries because results of some rat-feeding studies showed the substance to cause bladder tumours. Many scientists questioned the results of the original studies and this led to many follow-up studies in a variety of animal species. The prevailing opinion today is that neither cyclamate nor cyclohexylamine are likely to be carcinogenic to humans, especially at levels recommended for diet foods (see Table 1). The main reason now that cyclamate is not permitted is that during the follow-up feeding studies to evaluate its carcinogenicity it was observed that cyclohexylamine, the main metabolite of cyclamate, causes irreversible testicular atrophy in rats. Further research is required to study this effect in detail. The Food and Agriculture Organization/World Health Organization has determined an acceptable daily intake (ADI) value (the maximum amount that could be consumed daily for a lifetime without appreciable risk) for cyclamate to be 11 mg per kilogram of bodyweight. However, in the UK a temporary maximum ADI of only 1·5 mg per kilogram of bodyweight has been established until the results of further research are known.

Analysis

Methods for the determination of cyclamate in foods are not as simple nor as straightforward as for those sweeteners such as acesulfam-K, aspartame and saccharin which strongly absorb ultraviolet light. The latter can be measured by direct means (usually high-performance liquid chromatography) without recourse to chemical derivatization.

The most common analytical methods for cyclamate involve chemical conversion to cyclohexylamine followed by determination of the amine by gas chromatography with flame ionization detection. Several methods employing high-performance liquid chromatography have been evaluated which offer potential for cyclamate determination without the need to convert to cyclohexylamine or other product. These employ direct conductivity detection, indirect ultraviolet absorption detection or postcolumn ionpair extraction detection. *See* Acesulphame; Chromatography, High-performance Liquid Chromatography; Chromatography, Gas Chromatography

Bibliography

Franta R and Beck B (1986) Alternatives to cane and beet sugar. *Food Technology* 40: 116–128.
IARC (1980) *IARC Monographs on the Evaluation of the Carcinogenic Risk of Chemicals to Humans, Some Non-Nutritive Sweetening Agents* vol. 22. Lyon: International Agency for Research on Cancer.
Shaw JH and Roussos GG (1978) *Sweeteners and Dental Caries*. Washington, DC: Information Retrieval.

James F. Lawrence
Sir F. G. Banting Research Centre, Ottawa, Canada

CYSTIC FIBROSIS

Cystic fibrosis (CF), an autosomal recessive hereditary disease of exocrine gland secretion, is characterized by recurrent pulmonary infections, pancreatic insufficiency with maldigestion, malabsorption and abnormal levels of sweat electrolytes. The abnormal gene locus is localized on the long arm of chromosome 7, most commonly at $\Delta F508$ (in approximately 70% of cases). Biochemical studies have suggested that the defect occurs in the regulation of ion transport across epithelial cell membranes, resulting in abnormal exocrine function. This in turn results in a wide range of clinical effects (Fig. 1). Recent advances in therapy have greatly improved life expectancy of this common disorder (1 in 2200 live births in Caucasians) such that most patients now survive into adulthood. This has resulted in an increasing population of patients requiring long-term medical care. The adverse effects of CF on nutrition and growth have long been recognized and, with improving lifespan, the assurance of normal nutrition and growth has become an increasingly important aspect of management. Nutritional growth retardation continues to affect a substantial number of patients and is a major factor adversely affecting survival. Optimal nutritional management is, therefore, crucial in terms of growth, quality of life, and perhaps long-term outcome.

This article reviews the nature and causes of nutritional growth regardation in CF, explores the consequences

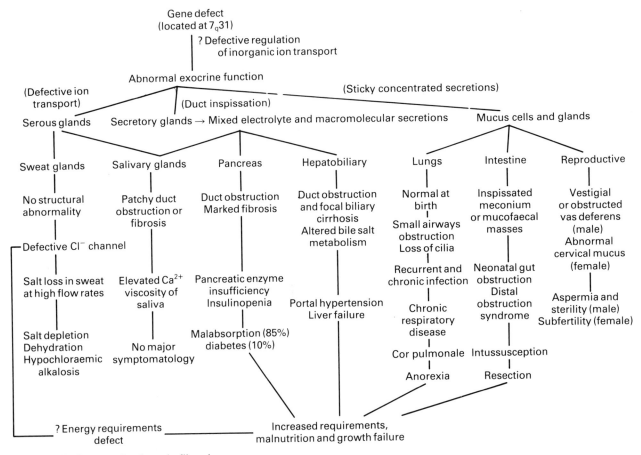

Fig. 1 Pathogenesis of cystic fibrosis.

and range of nutritional deficiencies documented in this disease, and describes current therapy.

The Nature of Malnutrition in Cystic Fibrosis

A wide range of nutritional deficits causing many deleterious effects have been described in CF. The heights and weights of many CF patients are markedly skewed towards the lower centile bands, particularly with increasing age. Body composition studies have suggested that underweight CF children have a deficit in body cell mass and body fat, with a reduction in mass, muscle mass and an excess of extracellular water compared to controls. Whole body protein turnover studies have suggested that many malnourished patients with severe lung disease are catabolic with a reduction in whole body protein turnover synthesis occurring during pulmonary exacerbations. The deficit of the body cell mass observed in CF from total body potassium counting can be present from the first few weeks of life, as judged by studies of newborn CF infants diagnosed by neonatal screening. Prior to neonatal screening, which has allowed the earlier introduction of therapy,

overt hypoproteinaemia was a common presenting symptom. Specific deficiencies of essential fatty acids, fat-soluble vitamins, some water-soluble vitamins, and specific micronutrients, including zinc, iron, and selenium, are well described. Another important consideration, particularly in tropical climates, is continuing specific loss of sodium chloride resulting from the sweat gland defect. *See* Body Composition; Protein, Synthesis and Turnover

The range of nutritional abnormalities occurring in CF seems likely to be caused by a combination of inadequate absorbed intake, nutrient losses and increased requirements (Fig. 2). Although many text-books describe voracious appetites in CF children, in reality, objective measurements often show an inadequate energy supply compared to recommended intakes, and such patients with strong appetites may be attempting to compensate for excessive requirements and excessive losses. A poor appetite may be due to malnutrition *per se*, but also appears to occur where there is poor pulmonary function and during active pulmonary infection. This latter problem may have a cumulative effect on nutritional status over years as lung disease progresses. *See* Energy, Energy Expenditure and Energy Balance

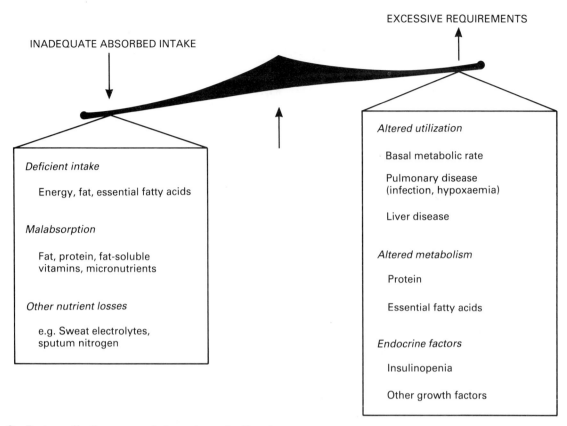

INADEQUATE ABSORBED INTAKE

EXCESSIVE REQUIREMENTS

Deficient intake

Energy, fat, essential fatty acids

Malabsorption

Fat, protein, fat-soluble
vitamins, micronutrients

Other nutrient losses

e.g. Sweat electrolytes,
sputum nitrogen

Altered utilization

Basal metabolic rate

Pulmonary disease
(infection, hypoxaemia)

Liver disease

Altered metabolism

Protein

Essential fatty acids

Endocrine factors

Insulinopenia

Other growth factors

Fig. 2 Factors affecting energy balance in cystic fibrosis.

Nutrient losses occur mainly from malabsorption, but in some cases excessive nitrogen loss in sputum, and excessive sodium losses from the sweat gland abnormality (Fig. 1) are also important. Fat and protein malabsorption are present in approximately 85% of patients because of pancreatic exocrine deficiency. The pancreatic abnormality involves both water–electrolyte (mainly bicarbonate) secretion as well as lipase–trypsin and amylase deficiency. Reduced bicarbonate secretion is universal, but a functional level of digestive enzyme capacity is retained in 10–15% of patients. In untreated cases where enzyme outputs are less than 10% of normal, steatorrhoea, azotorrhoea, starch intolerance and malabsorption of fat-soluble vitamins, some minerals, and vitamin B_{12} occur. *See* Sodium, Physiology

There has been a growing interest into the nature of energy and protein metabolism in CF since the recognition of an apparent maladaptation to undernutrition, and, more recently, the suggestion that there may be an energy-requiring basic defect in this disease. This complex area is confused at present and a division of opinion exists as to whether the observed discrepancies in energy balance are (1) secondary to abnormalities in intake or absorption, (2) secondary to the effects of chronic lung disease and infection, or (3) the result of a primary abnormality in energy use. It seems likely that, to a

variable degree, all of these factors may play a role in the energy defect in CF.

The Consequences of Malnutrition

The major effects of malnutrition in CF include nutritional growth retardation, delayed puberty, adverse effects on pulmonary disease, and, ultimately, a poorer prognosis. Patients dying of CF have marked nutritional failure in the 1–2 years prior to their death. Malnutrition *per se* can compromise absorptive and immune function, and all of the specific deficiencies mentioned above can have a wide range of secondary adverse effects. *See* Immunity and Nutrition

A close relationship exists between malnutrition and pulmonary disease in CF. Pulmonary disease apparently adversely affects energy requirements and whole body protein metabolism. As previously mentioned, CF patients who have chronic but stable pulmonary disease tend to have excessive protein catabolism, while those malnourished patients studied during acute pulmonary exacerbations have a significantly reduced level of whole body protein turnover. Acute and chronic pulmonary disease also appear to have a major effect on energy utilization. There is also evidence that malabsorption and malnutrition *per se* adversely affects the course of

Table 1. Nutrient requirements in cystic fibrosis

Nutrient	Requirement
Energy	120–150% RDA
Protein	120% RDA
Essential fatty acids	5% of total energy (kJ)
Vitamin A	5000–10000 iu per day (water-miscible)
Vitamin E	100–300 iu per day (water-miscible)
Vitamin K	5 mg, twice weekly
Vitamin D	800 iu per day in temperate zones
B vitamins	200% RDA
Vitamin C	200% RDA
Iron and zinc	120% RDA
Pancreatic supplements (as pH-sensitive microspheres)	Infants: 2000 μg of lipase per 120 ml of formula Older children: 12000 μg of lipase per meal

RDA, Recommended Dietary Allowance.

pulmonary disease. An improved respiratory prognosis has been observed in those patients with pancreatic sufficiency, and a number of specific effects of malnutrition on the respiratory system have been documented. Malnutrition can effect the central respiratory drive mechanism, the respiratory muscles and the growth of the lungs. Long-term studies of nutritional rehabilitation of malnourished patients have suggested that improved nutrition may favourably affect the course of pulmonary disease.

Nutritional Management in Cystic Fibrosis

The overall treatment of CF has become increasingly specialized and is most satisfactorily performed at major referral clinics where a comprehensive and intensive management programme is available. It would seem likely that early diagnosis by neonatal screening and the institution of an aggressive therapy programme, before irreversible lung damage and chronic nutritional deficits have occurred, may greatly prolong survival. Studies of neonatal screening programmes to date have indicated lower morbidity in those children diagnosed by neonatal screening compared with a clinically diagnosed group, and a recent study from Denmark has indicated that there may also be a lower mortality. The adverse effects of chronic pulmonary disease on nutritional status and, conversely, the adverse effects of malnutrition on pulmonary status, require an early aggressive approach to both aspects of the disease. Pulmonary therapy is beyond the scope of this discussion, but its importance in the prevention of malnutrition in CF cannot be overstated. Optimal nutritional therapy involves the restoration of energy balance by regular nutritional surveillance, and the maintenance of an adequate absorbed protein–energy intake with the prevention and

management of specific deficiencies (Table 1). Certain phases of the disease, such as those occurring in infancy, during and after pulmonary exacerbations, and during puberty, may be especially important for optimal nutritional therapy. Overtly malnourished patients can benefit from long-term enteral nutrition delivered via either nocturnal nasogastric feeding or a gastrostomy button. *See* individual nutrients

Surveillance

An important part of the routine management programme is the regular evaluation of protein-energy balance. This involves assessment of intake, absorbed energy, possible nutrient losses, and the recording of anthropometric data. An example of a computerized surveillance programme at the Royal Children's Hospital, Brisbane, is given in Fig. 3, showing the benefits of longitudinal evaluation. Certain noninvasive research techniques are deserving of wider application as markers of changing nutritional status in CF. Although many of these patients are within the normal centile bands for weight, measurements of total body potassium (which provide a much more sensitive indicator of the growth of the body cell mass) suggest many patients have lean body mass deficits. Body impedance, which can be measured by a simple bedside technique, correlates well with body potassium in CF and may serve as a reliable clinical tool for the surveillance of fat-free mass. The advent of the doubly labelled water technique to measure energy expenditure in free-living humans should also help to establish an evaluation of true nutritional requirements in this disease.

Dietary Therapy

Dietary counselling, and dietary and pancreatic supplements remain mainstays in preventive management of

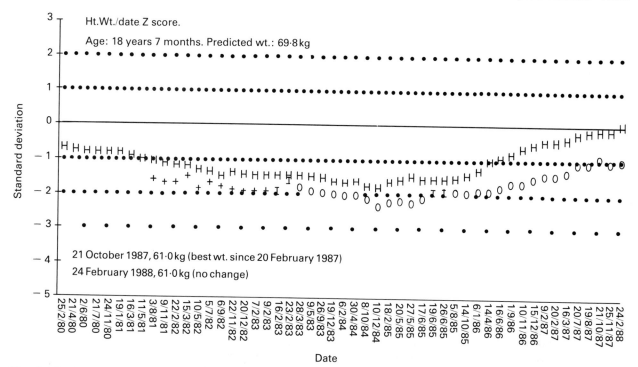

Fig. 3 Serial height and weight standard deviation scores from the computerized clinic data records of an adolescent with cystic fibrosis from the age of 10 to 18 years. Note the gradual decline in both height (H) and weight (I, weight as an inpatient; 0 or +, weight as an outpatient), until about the age of 14 years, when long-term enteral nutritional supplements were instituted by nocturnal intragastric feeding. By the age of 18 there was a gradual improvement in these parameters.

nutritional problems in cystic fibrosis. To achieve an adequate absorbed protein–energy intake (Fig. 2), daily intakes >130% of Recommended Dietary Allowance (RDA) are usually necessary to compensate for stool losses and increased requirements. In general, it is usually possible to achieve normal growth and nutrition in CF children with dietary counselling, pancreatic enzymes and high-energy supplements. Although in the past it has been standard practice in many CF clinics to prescribe low-fat, high-carbohydrate diets, low-fat diets offer no benefit to CF patients, impair total energy intake, and contribute to essential fatty acid deficiency. Since fibre has been shown to inhibit pancreatic enzymes *in vivo* and *in vitro*, fibre-enriched diets should be avoided. Patient tolerance of normal fat intakes of 40% of total energy is satisfactory, provided that appropriate enzyme preparations are used. Palatable and nutritious high-protein energy foods are encouraged and special milk drinks with added energy sources, such as chocolate-flavoured protein-enriched powders, glucose polymers and other foods, represent a good way of increasing total energy intake. A full range of vitamin and mineral supplements are necessary to prevent vitamin and mineral deficiency. In particular, fat-soluble vitamins presented in a water-miscible form are required in all patients with steatorrhoea, administered in a dosage twice the RDA. As mentioned previously,

where oral intake with supplements fails to achieve satisfactory height and weight gain, or if the patient is overtly malnourished, enteral supplements can be used. Studies of enteral supplementation using nocturnal intragastric feeding have demonstrated significant benefits in terms of weight gain, growth, body protein accretion and stabilization, and, perhaps, improvement of pulmonary function. High-energy defined semielemental formulae are most suitable for use in nutritional rehabilitation of malnourished CF patients, and are generally well tolerated. As illustrated in Fig. 3, surveillance of weight gain and growth provides a reasonable clinical indicator for nutritional intervention and the assessment of benefits derived.

Pancreatic Enzyme Replacement

Pancreatic enzyme replacement therapy needs to be tailored to individual requirements, according to the amount of food eaten and the degree of malabsorption. It is appropriate to assess quantitatively the degree of malabsorption and the ability of the therapy to correct this. Some measures to improve the efficacy of pancreatic enzyme therapy have been a recent area of study in CF, as conventional preparations rarely optimize absorption.

A bewildering number of pancreatic enzyme preparations are commercially available in the form of tablets, capsules, enteric-coated microspheres, granules and powders. Some products have not been designed specifically for the treatment of exocrine pancreatic insufficiency, but for patients with unspecified abdominal pain. Some contain bile salts; in general these should be avoided in patients with pancreatic insufficiency because high concentrations of bile salts may aggravate diarrhoea. Preparations that are protected against peptic acid inactivation are preferable to unprotected preparations: unprotected ingested enzymes are degraded to a significant degree as a result of increased gastric acidity, and lowered duodenal pH secondary to depressed bicarbonate secretion from the pancreas. The lipase content is the most important determinant of the effectiveness of these products. Between 80% and 90% of unprotected ingested lipase and trypsin is inactivated in the stomach. *See* Bile

It has been calculated that, in an adult, assuming there is no inactivation of enzymes in the stomach, approximately 30 000 iu of lipase is required to be delivered to the duodenum with an average meal for normal digestion. Mixing enzymes with food in the duodenum also seems to be important. Granulated preparations or microspheres are better than tablets in that they enable higher enzyme activities to reach the duodenum and mix with the food. The majority of enzyme preparations contain between 5000 and 12 000 iu of lipase. It can thus be calculated that for the average adult, if some defence against gastric inactivation is provided and there is an adequate enzyme–meal mix, approximately 6 to 12 capsules are required per meal to control steatorrhoea. Studies in children comparing conventional tablet enzyme therapy to enteric-coated microspheres of pancrelipase have shown that significantly less steatorrhoea and azotorrhoea occurred after using the microsphere preparation. In addition, there is an improvement in compliance because significantly fewer capsules are required.

Irrespective of the preparation used, there is good evidence that the enzymes need to be delivered appropriately and dispersed evenly thoughout a meal, in order to achieve maximum exposure of food to the ingested enzymes.

The success of enzyme therapy is assessed by bowel symptoms, quantitative absorptive tests, such as faecal fat analysis and the maintenance of normal nutrition. In children, assessment of growth is also essential. Azotorrhoea is more frequently abolished by pancreatic enzyme supplements than is steatorrhoea, possibly because trypsin secretion is better preserved than lipase secretion in pancreatic insufficiency, and because trypsin is not inactivated by acid but only by pepsin. Poor response to pancreatic enzyme preparations may result from poor compliance, inappropriate timing of administration, the presence of another condition causing steatorrhoea, (e.g. bacterial overgrowth), or the use of an unprotected, acid-sensitive enzyme preparation.

Adjuncts to Pancreatic Enzyme Therapy

Adjunctive treatment to neutralize or inhibit gastric acid and help to protect pancreatic enzymes against acid inactivation may be useful in selected cases. The use of antacids with pancreatic supplementation to neutralize gastric acid has achieved variable results, probably because some antacids form calcium soaps and precipitate glycine-conjugated bile salts. Histamine H_2-receptor antagonists are of theoretical value because many causes of pancreatic insufficiency (particularly cystic fibrosis) are associated with gastric hypersecretion. If there is adequate reduction of gastric activity, the addition of cimetidine does appear to be effective when used with enteric-coated, microsphere, pH-sensitive preparations. However, these enzyme preparations do not disintegrate and release their contents until encountering an alkaline pH, and despite acid suppression therapy, in some cases, complete correction of steatorrhoea has not been possible. Recently, a new approach to adjuvant therapy has been suggested with the use of misoprostol, a synthetic methylated prostaglandin E_1 analogue, which decreases secretion of gastric acid and increases duodenal bicarbonate secretion. This therapy may have inherent advantages over histamine H_2-receptor antagonists as adjuvant therapy for pancreatic insufficiency because of the latter effect.

Conclusions

Nutritional problems are common in CF and have an increasingly important role in management. Malnutrition is a major factor influencing survival, and may even influence the course of lung disease as there appears to be a close bilateral relationship between the progression of pulmonary disease and undernutrition, although the factors responsible for such a relationship are incompletely defined. Although it is widely recognized that factors such as nutrient losses from malabsorption, a variable but often inadequate intake, and chronic lung disease, contribute to malnutrition, recent studies have also suggested that the primary defect may require energy. A wide range of nutritional deficits occur in CF; many patients have deficits of body fat and body cell mass, and appear to be in a state of chronic catabolic stress. Whole body protein turnover would also appear to be abnormal in many CF patients, particularly during pulmonary exacerbations. Specific deficiencies of essential fatty acids, fat-soluble vitamins and some micronutrients also occur and may compromise pulmonary function and immunity. Optimal nutritional management in CF includes the provision of adequate absorbed energy by a diet containing adequate protein and extra energy as fat and carbohydrate, and an appropriate dosage of pancreatic enzyme supplements in a form which minimizes acid-peptic inactivation. Newer adjuncts to pancreatic enzyme therapy, such as prostaglandin analogues, show promise. Food supplements should provide extra energy, essential fatty acids, fat-soluble vitamins in a water emulsion, salt supplements in hot weather, and water-soluble vitamins and micronutrients. Routine surveillance of nutritional status and absorbed energy should be performed at regular intervals. Deviations from normal weight gain and growth may require nutritional intervention. Recent studies by a number of groups confirm that long-term supplementation can achieve sustained catch-up weight gain and growth, and provide support for the view that reversible nutritional factors may have an important influence on the course of pulmonary disease in those CF patients who have deteriorating lung function, and who are unable to sustain normal growth and nutrition by the oral route. Obviously, the overall goal should be to prevent this situation and provide the CF patient with as normal a lifestyle as possible, with management aimed at preventing progressive pulmonary disease, maintaining normal growth and nutrition, and preventing complications.

Bibliography

Gaskin KJ (1990) Hereditary disorders of the exocrine pancreas. In: Walker WA (ed.) *Pediatric Gastrointestinal Disease*, pp 1198–1202. Toronto: BC Decker Inc.

Shepherd RW and Cleghorn G (1990) *Nutritional and Gastrointestinal Problems in Cystic Fibrosis*. Boca Raton, Florida: CRC Press.

Shepherd RW, Holt TL, Thomas BJ, Ward LC, Isles A and Francis PJ (1984) Malnutrition in cystic fibrosis: the nature of the nutritional deficit and optimal management. *Nutrition Abstracts and Reviews* 54: 1009–1022.

Soutter VL, Kristidis P, Gruca MA and Gaskin, KJ (1986) Chronic undernutrition, growth retardation in cystic fibrosis. *Clinics in Gastroenterology* 15: 137–155.

Ross W. Shepherd
Royal Children's Hospital, Brisbane, Australia

DAIRY PRODUCTS – DIETARY IMPORTANCE

Dairy products are traditional dietary items in many parts of the world, in particular in regions such as Northern Europe where the cooler climate is especially suited to dairying. The history of milk as a food has been documented over the centuries and examples of early dairying are depicted in Egyptian friezes such as that from the sarcophagus of Queen Kawit from Der-al-Bahri, between Luxor and Karnack, dating back 4000 years. There is an even earlier Mesopotamian frieze from the temple of Nin-khasarg, near Ur, which is thought to be 1000 years older.

The popularity of milk as a staple food over the centuries must partly be due to its versatility. Early man discovered that it could be churned to make butter and fermented with bacterial cultures to produce cheese and yoghurt, all of which were methods of preserving some or all of the nutrients in milk for consumption at a later date. *See* Cheeses, Dietary Importance; Milk, Dietary Importance; Yoghurt, Dietary Importance

This article will summarize the nutritional contribution made by milk and milk products.

Variety

Today, the range of dairy products on the market is immense. In most countries, a range of milks with differing fat contents is available. For example, in the UK consumers can choose between Channel Islands milk, with 5·1 g per 100 g fat, through whole milk (3·9 g per 100 g) to semiskimmed (1·6 g per 100 g fat) and skimmed milk, which has virtually no fat. Similarly, a wide range of cheeses exists with varying fat contents: at one end of the spectrum are soft fresh cheeses, made with skimmed milk, and, at the other, hard cheeses such as Cheddar. Also available is cheese made with nonanimal rennet, suitable for vegetarians. In the UK alone, almost 200 different cheeses are produced, and cheese is particularly popular in countries such as France, where an even greater variety is available.

Fermented milk products such as yoghurt, smetana and kefir have always been popular in Middle Eastern countries, but their popularity, particularly that of yoghurt, is increasing dramatically in the UK. Again, a wide range of yoghurts exists, from the very-low-fat to the creamier, whole-milk or Greek-style product, including set yoghurts, stirred yoghurts, fruit yoghurts, frozen yoghurts and fromage frais. *See* Fermented Milks, Types of Fermented Milks; Yoghurt, The Product and its Manufacture

Traditional products such as cream and butter are still in demand, in spite of their relatively high fat content, and are being joined by other 'luxury' products, such as

Table 1.   Contribution of milk and milk products to daily nutrient intake in the UK

	Liquid milk		Cheese		All milk and milk products	
	Amount	Percentage of total intake	Amount	Percentage of total intake	Amount	Percentage of total intake
Energy (kJ)	613	7·3	265	3·2	1140	13·6
Protein (g)	7·2	10·6	4·0	5·9	15·2	22·4
Fat (g)	8·8	9·5	5·2	5·6	16·3	17·4
Saturates (g)	5·6	14·6	3·2	8·3	10·0	26·2
Monounsaturates (g)	2·4	7·2	1·4	4·2	4·4	13·1
Polyunsaturates (g)	0·3	1·9	0·2	1·3	0·6	4·3
Calcium (mg)	255	29·7	107	12·5	491	57·3
Iron (mg)	0·1	1·1	<0·1	0·4	0·3	2·5
Thiamin (mg)	0·08	5·5	<0·1	0·3	0·13	9·4
Riboflavin (mg)	0·37	22·2	0·06	3·9	0·64	37·9
Nicotinic acid equivalents (mg)	1·9	6·9	1·0	3·7	4·0	14·6
Vitamin C (mg)	1·5	2·5	—	—	2·9	4·8
Retinol equivalents (μg)	124	9·7	52	4·1	208	16·4
Vitamin D (μg)	0·06	2·1	0·04	1·3	0·29	9·2

Source: Ministry of Agriculture, Fisheries and Food (1989).

Dietary Importance

real dairy ice creams, fresh cream desserts and luxury mousses. To meet the demand for a spread with a buttery flavour, spreads have been developed which incorporate butterfat for taste but often have a lower fat and calorie content. *See* Butter, The Product and its Manufacture; Cream, Types of Cream; Ice Cream, Methods of Manufacture

A number of products also exist to which nutrients have been added, such as the calcium-enriched milks, and yoghurts fortified with additional vitamins.

Nutritional Value

Most dairy products offer a wide range of nutrients and this is reflected in the contribution made by milk and milk products to dietary intake in many countries. For example, in the UK, milk and milk products provide over half the calcium in the average diet and make a significant contribution to the needs of other nutrients (Table 1).

Nutritional Significance of Milk and Milk Products

In countries where dairying has traditionally been a strong industry, milk and milk product consumption tends to be widespread and makes a significant contribution to nutrient needs. For example, the average daily intake of milk in the UK is a little under half a pint per person (278 ml). Table 2 shows the contribution this quantity of whole milk makes to the nutrient and energy needs of a four-year-old girl and a man. Skimmed or semiskimmed milk would make smaller contributions to intake of energy and fat-soluble vitamins.

In Scandanavian countries, where dairying is also traditional, liquid milk consumption is typically higher than in the UK. However, in warmer climates, in particular the Indian subcontinent, Africa and South America, climatic conditions lend themselves less readily to cows' needs, so that the development of dairying and, hence, milk-drinking habits has been far more patchy. Exceptions exist, such as the Masai in Eastern Africa, whose culture is dominated by the cow. Similarly, in parts of India, cows have religious significance but have not, until recently, been intensively managed for their milk. Table 3 presents estimates of milk consumption in different countries.

Being rich in calcium needed for skeletal development and maintenance, milk has traditionally been seen as an important food during childhood, pregnancy and lactation, when calcium requirements are particularly high. This view is still supported today. A report from the British Dietetic Association (1987) recommended that children receive a pint of milk per day, and the

Table 2. Contribution of 285 ml (half pint) of whole milk to nutrient needs

	Percentage of UK Reference Nutrient Intake (RNI)	
	Girls (4–6 years)	Adult Men (19–50 years)
Energy*	12·5	7·6
Fat*	19·0	11·5
Saturates*	37·3	22·7
Monounsaturates*	14·3	8·6
Polyunsaturates*	2·7	1·7
Carbohydrate*	7·0	4·2
Protein	47·5	16·8
Nonstarch polysaccharide	—	—
Vitamin A	32·8	23·4
Thiamin	16·4	11·5
Riboflavin	62·5	38·5
Nicotinic acid equivalents	22·1	14·3
Vitamin B_6	19·4	12·5
Folic acid	17·5	8·8
Vitamin B_{12}	143·8	76·7
Calcium	74·8	48·1
Vitamin C	10·0	7·5
Sodium	23·9	10·4
Chloride	26·6	11·7
Copper	Trace	Trace
Iodine	44·0	31·4
Iron	2·4	1·7
Magnesium	26·7	10·7
Phosphorus	77·0	49·0
Potassium	37·3	16·4
Selenium	15·0	4·0
Zinc	17·7	12·1

Figures for milk composition from Holland B, Unwin ID and Buss DH (1989) *Milk Products and Eggs.* Fourth supplement of McCance and Widdowson's *The Composition of Foods* 4th edn. London: Royal Society of Chemistry and Ministry of Agriculture, Fisheries and Food.
Figures for RNIs from Department of Health (1979).
* There is no RNI for these components of food. For energy, the Estimated Average Requirement has been given; for fat and carbohydrate, the desirable average intake has been given.

importance of milk as a source of calcium (about 700 mg per pint) is emphasized to pregnant and lactating women. *See* Calcium, Properties and Determination; Children, Nutritional Requirements; Lactation

Claims of Adverse and Beneficial Effects to Health

Allergy or Intolerance to Cows' Milk

True milk allergy is typically seen in infants. Although estimates vary, it is thought that at its peak incidence in

Table 3. Estimates of liquid milk consumption in a selection of countries

	Liquid milk consumption (kg per person per year)
Australia	91·3
Canada	98·8
Chile	19·1
Czechoslovakia	103·6
Germany	70·7
Denmark	122·6
Finland	180·1
France	79·5
Ireland	184·6
Israel	68·5
India	51·1
Iceland	194·3
Italy	78·1
Japan	40·4
Netherlands	93·0
Norway	162·2
South Africa	102·6
Spain	139·8
Sweden	41·3
UK	122·5
USA	107·5

Source: International Dairy Federation (1991) Consumption statistics for milk and milk products, 1989. *Bulletin of the International Dairy Federation* 254.

1–3-year-olds, cows' milk allergy affects about 1% of infants. Most children outgrow this reaction to the protein in milk by their fifth birthday and in many instances it is short-lived, being brought on by a gastrointestinal upset.

Intolerance to the sugar in milk, lactose, occurs in those people who lack or who have low levels of the enzyme lactase, which digests lactose to its components, glucose and galactase. This enzyme is invariably present in the intestines of infants to enable them to digest their mother's milk, but levels fall off in some adults, particularly those who come from areas of the world where milk consumption is not traditional. Hence, in the UK, lactose intolerance is rare among Caucasians but is experienced by some ethnic groups of Indian, African or Chinese extraction. In many cases, sufferers have low levels of the enzyme and can thus tolerate small quantities of milk and larger quantities of foods such as cheese or yoghurt. In the case of cheese, the lactose has largely been lost with the whey in the cheese-making process. In the case of yoghurt, it is suggested that the β-galactosidase enzyme, present in the bacterial culture used to make yoghurt, may be able to digest some of the lactose. *See* Food Intolerance, Lactose Intolerances

Dietary Importance

Health Benefits of Yoghurt

A number of health benefits of yoghurt have been claimed, including an ability of certain types of bacteria used in the manufacture of yoghurt to colonize the gut and help fend off harmful bacteria.

Coronary Heart Disease

One of the risk factors for coronary heart disease (CHD) is a raised plasma cholesterol level. A number of factors, including genetic make-up, influence an individual's plasma cholesterol level. One such factor is thought to be intake of saturated fatty acids, particularly in genetically susceptible people who are less able to remove low-density lipoproteins (LDLs) from their bloodstream.

Many governments have issued guidelines on diet in relation to heart disease. In the UK, guidelines of energy and nutrient intake (Department of Health, 1991) include recommendations on total fat intake and on fatty acid intake. The guidelines on saturated fatty acids (saturates) has been set with a view to reducing average plasma cholesterol concentration by 0·4 mmol l^{-1}, thus bringing it down to a level associated with a substantially lower incidence of coronary heart disease than witnessed in the UK at present.

Currently, saturates provide an average of 17% of energy intake. The Department of Health report advises that average consumption is reduced to 10% of total energy (11% of food energy).

This advice does not apply to children under the age of two years, and for adults beyond middle age in whom the possible benefits of reducing fat intake will be less likely (DHSS, 1984).

Intake of specific foods has *not* been linked directly with (CHD) risk. However, a reduction in foods which contribute significant amounts of fat (Table 4), especially saturated fatty acids, to the diet has been recommended for those people with a high fat intake. Such advice calls for a reduction in foods such as whole milk and its products, fatty meats, fried foods, spreading and cooking fats, and baked goods such as biscuits, cakes and pies.

A wide range of lower-fat milks and milk products is now available, so that those people concerned about their fat intake can change to a lower-fat option rather than cutting down on dairy products and losing a valuable source of calcium and other essential nutrients.

Dairy Products and Dental Health

The frequency of sugar consumption and its concentration in food are positively related to the incidence of dental caries. Although lactose (milk sugar) is moder-

Table 4. Contribution of sources of fat and saturates in the household food supply of the UK (1988)

	Fat (g per day)	Fat (%)	Saturated fatty acids (g per day)	Saturated fatty acids (%)
Liquid milk (whole)	9·6	10·0	6·0	15·4
Cheese	5·3	5·5	3·2	8·1
Total milk, cream and cheese	**16·8**	**17·5**	**10·3**	**26·2**
Meat and poultry	15·3	16·1	5·9	14·9
Sausages and meat products	9·3	9·7	3·7	9·4
Total meat	**24·6**	**25·8**	**9·6**	**24·3**
Total fish	**1·6**	**1·7**	**0·4**	**0·9**
Total eggs	**2·1**	**2·2**	**0·6**	**1·6**
Butter	7·1	7·4	4·6	11·7
Margarine	13·1	13·7	3·8	9·6
Other fats and oils	12·6	13·2	4·0	10·1
Total fats and oils	**32·8**	**34·3**	**12·4**	**31·4**
Total vegetables	**3·1**	**3·2**	**0·8**	**2·0**
Total fruit	**1·3**	**1·4**	**0·3**	**0·9**
Cakes and pastries	2·0	2·0	0·8	2·0
Biscuits	5·0	5·2	2·4	6·1
Bread, flour and breakfast cereals	4·4	4·7	1·1	2·9
Total cereals	**11·4**	**11·9**	**4·3**	**11·0**
Other foods and beverages	**1·9**	**2·0**	**0·7**	**1·7**
Total all foods	**95·7**	**100·0**	**39·4**	**100·0**

Source: Ministry of Agriculture, Fisheries and Food (1989).

ately cariogenic if consumed in isolation, when it is consumed as part of milk any cariogenicity is counteracted by protective factors in milk (DHSS, 1989). Consequently, milk without added sugars can be considered to be virtually noncariogenic. *See* Dental Disease, Aetiology of Dental Caries

Cheese is also one of the least cariogenic foods. Dental caries result because of acid production on the tooth surface, following bacterial fermentation of sugar. If cheese is eaten either immediately before or after a sugary food, it results in much less acid production than would otherwise have been caused by the sugary food (Silva *et al.*, 1986).

A number of possible mechanisms have been offered to explain this beneficial effect of cheese. Eating cheese causes an increased flow of saliva, which is slightly alkaline and acts as a buffer to the acid. Also, cheese favours remineralization of any damage since it is rich in calcium and its consistency brings calcium and phosphorus into contact with the tooth surface.

Bibliography

British Dietetic Association (1987) *Children's Diets and Change.* A report of the Child Health and Nutrition Working Party. Birmingham: British Dietetic Association.

Department of Health and Social Security (DHSS) (1984) *Diet and Cardiovascular Disease.* Committee on Medical Aspects of Food Policy. Report on Health and Social Subjects 28. London: Her Majesty's Stationery Office (HMSO).

DHSS (1989) *Dietary Sugars and Human Disease.* Committee on Medical Aspects of Food Policy. Report on Health and Social Subjects 27. London: HMSO.

Department of Health (1991) *Dietary Reference Values for Food Energy and Nutrients in the UK.* Committee on Medical Aspects of Food Policy. Report on Health and Social Subjects 41. London: HMSO.

Ministry of Agriculture, Fisheries and Food (1989) *National Food Survey, 1988.* London: HMSO.

National Dairy Council (1988) *From Farm to Doorstep.* London: National Dairy Council.

National Dairy Council (1991a) *Coronary Heart Disease I.* Fact File 7. London: National Dairy Council.

National Dairy Council (1991b) *Coronary Heart Disease II.* Fact File 8. London: National Dairy Council.

Renner E (1983) *Milk and Dairy Products in Human Nutrition.* Munich: Volkswirtschaftlicher Verlag.

Renner E (1989) *Micronutrients in Milk and Milk-Based Food Products.* London: Elsevier Applied Science.

Silva MF de A *et al.* (1986) Effect of cheese on experimental caries in human subjects. *Caries Research* 20: 263–269.

Judy Buttriss
National Dairy Council, London, UK

Dietary Importance

DATE PALM*

The date palm is an evergreen tree that flourishes in dry hot climates found in desert regions of the world. It is a major crop in Iraq, Saudi Arabia, Egypt, Iran and Algeria; on a smaller scale, it is grown in countries of the Arabian peninsula, North Africa, the Indian subcontinent, Spain, Mexico and the USA. Climatic requirements for successful growth include a moderate winter and a hot summer, with little rainfall and low atmospheric humidity. Growth decreases with a decrease in environmental temperature and stops at temperatures below 10°C. Leaves are damaged at temperatures below −6·6°C. Heavy rain during blossoming and harvesting can cause damage to the crop. These climatic necessities restrict its zone of propagation; in order to extend the date palm beyond its natural habitat, studies aimed at developing new varieties, resistant to a wider range of climatic conditions, are under way.

Contrary to the common notion that date trees do not need much water, regular irrigation once or twice a week in summer and once a month in winter is recommended for maximum growth and fruit production. Irrigation involves adding water to a circular basin of 1–1·5 m radius around each tree. Freshwater irrigation promotes flavour and quality of the fruit, while saltwater has the opposite effect. The date palm also requires fertilizer applications, either once a year or once in 3 years, depending on the nature of the soil and judgement of the farmer. The time of application is soon after the harvest, and the fertilizer is mainly animal manure, although peats, composts and chemical fertilizers have recently been introduced. Fertilizer is applied by evenly spreading three to five donkey-loads of animal manure in the irrigation basin of each tree and loosening the soil, so that mixing of the fertilizer and soil is achieved. Pruning includes cutting off old leafstalks, offshoots and the remainders of fruit bunches, and removal of fibre between leafstalks and stem. It is done manually after the harvest and before the spring.

Propagation

The most favoured method is by cutting off the shoots grown on the mother tree, above or below the soil surface, and transplanting them. The offshoots are rich in nutrients which permit their growth after transplantation. This method is popular because the variety of the

transplant is known and it bears fruit after 3–4 years. However, it is expensive and limited in scope as the available offshoots are not enough for popular cultivars. A less attractive method of date palm propagation is by seed cultivation, which usually results in inferior varieties. The chance of dominant and recessive gene expression is, perhaps, responsible for the appearance of varieties that are inferior to the seed variety planted. Trees produced by seed cultivation are slow in bearing fruit, requiring about 12 years. Tissue culture techniques have been successfully applied to produce date palm trees, but efficiency, economics and the time required for fruit bearing by the tree remain to be worked out.

Pollination

Date palms produce flowers that are either male or female. In the spring, female and male flowers grow on fruit-producing and nonproducing trees, respectively. The male flowers are dull white in colour, clustered on short strands forming a bunch, and the entire bunch is covered by a long spathe. As the spathe grows, it opens spontaneously and pollinates the female flowers on adjacent trees. The spathe can be cut and sold in the market. The female flowers are greenish yellow in colour, forming clusters on long strands making a bunch. Although female flowers are spontaneously pollinated by the male pollen in nature, manual pollination is often practised and it is said to improve quality and fruit yield. The type of male flower used for pollination also affects the quality of the fruit. Manual pollination consists of placing three to four strands of male flowers in the middle of the strands of a female flower bunch and tying the female strands near the terminals with a strip cut from a date leaflet. After pollination, the entire bunch sometimes is covered with fibre from the palm trunk and tied to protect it against cold, birds, locusts and rats. It is left for about 3–6 weeks, then untied and spread over leafstalks for support, aeration and exposure to sunlight. Manual pollination before sunset leads to better fruit quality and yield than pollination carried out at any other time of the day. Spraying of unpollinated female flowers with growth regulators has yielded 70–79% seedless fruits.

Fruit Development Stages

After pollination, the female flowers grow rapidly. In the early stage, individual fruits appear yellowish green

---

* The colour plate section for this article appears between p. 1146 and p. 1147.

and turn dark green in about a month. Fruit thinning, which involves the removal of entire bunches leaving 12–16 bunches per tree, decreasing the number of strands per bunch, cutting the terminals of strands and removal of individual fruits from strands, is done at this stage. Ethepon has been tried as a chemical fruit thinner. Further growth continues for about 3 months, then the dark green fruits begin to change colour as the fruits reach maturity. According to variety, different colours are acquired. Bunches are often washed with a jet of water at this stage. Fruit ripening begins with the appearance of a characteristic soft brown spot at the tip; this progresses with time towards the disc joining the fruit to the strand. *See* Ripening of Fruit

Fruit Harvesting

The manner of harvesting varies with the size of the cultivar and intended use of the crop. Garden fruits are individually picked, collected in baskets made at the beginning of the ripening season from date leaflets, and eaten or sold fresh or dried. Towards the end of the season, entire bunches are cut and lowered to the ground with a rope. Fruits from bunches are picked up with discs, and allowed to cure, ripen and dry. In commercial cultivars, bunches of fruits are allowed to ripen and partially dry on the palm, then cut and lowered to the ground. Fruits are separated by shaking the bunches into large baskets made from palm leaflets. If the harvest has dried to a raisin-like consistency, it is sorted, packed and stored; if it is not sufficiently dry, it is spread on mats, exposed to the sun for about a week and then packed. The dried crop is traditionally packed in gasoline tins, or baskets made from date leaflets, or is sold unpacked. Automated sorting and packing facilities have been recently introduced, using cartons as packing material. *See* Drying, Drying Using Natural Radiation

Fruit Storage

Packed dry dates keep well without addition of preservatives. The high content of sugars serves as an effective preservative, allowing the dates to keep until the next harvest or longer, in the absence of added water. In the presence of water, harvested dates can easily be contaminated by microorganisms. Rinsing before consumption is harmless, but rinsed dates kept for several days run the risk of bacterial contamination. *See* Preservation of Food

Varieties of Date Palm

Extensive variation is known to occur in dates. More than 2000 varieties are estimated to exist in the Arabian peninsula, 600 varieties in Iraq, and unknown numbers in the rest of the world. In Saudi Arabia alone, 76 varieties in the eastern region, 104 varieties in the central region, and 207 varieties in the western region are documented. Criteria for classification include fruit shape, size, colour, flavour and ripening time, all these being remarkably variable. Fruit shapes vary from spherical to oval and from elongated to egg-shaped. Fruit sizes may differ by factors of two to five between varieties. Fruit colours among varieties include shades of white, yellow, brown, red and pink. Some varieties ripen early; others ripen late in summer, while some varieties ripen in autumn. This difference makes fresh dates available for about 8 months in a year. The flavour of some varieties is not acceptable to humans, and such dates are mixed with feed and given to animals. The purpose of growing dates also varies. Some varieties are grown mainly as local delicacies; others are ornamental trees; some are cultivated for traditional medical applications such as treatment for bone fractures, mental disorders, muscular defects and pain in childbirth; others are grown for commercial fruit production. Most of the date varieties have annual fruit-bearing habits, while some varieties bear fruits in alternate years.

Fruit Composition

It is a common experience that after eating 4–10 date fruits, with or without other foods, a unique feeling of satiety ensues. In addition, hunger and thirst are delayed in spite of continued manual work – a property not noticeable for other fruits. Explanation of these effects, and the role of dates in human nutrition in terms of nutrients they can supply, has been sought by measurement of the date's constituents.

Fruit varieties are often arbitrarily chosen for such analyses and results interpreted in a generalized form, often without recognition of factors that influence fruit composition to a significant extent. Factors demonstrated to affect the quality and composition of the fruit include the following: variety of the tree bearing the fruit; source of the pollen grain used for pollination; location and type of soil on which trees are grown; fertilizer application; nature of irrigation water; use of growth regulators; exposure to dusty winds, and diseases of the plant.

Although comprehensive data from well-planned programmes on the nutrient constituents of date varieties are not available, by collecting data from isolated analyses, a clear picture emerges, indicating the importance of dates in human nutrition. The fruit contains carbohydrates, minerals, dietary fibre, vitamins, lipids and proteins. In general, the quantities of carbohydrates, minerals, fibre and vitamins per 100 g of the dry fruit, make a significant contribution to human

Table 1. Carbohydrate content (% on a dry-weight basis) in dry date varieties

Variety	Place of growth	Total sugars	Reducing sugars (glucose and fructose)	Nonreducing sugars (sucrose)	Pectin	Crude fibres	Ash (minerals)
Sakhi		79·82	39·67	40·15	2·07	4·57	4·12
Safawi	Saudi	78·30	45·60	32·70	1·14	3·10	2·55
Shalabi	Arabia[a]	77·95	38·45	39·50	1·62	3·85	3·90
Sukkari		81·75	36·05	45·70	1·32	3·97	4·40
Al-Halawi		87·91	82·72 (43·69 + 37·21)	4·80	~2		
Al-Sayer	Iraq[b]	86·10	82·6 (44·79 + 38·04)	3·50	~2		
Al-Khadrawi		87·74	81·91 (44·73 + 38·48)	5·4	~2		
Al-Zuhdi		86·80	73·40 (32·77 + 39·15)	12·70	~2		

[a] Data from Hussein F (1975).
[b] Data from Al-Saeed A (1985).

requirements, while the amounts of lipids (2–3·5%) and proteins (1–6%) contribute little to human requirements. The amounts of nutrients per 100 g of dry fruit show significant variations among varieties.

Carbohydrates

Carbohydrates constitute the major component of the date, and consist mainly of reducing sugars, in the form of glucose and fructose, nonreducing sugars (primarily sucrose), and small amounts of polysaccharides (e.g. cellulose and starch, and carbohydrate-derived substances such as pectin and crude fibre. Table 1 shows the variation in amounts of these elements in dry date varieties. *See* Carbohydrates, Classification and Properties

The presence of dietary fibre can be anticonstipatory, and the presence of pectin adds a plasma-cholesterol-lowering property to the fruit. *See* Dietary Fibre, Physiological Effects

Minerals

The four varieties of Iraqi dates, named in Table 1, have been analysed and the following minerals have been found in the fruit (figures in brackets indicate the lowest and highest levels, in mg per 100 g of fruit): calcium

Table 2. Iron content of date varieties

Variety	Place of growth	Number of fruits in 100 g of seedless fruit	Iron content (mg per 100 g of fruit)
Duhni	Riyadh	13	7·0
Khidri		14	18·15
Rushudi	Qaseem	14	0·9
Rothana		15	10·65
Birhi	Madina	22	10·7
Gondela	Sudan	20	31·62
Zuhdi	Iraq	14	4·75
Sellage		17	12·5
Seki	Riyadh	14	6·15
Razez		10	5·0
Ekhlas		18	4·0

Data from Shinwari MA (1987).

(123–207); phosphorus (13–16); potassium (833–894); sulphur (10–21); sodium (5–16); chlorine (260–342); magnesium (56–60); iron (2·56–10·37); manganese (5·14–5·86); copper (2·54–2·89); cobalt (0·76–0·95); zinc (0·74–1·82) and fluorine (0·12–0·2). *See* individual minerals

The iron content of different varieties of dates has been further investigated, and the results obtained are shown in Table 2.

Data in Table 2 indicate that the iron content of the fruit is probably genetically determined, since different varieties grown in the same area have different amounts of the metal in fruits, although the ultimate source of iron for the tree is the soil. Further support for this observation is provided by experiments in which iron, introduced by injection into the tree or by soil supplementation, did not alter the iron content of fruits.

The iron content per 100 g of fruit in date varieties is of special interest as the range covers human needs for the metal, in all situations. It offers a practical method of iron supplementation in cases of iron deficiency anaemia during childhood, in pregnancy and in cases of haemorrhages occurring as a result of menstruation, parturition or wounds. This method appears to be superior to iron supplementation in the form of iron tablets, which produce reactions like nausea, headache and anorexia, while date intolerance is unknown in humans. Furthermore, absorption of iron from dates is expected to be more efficient because of the presence in the fruit of glucose, fructose and vitamin C – each known for promoting iron absorption. Dosage and administration do not require a physician's help, and dates are not expensive. *See* Anaemia, Iron Deficiency Anaemia; Iron, Physiology

Vitamins

Analytical work on vitamins in dates is limited and patchy. The four Iraqi date varieties, named in Table 1, are reported to contain the following vitamins (figures in brackets indicate lowest and highest amounts, in μg per 100 g of fruit): thiamin or vitamin B_1 (80–130); riboflavin or vitamin B_2 (135–173); biotin (4·09–6·48); folic acid or folacin (43–70), and ascorbic acid or vitamin C (2510–3560).

The Iraqi Society for Dates has estimated vitamin A (as carotene) occurrence in dates to range from 80 to 100 iu per 100 g of fruit. *See* individual vitamins

Energy Content

The energy content of fresh dates (86% water) has been found to be 406·14 kJ (96·7 kcal) per 100 g of fresh fruit. The same weight of dry dates, of raisin-like consistency (less than 20% water), would contain about 1470–1680 kJ (350–400 kcal). This means that 100 g of dates alone can provide about 14–17% of the daily energy allowance of a reference man (70 kg) and reference woman (55 kg). *See* Energy, Measurement of Food Energy

In the light of the analytical information, it may be concluded that dates are a natural mixture of nutrients and a rich source of energy; they contain variable amounts of minerals and vitamins, and therefore have an important place in human nutrition.

Eating a moderate amount of dates, perhaps an hour before the meal, does not cause obesity. However, eating large quantities of dates, especially after the meal, can be fattening because the excessive energy introduced into the system is stored as body fat.

Manner of Eating Dates

Fresh dates are eaten before the meal as an appetizer, after the meal as a dessert, or between meals as a snack. Dried dates are eaten in various ways. Traditionally, Arabs eat them with tea or Arabian coffee, or with milk, buttermilk or thick yoghurt. Consumption of dates with dairy products raises the fruit's nutritional value to the level of a complete meal, as high-quality proteins and lipids, in which dates are deficient, are introduced, together with other nutrients in milk products.

Dried dates are sometimes pitted, mixed with crushed aniseed, cardamom or other spices, stored in chocolate cans, and served on special occasions as delicacies. Pitted, dried dates are also eaten in combination with other foods; the popular forms include dates stuffed with almonds, walnuts or pistachios. Pitted dates are sometimes transformed into chocolate-like bars, sprinkled with white sesame seeds to cover the surface, wrapped with paper, and eaten as snacks. Fortification of dates with sesame seeds, which are rich in polyunsaturated fatty acids and proteins, also raises their nutritional value to the level of a meal. Another combination involves mixing of pitted dates with other food materials, transforming them into salami-like rolls, and serving them as slices. Pitted dates are also used in preparation of fruit cakes and biscuits.

Fruit-based Products

A number of date-based dishes, fluids and manufactured products are common among people of the date-growing regions. The following are selected examples.

Dibs

Dibs is a thick fluid, made by putting fresh, ripe dates in a funnel-like container and placing a heavy load on the top to cause exudation of the juice, which is tapped from the bottom and collected in storage bottles. It keeps well without the addition of preservatives, and is used in the preparation of sweet dishes, as a substitute for sugar in tea or coffee, or eaten directly with bread and rice.

Syrups

A variety of syrups and date honey, with different degrees of fluidity, flavour and colour, are made from the fruit and sold. They keep for up to 8 months without the addition of preservatives.

Alcohol

Fermentation of dates by yeast has been a classical method of liquor manufacture which can be adapted for the large-scale production of alcohol for industrial purposes. *See* Fermented Foods, Origins and Applications

Vinegar

Alcohol obtained from fermentation of dates is oxidized to yield vinegar. *See* Vinegar

Sugar

Manufacture of sucrose from a sucrose-rich variety of dates has been reported to be economically feasible. *See* Sugar, Palms and Maples

Glucose and Fructose

Two methods have been developed for the manufacture of glucose and fructose from dates. A syrup containing glucose and fructose is extracted from the fruit. In the first method, the temperature and concentration of the syrup are raised to 80°C and 75%, respectively. Allowing its temperature to fall slowly results in the formation of irregular solid crystals of glucose, leaving fructose in the aqueous phase. In the second method the hot syrup is treated with calcium oxide, which combines with the glucose and fructose. The calcium derivative of glucose crystallizes upon slowly lowering the temperature and leaving the calcium derivative of fructose in the aqueous phase. Treatment with carbon dioxide results in formation of calcium carbonate, leaving solutions of free glucose and free fructose. *See* Fructose

If the manufacture of fructose from dates were cost-effective, it would perhaps be useful for patients with diabetes mellitus, because a large part of fructose in tissues is transported by a passive mechanism. Substitution of fructose for sugar may permit diabetics to enjoy its sweetness and obtain energy from it, without raising blood glucose. The separated glucose can be utilized for dextrose drips for hospital use.

Date Seeds

Large quantities of date seeds (date stones) can accumulate as a result of pitting the fruit in commercial farms; these can be put to use. Chemically, they contain up to 8·4% lipids, 5·2% proteins, 62·5% carbohydrates, and variable amounts of minerals and fibre. This indicates their suitability for use in animal feeding and oil extraction. In animal feeding, the seeds are crushed and mixed with feeds. Oil extracted from date stones is reported to be good for human consumption, and it contains linolenic acid, among other fatty acids. *See* Fatty Acids, Gamma Linolenic Acid

The Wood

Date trees grow vertically, forming a straight trunk, bearing the leafstalks like a crown. Old tree trunks can be 15–25 m long and be 20–40 cm in cross-section radius. It is made of strong cellulose fibres, making a tough log. Traditionally, the log has been used in house roofs, in bridges and as support pillars and poles. As a result of improved economies it has lost these roles to reinforced concrete and metal pylons. The log can be used in making plywood. Date fibre is suitable for nonabrasive cleaning materials.

Economic Importance

Date cultivation has nutritional, economic, aesthetic and environmental benefits. Planting the trees along city roads is primarily to purify air pollution and beautify the scenery, with fruit and shade being secondary objectives. Growing dates in domestic gardens is mainly for nutritional, aesthetic and economic reasons, while air purification and shade are additional benefits. In commercial situations, economic return is the major consideration. Investment of resources in the form of land, water, fertilizers and labour is a long-term commitment with profitable annual returns. Fruit yield per tree varies between 400 and 600 kg of fresh crop (100–150 kg of dry crop). The tree can produce at this rate up to and beyond 60 years, if properly tended. The 1990 price in Riyadh market for fresh, high-quality Nabute Seif and Sellage varieties was 12–15 and 8–10 Riyals per kg respectively, while cheaper varieties were sold at 4–6 Riyals per kg ($1 = 3·75 Riyals). Even if 25% of these prices is realized, date farming appears to be a profitable investment. The profit is further boosted by the secondary crop, grown under date trees, which varies with local preferences and conditions. The secondary crop includes rice (eastern region of Saudi Arabia), alfalfa for animals (central and western regions of Saudi Arabia), and others such as parsley, spinach, tomatoes, onions, squashes, mint, cilantro, carrots and many more. Sale of produce from the secondary crop significantly boosts the annual return.

Fruit Potential

Reclamation and better utilization of land via date cultivation in suitable regions of the world seem to offer reasonable prospects for fighting hunger and disease.

Cheap varieties of dates can be used as a substrate for microorganisms to produce a whole range of pharmaceutical and industrial products.

Dates can be used as a basic food substance in two ways: (1) in clinical nutrition for patients with diseases of the heart, kidneys or liver, for arterioslcerosis and for obesity control, or to be eaten in combination with specific foods – rich or deficient in energy, proteins and lipids, and lacking cholesterol; (2) in the preparation of special foods for patients with disorders of metabolism, such as galactosaemia and lactose intolerance, by fortification with desired nutrients and transformation into suitable forms. *See* Liver, Nutritional Management of Liver and Biliary Disorders; Obesity, Treatment

Pests and Diseases of Date Palm

Although comprehensive information on date pests and diseases, and the extent of damage caused annually to the crop, is not available, the following are some of the recognized hazards:

1. The migratory locust (*Schistocerca gregaria* Forsk) feeds on the leaves and can defoliate the tree.
2. Parlatoria date scale (*Parlatoria blanchardii*-Targ) infects some date palm trees and leaves.
3. Date mite (*Paratetranychus afrasiaticus* McGregor) causes drying and reddening of young date fruits which drop between the time of pollination and the beginning of summer. Covering the inflorescence after pollination with the fibre from the tree trunk gives some protection against date mite.
4. Lesser date moth (*Bracheda amydraula* Meyer) larvae feed upon young date fruits which then drop.
5. A large beetle (*Pseudophilus testaceus* Gahn) bores into the trunk of the palm tree. Borers reduce both yield and life of the tree.
6. Graphiola leaf spot or false smut (*Graphiola phonicus* (Moug) Piot) is a fungal disease which produces a reduction in leaf surface.
7. Black scorch (*Thielaviopsis paradoxa* (De Seyn) Hoehn) occurs sporadically in date palms.

8. Infection by *Fusarium oxysporum* var. *albidins* has caused widespread damage to date palms in Morocco.
9. 'Al-Wajam' is an Arabic name given to a disease of date palm which causes stunted growth, reduced fruiting and declining vitality; the affected tree eventually dies.

Bibliography

Abo-Rady MDK, Jehjeh MA and Ahmad HS (1986) *Response of date palm to iron fertilization by soil application and injection II: Effect on fruit quality.* Proceedings of the Second Symposium on Date Palm, March, Al-Hassa, Saudi Arabia.

Al-Ghamdi AS, Al-Hassan GM and Jehjeh M (1988) Evaluation of eight seedling date palm males and their effects on fruit character of three female cultivars. *Arab Gulf Journal of Scientific Research* (*B: Agriculture and Biological Sciences*) 6: 175–187.

Al-Saeed A (1985) Fresh dates and date trees. (In Arabic.) Jeddah/Dammam/Riyadh: Saudi House for Publication and Distribution.

Bacha MA and Abo-Hassan AA (1982) *Effects of soil fertilization on yield, fruit quality and mineral content of Khudari date palm variety.* Proceedings of the First Symposium on Date Palm in Saudi Arabia, March, Al-Hassa, Saudi Arabia.

Bacha MA, Nasr TA and Shaheen MA (1988) *Effects of different male types on mineral composition of some date cultivars.* Proceedings of the Eleventh Symposium on the Biological Aspects of Saudi Arabia, May Yanbu, Saudi Arabia.

Dowson VHW and Aten A (1987) *Dates: Handling, Processing and Packing.* Rome: Food and Agriculture Organization.

Hussein F (1975) *Date Culture in Saudi Arabia.* Riyadh: Kingdom of Saudi Arabia Ministry of Agriculture and Water, Department of Research and Development.

Moustafa AA, El-Hennawy HM and Shazly SM (1986) *Effect of different day time pollination on fruit setting and fruit quality of 'Seewy' date palm in Fayoum (Egypt).* Proceedings of the Second Symposium on Date Palm, March, Al-Hassa, Saudi Arabia.

Nasr TA, Bacha MA and Shaheen MA (1988) Effects of some plant growth regulators on induction of seedless fruits in some date palm cultivars. *Journal of the College of Agriculture, King Saud University* 10: 129–138.

Shinwari MA (1987) Iron content of date fruits. *Journal of the College of Science, King Saud University* 18: 5–12.

Sood DR, Wagle DS and Dhindsa KS (1982) Compositional variations in dried date palm fruit varieties. *Indian Journal of Nutrition and Dietetics* 19(5): 146–148.

Mohammad Anwar Shinwari
King Saud University, Riyadh, Saudi Arabia

DEGRADATION

See Spoilage and Storage Stability

DEHYDRATION

Definition

Dehydration strictly means lack of water, but has come to be used more colloquially to mean salt and water depletion, and, even more loosely, to mean a deficit in body fluid of any kind. It is unfortunate that such loose terminology leads to loose thinking, imprecise diagnosis and, in some cases, inappropriate treatment. In contrast, the terms 'water depletion', 'salt and water depletion', and 'plasma volume deficit', have more precise diagnostic meaning and imply the appropriate treatment for their correction. Pure water depletion is in fact rare. The most obvious example is diabetes insipidus, caused by a lack of antidiuretic hormone. In contrast, salt and water depletion, or desalination, is extremely common. A prime example is that caused by diarrhoeal diseases, which kills millions of children throughout the world each year.

Physiology

The loss and gain of fluid by the body to and from its surroundings is normally small compared with the enormous daily flux between the different compartments within the body. Assuming the maximal concentrating ability of healthy kidneys, the volume of urine required to excrete waste products may be as little as 500 ml, although it is safer to allow 1–1·5 l. Insensible loss by evaporation from the lungs may be 500 ml, and from the skin surface 400 ml, although this may be greatly increased in hot climates or during fever, owing to sweating. The amount lost from the gastrointestinal tract as faeces is usually as little as 100 ml, but in the presence of diarrhoeal disease this may increase enormously. Thus the minimal daily input of fluid to maintain balance in a healthy adult in a temperate climate is approximately 1500 ml, although 2 l provides a safer margin. In warmer climates this requirement is increased considerably. *See* Kidney, Structure and Function

The distribution of body fluids in an adult between different compartments is shown in Fig. 1. Total body water is approximately 60% of the bodyweight (more in small children, less in the obese). The intracellular fluid (ICF) is just over 40% of bodyweight and extracellular fluid (ECF) just under 20% of bodyweight; 25% of the ECF is within the intravascular space, i.e. plasma; the remaining 75% is termed the 'interstitial fluid' and surrounds the cells. The integrity of these body fluid compartments is maintained by the properties of their separating membranes (e.g. the cell membrane with its sodium pump, and the capillary membrane and its pore size) and their osmotic or oncotic content (e.g. sodium ions Na^+, for ECF; potassium ions, K^+, for ICF; albumin for plasma). Not only is external fluid balance important, but also changes in fluid compartments, where shifts may be large. For example, the rate of exchange of albumin between the intravascular and interstitial spaces is normally 10 times its rate of synthesis. Fluid deficits may also have different effects on each compartment. In an average adult, a deficit of 2 l of pure water reduces the total body water evenly by 2 l (and, incidentally, the weight by 2 kg) with a 1400 ml reduction in ICF, a 600 ml reduction in ECF fluid, and a 150 ml reduction in plasma volume. However, a loss of 2 l of salt and water, at a concentration of 140 mmol Na^+ per l, reduces total body water by 2 l and weight by 2 kg, but causes a selective loss of 2 l from the ECF, with a consequent reduction in plasma volume of nearly 500 ml. The clinical problems presented by these two situations are of an entirely different order. *See* Potassium, Physiology; Sodium, Physiology; Water, Physiology

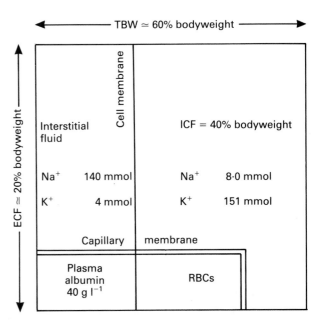

Fig. 1 Diagrammatic representation of body fluid compartments and concentrations of sodium ions (Na^+), potassium ions (K^+) and albumin. TBW, total body water; ICF, intracellular fluid; ECF, extracellular fluid; RBCs, red blood cells.

Table 1. Approximate electrolyte content of gastrointestinal secretions

Secretion	Sodium (Na$^+$) (mmol l^{-1})	Potassium (K$^+$) (mmol l^{-1})	Chloride (Cl$^-$) (mmol l^{-1})
Saliva	44	20	
Gastric	70–120	10	100
Small intestine	110–120	5–10	105
Bile	140	5	100
Pancreas	140	5	75
Diarrhoea			
Cholera (adult)	120	15	90
Cholera (child)	100	27	90
Nonspecific (child)	56	25	55

To understand the problems of fluid deficit it is also necessary to consider the large daily volume of secretions, particularly those into the gastrointestinal tract (Table 1). Under normal circumstances, these are almost entirely reabsorbed, with a minimal daily loss of 100 ml in the faeces. With gastrointestinal disease, e.g. vomiting, diarrhoea or fistula, large volumes of water and electrolytes may be lost to the outside or, in the case of intestinal obstruction or ileus, pooled in the gut and lost to the functional compartments. In an adult, during a normal day, 8000 ml of fluid enter the small bowel; 500 ml as saliva, 1200 ml as gastric fluid, 600 ml as bile, 1200 ml as pancreatic juice, 2000 ml as small bowel secretion and the remainder as ingested fluid. All but 1·5 l is reabsorbed in the small intestine, and a further 1·4 l is reabsorbed in the colon with much of the remaining sodium chloride. Approximate electrolyte content of gastrointestinal secretions is shown in Table 1.

Diagnosis and Monitoring

In common with most diagnoses, that of dehydration depends mainly on the history and examination. The history, combined with a knowledge of the natural history of the presenting condition, provides the main clues to the presence of salt and water depletion, the likely progress of the condition and the necessary treatment.

The physical signs are helpful but none are pathognomonic. The facies and eyes appear sunken, but this is also seen in cachexia. The mouth and tongue are dry, but this can also be caused by mouth breathing. The skin turgor, assessed by pinching up a fold of skin and observing its recoil, is diminished with salt depletion, but also in old age, cachexia and extreme cold. A marked fall in blood pressure between the lying and sitting or standing positions is also characteristic of salt and water depletion, as is tachycardia. A low output of

concentrated urine, associated with a rise in blood urea owing to prerenal failure, is also seen.

Other biochemical indices are less useful in diagnosis. The plasma sodium concentration gives no clue to the total body sodium content unless water balance is also known. It merely reflects the relative proportion of sodium and water in the extracellular space. Thus, with pure water lack, the plasma sodium concentration increases. With a mixed deficit of sodium and water, the plasma sodium reflects the relative proportion of the two which are lost.

Progress is first monitored by observing the improvement in the appearance of the patient; guard against fluid overload by watching for oedema, a raised jugular venous pressure, or pulmonary oedema. A fluid balance chart is valuable, but water balance is best measured by changes in weight which should be monitored at least daily. Plasma sodium concentration changes can then be interpreted in the light of water balance.

Conditions associated with Water and Salt Depletion

Diarrhoea

Worldwide, diarrhoea is by far the most important numerically, causing large numbers of childhood deaths from dehydration. Its severity varies from cholera, in which the stool output may be up to 1 l h^{-1} (for electrolyte losses see Table 1), to other infective conditions in which stool losses are smaller, although potentially life-threatening. Treatment is usually by oral rehydration therapy (see below), although severe cases require intravenous or subcutaneous fluid replacement where logistically possible. Formulae are shown in Table 2 and are based on the principle that small bowel sodium absorption is linked to that of glucose. The presence of starch, polysaccharide or glucose in such formulae is vital. Amino acids and peptides also enhance sodium reabsorption.

Vomiting or Nasogastric Aspiration

An examination of Table 1 will show the likely loss of electrolytes from vomiting or nasogastric aspiration and the logical replacement requirements. Aspirate volumes must be measured and replaced appropriately.

Intestinal Fistula or Short Bowel Disease

Up to 4 l per day may be lost from an upper jejunal or duodenal fistula. Parenteral nutrition is almost mandatory in this situation and must be combined with

Table 2. Concentration of electrolytes in oral rehydration solutions

	Sodium (Na$^+$) (mmol l^{-1})	Potassium (K$^+$) (mmol l^{-1})	Chloride (Cl$^-$) (mmol l^{-1})	Citrate or bicarbonate (mmol l^{-1})	Glucose[a] (mmol l^{-1})
For mild to moderate diarrhoea	35–60	13–25	50	10–20	100–200
For severe diarrhoea	90	20	80	10	111

[a] Glucose may be substituted by sucrose, maltose or rice water according to local availability.

adequate salt and water replacement guided by measured losses, daily weight changes, plasma electrolyte measurements and a knowledge of electrolyte concentrations in the fluid lost. Lower bowel fistula or short bowel can be treated by the enteral route, enhancing water and salt absorption using principles similar to those used in oral rehydration therapy. If enteral tube feeding is employed, a feed with sodium content less than 90 mmol causes net sodium secretion into the jejunum, whereas levels greater than this are associated with net absorption. The presence of carbohydrate and protein ensures the additional effect of glucose and amino acids on sodium absorption. The rate of administration may also be important. Too rapid rates may overwhelm the capacity of a shortened bowel to absorb all the fluid presented to it. Total osmolar content should also be considered, although the number of osmoles administered per unit time is more important than concentration.

Metabolic and Renal Disorders

The hyperglycaemia of diabetes mellitus causes an osmotic diuresis, leading to large deficits of water, sodium and potassium during acute loss of control, e.g. diabetic ketoacidosis. An osmotic diuresis may also result from excessive urea production owing to excessive protein administration. Hypercalcaemia poisons distal tubular function, leading to excessive production of dilute urine. Diabetes insipidus due to lack of antidiuretic hormone (ADH) has already been referred to. Alcohol excess dehydrates through inhibition of ADH. Acute or chronic renal damage may be associated with tubular dysfunction, loss of renal concentrating capacity, and water and salt deficit. This may be observed most strikingly in the polyuric phase of recovery from acute renal failure or following relief of obstructive uropathy. Treatment consists of the appropriate administration of water and electrolytes either orally or intravenously.

Excessive use of Diuretics

Excessive use of diuretics is a common cause of water, sodium and potassium depletion in the elderly and results from regimens that are too rigid and from lack of patient education. Patients need to know, for example, that if they fall ill from some condition that prevents salt and water intake or leads to excess loss, they should stop their diuretics.

Excessive Sweating

Excessive sweating, e.g. in the tropics, merits appropriate replacement. Before adaptation takes place, those going from temperate to hot climates are particularly prone to dehydration and heat stroke. A liberal water intake, combined, if necessary, with additional salt, should be taken prophylactically.

Errors in Diagnosis

Errors in diagnosis are particularly common in already hospitalized patients who are more often the victims of excess fluid administration than of dehydration. This results commonly from a naive interpretation and reliance on one or more physical signs, e.g. dry mouth, or from a failure to understand the compartmental distribution of body fluids and how these are affected by disease. A proper understanding of simple fluid balance concepts is a prerequisite for managing the many conditions in which dehydration or salt and water depletion are common. Salt and water are also intrinsic components of food and of the regimens used in the nutritional support of the sick.

Oral Rehydration Therapy

Solutions enhance the absorption of water and electrolytes through their substrate content, e.g. glucose, while replacing electrolyte deficit safely, e.g. avoiding hypernatraemia in infants. They should be palatable and acceptable to children, readily available and simple to use under all conditions. An alkalizing agent to counter acidosis may be advantageous. Solutions used in the UK for mild to moderate diarrhoea contain less sodium and more glucose than the World Health Organization (WHO) formula which is used for severe diarrhoea, e.g.

cholera. Dose is according to fluid loss, but a rough guide for adults is 200–400 ml for every loose stool, for children 200 ml per motion, and for infants 1–1·5 times usual feed. In severe cases, doses may be higher. The WHO policy is to promote its own single oral rehydration solution and to prevent hypernatraemia in children by giving extra water between doses. For further details, see *British National Formulary*.

Bibliography

Guyton AC (1991) *Textbook of Medical Physiology*. Philadelphia: WB Saunders.

Hladky SB and Rink TJ (1986) Body fluid and kidney physiology. *Physiological Principles in Medicine Series*. London: Edward Arnold.
Turnberg LA (1992) Pathophysiology of secretory diarrhoea. *Hospital Update* 18: 93–104.
Walters G (1983) Disorders of fluid and electrolyte balence. In: *Scientific Foundations of Clinical Biochemistry: Biochemistry in Clinical Practice* (Williams DL and Marks V, eds) pp 1–23. London: Heinemann.

S. P. Allison
University Hospital, Nottingham, UK

DENTAL DISEASE

Contents

Structure of Teeth*

The teeth comprise the hardest structures of the human body and as such, once fully formed, change little throughout life. Their resistance to destruction is such that they play a major role in archaeological and forensic studies. Teeth as archaeological remains are well known to survive for thousands, if not millions, of years after the death of the animal of which they were a part.

Despite their apparent indestructibility in relation to physical damage, and the ravages of time as skeletal remains, the teeth are susceptible to chemical damage during life by acid dissolution, the process of which is known as dental caries. This disease has occurred in humans for as long as they have existed. Even in the earliest human skull specimens the teeth show signs of dental decay, albeit of a limited extent, with only one or two cavities occurring in the mouth of an individual. The susceptibility of the teeth to dental caries has therefore always been present, but the prevalence and incidence of the disease has varied. This will be discussed more fully in latter articles, but an understanding of the dental caries process is based upon a knowledge of the structure of the teeth, which is discussed in this article in

overall terms of the teeth and the components that make up a tooth.

Teeth

In all mammals there are two sets of teeth; in humans a primary (baby) or deciduous set of 20 teeth is replaced between the ages of 6 and 12 by a secondary or permanent set of up to 32 teeth.

Primary Teeth

The primary teeth are laid down *in utero* and commence calcification at or immediately after birth. The first teeth to erupt are usually the incisors at about 6 months of age and the final primary teeth to come into the mouth are the second molars between the ages of 2 and 3 years.

The primary teeth have the same basic structure as the permanent teeth, i.e. enamel, dentine, cementum and pulpal (nerve) tissue. However, the overall morphology of a primary tooth does differ somewhat from the permanent successor. The major difference lies in the crown, particularly of the primary molars, which are more bulbous. The bulbosity is most pronounced on the first primary molar in the lower jaw, or mandible.

The roots of the primary teeth are shorter, smaller and in the molar more curved than the permanent succes-

---

* The colour plate section for this article appears between p. 1146 and p. 1147.

sors. There is therefore less dentine in a primary tooth. As the enamel is also thinner than in permanent teeth, so dental caries progresses through to the nerve faster in primary teeth. Furthermore, as the nerves or pulps of the primary teeth are relatively larger and more prominent, so the risk of abscess, as a result of caries penetrating through to the pulp, is that much greater.

Permanent Teeth

In a full set of permanent teeth there are 32, although not all teeth always develop so that from one to many teeth may be missing. The commonest tooth to be absent is the third molar, or wisdom tooth.

The morphology of the permanent teeth is very similar to the primary teeth, but larger and with much bigger roots relatively to crown size. The enamel is also much thicker. The dentine comprises the bulk of a permanent tooth and becomes thicker with age. This is because, as teeth age, the wear on the outside of the enamel caused by eating slowly removes the enamel. In wearing away the tooth the masticated foods produce a response in the nerve, which is slowly reduced as dentine is produced by the odontoblasts. In time, the nerve can shrink to the extent that the pulp chamber almost disappears. Where a coarse, abrasive diet is used, this process of laying down secondary dentine can occur earlier in life and at a much faster rate.

Structure of Teeth

The differences in the structure between primary and permanent teeth are therefore those of size and thickness. The chemical compositions of the enamel, dentine and cementum of primary and permanent teeth are essentially the same. As the chemistry of their structure affects their subsequent resistance or susceptibility to dental caries, it is appropriate to discuss their structure in detail.

Enamel

Tooth enamel comprises a hard, porcelain-like cap covering the whole of the clinical crown of a primary or permanent tooth. The crown is defined as that part of a tooth which is erupted and is visibly present in the mouth. It is distinct from the anatomic crown, as shown in Plate 18. However, with age, as the tooth continues to erupt, the clinical crown becomes the same as the anatomic crown.

The enamel comprises calcium, phosphate, water (as OH) of a form known as hydroxyapatite $[Ca_{10}(PO_4)_6.2OH]$. This basic chemical structure is widespread in the animal kingdom and is the building block of all calcified tissue. Where enamel is unique is that the percentage of inorganic component making up enamel is higher than any other tissue. Analysis of enamel shows that an average of 98% is made up of the inorganic component, largely the hydroxyapatite. *See* Calcium, Physiology

Developing enamel, which is of ectodermal origin, is composed of up to 18% calcium and heterogeneous proteins. The majority of the developing enamel matrix consists of amelogenin, which is protein-rich. The remainder of the enamel protein is a high-molecular-weight phosphoprotein, known as enamelin. As the enamel continues to develop, the amelogenin is replaced as the enamel calcifies and then matures. During this process over 90% of the amelogenin is removed. If this process does not occur properly, e.g. during some metabolic disorders, then enamel hypoplasia occurs. At a later stage, if calcification does not proceed properly during maturation, hypocalcification results. In both instances, the tooth may be more susceptible to dental caries.

Mature enamel consists of enamel crystallites of the aforementioned hydroxyapatite. These crystallites mature rapidly in width but slowly in thickness. The end result is a crystallite of large size.

The crystallinity of enamel varies depending on its purity and the degree of incorporation of other elements. However, enamel is never a pure substance and always includes other inorganic or organic components during the developmental stage. The main one of interest is fluoride, which may be substituted for part of the hydoxyl ion to form fluorapatite. This is of considerable interest in dentistry as this change produces an enamel which has much greater resistance to acid dissolution. The incorporation of fluoride in the enamel will also provide a reservoir of fluoride ion which plays a role not only in resisting dissolution, but more importantly in remineralization.

The crystallinity is affected not only by incorporation of other ions, but also in surface enamel and in physicochemical ionic exchanges. Posteruptively, these changes in enamel chemistry are notably influenced by the uptake and release of fluoride and a reduction in carbonate. The latter is about 2·5% by weight, compared with calcium at 36% and phosphorus at 18%. However, it is felt that the carbonate component, as it is less stable than pure hydroxyapatite, may lead to a disruption of the enamel crystallinity and probably play an important role in enamel maturation. It is felt that as carbonate is more acid-labile than other components, it is lost during early caries, or may make a high-carbonate enamel more susceptible to acid dissolution.

Enamel is laid down during development by specialized cells called ameloblasts, and if a higher concentration of fluoride is available in the bloodstream, this trace element becomes incorporated by the ameloblasts in the developing enamel. This mechanism is important when discussing the resistance of enamel to dental caries, but also in the formation of mottled enamel associated with high fluoride intake.

As mentioned above, enamel is laid down by ameloblasts by a process of secretion of an enamel matrix, which then becomes calcified. Further calcium and phosphate salts are laid down as the enamel matures prior to and soon after eruption in the mouth. During this period of maturation, the enamel appears to be more susceptible to acid dissolution, demineralization, and the development of carious cavities. The carbonate content of such enamel is high; carbonate is subsequently lost during maturation, but this will be offset by incorporation or the presence of fluoride in the oral environment.

The enamel surface of the outermost layers of 10 μm are of a slightly different histological structure. During the formation of the enamel the ameloblasts lay down an outer 'surface layer' of different, higher mineral composition. If an increased level of fluoride is incorporated in this layer then that tooth will have a greater resistance to subsequent decay. Even during the process of early demineralization this 'surface zone' remains intact, probably by a process of continuous remineralization by inorganic ions released from the inner layers of enamel as it dissolves. During the early stages of demineralization (caries), when the inner layers of enamel are dissolved, the outer layer retains its structure but becomes whitish in appearance when seen clinically. This is known as a 'white spot' or 'incipient caries' and it is the first clinical sign of decay, but can be reversed by remineralization. The rate at which demineralization occurs, will depend not only on the level and frequency of acid attack, but also on the resistance of the enamel. This in turn will depend on the degree of mineralization, maturation, and fluoride and carbonate content.

Dentine

The major part of a tooth is dentine (Plate 18). The structure is laid down by cells called odontoblasts, which secrete tubules of dentine from the junction with the enamel to the nerve or pulp of the tooth. The odontoblasts are mesenchymal in origin and the structure they lay down has a lower level of mineralization, as well as smaller crystallites than enamel.

The dentine differs from the enamel in composition, being only 79% inorganic, although this inorganic material is the same hydroxyapatite as in the enamel and resembles bone in composition. The higher organic component consists of collagen type I, making up the walls of the dentine tubules and the dentine process in the centre of the dentinal tubules.

Unlike enamel, dentine has an innervation by means of nerve endings located at the pulpal end of the dentinal tubules. It is for this reason that pain is experienced when dentine is exposed in the mouth. This exposure may occur as part of the carious process when weak or undermined enamel breaks away to form a cavity. Alternatively, when a cavity is drilled by a dentist, in the process of removing decay, the sensitive dentine is cut, also causing pain unless some form of anaesthesia is used.

Because of the higher organic content of the dentine the process of dental decay is somewhat different to that of the enamel. While the caries in enamel is almost entirely a chemical dissolution by acids produced by bacteria, such as *Streptococcus mutans*, a secondary process of proteolytic removal of the collagen occurs in dentinal caries.

Although most dental caries originates with dissolution of the enamel, the structure of the teeth is such that should the gingival tissues or gums recede then the neck of the tooth may be exposed. If this occurs dentine is quickly exposed, leading to sensitivity of the tooth and, subsequently, dentinal or root caries. As receding gingiva occurs with age, so root caries is associated with the ageing dentition and is seen mostly in patients over 50 years of age.

Cementum

The dentine of the root of the tooth is covered by a thin layer of cementum (Plate 18). This structure, also of mesenchymal origin, is again composed of inorganic and organic material, but is closer to bone in the proportion of the two components. *See* Bone

Cementum provides a mean of bonding the teeth into the bony sockets of the jaws by means of strands of collagen, known as periodontal fibres. The whole root is surrounded by many of these fibres, attaching the tooth to the bone, and providing a system of 'elastic bands', or a hydraulic system, so that the tooth can be pressed deeper into its socket under biting forces. This mechanism takes up heavy forces on the tooth without them being transferred directly to the bone, which would be very uncomfortable on biting.

The cementum may break down as part of the dental caries process or during gum disease, or be worn away by excessively hard tooth brushing. Because of its lower inorganic content, its resistance to decay or wear is far less than either enamel or dentine and, if exposed ,it can wear away quite quickly.

Bibliography

Nikiforuk G (1985) *Understanding Dental Caries: 1. Etiology and Mechanisms. Basic and Clinical Aspects.* Basel: Karger.
Thylstrup A and Fejerskov O (1986) *Textbook of Cariology* 1st edn. Copenhagen: Munksgaard.

M. E. J. Curzon and M. S. Duggal
University of Leeds, Leeds, UK

Aetiology of Dental Caries

Dental caries or tooth decay is a pathological process of localized destruction of tooth tissues. It is a form of progressive loss of enamel, dentine and cementum initiated by microbial activity at the tooth surface. Loss of tooth substances is preceded by a partial dissolution of mineral ahead of the total destruction of the tissue. It is because of this characteristic that dental caries can be differentiated from other destructive processes of the teeth, such as abrasion through mechanical wear and erosion by acid fluids.

Current Concepts of Caries Aetiology

There is overwhelming evidence that the initial phase of dental caries involves demineralization of the tooth enamel by localized high concentrations of organic acids. These acids are produced by the fermentation of common dietary carbohydrates by bacteria that accumulate in dental plaque on the teeth. This concept of dental caries aetiology is based essentially on the interplay of four principal factors: a susceptible host (the tooth), microflora with an acidogenic potential, a suitable substrate available locally to the pathodontic bacteria (carbohydrate) and a fourth important dimension, time (Fig. 1). Because of the multiplicity of factors which influence the initiation and progression of dental caries it is often referred to as a disease of a 'multifactorial aetiology', an old but appropriate descripton. In this article the role of microflora and the host susceptibility are discussed. The role of carbohydrates in the diet is discussed later. *See* Carbohydrates, Digestion, Absorption and Metabolism; Carbohydrates, Requirements and Dietary Importance

The Role of Microorganisms

Considerable difference of opinion exists within the dental research community as to which microorganisms cause dental caries and whether indeed a specific strain of bacteria is responsible in its causation. However, there is evidence that microorganisms, which accumulate in dental masses (dental plaque) on the teeth, cause fermentation of dietary carbohydrates, producing organic acids which cause demineralization of the tooth enamel. This concept is a combination of Miller's acidogenic theory of 1889 and that of dental plaque introduced by Williams in 1897. Subsequent research has supported this original view and the evidence implicating oral microorganisms in the aetiology of dental caries is summarized below:

1. Germ-free animals do not develop dental caries.

2. Addition of penicillin to the diet of rats prevents caries.
3. Plaque bacteria can demineralize enamel *in vitro* when incubated with dietary carbohydrates.
4. Microorganisms can be found invading carious enamel and dentine.
5. Animals in which diet or dietary carbohydrates are delivered directly into the stomach through a tube do not develop caries.

Role of Dental Plaque

Dental plaque is the name given to the aggregations of bacteria and their products which accumulate on the tooth surface. Plaque collects rapidly in the mouth although the actual rate of formation varies from one individual to another. When plaque accumulates on the crowns of teeth the natural, smooth, shiny appearance of the enamel is lost and a dull, matt effect is produced. As it builds up, masses of plaque become more readily visible to the naked eye. In direct smears, the early plaque is dominated by cocci and rods, most of which are Gram-positive. In the mature plaque (after about 7 days) the percentage of cocci in the plaque decreases rapidly and filaments and rods constitute about 50% of organisms in plaque. The ecological term for this shift from a predominantly coccal type in the beginning to a predominantly mixed, filamentous flora a few days later is 'bacterial succession'.

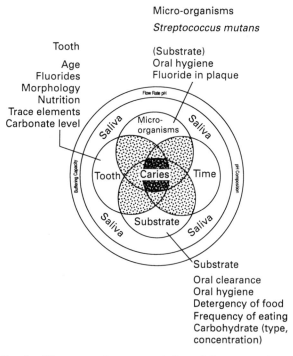

Fig. 1 Diagrammatic representation of the parameters involved in the carious process. All factors must be acting concurrently for caries to develop.

Table 1. Factors influencing pH of dental plaque

Carbohydrates	Saliva	Plaque
Quantity of intake	Flow rate	Bacterial mass
Frequency of intake	Buffer capacity	Bacterial composition
Retentiveness	Other factors, e.g. urea, ammonia	Acid production
Modifying effects of other ingredients of foodstuffs		Acid tolerance
		Acid retention

There is no doubt that the presence of plaque is required for caries development in humans. The best available evidence suggests that a carious lesion results from the action of bacterial metabolic end products localized to the enamel surface by dental plaque. It is therefore the acidity generated by the microorganisms in the plaque after exposure to carbohydrates that is directly responsible for causing demineralization. This is under the influence of many factors.

Regulators of Plaque Acidity

Various parameters have been studied for their effect on plaque acidity, and hence their effect on caries; these are listed in Table 1. The role of saliva will be discussed later, and carbohydrates as regulators of plaque pH are discussed elsewhere.

Bacterial Mass in relation to Caries

Plaque is required for caries initiation, although the relationship between the plaque quantity and dental caries activity is unclear. Some earlier studies, using a crude methodology, showed a positive correlation between caries increment and oral hygiene, but more controlled investigations failed to establish this finding. Many individuals remain caries-free in spite of an unfavourable oral hygiene. This lack of a clear-cut relationship between amount of plaque and dental caries suggests that plaques vary in their microbial composition and, although present in equal amounts, might vary in their cariogenicity. Impressive evidence indicates that the qualitative nature of the plaque flora determines the metabolism and the potential for caries production. This view has been referred to in the literature as the *specific plaque hypothesis*.

Bacterial Composition of Plaque and Caries

Most published data on gnotobiotic animals have concentrated on the cariogenic potential of streptococci, especially *Streptococcus mutans*. However, several organisms have been found capable of inducing carious lesions when used as monocontaminants in gnotobiotic rats. These include *S. mutans*, *S. salivarius*, *S. sanguis*, *S. milleri*, *Lactobacillus acidophilus*, *Peptostreptococcus intermedius*, *Actinomyces viscosus* and *A. naeslundii*. However, not all organisms are equally cariogenic. Table 2 shows the acidogenicity and acid tolerance of plaque bacteria. In evaluating data shown in Table 2 it should be noted that the final pH represents the pH observed after incubation of pure bacterial cultures in broth with excess carbohydrates. Table 2 also indicates the tolerance of bacterial systems of plaque to acid. Though these data do not reveal the rate at which acid is produced or the pH at which growth ceases, they give some insight into the relative acidogenic, i.e. cariogenic, potential of plaque bacteria.

Bacterial Specificity and Dental Caries

Investigations into the relationship between various plaque organisms and dental caries have mainly focused on streptococci, lactobacilli and filamentous bacteria.

Table 2. Acidogenicity and acid tolerance of some plaque bacteria

	pH				Initiation of growth
	<4·0	4·1–4·5	4·6–5·0	>5·0	
Streptococcus mutans	+	+			5·2
S. sanguis		+	+		5·2–5·6
S. salivarius	+	+			5·2
S. mitis		+	+		5·2–5·6
Lactobacillus	+	+			<5·0
Actinomyces			+	+	?
Enterococci		+	+	+	?

Adapted from Van Houte J (1980).

Streptococci

Studies of *S. mutans* strongly suggest its active involvement in the initiation and progression of dental caries. Members of this species are nonmotile, catalase-negative, Gram-positive cocci. On *mitis salivarius* agar they grow as highly convex colonies. When cultured with sucrose they form polysaccharides which are insoluble. This property of forming insoluble polysaccharides from sucrose is regarded as an important characteristic contributing to the caries-inducing properties of the species. *Streptococcus mutans* can invariably be isolated from incipient lesions as well as lesions that have cavitated on pits and fissures, approximal and smooth surfaces. It can also be isolated with highest frequency from plaque over carious lesions, and the isolation frequency decreases when the samples are taken further away from the lesions.

Streptococcus sanguis is also one of the predominant groups of streptococci which colonize the tooth surface. Evidence suggests that caries from this strain is significantly less extensive than that from *S. mutans* and occurs primarily in pits and fissures, whereas *S. mutans* causes smooth surface caries as well.

It would therefore appear that *S. mutans* is the most cariogenic of the family of streptococci. Its cariogenicity is attributed to several important properties:

1. It synthesizes insoluble polysaccharides from sucrose.
2. It colonizes all tooth surfaces.
3. It is a homofermentative producer of lactic acid.
4. It is more acidogenic than other streptococci.

Lactobacilli

Lactobacilli have also been implicated in the aetiology of dental caries for many decades. Although a few studies have suggested their involvement in the initiation of caries, they are most often found in large numbers in carious cavities. This and the fact that lactobacilli have a relatively low affinity for the tooth surface suggest that they might have a more important role to play in the progression rather than initiation of dental caries.

Filamentous Bacteria

Filamentous bacteria, especially actinomycetes, have been found to be associated with root surface caries. *Actinomyces viscosus*, an acidogenic bacterium, is almost always isolated from plaques overlying root lesions. The role of *A. viscosus* in the initiation of root lesions is difficult to assess because they are often predominant on the sound root surfaces in subjects experiencing and resisting root caries. More definitive studies are needed to determine the association of *A. viscosus* and root caries.

It must be remembered that most of the microorganisms implicated in dental caries aetiology are indigenous organisms and exist in a dynamic relationship with the host. Disease is not a necessary outcome of this association but it may ensue when the balance is greatly disturbed. With *S. mutans* this may occur, for example, when its numbers on teeth are increased owing to a higher or more frequent consumption of carbohydrates.

The Host Factors

Saliva

Saliva significantly influences the carious process. For example, removal of the salivary glands of hamsters greatly enhanced the caries activity when they were fed a high-sucrose diet. Human studies have demonstrated the same results and have shown that if the exposure of teeth to saliva is restricted by blocking the opening of the salivary glands the pH values of plaque, after exposure to carbohydrates, are lower.

Salivary Flow and Caries Rate

Humans suffering from xerostomia or decreased secretion of saliva as a consequence of a pathological condition such as sarcoidosis, Sjogren's syndrome, etc., often experience a higher rate of caries. The tooth destruction as a result of desalivation is typically quite rapid. Rampant caries has been demonstrated in patients who have been treated by radiotherapy to the head and neck as irradiation of the salivary glands leads to decreased salivary flow and usually leads to extensive caries in the cervical region of the teeth. These observations have led to the conclusion that saliva is in some way important to maintain the integrity of the tooth substance.

Salivary Buffering and Dental Caries

Saliva contains bicarbonate–carbonic acid and phosphate buffer systems. The buffering capacity acquired by saliva by the virtue of these ion systems tends to correct pH changes caused by concentration changes of acidic ions produced by fermentation of carbohydrates. A typical reaction of plaque to carbohydrate challenge is an immediate drop in plaque pH followed by a gradual rise to the resting value. However, if plaque and teeth are isolated from the influence of saliva the pH of plaque drops further and remains low for prolonged periods. Thus the buffering capacity of saliva is an important factor in reducing the time the tooth enamel is exposed to the acidogenic challenge.

Other Protective Factors in Saliva

Saliva contains a number of factors of glandular origin, including lysosymes and a peroxidase system. Interest has also been focused on the immunological aspect of caries, and specific IgA (immunoglobulin A) antibodies to *S. mutans* have been detected in saliva by immune assays. The concentration of secretory IgA in whole saliva has been reported to be significantly less in subjects with a high caries rate as compared with those with a lower caries experience. Although substantial evidence suggests that the aforementioned factors form an antibacterial system in saliva, the extent to which they contribute to caries resistance of the host is not yet clear. *See* Immunity and Nutrition

Tooth

Tooth Morphology and Dental Caries

A susceptible host is one of the factors which is required for caries to occur. The morphology of the tooth has long been known to be one of the major determinants of its susceptibility. Clinical observations have suggested that pits and fissures of posterior teeth are highly susceptible to caries. This is thought to result from impaction of food and microorganisms in the fissures which are also difficult to reach with routine oral hygiene aids. An interesting observation is that there is a positive correlation between the depth of the fissures and caries susceptibility.

It has also been observed that certain surfaces of a tooth are more prone to caries than other surfaces. For example, the occlusal surface and the buccal surface of the lower first permanent molar are more likely to develop caries as compared with the lingual, mesial or the distal surfaces, probably because of the presence of the fissures on the occlusal surfaces and the buccal pit on the buccal surface. Similarly an intraoral variation in the susceptibility to caries exists between different teeth. The caries susceptibility by tooth type, in descending order, is as follows: first permanent molar, second permanent molar, second premolar, upper incisor, first premolar with the lower incisors and canines least likely to develop caries.

Arch Morphology and Caries

Irregularities in the arch form and imbrication of the teeth also favour the development of caries. It has been shown experimentally that enamel in stagnation areas is more likely to develop demineralization, which is manifested as white spot lesions.

Tooth Composition and Dental Caries

It is well known that the surface enamel is more resistant to caries attack than the subsurface. This is attributed to a higher concentrtaion of fluoride and other trace metals, such as zinc and lead, which are thought to protect the surface enamel from demineralization. It is because of this that dental caries is often said to be subsurface in origin. Although there is plenty of evidence to support the direct relationship between the fluoride content of the surface layer of enamel and its resistance to caries attack, the relationship of other trace elements is unclear and still being investigated.

Bibliography

Newbrun E (1979) *Cariology*, 2nd edn. Baltimore: Williams and Wilkins.
Silverstone LM, Johnson NW, Hardie JM and Williams RAD (1981) *Dental Caries – Aetiology, Pathology and Prevention.* London: Macmillan.
Thylstrup A and Fejerskov O (1986) *Textbook of Cariology* 1st edn. Copenhagen: Munksgaard.
Van Houte J (1980) Bacterial specificity in the etiology of dental caries. *International Dental Journal* 30: 305–325.

M. S. Duggal and M. E. J. Curzon
University of Leeds, Leeds, UK

Role of Diet

The driving force for the development of preventive dentistry and its effective use in patient management has been the expanding understanding of the disease of dental caries itself. As already discussed, dental caries is now recognized as a disease of altered ecology in which the host, oral microflora and diet interact to present a challenge too strong for the normal defence mechanisms. It is wrong, however, to regard caries as a simple, continuing acid demineralization of the tooth enamel. Although teeth may be frequently exposed to acid environment, caries does not always arise as it is a result of a dynamic interaction of demineralization and remineralization. These are under the influence of a whole range of both cariogenic and protective factors (Fig. 1). It is clear from this model that diet forms a part of a large spectrum of aetiological factors involved in the caries process. Sugar and other fermentable carbohydrates in the diet constitute an essential aspect of cariogenic potential of food, with other factors, such as the frequency of intake, retentiveness and buffering potential of foods, also playing an important part. These are in addition to the tooth structure, saliva flow and composition and the presence of oral bacteria. This article is concerned with the discussion of the dietary considerations related to the aetiology of dental caries.

The Role of Diet in the Aetiology of Dental Caries

Epidemiological studies have been used to try to establish the relationship of various types of diets and dietary components to caries incidence. Circumstantial evidence linking sucrose consumption and prevalence of dental caries can be readily found in several epidemiological surveys. For example, the prevalence of caries among the native population of Tristan da Cunha, and among Eskimos and Australian Aborigines, was low before Western-type food was introduced into their diets. Controlled human studies, mostly on institutionalized subjects, also indicated that sucrose-containing diets were cariogenic. *See* Sucrose, Dietary Sucrose and Disease

It is well known that when eating foods containing fermentable carbohydrates the pH of plaque drops, implying localized generation of acid. The drop in the pH is the result of fermentation carbohydrates by the plaque bacteria, producing lactic and other organic acids, and is followed by a gradual return to the resting or near resting pH. This recovery depends on a number of factors, including the buffering potential of plaque and the food, retention or the rapidity of clearance from the mouth. The whole cycle of pH drop and recovery was first described by Stephan in 1940 and is commonly known as the Stephan curve (Fig. 2). *See* Carbohydrates, Digestion, Absorption and Metabolism; Carbohydrates, Requirements and Dietary Importance

It is agreed that foods which produce a pH drop below pH 5·5, known as critical pH, are considered detrimental

to teeth. The pH value 5·5 is considered 'critical' because it is thought that enamel demineralization occurs below this point. Some authors regard values below 5·7 as being cariogenic. Foods giving a pH drop between 5·5 and 6·0 are also dubious. This form of ranking is referred to as 'relative potential cariogenicity'. Of greater importance is the relative cariogenic potential of foods compared with known foods of high cariogenicity (sucrose) and low cariogenicity (sorbitol), as agreed at the international conference on cariogenicity of foods at San Antonio in 1985.

Edgar *et al.* (1975) using the plaque harvesting method, removed a representative sample of plaque from human mouths before and after consumption of foods, and the pH response of that plaque was assessed. The response followed a typical Stephan curve and the potential acidogenicity of the foods was compared by measuring the minimum pH recorded and the area enclosed by the curve under the resting pH value. Acidogenicity in a range of snack foods is assessed in Table 1. Interestingly, some foods which are perceived to be 'better for teeth' actually fare quite badly in such a ranking, compared with foods traditionally thought of as 'bad for teeth', such as chocolate.

This study bore out the work of Rugg-Gunn *et al.* (1978), who demonstrated that ingestion of chocolate or even apples resulted in a similar pH response. Later work by Edgar *et al.* (1981), using the same test procedure, also showed that a wide range of foods containing either sugar or starches, or combinations thereof, are potentially acidogenic and thus possibly cariogenic.

It is important to note that the *concentration* of fermentable carbohydrate in a food does not affect the

---

Total cariogenic load

Carbohydrates
Retention/clearance
Frequency
Cariostatic factors
Buffering

Demineralization

Sound enamel → Dental caries

Remineralization

Total protective factors

Salivary components
Host susceptibility
Fluorides
Fissure sealants
Oral hygiene

Fig. 1 A dynamic model of caries.

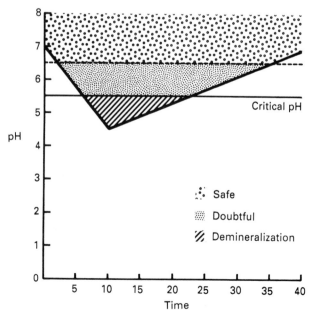

Fig. 2 A typical Stephan's curve.

Table 1. Acidogenic potential of carious snack foods (US) grouped by category and acidogenicity

Group	Beverages	Fruit, etc.	Baked goods	Sweets
Least acidogenic	Milk Chocolate milk	Peanuts Crisps Apple	Bread and butter Graham crackers	Caramels Sugared gum Chocolate Liquorice Sugarless gum
	Carbonated beverages Apple juice Orange juice	Banana Dates Raisins Sweetened cereal	Cream-filled cakes Sandwich cookies Doughnut Bread and jam Whole-wheat bread Plain sweet biscuits/Cakes Apple pie Chocolate Graham Angel food cake	Orange jellies Rock candy Clear mints
Most acidogenic				Sourballs Fruit gums Fruit Lollipops

After Edgar WM (1981).

pH drop in the mouth, although the period of time taken to return to normal pH levels may be related to concentration. This return to resting pH is as much related to the buffering capacity of the saliva or plaque, buffering capacity of the foods and the physical properties of the food itself. The retentiveness, and hence clearance rate, of a food is therefore an important determinant of the cariogenic potential of that food. The concentration of a single ingredient of a food has little relation to the cariogenicity; it is the ability of the whole food to promote caries that is important.

Tests for Cariogenicity of Foods

Animal experiments have been used to rank different foods in the order of their cariogenicity. In one such study a selection of human snack foods was ranked by their 'cariogenic potential index' (CPI) by feeding laboratory rats via a gastric tube, thus bypassing the mouth. Sucrose was used as a reference food and given a CPI of 1·0. Foods with a score of less than 1·0 were considered less cariogenic than sucrose, while those with a score above 1·0 were thought to be more cariogenic. Interestingly, the concentration of sucrose in a breakfast cereal made little or no difference to the CPI. The results, given in Table 2, show that potato chips (crisps) actually score higher than chocolate bars. Comparable results were obtained by Navia et al. (1983). It is clear from

Table 2. Selected rankings of cariogenic potential index (CPI) in rats using human food as snacks

Food tested	CPI
Sucrose	1·0
Filled chocolate cookie	1·4
Cereal (14% sucrose)	1·1
Cereal (8% sucrose)	1·0
Cereal (60% sucrose)	0·9
Coated chocolate candy	0·9
Potato chips	0·8
Caramel	0·7
Chocolate bar	0·7
Cereal (2% sucrose)	0·5
Starch	0·5
Sucrose plus 5% Dical	0·4
No meals by mouth	0·0

After Bowen WH et al. (1980).

most of these experiments that any foodstuff containing carbohydrate has the potential to cause significant amounts of acid to be produced at certain sites in the dentition, which can be followed by demineralization of the enamel and subsequent caries. However, it must be remembered that not all occasions of a drop in plaque pH are accompanied by demineralization of the enamel. This has prompted many investigators to question the significance of acid production as a measure of the cariogenicity of the foods. It has also been shown that the total amount of titratable acid produced by the foods does not neccessarily parallel the amount of enamel it will dissolve. It is now well accepted that the cariogenic potential of a food is influenced by a number of other factors, including the ability of the foods to remain in the oral cavity and, in some cases, the sequence of food intake. Thus studies on the relationship between food and dental caries should consider not only foods in themselves but also their relationship with other items of diet with regard to their nature, timing and order of usage.

Cariostatic Factors in Food

Some components of foods may be cariostatic. Proteins may assist remineralization of enamel or reduce the rate of crystal dissolution. Some fatty acids have been shown to reduce caries in rat studies while phosphates have been shown to have a marked protective effect. Inorganic phosphates have been demonstrated to have a protective influence when added to a cariogenic diet. Organic phosphates such as phytates and glycerophosphates also have a cariostatic action and are thought to reduce the cariogenicity of diets. Although the exact mechanism of action is unknown, studies have indicated that it might be a local modifying influence in the oral cavity, rather than a systemic effect through ingestion. The local effects of phosphates can be attributed to various properties:

1. Phosphates are good buffers; thus they can buffer organic acids produced by plaque flora.
2. Phosphates are known to reduce the rate of dissolution of hydroxyapatite.
3. Phosphates can desorb proteins from the enamel surface; thus they can possibly have a modifying influence on acquired pellicle.

The protection afforded by fluoride is well documented and has led some researchers to refer to dental caries as a fluoride deficiency disease. These materials are all components of various foods. Furthermore, some cariostatic agents have been isolated from cereals and cocoa and these factors may all influence the level of caries caused. Accordingly the level of fermentable carbohydrate in a food will not be *directly* related to the degree of caries caused.

Food Retention

Tests carried out by Bibby (1981) illustrated that, contrary to popular opinion, foods that are perceived to be 'sticky', such as caramel, tend to clear from the oral

Table 3. Representative figures (mg) for food retention in mouth after eating

Food	Food retention (mg) after:		
	5 min	15 min	30 min
Peanuts	4·9	3·3	2·6
Dentyne gum	5·0	3·9	3·1
7-Up	6·3	2·4	2·1
Chocolate milk	7·4	3·8	1·9
Potato chip	12·3	4·9	2·5
White bread	16·1	10·0	3·6
Raisins	16·8	5·7	3·0
Sponge cake	18·8	6·0	4·2
Caramel	19·0	4·2	2·5
Milk chocolate	19·0	6·8	3·0
Cracker (oil-sprayed)	23·8	8·5	3·7
Hard mint	31·9	9·4	2·5
Cracker (plain)	33·6	10·4	3·3
Sandwich cookie	35·0	8·4	4·9

After Bibby BG (1981).

cavity faster than many other foods considered cariogenic. As Table 3 shows, after 15 min, white bread was retained in higher quantities in the oral cavity than cake, chocolate or hard mint. After 30 min, there was more residue from raisins than from caramel. Raisins have been consistently shown to be highly cariogenic.

Beverages, which are perceived to clear quickly from the mouth, actually sustain a low pH level for the same period as a 'sticky' confectionery. In a recent study a range of fruit drinks which were advertised as 'sugar-free' or as 'no added sugar' were assessed on the basis of their ability to drop the pH of plaque. It was found that the fact that most of these drinks had little natural sugar (sucrose) did not affect their ability to drop the pH of plaque; when compared with a standard 10% sucrose rinse they were equally acidogenic. This was attributed to the presence of natural sugars – fructose and glucose – in these drinks. These so-called 'natural sugars' are also fermentable by oral bacteria and their presence instead of sucrose does not render the drinks any safer for teeth. In fact, when the fruit drinks were compared with 10% sucrose it was obvious that the pH recovery was slower after consumption of fruit drinks and the pH remained below 5·5 for a longer time (Fig. 3). This is because of an inherent buffering potential of fruit drinks which gives them an ability to resist any attempts by saliva to buffer the acid. These drinks can therefore be deemed to be more cariogenic than a pure 10% sucrose solution. This research highlighted the fact that the concentration of sugars alone is not the sole determinant of the acidogenicity, and hence cariogenicity, and other factors discussed above are equally important. *See* Carbohydrates, Metabolism of Sugars

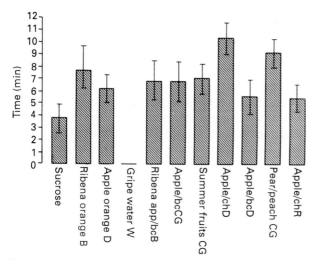

Fig. 3 Bar graph showing mean time spent below pH 5·5 for fruit drinks compared with a 10% sucrose rinse.

Eating Pattern and Frequency

On a population level, the average amount of sucrose consumed per capita relates to the average level of caries in the population. However, more detailed studies show the relationship to be less consistent and of low statistical significance. In the classical study often referred to as the Vipeholm study, inmates of a Swedish Medical Institute were fed increased sucrose or other foods in different patterns and caries experience was monitored. Groups of patients receiving high levels of sucrose (up to 330 g per day) with their meals experienced minimal increase in caries. But if smaller quantities of sucrose were consumed between meals, very high levels of caries ensued. The relationship was not therefore between quantity of sucrose and caries but rather frequency of intake and caries experience. This relationship, which has been confirmed in human and animal research, sheds light on why population studies do not demonstrate a clear and consistent relationship between sugar consumption and caries. For example, long-term diet–caries studies carried out in the UK showed that statistical correlation of sugar concentration to caries was 0·16 and explained only 4% of the caries variance.

Experience from primitive and developing cultures with little access to sucrose but abundant access to starch is often cited as evidence that sucrose and not starch results in dental caries. This evidence purports to be strengthened by the fact that introduction of Western diet (including sucrose) immediately results in development of dental caries. It can be argued that introduction of a Western diet is accompanied by increased affluence and an altered eating pattern. Such changes also include differences in the use of cooked starches as much as differences in use of sucrose. Frequency of intake of any food increases dramatically, along with the potential

incidence of dental caries. It is also interesting to note that caries has been shown to be associated with a diet consisting of sago starch, as in the Sepik villages in Papua New Guinea.

Sugars and their Role in Caries

In Western society, eating frequency has generally increased and snacking has become an accepted aspect of life. This change took place over a long period of the nineteenth and early twentieth centuries when the incidence of dental caries increased. However, in the past 20 years while the sucrose usage has not changed, dental caries has dramatically decreased. In the case of 5-year-olds, the percentage with tooth decay fell from 73% in 1973 to 48% in 1983.

Reducing the frequency of eating just one of these foods, or reducing the concentration of sugars in a food, is unlikely to have a significant effect on the incidence of caries as nearly all foods contain some fermentable carbohydrate. It has been assumed tacitly both by practising dentists and by too many dental investigators that the cariogenicity of an individual food is directly proportional to its content of sucrose of other fermentable carbohydrates. There is no quantitative data to support this belief. The effects of high sucrose concentrations in increasing the rate of food clearance of some foods from the mouth and in inhibiting the fermentation process make it seem improbable that high sugar content of itself would be particularly damaging to teeth. The Vipeholm study has been mentioned as evidence for the cariogenicity of sucrose, although investigators have questioned the reliability of a single clinical study from a mental institute. There are a number of contradictory studies that have not been widely recognized. For example, King et al. (1955), studying English children, found that they could substantially increase sugar as sucrose in the children's diet without increasing the incidence of caries.

It is the frequency of consumption rather than the amount consumed which is associated positively with dental caries incidence. Considering the already substantial decline in the incidence of dental caries in the West, where frequency of eating has generally increased, and given the fact that dietary manipulation is difficult to achieve, it is reasonable to assume that alternative preventive measures such as the use of fluoride would be more effective in prevention of caries. It would be unfortunate if the public hopes were raised to believe that dietary control alone would solve the problem of dental caries.

Bibliography

Bibby BG (1981) Foods and dental caries. In: Hefferren JJ (ed.) *Foods, Nutrition and Dental Health*, vol. 1, pp 257–278. Illinois: Pathotox.

Bowen WH, Amsbaugh SM, Monnel-Torrens S *et al.* (1980) A method to assess cariogenic potential of foodstuffs. *Journal of the American Dental Association* 100: 677–681.

Duggal MS and Curzon MEJ (1989) An evaluation of the cariogenic potential of baby and infant fruit drinks. *British Dental Journal* 160: 327–330.

Edgar WM, Bibby BG, Mundorff S and Rowley J (1975) Acid production in plaques after eating snacks: modifying factors in foods. *Journal of the American Dental Association* 90: 418–425.

Edgar WM (1981) Plaque pH assessments related to food cariogenicity. In: Hefferren JJ (ed.) *Foods Nutrition and Dental Health*, vol. 1, pp 137–150. Illinois: Pathotox.

Gustafsson BE, Quensel CE, Lanke LS *et al.* (1954) The effect of different levels of carbohydrate intake on caries activity in 436 individuals observed for five years. The Vipeholm Dental Caries Study. *Acta Odontologica Scandinavica* 11: 232–364.

King JD, Mellanby M, Stones HH and Green HN (1955) The effect of sugar supplement on dental caries in children. MRC Special Report Series, No. 288. London: Her Majesty's Stationery Office.

Navia JM *et al.* (1983) Nutrition in oral health and disease. In: Stallard RE (ed.) *A Textbook of Preventive Dentistry*, pp 90–146. Philadelphia: WB Saunders.

Rugg-Gunn AJ, Edgar WM and Jenkins GN (1978) The effect of eating some British snacks upon the pH of human dental plaque. *British Dental Journal* 145: 95–100.

Stephan RM (1940) Changes in hydrogen ion concentration on tooth surfaces and in carious lesions. *Journal of the American Dental Association* 27: 718–723.

M. S. Duggal and M. E. J. Curzon
University of Leeds, Leeds, UK

Fluoride in the Prevention of Dental Decay

Since the mid-1940s fluoride has become increasingly important for the prevention of a substantial proportion of dental caries. The major reductions in dental caries incidence reported for the last two decades in several industrialized countries are generally attributed by dental investigators to the widespread use of fluoride.

What is Fluoride?

The element, fluorine, is number 9 in the periodic table, the lightest and most chemically reactive of the four halogen elements. Fluorine is never found in free form in nature because of its high reactivity. It is chemically bound to other elements in various simple and complex forms. The best known are the simple salts, sodium and calcium fluoride, and the more complex fluorophosphates and fluorapatite. In bone mineral, partial replacement of the hydroxyl ion in hydroxyapatite occurs during mineralization. The most common fluorides in the earth's crust are fluorspar (calcium fluoride) and cryolite (sodium aluminum fluoride). Fluoride compounds comprise about 0·1% of the earth's crust and are ubiquitous, albeit in small and varied amounts, in all natural sources of water and foodstuffs.

Fluoride dissolves in water from the rock and soil through which the water percolates. The fluoride concentration of water is dependent upon the fluoride concentration and relative solubility of the compounds in the rock strata.

Fluoride in foods of plant origin is obtained from the soil in which the plants are grown. With rare exceptions, such as tea, food plants do not concentrate fluoride from the soil. Plants grown near industrial sites where fluoride in particulate form is produced in the airborne effluent, may have measurable amounts of fluoride deposited on their leaves. Such concentrations may be sufficiently high to be toxic for grazing animals. Fluoride concentrations in animal tissues, especially in bones, are proportional to the amount of fluoride consumed.

History of Fluoride and Human Health

Fluoride was observed in bones and teeth in 1805, decades before fluorine was isolated in pure form. In 1901, a dentist in the US consulate in Naples, Italy, described discolorations of tooth enamel in older applicants for visas. This condition, which became known as mottled enamel, was absent in younger individuals and was attributed to a change in the water supply before the teeth in these younger individuals had formed. Mottled enamel was also evident in several portraits painted in that area in preceding decades.

In subsequent years numerous descriptions of mottled enamel were published in the USA and other countries. Experiments with rats, as well as human epidemiological studies, indicated that the cause of mottled enamel was ingestion of excess fluoride from communal water during tooth development. The condition is also called chronic endemic dental fluorosis, or simply dental fluorosis; it is related to protein removal from the matrix of enamel and to mineralization during tooth development.

Until the cause of mottled enamel was identified, numerous investigators suggested that teeth with mottled enamel were no more susceptible to dental caries than normal teeth. In 1928, however, clear evidence was provided that dental caries was particularly rare in the children of Minonk, Illinois; the teeth of these children had mild evidence of mottled enamel.

In the late 1930s and early 1940s, surveys on mottled enamel and dental caries in permanent teeth among teenage children in numerous communities in Illinois clearly established that the higher the level of fluoride in the communal water supply, the lower the number of decayed, missing and filled (DMF) teeth in a dose-related response up to a fluoride concentration of approximately 1·2 ppm. Children who did not reside in these communities during tooth development, but had moved from low-fluoride communities had higher numbers of DMF teeth than those whose residence had been continuous. No evidence of mottled enamel was observed among children who moved into high-fluoride communities after tooth development was complete.

Mild degrees of mottled enamel, at optimal fluoride levels in the water supply for caries prevention occurred in a small percentage of the children but were not of aesthetic significance. The manifestations of mottled enamel in these communities were much less severe than had been reported, and reflected the lower levels of fluoride being ingested by these Illinois children in comparison to those ingested by the residents of Naples.

The optimal fluoride concentration in drinking water for the relatively temperate Illinois region was considered to be 1·2 ppm, which was later reduced to 1·0 ppm. In warmer regions, where more water is consumed, the optimal fluoride concentration is proportionately lower. Dental fluorosis prevalence is increasing slightly in the USA but not sufficiently to be of aesthetic concern.

Dental caries reductions reported in various early, epidemiological surveys of areas where optimal fluoride was present in communal water varied from 50% to 65%. The benefits were greatest for smooth surface lesions and least for occlusal lesions. Caries reductions were not limited to children but were reported for middle aged adults who had lived continuously in communities where fluoride had been present in their water during tooth development. Individuals who moved from optimal-fluoride areas to low-fluoride areas had higher DMF scores than those who lived continuously in optimal-fluoride areas. Root caries is also rarer in older individuals in high-fluoride areas.

After many epidemiological surveys and studies with experimental animals, the medical and dental communities in the USA and Canada concluded that fluoride addition to communal water to attain an optimal fluoride level was a safe, inexpensive and worthwhile public health procedure to reduce the occurrence of dental caries.

In 1945 the first three water fluoridation trials were begun. Trial communities in (1) Grand Rapids, Michigan, (2) Newburgh, New York, and (3) Brantford, Ontario, were compared with suitable control communities with low fluoride levels. Reductions in DMF teeth were reported in each trial community. Within 10 years, the DMF values for teeth formed during the trial period were similar to those in communities where optimal fluoride was present from natural sources. Permanent teeth formed before fluoridation was begun had 10–15% DMF reductions.

When these first water fluoridation trials began, the major fluoride source was the water supply. Relatively small additional amounts of fluoride were consumed in foods, which had low and relatively constant fluoride concentrations. Only tea, and bones in canned fish, contributed significantly more fluoride to those who consumed these items. Recent food analyses in the USA have indicated that food fluoride has not increased significantly in the last 40 years.

Fluoride Provision for Human Use

Since the mid-1940s many additional fluoride sources have been introduced. While some were intended as systemic fluoride sources, others were designed for topical use in the mouth, on the assumption that they would not have systemic influences. Inevitably, some products developed for topical use are absorbed through the mouth, or swallowed, contributing to ingested fluoride.

Procedures for fluoride administration include the following:

1. Intended systemic routes: addition of fluoride to municipal or school water supplies to obtain optimal fluoride concentrations for partial prevention of dental caries; and inclusion of higher amounts of fluoride in table salt, provision of appropriate fluoride levels in drops or tablets.
2. Intended topical applications: inclusion of fluorides at relatively high levels in toothpastes and mouthrinses for individual use; and inclusion of fluoride at higher amounts in gels and solutions for application under supervision.

Physiology of Fluoride

Most fluoride provided by a systemic route is absorbed, and rapidly and widely distributed throughout all body tissues, fluids and secretions. Ingested fluoride may exert its influences through one or more systemic routes, or through topical routes, or through some combination of systemic and topical routes. Mineralizing tissues incorporate fluoride actively into the hydroxyapatite which is crystallizing at the time of ingestion. Developing bones and teeth, and remodelling Haversian systems in the long bones, incorporate elevated fluoride levels roughly proportional to the amounts in blood plasma and extracellular and intracellular fluids. Since absorbed fluoride is distributed widely in tissues and fluids, duct saliva and gingival crevicular fluid contain measurable amounts of fluoride. Mixed saliva bathing tooth surfaces contains fluoride from these sources in addition to the fluoride which is passing through the mouth in ingested fluids and foods. As a results, fluoride provided by a systemic route is also available to exert local (topical) effects in the mouth.

Fluoride in the Prevention of Dental Decay

Unabsorbed fluoride, largely attributable to fluoride ingestion in forms which are not readily soluble, is excreted in the faeces. Absorbed fluoride which is not incorporated into tissues is excreted in the urine. Urinary fluoride excretion is highly pH-dependent, with the rate increasing as the urine pH increases. The percentage of ingested fluoride in urine is lower after a steady rate of intake in growing individuals than in adults because of incorporation into mineralizing tissues. When fluoride intake is sharply increased, the proportion of ingested fluoride excreted in the urine is reduced until equilibration with the skeletal system has been attained. When fluoride intake is sharply reduced, higher urinary excretion continues for prolonged periods, indicating that fluoride is being lost from the remodelling skeletal system.

The average fluoride concentrations of enamel and dentine in teeth, developed while the individual is consuming optimal amounts of fluoride, are proportionately higher than for individuals in low-fluoride communities. Dentine fluoride concentrations are routinely two to three times higher than those in enamel, regardless of the amount of fluoride ingested.

Mechanisms of Fluoride Action

This subject is characterized by continuing controversy and little agreement among dental investigators. When the fluoride–dental caries relationship was first recognized, the mechanism of action was considered to be related to the incorporation of increased fluoride levels in enamel and dentine during tooth development. Various hypotheses revolved around the increased fluoride in tooth mineral and especially in the surface layer. The slightly larger and more perfect crystals of hydroxyapatite with higher levels of fluoride were considered to be slightly less soluble in acid. Other investigators believed that the dissolution of these crystals in early carious lesions released sufficient fluoride into the medium to have adverse influences on the metabolic capabilities of the plaque bacteria.

The concept of remineralization of early lesions during periods of microbial quiescence, and the relation of increased fluoride to remineralization, were unknown then. Several recent observations tend to focus attention on the local pathways by which fluoride can act to reduce caries. Saliva contains important, although low, fluoride concentrations; plaque has been shown to contain higher than expected fluoride concentrations, mostly bound; and low fluoride concentrations in mineralizing solutions increase the rate of crystal formation, which probably improves the ability of early carious lesions to remineralize. Low fluoride concentrations inhibit the enzyme enolase and decrease plaque pH after carbohydrate ingestion by as much as 0·1–0·2

units, which represent an appreciable decrease in hydrogen ion concentration since pH is a logarithmic function.

The following observations support the likelihood that systemic pathways are important:

- After initiation of fluoridation of a water system it is several years before maximum caries reduction is observed.
- Cessation of a water fluoridation programme, even in recent years when other fluoride sources are readily available, results in an increase in caries incidence.
- Communities with optimal water fluoride continue to have a lower incidence of caries than communities with low water fluoride.
- Children moving into a community during an optimal water fluoridation trial do not receive the same level of benefit as children residing in the community for the full period.
- Individuals moving from an optimal fluoride community retain some benefits when living in a low fluoride community.

The following observations support the likelihood that local mechanisms of fluoride action are involved.

- Application of fluoride by numerous local (topical) procedures cause significant reductions in dental caries.
- In several countries where widespread caries reductions have been reported in the last 20 years, fluoride was not provided by systemic routes (it is improbable that sufficient fluoride had been absorbed locally or swallowed during topical use of any products to cause the observed reductions).
- Teeth erupted at the time that water fluoridation was initiated were partially protected against caries.
- Topical use of fluoride in communities with water fluoridation resulted in additional caries reductions.

The logical hypothesis is that both systemic and local influences are involved in reduction in dental caries incidence. In view of the complicated interrelationships in dental caries aetiology and fluoride metabolism, the mechanism(s) of action of fluoride may never be precisely defined.

For continuation of the current downward trend in dental caries, which transcends national boundaries, emphasis needs to be maintained on optimal use of fluorides from all sources. However, continued attention must be given to ensure that aesthetically disfiguring levels of mottled enamel are not allowed to occur because of excess fluoride ingestion.

Fluoride in the Prevention of Dental Decay

Benefits and Costs of Fluoride Use

Current Effectiveness of Communal Water Fluoridation

In 1989, the available data for surveys comparing fluoridated and nonfluoridated communities in the previous decade were reviewed. 30–60% less caries in deciduous teeth in fluoridated communities, 20–40% less caries in the mixed dentition (ages 8–12), and 15–35% less caries in adolescents (ages 14–17) and in adults and seniors was reported. Newbran noted the need for lifetime residence in the designated communities and the increasing difficulties of conducting such surveys in view of the high mobility in society and the numerous fluoride sources compared to the 1940s and 1950s. Fluoride benefits have spread to communities which do not have fluoridation of community water supplies because of the availability of numerous fluoride sources other than communal water supplies.

The cost of water fluoridation was reviewed based on existing equipment and found ranges between $0·12 and $1·16 per person per year, with a median value of $0·24 and a mean of $0·49. These values become somewhat higher when costs to replace equipment are included.

Effectiveness of School Water Fluoridation

Fluoridation of school water supplies is appropriate where the community is too small for communal fluoridation, where adamant political opposition prevents fluoridation of the water supply and where the children come from homes with individual water supplies. Since the children are in school for only part of the day and little more than half of the days in a year, the optimal fluoride levels are about 3 to 4·5 times the optimal concentration for communal fluoridation. Caries reductions of about 40% are typical for school water fluoridation.

The cost for school water fluoridation is higher and more variable because of the smaller installations. Based on existing equipment, the costs ranged from $0·85 to $9·88 per child per year, with a mean of $4·60 and a median of $4·29.

Effectiveness of Dietary Fluoride Supplements in School Programmes

Horowitz indicates that reductions of 30%, with a range of 17–69%, have been reported in school-based fluoride tablet programmes. Dosages varied from 0·75 to 2·0 mg of fluoride for 2 to 6 years. The cost of school-based fluoride tablets or drops varied from $0·89 to $5·40 per child per year, with a mean value of $2·53 and a median of $2·26.

Effectiveness of Mouthrinsing with Fluoride Solutions

Nearly 36 mouthrinsing studies were conducted in the past 30 years with various products and protocols, some without placebo controls when the secular rate of dental caries was declining. Most studies reported statistically significant reductions in dental caries. Leverett concludes that at current low caries incidences, reductions of about 0·4 carious surfaces per year can be expected for mouthrinse users of all ages. The direct costs of mouthrinsing programmes range from $0·52 to $1·78 per person per year, with a mean and median of $1·30.

Effectiveness of Professionally Applied and Self-applied Topical Fluoride Gels

In low-fluoride communities caries was reduced about 26% with either a professionally or self-applied fluoride gel. This level of reduction can be expected in communities with fluoridated water supplies with topical gel programmes but the absolute reduction will be lower because of the lower baseline. Gel programmes appear to be especially appropriate for the small percentage of children with high caries susceptibilities and for medically compromised individuals with xerostomia. Costs for topical gel use can be expected to be higher than other programmes because of the costs of the materials and, especially in professionally applied situations, the high personnel costs.

Bibliography

Adler P (ed.) (1970) *Fluorides and Human Health*. Geneva: World Health Organization.

Burt BA (ed.) (1989) Proceedings for the workshop: cost effectiveness of caries control in dental public health. *Journal of Public Health Dentistry* 47: 252–344.

Horowitz HS (ed.) (1991) Symposium on appropriate uses of fluoride in the 90s. *Journal of Public Health Dentistry* 51: 20–63.

Johansen E, Taves DR and Olsen TO (eds) (1979) *Continuation Evaluation of the Use of Fluorides*. American Association for the Advancement of Science Selected Symposium 11. Boulder, Colorado: Westview Press.

McClure FJ (1970) *Water Fluoridation, the Search and the Victory*. Bethesda: United States Department of Health, Education, and Welfare, National Institutes of Health, National Institute of Dental Research.

Murray JJ (ed.) (1986) *Appropriate Uses of Fluoride for Human Health*. Geneva: World Health Organization.

Whitford GM (1989) The metabolism and toxicity of fluoride. *Monographs in Oral Science*, Vol. 13. Basel: Karger.

Whitford GM (ed.) (1990) Joint IADR/ORCA International symposium on fluorides: mechanisms of action and recommendations for use. *Journal of Dental Research* 69 (special issue): 506–835.

James H. Shaw
Harvard School of Dental Medicine, Boston, USA

Fluoride in the Prevention of Dental Decay

DETERGENTS

See Cleaning Procedures in the Factory

DETOXIFICATION

See Plant Toxins

DEXTRAN

Source, Structure and Properties

Dextran is a generic term for a family of glucans made by polymerization of the α-D-glucopyranosyl moiety of sucrose. The responsible enzyme is dextransucrase. The common feature is a preponderance of 1,4-linked α-D-glucopyranosyl units. *See* Sucrose, Properties and Determination

A number of microorganisms produce dextrans with ranges of molecular weights and with structures varying from slightly to highly branched. Commercial dextran is biosynthesized by the nonpathogenic organism *Leuconostoc mesenteroides* NRRL B-512. The basic reaction catalysed by dextransucrase is n sucrose→(α-D-glucopyranosyl unit)$_n$+n D-fructose. Branches arise from position 3 of the glucosyl units. The degree of branching of commercial dextran is about 5%. About 40% of the side-chains are single α-D-glucopyranosyl units; about 45% are two units long, and about 15% contain more than 30 units. The molecular weight of native *L. mesenteroides* NRRL B-512 dextran is 9 million to 500 million daltons. Dextran of lower molecular weight is produced for clinical applications.

Dextran is a very flexible polymer. It differs from other neutral polysaccharides in producing low-viscosity solutions in spite of its high molecular weight and in having very few primary hydroxyl groups.

Food Uses

Many applications of dextrans in the production of foods have been described and patented, but the toxicological studies required to gain approval for food use have not been carried out. As a result, dextrans are not permitted as foodstuff additives in the USA or Europe and have not been considered by the Joint Food and Agriculture Organization/World Health Organization Expert Committee on Foodstuff Additives. The generally recognized as safe (GRAS) status was removed by the US Food and Drug Administration in 1977 because dextran was not being used in foods. The principal potential uses of dextran in foods appear to be related to its capacity to prevent crystallization, retain moisture and provide body.

Dextran formation is detrimental to sugar (sucrose) production, as dextran inhibits crystallization, increases viscosity and, hence, decreases filterability and heat transfer in evaporators, crystallizers, and pans, and results in poor clarification. As a result, dextran formation by contaminating bacteria is to be avoided. Dextranases may also be employed to break down any dextran that is introduced. If approved for use, dextran could be used by confectioners to prevent crystallization of sugar.

Small amounts of dextran, primarily produced by species of *Leuconostoc* and *Lactobacillus*, are likely to be present in fermented foods that originally contained sucrose.

Metabolism

Dextrans are not broken down by human digestive enzymes. They are degraded by enzymes from bacteria in the large intestine and the released glucose can be absorbed as well as fermented anerobically.

Medical and Other Uses

L. mesenteroides NRRL B-512(F) dextran of average molecular weight of 70 000 is used clinically as a plasma volume expander for the treatment of shock or impending shock. The antithrombic effect of a preparation of average molecular weight of 40 000 provides a prophylactic treatment for venous thrombosis and pulmonary emboli. These and other applications reveal that dextrans of various molecular weights can be safely injected into the bloodstream. Strains of *L. mesenteroides* NRRL B12(F) are used for the manufacture of clinical dextrans outside Europe and the USA.

A complex of ferric hydroxide and dextran is used in the treatment of neonatal anaemia in pigs. Dextran sulphate improves photographic emulsions. Dextran and its derivatives can also be used as adjuvants, carriers and stabilizers in cosmetic preparations.

A principal use is in the preparation of gels in bead form for size exclusion, ion exchange and hydrophobic chromatography.

Bibliography

DeBelder AN (1992) Dextran. In: Whistler RL and BeMiller JN (eds) *Industrial Gums*. New York: Academic Press.

J.N. BeMiller
Purdue University, West Lafayette, USA

DEXTRINS

Dextrin is a generic term applied to a variety of products obtained by heating a starch in the presence of small amounts of moisture and an acid. Dextrins are generally classified as white dextrins, yellow (or canary) dextrins and British gums. Each is more water-soluble and produces less viscous solutions or dispersions as compared to the parent starch. Each is produced by combinations of depolymerization, i.e. hydrolysis of glycosidic linkages, and transglycosylation, which produces more highly branched structures and forms glycosidic linkages not found in native starches. Most dextrins are used as adhesives for products such as envelopes, bottle labels and postage stamps. Only a small amount of white dextrin is used in prepared foods. A white dextrin is essentially an acid-thinned starch prepared by heating a dried, acidified starch. *See* Starch, Structure, Properties and Determination

Hydrolytic breakdown products from starch are often characterized by their dextrose equivalency (DE), which is the percentage of reducing power compared to anhydrous D-glucose (dextrose). The DE value is inversely related to molecular size, i.e. the degree of polymerization (DP), and is, thus, an indicator of the degree of hydrolysis. The DE value of anhydrous D-glucose is 100. The DE value of native starch is 0.

Maltodextrins are those products having a DE value of less than 20, generally 5–19. A separate designation of (corn) syrup solids is used by some to designate those products of starch hydrolysis with DE values above 20 that are available as dry powders; in other words, they are dried glucose (corn) syrups.

While dextrins are little used in foods, maltodextrins and (corn) syrup solids are used extensively. Both are produced from starch by hydrolysis only, i.e. without molecular rearrangement (transglycosylation), and are of lower average molecular weight than either dextrins or acid-thinned (thin-boiling) starches, which are slightly depolymerized starches that remain in granular form. The primary difference between thin-boiling starches, maltodextrins and syrups/syrup solids is the degree of depolymerization. The primary difference between dextrins and thin-boiling starches is the method of preparation.

Production

Dextrins are prepared by heating starch moistened with dilute hydrochloric acid until it is cold-water soluble.

Maltodextrins and (corn) syrup solids are prepared in basically the same way as are starch-based glucose syrups (corn syrups in the USA), except that the process is stopped at an earlier stage to keep the DE value low. Depolymerization can be effected with either an acid or an enzyme or by combination treatments. These processes are referred to as acid conversions, enzyme conversions and combination conversions, respectively.

Starch conversion to produce maltodextrins is usually done in a continuous process. A typical process is as follows. A starch slurry is pasted, generally in a jet cooker followed by an atmospheric flash. Conversion (dextrinization, liquefaction) is accomplished with an exceptionally thermostable bacterial α-amylase. Depolymerization is stopped by enzyme inactivation and the pH is adjusted. The solution is filtered, treated with carbon, concentrated and spray dried to give a maltodextrin or (corn) syrup solid preparation. In this process, a starch slurry as obtained from the mill at a concentration of 30–40% dry solids (17–22 Bé) is used; the pH is 6·0–6·5; the temperature for pasting is 105°C; the temperature of conversion is 95–100°C; an α-amylase such as that from *Bacillus licheniformis* or *B. stearothermophilus* is used; the time of pasting is about 5 min; and the time of conversion is 60–120 min.

In a lower-temperature batch process, steam is introduced into a starch slurry for pasting. Conversion is accomplished with a thermostable bacterial α-amylase such as that from *B. subtilis* in the same, stirred tank. In this process, the starch concentration is 30–40% dry solids (17–22 Bé); the pH is 6·0–6·5; the temperature is 80–90°C; and the reaction time is 60–120 min. A debranching enzyme may also be used in this process.

For an acid conversion, a starch slurry is acidified, generally to a pH of about 2. (Both hydrochloric and sulphuric acids are allowed, but the former is preferred because of the preference for sodium chloride in the final product.) The slurry is passed through a jet cooker and converter to paste and dextrinize the starch. Alternatively, the pH can be adjusted after pasting or a starch paste can be converted in a batch process. The degree of hydrolysis, i.e. the DE value, is controlled by the combination of time, temperature and acid concentration. The process is terminated via cooling and neutralization. The resulting liquor is clarified, treated with carbon, concentrated and spray dried. Combinations of acid and enzyme(s) are also used in conversions. Maltodextrins may also be obtained as concentrated solutions but are not often sold as such.

A variety of maltodextrins can be produced. The variables in the process are the starch source, the means of conversion (i.e. the use of an acid and/or an enzyme preparation), and the extent of breakdown (i.e. the DE value of the product). In general, DE values range from 5 to 19; the amount of D-glucose (dextrose) ranges from 0·5 to 3%; and the moisture level is 4–6% (Table 1). As much as 98% of the components can be of DP 3 or higher (Table 2).

Table 1. Typical analysis of maltodextrins (dry weight basis)

Carbohydrate	>99%
Moisture	5–6%
Solution pH	4·5
Ash	0·1–0·5%
Chloride	1500 ppm
Sodium	750 ppm
Calcium	200 ppm
Magnesium	100 ppm
Phosphorus	50 ppm
Potassium	50 ppm
Sulphite	<5 ppm
Iron	<1 ppm
Zinc	<1 ppm
Manganese	<1 ppm
Protein	0·05%
Fat	0·01%
Crude fibre	0·01%

Table 2. Typical maltodextrins

Approximate DE	Average DP	1	2	3	4	5	6	7	8	9	10	>10	Bulk density (g cm^{-3})	Description
5	22·1	0·3	0·9	1·4	1·4	1·3	1·8	2·4	2·0	1·8	1·7	85·0	0·51	Excellent film-forming characteristics. Produces viscosity at 20–40% solids, clear solutions at 15% solids. Extremely low hygroscopicity. Very minimal sweetness
10	11·1	0·8	2·9	4·4	3·8	3·4	5·7	6·8	4·5	3·1	2·5	62·1	0·56	Forms clear solutions at 30% dry solids at room temperature. Very low hygroscopicity. Low browning tendency. Low sweetness
15	7·4	1·3	4·8	6·7	5·5	4·7	8·4	9·1	4·8	2·9	2·1	49·7	0·58	Forms clear solutions at 50% dry solids at room temperature. Low hygroscopicity. Low browning tendency. Slight sweetness

The "Saccharide distribution, DP (average % by weight)" header spans columns 1 through >10.

Table 3. Some typical applications of maltodextrins

Product	DE types	Reasons for use
Dry beverage mixes		
Cold	10, 15	Resistance to caking, good dispersibility and solubility, low dustiness,
Cold, diet	5, 10, 15	bulking agent/diluent, development of body and mouth feel, sweetness
Hot	1, 5, 10, 15	control, faster drying, flavour retention
Infant formulae	15	Dispersibility and solubility, easy digestibility, nutritive value, control of osmolality
Milk flavouring mix	1, 5, 10	Bulking agent/diluent, development of body and mouth feel
Soup and sauce mixes	5, 10, 15	Bulking agent/diluent, development of body and mouth feel, resistance to caking, fat dispersibility
Spice blends	10, 15	Decreased caking, longer shelf life, bland flavour, high solubility, bulking agent/diluent
Artificial sweetener	5, 10, 15	Bulking agent/diluent, resistance to caking, bland flavour, quick dispersion
Coffee whitener	10, 15	Bulking agent/diluent, development of body and mouth feel, improved flavour, fat dispersibility
Imitation cheeses	10	Processing aid, browning control, texture control, bland flavour, heat-reversible gel formation
Imitation sour cream	5	Good solubility, bland flavour, builds solids/body, smooth mouth feel
Cheese sauces and dip mixes	5, 10	Adhesion, viscosity control, freeze–thaw stability, smooth mouth feel, bland flavour
Granola bars	10, 15	Binding, moisture control
Cream-type fillings	10	Rapid solubility, smooth texture, fat dispersion, flavour control
Fruit leather	5	Film formation, moisture control, crystallization inhibition, low stickiness
Glazes, frostings and icings	5, 10, 15	Crystallization inhibition, moisture control, viscosity, smooth texture, adherence, bland flavour
Snacks	10	Binding, low stickiness, bland flavour
Nut and snack coatings	10, 15	Film formation, flavour carrier, partial oxygen barrier, sheen, extended shelf life
Compressed confections	10, 15	Adhesion, sheen, binding, low hygroscopicity, compressibility
Chewy confectionery	5, 10	Good solubility, high viscosity, low flavour masking, plasticizer
Pan coatings	5, 10	Film formation, adhesion, binding, good solubility, bland flavour, sheen
Hard confectionery	10	Low hygroscopicity, less stickiness, slower meltdown
Frozen foods	10	Viscosity formation, crystallization inhibitor, film formation, moisture control
Frozen novelties	10	Viscosity formation, crystallization inhibition, high freezing point, smooth texture, addition of body, slower meltdown
Carrier for essential oils and other flavours	1, 5, 10, 15	Bulking agent, encapsulating agent
Spray-drying aid for cheese, fats, flavours, fruit juices and syrups	10	High dispersibility and solubility, fat dispersion, low hygroscopicity, free-flowing products, bland flavour
Agglomerating agent for water-soluble gums	10	Good dispersibility and solubility, low hygroscopicity, standardization of viscosity grades

Properties

Dextrins are cold-water soluble. Upon drying of a dextrin solution, clear films are obtained. Maltodextrins are quite soluble; depending on the type, 15–60% solutions can be made easily at room temperature. Syrup solids (dried glucose or corn syrups) are granular, semicrystalline or powdery amorphous products. They are mildly sweet. Because of their moderate hygroscopicity, they must be packaged in moisture-proof bags.

Maltodextrins are less hygroscopic because of their lower monosaccharide content. They are usually white, free-flowing powders.

Maltodextrins are available as spray-dried powders, in agglomerated form, and as products with an even lower bulk density and even larger surface area. They have the ability to absorb flavour oils and other nonaqueous liquids. Their flowability, compressibility and low hygroscopicity make them excellent excipients. They provide good to excellent solution clarity. They provide moderate to very low solution viscosity, and low to extremely low browning. They are generally bland and generally resist caking. They form protective films with oxygen barrier properties and provide binding, surface sheen and high solids content without affecting freezing points.

The characteristics and properties that increase as the DE increases are bulk density, hygroscopicity, ability to participate in the browning reaction, solubility, clarity of solutions, osmolality, freezing point depression, sweetness and particle size. The characteristics and properties that decrease as the DE increases are the abilities to form films, build viscosity, bind and provide body. *See* Browning, Nonenzymatic

Especially prepared, low-DE, more crystalline malto-dextrins produce a fatty mouth feel. They are most often made from potato or tapioca starch; oat flour and bran is another source; rice flour has also been used for their preparation. These products, when hydrated, form soft, spoonable gels with a creamy texture. They generally have DE values less than 3.

Uses

Dextrins are usually used to produce protective coatings such as those applied to panned confections.

Maltodextrins and (corn) syrup solids are used as: carriers for vegetable oils, butter fat, flavour oils, fatty acids, resins and emulsifiers such as lecithin; spray-drying aids; and bulking agents for flavouring materials and artificial sweeteners. In confections, they prevent sugar crystallization, improve chewiness in soft confectionery, increase shelf life and maintain moisture levels in hard confectionery, and speed up the panning process. They are effective binders and excipients for direct compression confectionery (and pharmaceutical tablets). They are widely used as spray-drying aids. They control the freezing point and ice crystal growth in frozen dairy products. They control sugar crystallization, control sweetness and add solids to bakery fillings, frostings and glazes. They provide a chewy texture and extend the shelf life of fruit leathers and granola bars. *See* Drying, Spray Drying; Sugar, Handling of Sugar Beet and Sugar Cane

Maltodextrins are excellent flavour carriers and dispersants for instant dry mixes. In cereals and snacks, they give uniform coatings, bind, and function as a carrier for sweeteners, flavours, spices and seasonings.

They also provide lubricity and control expansion in the preparation of extruded snack products. They are bulking agents for frozen desserts and novelties. They provide viscosity and mouth feel in diet gelatin desserts made from mixes. Some typical applications of malto-dextrins are given in Table 3. Corn syrup solids are generally used alone or in combination with maltodextrins when one or more of the following characteristics is desired: browning, freezing point depression, greater solids content, increased solubility, some sweetness, increased clarity.

The more crystalline maltodextrins are effective fat sparers and replacers in low-fat or non fat dairy products such as: ice milks, frozen yoghurt, frozen desserts, dips, margarine spreads, cheese-type spreads; creamy dressings; spoonable dressings; and baked goods, including frostings and fillings. They have a energy value of about $3 \cdot 8$ kcal g^{-1} as compared to about 9 kcal g^{-1} for a fat or oil.

Digestion and Metabolism

All products made by simple depolymerization of a starch (food dextrins, thin-boiling starches, maltodextrins, dried syrups, syrups) are nutritive saccharides. They are generally recognized as being safe and non-toxic. Human digestive enzymes (pancreatic α-amylases and maltooligosaccharidases of the epithelium of the small intestine) convert each into D-glucose, which is absorbed, raising blood sugar levels. The D-glucose is then metabolized in the usual ways. So each provides approximately 4 kcal g^{-1}.

Maltodextrins and syrup solids are the carbohydrates of choice for sport drinks and liquid diet formulations because of the low osmolality of their solutions. These properties and their easy digestibility make them suitable for infant formulae.

Bibliography

Van Beynum GMA and Joels JA (eds) (1985) *Starch Conversion Technology*. New York: Marcel Dekker.

J. N. BeMiller
Purdue University, West Lafayette, USA

DEXTROSE

See Glucose

Dextrins

DIABETES MELLITUS

Contents

Aetiology

Definition and Classification

Diabetes mellitus is a complex disorder of metabolism (fat and protein as well as carbohydrate) caused by either a deficiency of or defective action of insulin. It is not a single disease entity, but rather a syndrome of variable clinical presentation and aetiology:

1. Primary diabetes mellitus (DM)
   Insulin-dependent, type I (IDDM)*
   Non-insulin-dependent, type II (NIDDM)*
   Obese
   Nonobese
   Gestational diabetes
2. Diabetes secondary to other conditions
   Pancreatic disease
   Endocrine diseases (Cushing's syndrome, acromegaly, glucagonoma, phaeochromocytoma)
   Metabolic disorders
   Haemochromatosis
   Insulin receptor antibodies
   Drug-induced (e.g. glucocorticoids, thiazide diuretics, ethanol)
3. Impaired glucose tolerance (IGT)

Basic Features of Diabetes

Type I (insulin-dependent) and II (non-insulin-dependent) diabetes account for the great majority of patients. They differ in terms of their clinical presentation, aetiology and basic metabolic defect, type I diabetes being characterized by absolute insulin deficiency owing to B-cell destruction, and type II diabetes by relative insulin deficiency due either to resistance to insulin or dysfunctional insulin secretion. Although it is probable that neither type represents a single disease entity, the majority of patients with type I diabetes, at least, appear to share a common aetiology.

Successful treatment of diabetes, with diet, oral hypoglycaemic drugs or insulin, enables the majority of patients to lead long and near-normal lives. Increasingly, it is the long-term complications of the disease which are the major challenge in the treatment of diabetes. The most important of these are the microvascular complications (retinopathy and nephropathy), the macrovascular complications (atherosclerosis, coronary artery and peripheral vascular disease), and hypertension and the neuropathies. These complications are uncommon in type I diabetes of less than 10 years' duration but are not uncommon at presentation in type II diabetes, possibly because of the long period of asymptomatic hyperglycaemia which may precede the clinical diagnosis. In the majority of patients it is relatively easy to achieve good or at least reasonable health in the short term. However, with increasingly convincing evidence that the incidence of long-term complications can be reduced by maintaining good diabetic control, this has become the major area of concern and emphasis in the clinical monitoring and management of diabetes.

The major differences between types I and II diabetes are shown in Table 1.

Clinical diabetes represents a continuous spectrum from the young, underweight, ketotic and sometimes comatose patient on the one hand to the elderly, obese and frequently asymptomatic patient on the other. While the majority of patients with types I and II diabetes conform to the patterns in Table 1, there are frequent exceptions, particularly in the elderly, in whom weight loss may be a presenting feature and in whom treatment with insulin is often necessary. There is more uniformity in young patients, almost all of

---

* These terms have largely replaced the older nomenclature of juvenile- and adult-onset diabetes. Strictly speaking, the terms type I and insulin-dependent, and type II and non-insulin-dependent are not synonymous, type I originally applying to diabetes with specific HLA and auto-immune associations. However, the terms are often used interchangeably in a clinical context. In this text, the terms IDDM and NIDDM are preferred except when referring specifically to type I diabetes as originally defined.

Table 1. Features of types I and II diabetes

	Type I (IDDM)	Type II (NIDDM)
Age at onset (years)	Usually < 30	Usually > 40
Weight	Weight loss	Normal or overweight
Rate of onset	Rapid	Slow
Ketosis	Usual	Absent
Complications at presentation	Rare	Common
HLA association	Usual	Absent
Islet cell antibodies	Usual	Absent

HLA, human lymphocyte antigen.
Adapted from Home PD et al. (1989).

whom require insulin. A well-defined exception is the syndrome of maturity-onset diabetes of the young (MODY) which usually presents before the age of 25 years, is generally inherited as an autosomal dominant gene, and does not usually require treatment with insulin.

Diagnosis

Although insulin deficiency results in abnormalities of fat, protein and carbohydrate metabolism, it is upon the changes in blood *glucose* levels that both diagnosis and monitoring are primarily based*. The diagnosis of diabetes is based upon the criteria set by the World Health Organization (1985) and these largely depend on the standard 75-g oral glucose tolerance test (GTT). However, if in symptomatic patients the fasting blood glucose level is above 6.7 mmol l^{-1} or a random level above 10.0 mmol l^{-1} (7.8 or 11.1 mmol l^{-1} respectively for plasma glucose), the diagnosis is confirmed and a formal GTT is unnecessary. The fasting blood glucose may be normal in early diabetes and, therefore, although the diagnosis is unlikely if the fasting blood glucose is between 4.4 and $6–7 \text{ mmol l}^{-1}$ (plasma glucose $5.5–7.8 \text{ mmol l}^{-1}$) it cannot be excluded with certainty in a patient with appropriate symptoms unless a GTT is performed. The criteria for interpretation of the oral glucose tolerance test are shown in

---

* The criteria are complicated by the fact that glucose can be measured on either plasma or whole blood, and on either a venous or a capillary specimen. The blood glucose level is approximately 1 mmol l^{-1} higher in plasma than in whole blood, and while there is no difference between glucose levels in capillary or venous blood in the fasting state, capillary (arterialized) levels are, again, about 1 mmol l^{-1} higher than venous levels in the postprandial state (which includes the 2-h post-glucose-load sample). It is therefore essential to define the diagnostic criteria according to the methodology used locally.

Table 2 and are based upon the blood glucose level measured in the fasting state and 2 h after a 75-g glucose (or equivalent) load; neither the glucose level measured 1 h postload, nor measurements of plasma insulin levels are of diagnostic use. The glucose load should be dissolved in 250–300 ml of water and drunk within 5 min after an overnight fast; dietary carbohydrate should not have been restricted during the 3 days prior to the test. *See* Glucose, Maintenance of Blood Glucose Level; Glucose, Glucose Tolerance and the Glycaemic Index

Although individuals classified as having impaired glucose tolerance (IGT) do not, by definition, have diabetes, they are at increased risk of developing diabetes (10–25% within 5 years) and, importantly, at risk of developing the syndrome of obesity, hypertension, and hyperlipidaemia as well as the macrovascular complications of diabetes. They should therefore be monitored carefully and treated with dietary restriction and weight loss where appropriate. *See* Hyperlipidaemia; Hypertension, Nutrition in the Diabetic Hypertensive

Epidemiology

Type I (Insulin-Dependent Diabetes Mellitus (IDDM))

There are dramatic differences in the prevalence of IDDM both racially and geographically. The annual incidence rate in young people below the age of 20 years varies from almost 30 per 100 000 per year in Finland and Scandinavia to less than 1 per 100 000 per year in oriental populations such as the Koreans and the Japanese. Rates are generally much higher in northern than southern Europe, and higher in Whites than Blacks from the same geographical area. Racial differences in the prevalence of IDDM may relate to differences in the frequencies of human lymphocyte antigen (HLA) genotypes in the population.

The peak age of onset of IDDM is between the ages of 11 and 13 years. Thereafter, the incidence rate is low during middle life but there is a further peak in the elderly, in whom the presenting features of the disease may be similar to those seen in children, although the aetiology is probably different. In addition to age-related differences in incidence, there is also a seasonal variation, seen only in older children, with a maximum during the winter months, possibly related to seasonal variations in viral illnesses involved in the aetiology of the disease. Of particular concern is the fact that the incidence of children appears to be increasing steadily in some countries, including the UK.

Table 2. Diagnostic values for the oral glucose tolerance test

	Glucose concentration (mmol l^{-1})			
	Whole blood		Plasma	
	Venous	Capillary	Venous	Capillary
Diabetes mellitus				
Fasting value, *or*	>6·7	>6·7	>7·8	>7·8
2 h after glucose load	>10·0	>11·1	>11·1	>12·2
Impaired glucose tolerance				
Fasting, *and*	<6·7	<6·7	<7·8	<7·8
2 h after glucose load	6·7–9·9	7·8–11·0	7·8–11·0	8·9–12·1

Type II (Non-Insulin-Dependent Diabetes Mellitus (NIDDM))

There are also marked differences in the prevalence and incidence of NIDDM. The lowest rates are found in underdeveloped, rural communities in Africa and Asia. The prevalence in most European countries is between 1% and 3%. Unlike IDDM, surveys in the USA show that the prevalence of NIDDM is higher among the Blacks than among the Whites.

Extremely high rates are found in certain ethnic groups when subjected to rapid 'Westernization'. The most extensively studied are the Pima Indians in Arizona and the Micronesian population of the Pacific island of Nauru where inheritance appears to be autosomal-dominant and the prevalence in adults may be as high as 80%. Recently, high rates have also been found in a number of migrant populations, particularly in those from the Indian subcontinent to the West. It has been suggested that these peoples possess a 'thrifty genotype' which confers the advantage of metabolic efficiency when food is in short supply but which leads to obesity, insulin resistance and NIDDM when food becomes plentiful.

Complications and Mortality

The pattern of complications varies between IDDM and NIDDM. In both, the major cause of death is from cardiovascular disease, but in IDDM, microvascular complications (nephropathy and retinopathy) are the dominant complications, with a significant increase in deaths from renal disease and its sequelae. In NIDDM, the increased mortality is largely attributable to deaths from cardiovascular disease. These differences probably reflect fundamental differences in the pathophysiology of the two conditions, particularly in the levels of circulating insulin, proinsulin and insulin intermediates.

Causes

The underlying lesions in types I and II diabetes are different and almost certainly result from different pathogenic processes. Type I diabetes is characterized by loss of insulin secretion owing to autoimmune destruction of B cells, while in type II diabetes there is minimal loss of B cells but evidence of dysfunctional insulin secretion and peripheral insulin resistance. In both cases the disease process appears complex and almost certainly involves genetic, environmental and possibly dietary factors.

Type I, Insulin-Dependent Diabetes

Genetic Factors

About 60% of the genetic predisposition to IDDM is accounted for by genes of the major histocompatibility complex (MHC). These genes, which are located on the short arm of chromosome 6, encode for a number of proteins, many of which are involved with immune function and susceptibility to autoimmune disease. The most important of these are the HLAs. The HLA region can be subdivided into four subregions (classes):

1. Class I: HLA-A, -B, -C and -E.
2. Class II: HLA-DP, -DQ, -DR (also HLA-DN, -DO and -DV).
3. Class III: Properdin Bf, complement components 2 and 4, and 21-hydroxylase.
4. Class IV: Tumour necrosis factor (TNF) and heat shock proteins.

Class I proteins are expressed on the surface of most nucleated cells and are involved in the presentation of processed antigens to cytotoxic T lymphocytes. Class II proteins are expressed on B lymphocytes, macrophages and activated T cells and are involved in the presentation of antigens to activated T cells. Each of the class II

Table 3. Human lymphocyte antigen (HLA) associations and the relative risk of IDDM

HLA-DR antigen	Relative risk of IDDM	95% confidence limits
DR2	0·1	0·05–0·3
DR3	5·0	2·9–8·8
DR4	6·8	3·8–12·1
DR3 and DR4	14·3	6·3–32·4

Data from the Barts–Windsor Study (1983).

alleles can be further subdivided into the genes encoding for the α and β chains.

The major association with Type I diabetes is with possession of the alleles DR3 and DR4. The relative risks of IDDM associated with these HLA genes are shown in Table 3. More recently, an even stronger association with a particular HLA-DQ marker has been described.

The overall risk for diabetes in siblings who are HLA-identical but otherwise genetically nonidentical is around 15%, considerably less than the risk in identical twins (30–50%); this indicates a role for genetic factors other than MHC or HLA genes in susceptibility to IDDM. Non-MHC markers are controversial and much less well understood, but there is some suggestion that non-MHC genetic factors may be involved in the development of insulitis.

An alternative, but less well-developed hypothesis, is that predisposition to IDDM is attributable to the lack of a protective genotype rather than possession of at-risk alleles, for example, the negative association with HLA-DR2.

Environmental Factors

Since only a small proportion of individuals possessing a susceptible genotype develop diabetes, it is clear that other factors are also involved in triggering the autoimmune process. The most likely of these is viral infection, and several candidate viruses have been identified; the best documented is congenital rubella, with IDDM developing in 10–20% of affected individuals. Other possible viral infections include mumps, and Coxsackie B, echovirus and cytomegalovirus infections.

The earliest change in the islet Type I diabetes is the appearance of activated macrophages and increased production of class I antigens. The sequence of events which follows is not fully understood but it seems likely that a triggering event (probably a viral infection) stimulates the production of cytokines such as TNF and γ-interferon which are capable of inducing aberrant expression of class II antigens on B cells, thus enabling B

cells to act as antigen-presenting cells, and to present their own surface autoantigens directly to T cells. Neither A nor D cells appear to be capable of being induced to express class II antigens and are therefore spared. *See* Immunity and Nutrition

Of interest is the fact that there are variations in susceptibility genotypes in different racial and ethnic groups, the association with DR3, DR4 and DQ being strongest in White Caucasians. These variations may reflect differences in the environmental antigens which trigger the autoimmune process in different populations.

The result of the autoimmune process is the production of autoantibodies which can be detected in the circulation of almost all newly diagnosed cases of IDDM. Antibodies may be directed against either cytoplasmic antigens (islet-cell antibodies, ICAs) or against surface antigens (islet-cell antibodies, ICSAs) and even against insulin itself (insulin autoantibodies, IAAs). They may be complement-fixing and therefore cytotoxic. Recently, antibodies to a protein of molecular mass 64 000 which is probably identical to the enzyme glutamate dehydrogenase have been found in a high proportion of patients and first-degree relatives.

Autoantibodies may be present in the circulation for months or even years before the clinical presentation of the disease during which time insulin secretion may decline gradually. There may then be a final event which precipitates the development of clinical diabetes, either a further viral infection or re-exposure to the original triggering infection, thus explaining the seasonal peaks in the incidence of new cases of type I diabetes.

Type II, Non-Insulin-Dependent Diabetes

The factors involved in the pathogenesis of type II diabetes, several of which may be interrelated, are summarized as follows:

1. Genetic factors
   Ethnic or racial: thrifty genotype
   Specific genes: insulin, insulin receptor, glucose transporter, HLA
2. Dysfunctional insulin secretion
3. Insulin resistance
4. Obesity
5. Lack of exercise
7. Dietary factors?

As is clear from the prevalence patterns, certain ethnic groups are highly susceptible to diabetes when exposed to an affluent, 'Western' life style. A similar phenomenon is being recognized with increasing frequency in a number of other ethnic groups, often associated with other features of so-called 'syndrome X' (or Reaven's syndrome) such as hypertension, hypertriglyceridaemia and premature ischaemic heart disease.

Genetic factors are clearly much stronger in NIDDM than in IDDM. Concordance is greater than 90% for NIDDM in monozygotic twins compared with around 40% for IDDM. In high-risk populations, the risk of diabetes in offspring when both parents have NIDDM may be greater than 50%, and as high as 80% in Pima Indians and Nauru islanders when parents develop the disease before the age of 45 years. Despite these figures, much less is known about the genetic associations of NIDDM than those of IDDM. In particular, there is only weak evidence for association with MHC or HLA markers, although there is some evidence for an association with the hypervariable region of the insulin gene with predisposition not only to NIDDM but also to other features of 'syndrome X'. Other postulated associations include the insulin receptor and glucose transporter genes but the significance of these is unclear.

An important factor in the pathogenesis of NIDDM is insulin resistance. The precise cause of this is uncertain, although a number of factors, including genetic predisposition, obesity, lack of physical exercise and possibly diet, probably contribute to its development. The nature and consequences of insulin resistance are discussed in the following article.

Increasing obesity is associated with deterioration in glucose tolerance, and the majority of patients with NIDDM are overweight, around 75% having a body mass index (BMI) of over 25 kg m^{-2}. If obesity has a role in the *cause* of NIDDM, it is probably in modulating the speed of progression to symptomatic disease, possibly by contributing to the development of insulin resistance and the earlier onset of B-cell exhaustion. The risk of developing NIDDM is related to both the degree and the distribution of obesity. The greatest risk is seen with male-pattern, central obesity which is also associated with hypertriglyceridaemia, hypertension and an increased risk of ischaemic heart disease.

Lack of physical exercise also probably modulates the rate of development of IDDM, particularly in women.

The role of dietary factors in the pathogenesis of diabetes is unclear. It is difficult to dissect out the contribution of the major macronutrients since the levels of fat and carbohydrate in the diet tend to alter in parallel. If anything, high-fat diets tend to be more diabetogenic, perhaps enhancing hyperinsulinaemia by increasing the levels of the hormones of the enteroinsular axis such as gastric inhibitory polypeptide and glucagon-like polypeptide-1. In many countries where the prevalence of diabetes is low, dietary fat intake is also low. In most of these, the high dietary carbohydrate intake tends to be unrefined, with a higher proportion of soluble and insoluble fibre, both of which may mitigate against the development of diabetes. As far as refined sugar is concerned, although it may exacerbate hyper-

glycaemia in frank diabetes, there is very little evidence that it plays a causative role except by contributing to overall energy intake and thus obesity.

Screening and Prevention

Insulin-Dependent Diabetes

Different arguments can be advanced for screening for the different types of diabetes. Screening for susceptible individuals or for preclinical type I diabetes might be justified as part of a prevention programme if means were available to avert or delay for a significant time the onset of clinical disease. Once glucose intolerance starts to develop, the progression to clinical disease is usually rapid. Measurement of blood or urine glucose is therefore useless, and screening would, of necessity, be limited to testing for susceptible genotypes or the presence of autoantibodies in children or young people with a family history of the disease; sporadic cases would, of course, remain undetected. Such a programme would be extremely costly and at present there is insufficient evidence that early intervention might be effective. Further experience is required with measures such as immunosuppressive therapy with cyclosporin, which has been used to induce remission in newly diagnosed cases, or with nicotinamide treatment, which has recently been found to have some effect in slowing the rate of deterioration of B-cell function. A further possible approach is to immunize high-risk individuals against viruses capable of precipitating diabetes but this, too, remains an unproven strategy.

Ultimately, preventative measures might include genetic engineering, e.g. to select from parents only those gametes which do not contain susceptibility genes, but such methods clearly raise ethical as well as practical problems.

Non-Insulin-Dependent Diabetes

Below the age of 45 years, the prevalence of NIDDM in the population is around 3%, and screening on a large scale is probably not cost-effective. However, the nature of NIDDM (frequently asymptomatic), the high prevalence of diabetes (predominantly NIDDM) in older age groups (see Table 4) and the high prevalence of complications, both at presentation and in the early years after diagnosis, provide some justification for the establishment of screening programmes in the older population. Problems arise in deciding when to rescreen subjects who were initially negative since the pick-up rate will clearly be lower on retesting. In addition to the elderly, screening may be justified in those ethnic groups in whom there is known to be a high incidence of NIDDM.

Aetiology

Table 4. Age-related prevalence of diabetes in White Caucasians

Age-group (years)	Prevalence of DM
0–9	0·5
10–19	1·8
20–29	4·0
30–39	4·6
40–49	7·5
50–59	13·8
60–69	21·3
70–79	37·1
80+	35·6

Modified from Singh BM *et al.* (1988).

To some extent, however, the question of establishing specific screening programmes is becoming redundant as testing for diabetes forms part of a more general health screen which general practitioners are encouraged to provide.

Screening can be based upon testing for glycosuria, measuring fasting or random blood glucose levels or upon measurements of glycated haemoglobin (HbA₁). Of these, blood glucose measurements are more precise and probably to be preferred, provided that they are interpreted in relation to the time of meals.

Bibliography

Alberti KGMM, Boucher BJ, Hitman GA and Taylor R (1990) Diabetes mellitus. In: *The Metabolic and Molecular Basis of Acquired Disease* (Cohen RD, Lewis B, Alberti KGMM and Denman AM, eds), pp 765–840. London: Ballière Tindall.

Atkinson MA, Maclaren NK, Scharp DW, Lacy PE and Riley WJ (1990) 64,000 Mᵣ autoantibodies as predictors of insulin-dependent diabetes. *Lancet* 335: 1357–1359.

Home PD, Johnston DG and Alberti KGMM (1989). Diabetes mellitus. In: *Fundamentals of Clinical Endocrinology* (Hall R and Besser G, eds), pp 318–361. Edinburgh: Churchill Livingstone.

Nattrass M and Hale PJ (eds) (1988) Non-insulin-dependent diabetes. *Clinical Endocrinology and Metabolism* 2(2).

Pickup JC and Williams (eds) (1991) *Textbook of Diabetes.* Oxford: Blackwell.

Reaven GM (1988) Role of insulin resistance in human disease. *Diabetes* 37: 1595–1607.

Singh BM, Rutter JD and Fitzgerald MG (1988) The natural history of non-insulin-dependent diabetes mellitus. *Clinical Endocrinology and Metabolism* 2: 343–358.

WHO Expert Committee on Diabetes Mellitus (1980) Technical Report Series 646. Geneva: WHO.

Wolf E, Spencer KM and Cudworth AG (1983) The genetic susceptibility to Type I (insulin-dependent) diabetes: an analysis of the HLA-DR association. *Diabetologia* 24: 224–230.

J. Wright
University of Surrey, Guildford, UK

Chemical Pathology

Chemical Pathology

Morbid Anatomy of the Pancreas

The Normal Pancreas

Insulin is secreted from the B cells of the islets of Langerhans. There are approximately one million islets distributed throughout the pancreas. Individual cells can be identified using immunocytochemistry, whereby cells are stained using antibodies directed at their secretory products. The B cell is the dominant cell type of the islet but there are a number of others, as shown in Table 1. There is a complex interrelationship between the cells of the islet and their products, with glucagon and somatostatin acting as paracrine factors and, respectively, enhancing and inhibiting the insulin response to stimuli. (The function of pancreatic polypeptide is not known.)

Type I Diabetes (IDDM)

Type I diabetes is caused by autoimmune destruction of B cells, possibly triggered by a viral infection in genetically susceptible individuals (see previous article). The first stages in this process involve the appearance of macrophages within the islets and the establishment of a typical chronic inflammatory reaction with lymphocytic infiltration; this is termed 'insulitis'. Loss of B cells is a gradual process which may first be detectable several years before the development of clinical diabetes. In some patients, residual B-cell function persists for many years after the onset of diabetes, with persistence of insulitis in remaining B cells. Continuing insulin secretion (as assessed by a positive C-peptide response to glucagon stimulation) is characteristically associated with easier glycaemic control.

In established insulin-dependent diabetes mellitus (IDDM), there is almost total loss of B cells. As a result, the islets appear atrophic, although the number and distribution of A, D and PP cells remains almost normal.

Table 1. Cell types and secretory products of the islet of Langerhans

Cell type	Secretory product
A	Glucagon
B	Insulin
D	Somatostatin
PP	Pancreatic polypeptide

Table 2. Major physiological stimuli to insulin secretion

Metabolites	Glucose
	Amino acids
	Ketone bodies
Gastrointestinal hormones	GIP
	GLP-1
	Glucagon
Neural	Vagal stimulation

GIP, gastric inhibitory polypeptide; GLP-1, glucagon-like polypeptide-1

Type II Diabetes (NIDDM)

Unlike type I diabetes, the gross morphology of the islet is normal. The extent of B-cell loss is variable and usually only minimal, although there is occasionally a loss of up to 50% of B cells, with a similar reduction in total islet volume and a small increase in the number of A cells. The one abnormality which has attracted considerable attention is the presence of amyloid material within the islet. This differs from the substance derived from immunoglobulin light chains and found in systemic amyloidosis and plasma cell dyscrasias. Islet amyloid contains a novel 37 amino acid peptide ('amylin') which is similar to calcitonin-gene-related peptide (CGRP, 45% sequence homology). It is found in association with secretory granules and may be cosecreted with insulin. Amylin is subsequently transformed or incorporated – by a process which is not understood – into amyloid fibrils which are found between the B cells and the adjacent capillaries. Although the gene for amylin is probably on chromosome 12, it may share a common evolutionary origin with the gene for CGRP which is found (along with the genes for both calcitonin and insulin) on chromosome 11.

The precise relationship between islet amyloid and non-insulin-dependent diabetes mellitus (NIDDM) is unclear. It is not seen in the islets of patients with type I diabetes, and although small amounts may be found in normal islets, it is only present in large amounts in association with NIDDM. There is some evidence that amylin secretion or accumulation may impair insulin secretion, and even that amylin may have a hormonal role and may induce insulin resistance in muscle.

The Metabolic Effects of Insulin Insufficiency

The major stimulus to insulin secretion is an increase in blood glucose concentration. A number of other physiological factors also stimulate insulin secretion (see Table 2), in particular the hormones of the enteroinsular axis which augment the insulin response to feeding but only in the presence of a raised blood glucose level. The 'cephalic phase' of insulin secretion, which occurs prior to eating, is mediated by the vagus nerve.

Insulin is thus the hormone of the fed state with low circulating levels in the post-absorptive state, and its metabolic actions (see Table 3) are primarily concerned with the coordinated disposal, metabolism and storage of the major nutrients. The major effects are upon carbohydrate metabolism, with control of blood glucose level being the most obvious of these. This depends on a balance between output from the liver and peripheral uptake, utilization and storage of glucose, and this balance is largely dependent on those tissues which require insulin for intracellular transport of glucose (i.e. muscle and adipose tissue). *See* Glucose, Maintenance of Blood Glucose Level

Since diabetes is characterized by the *absence of effective insulin activity*, it is possible to view the major metabolic features of diabetes as a reversal of the actions in Table 3. This may be due to absolute insulin deficiency (IDDM) or to insulin resistance (NIDDM). The precise definition and criteria for establishing the presence of insulin resistance are controversial. It is usually based upon the finding of high fasting and postprandial plasma insulin levels, but there may be difficulties in interpreting these findings. When the high blood glucose level is taken into account, the concomitant insulin level may, in fact, be relatively low. The rise in insulin level with blood glucose parallels that seen in nondiabetics, suggesting a change in the 'set' of insulin level. Finally, recent highly specific two-point immunoassays for insulin have suggested that much of what has hitherto been measured and called 'insulin' may be either proinsulin, or insulin/proinsulin intermediates and that the level of true, bioactive insulin may, in fact, be low rather than high. This suggestion is clearly a challenge to the traditional concept of NIDDM and requires further investigation.

The insulin resistance of NIDDM is demonstrable both in liver and skeletal muscle. Although there is continuing uncertainty about which of these is the more important, hepatic resistance (leading to increased glucose output) appears to be the major cause of fasting hyperglycaemia, while muscle resistance (impaired glucose uptake) is probably the major determinant of postprandial hyperglycaemia. Both are believed to be associated with a reduction in the number of insulin receptors.

Although plasma levels of free fatty acids may be slightly elevated in IDDM, the adipocyte appears to be more sensitive to the action of insulin than either muscle or liver, and inhibition of lipolysis is relatively normal. As a result, ketosis is not a feature of NIDDM. In contrast, in untreated IDDM resulting from absolute insulin deficiency, not only is lipolysis uninhibited, but re-esterification of free fatty acids to form triglycerides cannot take place because of the reduction in supplies of

Table 3. The metabolic actions of insulin

Metabolism	Action	Site (tissue) of action
Carbohydrate metabolism	Stimulates glucose transport,	MF
	glucose phosphorylation,	MFL
	glycolysis, and	MFL
	glycogen synthesis	ML
	Inhibits gluconeogenesis and	L
	glycogen breakdown	ML
Fat metabolism	Stimulates fatty acid synthesis and	LF
	triglyceride synthesis	LF
	Inhibits lipolysis	LF
Protein metabolism	Stimulates amino acid transport and	LM
	protein synthesis	LM
	Inhibits protein breakdown	LM

M, muscle; F, fat; L, liver.

α-glycerophosphate from glycolysis. In the liver, glycolysis is not insulin-dependent and triglyceride synthesis is unimpaired and may even be increased because of an increased supply of free fatty acids. *See* Fatty Acids, Metabolism

Insulin is the only major anabolic hormone in the body (growth hormone also has anabolic properties but these are only manifest in the presence of insulin). The action of insulin is opposed by a number of other counterregulatory hormones, including glucagon, cortisol, catecholamines, vasopressin and growth hormone. The action of these hormones is essential in maintaining fuel supplies (fatty acids and ketones as well as glucose) in the fasted state. These actions are unopposed in the absence of insulin, and in the extreme situation of diabetic ketoacidosis they are probably responsible for many of the metabolic abnormalities. Their importance otherwise in the pathogenesis of diabetes is uncertain; the ratio of hepatic insulin to glucagon may be an important metabolic determinant but it is interesting that diabetes which occurs as a result of tumours secreting an excess of any one of the counterregulatory hormones is usually mild, indicating the relatively greater importance of insulin. *See* Hormones, Adrenal Hormones; Hormones, Pituitary Hormones

Hyperglycaemia and Glycosuria

Blood glucose concentration is normally carefully controlled and maintained between fairly narrow limits as a result of a balance between hepatic output and peripheral uptake of glucose. Even following carbohydrate feeding, around 60% of absorbed glucose is extracted during the first pass through the liver under the influence of insulin, such that the postprandial rise in blood glucose is normally modest.

A number of tissues in the body have an obligate requirement for glucose and are unable to use fatty acids or ketones as an energy source. These tissues include the retina, renal medulla and erythrocytes; the brain is also normally dependent upon glucose but can adapt to using ketone bodies during prolonged starvation. The total glucose requirement of these tissues is approximately 150 g per day. In the early fasted state (24–36 h), these demands are met by glucose release from hepatic glycogenolysis (muscle does not possess the enzyme glucose-6-phosphatase and therefore cannot release the glucose produced from the breakdown of muscle glycogen). When glycogen stores are exhausted, glucose supply is maintained by synthesis (gluconeogenesis) in the liver and, during prolonged starvation, the kidney. The main substrates for gluconeogenesis are glycerol (from triglyceride breakdown), alanine and glutamine (from muscle protein), and lactate and pyruvate (recycled from glycolysis). The factors controlling gluconeogenesis include substrate supply, hormones (cortisol, growth hormone, catecholamines and vasopressin) and, in particular, the insulin : glucagon ratio in the liver. As a result, hypoglycaemia (conventionally defined as a blood glucose level of less than 2·2 mmol l^{-1}) does not usually develop, even during prolonged starvation or strenuous exercise, in the nondiabetic. *See* Hypoglycaemia for Nutrition

Hyperglycaemia arises as a result of an imbalance between the supply and the removal of glucose, in particular because of continued glucose production despite hyperglycaemia, and the failure of peripheral glucose uptake and utilization. Both result from the absence of effective insulin action. In itself, hyperglycaemia is asymptomatic, and patients who do not carry out blood glucose monitoring because they know when their blood glucose is high must be treated with some scepticism.

Glucose is freely filtered by the glomerulus and reabsorbed by an active transport system in the proximal tubule. Under normal circumstances, the urine contains virtually no glucose as the capacity of the renal tubules to reabsorb glucose exceeds the filtered load. However, as the blood glucose rises, there comes a point at which the filtered load of glucose in the renal tubule exceeds the absorptive capacity, and glucose appears in the urine; this is the 'renal threshold' for glucose. The normal renal threshold is between 6 and 7 mmol l^{-1}. It is lower in those individuals with idiopathic renal glycosuria and during pregnancy. The presence of glucose in the urine exerts an osmotic effect in the distal and collecting tubules of the kidney, countering physiological mechanisms for urine concentration, resulting in an increase in urine volume (polyuria). The resultant loss of water from the body (plus the direct effect of hyperglycaemia on osmoreceptors in the hypothalamus) results in polydipsia (excess thirst) and, if fluid intake is inadequate, dehydration. *See* Kidney, Structure and Function

Clinical Features and Symptoms

Type I Diabetes

The classical features of type I diabetes are weight loss, polydipsia and polyuria. The latter are the direct result of the osmotic diuresis which results from hyperglycaemia; the weight loss results from the catabolism which occurs in the absence of insulin and which affects fat and protein as well as carbohydrate metabolism. In addition to these specific symptoms, there is frequently a history of increasingly severe, nonspecific symptoms such as tiredness, lack of energy, muscle cramps and general ill health, over a period of some months, which may only be recognized retrospectively after the development of full-blown diabetes. In children particularly, the onset may be more rapid with ketoacidosis supervening before the diagnosis is established.

Type II Diabetes

In contrast to type I, the symptoms of type II diabetes are very insidious, frequently very mild and often absent altogether. Weight loss is unusual except in older patients, who often require treatment with insulin from the outset; indeed, most patients are overweight. Polyuria and polydipsia may be noticed, and a history of urinary tract infection and vulval candidiasis can frequently be elicited. Ketoacidosis does not occur but occasional patients present with hyperosmolar, nonketotic coma (see below).

Complications such as neuropathy, peripheral ischaemia and retinopathy are more likely to be present at diagnosis than in type I diabetes and may be a presenting feature. In many patients, however, the condition remains asymptomatic and is only detected on routine screening.

Coma in Diabetes

Three types of coma occur in diabetes:

- Hypoglycaemic coma.
- Hyperglycaemic coma, *either* ketoacidotic coma (diabetic ketoacidosis, DKA) *or* hyperosmolar, nonketotic coma.

Hypoglycaemic Coma

Hypoglycaemia occurs predominantly in patients taking insulin but also in patients taking suphonylureas, particularly long-acting preparations such as chlorpropamide and glibenclamide. The factors which commonly predispose to hypoglycaemia, either alone or in combination, are as follows:

- Too much insulin or sulphonylurea.
- Too little food or delayed meal.
- Too much physical exercise.

In addition to simple overdosing with insulin, variations in absorption from different injection sites, or even inadvertent intravenous injection, can also precipitate hypoglycaemia. Similarly, exercise, as well as lowering blood glucose in its own right, may provoke hypoglycaemia by increasing the rate of absorption of insulin from an injection site. A further important cause of hypoglycaemia is alcohol which, by inhibiting gluconeogenesis, potentiates the action of insulin and delays the recovery from hypoglycaemia.

The onset of hypoglycaemic symptoms is usually rapid. The pattern of symptoms varies from patient to patient but is usually constant for any individual. The symptoms are those of neuroglycopenia (incoordination, impaired intellectual function, confusion, inability to concentrate, blurring of vision) and of sympathoadrenal activity (sweating, anxiety, tremor, hunger, palpitations). Unless treated by immediate ingestion of carbohydrate (preferably sucrose or glucose), the patient may lose consciousness. Untreated, the resultant coma may last for several hours, but spontaneous recovery owing to counterregulatory hormone (adrenaline, glucagon, cortisol and vasopressin) and sympathetic stimulation of gluconeogenesis is the rule. Treatment of the comatose patient consists of glucose gel smeared inside the mouth, intramuscular glucagon (1 mg) or intravenous glucose. It is important to avoid giving excess intravenous glucose, particularly in young children in whom the resultant *hyper*glycaemia can result in cerebral damage. The dose of intravenous glucose in an adult should not normally exceed 50 ml of a 20% solution. Prolonged coma is occasionally seen in association with massive (sometimes intentional) insulin overdosage, with alcohol and with sulphonylurea-induced hypoglycaemia, and may require prolonged intravenous glucose infusion.

Particular care should be taken to identify nocturnal hypoglycaemia. This frequently occurs during sleep without waking the patient and therefore may not give rise to typical symptoms. It commonly causes restlessness or sweating at night, vivid dreams or nightmares, and morning headaches or 'hangover'. It is often associated with paradoxically high and/or rising morning blood glucose levels. This phenomenon (the Somogyi effect) is probably caused by a combination of declining insulin levels and a marked counterregulatory (particularly growth hormone) response.

A distressing experience of some patients is that of hypoglycaemic unawareness, which can be both alarming and potentially dangerous. This is known to occur in over 20% of patients after 20 years of diabetes and is frequently associated with autonomic neuropathy and impaired counterregulatory response to hypoglycaemia. It is also encountered in patients taking nonselective β-blocking drugs. More recently, it has been attributed (controversially) to a change in treatment from animal to human insulin. The reasons for this phenomenon (if, indeed, it is real) are unclear. Human insulin given by subcutaneous injection, produces a slightly faster fall in blood glucose than animal insulin but the pattern of both glycaemic and counterregulatory response is otherwise virtually identical. Part of the explanation for the loss or, at least, change in symptoms may be attributable to the fact that when patients were transferred to human insulin the opportunity was taken to review and, frequently, to encourage stricter glycaemic control which is known to be associated with a reduction in hypoglycaemic awareness.

Hypoglycaemia is unpleasant and distressing for patients and their families. It also causes 'swings' in blood glucose control because of both the physiological response and overcompensation by the patient. It should be avoided as far as possible but not at the expense of abandoning attempts to obtain good control.

Diabetic Ketoacidosis

Diabetic ketoacidosis is the most serious metabolic emergency associated with IDDM. It is the largest single cause of death in young diabetics and, although uncommon in older patients, it has a very high mortality in this age-group. The fundamental cause is either absolute insulin deficiency or, less commonly, relative deficiency associated with an acute physiological 'stress'. The resultant metabolic effects consist of the following:

(1) Hyperglycaemia, owing to grossly impaired peripheral glucose uptake and utilization, plus continuing, uninhibited gluconeogenesis, leading to increased polyuria and severe fluid and electrolyte loss.

(2) Ketoacidosis, owing to accelerated lipolysis and ketogenesis, with production of excess acetyl coenzyme A (acetyl CoA) which is partially oxidized to the ketoacids, acetoacetic and β-hydroxybutyric acid. Along with acetone derived from acetoacetate, these 'ketone bodies' accumulate in larger amounts than can be metabolized, and are excreted unchanged in urine and on the breath. Both acetoacetic and β-hydroxybutyric acids are weak acids, but in the amounts produced lead to a metabolic acidosis with a concomitant rise in hydrogen ion concentration.

Precipitating causes include infection (in about one third of cases), inappropriate insulin treatment (frequently resulting from the erroneous advice to reduce insulin dosage when unwell and not eating) and, uncommonly, myocardial infarction. Diabetic ketoacidosis is occasionally the presenting feature in new cases of IDDM, but in a high proportion of cases (30–40%) no precipitating factors can be identified.

Diabetic ketoacidosis develops relatively slowly (compared with hypoglycaemic coma), usually over a period of 24–36 h. Symptoms include an increase in thirst and polyuria, general ill health, nausea, vomiting, drowsiness and eventually coma. Clinically, the patient is often febrile, with evidence of dehydration (thin, rapid pulse, postural hypotension). Hyperventilation (owing to the metabolic acidosis) is an important feature, and there is frequently a strong smell of acetone on the breath. Treatment should be instituted as a matter of urgency as soon as the diagnosis is confirmed by the finding of hyperglycaemia and ketonuria without waiting for the results of other laboratory tests (blood gases; plasma sodium, potassium and creatinine or urea; urine, sputum and blood cultures.

Treatment consists of replacement of fluid and electrolyte deficits which, in established DKA in adults, are in the order of 5 l of fluid and 500 mmol each of sodium, chloride and potassium. (It is important to remember that plasma potassium levels may not reflect this and may even be paradoxically high due to the effects of acidosis). Although there may be a similar theoretical deficit of bicarbonate, replacement is unnecessary and even counterproductive; small amounts only should be given as required to raise the blood pH above 7·0. Insulin is given in relatively small doses (6–10 units per h) either by intravenous infusion or intramuscular injection.

Nonketotic Hyperosmolar Coma

Nonketotic hyperosmolar coma occurs only in NIDDM, sometimes as a presenting feature, and consists of gross hyperglycaemia and dehydration but without ketosis. The mechanism of this is uncertain. The condition develops more insidiously than DKA, allowing time for a greater degree of dehydration to develop. Treatment consists of fluid replacement and low-dose insulin therapy. The prognosis is poor with a mortality of around 30%.

Bibliography

Alberti KGMM, Boucher BJ, Hitman GA and Taylor R (1990) Diabetes mellitus. In: *The Metabolic and Molecular Basis of Acquired Disease* (Cohen RD, Lewis B, Alberti KGMM and Denman AM, eds), pp 765–840. London: Ballière Tindall.

Berger W and Keller U (1992) Treatment of diabetic ketoacidosis and non-ketotic hyperosmolar coma. *Clinical Endocrinology and Metabolism* 6: 1–22.

Gale EA (1989) Hypoglycaemia and human insulin. *Lancet* ii: 1264–1266.

Home PD, Johnston DG and Alberti KGMM (1989) Diabetes mellitus. In: *Fundamentals of Clinical Endocrinology* (Hall R and Besser G, eds), pp 318–361. Edinburgh: Churchill Livingstone.

Johnson KH, O'Brien TD, Betsholtz C and Westermark P (1989) Islet-amyloid, islet-amyloid polypeptide and diabetes mellitus. *New England Journal of Medicine* 321: 513–518.

Moller DE and Flier JS (1991) Insulin resistance – mechanisms, syndromes and implications. *New England Journal of Medicine* 325: 938–948.

Nattrass M and Hale PJ (eds) (1988) Non-insulin-dependent diabetes. *Clinical Endocrinology and Metabolism* 2(2).

Pickup JC and Williams (eds) (1991) *Textbook of Diabetes*. Oxford: Blackwell.

Temple RC, Carrington CA, Luzio SD *et al.* (1989) Insulin deficiency in non-insulin-dependent diabetes. *Lancet* i: 293–294.

J. Wright
University of Surrey, Guildford, UK

Treatment and Management

Aims of Treatment

The main objectives in the treatment of diabetes can be summarized as follows:

1. The alleviation of symptoms;
2. The maintenance of good general health;
3. The prevention of long-term complications.

It is relatively easy to achieve the first of these objectives and, in the majority of patients, reasonable or good general health can be maintained in the short or medium term without necessarily achieving good diabetic control. The major question, which has stimulated an enormous amount of research and debate in recent years, concerns the relationship between glycaemic control and the so-called long-term complications of diabetes. It now seems clear that the development of *microvascular* complications (nephropathy and retinopathy) is closely related to the degree of diabetic control, but as far as *macrovascular* disease is concerned, the situation is more complicated. Ischaemic heart disease is the major cause of death in long-standing type I diabetes, and in type II diabetes of relatively short duration. The risk of atherosclerosis appears to be less obviously related to glycaemic control and more to other risk factors, such as ethnic origin, smoking, hypertension, dyslipidaemia (raised very-low-density lipoprotein (VLDL)-triglycerides and reduced high-density lipoprotein (HDL)-cholesterol), male pattern obesity and hyperinsulinaemia. Microalbuminuria is a particularly good marker of risk from ischaemic heart disease. *See* Atherosclerosis; Coronary Heart Disease, Intervention Studies

Thus it is clear that, if a major objective of treatment is to prevent long-term or associated complications, attention must be paid not only to control of blood glucose but also (and in some situations, primarily) to these other risk factors.

Choice of Treatment Regimen

Diet, oral hypoglycaemic agents and insulin remain the cornerstones of treatment of diabetes. Dietary advice is required by all patients, but the selection of other treatment measures is largely based on individual clinical assessment along with measures of glycaemic control. The criteria used in the selection of treatment are summarized in Table 1.

With the exception of pregnancy, in which strict criteria are generally agreed, the classification of hyperglycaemia into mild, moderate or severe is personal to both the physician and the individual patient. A common dilemma is the overweight patient with uncontrolled hyperglycaemia in whom treatment with insulin, while improving glycaemic control, frequently results in increasing weight gain and little in the way of symptomatic improvement. *See* Glucose, Maintenance of Blood Glucose Level; Pregnancy, Nutrition in Diabetic Pregnancy

Diabetic Diet

Although the importance of diet in the treatment of diabetes has been recognized for centuries, fashions have changed considerably even in recent years. Carbohydrate restriction and even semistarvation (leading to such gross reduction in body fat that keto-acidosis could not occur) were in vogue prior to the introduction of insulin. With insulin, it became possible to liberate energy consumption but, with continuing carbohydrate restriction, diets were inevitably high in fat. Major changes in the dietary recommendations for diabetics were introduced in the 1980s in the UK, continental Europe and the USA. Following both epidemiological and experimental studies which showed that a high-carbohydrate diet does not have a deleterious efect on diabetic control, there has been a swing away from carbohydrate restriction, and the promotion of diets *high* in carbohydrate (particularly complex carbohydrate and fibre) and lower in fat than previously. These recommendations have been widely implemented; they have the advantage of being similar to those which are currently believed to be desirable for the population at large and, therefore, more acceptable socially, but as yet there have been no studies comparing the efficacy of high- and low-carbohydrate diets in the long term.

The concept of the glycaemic index of foods has some attraction and validity, but it is generally considered too complicated to be of practical use in the detailed design of individual diets. Nevertheles, recognition of the principle is reflected in the recommendation that dietary carbohydrate should be predominantly unrefined (although it has recently been accepted that a small increase in the proportion of sucrose in the diet has little effect on glycaemic control). *See* Glucose, Glucose Tolerance and the Glycaemic Index

Controversy still surrounds a number of associated areas, in particular those concerned with reducing the incidence or rate of progress of complications, e.g. salt and hypertension, fat and cardiovascular disease, protein and renal impairment. Similar arguments apply in diabetics as in the nondiabetic population. *See* Hypertension, Nutrition in the Diabetic Hypertensive

The main dietary recommendations are summarized below. (NB. There are no great differences between the general principles of dietary treatment in insulin-dependent diabetes mellitus (IDDM) and those in non-insulin-dependent diabetes mellitus (NIDDM), although there is frequently more emphasis on weight loss in NIDDM, while meal distribution may be more important in IDDM.)

Energy

Overall energy content should be determined on an individual basis, and the diet designed to achieve and maintain desired bodyweight. *See* Energy, Energy Expenditure and Energy Balance

Carbohydrate

At least 50% of dietary energy should be obtained from carbohydrate, the majority of which should be complex (i.e. polysaccharides). Up to 25 g of sucrose per day may be allowed, provided that it substitutes for other carbohydrate. *See* Carbohydrates, Requirements and Dietary Importance

Fat

Fat should account for no more than 35% of dietary energy and preferably no more than 30%, especially in patients at high risk of cardiovascular disease. The type of fat advocated remains controversial, with recent evidence that monounsaturated fat may be preferable to a high intake of polyunsaturated fat. The place of fish oils (high in long-chain n − 3 fatty acids) in the diabetic diet is unclear. Cholesterol intake should be less than 300 mg per day. *See* Fats, Requirements; Fish Oils, Dietary Importance

Distribution of Carbohydrate

In patients treated with insulin, the importance of timing of meals and of taking snacks between meals in order to prevent hypoglycaemia should be stressed.

Fibre

Foods high in soluble fibre are encouraged. *See* Dietary Fibre, Fibre and Disease Prevention

Salt

High salt intake should be discouraged, particularly in hypertensive patients. At the same time, a relatively high

Table 1. Treatment options in diabetes

Treatment option	Criteria
Diet alone	Moderate hyperglycaemia only
	Obesity
Oral hypoglycaemic drugs[a]	
Sulphonylureas	Moderate to severe hyperglycaemia
	Near-normal bodyweight
Biguanides	Moderate to severe hyperglycaemia
	Obesity
Insulin[a]	Severe hyperglycaemia
	Ketosis
	Unintentional weight loss
	Nonspecific symptoms (general ill health, tiredness)
	Specific symptoms (painful neuropathy, amyotrophy)
	Pregnancy
	Intercurrent illness, surgery, myocardial infarction

[a] Plus diet.

Treatment and Management

potassium intake should be encouraged. *See* Potassium, Physiology; Sodium, Physiology

Protein

In patients with early nephropathy, protein intake should not exceed 12% of total dietary energy. *See* Protein, Requirements

Alcohol

Guidelines are similar to those for the general adult population, i.e. a maximum of 30 g (3 units) per day for men, and 20 g (2 units) per day for women. Patients taking insulin need to be especially careful since alcohol, by inhibiting gluconeogenesis, can predispose to severe hypoglycaemia. *See* Alcohol, Alcohol Consumption

Special Foods

In general, special 'diabetic' foods are not recommended. Artificial sweeteners are acceptable in moderation.

Individualization

The most important of all the recommendations is that diets should be specifically tailored for individual patients. This is critical in certain groups, such as growing children, pregnant women and the elderly, in whom restrictive diets may be inappropriate.

Oral Hypoglycaemic Agents

Oral hypoglycaemic agents rely on residual insulin secretion for their action. Their use is therefore almost exclusively restricted to the management of NIDDM. Two groups of drugs are in use, the biguanides and the sulphonylureas. The two are chemically dissimilar, have different modes of action and are used in different clinical situations.

Biguanides

The two drugs in this group are phenformin and metformin. Phenformin has now been withdrawn in most countries because of its association with severe and occasionally fatal lactic acidosis.

Metformin reduces both fasting and postprandial blood glucose levels in diabetics but rarely causes hypoglycaemia. The precise mechanism of its action is uncertain but the major effect appears to be an increase in peripheral uptake of glucose by muscle, possibly by increasing insulin receptor binding. Metformin also reduces hepatic glucose output, probably by inhibiting

Table 2. Examples of sulphonylurea drugs

Drug	Half-life (h)
First generation	
Tolbutamide	3–8
Chlorpropamide	35
Acetohexamide	6–8
Second generaton	
Glibenclamide	5
Glibornuride	8
Glipizide	4
Gliclazide	12
Gliquidone	4

gluconeogenesis. (This results in a small increase in blood lactate concentration but less than that produced by phenformin and insufficient to cause significant lactic acidosis.) Unlike the sulphonylureas, metformin does not cause weight gain; in fact, it often helps with weight loss, and is therefore most suitable in overweight patients. The drug is not metabolized but is excreted unchanged via the kidney and must therefore be used with caution in patients with renal impairment. The major side-effects of metformin are dose-related and include gastrointestinal discomfort and diarrhoea.

Sulphonylureas

The sulphonylurea group comprises a large number of closely related compounds. The important differences between individual drugs are related to differences in half-lives, and in route of metabolism and excretion (see Table 2).

The major effect of the sulphonylureas is to stimulate insulin secretion which can be demonstrated following acute administration either intravenously or orally. Enhanced insulin secretion appears to be maintained during long-term treatment and is probably responsible for the therapeutic effect of the drugs. It is possible that the sulphonylureas also exert a peripheral 'postreceptor' effect on insulin sensitivity.

The fact that the sulphonylureas increase insulin secretion means that they tend to encourage weight gain. They are therefore most suitable for lean patients and should be used sparingly in the obese. Weight gain may be less marked with those drugs which have shorter half-lives; if given before meals, these have been claimed to enhance the insulin response to food without inducing sustained hyperinsulinaemia.

The major adverse effect of the sulphonylureas is hypoglycaemia which may be both profound and prolonged. This is seen particularly with those drugs which have a longer half-life or where this is prolonged by hepatic or renal dysfunction. Chlorpropamide, for

Table 3. Major available insulin preparations

Formulation	Time of action (h)[a]			Other names
	Onset	Peak	Duration	
Crystalline	0·5–1	2–4	8	Regular, soluble, neutral
Zinc				
Amorphous	1–2	4–6	8–12	Semilente
Crystalline	2–4	14–20	24–36	Ultralente
Mixed	2–4	6–10	12–24	Lente
Protamine	2–4	6–10	12–24	Isophane
Premixed[b]	Dependent on ratios			
Protamine–zinc insulin	3–4	14–20	24–36	
Biphasic[c]	0·5–1	2–10	12–24	Rapitard

[a] Approximate times following subcutaneous injection.
[b] Available mixtures contain crystalline and isophane insulin in the ratios 1:9, 2:8, 3:7, 4:6 and 5:5.
[c] Neutral suspension of porcine amorphous insulin in a solution of crystalline bovine insulin.

example, should be used with caution in the elderly and should be avoided in patients with renal impairment. Other adverse effects are uncommon and include nausea, dizziness, skin rashes and water retention. Flushing with alcohol (probably owing to inhibition of acetaldehyde metabolism) is common in patients taking chlorpropamide and can frequently be improved by transfer to an alternative sulphonylurea preparation. *See* Hypoglycaemia for Nutrition

Insulin

Prior to the isolation of insulin in 1922, juvenile-onset diabetes was an untreatable and rapidly fatal condition. With well-managed insulin treatment, such patients can now expect to live a full and virtually normal life. Until recently, insulin was extracted from either beef or pork pancreas. The resulting bovine and porcine insulins differ from human insulin by two and one amino acids respectively. The majority of insulin is now bioengineered using recombinant deoxyribonucleic acid (DNA) technology. The proinsulin thus produced is cleaved to give insulin which is identical in its amino acid sequence to human insulin.

Regular, soluble neutral insulin is relatively short-acting and a number of techniques have been used to produce preparations with longer duration of action. The most successful of these are the complexing of insulin with either zinc or a protein (protamine) to produce zinc and isophane insulins respectively. Within the range of zinc insulins, further variations in duration of activity are achieved by varying the pH and, therefore, the particle size from amorphous (microcrystalline) medium-acting (semilente) to crystalline, long-acting (ultralente) preparations. Lente insulin is a mixture of these two in the ratio 30% semilente to 70% ultralente.

Isophane insulin is of standard formulation and duration of action. However, a range of premixed insulins, containing from 10% soluble and 90% isophane to 50% of each, is available. (Such premixtures are not possible with zinc insulins owing to the loss of the short-acting, soluble component which results from complexing with any excess zinc present.)

With the continuing availability of animal (pork and beef) insulins, a bewildering range of preparations is now available. The most important of these are listed in Table 3.

Choice of Insulin Regime

The decision to start insulin treatment is made on clinical grounds. In younger patients with evidence of ketosis, the decision is usually unambiguous. Difficulties arise in older patients in whom there is frequently considerable reluctance and, moreover, little immediate benefit on starting insulin. However, age is certainly not an absolute criterion and, indeed, many newly diagnosed elderly patients need insulin treatment from the outset. Unfortunately, there are no objective biochemical criteria (apart from glucose and ketones) on which to base treatment decisions. In particular, measurement of endogenous insulin secretion (e.g. C-peptide response to glucagon stimulation), while of interest for research purposes, should not be used in the decision to treat with insulin or not.

Insulin is given by subcutaneous injection. Examples of injection regimes in current use are shown in Table 4. A once-daily regime may be used in the elderly but for the majority of patients, good control can only be achieved by using at least twice-daily injections. A number of 'pen' injector devices are now available for the administration of both soluble insulin and soluble–

Table 4. Examples of insulin regimes

Regime	Formulation
Once daily	Lente, ultralente, PZI
Twice daily	Soluble plus lente
	Soluble plus isophane (premixed or variable)
Multiple injections	Soluble two or three times daily before meals plus either ultralente or isophane at night

PZI, protamine–zinc insulin.

isophane mixtures. An alternative to intermittent insulin injections is the technique of continuous subcutaneous insulin infusion (CSII) whereby insulin is infused continuously (with boosts at meal times) via an indwelling subcutaneous cannula from a pump which is worn or carried permanently by the patient. Although impeccable glycaemic control can be achieved with CSII, enthusiasm for the technique has waned because of the problems involved and the degree of supervision required.

Of the other alternative methods of insulin administration (intraperitoneal injection, nasal spray, implantable programmed infusion devices, etc.), some have been abandoned while others are still under evaluation. Although new insulin analogues with more convenient pharmacokinetic profiles may soon become available, and other therapeutic strategies such as pancreatic transplantation hold some promise, the prospects for a practical alternative to insulin injections in the near future seem remote.

Patient Education

Perhaps more than in any other disease, the person with diabetes needs to participate in treatment and to take responsibility for the day-to-day management of the condition. This cannot be successfully accomplished without a clear understanding of treatment objectives and the means of achieving them.

A successful educational programme needs to be carefully planned and coordinated, with opportunities for individual as well as group sessions, and a commitment to long-term reinforcement. The contribution of the diabetes nurse specialist, who is usually the ideal person to undertake much of the responsibility for patient education, has proved invaluable. The traditional hospital diabetic clinic is by no means the best environment for teaching and in many areas dedicated diabetic centres have been established for this purpose. A vast array of literature and audiovisual aids is available both from support organizations, such as the British Diabetic Association, and from commercial firms.

An essential part of any educational programme is long-term evaluation. Despite the apparently obvious need for education, the results, when formally assessed, have not been uniformly encouraging. A reduction in hospital admissions can be achieved but this might simply reflect an improvement in care and support services in general. Furthermore, the effects may not be sustained in the long term. As yet, there is no conclusive evidence that improvements in knowledge lead to better metabolic control; poor compliance is usually attributable to factors other than simple ignorance. Successful self-treatment requires, in many people, fundamental changes in attitude and behaviour. It is these benefits rather than the acquisition of knowledge that educational programmes may provide.

Assessment of Diabetic Control

Glycaemic Control

Regular monitoring of diabetes is essential in order to make short-term adjustments to treatment (particularly insulin dosage) and in order to assess control in the longer term.

Short-term assessment is achieved by monitoring glucose in urine or blood, and long-term assessment by measurement of glycated (glycosylated) proteins. Monitoring diabetes by means of urine tests was for a long time the only practical method available, but must now be considered crude and often misleading. The renal threshold for glucose varies widely in diabetes but is frequently well above target levels for blood glucose; the urine may therefore be free of glucose when the blood glucose is higher than desired. At the same time, urine tests are of no value in detecting hypoglycaemia. Persistent, heavy glycosuria is probably an indication of poor control (except in those with a very low renal threshold) but more subtle interpretation of tests is usually impossible.

Occasional, single measurements of blood glucose are also of very limited value in monitoring control since there are wide variations in blood glucose throughout the day in both IDDM and NIDDM. Once a common feature of diabetic clinics, 'one-off' blood glucose measurements have been abandoned in many centres. Regular measurement of blood glucose by patients ('home monitoring') has become commonplace and is essential in managing changes in insulin treatment, and in making day-to-day adjustments in insulin dosage (especially with multiple injection regimes) particularly during periods of metabolic instability such as intercurrent illness or pregnancy. A number of test 'sticks' are available (most of which employ dry-reagent chemistry

Treatment and Management

based upon glucose oxidase) and these can be read visually or using one of the many meters designed for the purpose.

Measurement of glycated proteins has become the standard method of monitoring medium-term glycaemic control. These compounds result from the nonenzymatic attachment of glucose to proteins (in the case of haemoglobin, to the N-terminal valine residue of the β chain). The initial aldimine linkage undergoes an Amadori rearrangement to form a stable ketoamine product. The rate of glycation depends on the prevailing glucose concentration, and the extent of glycation of any protein is therefore a function of the average glucose concentration during its lifetime. Glycated haemoglobin is most commonly used because of its availability and because the half-life of the red blood cell (around 8 weeks) is a convenient period of time over which to assess control. Different analytical methods measure either total haemoglobin A_1 (HbA_1) or the more specific HbA_{1C} fraction. The level of HbA_1 in nondiabetics is around 5–7%; in well-controlled diabetes the level should be below 10%, while, in poorly controlled diabetes, levels of up to 20% may be found. Low values may be found in patients who are experiencing frequent hypoglycaemia. Spuriously low values are found in conditions associated with reduced red-cell survival (e.g. haemolytic anaemias), while high values are found in renal failure (owing to the presence of carbamylated haemoglobin) and in certain haemoglobinopathies (e.g. thalassaemia).

In situations such as pregnancy, the half-life of haemoglobin is too long for HbA_1 to be useful in monitoring glycaemic control as closely as is required. Glycated albumin (half-life of around 19 days) would be ideal for this purpose and suitable methods are awaited. Measurement of glycated serum proteins or 'fructosamine' (mostly albumin and, therefore, of similar half-life) has gained some acceptance but suffers from lack of accurate standardization and from variations in albumin levels which occur in a number of disease states.

Nonglycaemic Control

In addition to measures of glycaemic control, it is clearly essential to monitor a large number of other biochemical and clinical parameters on a regular basis in an attempt to anticipate and, if possible, prevent the development of complications. Such monitoring is best done as part of a regular (usually annual) formal review (see Table 5).

Prognosis

Despite the advances which have been made over the last 70 years, life expectancy is still reduced in both

Treatment and Management

Table 5.   Parameters to be reviewed at annual follow-up

Biochemical	
Blood	HbA₁, creatinine, potassium, lipids (cholesterol, HDLC, triglycerides)
Urine	Albumin excretion rate, ketones
Hypoglycaemia	Occurrence, severity, adequacy of warning symptoms
Anthropometric	Weight, body mass index, height (children)
Clinical	
Cardiovascular	Blood pressure, peripheral pulses
Eyes	Visual acuity, fundoscopy
Neurological	Vibration threshold, tendon reflexes, peripheral sensation
Chiropody	Feet inspection
Treatment	Diet
	Insulin or oral agents
	Injection sites
	Other drugs
Social factors	Smoking, alcohol consumption

HbA₁, haemoglobin A₁; HDLC, high-density lipoprotein cholesterol.

IDDM and NIDDM. This is largely attributable to arterial disease (especially coronary artery and peripheral vascular disease) which occurs at an earlier age than in the nondiabetic population, and to those complications which are peculiar to diabetes, i.e. microvascular disease (particularly nephropathy) and both ketoacidosis and hyperosmolar coma. In IDDM, life expectancy is reduced by about 25%, with a peak in mortality occurring between 15 and 25 years after diagnosis.

There is a common misconception that the situation is less serious in NIDDM but this is clearly not so. Overall life expectancy is reduced by between 5 and 10 years, largely owing to the very high incidence of coronary and cerebrovascular disease. Nephropathy is relatively uncommon in NIDDM, but visual loss resulting from maculopathy is as common as in IDDM and frequently occurs early in the course of the disease. It is important to remember that NIDDM may be only a single aspect of a syndrome which comprises, in addition to carbohydrate intolerance, hypertension, dyslipidaemia, obesity and marked insulin resistance. The diabetes itself may be mild, but patients should not be dismissed lightly in view of the high mortality associated with the syndrome. *See* Lipoproteins

Bibliography

Alberti KGMM, Boucher BJ, Hitman GA and Taylor R (1990) Diabetes mellitus. In: *The Metabolic and Molecular Basis of Acquired Disease* (Cohen RD, Lewis B, Alberti KGMM and Denman AM, eds), pp 765–840. London: Ballière Tindall.

British Diabetic Association (1992) Dietary recommendations for people with diabetes: an update for the 1990s, *Diabetic Medicine* 9: 189–202.

Home PD, Johnston DG and Alberti KGMM (1989) Diabetes mellitus. In: *Fundamentals of Clinical Endocrinology* (Hall R and Besser G, eds), pp 318–361. Edinburgh: Churchill Livingstone.

Keonig RJ, Peterson CM, Jones RL, Saudek C, Lehrman M and Cerami A (1976) Correlation of glucose regulation and hemoglobin A_{1c} in diabetes mellitus. *New England Journal of Medicine* 295: 417–420.

Nattrass M and Hale PJ (eds) (1988) Non-insulin-dependent diabetes. *Clinical Endocrinology and Metabolism* 2(2).

Pickup JC and Williams (eds) (1991) *Textbook of Diabetes.* Oxford: Blackwell.

Singh BM, Rutter JD and Fitzgerald MG (1988). The natural history of non-insulin-dependent diabetes. *Clinical Endocrinology and Metabolism* 2: 343–358.

J. Wright
University of Surrey, Guildford, UK

Problems in Treatment

Children and Young People

The diagnosis of diabetes in a child is a traumatic event for the entire family, and parents usually take far longer than the child to adapt to the situation. Diet is often one of the major worries and a high level of support and reassurance from professional advisers is essential in the early stages.

Fortunately, recent changes in thinking mean that the diabetic diet is no longer as restrictive or disruptive to family life as it used to be. The objective of dietary management – to prevent wide swings in blood sugar by balancing food consumption against injected insulin – is unaltered, but the way in which this is achieved has changed considerably. In the past, children were given a diet restricted in carbohydrate content, virtually devoid of sugar, and high in fat and protein. Such a diet is now considered to be neither necessary nor desirable. To a large extent, the modern diabetic diet can be accommodated within ordinary family meals; children with diabetes should no longer grow up feeling that they have to eat differently from everyone else.

Dietary Composition

The basic nutritional requirements of children with diabetes are the same as those of nondiabetic children of a comparable age. Children with diabetes should also, like their peers, be encouraged to develop healthy eating habits which may be of benefit in later life. Although the presence of diabetes imposes certain dietary constraints, the composition of the diet now recommended for the diabetic is largely compatible with the healthy eating guidelines advocated for the rest of the population.

The diet for a diabetic child should contain sufficient energy to permit growth but prevent obesity. The proportion of energy derived from carbohydrate should certainly not be less than average (i.e. around 45% of dietary energy) and most of this carbohydrate should be in an unrefined (fibre-containing) form. More dietary energy from carbohydrate enables the proportion of energy from dietary fat, particularly saturated fat, to be reduced, a measure which may be of long-term benefit to the atherogenically at-risk diabetic.

However, in practice the proportion of nutrients in a child's diet must be determined on an individual basis, taking factors such as age, appetite and food preferences into account. If children who eat little are offered only bulky, relatively low-energy foods, their nutritional needs are unlikely to be met. Equally, trying to force a child to eat foods which are actively disliked will also be counterproductive. The change to a healthy pattern of eating should therefore proceed slowly and ideally be adopted by all the family. *See* Children, Nutritional Requirements

Energy

In practical terms, ensuring that the diet contains an appropriate amount of energy is the cornerstone of good dietary management. If the dietary energy content is too low, growth will be impaired; if it is too high, diabetic control will be jeopardized and obesity may result. Energy needs of children vary widely and cannot be accurately assessed from tables of average needs alone; the child's habitual energy intake (which can be assessed by dietary enquiry) should also be taken into account. *See* Energy, Measurement of Food Energy

Carbohydrate

The proportion of dietary energy from suitable carbohydrate can gradually be increased by measures such as substituting high-fibre breakfast cereals for low-fibre (especially the sugar-coated) varieties. Wholemeal bread should be offered instead of white bread but, if the child refuses to eat it, white bread is better than no bread at all. Alternatively, one of the white breads containing added fibre may be an acceptable compromise. Potatoes, pasta, rice, baked beans and fruit are sources of suitable carbohydrate which tend to be liked by children. *See* Carbohydrates, Requirements and Dietary Importance

Since virtually all children and young people with diabetes will require insulin, the quantity and timing of carbohydrate intake is important. A regular meal pattern is essential but, with the wide variety of insulins currently available, it is now possible to devise an insulin regimen which suits the child's (and the family's) eating habits rather than forcing the child to eat at unaccustomed times to accommodate the insulin. Parents generally find it easier to regulate the amount of carbohydrate consumed at each meal by means of a food exchange system, but precise weighing is no longer thought necessary; handy measures are quite sufficient.

Sugar and Sweeteners

The amount of sugar in the diet should be kept to a sensible minimum but its avoidance should not become an obsession. Isolated sources of readily absorbed carbohydrate, such as sugar-rich drinks, should be avoided (apart from when needed to prevent or treat hypoglycaemia) and can easily be substituted by sugar-free or low-energy alternatives.

Noncaloric sweeteners such as aspartame, acesulfame K or saccharin should be used in preference to table sugar on foods such as breakfast cereals, but small amounts of sucrose present in manufactured foods (e.g. jam or flavoured yogurt), or incorporated into home-made desserts, do not pose a hazard as long as they are consumed as part of a mixed meal. Provision for sweets and chocolate can be made either by incorporating them as part of the carbohydrate allowance at the end of a meal, or as a carbohydrate boost prior to exercise. *See* Acesulphame; Aspartame; Saccharin; Sweeteners – Intense

The use of nutritive sweeteners such as sorbitol and fructose, and specially manufactured 'diabetic foods' containing them, are not recommended. These products are expensive and unnecessary, and chldren may be especially sensitive to their ability to cause osmotic diarrhoea. Regulated quantities of the conventional product they are designed to replace are preferable.

Fat

There are several relatively painless ways in which fat intake can be limited. Unnecessary use of fat when cooking should be avoided. Foods should be grilled or baked rather than fried, and items such as chips should be an occasional treat, not a daily occurrence. Smaller quantities of leaner meat should be purchased in preference to larger amounts of fatty meat, and any obvious fat or poultry skin discarded before cooking. If children are unwilling to forego relatively high-fat foods such as sausages or burgers, those products which have a reduced-fat content are preferable (but care should be taken to avoid overuse of these foods). The entire family, including any children over the age of 2 years, can change to the use of semiskimmed milk as long as the rest of the diet is nutritionally adequate. However, skimmed milk is unsuitable for the under-fives because it contains insufficient vitamin A and energy. *See* Fats, Requirements

Protein

Protein intake should not be excessive. In the era of carbohydrate restriction, liberal consumption of carbohydrate-free foods such as meat, cheese and eggs was encouraged. This is not only unnecessary and expensive but may also be unwise in terms of the later development of diabetic nephropathy. Instead, carbohydrate foods should be the main component of the meal and any hunger pangs met with extra helpings of vegetables or fruit. A child who is persistently hungry should be referred back to the dietitian as an increase in dietary carbohydrate content may be needed. *See* Protein, Requirements

Vitamins

Children with diabetes have no additional requirements for vitamins. The under-fives should be given the supplements which are advised for all members of this age-group. *See* Vitamins, Overview

Role of the Dietitian

The expertise of a dietitian is essential for optimal dietary management of a child with diabetes. Dietary advice must be constructed on an individual basis in accordance with the nutritional needs, the insulin treatment and the usual eating habits of the family. Few families are able to comprehend and implement all the dietary and other aspects of diabetic management immediately after diagnosis, and the process of education and adaptation should proceed at a pace which both parents and child can cope with. Continuing dietetic support is likely to be needed for some time. *See* Dietetics

Children with established diabetes still require frequent (at least annual) review of dietary and insulin needs. The fact that children grow and their dietary requirements change can sometimes be overlooked.

Dietary Considerations of Particular Age-groups

The Preschool Child

The combination of erratic food habits and unpredictable levels of activity mean that hypoglycaemia is a constant threat in this age-group. Most parents find food refusal and food fads exasperating, but the parents of a diabetic toddler also find such behaviour extremely worrying because they feel that they have lost some of their ability to control the diabetes. However, sensible dietetic guidance can usually avert disaster. The risk of hypoglycaemia can be minimized by dividing the day's diet into smaller but more frequent meals – a dietary pattern which in any case tends to be preferred by young children. Refusal of food should be treated with calm detachment and, if necessary, the missed carbohydrate unobtrusively replaced in the form of a glucose-containing drink. As in any family, meal-times should not be allowed to develop into a battleground since this will only make the problem worse. *See* Glucose, Maintenance of Blood Glucose Level

A home blood glucose monitor can provide valuable reassurance to parents of children in this age-group.

The School-age Child

Children of this age-group usually adapt to the demands of diabetes with remarkable equanimity. Most prefer to inject their own insulin and quickly learn that they need to eat certain foods at certain times.

It is vital that the school staff are given clear instructions about the diet and other aspects of diabetic management and that they understand the problems which may arise. Staff need to be aware of the amounts of carbohydrate required at lunch time and other times of the day, and what this means in terms of food. However, it is also crucial that they are aware that these are guidelines, not inflexible rules – a child who senses that hypoglycaemia is imminent must not be made to wait until the allotted time for his next carbohydrate snack. Additional carbohydrate will also be required before exercise and, if particularly strenuous or prolonged, possibly afterwards as well. Needs will vary from day to day and the person best able to gauge these needs is usually the child. However, even capable children do not always get the balance right and staff must also be taught how to recognize and treat early signs of hypoglycaemia, e.g. a sudden loss of concentration or uncharacteristic outburst of temper, as well as the emergency measures required if severe hypoglycaemia or loss of consciousness should result.

The Adolescent

Most adolescents have a desire to assert their independence and those with diabetes often use diet as a focus for rebellion. They may want to eat snack foods rather than conventional meals, eat out with friends instead of at home with the family, try new foods and reject familiar ones. *See* Adolescents, Nutritional Problems

Energy requirements will also change during these years. Sudden growth spurts, especially in boys, may necessitate a dramatic increase in energy and carbohydrate requirements. Energy expenditure may be altered by changes in the level and nature of sporting activities. Some adolescents may take up physically demanding new activities such as squash or jogging. Others may give up sport altogether.

This period of transition need not be difficult if these near-adults are treated in an adult way and shown how they can take responsibility for their own wellbeing. The reasons why good glycaemic control is important and how this can be maintained in different circumstances should be explained. A pronouncement by teenagers that they wish to slim or adopt vegetarianism should not be met with straight opposition but with the encouragement to find out how this can be done in a sensible way. The hazards of alcohol for those who take insulin must be clearly set out and guidance given on its sensible and safe use. *See* Vegetarian Diets

Above all, adolescents should be encouraged to seek professional guidance from their doctor or dietitian for their own particular needs and to regard these advisers not as people telling them 'what to do' but 'how to do it'.

Pregnancy

There are two distinct groups of women who may be both pregnant and diabetic: those with pre-existing diabetes who become pregnant, and previously normal women who develop a form of diabetes (gestational diabetes) during pregnancy. There are some differences between these groups in terms of the effects of the diabetes and its management. *See* Pregnancy, Nutrition in Diabetic Pregnancy

Pregnancy in Women with Pre-existing Diabetes

It is only relatively recently that women with diabetes have been able to look forward with any degree of confidence to the safe arrival of a healthy child. A few decades ago, the combination of diabetes and pregnancy was associated with a greatly increased risk of pre- or perinatal death, congenital malformations and maternal death. However, the incidence of these has now fallen dramatically as a result of better management during pregnancy and advances in postnatal care, although the risks remain slightly higher than for the nondiabetic population.

Strict control of glycaemia is now recognized as vital in order to minimize the problems associated with a diabetic pregnancy. There appear to be strong links between maternal hyperglycaemia and the development of congenital malformations, which are still three times more likely to occur in the children of diabetic mothers. The time of greatest risk appears to be during the first trimester when organogenesis is taking place. Since damage may occur even before pregnancy is suspected, it is essential that diabetic control is optimized before attempting to become pregnant as well as during the pregnancy itself.

Problems in Treatment

During the second and third trimesters, elevated glucose levels in the maternal circulation will tend to enhance insulin production by fetal β-cells. This results in disordered growth and the development of a child who is longer, larger and more obese than average (macrosomia). Delivery of the macrosomic child inevitably causes greater problems for the mother and the hospital team.

Maternal hyperglycaemia may also increase the risk of respiratory distress syndrome, the major cause of perinatal death in infants of diabetic mothers.

Pregnancy tends to exacerbate some of the complications associated with diabetes. Retinopathy may worsen and renal function tends to deteriorate, sometimes leading to nephropathy. Good diabetic control during pregnancy may help to minimize some of these effects.

Dietary Management

The ability to improve the degree of glycaemic control has largely resulted from the advent of multiple insulin regimens, continuous subcutaneous insulin infusion (CSII) and the availability of home blood glucose monitoring. However, diet remains an important aspect of management. A stable, regular meal pattern is essential and the change to more frequent insulin administration usually means that meals will also need to be smaller and more frequent.

Energy intake will need to be increased slightly to meet the increased requirements of pregnancy but must not be excessive. The adequacy of the energy intake can be assessed from the rate of weight gain; on average, nondiabetic and well-controlled diabetic women gain about 10–12 kg during pregnancy. Dietary measures may be needed to slow the rate of weight gain, but active weight reduction should not be attempted during pregnancy itself.

An increased energy intake means that the quantity of nutrients consumed will increase in absolute terms, but the overall composition of the diet in terms of the proportion of energy supplied by each of the major nutrients should not change. As in any diabetic diet, more of the dietary energy should come from unrefined carbohydrate (the consequent high fibre content also helping to prevent constipation, so often a problem in pregnancy) and less from fat. The proportion of energy from protein should remain unchanged. Requirements for vitamins and minerals are the same as for the nondiabetic pregnant woman, and iron and folate supplements should be provided as necessary.

As in any pregnancy, nausea and morning sickness can be a problem in the early weeks. Carbohydrate snacks such as biscuits or crispbread may be helpful and, if solid foods cannot be faced at all, carbohydrate needs can be met on a short-term basis by glucose-containing drinks.

As pregnancy advances, appetite usually increases and the consequent hunger, and in some cases an overwhelming desire for particular foods, can lead to erratic food intake and seriously disturbed control. Patients should see a dietitian regularly during their pregnancy so that these problems can be identified and countered at an early stage.

Following delivery, the characteristic insulin resistance of pregnancy rapidly disappears and insulin requirements return to the prepregnancy state. Dietary needs will return to normal, except in those who decide to breast-feed; these women will need to maintain, and possibly even increase, their energy intake. Patients will wish to lose weight following pregnancy; they must be strongly discouraged from drastic dieting and given guidance on how weight loss may be achieved gradually and safely.

Gestational Diabetes

Gestational diabetes is an impaired glucose tolerance which occurs during pregnancy. Because it usually only develops after about 20 weeks, when the embryonic stage of pregnancy has been completed, gestational diabetes is less likely to cause congenital malformations. However, the fetus is still at risk from the effects of hyperglycaemia in the later stages of pregnancy, and the gestational diabetic pregnancy can also result in a macrosomic child and an increased likelihood of birth trauma or stillbirth.

Since gestational diabetes is usually asymptomatic, it is vital that all pregnant women are properly screened for this condition and at the appropriate time (e.g. a preprandial blood glucose measurement midway through pregnancy). Many cases are likely to be missed if screening only comprises a test for glycosuria at the first antenatal visit.

Dietary Management

Many patients with gestational diabetes are obese and can be treated by dietary measures alone. A moderate reduction in energy intake, achieved by a diet relatively low in fat and high in unrefined carbohydrate, and the avoidance of concentrated sources of simple sugars may be all that is required.

However, patients with severe hyperglycaemia will require insulin. Oral hypoglycaemic agents cannot be given as they stimulate fetal insulin secretion and so increase the likelihood of macrosomia. A combination of short and intermediate regimen of insulin is usually given together with appropriate dietary measures. Regular monitoring of blood glucose levels is desirable.

Gestational diabetes usually disappears after childbirth but often recurs in subsequent pregnancies. A

Problems in Treatment

significant proportion of women with gestational diabetes will develop diabetes in later life, particularly if they are obese. The latter should therefore be encouraged to make a permanent effort to lose weight in order to lessen this risk.

Surgery

Surgical procedures pose a potential hazard to the diabetic as they tend to make the diabetes more unstable and increase the risk of ketoacidosis. These problems will be minimized by close collaboration between physician, surgeon, anaesthetist and nursing staff.

The way in which the diabetes is managed will depend on individual circumstances, including the type and stability of the diabetes, the nature of the surgical problem and whether or not it has caused associated debilitating illness, and whether the surgery to be performed is major or minor.

Prior to surgery, the major aim is to minimize the risk of hypoglycaemia since the symptoms of this may not be apparent in a sedated or semiconscious patient. Patients on a long-acting insulin should be changed to one of shorter duration so that there is no hypoglycaemic action during preoperative starvation. For the same reason, patients on oral hypoglycaemics with a long half-life (such as chlorpropamide) should be changed to a shorter-acting oral agent.

During the surgery itself, insulin-dependent diabetics will be controlled by the intravenous infusion of glucose and insulin (usually with additional potassium, the so-called GKI system). Non-insulin-dependent diabetics will usually have sufficient insulin reserves to maintain them during the surgical procedure and require no special measures; however, those undergoing prolonged surgery may also require glucose–insulin infusion.

As soon as the patient can eat normally following surgery, the usual treatment is restarted. However, frequent blood glucose monitoring is essential as the stress effect of surgery is liable to worsen diabetic control and increase insulin requirements. If the patient is anorexic, carbohydrate needs can be met from liquid or semiliquid sources (e.g. soups, glucose drinks, yoghurt, ice cream) until appetite is restored.

Dietary Compliance

In recent years the ideal dietary composition for people with diabetes has been the subject of much debate but there has also been growing awareness that even the best diet is useless if it is not followed.

Compliance with the traditional low-carbohydrate diabetic diet was known to be poor. Since diet is an integral part of diabetic management, either to balance the effects of insulin or hypoglycaemic drugs, or as a treatment in itself, it seemed reasonable to assume that poor dietary compliance would lead to poor diabetic control and ultimately increase the risk of long-term complications.

In practice, this has been difficult to prove. Many studies have failed to demonstrate that noncompliers have worse control or more complications than those who closely follow the prescribed diet. Few would suggest that this means that dietary measures are unimportant – diet is clearly relevant to diabetic health. It seems more likely that these findings reflect the difficulties of assessing 'compliance' in a quantifiable way. For example, a commonly used yardstick is a comparison of the amount of carbohydrate prescribed and consumed, but there are a number of reasons why this may be misleading:

1. The amount of carbohydrate prescribed may not have been appropriate in the first place. Carbohydrate prescriptions are calculated from the energy content of the diet. However, the energy content of the diet is often decided on the basis of average energy needs, despite the fact that individual requirements may vary widely from this mean. A subsequent dietary intake which differs from the prescribed figures may be defined as 'noncompliance' whereas, in reality, some patients might be consuming a diet which more closely matches their energy needs.

2. Not all carbohydrates, even unrefined carbohydrates, have the same effects on blood glucose levels. The amount, type and structural integrity of dietary fibre associated with the carbohydrate, and even the presence or absence of other nutrients such as fat influence the relationship between carbohydrate consumed and subsequent glycaemia. The total amount of carbohydrate eaten may therefore bear little relation to the effect which it has had on glycaemia.

3. A dietary prescription implies that the amount of energy and carbohydrate required each day will remain constant; in practice these needs will vary according to the activity level. If carbohydrate intake is increased on a particular day in order to balance an increased level of exercise, this is not 'poor compliance'.

Dietary knowledge has also been used as a measure of compliance on the (not unreasonable) grounds that if people do not understand basic concepts of their diet, they are unlikely to be able to follow it. However, results from such studies also need to be interpreted with caution. What people know is not necessarily the same as what they do. Some patients will follow a diet sheet to the last detail, yet remain totally ignorant of the difference between calories and carbohydrate. Others can recite their dietary prescripton with ease yet freely admit they take little notice of it. The significance of dietary knowledge also differs between groups of patients; it may not matter if a non-insulin-dependent diabetic does not know which foods will stave off imminent hypoglycaemia, whereas such lack of knowledge in an insulin-dependent patient could be disastrous.

Different aspects of compliance may affect different aspects of control and the progression of different complications. Microvascular complications such as retinopathy are closely linked with the degree of hyperglycaemia over a period of time. People whose diet varies because they have a casual attitude to its importance may be more at risk than those who closely monitor their blood glucose levels and vary their diet as a way of maintaining near-normal glycaemia. Other complications, such as cardiovascular disease, may be more closely linked with lipidaemia than with glycaemia, and more influenced by the amount of saturated fat consumed.

Ultimately, the effectiveness of a dietary regimen – and, by implication, compliance with it – can only be assessed by evaluating the degree to which diet and any other treatment have achieved good diabetic control. This may depend not so much on whether nutrient intake in absolute terms has matched pre-ordained targets but on less quantifiable factors such as dietary attitude and application. These will be influenced by the following:

1. People must be motivated to follow the diet. Changing the established eating habits of a lifetime is not easy and people will only make the effort to to do so if they are convinced that it is both necessary and important.
2. People must be given some explanation of how the diet works and what it is trying to achieve, but at a level which each individual can understand. Some people like to be given as much information as possible; others get confused by too much detail and need a simpler message.
3. The diet must be based on individual rather than average dietary needs and should, as far as is possible, be compatible with the habitual eating pattern and lifestyle. A standardized meal plan handed out to all-comers will suit no-one and be doomed to failure.
4. Initial dietetic support and regular follow-up are essential, not only so that dietary problems can be discussed but also so that patients do not forget that diet is a vital part of their treatment.

Unfortunately perhaps, the penalties for noncompliance are not immediately obvious to the patient unless deviation is so severe that diabetic symptoms such as thirst and polyuria reappear. It is also difficult to maintain motivation when people are striving for a negative objective – freedom from complications. Furthermore, the rewards for their efforts will not be apparent for many years and even then cannot be guaranteed.

That there are benefits from compliance with the appropriate dietary regimen cannot be doubted. The goal of metabolic normality – essential for the minimization of complications – cannot, at present, be achieved by clinical means alone; for many diabetics, diet remains the only suitable form of treatment. The mistakes made in the past were that dietary treatment was not always the most suitable in terms of composition, it was often implemented in an inappropriate way, and it was often regarded as an adjunct to treatment rather than an integral part of it. The recent change to a diabetic dietary regimen containing less fat and more carbohydrate offers many theoretical benefits to the diabetic. Whether or not these are realized in practice depends to a large extent on whether or not the associated factors that determine compliance are addressed as well.

Bibliography

Baum JD and Kinmonth AL (1986) *Care of the Child with Diabetes.* Edinburgh: Churchill Livingstone.

British Diabetic Association (1982a) Dietary recommendations for diabetics for the 1980s – a policy statement. *Human Nutrition Applied Nutrition* 36A: 378–394.

British Diabetic Association (1982b) The role of the dietitian in the management of the diabetic. *Human Nutrition Applied Nutrition* 36A: 395–400.

British Diabetic Association (1989) Dietary recommendations for children and adolescents with diabetes. *Diabetic Medicine* 6: 537–547.

British Diabetic Association (1991) Dietary recommendations for people with diabetes: an update for the 1990s. *Journal of Human Nutrition and Dietetics* 4: 393–412.

Brudenell JM and Doddridge M (1989) *Diabetic Pregnancy.* Edinburgh: Churchill Livingstone.

Day JL (1986) *The Diabetes Handbook: Insulin Dependent Diabetes.* Wellingborough and London: Thorsons and the British Diabetic Association.

Gill GV (1991) Surgery and diabetes mellitus. In: Pickup J and Williams G (eds) *Textbook of Diabetes,* pp 820–826. Oxford: Blackwell Scientific Publications.

Husband DJ, Thai AC and Alberti KGMM (1986) Management of diabetes during surgery with glucose–insulin–potassium infusion. *Diabetic Medicine* 3: 69–74.

Keen H and Thomas BJ (1988) Diabetes mellitus. In: Dickerson JWT and Lee HA (eds) *Nutrition in the Clinical Management of Disease* 2nd edn, pp 167–186. London: Edward Arnold.

Lowy C (1991) Pregnancy and diabetes mellitus. In: Pickup J and Williams G (eds) *Textbook of Diabetes,* pp 835–850. Oxford: Blackwell Scientific Publications.

Moran A, Hessett C, Pooley J and Boulton AJM (1989) An assessment of patient knowledge of diabetes, its management and complications. *Practical Diabetes* 6: 265–267.

Sutherland HW and Stowers JM (eds) (1984) *Carbohydrate Metabolism in Pregnancy and the Newborn.* Edinburgh: Churchill Livingstone.

Thomas BJ (1981) How successful are we at persuading diabetics to follow their diet – and why do we sometimes fail? In Turner M and Thomas B (eds) *Nutrition and Diabetes*, pp 57–66. London: John Libbey.

Thomas B (ed.) (1988) Dietary management of children with diabetes mellitus. *Manual of Dietetic Practice*, pp 366–367. Oxford: Blackwell Scientific Publications.

Thompson AV, Neil HAW, Thorogood M, Fowler GH and Mann JI (1988) Diabetes mellitus: attitudes, knowledge and glycaemic control in a cross-sectional population. *Journal of the Royal College of General Practitioners* 38: 450–452.

Watkins PJ, Drury PL and Taylor KW (1990) *Diabetes and its Management* 4th edn. Oxford: Blackwell Scientific Publications.

West KM (1973) Diet therapy of diabetes: an analysis of failure. *Annals of Internal Medicine* 79: 425–434.

Briony Thomas
Dorking, Surrey, UK

Secondary Complications

Types of Complications

As the life expectancy of people with diabetes has increased, the secondary consequences of diabetes over a long period of time have become more apparent. Management of diabetes is no longer confined to the short-term relief of symptoms but is increasingly focused on measures which will prevent or minimize its long-term effects.

Complications of diabetes can be divided into two main categories: arterial disease of large or medium-sized blood vessels (macrovascular or 'large-vessel' disease), and damage to the microvascular circulation of the retina and kidneys and to peripheral nerves (microvascular or 'small-vessel' disease).

There are differences in the pathogenesis of these two types of complications. Microvascular complications are unique to diabetes, and their development appears to be associated with prolonged exposure to hyperglycaemia and other metabolic disturbances associated with diabetes. In contrast, large-vessel disease affects both diabetic and nondiabetic populations alike, although the prevalence of the disease is greatly increased in people with diabetes. However, there are some links between diabetic complications: retinopathy and nephropathy often develop together and patients with diabetic nephropathy have a greatly increased risk of cardiovascular mortality.

Macrovascular Disease

Macrovascular disease results from atheromatous changes in large and medium-sized blood vessels which may become partly or totally blocked. The resulting impairment can affect the cardiovascular system (causing angina and coronary thrombosis), the cerebrovascular system (causing strokes), and the peripheral blood supply to the lower limbs (causing claudication and tissue damage).

People with diabetes have an increased risk of developing all types of vascular disease, but their susceptibility to cardiovascular disease is perhaps of greatest concern. Diabetic cardiovascular mortality rates are considerably higher than in the general population, and the disease tends to strike at a younger age and at both sexes.

The fact that diabetes enhances the atherogenic process has not been fully explained, but it is probably attributable to a combination of factors. Hyperglycaemia may have some directly damaging effect on arterial walls, but other biochemical disturbances associated with diabetes – notably hyperlipidaemia – may be of greater significance. Elevated levels of blood cholesterol, particularly cholesterol carried by low-density lipoproteins (LDLs), are known to enhance the risk of vascular disease. The LDL-cholesterol level is primarily determined by dietary and genetic factors but diabetes tends to have an additional elevating effect, possibly as a result of reduced LDL clearance at the cellular level. *See* Atherosclerosis; Cholesterol, Role of Cholesterol in Heart Disease; Hyperlipidaemia; Lipoproteins

Hypertriglyceridaemia and raised levels of very-low-density lipoprotein (VLDL) are also common features of diabetes. Poor metabolic control and associated insulin insufficiency impair lipoprotein lipase activity and consequently reduce the clearance of VLDL. In the non-insulin-dependent diabetic this may be compounded by insulin resistance and overproduction of VLDL. Hypertriglyceridaemia causes concern because it tends to depress levels of the atherogenically protective high-density lipoprotein (HDL).

Thrombogenic factors, such as the fibrinogen level or degree of platelet stickiness, may also be adversely affected by diabetes, leading to an increased likelihood of thrombosis and blood vessel occlusion.

Optimizing diabetic control is a vital part of reducing the cardiovascular risk. The risk from factors such as hypertension and cigarette smoking should also be minimized. Secondary risk factors such as obesity (which causes hypertension, hyperlipidaemia and insulin resistance) and lack of exercise should also be identified and corrected. *See* Coronary Heart Disease, Intervention Studies; Exercise, Metabolic Requirements; Smoking, Diet and Health

Diet plays an important part in achieving many of these objectives. The modern diabetic diet which encourages the consumption of unrefined carbohydrate at the expense of dietary fat is more likely to be atherogenically protective than its low-carbohydrate, high-fat predecessor. Both the blood cholesterol level and the lipid profile (e.g. the LDL:HDL ratio) will be considerably improved by a restriction in fat intake to around 30–35% of dietary energy. A smaller proportion of dietary fat should come from saturated sources (such as fat derived from meat and dairy products) and more from monounsaturated and polyunsaturated sources (such as cooking oils and fats derived from some vegetable oils). *See* Fats, Requirements

An increased intake of dietary fibre, a consequence of an increased consumption of unrefined carbohydrate, may also have beneficial effects on blood lipids, particularly if the fibre is of the soluble type (i.e. that derived from oats, pulses, fruit and vegetables). *See* Dietary Fibre, Fibre and Disease Prevention

High sodium intakes may exacerbate or contribute to hypertension (a primary risk factor for cardiovascular disease) and excessive amounts should be avoided. In some patients, reducing dietary sodium from 6 g per day to 3 g per day may correct hypertension without the need for antihypertensive drugs (some of which have undesirable side-effects on serum lipids). *See* Sodium, Physiology

For those who are overweight, loss of weight is an important objective. Losing excessive weight will reduce the risk from other factors, such as elevated blood pressure and an abormal lipid profile. Weight loss is the only form of management in non-insulin-dependent diabetes which has been related to improved life expectancy. In general, a low-energy diet relatively high in fibre-containing carbohydrate and low in fat is the most suitable for weight loss as it has a high satiety value. *See* Obesity, Treatment

Microvascular Disease

Nephropathy

Diabetic nephropathy results from damage to the microvascular circulation of the kidney. It is characterized by persistent proteinuria, rising blood pressure, and progressive decline in renal function which may eventually result in renal failure. *See* Kidney, Structure and Function

In insulin-dependent patients, nephropathy most commonly appears after about 15 years of diabetes and may affect as many as one third of diabetics. Non-insulin-dependent patients appear to be less susceptible to this complication, but when it does develop it usually occurs after a much shorter duration of the diabetes. Since there are so many more patients with the non-insulin-dependent form of the disease, nephropathy is commonly encountered in this group as well.

Prior to the development of overt diabetic nephropathy, damage to the glomerular capillaries results in leakage of albumin into the urine. These losses are small and symptomless but appear to be an important predictor of the subsequent development of clinical nephropathy. Identification of patients with 'microalbuminuria' (urinary albumin excretion in the range of 30–300 mg per day) may be an important way of ensuring that preventive measures are applied at an early stage to those most at-risk.

The development of microalbuminuria appears to be linked with the quality of diabetic control; the level of hyperglycaemia during the first 15 years of diabetes has been shown to be directly related to the risk of developing persistent proteinuria. However, genetic susceptibility also plays a part, and there appears to be an increased risk in people of Afro-Caribbean and Asian Indian origin.

In the early stages of the disease, strict glycaemic control and effective antihypertensive treatment can reduce microalbuminuria and restore the glomerular filtration rate (GFR) to the normal range. There is evidence that the progression to clinical nephropathy can be slowed and associated mortality reduced if these measures are started early enough.

Recently, there has also been interest in the possible role of protein restriction in the prevention of this complication. Dietary protein intake is known to influence renal function, and a low-protein diet retards the progression of chronic renal failure. There is some evidence that a diet which includes moderate dietary protein restriction (to about 45 g per day or 0·6–0·7 g per kg of ideal bodyweight) may also slow the rate of decline in GFR and reduce urinary protein excretion in some patients, particularly if started before renal impairment is too advanced. Further research is required to determine precisely which dietary components are important, at what stage protein restriction should be introduced and at what level. Too severe a protein restriction (e.g. 20–25 g per day) may be counterproductive in terms of nutritional adequacy and dietary acceptability. All patients should certainly be discouraged from consuming an above-average protein intake. In the era of carbohydrate avoidance, diabetic patients were encouraged to increase their consumption of protein-rich foods such as meat, cheese and eggs. This is now seen as unnecessary and, in terms of renal function, may have been unwise. Current recommendations in the USA are that diabetics should not exceed a protein intake of 0·8 g per kg of bodyweight. Reduction in protein intake to this level may be sensible for all patients with proteinuria and a reduced GFR or raised creatinine level. The type of protein may be relevant too; there is some evidence that vegetable protein may have less deleterious effects on renal function than animal protein. *See* Protein, Requirements

Moderate protein restriction can be achieved by reducing portion size of foods such as meat, poultry, fish and cheese. Such a measure will also help to decrease the consumption of saturated fat. Hyperlipidaemia is especially common in patients with diabetic nephropathy, and most die of heart disease. It is therefore particularly important that dietary aspects which may minimize this risk, e.g. fat modification, weight reduction and salt restriction, are given full consideration.

Retinopathy

Diabetic retinopathy is the most common cause of blindness in the UK. Damage to retinal capillaries causes oedema, new vessel formation and haemorrhages which, if unchecked, can result in visual impairment. There is also an increased risk of cataracts.

Retinal changes usually remain mild and asymptomatic for many years, so-called 'background retinopathy'. However, in time, 'proliferative retinopathy' may develop; new blood vessels appear and eventually lead to retinal detachment or vitreous haemorrhage and loss of sight.

The development of background retinopathy is closely associated with the duration of diabetes and, by implication, the degree of exposure to hyperglycaemia. Virtually all diabetic patients, whether insulin- or non-insulin-requiring, will have background changes after 15–20 years of diabetes. However, not all will develop the sight-threatening proliferative changes, the peak incidence of which occurs after about 15 years of diabetes and remains constant at about 3% per annum thereafter. It is unclear which factors trigger this effect. Poor control is a contributory factor (although a sudden improvement in diabetic control often leads to an abrupt deterioration in retinopathy for a period).

Good diabetic control is of prime importance in minimizing the development of retinopathy, and the advent of laser photocoagulation has dramatically improved the prognosis of retinopathy once it has appeared. This technique uses a laser beam to burn away any extra blood vessels which have developed on the retina, thus preventing them from spreading and threatening sight. The operation of vitrectomy can restore vision and prevent further vitreous haemorrhage from new vessels.

Early retinopathic damage is asymptomatic, so that regular screening is important. Insulin-dependent patients should have annual ophthalmological examinations once they have had diabetes for about 5 years. Non-insulin-dependent patients should be screened from the time of diagnosis, since some of them may have had sub-clinical diabetes for a number of years.

Neuropathy

Diabetes may result in damage to nerves, causing disordered motor, sensory and autonomic function. Relatively little is known about the incidence and prevalence of this complication because its effects are so diverse and difficult to classify.

Between 10–20% of insulin dependent patients may have evidence of peripheral neuropathy. Peripheral nerve damage is characterized by 'pins and needles', numbness or pain in the lower limbs and is particularly likely to contribute to problems in the diabetic foot. Loss of sensitivity to pain can result in unfelt injuries which, if associated with poor control or peripheral vascular disease, may become infected leading to ulcers and, possibly, gangrene.

Symptomatic autonomic neuropathy is more rare but when it does occur it may cause severe problems, including postural hypotension, incontinence and impotence. Neuropathy affecting the gastrointestinal tract can cause diarrhoea or constipation. Gastric neuropathy may reduce gastric secretion and delay gastric emptying, causing unpleasant sensations of bloating and resulting in anorexia, or even nausea and vomiting. These problems can seriously affect dietary management.

As with other microvascular complications, hyperglycaemia appears to promote neuropathy, and its development is related to the duration of diabetes. There is some evidence that improved glycaemic control benefits nerve function.

Recently it has been suggested that dietary supplementation with γ-linolenic acid may improve nerve conduction in diabetic subjects, possibly by normalizing the metabolism of the long-chain essential fatty acids derived from linoleic acid. However, this finding requires further evaluation.

Prevention

Some of the measures which may help to lessen the risk and the consequences of specific diabetic complications have been outlined above. However, general preventative measures should be applied to all patients.

Good control of blood glucose is paramount in minimizing the risk of all complications. The effects of hyperglycaemia cannot be predicted with absolute certainty; some well-controlled diabetics develop severe complications, while a few patients break all the rules but escape relatively unscathed. It appears that other factors, possibly genetic ones, affect individual susceptibility. However, since such factors cannot be identified in advance, aiming to approach normoglycaemia in all patients is sensible. Furthermore, this objective must be pursued with equal vigour in both insulin- and non-insulin-requiring patients. Although non-insulin-dependent diabetes is sometimes called 'mild' diabetes, it is anything but mild in its effects.

The best means of optimizing diabetic control in an

individual is a matter of clinical judgement dependent on individual medical needs and circumstances. The development of multiple injection regimens and techniques such as continuous subcutaneous insulin infusion have greatly improved the ability to achieve strict blood glucose control.

Good dietetic management is essential. A diet containing a relatively high proportion of its energy as unrefined carbohydrate and a low proportion from saturated fat, and not excessive in its content of protein, salt or simple sugars, is believed to be of most benefit in terms of both glycaemic control and atherogenesis. However, the practical means by which this is achieved must be determined in accordance with individual preferences; a diet which is disliked will not be followed and will be of no benefit. All patients need expert dietetic guidance in the early stages in order to achieve the best dietary compromise, and regular follow-up thereafter in order to identify and eliminate any problems which have arisen.

Those who need to lose weight will require particular support and encouragement. Achieving effective weight loss is a notoriously difficult task but the potential health benefits to those with diabetes justify the efforts required from both the advisors and the advised. *See* Slimming, Metabolic Consequences of Slimming Diets and Weight Maintenance

The availability of the home blood glucose monitor has greatly improved the patient's ability to keep his or her diabetes under tight control. However, other blood parameters, such as lipids, should also be regularly checked by the diabetic clinic and treated if necessary.

Patients should be regularly screened for signs of retinopathy or renal damage so that problems can be identified at an early stage and minimized. Blood pressure should be measured regularly and hypertension treated. Any associated risk factors to health, such as smoking or lack of exercise, should also be tackled.

Prevention of diabetic complications depends first on achieving the best possible control of the diabetes and, second, on early diagnosis of any problems which do arise. Diabetic care which consists solely of brief routine visits to an overworked doctor in a busy outpatient clinic may be sufficient to maintain short-term control of diabetes but is unlikely to be adequate to identify small problems until they have turned into large and possibly serious ones. Effective prevention depends on utilizing the skills of a number of members of the diabetic care team – physicians, nurses, dietitians, chiropodists, ophthalmologists, and biochemists – in a way which ensures that all patients are regularly reviewed and given the best possible continuing care.

Bibliography

Barsotti G, Ciardella F, Morelli E *et al.* (1988) Nutritional treatment of renal failure in Type 1 diabetic nephropathy. *Clinical Nephrology* 29: 280–287.

Betteridge J (1984) Diabetes, lipids and atherosclerosis. *Practical Diabetes* 1: 26–30.

Borch-Johnsen K and Kreiner S (1987) Proteinuria: value as a predictor of cardiovascular mortality in insulin dependent diabetes mellitus. *British Medical Journal* 294: 1651–1654.

Brenner BM, Meyer TW and Hostetter TH (1982) Dietary protein intake and the progressive nature of kidney disease. *New England Journal of Medicine* 307: 652–660.

Dahl-Jorgensen K, Bringhmann I, Hanson O *et al.* (1986) Effect of near-normoglycaemia for two years on progression of early diabetic retinopathy, nephropathy and neuropathy: the Oslo study. *British Medical Journal* 293: 1195–1199.

D'Antonio JA, Ellis D, Doft BH *et al.* (1989) Diabetes complications and glycaemic control. The Pittsburgh prospective insulin dependent diabetes cohort study status report after 5 years of IDDM. *Diabetes Care* 12: 694–700.

Dodson PM, Beevers M, Hallworth R *et al.* (1989) Sodium restriction and blood pressure in hypertensive Type 2 diabetes: randomised blind controlled and crossover studies of moderate sodium restriction and sodium supplementation. *British Medical Journal* 298: 227.

Fuller JH, Shipley MJ, Rose G, Jarrett RJ and Keen H (1983) Mortality from coronary heart disease and stroke in relation to the degree of hyperglycaemia: the Whitehall study. *British Medical Journal* 287: 867–870.

Jarrett RJ (ed.) (1984) *Diabetes and Heart Disease.* Amsterdam: Elsevier Science Publishers BV.

Kannel WB and McGee DL (1987) Diabetes and glucose tolerance as risk factors for cardiovascular disease: the Framingham study. *Diabetes Care* 2: 120–126.

Keen H and Jarrett RJ (eds) (1982) *Complications of Diabetes.* London: Edward Arnold.

Levine SE, D'Elia JA, Bistrian B *et al.* (1989) Protein-restricted diets in diabetic nephropathy. *Nephron* 52: 55–61.

McCance DR, Hadden DR, Atkinson AB, Archer DB and Kennedy L (1989) Long term glycaemic control and diabetic retinopathy. *Lancet* ii: 824.

Pickup J and Williams G (eds) (1990) *Textbook of Diabetes*, vol. 2. Oxford: Blackwell Scientific Publications.

Porte D, Graf RJ, Halter JB, Pfeifer MA and Halar E (1981) Diabetic neuropathy and plasma glucose control. *American Journal of Medicine* 70: 195–200.

Service FJ, Rizza RA, Daube JR, O'Brien PC and Dyck PJ (1985) Near normoglycaemia improves nerve conduction and vibration sensation in diabetic neuropathy. *Diabetologia* 28: 722–727.

Stone DB and Connor WE (1963) The prolonged effects of a low cholesterol, high carbohydrate diet upon the serum lipids of diabetic patients. *Diabetes* 12: 127–135.

Teuscher A, Schnelle H and Wilson PWT (1988) Incidence of diabetic retinopathy and relationship to baseline plasma glucose and blood pressure. *Diabetes Care* 11: 246–251.

Walker JD, Bending JJ, Dodds RA *et al.* (1989) Restriction of dietary protein and progression of renal failure in diabetic nephropathy. *Lancet* ii: 1411–1415.

Briony Thomas
Dorking, Surrey, UK

Secondary Complications

DIALYSIS

See Membrane Techniques

DIARRHOEAL DISEASES

The diarrhoeal disease control programme of the World Health Organization (WHO) has estimated that $700-1000 \times 10^6$ cases of acute diarrhoea occur every year in children under 5 years of age in the developing countries. It is estimated that of these up to 5×10^6 die per year from diarrhoea. In addition, more than 500×10^6 people travel as tourists every year and as many as 20–50% of them suffer from some type of diarrhoea. Even in industrialized countries, foodborne diseases are still major causes of morbidity.

During the last decade there have been considerable advances in the understanding of the physiology of different diarrhoea syndromes and it is now customary to divide diarrhoea into three broad categories: acute watery diarrhoea, dysentery, and persistent diarrhoea.

Acute Watery Diarrhoea

The commonest syndrome is that of acute travellers' diarrhoea which has rather descriptive names according to the source of infection e.g. Hong Kong dog, Delhi belly, Aztec two-step, etc. The onset of symptoms can occur at any time during travel or soon after returning from abroad. Several microorganisms are capable of producing such an illness (Table 1). The main mechanism by which diarrhoea occurs involves the production of a toxin by the bacteria. These toxins bind to receptors on the intestinal mucosal cells. This stimulates activation of intracellular messengers, such as cyclic adenosine monophosphate (cAMP) or cyclic guanosine monophosphate (cGMP) which start a series of intracellular processes in which there is secretion of water and sodium from the body into the lumen of the intestine. Cholera is a particularly life-threatening watery diarrhoea which develops as a result of cholera toxin binding to the mucosal cells. *See* Parasites, Occurrence and Detection; Viruses and also individual bacteria

Other organisms may damage the mucosal cells (e.g. rotavirus) and decrease the surface area of absorption. In addition, they bring the secretory crypt cells to the surface and increase the total volume of secretion. In the early stages of infection with certain parasites, such as *Giardia lamblia* and *Trichuris*, there can be acute watery diarrhoea.

Dysentery

The term 'dysentery' is used to describe diarrhoea in which there is increased passage of mucus and blood. The prognosis is more serious than watery diarrhoea and – particularly in the elderly, the very young and the malnourished – if diagnosis and treatment are delayed the illness may be fatal.

The disease occurs as a result of pathogens (Table 2) invading the distal small bowel and large bowel where they cause inflammation, ulceration and haemorrhage. Certain pathogens cause a mild illness which may

Table 1. Pathogens causing acute watery diarrhoea

Type of pathogen	Examples
Bacteria	Enterotoxigenic *Escherichia coli* (ETEC)
	Salmonella spp.
	Shigella spp.
	Vibrio cholerae
	Bacillus cereus
	Vibrio parahaemolyticus
	Campylobacter jejuni
Viruses	Rotavirus
	Norwalk virus
	Enteric adenoviruses
Parasites	*Giardia lamblia*
	Strongyloides stercoralis
	Cryptosporidium
	Balantidum coli
	Entamoeba histolytica
	Coccidia

Table 2. Pathogens causing acute dysentery

Type of pathogen	Examples
Bacteria	*Shigella* spp.
	Salmonella spp.
	Campylobacter jejuni
	Enteroinvasive *Escherichia coli* (EIEC)
Parasites	*Entamoeba histolytica*
	Trichuris
	Schistosoma spp.

Table 3. Pathogens causing persistent diarrhoea

Type of pathogen	Examples
Bacteria	Enteroadherent *Escherichia coli* (EAEC)
	Campylobacter jejuni
	Shigella spp.
	Salmonella spp.
	Helicobacter pyloris
Parasites	*Trichuris*
	Giardia lamblia
	Cryptosporidium
	Strongyloides
	Capillaria
	Coccidia
Fungi	*Candida*

recover spontaneously; this occurs in many cases of infection with campylobacter. But others, such as bacillary dysentery, may involve infections with life-threatening organisms such as *Shigella* species. In addition, the parasite *Entamoeba histolytica* may damage the large intestine and even invade the liver and other organs. *See* Colon, Diseases and Disorders

Dysentery is often accompanied by severe systemic disturbances involving a high temperature, decrease in blood pressure and renal failure.

Persistent Diarrhoea

The term 'persistent diarrhoea' is usually used for diarrhoea which persists for more than 14 days. Many pathogens have been implicated (Table 3). It may involve disturbances of the upper intestine as a result of infections which characteristically cause persistent diarrhoea such as *Giardia lamblia* or *Strongyloides*. There are important interactions with host immune and nutritional status. Thus hosts who are malnourished may have more persistent symptoms than those who are

well nourished. This is attributable partly to decreased immunity leading to delay in clearing of the pathogen, and partly to a delay in recovery and replacement of the mucosal cells. In order for a pathogen to colonize the intestine and cause infection of the gastrointestinal tract, a number of host defence mechanisms need to be overcome. These include the following:

1. Gastric acidity. Most intestinal pathogens are inhibited by hydrogen ions and, conversely, patients with hypochlorhydria are more susceptible to cholera and salmonellosis.

2. Motility. Alterations in peristalsis, as a result of administration of various drugs such as ganglion blockers, are associated with increased bacterial numbers in the upper intestine. Antimotility drugs are contraindicated in the management of acute diarrhoea for this reason. *See* Malnutrition, The Problem of Malnutrition

3. Resident microflora. Soon after birth, the intestine becomes colonized by a variety of organisms. The pattern of this microflora is markedly influenced by the type of feeding. Breast-fed babies are characteristically colonized by large numbers of bifidobacteria, with low numbers of *Escherichia coli*. They tend to have a low faecal pH in comparison with bottle-fed babies, who have low numbers of bifidobacteria and higher numbers of anaerobic organisms. It is likely that the low pH of the intestines in the breast-fed baby facilitates production of metabolites that are toxic to certain enteropathogens. Volatile fatty acids, which are excreted in greater quantities by breast-fed babies than by bottle-fed babies, are inhibitors of *Shigella* species, for example. *See* Infants, Breast- and Bottle-feeding; Infectious Disease and Infant Feeding

4. Immunity. There is a highly developed series of immune reactions in the intestines, involving the production of immunoglobulin A (IgA) an an antibacterial layer and sensitized T lymphocytes. In general, these contribute to the resistance to colonization by enteropathogens, the speed of clearance of pathogens, and the manner in which the mucosa is damaged. In some illnesses, the invading pathogen damages the intestine directly. In others, an immunological reaction is set up whereby the lymphocytes react against the pathogen to cause localized damage. *See* Immunity and Nutrition

5. Breast milk. Many constituents of breast milk have potent antibacterial activities. Significant quantities of IgA are secreted in breast milk. This has marked antibacterial activity. Iron-binding proteins, including lactoferrin and transferrin, normally in the unsaturated state, are found in human milk. Combinations of these and the immunoglobulins produce powerful bacteriostatic and bacteriocidal activity.

Certain characteristics of the pathogens favour their colonization. Recent studies have demonstrated the presence of adherence characteristics on the plasmids of organisms. This is particularly important in children with persistent diarrhoea.

Clinical Features

The clinical features of diarrhoea vary considerably according to the pathogen and to the underlying host immune status. The simplest form is acute watery diarrhoea in which an incubation period of 1–5 days is followed by a sudden onset of severe diarrhoea, sometimes 10–20 times per day, accompanied by nausea, fever and mild abdominal pains. The stool is fluid and usually does not contain mucus or blood. In the majority of subjects there is marked improvement in symptoms within a few days, whatever treatment is given, and only a minority (less than 5%) go on to develop persistent diarrhoea.

In dysenteric illness there is a spectrum of symptoms from mild diarrhoea to fulminant dysentery with severe systemic features. After an incubation period of 1–5 days there is onset of diarrhoea. Sometimes this is sudden and voluminous from the start. In other patients it gradually worsens over several days as the bacilli invade the mucosa. Excessive quantities of mucus and blood may occur, and ulceration of the colon may develop. Appearances may be very similar to those of ulcerative colitis. There may be severe systemic features, including fever, leucocytosis and meningism (especially in infants and small children).

In persistent diarrhoea the symptoms may be mild, with loose stools persisting for several weeks following an initial acute watery episode. In other cases there may be features of malabsorption syndromes in which there are bulky stools which are characteristic of malabsorption of fat and other nutrients. Parasitic diseases causing persistent diarrhoea may be associated with long-term losses of blood and protein. In addition, there may be invasion of organs other than the intestine, such as the lungs and liver.

Nutritional Significance of Diarrhoeal Disease

It is quite clear that there is a close association between diarrhoea and malnutrition of different types. Acute and persistent diarrhoeal episodes are associated with growth faltering, frank clinical features of protein energy malnutrition, vitamin A deficiency, zinc deficiency and iron deficiency. Many reviews have emphasized the causal nature of diarrhoea in the development of nutritional disorders. *See* Iron, Physiology; Protein, Deficiency; Retinol, Physiology; Zinc, Deficiency

At the same time, there is clear evidence that subjects who are undernourished or vitamin-A-deficient in the first place have an increased prevalence and severity of diarrhoea. Thus the bidirectional relationship between diarrhoea and nutrition is complex and the term 'malnutrition infection syndrome' has been coined to describe this.

In recent years the relationship between undernutrition and diarrhoeal disease has been investigated by a series of longitudinal studies. Growth faltering, protein energy malnutrition or vitamin A deficiency are not associated with an increased attack rate of diarrhoea. Rather, it seems as though attack rates are attributable to the behavioural characteristics of the host, the environment in which the host lives and the characteristics of the pathogen which cause the diarrhoea. On the other hand, duration of diarrhoea is increased in malnutrition. Furthermore, mortality is significantly increased in individuals with moderate or severe malnutrition.

The relationship between diarrhoea and malnutrition has been studied intensively over the last decade. Acute watery diarrhoea can be associated with a decrease in food intake for a few days. However, if oral rehydration and general supportive treatment is given, dietary intake and absorptive function may recover rapidly, and catch-up nutritional rehabilitation can occur within a few weeks. Acute watery diarrhoea may be responsible for short-term impact on nutritional status but may have very little impact on long-term nutritional status. It appears that the value of oral rehydration as a nutritional strategy has been overemphasized in the past.

The situation with persistent diarrhoea is rather different. It is quite clear that children with persistent diarrhoea (who make up perhaps 5–10% of all diarrhoea cases) have severe problems with food intake, nutrient absorption and indigenous losses. They are the most likely to be affected by growth faltering and micronutrient deficiencies (especially vitamin A, iron, zinc and folic acid). *See* Folic Acid, Physiology

Subjects with dysentery may have marked nutrient losses, and, in addition to growth faltering, protein, iron and important micronutrients such as zinc may be lost in intestinal fluids, resulting in losses of plasma proteins and haemoglobin.

Current emphases on the interaction between intestinal disease and nutrition concentrate on two aspects: prevention of infection, and management of infection. Prevention of infection in the first place involves the following:

1. Promotion of breast-feeding, exclusively for the first 4–6 months wherever possible, together with promotion of improved personal hygiene, water supplies and sanitation.
2. Promotion of immunization within expanded programmes of immunization, especially concentrating on

measles, which may precipitate acute diarrhoea, persistent diarrhoea syndromes and dysentery.

3. Promotion of vitamin A, iron and zinc status.
4. Improvement of birthweight as it is known that a low birthweight is associated with an increased risk of diarrhoea.

The main interventions in the management of infection to prevent any nutritional deterioration include the following:

1. Promotion of breast-feeding, especially during diarrhoeal episodes.
2. Timely use of antibiotics and antiparasitic drugs in order to reduce the severity and duration of diarrhoeal episodes which compromise nutritional status.
3. Appropriate interventions to reduce body temperature during illness.
4. Frequent feeds during diarrhoeal illness, especially using low-viscosity feeds.
5. Promotion of local appropriate mixes for the dietary management of diarrhoea, especially in convalescence.

Oral Rehydration

Dramatic reductions in mortality from diarrhoea have been achieved since the introduction of simple successful rehydration regimes. This has been most striking in areas of the developing world which are endemic for cholera. Efficient village-health-centre-based regimes of oral rehydration have reduced the mortality from 50% to almost zero.

Oral rehydration depends on the stimulation of sodium and water transport from the lumen across the enterocyte membrane and into the mucosa as a result of the additional presence of glucose in the lumen. Initially, there was much concentration on the use of glucose electrolyte mixes which provided either 90 mmol of sodium per litre or 30 mmol per litre. More recently, there has been an interest in the use of cereal-based rehydration. In this approach the cereals such as millet or rice are mixed to provide a thin soup. The carbohydrates in the cereal are broken down by the intestine to glucose and this stimulates the absorption of sodium and water. Future developments will include the wider availability of glucose electrolyte mixes, both in health centres and homes, throughout the developing and industrialized world. They will also concentrate on the development, testing and promotion of local appropriate regimes of cereal based hydration.

Bibliography

Behrens R (1991) Persistent diarrhoea syndrome in Africa. *Health* July: 10–11.

Farthing NJG and Keusch GT (eds) (1989) Global impact and patterns of intestinal infection. *Enteric Infection: Mechanisms, Manifestations and Management*, pp 3–12. London: Chapman and Hall.

Frost JA, Rowe B, Vandepitte J and Threlfall EJ (1981) Plasmid, characterization in the investigation of an epidemic caused by multiple resistant *Shigella dysenteriae* type 1 in Central Africa. *Lancet* 2: 1074–1075.

Gorbach SL (1989) Infectious diarrhoea. In: Sleisinger MH and Fordtran JS (eds) *Gastrointestinal Disease: Pathophysiology, Diagnosis and Management* 4th edition, pp 1191–1232. Philadelphia: WB Saunders.

Tomkins AM (1989) Infections of the gastrointestinal tract. In: Warrell D and Wetherall D (eds) *Oxford Textbook of Medicine*. pp 12.129–12.139. Oxford: Oxford University Press.

Tomkins AM and Watson FM (1989) *Malnutrition and Infection*. Administrative Committee on Coordination/Subcommittee on Nutrition. WHO Nutrition Policy Discussion Paper No. 5, pp 1–137. Geneva: World Health Organization.

Tomkins AM, Bradley AK, Oswald S and Drasar BS (1981) Diet and the faecal microflora of infants, children, and adults in rural Nigeria and urban UK. *Journal of Hygiene* 86: 285–291.

Andrew Tomkins
Institute of Child Health, London, UK

DICING

See Comminution of Foods

DIET

The dictionary defines diet as 'food and drink regularly provided or consumed' or 'the kind and amount of food prescribed for a special reason'. In the first case, a diet is merely the usual food pattern practised by an individual, whereas the second situation refers to special food patterns that differ from the normal pattern in order to try to improve health. For others, 'diet' is synonymous with losing weight.

Meal and Diet Planning

Meal planning is a constructive and creative process to help ensure that an individual or family will be well nourished. Ideally, meals are planned within the framework of an entire day's dietary pattern, so that any dietary deficiencies or excesses can be detected and corrected. Greatest efficiency in planning, shopping, and preparing food can be achieved if meals are planned for a few days at a time. This makes it easy to see where economies can be made by creative use of leftovers, purchasing in suitable quantities, and buying foods that are in season.

It is sensible to use a format for breakfast, lunch and dinner when planning menus for several days. A typical breakfast pattern might include cereal, bread and beverage. An occasional variation could be an egg, sausage, or bacon to replace the cereal. Lunch might be a main dish or sandwich, salad, dessert (optional) and beverage. Dinner might be a meat (fish or poultry) entrée, potato or rice, two vegetables, salad and beverage, with dessert again being optional, depending on bodyweight. The diet pattern provided by the formats outlined above will generally ensure that the diet is nutritionally well balanced if a variety of foods are chosen.

Eating is one of the pleasures of life, yet food can become monotonous if little thought is given to its selection and preparation. Important considerations are colour, flavour, aroma, texture, temperature, size and shape, availability, and variety.

Menu planning should be tailored to the people eating the meals. Food is an excellent way of extending knowledge, both for children and adults. The inclusion of an unfamiliar food from another culture can add considerable interest to a meal. However, the meal is less enjoyable when almost all of the foods being served are unfamiliar or poorly prepared. Familiar foods should form the basis of meals, while occasionally introducing a new food. In this way children and adults can learn more about the world and its food. Fortunately, the increasingly diverse ethnicity of most populations is making it easier to buy the ingredients that are needed for some of these dishes.

For families in which both adults work, there is less time for food preparation. Frozen and pre-prepared foods can be time savers, and freezing home-cooked dishes for reheating can save considerably in food costs. *See* Convenience Foods, Definition and Classification

Factors Influencing Food Choices

The nutritional requirements of all family members need to be considered when making food choices in menu planning. If anyone is on a special diet prescribed by a dietitian or a physician, such requirements need to be met either in the plans for the entire family or via substitutions where the planned menu for the family does not meet the dietary guidelines. It is important that the actual requirements of the diet be understood and applied to the purchase of ingredients and the selection of recipes for menus.

Another factor which influences food choices is heritage. Foods that were considered special during childhood are likely to be favourites in adulthood. Such specialities may be specific recipes for fairly common foods, but they also may be foods that mirror the cultural and ethnic heritage of families. Most people like certain foods, such as chocolate, simply because of taste appeal or some other pleasurable aspect of the food. Sometimes people choose particular foods because of an element of status associated with them (caviar, for example). Cost is an important factor, strongly influencing food choice. When funds have to be stretched to cover a multitude of needs, less expensive food choices provide money-saving options without necessarily jeopardizing nutrient quality.

Optimal Nutrition

An important area of research in the field of nutrition is the quest for ways to eat to promote better health and longer life. Particular attention has been directed towards studying the possible interrelationship between diet and chronic diseases, including heart disease, cancer, and other nutrition-related conditions such as diabetes and osteoporosis. As information has accumulated regarding the dietary practices that may be effective in reducing the likelihood of developing serious health problems, the US government has taken an active role in developing and promoting dietary guidelines to benefit the nation as a whole. The third edition of these guidelines (*Dietary Guidelines for Americans, 1990*) provides the foundation needed for planning a healthy diet. This edition differs only slightly from the preceding editions published in 1980 and 1985. *See* Nutrition Education

There are seven dietary guidelines:

1. Eat a variety of foods.
2. Maintain a healthy weight.
3. Choose a diet low in fat, saturated fat, and cholesterol.
4. Choose a diet with plenty of vegetables, fruits, and grain products.
5. Use sugars in moderation.
6. Use salt and sodium in moderation.
7. If you drink alcoholic beverages, do so in moderation.

The first guideline recognizes that foods are the best sources of nutrients and that the nutrients vary markedly from one food to another. A wide variety of foods helps to assure that enough of all of the known nutrients (and no doubt some unknown ones) will be available to the body. *See* Cholesterol, Role of Cholesterol in Heart Disease; Fats, Requirements; Sucrose, Dietary Sucrose and Disease; Sodium, Physiology

Consumption of a wide variety of foods has been the main point of good nutrition for at least the past 50–60 years. At one time, nutritionists had divided the various foods into 11 basic food groups. These were then simplified to seven. In 1955, the Department of Nutrition at Harvard University simplified them still further to what are commonly referred to as the Basic Four Food Groups: fruits and vegetables; dairy foods, except butter; cereals and foods made primarily from them; and the protein group, including meat, fish, poultry, eggs, nuts and legumes. At least four or five servings of fruits and vegetables (any kind, but in variety) should be eaten each day, and that advice is appropriate for the cereal group. Depending upon the age of a person, between two and four servings of dairy foods are recommended. The protein group should be limited to two servings, each equal to about 85 g (3 oz) of cooked meat. Serving sizes, particularly of meats and whole-milk products, should be adjusted so that, in association with physical activity, a reasonable weight is reached and maintained. Extremely active people and teenagers who are growing rapidly will need to increase serving sizes. *See* Adolescents, Nutritional Problems; Children, Nutritional Requirements; Dietary Requirements of Adults

Sugars and fats are not included in the basic groups because these are constituents of the foods in the basic groups, and are used as ingredients in recipes. Nutritionists in other countries have developed similar basic food groups; the principle is the same – eat a variety of foods from each of the groups.

Alcoholic beverages generally are not considered as foods, but they are comparatively high in calories and essentially void of nutrients. Although alcohol provides 7 cal per g (compared with 9 cal for the same amount of fat), it is almost twice as high in calories as carbohydrates and proteins (both of which contribute approximately 4 cal per g). *See* Alcohol, Metabolism, Toxicology and Beneficial Effects

Vegetables and fruits provide vitamins, minerals and fibre. The three vitamins for which many of them are particularly noteworthy are vitamin C, folic acid, and vitamin A (as carotene). Whole-grain breads and cereals provide fibre, thiamin, riboflavin, nicotinic acid, iron, and some protein; enriched refined cereals are also sources of these nutrients, but provide less fibre. Milk and milk products are good-to-excellent sources of almost all nutrients, with the exceptions of iron and vitamin C. This group of foods is particularly important for its calcium content. The meats and meat substitutes group is valued for its complete protein, zinc, and B vitamins. Meats also are key sources of haem iron, the form of iron which is absorbed most readily. On the negative side, meats are a source of saturated fat, and this is why fatty cuts of meat should be limited. The legumes in the protein group are good sources of starch, a complex carbohydrate which also is found in abundance in breads, pasta and cereals. *See* individual nutrients

Role of Diet in Health, Wellbeing, and Longevity

Maintenance of a reasonable weight is an important element of eating for good health. The underweight are at increased risk of developing a variety of infectious diseases and also osteoporosis (literally 'porous bones') later in life. Excess weight also is unhealthy and is associated with a greater likelihood of developing heart disease, some types of cancer, adult-onset diabetes, and strokes, as well as other adult health problems.

Weight control is a matter of balancing the calories taken in with the calories expended. The key to controlling calories is to watch serving sizes, particularly of meats, while also making choices for low-fat or nonfat milk and cheeses and avoiding high-fat desserts. Fruits, vegetables and cereals are very low in fat and are high in nutrients in relation to the number of calories they provide. Even when eating a low-calorie diet, people should eat a variety of foods from all of the food groups. Omitting any of the basic groups will eliminate adequate intake of some essential nutrients.

Exercise is a facet of energy expenditure over which people have considerable control; moderately vigorous walking or comparable exercise for about 30 min or more at least three times a week (and preferably somewhat longer and more frequently) can be a key component for controlling weight and maximizing health.

In the USA, the guideline to choose a diet low in fat (particularly saturated fat) and cholesterol is interpreted to mean that adults should have a maximum of 30% of their calories from fat. However, children under the age of 2 should not be restricted to this level. The actual number of grams of fat a person could eat to stay within this level obviously is dependent on the total caloric intake; for women eating 2000 cal per day, maximum fat level is in the region of 67 g, a little more than 2 oz. No more than 10% of the day's total calories should be from saturated fatty acids, which would be 20 g, a little less than 1 oz, for a 2000-cal diet. Animal fats are comparatively high in saturated fat. Hydrogenated fat, such as shortening, should also be restricted. Dietary cholesterol is found in certain foods of animal origin, particularly egg yolk. Plant foods are not sources of cholesterol; despite the confusing proclamations on some vegetable oils and margarines, these products never did contain cholesterol. Thorough trimming of fat from meats, limited use of fried foods, selecting foods that are low in fat, and eating smaller portions of meats and whole-milk products that are high in fat are practical ways of ensuring that the menu provides a maximum of 30% of its calories from fat, and that the calorie content of the meal is modest for those with a weight problem.

Sugars are not essential in the diet, but they add a considerable amount of pleasure to eating. The suggestion to limit them, particularly in infants and children, is prompted by their propensity to cause dental caries and potential problems in weight control. The best way to reduce dental decay is to drink water that contains an adequate amount of the mineral nutrient fluoride. This usually involves adding fluoride to community water supplies, a process called fluoridation. *See* Dental Disease, Role of Diet

Current dietary advice is to use salt and sodium in moderation. This guideline can be implemented by salting foods lightly in preparation, eliminating the salt shaker from the table, and eating salted crackers, pretzels, chips, pickles, olives, and other condiments, such as soy sauce, less frequently. Food labels highlight products containing sodium (monosodium glutamate, for example) and can be helpful to people who should reduce their sodium intake because of high blood pressure or excessive accumulation of fluid in body tissues, particularly in the feet and ankles.

By following the dietary guidelines outlined above and utilizing the suggestions that were provided for planning nutritious and appealing meals, people can achieve optimal nutritional status. Together with exercise, these can help to improve the chances for a long and healthy life.

Bibliography

Guthrie HA (1989) *Introductory Nutrition* 7th edn. St Louis: Times/Mirror/Mosby.

McWilliams M (1986) *Nutrition for the Growing Years* 4th edn. New York: Macmillan.

McWilliams M (1991) *Fundamentals of Meal Management* 2nd edn. Redondo Beach, CA: Plycon Press.

National Research Council, US National Academy of Sciences (1989) *Recommended Daily Allowances* 10th edn. Washington DC:

Stare FJ and McWilliams M (1984) *Living Nutrition* 4th edn. New York: Macmillan.

Stare FJ, Olson RE and Whelan EM (1989) *Balanced Nutrition: Nutrition Beyond the Cholesterol Scare*. Holbrook, MA: Bob Adams.

Margaret McWilliams
California State University, Los Angeles, USA
Fredrick J. Stare
Harvard School of Public Health, Boston, USA

DIETARY FIBRE

Contents

Properties and Sources

Although dietary fibre has been known for more than 2000 years under various terms (e.g. bran), the term 'dietary fibre' appeared in 1953 and referred to hemicelluloses, cellulose and lignin. The term 'fibre' is confusing since only a fraction of dietary fibre has a fibrillar structure. Other terms (e.g. plantix) have been proposed to replace it but the term 'dietary fibre' has survived. The dietary fibre hypothesis has stimulated research in this field of food science since the early 1970s. The first part of this article deals with the definition of dietary fibre. This is followed by a description of its properties and sources.

Definition (Based on Function and Structure)

First Definition

Knowing Cleave's hypothesis on refined foods and Western diseases, Burkitt, Trowell, Southgate and collaborators hypothesized that a diet consisting of whole or lightly processed foods (cereals, fruits, vegetables and legumes) contains intact indigestible polymers which are beneficial for health. The first definition of dietary fibre in 1972 read as follows: 'that portion of food which is derived from the cellular walls of plants and is digested very poorly by human beings . . . Fibre is composed largely of cellulose, . . . hemicelluloses, pentosans, pectin and lignin'.

The widespread use of the crude fibre method, for the determination of crude fibre, had unfortunately led to equating fibre with cellulose, which has a fibrillar structure. The material retained by this method is mostly, but not entirely, cellulose, and it represents only a small part of total dietary fibre. Several reports have stressed differences between dietary fibre and crude fibre. *See* Cellulose; Hemicelluloses; Lignin

Definition of Dietary Fibre

Recent versions of the dietary fibre definition made it clear that 'alimentary enzymes' meant 'the endogenous

secretions of the human upper gastrointestinal tract' (secretions from mouth, stomach, gall bladder, exocrine pancreas and small intestine). Enzymatic digestion by colonic bacteria (fermentation) is not considered in the definition (HWC, 1985). It was also specified that dietary fibre is 'the endogenous components of plant material in the diet', emphasizing that undigestible materials formed during food processing, such as the products of the Maillard reaction, are not to be included. Dietary fibre has been identified as being predominantly nonstarch polysaccharides and lignin (HWC, 1985; Pilch, 1987; Trowell *et al.*, 1985; Van Soest, 1978) and possibly including associated substances such as undigestible structural protein (Dintzis, 1983; HWC, 1985; Selvendran, 1987). Although starch and dietary fibre are often intimately associated in whole foods and could share some common effects in the gastrointestinal tract, starch is not fibre (Trowell *et al.*, 1985). Cummings (1976) considered that dietary fibre is made of structural (cell wall) components and that the concept of dietary fibre should not be stretched to include various heterogeneous substances which are different from dietary fibre in terms of chemical composition, physical structure, and biological significance. The conceptual definition and original use of the term 'dietary fibre' should be kept in mind for discriminating between dietary fibre and other undigestible material (Southgate, 1986). These pieces of information are incorporated in the following definition of dietary fibre:

> The endogenous components of plant material in the diet which are resistant to the digestive secretions of the human upper gastrointestinal tract. These components are predominantly nonstarch polysaccharides and lignin, and may include associated substances such as undigestible structural protein.

More recently, the small contribution of lignin (in most foods) to dietary fibre has led to the recommendation that the term 'nonstarch polysaccharide' (NSP) should be used instead of dietary fibre (Department of Health, 1991). This recommendation is gaining more widespread acceptance but is not at present (1992) universally used. *See* Carbohydrates, Classification and Properties; Starch, Structure, Properties and Determination

Biological 'Activity' and Definition

The beneficial health effects of dietary fibre include normalizing serum lipid levels, attenuating the postprandial glucose response, and regulating the colonic function. A traditional source of dietary fibre can be altered by processing so that its ingestion may cease to be associated with beneficial effects. This does not comply with the original concept of dietary fibre. The structural integrity of the plant food cell wall is even considered more important than its resistance to digestive secretions. *See* Colon, Structure and Function; Glucose, Maintenance of Blood Glucose Level

The sources of undigestible material which have not been part of the human diet may not represent adequate substitutes for dietary fibre and they need to be comprehensively tested for their physical characteristics and their physiological effects, including the extent and rate of fermentation. Dietary fibre cannot be associated with inert materials such as wood cellulose.

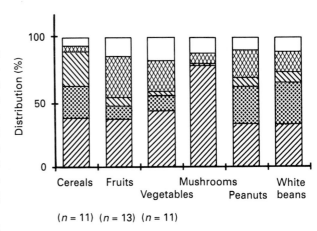

Fig. 1 Distribution of the main polysaccharidic constituents of dietary fibre from some foods and food categories. The number of foods in each category (*n*) is shown in parentheses. ▨ Glucose; ▦ arabinose; ▧ xylose; ▩ uronic acid; □ others.

Measurement of Dietary Fibre

For the majority of foods and food products, the dietary fibre methods are in relative agreement, but there are a few foods for which dietary fibre components may be undetected and nonfibre material may be included as fibre depending on each method. The exclusion of lignin from the definition of dietary fibre and the inclusion of some starches have been debated with regard to problems of analytical methodology.

Chemical Structure

The composition and structure of dietary fibre varies according to the type of plant and changes as the plant matures. It is made of interlinked polymers (hemicelluloses, pectic substances, phenolics, glycoproteins and proteoglycans) in a matrix of amorphous structure with some cellulose microfibrils enmeshed in it.

Table 1. Main macromolecular constituents of dietary fibre

Constituents	Fruits and vegetables	Cereals	Legumes
Polysaccharides			
Hemicelluloses			
Xyloglucans	X		X
Glucuronoxylans	X		
Arabinoxylans		X	
Glucuronoarabinoxylans		X	
Galactomannans			X
Cellulose	X	X	X
β-D-Glucans		X	
Pectic substances	X	X	X
Others			
Lignin	X	X	
Phenolic esters		X	
Protein		X	
Glycoproteins	X		X

Polysaccharidic Fibre Components

Dietary fibre comprises carbohydrate and non-carbohydrate polymers, most being structural components. Figure 1 shows the proportion of the monomer constituents of fibre polysaccharides from three food categories (11 cereals, 13 fruits and 11 vegetables), and from canned mushrooms, peanuts and baked white beans. Arabinose is a major component of the NSPs of cereals, peanuts and beans. Xylose is present in large amounts only in cereals. Pectic substances (uronic acids) represent a substantial part of the NSP of fruits, vegetables,

peanuts and beans. Mushroom NSP is mostly made of glucose. These results were based on the analysis of composites, made of up to 20 individual foods purchased over a 30-month period, using the Englyst GLC (gas–liquid chromatography) method. A more recent version of this method would have given a higher proportion of xylose relative to glucose.

The different monomers of NSP are part of macromolecular constituents of dietary fibre which are outlined in Table 1. Glucose is the major component of the cellulose and β-glucan fractions which are generally unbranched. β-D-Glucans have mixed β-1,3 and β-1,4 linkages and are a constituent of fibre from barley and oats. The glucose molecules of cellulose are β-1,4-linked. By contrast with the α-1,4 linkages of starch, the β-1,4 linkages favour hydrogen bonding within the linear polymer and between adjacent polymers which are tightly held together in crystalline regions. Some amorphous regions may include other sugars. Cellulose represents a minor fraction of cereal fibre and a major fraction of fibre in other food categories. This difference is not evident from their glucose content in Fig. 1 because glucose is also apparent in the primary chain of hemicelluloses. Gums may also contain glucose. Xylose is part of the primary chain of hemicelluloses and gums, and of the secondary chain of pectin and gums. *See* Gums, Properties of Individual Gums

Arabinose is in the primary chain of gums and the secondary chain of hemicelluloses and pectin. Hemicelluloses constitute a major fraction of dietary fibre; this fraction is largely made up of arabinose and xylose in cereals, and xylose and glucose in fruits and vegetables (Table 1). Pectic substances (polyuronides) are prevalent in citrus fruits. They are also present in vegetables, legumes and cereals in small amounts (Table 1). Other polysaccharidic constituents are mainly represented by galactose, or mannose in bananas. The nonstructural polysaccharides of fibre represent a small portion of dietary fibre. *See* Galactose

The monomer composition of the carbohydrate portion of dietary fibre is of limited usefulness in predicting the properties and functions of dietary fibre because these are also dependent on the structural architecture. Minor components, not apparent in NSP composition, may play an important structural role.

Nonsaccharidic Fibre Components

Table 1 shows the distribution of the nonsaccharidic polymers which are intimately associated with dietary fibre structure. They include glycoproteins (fruits, vegetables and legumes), protein (cereals), phenolic esters (cereals) and lignin (lignified tissues of fruits, vegetables and cereals). Edible plant tissues are consumed in a relatively immature stage and their cells are largely undifferentiated. Cell differentiation involves the deposition of lignin at the expense of water and pectin. This corresponds with increased rigidity of the cell wall. Wheat bran and the small seeds covering strawberries are examples of lignified tissue. In fruits and vegetables, lignin represents only a small part of dietary fibre. Lignin is a complex group of phenylpropane polymers formed by the condensation of some aromatic alcohols. Cutin, waxes, or suberin may be present in some tissues. More details can be obtained from comprehensive reviews. *See* Phenolic Compounds; Protein, Chemistry

Table 2. Effect of grinding on dry bulk of wheat brans (ml g^{-1})

Sieve aperture[a] (mm)	Bran A[b]	Bran B	Bran C	Bran D
As is	3·1[c]	3·4	5·1	3·5
2·0 (10 mesh)	2·7	2·4	2·8	2·1
1·0 (18 mesh)	2·2	2·1	2·4	2·0
0·5 (35 mesh)	1·8	1·8	1·9	1·7

[a] Using an M5 Wiley mill. Mesh sieve equivalence is indicated in parentheses.
[b] Bran A was American Association of Cereal Chemists (AACC)-certified soft white wheat bran; brans B–D were soft or hard wheat brans from other sources.
[c] Mean of duplicate measurements.

Structure

Models of primary cell walls of plants were often obtained from nonfood material such as wood and tobacco. Recent reports have provided structural information on the cell walls of plant food material. In carrots, for example, protein–protein or protein–polysaccharide linkages may contribute to the formation of a rigid, inextensible cell wall. Protein may form up to 10% of cell walls in immature plants and appears to be important for structural cohesion.

Physical Properties

The physicochemical properties of dietary fibre are dependent on both composition and structure. The *in vitro* properties of fibre isolates have been used to estimate their potential *in vivo* effect. However, *in vitro* data should be used with caution. The measurements are influenced by the method used and by the preparation of the fibre. The fibre residue obtained *in vitro* may have been altered by heat or chemicals or it may still contain residual digestible materials. *In vivo* conditions generally result in a more extensive digestion than that which occurs *in vitro*.

Another important consideration is that dietary fibre is concentrated and denuded only in the terminal small intestine. Along the small intestine, the fibre which is partially associated with digestible materials may show physical properties that are different from those of an entirely denuded fibre matrix. In the large intestine, most soluble fibre, and a large but variable portion of insoluble dietary fibre, is degraded by the colonic microflora. *See* Microflora of the Intestine, Role and Effects

Particle Size

Table 2 shows the effect of milling on the dry bulk volume of wheat bran as measured in a volumetric cylinder. While the volume of the coarse brans occupied up to 5 ml g^{-1}, this was reduced to less than 2 ml after grinding in an M5 Wiley mill using the 0·5 mm screen. Fibre from different sources, ground under the same conditions, may have different particle sizes. *See* Flour, Dietary Importance

Some collapsing of the fibre structure occurs during food preparation and/or mastication due to the reduction of particle size; in addition, the fibre structure of sources such as spinach may be modified by cooking. The particle size of unfermented wheat bran fibre has been related to colonic function and faecal characteristics in humans and laboratory animals. For example, when rats were fed diets containing 12% hard wheat bran, the faecal wet density was 0·796±0·010 (mean± SEM; $n=12$) in the coarse bran group (geometric mean particle size (MPS), 850 µm), but it was increased to 0·888±0·013 in the fine bran groups (MPS, 308 µm). This increase was due not to a change in the faecal weight but to a decrease in the volume, paralleling the effect observed in a volumetric cylinder. In ready-to-eat breakfast cereals, the MPS of the fibre has been found to vary between 350 and 2000 µm.

Attention should be paid to reduction of the particle size of fibre in the 7–70 µm range which could be associated with negative effects. For various reasons, the persorption (paracellular passage of small amounts of solid food components from the lumen of the intestine into the lymphatic and blood circulation, this occurring without structural changes) of a small amount of fibre particles may occur in some regions of the intestinal wall. Contrary to persorbed starch granules, fibre particles are not degraded in the blood and may impose an increased workload on the kidneys. Data on persorption are scarce and much work is needed on this subject.

Water-holding Capacity

Dietary fibre holds water by adsorption and absorption, and some is retained outside the fibre matrix (free water). The particle size, chemical composition and structure of dietary fibre influence its water-holding capacity. Methods for measuring water-holding capacity have been discussed by Dreher (1987). The *in vitro* water-holding capacity cannot be used to predict the impact of highly fermentable fibre on colonic function.

Although lettuce fibre isolates retain much water, the water-holding capacity expressed in grams of water held by fibre per gram of edible portion of food was higher for the fibre from wheat bran (4·5 g) than for that of lettuce and various other foods (0·3–1·3 g). The water-holding capacity of fibre from brans or ready-to-eat breakfast cereals has been positively correlated ($r \geq 0·85$, $P < 0·05$) with its MPS. A reduction of the MPS of wheat bran fibre from 800 to 180 µm has been associated with a 41% decrease of its water-holding capacity (Table 3). A

Table 3. Effect of grinding on properties of wheat bran insoluble fibre[a]

Mesh sieve	Aperture[b] (µm)	MPS[c] (µm)	HWC[d] (g per g)	Glycocholate binding g per 0·2 g[e]
As is		800	9·5±0·1	26·5±1·5
20	840	420	8·1±0·1	24·9±1·2
40	420	280	6·6±0·2	23·8±0·8
60	250	180	5·8±0·1	22·1±1·0
80	175	160	5·6±0·1	21·5±0·3

[a] Residue after neutral detergent and porcine pancreatic α-amylase treatments.
[b] Aperture size of sieve used with a Wiley mill, intermediate model.
[c] MPS, geometric mean particle size.
[d] HWC, water-holding capacity, g water per g insoluble fibre, using the centrifugation method; mean±SEM of three measurements.
[e] Glycocholate: g bound per 0·2 g insoluble fibre; mean±SEM of four measurements.

large portion of the water held by wheat bran fibre appears to be free water. *See* Water, Structure, Properties and Determination

Bile-salt-binding

The interest in measuring the bile-salt-binding capacity of dietary fibre has been to estimate its action in preventing the reabsorption of bile salts. Deconjugated bile salts are bound to pectic substances by hydrogen bonding. This property appears to be part of the mechanism by which certain fibres influence blood cholesterol levels. *See* Bile

In common cereal sources, glycocholate ($r = 0·90$, $P < 0·001$) and taurocholate ($r = 0·86$, $P < 0·05$) binding were positively correlated with the MPS of the neutral detergent fibre (NDF). Reducing the particle size of wheat bran NDF from 800 to 160 µm reduced its glycocholate binding by 19% (Table 3).

The bile-salt-binding capacity of fibre isolates, although method-dependent, could reflect events in the terminal small intestine. Purified fibre fractions may be poor (cellulose) or strong (lignin) binders. Some rice brans appear to have a high capacity to bind bile salts.

Cation Exchange Capacity

Cation exchange is partly dependent on the presence of uronic acid in the nonesterified form. The preparation of the fibre material may decrease the number of nonesterified carboxyl groups and the apparent cation exchange capacity. Wheat bran contains little uronic acid and its cation exchange capacity is mainly due to diffusion within the dietary fibre network.

The cation exchange capacity of fibre from different

sources is difficult to compare unless it is expressed per edible portion. According to the affinity of minerals for carboxylic acid groups, cabbage and coarse wheat bran showed a high cation exchange capacity compared with that of pectin.

The minerals (e.g. calcium ions, Ca^{2+}) entrapped in the cell wall matrix may not be absorbed in the small intestine, but they could be partially released and absorbed in the colon when the fibre is degraded by bacteria. This may explain why cation adsorption has not been consistently related to mineral bioavailability. On the other hand, wheat bran fibre appears to be able to bind permanently heavy metal ions and to decrease their toxicity. *See* Bioavailability of Nutrients

Viscosity and Gelling Properties

The viscosity of certain water-soluble dietary fibre components, such as oat β-D-glucans and pectin, influences gastric emptying and absorption rates in the small intestine. Based on concentrations likely to be used in diets, the viscosity in the lumen of the small intestine is little changed by low levels of methoxy pectin. It is slightly increased by wheat bran and highly increased by high levels of methoxy pectin. Some of the nonstructural dietary fibre components show viscous properties. Viscous materials may also show gelling properties. The viscosity, thickening and gelling properties of gums have been described by Dreher (1987).

Microbial Degradation (Fermentability)

Most dietary fibre remains undegraded until it reaches the large intestine where the extent of fermentation depends on the source, and probably several other factors (e.g. presence of specific components in the fibre matrix, nitrogen source, bacterial adaptation and transit time). The dietary fibre from most sources (e.g. fruits, vegetables, oat bran) is highly fermentable so that up to 80% of it in mixed diets is degraded by colonic bacteria.

Some data have suggested that fine bran is slightly more fermentable than coarse bran, but this has not been consistently reported. In rats fed purified diets containing 15% hard wheat bran with MPS varying from 1275 to 394 μm, the neutral detergent fibre (NDF) fermentability remained within $34.2 \pm 0.6\%$ and $35.8 \pm 0.8\%$. Similar conclusions were reached using soft and hard wheat bran from the American Association of Cereal Chemists (AACC) with various MPS values: 37·3–37·6% and 30·0–32·8% of NDF were fermented, respectively.

Soluble Fibre

Soluble fibre was initially considered to be insignificant in commonly eaten foods. Reports on pectin, guar, legume fibre and oat bran appeared in the early 1960s, but it was only in the mid-1970s that the implication of soluble fibre in the regulation of blood glucose and/or cholesterol levels received much attention. The mechanisms by which soluble fibre exerts its physiological effects are not fully understood, but viscosity and gelling properties appear to be associated with delayed digestion and absorption in the small intestine. The water-holding capacity is not related to effects in the large intestine since soluble fibre is mostly degraded by the microflora.

The soluble fibre content of a fibre source is influenced by the preparation of the food. Some polyuronides are susceptible to depolymerization caused by high temperature. The methods of analysis of dietary fibre utilize various conditions (e.g. time, temperature, pH, and type of buffer) for measuring the water-soluble fibre. The proportion of soluble fibre determined using one method differs from that of another. The consumption of a variety of foods containing dietary fibre (whole-grain products, fruits, vegetables and legumes) provides both soluble and insoluble fibre fractions in the ratio of 1:2 or 1:3.

Sources of Dietary Fibre

The actual contribution of plant food tissues in the diet to the dietary fibre intake depends on (1) the variety, (2) the maturity, and (3) the growing conditions of the plant, and (4) on the preparation of the food. Although methodology problems have not been completely resolved, there has been increasing agreement among the dietary fibre methods for a majority of foods.

The names of 49 sources of dietary fibre are provided in Table 4. Foods are classified in arbitrary categories according to their total dietary fibre (TDF) content, expressed on an 'as is' basis. The letters 'E', 'M', and 'P' in the right-hand column identify the methods agreeing with the TDF range shown. Other methods not included in the comparison are likely to agree with these figures. The letter 'E' refers to the NSPs (Englyst GLC), plus the potassium permanganate lignin value, measured separately; the letter 'M' refers to the Mongeau rapid method; and the letter 'P' refers to the Prosky method. The last two methods are gravimetric and include lignin. Table 4 shows 33 foods associated with the letters 'EMP', three foods with the letters 'MP' (E-method values are shown in parentheses), and 13 foods with the letters 'M'. The latter 13 foods were measured only with the Mongeau rapid method and each TDF value was based on winter and summer collections of up to 20 individual foods over 30 months in different locations.

Most fruits and vegetables were in the 1·0–2·2% TDF category, while cereals were distributed throughout all categories. Sources of dietary fibre with more than 4·3% TDF were generally cereal products and legumes.

Table 4. Sources of dietary fibre

TDF[a]	Foods	Methods[b]
0·1–0·5	White rice, cooked	M
	Orange juice from concentrate	M
0·6–0·9	Lettuce	M
	Cucumbers	EMP
	Pineapple, melons (cantaloupe)	EMP
1·0–2·2	White bread	EMP
	Corn kernel (canned), potatoes (boiled), green beans (boiled), cabbage (raw), celery (raw), onion (cooked), green peppers (raw)	EMP
	Cauliflower (cooked), tomatoes	M
	Apple, bananas, orange, pears, strawberries, cherries, grapefruit, plums	EMP
	Apple pie, blueberry pie, pasta (cooked)	M
2·3–3·0	Rye bread	M
	Mushroom (E = 2·0)	MP
	Beets (canned), rutabaga (raw), carrots (raw), broccoli (raw)	EMP
	Blueberries (E = 1·9)	MP
3·1–4·3	Brown rice	EMP
	Raisins (seedless)	M
4·4–6·4	Bran muffins, wheat cereal, wholemeal bread	EMP
	White beans (baked)	EMP
	Kidney beans (baked), peanut butter	M
6·5–7·3	Peanuts	EMP
	Green peas (boiled)	M
8·0–9·3	Oatmeal cereal	EMP
9·4–10·3	Shredded wheat	EMP
12·3–13·1	Bran flakes	EMP
15·5–15·8	Oat bran	EMP
40·6–40·9	Hard wheat bran (E = 36·4)	MP

[a] TDF, total dietary fibre range, g per 100 g, as is basis.
[b] Methods: E, Englyst GLC method plus potassium permanganate lignin; M, Mongeau rapid gravimetric method; P, Prosky gravimetric method.
From: Mongeau R and Brassard R (1989) A comparison of three methods for analyzing dietary fiber in 38 foods. *Journal of Food Composition and Analysis* 2: 189–199.
Mongeau R, Brassard R and Verdier P (1989) Measurement of dietary fiber in a total diet study. *Journal of Food Composition and Analysis* 2: 317–326.

The dietary fibre content of foods is greatly influenced by moisture content. Table 4 presents the foods as they are most often eaten; cereals are shown in their dry 'as is' form, unless contrary indications are provided. It is noteworthy that peanut products contain 1% moisture while some fruits and vegetables contain more than 90% moisture. The amount of dietary fibre provided by a source is also dependent on portion size, e.g. 30 g for breakfast cereals, 50 g for lettuce raisins, and 125 g for vegetables and fruits.

The word 'fibre' evokes fibrillar material but the fibrillar appearance of foods is not related to their dietary fibre content. Whole grains and legumes should certainly be part of the various sources of dietary fibre in a balanced diet.

Bibliography

Bainter K (ed.) (1986) *Intestinal Absorption of Macromolecules and Immune Transmission from Mother to Young.* Boca Raton, Florida: CRC Press.

Carpita NC (1990) The chemical structure of the cell walls of higher plants. In: Kritchevsky D, Bonfield C and Anderson JW (eds *Dietary Fiber: Chemistry, Physiology, and Health Effects*, pp 15–30. New York: Plenum Press.

Cummings JH (1976) What is fiber? In: Spiller GA and Amen RJ (eds) *Fiber in Human Nutrition*, pp 5–30. New York: Plenum Press.

Department of Health (1991) *Dietary Reference Values for Food Energy and Nutrients for the United Kingdom.* Department of Health Report on Health and Social Subjects No. 41. London: Her Majesty's Stationery Office.

Dintzis FR (1983) Dietary fiber analysis – concepts and problems. In: Lineback DR and Inglett GE (eds) *Food Carbohydrates*, p 326. Wesport, Connecticut: AVI Publishing.

Dreher ML (ed.) (1987) *Handbook of Dietary Fiber: An Applied Approach.* New York: Marcel Dekker.

Heaton KW (1990) Concepts of dietary fibre. In: Southgate DAT, Waldron K, Johnson IT and Fenwick GR (eds) *Dietary Fibre: Chemical and Biological Aspects*, pp 3–9. Cambridge: Royal Society of Chemistry.

HWC (1985) *Report of the Expert Advisory Committee on Dietary Fibre.* Ottawa: Health Protection Branch, Health and Welfare Canada.

Mongeau R and Brassard R (1982) Insoluble dietary fiber from breakfast cereals and brans: bile salt binding and water-holding capacity in relation to particle size. *Cereal Chemistry* 59: 413–417.

Pilch SM (1987) *Physiological effects and health consequences of dietary fiber.* Life Sciences Research Office, FASEB. Prepared for the Center for Food Safety and Applied Nutrition, Food and Drug Administration, Department of Health and Human Services, Washington, DC.

Selvendran RR and Robertson JA (1990) The chemistry of dietary fibre: an holistic view of the cell wall matrix. In: Southgate DAT, Waldron K, Johnson IT and Fenwick GR (eds) *Dietary Fibre: Chemical and Biological Aspects*, pp 27–43. Cambridge: Royal Society of Chemistry.

Selvendran RR, Stevens BJH and Dupont MS (1987) Dietary fibre: Chemistry, analysis and properties. *Advances in Food Research* 31: 117–209.

Southgate DAT (1979) The definition, analysis and properties of dietary fibre. In: Heaton KW (ed) *Dietary Fibre: Current Developments of Importance to Health.* Westport, Connecticut: Food and Nutrition Press.

Southgate DAT (1986) Food components that behave as dietary fibre. In: Spiller GA (ed) *Handbook of dietary fiber in human nutrition*, pp 21–22. Boca Raton, Florida: CRC Press.

Trowell HC, Burkitt DP and Heaton KW (1985) Definitions of dietary fibre and fibre-depleted foods. In: Trowell HC, Burkitt DP and Heaton KW (eds) *Dietary Fibre, Fibre-*

depleted Foods and Disease, pp 21–30. London: Academic Press.

Van Soest PJ (1978) Dietary fibers: their definition and nutritional properties. *American Journal of Clinical Nutrition* 31: S12–S20.

Roger Mongeau
Health and Welfare Canada, Ottawa, Canada

Determination

Although the integrity of the plant cell wall is important in the concept of dietary fibre and its physiological effects, methods for dietary fibre analysis only provide quantitative estimates. Procedures have been described for the isolation and detailed analysis of dietary fibre in specific foods, but the present article is focussed on practical methods which are applicable to the routine analysis of a range of foods. Most total dietary fibre (TDF) methods have optional procedures to estimate fibre fractions (e.g. soluble fibre, insoluble fibre, cellulose) but only the TDF versions are considered here. Modern methods of dietary fibre analysis have largely evolved from the work of Southgate and Van Soest and the method agreement for TDF values has constantly increased since the early 1980s. The complexity and variability of dietary fibre and the various food-processing techniques have contributed to the difficulties encountered in determining dietary fibre.

Ideal reference standards do not exist for dietary fibre analysis. Purified fibre components and unpurified standardized 'reference samples' are both used as standards of analysis, but the former group rarely represents the complex dietary fibre matrix and the latter group remains variable in composition, structure and properties.

The crude fibre method has been in use for more than 150 years and consists of sequential extractions with hot dilute acid and alkali. The residue, however, contains no soluble fibre and only about 15% hemicelluloses, 50–100% cellulose and 10–50% lignin. The crude fibre values do not represent an adequate estimation of dietary fibre. *See* Cellulose; Hemicelluloses; Lignin

Gravimetric Methods

In the gravimetric methods, the food sample is subjected to enzyme and/or chemical treatments to remove digestible material. The weight of the residue is corrected for ash and corrections may also be applied for incompletely digested components. The remaining weight is considered to be dietary fibre.

Gravimetric determinations involve weighing the residue retained on a filtering glass crucible of a specific porosity. In the preparation of the sample, care should be taken not to pulverize it into fine particles because some insoluble fibre may be lost during filtration; this is avoided by using a Wiley mill.

The Detergent System

The detergent system has been widely utilized for feed analysis and has represented a great improvement in the recovery of insoluble fibre, compared with the crude fibre method. The system includes the neutral detergent fibre (NDF) and the acid detergent fibre (ADF) procedures which consist of hot detergent treatments to remove digestible material (and soluble fibre). The system discriminates among the insoluble fibres in hemicelluloses, cellulose and lignin. A chelating agent present in the neutral detergent solution also solubilizes some insoluble pectin. When NDF and ADF are measured sequentially, the difference in weight between NDF and ADF is an estimation of the insoluble hemicelluloses. The ADF residue contains the lignin, cellulose and cutin, if any. The loss in weight of the ADF residue following the permanganate treatment represents the lignin content. A 72% sulphuric acid treatment removes the cellulose from cutin.

NDF and Porcine α-Amylase

Since most dietary fibre is water-insoluble, the simplicity of the NDF procedure has prompted its adaptation for the analysis of human foods. Starch, protein and artefact fibre remaining in the NDF residue are efficiently removed by a rapid treatment with α-amylase from porcine pancreas; the rapid treatment consists of 5 min and 60 min incubations at 55°C and is at least as effective as the 18 h treatment at 37°C originally proposed by Schaller. Unpurified porcine α-amylase (PA) has unique amylolytic and proteolytic activities if applied after (not before) the neutral detergent treatment. *See* Enzymes, Use in Analysis; Protein, Determination and Characterization; Starch, Structure, Properties and Determination

The α-amylase from *Bacillus subtilis* (ABS) has been used with the neutral detergent treatment, but this source may contain fibre-digesting enzymes. In addition, it does not remove the nonfibre material which causes overestimation of the lignin and possibly the hemicellulose fractions. Table 1 shows that, for shredded wheat, the NDF-ABS residue was 30% higher than the NDF-PA residue, with three times more apparent lignin and four times more protein. The same observation was made for bran flakes. The example of whole

Table 1. Effect of two sources of α-amylase on the apparent NDF and lignin contents of breakfast cereals and bread (g per 100 g, dry weight basis)

	Porcine pancreas (PA)[a]			Bacillus subtilis (ABS)		
	NDF	Lignin	Protein[b]	NDF	Lignin	Protein[b]
Shredded wheat	10·2	0·8	0·4	13·4[c]	2·7[c]	1·7[c]
Bran Flakes	10·1	0·9		15·8	2·4	
Whole wheat bread[d]	5·2	0·3		5·9	0·4	
Whole wheat bread toasted[d]	5·4	0·4		10·1	2·2	

[a] α-Amylase from porcine pancreas (Sigma Chemical Co., Cat. No. A-3176).
[b] Protein measured in NDF residue (N×6·25).
[c] From PJ Van Soest (1978) *Fiber Analysis Tables. American Journal of Clinical Nutrition* 31: S284.
[d] From R Mongeau and R Brassard (1980) Rapid digestion of starch and artifact fibre in the measurement of neutral detergent fibre of cereal products. *Getreide Mehl und Brot* 34: 125–127.

wheat bread shows that the mammalian amylase renders the NDF procedure quite independent from food processing (toasting), by comparison with the bacterial amylase which left apparent NDF and lignin values about two- and five-fold higher, respectively (Table 1). The efficacy of the NDF-PA treatments have been verified in various foods and food products; this has been confirmed by Marlett and coworkers. In addition, the NDF-PA treatments favour rapid filtrations and discriminate well between plant and bacterial cell walls; the latter interferes with the fibre analysis of faecal samples.

Other modifications from the original Van Soest NDF method include the deletion of decalin, 2-ethoxy-ethanol and sulphite (to maximize the recovery of lignin).

Rapid TDF Method

A soluble fibre procedure complementing the NDF-PA procedure provides an estimate of TDF. The development of the soluble fibre procedure was aimed towards practicality while maximizing the recovery of soluble fibre and the exclusion of protein and other precipitable materials. This latter characteristic is important to avoid the time-consuming protein determination. The soluble fibre procedure includes a gelatinization step in acetate buffer at pH 4·5 (121°C) followed by a treatment with heat-stable α-amylase (100°C). The soluble material is separated from insoluble fibre by filtration and is treated at 60°C with amyloglucosidase, and then with protease. The soluble fibre is precipitated in 80% ethanol at room temperature (RT).

Compared with extraction at higher pH values (e.g. phosphate buffer at pH 7), acetate buffer at pH 4·5 favours the exclusion of protein and appears to prevent

the degradation of fibre components at high temperature. If some fibre is not retained, the difference in TDF value is small according to method comparisons (Tables 2 and 3, Fig. 1). The method is considered 'rapid' compared to other fibre methods, particularly with the use of Fibertec E for soluble fibre and Fibertec I for insoluble fibre. For example, the maximum number of duplicate determinations using the Prosky TDF method is 20 per week, while 44 TDF duplicate determinations are possible using the rapid method within the same period of time. This evaluation takes into account the time for the analysis and the preparation of solutions (reagents), but not the time for preparing the samples (freeze drying, grinding).

This method has been carried out with the soluble and insoluble fractions measured either from two separate samples, or from one sample using sequential determination. In the latter case, the insoluble residue generated during the soluble fibre determination is treated with neutral detergent and porcine amylase, leaving insoluble fibre. Measuring TDF from one sample provides a better justification of the method since the same fibre component cannot be counted twice. Table 3 (far right column) indicates that TDF values are comparable in either ways. For 28 foods from various categories, the rapid sequential method was in agreement with the Prosky TDF method (Table 2) and with the Englyst gas-liquid chromatography (GLC) method (Fig. 1). With the latter, lignin was measured in each food and the value added to nonstarch polysaccharides (NSPs) to obtain the TDF value. In Table 2, the regression parameters suggest that the rapid method and the Prosky TDF method retain similar material with r^2 values of 0·98–0·998 and a slope close to unity. However, the negative intercept indicates that TDF values for low-fibre foods tend to be lower with the rapid method. *See* Carbohydrates, Classification and Properties; Chromatography, Gas Chromatography

Determination

Table 2. Regression analysis of TDF values in various foods using the rapid gravimetric method (Y) and the Prosky TDF gravimetric method[a] (X), ($Y=a+bX$) (fresh weight basis)

Foods	n	TDF range	a	b	r^2
Mostly cereals[b]	16	1–80	−0·39	0·98	0·994
Unprocessed and processed	25	1–89	−0·57	1·01	0·986
Total diet[c]	38	1–13	−0·13	1·02 (0·97, 1·07)	0·98
Total diet[d]	28	1–16	−0·11	0·99 (0·94, 1·04)	0·985

[a] Prosky et al. (1985) Determination of dietary fiber in foods and food products: collaborative study. *Journal of the AOAC* 68: 677–679.
[b] From Mongeau R and Brassard R (1986) A rapid method for the determination of soluble and insoluble dietary fiber: comparison with AOAC total dietary fiber procedure and Englyst's method. *Journal of Food Science* 51: 1333–1336.
[c] From Mongeau R and Brassard R (1989). The 95% confidence limits are shown in parentheses.
[d] Re-analysis of most of the above foods plus oat bran by the rapid method using sequential analysis of soluble and insoluble fibre fractions.

Table 3. Comparison of TDF values by GLC (NSPs+lignin) or gravimetric methods (dry weight basis)

				TDF (gravimetric)[d]		
					Rapid	
	NSPs[a]	NSPs[b]	L[c]	Prosky	Separate	Sequential
Apple	9·9–14·7	13·4	0·8	14·6	14·1	14·6
Beans, green	27·8–32·2	30·6	2·1	33·7	31·3	29·1
Bread, white wheat	2·6–3·3	3·0	0·6	3·5	3·0	3·9
Carrot	22·8–28·9	23·5	1·8	25·4	23·4	23·4
Corn kernels, canned	6·7–8·9	5·9	1·0	7·7	7·8	7·6
Corn flakes	0·7–2·4	1·1	<0·1	2·5	1·1	2·6
Flour, white wheat	3·0–3·7	2·6	<0·1	3·0	3·9	3·6
Oats, rolled	7·1–9·5	8·2	0·9	10·5	11·0	9·6
Peas, canned	20·4–22·3	—	—	—	23·3	20·9

[a] Range of values reported by Anderson and Bridges, Englyst et al. and Marlett (from Marlett JA, 1990).
[b] NSP using the Englyst GLC method, from Mongeau R and Brassard R (1989).
[c] L, permanganate lignin.
[d] Prosky TDF method; rapid, separate—separate (two samples) analysis of soluble and insoluble fractions (from Mongeau R and Brassard R, 1989); rapid, sequential—sequential (one sample) analysis of soluble and insoluble fractions.

Prosky Methods

The Prosky TDF method has also been referred as the AOAC (Association of Official Analytical Chemists) method since 1985. The Prosky and Asp methods are similar, but do not use exactly the same enzymes; their TDF values have been reported to be comparable. In the Prosky TDF method, duplicate samples are treated with amylase, protease and amyloglucosidase to remove digestible material. Four volumes of 95% ethanol are added and the precipitate is filtered. The residue contains a substantial amount of nitrogen. One of the duplicates is analysed for ash and the other for protein (nitrogen (N) content × 6·25). The total amounts of ash and calculated protein are subtracted from the residue weight. Englyst and Cummings believe that the use of this protein conversion factor leads to overestimation of dietary fibre. It is mainly the additional protein determination which prevents this method from being considered rapid. Some types of starch can also be retained

Determination

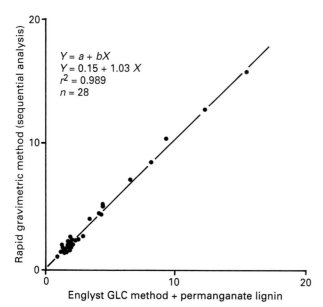

$Y = a + bX$
$Y = 0.15 + 1.03\ X$
$r^2 = 0.989$
$n = 28$

Fig. 1 TDF values in various foods: comparison of the rapid gravimetric method (Y) with the Englyst GLC method+lignin (X) (g per 100 g, fresh weight basis).

in the residue. A simplified version of the Prosky method deletes the protease step since protein is measured; a larger amount of protein is thus subtracted, compared with the original Prosky procedure. Another version of the Prosky method has been proposed for improving its precision. The method comparisons in Tables 2 and 3 were confined to the results obtained with the integral version of the Prosky method. The filtering aid used was celite C-211 (Fisher Scientific). The nature of the celite used in different laboratories has been considered as a source of variation in the results.

Jeraci Method

This method is also called the urea enzymatic dialysis (UED) method. The sample is treated with urea and heat-stable amylase and, after dialysis, with protease. After further dialysis, fibre is precipitated with four volumes of ethanol, filtered and weighed. Corrections are made for residual protein and ash. This method appears to remove essentially all starch from the fibre residue with minimal heat treatment. The corrections for crude protein and ash are smaller than in the Prosky method. This method requires only simple equipment. Little data are yet available for comparing with other fibre methods.

Complete Polysaccharidic Components (GLC Methods)

The Southgate method published in 1969 measures the TDF (NSPs + lignin) and provides values for hemicellu-

loses, cellulose and lignin. The alcohol (85% v/v) insoluble residue is gelatinized and treated with an enzyme to digest the starch. The takadiastase used originally had an amylolytic activity combined with a proteolytic activity; this enzyme became unavailable in the 1970s and the other enzymes used were often less effective, but the α-amylase from porcine pancreas appeared to be adequate. This method measures the hydrolysed fibre polysaccharides by colorimetry, which is less specific than GLC. *See* Spectroscopy, Visible Spectroscopy and Colorimetry

In the more recent chemical methods, the food sample is subjected to enzyme and/or chemical treatments to remove digestible material and the residue is hydrolysed by acid. The acid treatment needs to be severe enough to assure complete hydrolysis but mild enough to prevent degradation of the monomers released. The neutral polysaccharidic constituents of fibre are measured chemically, usually by GLC after transformation into a measurable form (e.g. alditol acetates). With high-performance liquid chromatography (HPLC), the latter transformation is not required. Acidic sugars (uronic acids) are measured colorimetrically. Appropriate calculations give the total NSPs. TDF is considered to be NSPs + lignin. The main GLC methods have been published by Anderson, Englyst and Theander and their coworkers. Marlett uses a modified Theander method. The GLC methods are different in several aspects, including the starch gelatinization step, enzyme treatments and conditions of acid hydrolysis. This explains why the methods may be in agreement for some foods, but not for others. *See* Chromatography, High-performance Liquid Chromatography

Englyst Method

The Englyst method measures NSPs (neutral sugars + uronic acids): the food sample is treated with dimethyl sulphoxide (DMSO) to disperse starch and then with a heat-stable α-amylase and a mixture of pullulanase-pancreatin in acetate buffer at pH 5·2. After precipitation in 80% ethanol and centrifugation, the residue is hydrolysed with sulphuric acid. Neutral sugars are measured by GLC as alditol acetates and uronic acids are measured by colorimetry. According to Englyst and Cummings, the times required to complete the Prosky TDF method and the Englyst GLC method (total NSPs) are very similar. This is true when the GLC instrument is equipped with an autosampler. In a rapid version of the Englyst method, the sugar components are measured colorimetrically, but the procedure requires about the same operator time as the GLC method with an autosampler.

One great advantage of the Englyst method is its applicability to processed foods due to the use of DMSO during the gelatinization step. However, care is needed when using this toxic chemical.

The Englyst method is the only dietary fibre method which does not include lignin. The role of the noncarbohydrate components (which include lignin) may significantly modify the behaviour of dietary fibre but they should be measured independently from NSPs.

Theander Method

In the Theander method, the food sample is first extracted with 80% ethanol. This extraction appears important to reduce the coprecipitation of simple sugars with fibre components. Starch is digested in acetate buffer at pH 5·0 by incubations with a thermostable α-amylase and then with an amyloglucosidase. DMSO is not used and starch may be less efficiently dispersed and removed. After precipitation in 80% ethanol and centrifugation, the residue is hydrolysed with sulphuric acid. Neutral polysaccharides are analysed as alditol acetates by GLC and uronic acids by decarboxylation with special equipment or by colorimetry.

Klason lignin is measured gravimetrically; this fraction may include other material which overestimates insoluble fibre. For example, the insoluble fibre of apple, peas or food composite retained by this method included 0·9–3·5% (dry weight basis) apparent lignin while no lignin was found in the corresponding NDF residue treated with the porcine α-amylase; the latter results are more likely. The sequential NDF-PA and ADF treatments prior to permanganate lignin determination leave a low lignin value which is quite independent from food processing (Table 1). The necessity to measure lignin and the problems related to its measurement have been discussed by Marlett.

Anderson Method

As in the Englyst method, the Anderson GLC method uses DMSO to disperse starch. Starch is digested with porcine α-amylase in acetate buffer at pH 5·2. After precipitation with four volumes of ethanol, the residue is extracted with water at 100°C. Following centrifugation, the soluble fibre from the supernatant and the insoluble fibre from the pellet are hydrolysed with sulphuric acid. Klason lignin is measured according to loss in weight of the nonhydrolysed residue upon ashing.

Comparison of GLC and Gravimetric Methods for TDF

For 25 foods, TDF values measured by the rapid gravimetric method were in agreement with those reported by Anderson's laboratory. Direct comparisons using the same samples are needed.

Table 3 compares the fibre values expressed on a dry weight basis to magnify differences which could appear negligible when expressed on a fresh weight basis. For the chemical methods, only the NSP value is shown (i.e. lignin excluded) and the lignin (L) value can be added to compare with the gravimetric TDF values. The far left column shows the NSP range provided by three laboratories (from samples which may vary). The results shown in columns two to six were obtained in one laboratory and the samples were composites based on winter and summer collections of up to 20 individual foods over 30 months in different locations. These results indicate that possible disagreements exist among GLC methods and that, when lignin is taken into account, there is not a definite gap between GLC and gravimetric methods for the TDF values of the foods compared. The latter view is supported by the results shown in Fig. 1.

Nutritional Labelling and Analysis

Measuring the dietary fibre content of food for regulatory purposes is a challenge to retain all fibre polymers and not contaminants. The proportion of soluble fibre with one method differs from that of another and the differences have not been related to physiological effects. Therefore, only the TDF methods are compared in regard to several characteristics deemed to be important for food labelling.

Equipment

A method requiring simple inexpensive equipment would have wide applicability. The gravimetric methods, particularly the Jeraci UED method, require simpler equipment than other methods. The Englyst colorimetric method may also be used with a simple spectrophotometer.

Operator Time

The rapid method requires less operator time per duplicate determination than all other methods because it is the only gravimetric method which does not include a protein determination. The method is practical in a well-organized laboratory (e.g. with a convenient hot water supply) and, if desired, semiautomatic equipment can be used. This equipment is not available for other gravimetric methods. The GLC methods greatly benefit from the use of an autosampler.

Determination

Lignin

The Englyst method is the only one which does not include lignin. Most other methods may include non-fibre material (e.g. Maillard products) in their lignin fraction. The NDF-PA and ADF treatments appear to be adequate preliminary steps for lignin determination.

Independence from Food Processing

Some starch has been reported to be included in dietary fibre using Theander or Prosky methods. With the latter, TDF values were higher for cooked rice and cooked potatoes than for the corresponding uncooked samples; problems also occurred for roasted peanuts where nonfibre material was included with TDF. The Englyst method is the most independent from food processing because it uses DMSO and excludes lignin. The rapid gravimetric method is also quite independent from food processing and includes lignin.

Precision

In a study in which 25 blind duplicate food samples were provided by the US Department of Agriculture, method variability pooled over all foods was measured. The coefficient of variation for the case of a single observation was 2·97% with the rapid method and 4·74% with the Prosky TDF method. This represents an estimation of the intralaboratory precision for selected unprocessed and processed foods. More interlaboratory work comparing precision of several methods is needed.

Remaining Problems

The general agreement between fibre methods is encouraging but many problems remain to be solved. First, only the defatting procedure of Bligh and Dyer would be efficient enough to defat some of the food products, although acetone or ether are sufficient for the great majority of samples. Secondly, during the alcohol precipitation step, it is possible that fibre components are not completely precipitated and that some sugars released by starch digestion are coprecipitated, this varying with the method used. Thirdly, structural fibre protein may represent up to 10% of dietary fibre in immature plant tissues and, although the rapid gravimetric method presumably includes it, none of the methods can specifically measure it. Fourthly, in vegetables, uronic acid values were higher by a decarboxylation method than by colorimetric determination; while most GLC methods measure uronic acid colorimetrically, this discrepancy remains to be explained. Fifthly, there appears to be a small number of foods for which a method disagreement occurs: the NSP value using the Englyst GLC method may be lower (e.g. for soya bean fibre isolate) than the TDF value measured gravimetrically.

Conclusion

In conclusion, measuring dietary fibre using any of the methods mentioned above should provide comparable TDF values for many foods. Inclusion of starch could be a cause of error. Another cause of error, particularly in processed foods, is Klason lignin. A lignin value exempt of nonfibre polymers should be obtained from the following sequential treatments: neutral detergent, α-amylase from porcine pancreas, acid detergent and permanganate solution. The latter lignin determination combined with NSPs determined by GLC provides a detailed composition of dietary fibre.

Among the gravimetric methods, the rapid method does not need a starch determination, and this also seems to be the case for the Jeraci UED method. The rapid method, including the neutral detergent and porcine α-amylase treatments, has several desirable characteristics for food labelling.

Bibliography

Bligh EG and Dyer WJ (1959) A rapid method of total lipid extraction and purification. *Canadian Journal of Biochemistry and Physiology* 37: 911–917.

Englyst H and Cummings J (1989) Dietary fibre and starch: definition, classification and measurement. *In:* Leeds AR (ed.) *Dietary Fibre Pespectives. Reviews and Bibliography*, pp 3–26. London: John Libbey.

Jeraci JL, Carr JM, Lewis BA and Van Soest PJ (1990) Evaluation of dietary fiber methods and the distribution of β-glucan among various fiber fractions. *In:* Southgate DAT, Waldron K, Johnson IT and Fenwick GR (eds) *Dietary Fibre: Chemical and Biological Aspects*, pp 119–129. Cambridge: Royal Society of Chemistry.

Marlett JA (1990) Analysis of dietary fiber in human foods. *In:* Kritchevsky D, Bonfield C and Anderson JW (eds) *Dietary Fiber: Chemistry, Physiology and Health Effects*, pp 31–48. New York: Plenum Press.

Mongeau R and Brassard R (1989) A comparison of three methods for analyzing dietary fiber in 38 foods. *Journal of Food Composition and Analysis* 2: 189–199.

Mongeau R, Brassard R and Verdier P (1989) Measurement of dietary fiber in a total diet study. *Journal of Food Composition and Analysis* 2: 317–326.

Theander O (1981) A review of the different analytical methods and remaining problems. In: James WPT and Theander O (eds.) *The Analysis of Dietary Fiber in Food*. New York: Marcel Dekker.

Selvendran RR and O'Neill MA (1987) Isolation and analysis of cell walls from plant material. *In:* Glick D (ed.) *Methods of Biochemical Analysis*, vol. 32. New York: Wiley.

Roger Mongeau
Health and Welfare Canada, Ottawa, Canada

Physiological Effects

The dietary fibre hypothesis, founded in the early 1970s by a group of colonial medical officers, chemists and gastroenterologists, contained a number of very novel propositions. The idea that the populations of wealthy industrialized countries were suffering from a form of chronic malnutrition was remarkable, as was the sheer number and variety of gastrointestinal and metabolic diseases which were attributed to this cause. Most controversial of all, however, was the assertion that, besides nutrients, the indigestible components of the diet might also be essential to human health. It is extremely difficult to examine directly the role of dietary fibre in the aetiology of disease, but the hypothesis has generated a considerable volume of physiological research concerned with the mechanisms by which fibre may act.

It has become clear that dietary fibre influences the function of the entire alimentary tract, and the metabolic processes with which it is linked. However, the various polysaccharides which comprise dietary fibre differ greatly in their biological and physical properties, and generalizations based on an analytical definition of dietary fibre are usually misleading. This brief review is concerned with the main physiological effects of cell wall components and other nonstarch polysaccharides in the small and large bowel.

Nutrient Absorption

The proximal small intestine is the main site of nutrient absorption, a process which includes hydrolysis of digestible polymers such as proteins, starch and triglycerides, and transport of the products by the mucosal epithelial cells that line the mucosa. The diverse group of polysaccharides which comprise dietary fibre are all resistant to hydrolysis by mammalian pancreatic enzymes. However, the complex architecture of plant cell walls is disrupted during food processing, mastication, and the gastric stages of digestion. Insoluble components are degraded to finer particles, and soluble polysaccharides, such as pectins and β-glucan, become dispersed in the aqueous phase. The possibility that the absorption of nutrients might be delayed by the presence of cell wall polysaccharides in the gut lumen was an early premise of the dietary fibre hypothesis. Subsequent physiological studies have confirmed this and clarified the various mechanisms involved. *See* Colon, Structure and Function; Colon, Diseases and Disorders

Barrier Effects

Cell walls contribute structural organization to plant tissues as well as mechanical strength. Once ingested as food, they constitute a barrier which separates digestive enzymes from substrate such as starch granules and intracellular lipids, and they can slow the diffusion of hydrolytic products through the partially digested matrix in the gut lumen. The susceptibility of cell walls to physical disruption during their passage through the alimentary tract varies considerably between foods. Where they survive relatively intact, they have been shown to slow the assimilation of nutrients considerably. For example, legume seeds have relatively thick cell walls which resist destruction during processing and cooking, and this is reflected in a slow rate of glucose absorption from beans and other pulses. This effect of dietary fibre is very difficult to predict from analytical values of fibre content because it is a function of the structural integrity of cell walls, rather than the absolute quantity of polysaccharides within the food.

Binding Effects

Many cell wall polysaccharides and associated lignin polymers have charged groups which can interact with ionized species in the aqueous phase of the gut contents. Such interactions can, at least in theory, restrict the bioavailability of nutrients for transport by the cells of the intestinal mucosa. Iron, zinc and calcium are relatively poorly absorbed from the human diet. The limiting factor is usually the formation of insoluble precipitates or nonabsorbable complexes in the intestinal lumen. Various forms of dietary fibre have been observed to bind metal ions *in vitro*, and nutritionists have long suspected that the consumption of diets rich in unrefined cereals might lead to a general reduction in the bioavailability of mineral nutrients. *See* Bioavailability of Nutrients

The use of isotopically labelled minerals has made it possible to undertake experiments in which minerals such as iron, zinc and calcium are fed to human subjects in conjunction with isolated components of dietary fibre, including cellulose, pectin and plant gums. In general, cell wall polysaccharides have been found to exert only a relatively small adverse effect on mineral absorption in humans. However, diets which contain a high proportion of legumes, oats or wholemeal products do have an adverse effect on the balance of mineral intake and excretion. This appears to be mainly an effect of phytate (myo-inositol hexaphosphate), which is a mineral-binding substance associated with plant cell walls. It is difficult to select diets which are rich in fibre but low in phytate, but dephytinization can be carried out commercially to improve mineral bioavailability in high-value products. *See* Phytic Acid, Nutritional Impact

Intraluminal binding of organic nutrients and bile acids has also been investigated in some detail, as a mechanism has been sought to explain the postulated protective effect of dietary fibre against heart disease. The consumption of diets rich in dietary fibre leads to an increase in the faecal excretion of lipids and protein. Much of this material is of endogenous origin, but a substantial proportion appears to be derived from dietary fat and proteins which have escaped digestion. This is probably partly the result of binding of fatty acids in the gut lumen. There is little evidence that such relatively minor faecal nutrient losses are of much nutritional significance, but they probably reflect changes in the rate and site of nutrient absorption which can have far-reaching metabolic consequences. *See* Coronary Heart Disease, Intervention Studies

Some forms of dietary fibre have been shown to reduce plasma cholesterol levels in man, at least under experimental conditions. The mechanism underlying this effect is still unclear, but the problem has prompted many studies on the effects of fibre on bile acid absorption. Bile acids are natural surfactants, synthesized from cholesterol in the liver, and released from the gall bladder into the small intestinal lumen, where they assist in the emulsification of fat and the formation of micelles. Bile salts are not absorbed in the proximal small intestine, but they are taken up by an efficient active transport system in the distal ileum. The bile salts then return to the liver via the portal vein and are re-secreted, often during the course of a single meal. This 'enterohepatic circulation' can be interrupted by the consumption of artificial sequestrants such as ion-exchange resins, which cause increased faecal excretion and a reduction in serum cholesterol. This principle is used clinically to treat some forms of hypercholesterolaemia. *See* Bile; Cholesterol, Role of Cholesterol in Heart Disease

Cell wall polysaccharides and lignin have been shown to bind bile acids *in vitro*, and it has been frequently proposed that dietary fibre acts as natural bile acid sequestrants. However, the balance of evidence suggests that this is not an important mechanism influencing human cholesterol metabolism. This is partly because the maximum binding of bile acids occurs at acid pH, whereas the distal ileum where bile salts are actively absorbed is at near neutral pH. Moreover, where a hypocholesterolaemic effect of dietary fibre in man has been established, it is the soluble polysaccharides such as guar gum and oat β-glucan which are most effective, whereas these components of fibre are relatively poor bile-acid sequestrants.

Rheological Effects

Diabetes mellitus is a common disorder which the advocates of the dietary fibre hypothesis have long regarded as a disease of fibre deficiency. Indeed it has been argued that the disease was virtually nonexistent before the introduction of milling techniques which facilitated the widespread consumption of white flour products. This hypothesis prompted a search for physiological mechanisms which could account for the protective effects of dietary fibre. Early studies were carried out with a variety of forms of fibre, given to normal or diabetic subjects in combination with a carbohydrate test-meal. The blood glucose response was then monitored over a period of hours. It soon emerged that only soluble polysaccharides with a high viscosity led to a significant reduction in post-prandial glycaemia.

Isolated polysaccharide gums such as guar gum and pectin slow the absorption of free sugars, or glucose derived from starch hydrolysis, by increasing the viscosity of the duodenal and jejunal contents. Glucose and fatty acids are rapidly absorbed by the cells of the intestinal mucosa, and this leads to depletion of nutrients in the luminal fluid immediately adjacent to the villi. Under normal circumstances the gut lumen is well stirred by peristaltic movements of the gut, but this process becomes much less efficient when the viscosity of the luminal contents is high. Under these circumstances physical mixing is replaced by diffusion as the main mechanism conveying nutrients through the boundary layer to the mucosal surface. Diffusion is a relatively slow process, and this stage can become the rate-limiting step in nutrient absorption and assimilation.

The high viscosity of water-soluble polysaccharides is caused by weak interactions within the dispersed network of carbohydrate polymers. Despite the very marked effects on the viscosity of the gut contents, polymer networks of this type seem to impose relatively little restriction on the diffusion of low-molecular-weight solutes. However, this is not true in the case of micelles, which are very large molecular aggregates containing fatty acids, bile salts and cholesterol. Diffusion of micelles is slowed by polysaccharide gums, presumably by a form of molecular sieving, and the effect contributes to the delayed absorption of fat and cholesterol. *See* Gums, Nutritional Role of Guar Gum

As nutrient absorption is slowed the process is extended, both in time and physically, along the length of the small bowel. This reduces the rate at which nutrients appear in the circulation, and increases the exposure of the gut surface to nutrients. In experimental animals these effects trigger the release of regulatory hormones, and stimulate the growth of mucosal cells.

Few Western foods contain viscous polysaccharides at high enough levels to make much difference to intraluminal viscosity, but oats, which are rich in β-glucan gum, are one important exception. Other foods, including legumes such as beans and lentils, also give a relatively flat postprandial blood-glucose curve, and this property has been expressed numerically as the 'glycaemic index'. European legumes are not rich in viscous polysaccharides, and the slow digestion of legume starch appears to be primarily caused by the survival of cell walls after cooking. *See* Glucose, Glucose Tolerance and the Glycaemic Index

The discovery that viscous polysaccharides can improve the postprandial glycaemic response in diabetics has led to the development of pharmaceutical products containing guar gum which can be added to food or taken with meals in the form of a drink. These products can assist in the management of some diabetic patients, but their usefulness appears to be limited by poor palatability.

Faecal Bulk and Intestinal Transit Time

The functions of the colon are the partial recovery of endogenous materials and food residues which escape digestion and absorption in the small bowel, and the formation and temporary retention of faeces. The ability of cell wall polysaccharides to increase faecal bulk and stool frequency is perhaps the most widely recognized physiological property of dietary fibre. References to the laxative effects of wheat bran are found in classical Greek literature, and the benefits of 'roughage' were widely debated in the nineteenth and early twentieth centuries. The founders of the dietary fibre hypothesis built upon this work, and argued that in Western societies a low intake of fibre leads to undesirably high intraluminal pressures in the colon and rectum, and to prolonged straining at stool. These chronic physical stresses are assumed to cause degenerative changes in the colorectal wall, and in the large veins of the lower abdomen and legs, and eventually to lead to disease such as colonic diverticulae, haemorrhoids and varicose veins.

There have been many well-controlled studies which have confirmed that supplementation with some forms of dietary fibre leads to increased faecal bulk, reduced intracolonic pressure, and more frequent stools. This principle is widely used in the management of some forms of constipation, although its effectiveness varies widely between individuals. Degenerative diseases of the large bowel are more common in societies eating refined cereal foods, but the aetiological relationship has not been established with any certainty. Nevertheless, a large body of supportive physiological data has been acquired.

Transit Time

Food traverses the oesophagus within a few seconds, but the head of a meal takes about 4 h to reach the colon in most individuals. Some residual components of a meal may appear in the faeces within about 12 h after consumption, but the total time needed for all traces of the meal to disappear from the alimentary tract can be several days. Transit times vary considerably, both between populations and between and within individuals, and there is little doubt that the type and quantity of dietary fibre consumed is partly responsible for such differences.

Complex plant foods which retain the integrity of their cell walls take longer to traverse the stomach and small intestine than do soluble nonabsorbable sugars such as lactulose. This is probably primarily attributable to slower gastric emptying of large particles. Viscous polysaccharides also delay gastric emptying and small intestinal transit time to some extent. However, in contrast to the proximal alimentary tract, a high intake of dietary fibre usually leads to faster transit through the colon. There is an inverse relationship between faecal bulk and transit time in the large bowel which is probably the result of an acceleration of colonic motility by increased intraluminal mass. It has often been stated that this reduces the time available for the synthesis and toxic effects of carcinogenic chemical species in the faecal stream but this hypothesis has not been rigorously tested. *See* Colon, Cancer of the Colon

Faecal Output

Wheat bran, which is a largely insoluble and highly lignified tissue, resists fermentation in the colon, thus increasing the dry matter content of the faeces. More importantly, it also retains water during transit through the bowel and thereby increases the moisture content of the faeces. Other sources of dietary fibre which have this property are rice bran, and isphagula husk, a mucilagenous material used pharmaceutically as a bulk laxative. However, not all forms of dietary fibre contribute significantly to faecal bulk. Polysaccharides such as pectin, guar and oat β-glucan, which are readily fermentable by anaerobic bacteria, are decomposed during transit through the colon. Some of the breakdown products contribute to faecal mass by virtue of their incorporation into bacterial cells, but this component is small compared to the original mass of cell wall polysaccharides. The other products of carbohydrate fermentation are volatile fatty acids and gases, which may increase the volume of faeces and perhaps stimulate colorectal motility, but do not contribute to total faecal mass.

Processing undoubtedly influences the physiological properties of dietary fibre to a significant extent. In general, the faecal bulking properties of large particles of wheat bran are greater than those of more finely divided material. Cooking also seems to reduce the ability of wheat bran to contribute to faecal bulk, perhaps by increasing its susceptibility to fermentation.

The mechanisms controlling faecal composition and bulk transit time remain poorly understood, and it is interesting to note that even finely divided plastic tubing can increase stool frequency and water content, perhaps by stimulating secretory receptors in the gut wall.

Colonic Microflora

The formation of faeces and the control of defecation are functions associated with the left or descending colon. The caecum and the right colon harbour a rich microbial flora commonly containing over 500 bacterial species. This substantial mass of bacteria undoubtedly makes an important contribution to the physiology of its human host, but the details are imperfectly understood. It has been suggested that the colonic bacterial mass should be looked upon as a single metabolic entity, or even as an organ in its own right. The colonic environment is poorly supplied with nutrients, and unabsorbed dietary carbohydrates provide most of the substrates for growth and metabolism of the intracolonic flora. One important side-effect of the dietary fibre hypothesis has been to stimulate interest in this problem and increase our knowledge of human colonic microbiology. *See* Microflora of the Intestine, Role and Effects

The faecal microorganisms degrade many components of dietary fibre, as well as undigested starch, to yield the volatile fatty acids, butyrate, propionate and acetate, which are transported across the colonic mucosa. Butyrate functions as a substrate for the growth and metabolism of the colonic mucosal cells. Propionate and acetate are absorbed and metabolized by the liver, and up to 75% of the energy value of the non-starch polysaccharides becomes available to the body by these routes.

The other major breakdown products of carbohydrate fermentation are hydrogen, methane and carbon dioxide, which together comprise flatus gas. The total volume of flatus produced by individuals varies considerably, as does its tendency to cause unpleasant symptoms of flatulence and abdominal pain. Some subjects report discomfort when consuming high-fibre diets, but much of this may be caused by oligosaccharides and other fermentable components in foods such as legumes, rather than to fermentation of cell wall polysaccharides.

Apart from the recovery of water, endogenous secretions and energy from food components which have escaped digestion, the major function of bacterial fermentation in the colon is to regulate the physical and chemical properties of the intraluminal environment. The colonic mucosa is much more susceptible to cancer than that of the small bowel and this may well be because it is exposed to faecal material throughout the lifetime of the individual. Fermentation of carbohydrate reduces the pH of the colonic contents, and increases the quantity of butyrate available to the mucosal cells. These changes may reduce the production of carcinogenic chemicals and lessen the susceptibility of the colonic mucosal cells to neoplastic change. On the other hand, in experimental animals, volatile fatty acids have been shown to stimulate the rate at which colonic mucosal cells are replicated, and this could have an adverse effect on the induction of genetic damage. Despite the epidemiological evidence for a protective effect of dietary fibre against colorectal cancer in man, the precise role and mechanisms of action of the particular cell wall polysaccharides in the Western diet remains uncertain. *See* Inflammatory Bowel Disease

Bibliography

Burkitt DP and Trowell HC (1975) *Refined Carbohydrate Foods and Disease. Some Implications of Dietary Fibre.* London: Academic Press.

Creutzfeldt W and Folsch UR (eds) (1983) *Delaying Absorption as a Therapeutic Principle in Metabolic Diseases.* Stuttgart: Georg Thieme Verlag.

Johnson IT (1990) Fibre sources for the food industry. *Proceedings of the Nutrition Society* 49: 31–38.

Southgate DAT, Waldron K, Johnson IT and Fenwick GR (eds) (1991) *Dietary Fibre: Chemical and Biological Aspects.* RSC Special Publication No. 83. Cambridge: Royal Society of Chemistry.

Trowell HC, Burkitt DP and Heaton K (1985) *Dietary Fibre, Fibre-Depleted Foods and Disease.* London: Academic Press.

I. Johnson
Institute of Food Research, Norwich, UK

Effects of Fibre on Absorption

The fibre hypothesis suggested that high dietary fibre intakes were protective against a range of metabolic disorders, including obesity, diabetes, gallstones and ischaemic heart disease. Controlled studies have indicated that fibre may have relevance in preventing these disorders by facilitating weight reduction on low-calorie diets, reducing blood glucose and lipid levels, and reducing the lithogenicity of bile. The mechanisms of these effects are not well understood, but are believed to be due directly or indirectly to the effects of fibre on the digestion, metabolism and absorption of nutrients in the small intestine and colon. The purpose of this chapter is to provide an overview of how dietary fibre influences the absorption of nutrients through its effects on small intestinal and colonic physiology.

Energy

Fibre does not have marked effects on overall energy absorption in healthy individuals, although malabsorption may be significant in subjects with pancreatic insufficiency or small intestinal disease. With the recent appreciation of the ruminant function of the colon, it is now realized that energy entering the colon may be salvaged and that fibre itself actually provides energy to humans. The exact implications of fibre on energy balance are not known since the extent of fermentation of most dietary fibres in the human colon is unknown. *See* Energy, Energy Expenditure and Energy Balance

Nonviscous fibres such as wheat bran, which increase the bulk of intestinal contents, increase the rate of gastric emptying and decrease small intestinal transit time (Table 1). This tends to decrease the time available for absorption and increase the amount of energy entering the colon. Viscous fibres tend to decrease the rates of transit and absorption from the small intestine by increasing the viscosity of intestinal contents, but this does not cause gross malabsorption because the reduced rate of transit allows more time for absorption to occur. Thus both viscous and nonviscous fibres shift the site of absorption of nutrients to the lower small intestine, with increased energy spilling into the colon. *See* Colon, Structure and Function

Carbohydrate

Viscous dietary fibres reduce the rate of absorption of glucose or other carbohydrates, resulting in a reduction of the blood glucose and insulin responses (Table 1). The effects of fibre naturally present in foods are not necessarily the same as those of purified fibres added to foods. There is only a weak relationship between the total fibre content of foods and their blood glucose responses, with no relationship between soluble fibre and the blood glucose response. This is most likely because the chemical measurement of fibre does not indicate its physical properties, and because many other food-related factors (e.g. type of starch, particle size, processing, antinutrients) affect the glycaemic responses. Normally, 2–10% of the available carbohydrate in refined food enters the colon, increasing to 15–20% for high-fibre foods. However, about 75% of the energy in the 'malabsorbed' carbohydrate is salvaged by absorption of the short-chain fatty acids produced by colonic bacterial fermentation of the carbohydrate. In addition, it has been estimated that up to 75% of the fibre in a normal diet is fermented and contributes to overall energy balance. *See* Carbohydrates, Digestion, Absorption and Metabolism; Glucose, Function and Metabolism; Starch, Resistant Starch

Protein

High-fibre diets increase faecal nitrogen output, a finding which has been interpreted to mean that fibre causes protein malabsorption. However, this is not necessarily the only interpretation. Animal studies suggest that much of the increase in faecal nitrogen on high-fibre diets is accounted for by bacterial cell protein. The increased amount of carbohydrate entering the colon on a high-fibre diet provides energy which stimulates colonic bacterial growth. Colonic bacteria meet their own protein requirements by synthesizing amino acids from ammonia, at least part of which is derived from the breakdown of blood urea which is freely diffusible into the colon. Thus high-fibre diets may redirect waste urea nitrogen from excretion in the

Table 1. Effect of various purified fibres on blood glucose and insulin responses and mouth-to-caecum transit time in healthy subjects

	Gum				
	Guar	Tragacanth	Pectin	Methyl cellulose	Wheat bran
Viscosity ($\times 10^{-4}$ m^2 s^{-1})	1·3	0·52	0·21	0·07	0·01
Glucose area (Percentage of control)	32	66	89	71	73
Insulin area (Percentage of control)	42	90	98	82	92
Transit time (Percentage of control)	183	133	117	100	62

Fibres were added to solutions containing 50 g of glucose. Data from Jenkins DJA, Wolever TMS, Leeds AR *et al.* (1978) Dietary fibres, fibre analogues and glucose tolerance: importance of viscosity. *British Medical Journal* 1: 1392–1394.

Effects of Fibre on Absorption

Table 2. Effect of 6 weeks' feeding on various fibres and cholestyramine on the absorption (percentage of control) of triolein(triglyceride) and cholesterol in rats

	Pectin	Wheat bran	Alfalfa	Cholesty-ramine	Cellulose
Triolein	87	88	68	53	47
Cholesterol	42	38	28	23	13

Data from Vahouny GV, Roy T, Gallo L *et al.* (1980) Dietary fibers III. Effects of chronic intake on cholesterol absorption and metabolism in the rat. *American Journal of Clinical Nutrition* 33: 2182–2191.

urine to excretion in the faeces in the form of bacterial cell protein. Evidence for this is that soluble fibre has been shown to decrease blood urea levels in patients with uraemia, and low glycaemic index diets, which increase colonic fermentation, decrease urine urea excretion in healthy subjects and diabetics. *See* Microflora of the Intestine, Role and Effects

Fat

Fat absorption is a complex process, dependent upon the emulsification of the fat by bile, the hydrolysis of triglycerides into free fatty acids and monoglycerides by pancreatic lipase, and the hydrolysis of cholesterol esters into free cholesterol by cholesterol esterase. The products of hydrolysis are absorbed into the intestinal mucosal cells, where they are re-esterified, and the resulting triglycerides and cholesterol esters are used to form chylomicrons which reach the blood stream via the intestinal lymph. A minority of dietary triglyceride, primarily that containing short- and medium-chain fatty acids, is absorbed directly into the portal blood. *See* Fats, Digestion, Absorption and Transport

There are several ways by which fibre has been suggested to influence fat absorption: (1) reducing the efficiency of micelle formation by binding components of bile or diluting their concentration via a bulking effect; (2) physically slowing the rate of fat absorption due to the formation of a viscous gel; (3) inhibiting lipase activity; and (4) acting as an emulsifying agent to enhance micelle formation.

The bile-acid-binding resin, cholestyramine, reduces the concentration of bile in the small intestine by about 50%, which significantly inhibits fat solubilization and absorption (Table 2). Many fibres bind components of bile to some extent and some studies suggest that the total amounts of phospholipid and bile acids in the aqueous phase of intestinal contents are significant predictors of the total amount of lipid solubilized. However, the extent to which various fibres bind bile components is not necessarily related to the slowing of fat absorption. For example, konjac mannan, guar and chitosan bind bile acids in the small intestine of the rat; chitosan bound phospholipids, whereas guar and konjac diluted the concentration of phospholipids by increasing the volume of intestinal contents. Guar and konjac mannan delayed cholesterol and triglyceride absorption, but chitosan had no effect. Thus, in the case of cholestyramine, the binding of micellar components is sufficiently strong to inhibit fat solubilization and absorption. In the case of fibre, the interactions are weaker and may not necessarily change lipid solubilization. The delay in the absorption of fat by the gums is probably related to their ability to increase the viscosity and volume of intestinal contents and inhibit micelle diffusion. Slowing fat absorption results in more lipid absorption from the lower half of the small intestine, but the implications of this with respect to gut endocrine responses are unknown. Although viscous fibre may slow the rate of fat absorption, there does not appear to be a major effect on the total amount of fat absorbed, except possibly in patients with pancreatic insufficiency. *See* Bile

Most studies of how fibre affects fat absorption have been done in experimental animals, with only a limited number in humans. Paradoxically, several studies in humans have shown that guar, pectin and oat bran may increase postprandial serum triglycerides after a fatty test meal. Such an effect could be caused by enhanced micelle formation, or by a reduced rate of fat clearance from the blood due to reduced postprandial insulin levels leading to reduced activation of lipoprotein lipase.

Cholesterol

The effects of various fibres on cholesterol absorption are in general related to their effects on triglyceride absorption (Table 2), except that an actual reduction in the total amount of cholesterol absorbed may occur. However, this does not explain the serum cholesterol lowering effects of fibre, since pectin, which lowers serum cholesterol, has an effect on fat absorption similar to that of wheat bran, which does not lower cholesterol (Table 3).

Minerals, Trace Elements and Vitamins

There is some evidence that certain types of dietary fibre reduce the rate or extent of absorption of some vitamins, but the reductions are small and unlikely to have an adverse effect on nutritional status.

There has been much more concern about the possible adverse effects of fibre on mineral and trace element absorption. Many types of dietary fibre bind minerals *in vitro* and, in short-term studies, have been shown to

Effects of Fibre on Absorption

Table 3. Effect of various fibres on serum cholesterol and stool weight in normal subjects

	Guar	Pectin	Apple	Carrot	Cabbage	Wheat bran
Serum cholesterol	−13%	−13%	−1%	−1%	+2%	−2%
Stool weight	+20%	+19%	+40%	+59%	+67%	+127%

Data from Jenkins DJA, Reynolds D, Leeds AR *et al.* (1979) Hypocholesterolemic action of dietary fiber unrelated to fecal bulking effect. *American Journal of Clinical Nutrition* 32: 2430–2435.

produce negative balance for several elements, including calcium, iron, zinc and magnesium. It is not always clear whether the reduction in mineral absorption is caused by the fibre itself or by other substances such as oxalate or phytate which are associated with the fibre. Nevertheless, there is concern that increasing fibre intake may result in trace element deficiency in the long term. A classical example occurs in Egypt, where severe zinc and iron deficiency, leading to hypogonadism and growth retardation, has been associated with the consumption of large amounts of unleavened wholewheat bread. However, a high-fibre intake is not the only cause of this syndrome; other relevant factors include low zinc and iron intakes, pica (i.e. the consumption of soil) and the high phytate level in unleavened bread (the phytate in wholewheat flour is mostly destroyed by yeast phytase). There is no evidence that populations consuming high levels of fibre and with adequate nutrient intakes, such as North American vegetarians, have an increased incidence of any nutrient deficiency. *See* Phytic Acid, Nutritional Impact and also individual nutrients

Nevertheless, there is concern that high levels of fibre supplementation may cause mineral deficiencies, especially in susceptible populations, such as elderly women who tend to have low calcium and iron intakes and are at increased risk of osteoporosis. In general, the concern is confined to insoluble fibres such as wheat bran, at intakes of over 25 g of insoluble fibre per day (equivalent to about 70 g of wheat bran). There is no evidence that supplementation with soluble fibres such as guar or pectin has long-term effects on mineral status. It has been suggested that soluble fibres do not lead to mineral deficiencies because, unlike insoluble fibres, they are highly fermented in the colon, thus releasing the bound minerals for potential absorption. Several minerals, including calcium, zinc and magnesium, can be absorbed from the colon, and their absorption may be enhanced by the short-chain fatty acid products of fibre fermentation. *See* Osteoporosis

Alcohol and Drugs

There are not many studies of the effects of fibre on alcohol and drug absorption, but they tend to show that the viscous fibres which delay carbohydrate absorption have similar effects on drug and alcohol absorption. For most drugs, slowing absorption is unlikely to have significant therapeutic implications. However, purified viscous fibres, if taken with large amounts of alcohol, may have the potentially dangerous effect of prolonging the duration of intoxication.

Composition of Bile

Wheat bran consistently reduces the cholesterol saturation index of bile when the initial saturation index is over 1·0, i.e. the bile is supersaturated. Supersaturated bile predisposes to the precipitation of cholesterol out of solution, cholesterol being the major component of 60–80% of gallstones. The mode of action of bran is not proven, but it has been suggested that the most likely explanation is via a reduction in the circulating pool of the secondary bile acid, deoxycholic acid (DCA). DCA is formed in the colon by the bacterial dehydroxylation of cholic acid. Wheat bran may reduce the DCA content of bile by adsorbing DCA and preventing its absorption, or by inhibiting its formation, either by lowering colonic pH or by reducing transit time. Paradoxically, pectin and a diet rich in fruit and vegetable fibres increase the DCA content of bile but do not elevate the cholesterol saturation index.

Intestinal Adaptation to a High-fibre Diet

Although the number of studies in this area is limited, fibre appears to have a number of long-term effects on intestinal structure and function. Most studies have been conducted in experimental animals, where the effects may be different from those in humans as a result of the higher amounts of fibre used in the experimental diets. Adaptations of the large intestine to fibre which influence the development of cancer are dealt with in other chapters and will not be covered here in detail. *See* Colon, Cancer of the Colon

Effects of Fibre on Absorption

Small Intestinal Anatomy

Long-term feeding of pectin has been shown to alter the morphology of the small intestinal villi in rats. The villi in the proximal intestine (duodenum and jejunum), normally long and fingerlike, become shorter and more leaflike, while the villi in the distal intestine (ileum), normally short and leaflike, become longer and more fingerlike. The duodenal villous architecture of rats on long-term pectin is similar to that in healthy rural Africans, in whom the blunted villi would be classified as abnormal if seen in Western populations. One possible interpretation of these findings is that the villous architecture in any segment of the intestine responds to the rate and amount of nutrients being absorbed. On a refined, low-fibre diet, the availability of nutrients in the proximal intestine is high and the villi are long and fingerlike, giving them a maximum surface area to facilitate absorption. In the distal intestine there is very little nutrient left to be absorbed and the villi have a small surface area, being blunted and leaflike. When the rate of nutrient absorption is reduced by fibre or an unrefined diet, nutrient availability is reduced in the duodenum and jejunum and increased in the ileum; the intestinal villi respond by decreasing their surface area proximally and increasing it distally.

Large Intestinal Anatomy

Numerous studies show that dietary fibre increases the weight of the colon in experimental animals. The changes are particularly marked in the caecum and are probably related to the degree of fermentability of the fibre, since lactulose, an unabsorbed sugar, also increases caecal weight. Fermentable carbohydrate entering the caecum provides energy to colonic bacteria, which stimulates their growth, and provides energy to the host in the form of the short-chain fatty acids, acetic, propionic and butyric acids. Butyric acid is believed to be utilized by the colonic mucosa itself, whereas acetic and propionic acids are utilized by the liver and by peripheral tissues.

Fibre produces a marked increase in colonic blood flow, but it is not known if this is due to vasoactive effects of short-chain fatty acids or simply to the increase in large intestinal weight. Increased blood flow, in turn, may account for the increased flux of urea and ammonia across the caecal wall. Blood urea is freely diffusable into the colon, where it is hydrolysed by colonic bacterial urease into ammonia. Increased blood flow delivers an increased load of urea, resulting in increased production of ammonia. However, nitrogen balance across the colon is positive because some of the ammonia is utilized by colonic bacteria to synthesize

Table 4. Effect of luminal mucus (mucin units per μg of protein) in rats fed 5% guar or 5% citrus fibre diets for 4 weeks

	Control	Guar	Citrus
Stomach	43	80[a]	181[a]
Small intestine	106	182	232[a]
Colon	49	51	74

[a] Significantly different from control.
Data from Cassidy MM, Satchithanandam S, Calvert RJ et al. (1990) Quantitative and qualitative adaptations in gastrointestinal mucin with dietary fiber feeding. In: Kritchevsky D, Bonfield C and Anderson JW (eds) *Dietary Fiber: Chemistry, Physiology, and Health Effects*, pp 67–88. New York: Plenum Press.

amino acids to meet their protein requirements. Positive nitrogen balance across the colon is increased on a high-fibre diet because the increased amount of carbohydrate entering the colon provides energy for bacteria and stimulates their growth.

Intestinal Mucus Production

Long-term fibre feeding in rats increases total mucin production in the stomach and small intestine but has no significant effect in the colon (Table 4). A pure soluble fibre, guar gum, had a much smaller effect in the stomach and small intestine than citrus fibre consisting of a mixture of cellulose plus lignin, hemicellulose and pectin (1:1:1·5). However, all sources of fibre tested increased the proportion of sulphated goblet cells in the terminal ileum and the mid- and distal colon. These changes in intestinal mucus may, in part, be mechanisms by which fibre reduces the rate of absorption of nutrients and inhibits experimental colon carcinogenesis.

Bibliography

Kritchevsky D, Bonfield C and Anderson JW (eds) (1990) *Dietary Fiber: Chemistry, Physiology, and Health Effects.* New York: Plenum Press.

Spiller G (ed.) (1985) *Handbook of Dietary Fiber in Human Nutrition.* Boca Raton, Florida: CRC Press.

Royall D, Wolever TMS and Jeejeebhoy KM (1990) Clinical significance of colonic fermentation. *American Journal of Gastroenterology* 83: 1307–1312.

Thomas M. S. Wolever
University of Toronto, Toronto, Canada

Effects of Fibre on Absorption

Bran

For many years, the term 'bran' referred only to wheat bran. With the growth of interest in dietary fibre since 1970, the term is now used to describe the outer layer of any cereal grain, external to the starchy endosperm, but beneath the hull, if the grain is encased in a hull. In recent years, considerable interest has been generated in a variety of brans, most specifically wheat bran, oat bran, corn bran and rice bran.

Bran as a Component of the Cereal Grain

Because the structure of cereal grains varies from one species to another, the component which constitutes bran is obtained and described differently. For the wheat kernel, the bran layer is easily distinguishable and is separated from the endosperm by the aleurone layer. For this reason, there is little contamination of wheat bran with starch or components of the germ. For oats, however, the bran layer is not as clearly separated from the underlying kernel, and because of the high fat content of oats, separation of the bran from the rest of the grain is difficult. For this reason, oat bran composition varies considerably depending on the exact separation conditions used. *See* Wheat, Grain Structure of Wheat and Wheat-based Products; Oats; Wheat

Corn bran resembles wheat bran in relation to its separation from the rest of the grain, as does rice bran, except that more starch is removed because of the elongated shape of the rice kernel, necessitating greater removal of starch at the ends of the kernel. The same is true for barley bran, one of the most recent additions to the bran family in terms of nutritional interest. *See* Barley

Chemical Composition of Brans

The fibre content of oat bran is considerably lower than that of the other brans. This is attributable to the higher content of fat, starch and protein, a result of the difficulty in removing the bran layer. These figures can vary considerably with separation procedures and are only broad averages.

Oat bran differs from the other brans in being largely soluble nonstarch polysaccharide (NSP), while the others are mainly insoluble. This is in part attributable to the presence of a hull on the oat grain; for the other cereals, the bran is the outermost layer of the kernel, and clearly a layer which is insoluble and lignified is required to resist environmental damage in the field. The major constituent of oat bran is β-glucan, a soluble and viscous component, which is considered of great importance in the physiological effects of oat bran. The major polysaccharides in the other brans are cellulose and arabinoxylans, both of which contribute to their insolubility and resistant nature.

Physiological Effects of Bran

With the enthusiasm for research into dietary fibre in the 1970s and 1980s there is now a considerable volume of literature on the physiological effects of bran, particularly wheat bran. Numerous experiments were conducted with wheat bran in the 1970s, and it was always found to be the most effective bulking agent in human subjects. It remains the most reliable and effective natural laxative known. The extent of the effect of wheat bran on faecal weight depends on its fibre content, and also on its particle size, with larger particles having a greater effect.

When consumed, wheat bran passes largely unchanged through the entire gastrointestinal tract. The protein and starch that may be contained in it will be degraded, but the fibre is virtually unchanged, with only about 20% being fermented by the intestinal microflora resident in the human colon. Scanning electron micrographs of wheat bran that has passed through the human body show bacteria attached to the inner layer of the cells, but the cells themselves remain intact. They are therefore capable of holding water, and this property, along with the bulk of bacterial cells excreted in the stools, explains the considerable bulking effect of wheat bran. Many other materials are fermented by the intestinal microflora and do not survive to the stool, any bulking effect being limited to the growth of the bacterial population as a result of fermentation. Since corn bran and rice bran are also largely insoluble, it is assumed that they bulk in the same way. One study comparing corn bran and wheat bran has shown similar effects, but the dose was too small for statistical significance. Oat bran, with its soluble NSP, is likely to be fermented in the large intestine and, therefore, to exert a lesser effect on bulking. Again, the bulking effects of oat bran have been investigated very little.

Another area of interest has been the influence of particular sources of fibre on serum lipids. Some fibre-containing materials lower cholesterol, but wheat bran is not one of them. In numerous studies, it has not shown any effect on serum lipids. Oat bran, however, does have an effect on serum cholesterol levels, although a small number of very recent studies have found no effect. The controversy surrounding the effectiveness of oat bran in reducing serum cholesterol levels, and hence its role in heart disease prevention, has resulted in considerable confusion, both for the scientific world and the public. A major part of the problem is in the design of some of the studies and any other dietary changes that may have occurred as a result of feeding oat bran to subjects with otherwise free food choice. The weight of evidence suggests that oat bran has a modest effect in reducing serum cholesterol, owing to the presence of the soluble β-glucan within it. The mechanism of this effect is not clear, but may involve fermentation of the soluble NSP, resulting in the production of short-chain fatty acids which are absorbed and may have effects on lipid metabolism in the liver. These possibilities are being investigated by a number of laboratories. *See* Cholesterol, Role of Cholesterol in Heart Disease; Fatty Acids, Dietary Importance

Another problem with some of the studies investigating the effects of oat bran in serum lipids is that healthy individuals with normal cholesterol levels were used as subjects. The cholesterol-lowering effect of oat bran depends on the initial cholesterol levels and it may only have a substantial effect in those whose blood cholesterol is elevated.

Other brans have not been investigated to nearly the same extent as wheat and oat bran. There have been a number of animal studies on most brans, but the number of human investigations is small. The evidence to date, however, suggests that corn bran does not lower cholesterol but has a bulking effect, whereas barley bran lowers cholesterol. Early studies on rice bran suggested that it also lowered cholesterol, but more recent work disputes this.

Further to the two mechanisms given above for the effect of oat bran, a third proposed mechanism relates not to the fibre content of the bran, but to the fat component, either the polyunsaturated fatty acids themselves, or through some fat-soluble component which is absorbed and has effects on lipid metabolism in the liver. This mechanism has also been suggested for rice bran and is substantiated by Japanese studies of the 'rice bran oil' which has been shown to be effective in lowering cholesterol. The insoluble nature of the NSP in rice bran would suggest no effect on serum lipids, and the fat component theory may therefore be plausible. Considerable work still needs to be done in this area.

Negative Aspects of Brans in the Human Diet

The major concern about overconsumption of dietary fibre in the Western world has been in relation to balance of certain minerals, in particular iron, calcium and zinc. Numerous studies have shown that wheat bran significantly increases faecal calcium excretion. In most cases, this is compensated for by a decrease in urinary excretion, such that balance is maintained, but there remains a concern, particularly in specific groups, such as the elderly, that mineral status is deleteriously affected by wheat bran. *See* Calcium, Physiology; Iron, Physiology; Zinc, Physiology

One of the problems is in knowing what component in the bran is responsible for the increased faecal excretion. It is often assumed to be the fibre, but wheat bran also contains considerable amounts of phytate, which is known to bind calcium *in vitro* and *in vivo*. *See* Phytic Acid, Nutritional Impact

In order to determine more firmly what component in the bran might be responsible, studies have been carried out with dephytimized wheat and also with phytate added to control diets to equalize the phytate content. These studies have clearly shown that it is the phytate in the bran which is responsible for the effect on the minerals.

Bibliography

Anderson JW, Story L, Sieling B *et al.* (1984) Hypocholesterolaemic effects of oat-bran or bean intake for hypercholesterolaemic men. *American Journal of Clinical Nutrition* 40: 1146–1155.

Davidson MH, Dugan LD, Burns JH *et al.* (1991) The hypocholesterolemic effects of beta-glucan in oatmeal and oat bran. *Journal of the American Medical Association* 265(14): 1823–1829.

Findlay JM, Smith AN, Mitchell WD *et al.* (1974) Effects of unprocessed bran on colon function in normal subjects and in diverticular disease. *Lancet* i: 146–149.

Kritchevsky C *et al.* (eds) (1990) *Dietary Fiber – Chemistry, Physiology and Health Effects.* New York: Plenum Press.

Leeds A and Avenell A (eds) (1985) *Dietary Fibre Perspectives: Reviews and Bibliography.* London: John Libbey.

Sandstron B, Kivisto B and Cederblad A (1987) Zinc absorption in humans from meals based on rye, barley, oatmeal, triticale and whole wheat. *Journal of Nutrition* 117: 1898–1902.

Simpson KM, Morris ER and Cook JD (1981) The inhibitory effect of bran on iron absorption in man. *American Journal of Clinical Nutrition* 34:1469–1478.

Vahouny G and Kritchevsky D (eds) (1986) *Dietary Fiber: Basic and Clinical Aspects.* New York: Plenum Press.

Vorster HH, Lotter AP and Odendall I (1986) Effects of an oat fibre table and wheat bran in healthy volunteers. *South African Medical Journal* 69: 435–438.

Alison Stephens
University of Saskatchewan, Saskatoon, Canada

Fibre and Disease Prevention

The impetus behind the front of research into dietary fibre (nonstarch polysaccharides) over the past 20 years has been the suggestion that many medical conditions common in Western countries might be prevented by a simple dietary change increasing fibre intake. The diseases cited as being affected by the dietary fibre content of diets range from those associated with the physiological function of the upper gastrointestinal tract, such as obesity, diabetes and heart disease, to several disorders of the large bowel. Analysis and definition of dietary fibre has been a stumbling block in many studies. Nonstarch polysaccharide (NSP) is a defined and measurable index of the main structural components of the plant cell wall and is used in this section. Despite well-documented physiological effects of NSP throughout the gastrointestinal tract, overall evidence for a protective role is most compelling for disorders of the large bowel. *See* Diseases, Diseases of Affluence

Obesity

Documented short-term effects of NSP in enhancing early satiety suggest that NSP would prevent overconsumption of food, and hence assist in the maintenance of energy balance. For example, in controlled trials, satiety is delayed when food with the NSP removed, such as apple juice, is fed compared with fresh apples. In controlled trials, supplements of NSP, as tablets or as special foods, have also consistently resulted in a decrease in weight. However, studies of individuals consuming high- and low-NSP diets when free-living give inconsistent results. This may be because high-NSP diets are characteristically more bulky and low in fat, so that it is difficult to ascribe any effect on appetite directly to NSP. UK Department of Health recommendations published in 1991 were unable to make specific proposals concerning the amount of NSP in ordinary diets that would be effective in reducing appetite and hence controlling the development of obesity. Despite the popularity of high-NSP diets, there are no controlled studies of their efficacy when compared with other regimens. *See* Obesity, Treatment

Non-Insulin-Dependent Diabetes Mellitus (NIDDM)

Gel-forming NSPs have been shown to lower blood glucose and insulin in both healthy and diabetic volunteers, and foods containing NSP often have a low glycaemic index. This may be due to a number of factors, including starch availability in high-fibre foods, and short-chain fatty acid production. However, other factors influence glycaemic index, and over a broad range of foods there is no correlation with NSP content. In general, weight reduction that may be brought about by a reduced-fat diet containing NSP is more important in the control of NIDDM than NSP *per se*. On the available evidence, authors of recent panel reports have been unable to find sufficient justification for increasing levels of NSP in order to lessen the risk of NIDDM.

Ischaemic Heart Disease (IHD)

It is now well established that soluble forms of NSP, such as β-glucan in oat bran, pectin and gum, lower serum cholesterol, particularly LDL (low-density lipoprotein) cholesterol. In controlled feeding trials, 60–100 g oat bran per day, for example, lowers LDL cholesterol by 8–23%. This effect may be brought about by decreased absorption of bile acids and cholesterol, or by enhanced LDL receptor activity, and LDL catabolism. The short-chain fatty acid, propionic acid, may also inhibit 3-hydroxy-3-methylglutaryl (HMG) CoA reductase, leading to a reduction in cholesterol synthesis. Insoluble NSPs, such as bran and cellulose, do not affect serum cholesterol.

In five prospective studies, there is some evidence that individuals consuming less fibre are at enhanced risk for IHD, although the relationships with soluble (vegetable) NSP and cereal (insoluble) NSP have not been consistently measured. Recent recommendations for Dietary Reference Values acknowledge that an increase in NSP from all dietary sources may lower LDL cholesterol and, hence, might assist in the prevention of IHD. However, NSP is not the major factor in IHD prevention.

The Large Intestine

NSPs have been shown to exert a profound effect on large bowel function, via fermentation, short-chain fatty acid production, decreased transit time and increased stool weight. There is a linear relation between NSP intake and daily stool weight in experimental studies of healthy people, stool weight increasing by 5 g per g of NSP consumed on an average basis. On an individual basis, there is considerable variation in the response of bowel habit to NSP intakes, partly because not all sources of NSP increase stool weight to the same extent. In general, NSPs found in wheat are more effective than the NSPs found in fruit and vegetables. The response to NSP is also moderated by factors affecting large bowel function, e.g. transit time, hormones and lifestyle factors. *See* Colon, Diseases and Disorders

The effect of NSP on bowel habit is probably not unique, and other sources of carbohydrate, such as starch, reaching the large bowel, are able to stimulate fermentation. Nevertheless, NSPs are generally the most effective. Recent guidelines published by the World Health Organization (WHO) and the UK Department of Health recommend a population average of 18 g of NSP per day, in order to achieve a stool weight of around 150 g per day. Present levels of 12 g of NSP intake in the UK, for example, are related to average stool weight of only 100 g per day, which is associated with increased risks of several bowel diseases discussed below. Evidence relating NSP to other diseases such as appendicitis and varicose veins is weak.

Constipation

Constipation impairs the quality of life of about 20% of people aged over 65 years and around 10% of the adult population. It is commoner in women. Constipation is characterized by infrequent bowel habit (less than three times a week), transit time of five days or more and stool weight below 50 g per day, although in healthy volunteers complaints of constipation became common when stool weights fell below 100 g per day. In the UK, less than 18% of the population pass less than 50 g stools per day, and less than 46% pass less than 100 g per day.

It is generally agreed that NSP, particularly in its insoluble form, is useful in the treatment and prevention of constipation. Although some pathological forms of constipation may not respond, in otherwise healthy individuals, it can be predicted that an increase of NSP intake to 18 g per day would reduce by half the proportion of adult individuals within the UK with stool weights of less than 100 g per day. UK recommendations stipulate that these levels, average of 18 g, range 12–24 g, should be achieved from a variety of foods whose constituents contain NSP as a naturally integrated component, and not from supplements.

Diverticular Disease

The frequency of diverticular disease is thought to have increased over the past 30 years in Western countries. Although rare before the age of 30 years, it is found in about 33% of people over the age of 60. Constipation may be a symptom, and low stool weight is associated with increased risk. Geographical comparisons suggest that it is more common in areas of the UK where fibre intake is low. It is less common in vegetarians, whose stool output and NSP intake is greater. *See* Inflammatory Bowel Disease

Major reviews have concluded that the primary treatment of diverticular disease is with diets high in NSP. All trials have shown that NSP relieves constipation and, in all but one trial, other symptoms, such as pain, were reduced. When measured, intracolonic pressures were reduced as a result of NSP supplementation.

Evidence that NSP may be important in the prevention of diverticular disease is circumstantial. Rats fed high cereal fibre intakes over their lifetime developed smaller diverticula, and at a later age, than rats fed a low-fibre diet. In humans, there is some evidence from case control studies of a protective effect of fibre-containing food. NSP may prevent the development of diverticular disease, but there has been little epidemio-

logical testing of the hypothesis. Populations at low risk, such as Japanese, Africans and Maoris, have not been shown to consume more NSP than Western populations. It is possible that high intakes of starch are equally protective.

Irritable Bowel Syndrome (IBS)

Irritable bowel syndrome comprises a variety of disorders of gastrointestinal function. It is thought to be a result of an inappropriate response to normal amounts of intestinal gas and luminal irritants, and it may be aggravated by lifestyle stresses. Symptoms can include abdominal pain, diarrhoea, or constipation, frequently accompanied by depression or anxiety. Food intolerance, acquired or inherited disorders of motility, and psychological disorders, have been suggested as causes. Little work has been done to examine the diets of patients with this syndrome, but in one study there were no differences between patients and controls for intake of total cereal fibre or fruit fibre. Vegetable fibre intake, however, was significantly lower in patients. Clinical trials of NSP supplementation in patients have partly shown benefits in its treatment, although no improvements in symptoms have been reported in half of the trials conducted so far. This may be the result of classifying a variety of disorders with no known cause into a single condition, and to the fact that most trials have shown a marked placebo response. Present evidence suggests that patients with IBS who are most likely to benefit from an increased intake of dietary fibre (as wheat bran) are those whose chief complaint is constipation.

Gallstones

In Western societies, gallstones are twice as common in women as in men, and they increase in prevalence with age. They occur more frequently in obese people and multiparous women. Obesity, diabetes and hypertriglyceridaemia are conditions which have been associated with gallstones. They are rare in rural African societies, but there have been few epidemiological studies related to diet. Case control studies are suggestive of a protective effect of NSP from vegetables.

Gallstones can be produced in hamsters, mice, rabbits, prairie dogs or monkeys, by using semipurified diets. In the hamster, the diet loses its stone-forming effect if it is supplemented with lignin, lactulose or bulking agents. In rabbits fed ordinary chow, stones dissolve rapidly. In humans, supplements of bran, lactulose, gum, pectin and oats have shown that deoxycholic levels and, hence, lithogenicity can be reduced, possibly by inhibiting bacterial secondary bile acid

Table 1. Regional studies of fibre intake and colorectal cancer

Area	Item	Correlation (r)	Probability (P)
Finland, Denmark	NSP	−0·78	0·05
Sweden	Fibre	−0·70	0·001
UK	NSP	−0·72	0·05

Table 2. Case control studies of dietary fibre (30 studies, 1969–1989)

	Number of studies	Reduced risk	Enhanced risk	No effect
Fibre	22	11	2	9
Vegetables	19	12	1	6
Cereals	13	3	3	7
Starch	2	1	0	1

(deoxycholate) formation by a reduction in caecal pH, or by hastening transit. Constipation is also associated with high deoxycholate levels in bile. *See* Gall Bladder

In general, there is suggestive evidence that NSP may be a protective factor in the development of gallstones. However, intervention with bran supplements to prevent their recurrence has not been successful.

Large Bowel Cancer

In 1960, Higginson and Oettle were among the first to document differences in colorectal cancer incidence amongst different groups in South Africa, and to attribute the low rates in the Bantu to the fact that 'in the Bantu a large amount of roughage is consumed and constipation in the Western sense is rare'. In 1969, Burkitt suggested a mechanism for the protective action of dietary fibre, stating that 'with regard to bowel tumours ... with the Western diet, the greatly delayed transit time (most of the delay occurring in the distal colon), together with the concentration associated with diminished stool bulk, might enhance the action of any carcinogen by the multiple of these factors'. *See* Colon, Cancer of the Colon

Since that time, attempts have been made to study the epidemiology of NSP intake and colorectal cancer. Worldwide, intakes of indicators of dietary fibre tend to be higher in countries at low risk of colorectal cancer. Although this inverse association is substantially reduced on controlling for meat and fat consumption, three studies within defined Western areas, where meat and fat consumption is high, also suggest that NSP intakes are lowest in areas where cancer occurrence is highest (Table 1). However, anomalies have been reported; for example, age-standardized colorectal cancer rates of the Maoris in New Zealand are approximately half those of New Zealand whites, yet intakes of dietary fibre are virtually the same. In South Africa, different racial groups are also at very different risks of bowel cancer, yet recent reports suggest that fibre intakes in these groups are also very similar. These anomalies support the suggestion that starch may be as important as NSP in protecting against colorectal cancer.

Thirty case control studies have been carried out in Europe, Australasia, North and South America, and Africa, over the past 20 years. Values for 'fibre' were derived from various indices of 'fibre-rich' foods, crude fibre, or dietary fibre using the British food tables. Several of these studies were very small-scale and tended to yield nonsignificant results. Table 2 summarizes these studies and shows that, where it has been measured, fibre has tended to be associated with a reduction in risk. For example, 11 out of 22 studies have shown that cases reported lower 'fibre' intakes than controls, and in only two studies had they reported eating more. In nine studies, there were no significant differences.

Much of this apparent protective effect of fibre is accounted for by the fact that in 12 out of 19 studies, cases reported eating smaller amounts of vegetables than controls. In the 13 studies in which cereal consumption was reported, risk was reduced by cereal consumption in three, but risk was increased in three other studies. However, in the largest study of 818 cases in Belgium, starch, fibre, and vegetable consumption were all protective factors, with relative risks for colorectal cancer being reduced to 0·71, 0·37, 0·82 and 0·67, respectively, for the highest levels of cooked vegetable, raw vegetable, starch and fibre consumption. Peas and beans were associated with increased risk. These findings of an apparent protective effect of NSP in colorectal cancer require confirmation with well-controlled prospective studies. To date, one study of this type in US nurses has not demonstrated a reduction in colorectal cancer risk in individuals with higher NSP intake.

The effect of purified sources of dietary fibre on chemically initiated colorectal cancer has been investigated in a large number of studies over the past decade. In these studies, the numbers of tumours induced by the administered carcinogen whilst the animals are fed on 'control' diets are compared with those found in animals fed on the same diets with fibre supplements. Although at first sight these types of experiments are easily standardized, comparisons between different studies are complicated by differences in age, sex, strain and type of animal used, the chemical carcinogen used and its route of administration, the timing of carcinogen dosage (whether before or during fibre supplementation) and

Fibre and Disease Prevention

Table 3. Effect of fibre on protection against chemical carcinogens

Type of fibre	Number of studies	Protective against carcinogenesis	No effect on carcinogenesis	Enhanced carcinogenesis
Wheat bran	17	13	3	1
Cellulose	9	6	3	0
Pectin	7	1	3	3

the levels of dosage. These animal models are highly susceptible to nutritional factors, such as the level of fat and energy in the control and experimental diets, and the type of fat used. Both increased levels of fat and energy are promoters of colon carcinogenesis, as are the ω6 polyunsaturated fatty acids. Further experimental variables are the level of fibre fed in the experimental diet and the level of fibre in the control diet. Some studies have been carried out with chow as the control, and others use a 'fibre-free' diet.

The overall findings of experimental studies were collated by the Federation of American Societies for Experimental Biology (FASEB) in 1987. Table 3 shows a summary of these studies for wheat bran, cellulose and pectin. In general, bran appears to have a consistently protective effect against chemical carcinogenesis. Bran decreased the number of tumours in 13 out of 17 studies, and increased the number of tumours compared with control levels in only one study. Cellulose also appeared to be protective in six of nine studies, with no significant difference in three. In three of seven studies, pectin apparently enhanced carcinogenesis, possibly as a result of the variety of experimental variables in these studies. No consensus was possible for the gums, guar gum and carrageenan.

The mechanism behind the effect of bran in reducing chemically induced tumour incidence is likely to vary with different carcinogens used. In humans, some support for the hypothesis that dilution and reduced transit time is important comes from studies in which faecal mutagenicity has been consistently reduced by bran supplementation.

Bibliography

Bingham S (1990) Evidence relating NSP and starch to protection against large bowel cancer. *Proceedings of the Nutrition Society* 49: 153–171.
British Nutrition Foundation Task Force (1990) *Complex Carbohydrates in Foods*. London: Chapman and Hall.
Dietary Reference Values for Food Energy and Nutrients for the United Kingdom (1991) Report for COMA, Department of Health. London: Her Majesty's Stationery Office.
Pilch S (ed.) (1987) *Physiological Effects and Health Consequences of Dietary Fiber*. Federation of American Societies for Experimental Biology. Washington, DC: US Food and Drug Administration.
World Health Organization (1990) *Diet, nutrition and the prevention of chronic disease. WHO Technical Report Series* 797.

S. A. Bingham
MRC Dunn Nutrition Unit, Cambridge, UK

DIETARY GOALS

See Community Nutrition and National Nutrition Policies

DIETARY REFERENCE VALUES

Assessment of Requirements

Although a sufficient supply of food is an essential prerequisite for life and health, quantification of the amounts of food necessary for individuals or groups of individuals has only been attempted in the last 100 years. Originally, ignorance of the chemical composition of food and of the nature of the micronutrients and their physiological roles limited such calculations to quantities of foodstuffs. Over the last century, knowledge of food composition and of nutritional physiology and biochemistry, although still incomplete, has enabled at least some assessment of people's needs for all known nutrients.

For most nutrients these assessments of needs have been imprecise for a number of reasons. First, there is usually no single universally agreed measure, and often many different ones, of physiological adequacy. Although absence of essential nutrients from the diet results in a syndrome characteristic of the particular deficiency, it is less easy to define clinical, physiological or biochemical parameters which reflect an integrated measure of body status for a particular nutrient. Indeed, there is no prima-facie reason to suppose that such an integrated measure actually exists. Second, it is clear that requirements for any nutrient vary, both within and between individuals. However, the magnitude of that variation, and its relationship with other factors, such as intakes of other nutrients, gender and body size, are often unclear. Consequently, it is extremely difficult to predict an individual's requirement for a nutrient with any degree of accuracy.

In spite of these uncertainties, assessments have been used in a number of ways. The US authorities tabulated in 1941 the amounts of food energy and nutrients which were deemed to be sufficient for the population of the USA. Adequacy at that time usually meant the avoidance of deficiency. Since then the sophistication of the tabulations has increased. For example, the 1991 UK Dietary Reference Values (DRVs; Department of Health, 1991) provide an estimate of the range of requirements for energy and most nutrients, together with an assessment of 'desirable' intakes of fats and carbohydrates. Over the years, most nations have used assessments of requirements to make tabulations under various titles:

1. *Recommended Nutrient Intakes* (RNIs) are usually said to be derived from estimates of individual physiological requirements plus an added safety margin, of variable size, to take account of the range of individual variation (Department of Health, 1991).

2. *Recommended Daily Intakes* (RDIs) are the amounts sufficient, or more than sufficient, for the nutritional needs of practically all healthy persons in a population (Department of Health and Social Security, 1969).

3. *Recommended Dietary Allowances* (RDAs) are the levels of intake of essential nutrients that, on the basis of scientific knowledge, are judged by the US Food and Nutrition Board to be adequate to meet the known nutrient needs of practically all healthy persons (National Research Council, 1989).

4. *Recommended Daily Amounts* (RDAs) are the average amounts of nutrients which should be provided per head in a group of people if the needs of practically all members of the group are to be met (Department of Health and Social Security, 1979).

5. *Estimated Safe and Adequate Daily Dietary Intakes* (ESADDIs) form a category of safe and adequate intakes for which data are sufficient to estimate a range of requirements but insufficient to develop Recommended Dietary Allowances (National Research Council, 1989).

Most tabulations, however, have set a single figure for each nutrient around the upper end of the range of requirements. Unfortunately, the uncertainties surrounding the estimates of adequacy and different interpretations of what is desirable, often varying with sociocultural factors as much as scientific data, have led to wide disparities in the figures which belie the general agreement on the data from which the figures are derived. The amount of each nutrient that anyone requires for health can, in theory at least, be measured, but in practice accurate quantification is almost impossible and considerable judgement is required. Nutritional health can also be defined in different ways. Nevertheless, the evidence demonstrates that requirements for many, if not all, of the nutrients differ somewhat with age, sex, size, physical activity and physiological state (e.g. menstruation, pregnancy or lactation). They also depend to some extent on nutrient interactions. If all these factors are taken into account the requirements of apparently similar individuals can easily differ twofold. *See* Food Composition Tables and also individual nutrients

Basis of DRVs

Figure 1 represents an idealized distribution of requirements for a nutrient within a homogeneous population

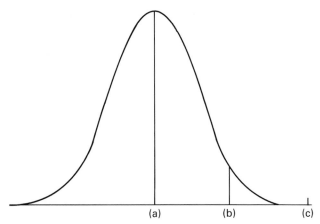

Fig. 1 Representation of the distribution of nutrient requirements, with three possible recommended intakes that might be based on it: (a) at the mean requirement; (b) at the mean plus 2 sd; (c) at the mean plus 4 sd.

and indicates four levels on which recommendations might be based. Recommendation (a) is the same as the average requirement. Recommendations of this kind are usually confined to energy and should differ between countries only in so far as some populations are physically larger or more active than others. Widely different recommendations have nevertheless been made.

In 1969 in the UK the RDIs were defined as the amounts sufficient, or more than sufficient, for the nutritional needs of practically all healthy persons in a population. This is usually equated with the mean requirement plus two standard deviations, or point (b) in Fig. 1. Theoretically, the residual 2·5% of the population represents a substantial number of people so that a safety margin is often added. Such margins are variable in their size and application, and if every other uncertainty in the evidence is a reason for adding a further safety margin, recommendations may well be made that are higher than any possible needs, at point (c) (Fig. 1). Some of these higher values, such as those of the USA, may be hard to meet, even in developed countries. This is not to say that recommendations and reference values should necessarily be lower in developing countries, but it demonstrates the importance of non-nutritional factors in determining what the reference value is intended to achieve. Consequently, the usual lack of any guidance as to the objectives or target audience of the tabulations has led to considerable confusion regarding their purposes and use.

International Differences

There are more similarities than differences between the reference values of different countries, although it is the differences that are often given more prominence. This is because a majority of the countries producing reference values opt to use either the RDAs of the USA which, for the reasons of differing definitions already given, tend to be on the high side, or the recommendations of the Food and Agriculture Organization (FAO) and World Health Organization (WHO) which, being designed mainly for Third World countries, tend to be among the lowest values. Most of the more obvious international differences occur for the following reasons:

1. There are different definitions and different uses of reference values.
2. Populations are subdivided in different ways by age, sex and physiological groups. In the UK there are 17 age and sex groups, including pregnant and lactating women, whereas in Japan there are 58 age and sex groups.
3. Different criteria of nutritional adequacy can be used for many nutrients.
4. Reference values, being country-specific, have to take account of the different foods available and preferred in each country, as well as the local socioeconomic culture.

The UK is unique in having separated the scientific discussion of *requirements* from the more political element of *recommendations*. In most countries, it is not clear to whom the 'recommended' amounts of nutrients are addressed.

As there are imprecise data and much uncertainty concerning many nutrients, the setting of *recommendations* based on the scientific data inevitably requires the exercise of judgements. For example, in assessing vitamin C requirements the major dilemma surrounds the 'desirable' level of tissue saturation. The USA now recommends 60 mg per day for men in order to maintain adequate reserves as well as to prevent scurvy. In the UK the RNI is now 40 mg per day, but in the past the UK, Canada and FAO/WHO, among others, have recommended only 30 mg per day on the basis only of preventing deficiency. Other countries have had other values, as shown in Table 1. For vitamin D the uncertainty surrounds estimates of exposure to sunlight; for calcium the area of uncertainty is the possible adaptation to low intakes; for folate it is the biological activity of various conjugated forms in foods; for iron it is the very considerable variation in the menstrual blood losses among women, and in absorption between different individuals and from different diets.

Determination of Reference Values

Requirements for a nutrient differ from one individual to another and may change with alterations in the composition and nature of the diet as a whole, because

Table 1. The recommended intakes of vitamin C for young men in selected countries[a]

Country	Recommended intake (mg per day)
Argentina, Uruguay, Venezuela	30
Bolivia, Colombia	40
Spain	45
Mexico	50
The Philippines, Portugal	75
UK	30
GDR	45
USA	60[b]
FRG	75
Bulgaria	95

[a] From International Union of Nutrition Sciences (1983).
[b] 75 mg in 1941; 60 mg in 1989. From reports from the (US) National Research Council, National Academy of Sciences, Washington, DC.

such alterations may affect the efficiency with which nutrients are absorbed and/or utilized. Classically, the requirement of an individual for a nutrient has been the amount of that nutrient required to prevent clinical signs of deficiency. While this must always be an important element in defining a requirement, it can be argued that societies should expect more than the basic need to avoid deficiency, and that some allowance should be made, where appropriate for a degree of storage of the nutrient to allow for periods of low intake or high demand without detriment to health. Claims have also been made that very high levels of intake of some nutrients have especially beneficial or therapeutic effects but these effects have not fallen within the definition of requirement. However, in future, better data relating to any such effects may allow useful quantification.

The information from which estimates of requirements have been made can be categorized as follows:

1. The intakes of a nutrient needed to maintain a given circulating level or degree of enzyme saturation or tissue concentration.
2. The intakes of a nutrient – by individuals and by groups – which are associated with the absence of any signs of deficiency diseases.
3. The intakes of a nutrient needed to maintain balance – noting that the period over which such balance needs to be measured differs for different nutrients, and between individuals.
4. The intakes of a nutrient needed to cure clinical signs of deficiency.
5. The intakes of a nutrient associated with an appropriate biological marker of nutritional adequacy.

No single criterion can define requirements for all nutrients. Some nutrients may have a variety of physio-

logical effects at different levels of intake. Which of these effects should form the parameter of adequacy is therefore to some extent arbitrary. When setting reference values the particular parameter or parameters which were used to define adequacy for each nutrient must be given. None of these criteria is perfect. In some cases the evidence on which they are based is reliable experimental data; in others it is from associations, often epidemiological, and in others evidence may be limited to anecdotal data of variable persuasiveness. *See* Dietary Surveys, Measurement of Food Intake; Dietary Surveys, Surveys of National Food Intake; Dietary Surveys, Surveys of Food Intakes in Groups and Individuals

There are inherent errors in some of the data, e.g. in individuals' reports of their food intake, and the day-to-day variation in nutrient intakes also complicates interpretation. Even given complete accuracy of a dietary record, its relation to habitual intake remains uncertain, however long the recording period. The food composition tables normally used to determine nutrient intake from dietary records contain a number of assumptions and imperfections. Furthermore, there is uncertainty about the relevance of many biological markers, such as serum concentrations of a nutrient, as evidence of an individual's 'status' for that nutrient. Thus uncertainties relating to the appropriate parameter by which to assess the requirement, to the completeness of the database for any nutrient, and to the precision and accuracy of dietary intake data lead to the need to make judgements.

Equally, when nutrient intakes are measured there is demonstrable interindividual variation, which is not necessarily related to the variation in requirements. Whatever parameter is used, the risk of deficiency in an individual at a given intake within the distribution of requirements will vary from virtually zero to virtually 100%. It should be recognized that the time course of the relationship between intake and status varies between different nutrients. For example, daily energy intakes should approximate daily requirements, while assessment of intakes of some micronutrients must be integrated over days, weeks, or even longer periods. Furthermore, not only may nutrients have effects on health at the time they are eaten, but also there is growing evidence that diet may be one of the factors in early, even intrauterine life which has an influence on later health in adult life. Arguably such factors should be taken into account in deriving reference values but the qualitative nature of much of the data is not helpful to deriving precisely quantified recommendations.

Many countries update their reference values at regular 5- or 10-year intervals. It is therefore not helpful to give current values for the 40 or so countries and organizations which have set them, especially as there are so many and varied age and sex groups. A committee of the International Union of Nutrition Sciences (IUNS) reviewed the reference values for all age and sex groups in all countries in 1983. Since then many countries have carried out routine reviews of their reference values, and others have started to set their own. The most recent values for each country can be obtained by contacting the official body responsible for their formulation, using the addresses in the 1983 IUNS report. The most up-to-date national reviews, however, are those of the USA and the UK. The current knowledge of the requirements for all nutrients can be obtained from these reports, along with the most recent philosophy underlying the definitions of the US RDAs and the UK DRVs.

The term 'Dietary Reference Value' covers the following:

1. Estimated Average Requirement (EAR). Of a group of people, about half will usually need more than the EAR for energy, protein, vitamin or mineral, and half will need less.
2. Lower Reference Nutrient Intake (LRNI) is an amount of the nutrient that is enough for only a few people in a group who have low requirements.
3. Reference Nutrient Intake (RNI) is an amount of the nutrient that is enough, or more than enough, for about 97% of the people in a group. If average intake in a group is at the RNI, then risk of deficiency in the group is small (cf. RDI, p 000).
4. Safe Intake is a term used to indicate intake, or a range of intakes, of a nutrient for which there is not enough information to estimate RNI, EAR or LRNI. It is an amount that is enough for almost everyone but not so large as to cause undesirable effects.

The current UK DRVs are unique in that they cover macronutrients other than protein, i.e. total fat, saturated fatty acids, unsaturated fatty acids, polyunsaturated fatty acids (including $n-3$ and $n-6$), *trans* fatty acids, total carbohydrate, nonmilk extrinsic sugars, intrinsic and milk sugars, and starch and nonstarch polysaccharides. Apart from the essential fatty acids, there is no absolute requirement for any of these nutrients in isolation, but an attempt was made to derive useful figures, as a proportion of energy, for specified purposes as pragmatic judgements based on an assessment of desirable intakes within the sociocultural context in the UK.

Purpose and Use of Reference Values

Reference values have been taken up by economists, food manufacturers, sociologists, politicians, journalists and others for a variety of uses. There have been at least five different purposes underlying their derivation, discussed below.

For Assessing Food Intake of Groups or Individuals

Any reference value provides a yardstick against which the diets of different sections of a community can be measured. In nutrition surveys, the single reference value has often been used as the cut-off point between inadequate and adequate group average intakes. The values can also be used by dietitians for assessing the diets of individual patients, but the diagnosis of deficiency must always rest with clinical, biochemical or physiological measurements. Reference values can only aid the assessment of risk of deficiency. *See* Dietetics

For Planning Individual Diets, or Meals in Institutions

Reference values provide a guide for dietitians prescribing diets for individuals. Use of recommendations at the upper end of the range of requirements minimizes risk of deficiency in any group of individuals. Caterers in hospitals (for patients not on special diets) and housekeepers in long-stay homes, boarding schools, colleges and other institutions usually work from menu cycles that are often passed from one person or place to another, with modifications from time to time. Reference values have sometimes been used in calculating the nutritional standards for school meals. The 1975 British standards for the school lunch were based on 33% of the recommended intake for energy and 42% (half-way between 33% and 50%) of the recommended protein intake.

For Planning and Assessing National Food Supplies

Reference values can provide a basis for setting targets in planning food supplies and policies for a nation. They are used by international agencies for assessing the adequacy of the diet in different underdeveloped countries, which helps to determine their relative need for aid. Thus reference values provide common ground between economists and nutritionists. The recommended intakes are an objective basis for calculating rations for use in time of food shortage, although in famine the definition of 'adequacy' may need revision.

As the Denominator for Nutrition Labelling

In nutrition labelling, the major components in an amount of food, usually a standard serving, need to be compared with a standard. In the USA, where nutritional labelling is more advanced than in other countries, the labelling standards laid down by the Food and Drug Administration are based on the US RDAs for particular age and sex groups. For adults the highest values for males have been used in the past, although currently proposals for reference figures based on the weighted national average age and sex distribution of the US population are in development. Commonly, the amount of nutrient in a standard serving is expressed as a percentage of the reference value. One serving (30 g) of a breakfast cereal, for example, may be seen to contribute 28% of the recommended intake of thiamin and 36% of the riboflavin recommendation. *See* Legislation, Labelling Legislation

Nutrient Density Index to Express the Nutritional Quality of Foods

The 1983 IUNS report suggested the use of reference values to determine a nutritional index of the quality of foods. Nutrient density (the ratio of a food's content of a nutrient to its energy content) is a useful concept for nutrition education and for trying to compare the nutritional quality of food. When the ratio of a nutrient content to the energy content of a food is the same as the respective recommended intakes, the density index of the food for that particular nutrient is said to be 1. The index can differ with age and physiological state. For men aged 18–35 years, the Australian recommendation for vitamin C is 30 mg and for energy 11·6 MJ (2700 kcal); a food containing 11 mg of ascorbic acid per 1000 kcal (4·2 MJ) therefore has a nutrient density index of 1. If a food contains more ascorbic acid per unit energy, then it is, as it were, a net contributor of vitamin C to the diet. Foods rich in sugar and fats, and alcoholic beverages tend to have nutrient density indices less than 1, and therefore contribute proportionately more energy than nutrients to the diet. The same concept can be used to evaluate new types of manufactured foods and the enrichment of foods with synthetic nutrients. In this way formulated foods that cannot be easily compared with a conventional food can be prepared so that, per serving, the major nutrients are obtained in about the same ratio to energy as in the reference values.

Limitations of Reference Values

There are many limitations to the use of any set of reference values. Most recommendations are only for nutrients as eaten after food processing and cooking. They are for healthy people and do not allow for illnesses. They are more than enough for almost everybody and are therefore too high to be sensitive criteria for inadequate food intake. The UK DRVs uniquely provide a guide to the *range* of requirements in a population.

Most nutrients do not have to be eaten every day or even every week, so that a low measured intake may be balanced by eating more later. Reference values do not indicate at what higher level toxic effects might arise. They make assumptions about a certain nutritive quality, biological value, or availability in the body (which is usually stated somewhere in the text of the report) and assume that enough of other major nutrients and energy are consumed. They are for standard body sizes (e.g. weight) and range of usual exercise (usually stated somewhere in the report).

Reference values may not cover minor vitamins and trace elements; assuming that if the intake of the main nutrients is adequate and the diet is mixed, intake of the minor nutrients will automatically be adequate. They cannot fully allow for adaptation that can occur to high or low intake of some nutrients, e.g. energy, iron and calcium. Apart from the current UK DRVs, other reference values only tell us about some 15% of the energy intake – protein plus essential fatty acids – and not how the rest of the dietary energy should be distributed between different carbohydrates and fats (and alcohol). They do not allow for interactions between nutrients and may be affected by a variety of drugs.

Nevertheless, reference values provide a valuable yardstick for the purposes specified in most reports. Their use or misuse for purposes other than those for which they have been derived is fraught with danger. *See* Bioavailability of Nutrients

Bibliography

Department of Health (1991) *Dietary Reference Values for Food Energy and Nutrients for the United Kingdom*. Report on Health and Social Subjects 41. London: Her Majesty's Stationery Office (HMSO).

Department of Health and Social Security (1969) *Recommended Intakes of Nutrients for the United Kingdom*. Report on Public Health and Medical Subjects 120. London: HMSO.

Department of Health and Social Security (1979) *Recommended Daily Amounts of Food Energy and Nutrients for Groups of People in the United Kingdom*. Report on Health and Social Subjects 15. London: HMSO.

International Union of Nutrition Sciences (1983) Recommended dietary intakes around the world. *Nutrition Abstracts and Reviews* 53: 939–1015: 1075–1119.

National Research Council (1989) *Recommended Dietary Allowances* 10th edn. Washington, DC: National Academy Press.

Trichopoulou A (ed.) (1990) Recommended dietary intakes in the EEC: scientific evidence and public health considerations. *European Journal of Clinical Nutrition* 44(Supplement 2): 1–125.

WHO (1985) Energy and protein requirements: report of a joint FAO/WHO/UNU meeting. *World Health Organization Technical Report Series* 724.

Robert W. Wenlock and Martin J. Wiseman
Department of Health, London, UK

DIETARY REQUIREMENTS OF ADULTS

In this article adults will be considered to be healthy males and females between the ages of 18 and 55 years of age. Dietary requirements will be considered to be the recommended amount of nutrients that must be ingested to meet the nutritional needs of these individuals. The data on which requirements are established, and the approach used in interpreting these data will be reviewed.

Determination of Requirements

The data on which nutrient requirements are based are derived from a variety of sources.

Analysis of the Nutrient Content of the Reported Food Intake of Apparently Healthy People

This information is derived primarily from large-scale surveys of population groups, supplemented by data from studies of smaller, more homogeneous population groups. If nutritional status data are available for respondents for any nutrients, it is possible to relate certain intake levels with the presence or absence of any evidence of a nutrient deficiency. Where only dietary data are available, it is assumed that if the participants are in good health the usual intake is sufficient to at least maintain health with no clinical evidence of a deficiency. *See* Dietary Surveys, Measurement of Food Intake

Experimental Repletion–Depletion Studies

A limited number of healthy subjects are fed a diet deficient in a specific nutrient under carefully controlled conditions until biochemical or physical symptoms of a deficiency become evident. At that point graded amounts of the missing nutrient are added to the diet to determine the amount necessary to alleviate the symptoms and restore normal metabolic functioning – an amount that is considered the minimum requirement. In the past, such studies have provided information on the needs for thiamine, riboflavin, nicotinic acid, vitamin B_6, vitamin E and folate. In most countries, current regulations regarding the protection of human subjects preclude the use of a diet that will induce even marginal deficiency symptoms. Thus investigators can obtain comparable data only by identifying people who have self-selected a diet that has caused deficiencies, and monitoring their recovery on graded amounts of the nutrient.

Balance Studies

These studies, which are expensive and demand a high degree of cooperation from the subjects, involve feeding a diet of known composition of a particular nutrient to a small group of subjects under very controlled conditions and collecting and analysing all nutrient losses from the body for periods of time ranging from 4 to 28 days. This includes losses in the urine and faeces and, in the case of some nutrients, losses in perspiration, menstrual flow, semen, hair, skin and nails. The amount fed is reduced until the subjects are in negative balance, i.e. loss of nutrients exceeds intake, indicating that the amount fed is insufficient to meet needs. The requirement for the nutrient is the smallest amount, above that which resulted in a negative balance, that results in either a balance between intake and excretion (i.e. there is neither a gain nor a loss of the nutrient) or a positive balance, which indicates that the amount in the body is increasing, representing either growth or an increase in body stores. In an alternative balance approach, the slope of the line relating balance at various dietary intakes is used to predict the level at which subjects will be at zero balance, i.e. intake equals need. Balance data have been used to assess dietary needs for protein, calcium, zinc, copper and selenium.

Use of Stable Isotopes

By feeding a known amount of a nutrient labelled with a stable isotope, and following (1) its retention in body tissues, (2) the extent to which it dilutes unlabelled nutrients in the same samples, and (3) its excretion from the body, it is possible to make estimates of the amount of nutrient required to meet metabolic needs.

Factorial Method

The amount of the nutrient needed for growth, for maintenance of body stores, and for replacement of losses in the skin, urine and faeces, are each estimated separately. They are then added together to estimate the minimum requirement, which is then increased to account for any inefficiencies in the absorption of the nutrient from food. This amount is considered the dietary requirement.

Extrapolation from Animal Studies

Much valuable information on nutrient needs can be obtained from data from experimental animal studies if sufficient consideration is given to differences in metabolism between the animal species and the human.

Establishing Standards

In most countries, estimates of nutrient requirements are made by a group of scientists knowledgeable about the metabolic nutrient needs of population groups and individuals. Before beginning their task it is customary for them to establish a philosophy to guide their interpretation of the diet. Most countries have set nutrient recommendations at a level which will protect the health of essentially all persons. As a result the values are generous for a large segment of the population and minimal for a small but important number of people. These standards do not include allowances for any possible pharmacological action of nutrients used in non-physiological amounts. Until recently, such committees of scientists were concerned only with standards that reflected the desired intake of essential nutrients. Countries such as Canada have now set standards that combine our information on the minimum intakes of essential nutrients with the growing body of information suggesting that diet plays an important role in the course and prevention of chronic diseases such as coronary heart disease, cancer, hypertension and osteoporosis. In several cases this involves establishing upper limits of intake of nutrients such as lipid, cholesterol and sodium. *See* Cancer, Diet in Cancer Prevention; Hypertension, Physiology; Osteoporosis; Sodium, Physiology

For most nutrients, committees have attempted, via one of the previously discussed methods, to identify the average requirement for a specific age- and sex-group, and the standard deviation (SD) of that requirement (assumed to be 15% of the mean observed for most biological parameters when no more precise information was available). By increasing the mean requirement by two standard deviations to set the recommended dietary intake, they assumed that these levels of intake would be sufficiently high to meet the needs of 97·5% of that population. When data on which to make judgements about specific age-groups were lacking, the values were extrapolated from values for other age-groups, taking into account body size, energy expenditure, protein intake or any other physical or dietary measure to which the need for the nutrient is related. In cases where the recommended intake is set at the mean + 2SD, the average requirement for the group will be $(100/130) \times 100$, or 77% of the recommended intake. Thus, if the average intake of a population group is 77% of the recommendation, assuming that intakes are also normally distributed, at least 25% and up to 50% of the group will have an intake adequate to meet their needs. If the average intake equals the recommended intake then the needs of a substantially higher proportion of the population will be met.

For some minerals for which the SD is quite large and for which there is no evidence of a deficiency, committees have been reluctant to add 2SD to the mean values since to do so would increase the recommended intake to a level that could not be provided by the diet and would necessitate the use of supplements. Assessing precise dietary requirements of many mineral elements is more difficult because of the extent to which many other dietary components and other mineral elements influence the bioavailability of mineral elements. *See* Bioavailability of Nutrients

For several vitamins, as our abilities to measure the amount in both food and body tissues with greater sensitivity, and to identify the bioavailability of the nutrient in various food sources have been enhanced, there has been a decline in the amounts recommended with each revision of the allowances. This is illustrated in changes in recommendations for zinc over time. Another point of discussion in setting requirements has been the question of the appropriate size of the body pool of nutrients such as vitamins A and C. Most investigators agree that it is not necessary to saturate tissues and body storage sites but rather to set the intake at a level that will provide a reserve of the nutrient to last for a period of 2 to 3 months on a marginal intake or under other metabolic stress. For vitamin A this has been set by most committees at 20 μg per g of liver, and for vitamin C 600–900 mg. There appears to be no evidence of any health advantage in maintaining a pool any greater than this. Moreover, for several nutrients, such as vitamins A and D, there is concern that the recommended level not be set so high that there would be a danger of toxicity in individuals who had a very low threshold for the nutrient. The bioavailability of the nutrient from the dietary food sources has a marked effect on the amount that must be provided in order for the body to 'net' adequate amounts. Other dietary components, such as phytates in cereals, tannins in tea and coffee, caffeine, oxalates in vegetables, and other substances that either inhibit or facilitate the absorption or retention of a nutrient, or any metabolic phenomena that influence the retention and excretion of a nutrient, add to our difficulty in recommending intakes and assessing the adequacy of observed intakes. *See* Ascorbic Acid, Physiology; Cholecalciferol, Physiology; Retinol, Physiology

Recommendations

The recommended intakes for adult men and women age 19, 35 and 55 suggested by the Food and Agriculture Organization and the World Health Organization (FAO/WHO), by Australia, Canada and the USA are given in Table 1. These ages were selected as representative of the varying age groupings used in these standards. The standards given by WHO/FAO are described

Table 1. Recommended Dietary Allowances (RDAs) from the WHO, USA, Canada and Australia

Nutrient	Age 19 years								Age 42 years								Age 55 years							
	WHO[a]		USA[b]		Canada[c]		Australia[d]		WHO		USA		Canada		Australia		WHO		USA		Canada		Australia	
	M	F	M	F	M	F	M	F	M	F	M	F	M	F	M	F	M	F	M	F	M	F	M	F
Energy (kcal)	2870	2550	2900	2200	3000	2100	2800	2000	2700	2500	2900	2200	2700	1900	2470	1850	2700	2500	2300	1900	2300	1800	2100	1520
Protein (g)	53	45	58	46	61	50	70	58	53	45	63	50	64	51	70	58	53	45	63	50	63	54	70	58
Calcium (mg)	500–600	500–600	1200	1200	800	700	400–800	400–800	400–500	400–500	800	800	800	700	400–800	400–800	400–500	400–500	800	800	800	800	400–800	400–800
Phosphorus (mg)			1200	1200	1000	850					800	800	1000	850					800	800	1000	850		
Iron (mg)	5–9	14–28	10	15	9	13	10	12–16		14–28	10	15	9	13	10	12–16		14–28	10	10	9	8	10	10
Zinc (mg)			15	12	12	9	12–16	12–16			15	12	12	12	12–16	12–16			15	12	12	9	12–16	12–16
Iodine (μg)	150	150	150	150	160	160	150	120	150	150	150	150	160	160	150	120	150	150	150	150	160	160	150	120
Copper (mg)			1·5–3·0	1·5–3·0							1·5–3·0	1·5–3·0							1·5–3·0	1·5–3·0				
Vit C (mg)	30	30	60	60	40	30	30	30	30	30	60	60	40	30	30	30	30	30	60	60	40	30	30	30
Vit A (μg RE)	600	500	1000	800	1000	800	750	750	600	500	1000	800	1000	800	750	750	600	500	1000	800	1000	800	750	750
Vit D (μg)	2·5	2·5	10	10	2·5	2·5			2·5	2·5	5	5	2·5	2·5			2·5	2·5	5	5	5	5		
Vit E (mg)			10	8	10	7					10	8	9	6					10	8	7	6		
Vit K (μg)			70	60							80	65							80	65				
Thiamin (mg)	1·2	1·2	1·5	1·1	1·2	0·8	1·1	0·8	1·2	0·9	1·5	1·1	1·1	0·8	1·0	0·8	1·2	0·9	1·2	1·0	0·9	0·8	1·0	0·8
Riboflavin (mg)	1·8	1·8	1·8	1·3	1·5	1·1	1·4	1·0	1·8	1·3	1·7	1·3	1·4	1·0	1·2	1·0	1·8	1·3	1·4	1·2	1·2	1·0	1·2	1·0
Nicotinic acid (mg)	20·3	20·3	20	15	22	15	18	13	19·8	14·5	19	15	19	14	16	12	19·8	14·5	15	13	16	14	14	10
Pyridoxine (mg)			2·0	1·6			1·3–1·9	0·9–1·4			2·0	1·6			1·3–1·9	0·9–1·4			2·0	1·6			1·3–1·9	0·9–1·4
Folate (μg)	200	200	200	180	210	180	220	200	200	200	200	180	230	185	220	200	200	200	200	180	230	195	200	200
Vit B12 (μg)	2·0	2·0	2·0	2·0	1·0	1·0	1·0	1·0	2·0	2·0	2·0	2·0	1·0	1·0	1·0	1·0	2·0	2·0	2·0	2·0	1·0	1·0	2·0	2·0

[a] FAO/WHO (1985) *Energy and Protein Requirements* TRS no. 724; (1962) *Calcium Requirements* TRS no. 230; FAO (1988) *Requirements of Vitamin A, Iron, Folate and Vitamin B12*. FAO Food and Nutrition Series No. 23.
[b] National Research Council (1989).
[c] Health and Welfare, Canada (1990).
[d] National Health and Medical Research Council (1984) *Dietary Allowances for use in Australia*. Canberra: National Health and Medical Research Council.
RE, retinol equivalents; M, male; F, female.

as 'practical' nutrient recommendations, which can be met by people in most of the developed and developing countries. The standards given by Australia, Canada and the USA are described as standards that will meet the needs of essentially all healthy people in the population. For some nutrients the figures are essentially the same in all standards, while for others, such as calcium, they vary up to threefold, reflecting variations in the interpretation of existing data by the 'experts' in each country. The availability of the nutrient in the country's food supply may also influence the final decision. In all cases those setting recommended levels point out that the need for nutrients directly involved in energy metabolism – thiamin, riboflavin, nicotinic acid and pantothenic acid – increase as energy expenditure increases. *See* Energy, Energy Expenditure and Energy Balance; Dietary Reference Values

Environmental and Physiological Influences

While dietary requirements for most healthy people are adequately met by recommended intakes, there are environmental and dietary factors which predispose an individual to enhanced need which may amount to a 10–40% increase over those of most people. For example, the need for ascorbic acid is higher among smokers than among nonsmokers; vitamin E requirements increase as the amount of polyunsaturated fat in the diet and exposure to free radicals in the environment increase; vitamin B_6 needs are higher among users of oral contraceptives; zinc requirements of endurance athletes are enhanced; iron needs are elevated at high altitudes; thiamin and nicotinic acid requirements increase as the use of alcohol increases. Stress is generally believed to result in slightly elevated requirements for several nutrients but there is little data on which to base recommendations. In most cases, however, there is a sufficient margin of safety in current standards that there is little danger of a deficiency if the nutrient is consumed at the recommended level.

There is currently very little data on which to base requirements of people over 50 years of age. As the population ages it becomes increasingly heterogeneous in regard to nutritional requirements, as a result of a complex interaction of genetic influences, state of health throughout life, environmental and health stresses, and physical fitness. At the same time that the need for some nutrients declines as a result of decreased energy expenditure, the decline in metabolic efficiency and poorer nutrient absorption suggest that intakes should be increased. The two influences may well counterbalance each other. *See* Elderly, Nutritional Status

Both pregnancy and lactation result in increased nutrient requirements. In pregnancy, for almost all nutrients, this occurs during the second and third trimester with increments varying from one nutrient to another but ranging from 10–15% for energy to 100% for folate. As a result, pregnant women must make careful and nutritious food selections to meet the added requirements within a very limited increase in energy. During early lactation, when breast milk is the sole source of nourishment for a rapidly developing infant, it is expected that the mother's needs will be met by increased dietary intake and from reserves established during pregnancy. *See* Lactation

As our knowledge of metabolism, of the interaction of the nutrients both during ingestion and in metabolism, and of the factors affecting bioavailability of nutrients from food sources and in specific dietary patterns increases, as a result of enhanced sensitivity in our analytical techniques and as molecular biologists shed light on the role of nutrients at the cellular level, it is anticipated that we will be able to set dietary requirements with an ever increasing degree of confidence. It is important, however, to keep in mind that our dietary requirements must relate to the needs of the total human rather than to the needs of the smallest cellular component.

Bibliography

Buss DH (1986) Variations in recommended nutrient intakes. *Proceedings of the Nutrition Society* 45(3): 345–350.

Food and Nutrition Board (1986) Recommended dietary allowances: scientific issues and process for the future. *Journal of Nutrition* 116(3): 482–488.

Harper AE (1987) Evolution of recommended dietary allowances – new directions? *Annual Review of Nutrition* 7: 509–537.

Harper AE (1990) Standards and dietary guidelines. In: (M. Browne ed.) *Present Knowledge of Nutrition* 6th edn, pp 491–501. Washington DC: International Life Sciences Institute, Nutrition Foundation.

Health and Welfare, Canada (1990) *Nutrition Recommendations*. The Report of the Scientific Review Committee, Ottawa, Canada.

Horwitt MK (1986) Interpretations of requirements for thiamin, riboflavin, niacin-tryptophan, and vitamin E plus comments on balance studies and vitamin B_6. *American Journal of Clinical Nutrition* 44(6): 973–985.

Murray TK and Beare-Rogers JL (1990) Nutrition recommendations, 1990. *Journal of the Canadian Dietetic Association* 51: 391–395.

National Research Council (1989) *Recommended Dietary Allowances* 10th edn. Washington DC: National Academy Press.

Olson JA (1986) Recommended nutrient intakes: guidelines for the prevention of deficiency or prescription for total health. *Journal of Nutrition* 116(8): 1581–1584.

Truswell AS (1987) Evolution of dietary recommendations, goals and guidelines. *American Journal of Clinical Nutrition* 45: 1060–1072.

Helen A. Guthrie
The Pennsylvania State University, Pennsylvania, USA

DIETARY SURVEYS

Contents

Measurement of Food Intake
Surveys of National Food Intake
Surveys of Food Intakes in Groups and Individuals

Measurement of Food Intake

Measuring food consumption is a complex and difficult task. There are many reasons for carrying out this task, including the following: to determine the level of adequacy of food and nutrient available to an entire country or to a selected group of individuals; to establish levels of food self-sufficiency in the development of agricultural policy; to examine the relationship between diet and health in groups or individuals; as part of fundamental research on nutrient metabolism. It is fair to say that there is *no* method available which provides an entirely accurate measure of food consumption or nutrient intake, at whatever level the measurement is being made. It is impossible at the national or regional level to make a complete measurement of all food production, and to take into account all food and production losses and wastage; at the household level, people alter their purchasing or food use habits while being observed; at the individual level, people change their eating habits during a survey, or fail to give an accurate description ot their eating habits. Awareness of the likely sources of error, however, allows for sensible interpretation of results from studies of dietary assessment.

The type of measurement made, whether at national, regional, household or individual level, will be dictated by the purpose of the study being undertaken. This article outlines the points in the food chain at which measurements of food consumption can usefully be made, and highlights the strengths and weaknesses of the techniques available. It also considers the validity and reliability of these techniques when trying to relate diet and disease. Recent publications that review methods for measuring food consumption include Bingham (1987), and Cameron and Van Staveren (1988). Interpretation of dietary assessments in epidemiological studies is discussed by Margetts and Nelson (1991). *See* Dietary Reference Values

Methodology

Figure 1 shows the points in the food chain at which food consumption is commonly measured. Point I is at the level of domestic food production. In virtually all countries, a Department or Ministry of Agriculture requires food producers to report the amount of food produced. This information is useful in establishing

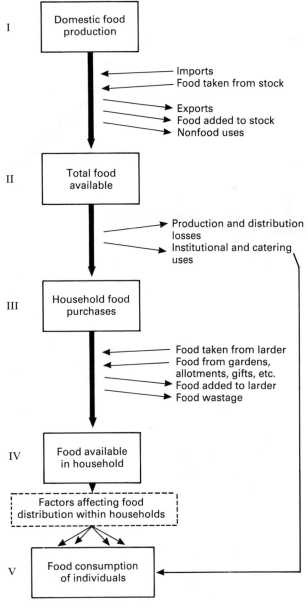

Fig. 1 Measuring food consumption.

Table 1. Main applications of the different dietary survey methods for measuring food consumption or nutrient intake in human populations

Application	Food balance sheets	Household surveys (with or without larder inventories)	Surveys of individuals					
			Prospective			Retrospective		
			Duplicate diet	Weighed inventory	Household measures	Diet history	24-h Recall	Questionnaires
National	+ + +	+ + +	−/+(C)	+	+	+	+	+
Regional	−	+ + +	−/+(C)	+	+	+	+	+
Institution or group	−	+ + +	+	+ +	+ +	+ +	+ +	+ +
Household	−	−/+(L)	+	+ +	+ +	+ +	+ +	+ +
Individual	−	−/+(D)	+ + +	+ + +	+ + +	+ + +	−/+ +(R)	+ +
Epidemiological studies	+ +	+ +	+	+ +	+ +	+ +	+	+ + +
Clinical studies	−	−	+ +	+ +	+	+	−/+ +(R)	+
Metabolic studies	−	−	+ + +	+	−	−	−	−

(C) Composite diet technique; (D) may be used if estimates of the distribution of foods and nutrients to groups of similar individuals within groups of households are known; (L) indicates the need for larger inventory; (R) indicates the need for repeat measures.

levels of food self-sufficiency, but cannot be used alone to estimate the average consumption in the population.

Measurements at point II are used by the Food and Agricultural Organization (FAO) to establish food balance sheets. These measurements reflect domestic production, plus food imports and food taken from stocks, minus food exports, food moved into stocks, and food used for animal feed or nonfood purposes (e.g. sugar used in the brewing industry). They can be used to show the average amount of food available per person in the population.

The next point of measurement (III) is often the household. Typically, the weights and costs (or imputed value) of all food acquisitions (purchases, gifts, food from gardens and allotments, payments in kind, etc.) are recorded over a set period, usually one week. In addition, an inventory of the larder contents may be carried out at the beginning and end of the survey period in order to determine changes in food stocks, and allowances made for estimated food wastage, to yield an estimate of the amount of food available for consumption in the household (point IV). Alternatively, respondents may be interviewed and asked to recall their purchases and food use over the previous week, usually having been forewarned and asked to keep receipts and other informal records of food use and acquisition. Household surveys do not usually include records of food purchased and eaten away from home, nor of household members' consumption of items not directly under the purview of the respondent, such as alcoholic beverages, sweets and soft drinks.

The final point of measurement (point V) is at the level of the individual. Briefly, there are two approaches, prospective and retrospective. Prospective methods include the following: the *duplicate diet*, in which an individual collects, for chemical analysis, an exact duplicate or fixed aliquot of all food and drink actually consumed (the aliquot technique is also suitable for households or institutions); the *composite diet* technique, in which representative local foods are combined into a single sample in proportion to the foods consumed (assessed using other techniques) – the sample is then analysed chemically for its nutrient content; the *weighed inventory*, in which the subject records and weighs all food and drink consumed; and *household measures*, in which the subject keeps a record of what is eaten and drunk, recording amounts in units of common household measures such as cups, spoons, bowls, etc. The period of recording for weighed inventory and household measures surveys will depend on the reliability with which individual food or nutrient intakes need to be assessed. Retrospective methods include the following: the *diet history*, in which the subject is asked by a trained interviewer about usual consumption habits in an extended interview lasting 1–2 h; *24-h recall*, in which a trained interviewer asks quantitatively about consumption of food and drink over the previous 24 h; and *questionnaires*, completed either by the respondent or with the help of an interviewer, which ask about the usual frequency and quantity of consumption of a wide range of food and drink, or which focus on the consumption of a limited range of items to estimate the intake of a specific nutrient.

Table 1 summarizes the principal applications of these different techniques. Food balance sheets are appropriate for estimating national consumption levels, and are therefore of use in epidemiological studies comparing diets between countries. They cannot be used for assessing consumption at regional, household or individual level. Household surveys lend themselves to a wide variety of uses. If, for example, a nationally representative sample of households is used, then it will be possible to estimate consumption levels nationally as well as in regional, socioeconomic, and other subgroups within the population. Some household surveys include larder inventories at the beginning and end of the survey period, which allow estimates of consumption at the level of single households. Techniques are available to estimate the distribution of food and nutrient to individuals of similar age and sex within groups of households, and household surveys may therefore have application in some epidemiological surveys where a knowledge of the *pattern* of consumption to individuals, but not individual intakes *per se*, is required.

Duplicate diet techniques are most suitable for metabolic studies of individuals, where a precise knowledge of nutrient intake is required. The composite diet technique is particularly suitable for estimating the nutrient content of foods eaten by a group of people where food composition tables are likely to be inadequate. The weighed inventory is again very suitable for assessment of individual food consumption or nutrient intake (using food composition tables), and thus lends itself to a wide variety of uses, in that accurate estimates of dietary intake for groups of people can be built up from individual data. Where a limited range of foods of accurately known composition is being consumed, the weighed inventory may also be used in metabolic studies. Because the household measures technique, like the weighed inventory, focuses on the individual as the unit of assessment, it can also be used in a wide variety of studies, but with some loss of precision in comparison with weighed inventories.

The retrospective techniques, because they rely on memory, are regarded as being less objective than the prospective techniques, but they may free the respondent of factors likely to distort the recording of diet (see Table 2). The diet history, in particular, may be used to assess the 'usual' diet of an individual more effectively than other techniques, in that seasonal variations in diet can be taken into account more readily. A single 24-h recall from one individual cannot be used to assess that individual's diet because of day-to-day variations in intake. Single 24-h recalls collected from a large number of subjects, however, may be useful for estimating the intake of a group. Repeat 24-h recalls collected from an individual may provide a more accurate assessment of that individual's diet. Questionnaires are of particular value in epidemiological studies, in that they can provide information economically from a large number of subjects.

Strengths and Weaknesses

Table 2 summarizes the main strengths of the methods available.

When conducting a survey of diet, it is important to ensure that the technique chosen is sufficiently robust to enable the original hypothesis to be tested adequately. It is likely that many studies which fail to show a relationship between diet and disease do so not because no relationship exists, but because the inaccuracies of the techniques used to assess diet were too great. It is equally important to realize that if the aim of a study is to relate diet and health in groups of people, e.g. by comparing diet and health status between countries or regions, then there is little point in spending resources on expensive and labour-intensive surveys which characterize the diets of individuals.

It must be decided at the outset whether measurements of food consumption, or nutrient intake, or both, are required. The reliability (standard error) of the measurements will determine the number of subjects and the number of measurements per subject required, or the number of regions or countries to be included in a regression analysis. If ranking of subjects or groups will suffice, then a technique which has a systematic bias or non-differential misclassification may be acceptable, but if absolute measures of consumption or intake are required then techniques with greater validity will be needed. Most prospective methods (apart from duplicate or composite diet techniques) and all retrospective methods rely on food consumption tables for estimating nutrient intake, and the weaknesses associated with their use should be considered.

The time of year (summer or winter, wet season or dry season, holy days, festival days), the time of week (weekdays or weekends), even the time of day (interview responses may differ before and after meals) and the period of interest (present or past consumption) will all affect the measurements made and the representativeness of the findings.

In studies of individuals, the skills which are needed to complete satisfactory records of diet differ between techniques and between subjects. For example, very young or very old subjects may be unable to recall diet accurately; people without literacy and numeracy skills will be unable to keep adequate records.

Food Balance Sheets

Food balance sheets are eminently suitable for comparing diets between countries, and are readily available, thereby reducing the cost of such studies. They do, however, show significant bias, in that the estimated availability of foods and nutrients may be considerably greater than the actual levels of consumption; in the UK, for example, food balance sheet estimates of energy intake are 25% greater than the estimated energy requirement in the population. More important, this bias is probably not constant between countries, and

Table 2. Main attributes of the different dietary survey methods for measuring food consumption or nutrient intake in human populations

Type of Survey	Strengths	Weaknesses
Food balance sheets	Determine national food consumption Compare diets between countries	National only Overestimation Bias with affluence
Household surveys	National, regional, or group data Useful where individual data hard to obtain Time trends	Home food only No meals away, sweets, soft drinks, alcohol No individual data
Without larder inventory	Lower respondent burden	Bias, especially with affluence Food acquisition, not consumption
With larder inventory	Consumption data	Distorts food purchasing pattern Higher respondent burden
Prospective surveys of individuals	Current diet Direct observation of diet Vary duration of survey according to needs	Labour-intensive Requires literacy and numeracy skills High motivation needed Distortion and/or omission owing to 'health' issues, body size, poor recording
Duplicate diet	Direct analysis of nutrient content of diet (no food tables needed)	Very expensive Intensive supervision required
Weighed inventory	Widely used; facilitates comparisons between studies or groups	Dependent upon food tables
Household measures	No scales needed	Loss of precision
Retrospective surveys of individuals	Inexpensive Quick Low subject motivation needed Good cooperation Current or past diet	Bias: memory, conceptualization, interviewer Daily variation not usually assessed Depends on regular eating habits
Diet history	Assesses 'usual' diet	Tends to overestimate nutrient intake
24-h Recall	Very quick Repeat observations to obtain daily variation	Tends to underestimate nutrient intake Does not reflect individual intake unless repeated
Questionnaires	Suitable for very large number of subjects Can be posted Focus on particular nutrients	Requires validation Literacy and numeracy skills needed if self-completed

more affluent countries are more likely to overestimate consumption than poorer countries. This may be attributable in part to more efficient recording of food production in affluent countries, and in part to the presence of smallholdings and subsistence farms where production is underrecorded in poorer countries.

Household Surveys

Household surveys of nationally representative samples are regularly conducted by many governments. The results provide a ready-made data base for analysis of food trends across time, and between regions or subgroups within the population. Where it is difficult to obtain individual data (such as in cultures where families eat communally from large serving vessels), then household surveys may provide a valuable way of characterizing diet.

Their principal disadvantage is that foods eaten away from home are rarely recorded. These usually include a high proportion of sweets, soft drinks, alcoholic beverages, and snack foods. In addition, individual intakes cannot be estimated, which may be a particular disadvantage in epidemiological studies where it is important to relate disease outcome in individuals to diet. *See* Epidemiology

Some household surveys are conducted without a larder inventory so as to reduce the respondent burden. The assumption is that over a sufficient number of households (say 20), the differences within individual households between purchases and actual consumption will balance out, giving an overall estimate of consumption close to the true level. In practice, it has been observed that surveys of food purchases in developed countries tend, on average, to stimulate purchasing in excess of actual consumption by as much as 15%. This bias is greater in lower-income than upper-income households, and as lower-income-group consumption levels are generally lower, comparisons of the food purchases or estimated nutrient intakes are likely to underestimate the true differences between income groups. Comparison of food or nutrient *profiles* (percentage of income spent on certain foodstuffs, or nutrient intakes per MJ) may be more reliable. This problem is less pronounced in surveys where the variety of food purchases is limited (as in many developing countries), or where purchases are reported retrospectively rather than recorded prospectively. Reported household food purchases may also include consumption by individual household members of foods eaten outside the home, but are more likely to be subject to errors of omission.

Household surveys conducted with larder inventories give a more precise estimate of levels of food consumption and nutrient intake, but they tend to distort usual purchasing patterns when respondents' attention may be drawn to the larder contents. They also have a higher respondent burden.

Prospective Surveys of Individuals

Prospective surveys of individuals have the advantage of direct observation of current diet. They can be varied in duration to improve the accuracy of classification of individuals' nutrient intakes, i.e. the greater the number of days of information recorded, the more likely it is to reflect the true intake of the individual. Thus carbohydrate intake may be estimated within a few days, whereas energy intake may require a week, and fatty acid intake 2 weeks. Where a large number of days is needed, problems of respondent fatigue can be overcome by having a series of shorter periods (e.g. four 4-day periods).

The principal disadvantage of prospective techniques is the level of literacy and numeracy skills required to complete the surveys. This can be overcome to some extent by having an interviewer do the recording and measuring, but this is very invasive for the subject and expensive in terms of staff time. Prospective methods may also encourage distortion of diet and avoidance of foods regarded as unhealthy, particularly sweets and alcoholic beverages, or there may be a simple omission of items owing to poor recording techniques. A particular problem that has come to light with the advent of the doubly labelled water method for estimating energy expenditure is that overweight subjects are more likely to underrecord their intake than normal weight subjects. *See* Energy, Energy Expenditure and Energy Balance

The duplicate diet technique is appropriate almost exclusively for metabolic studies, as it is very expensive and time-consuming. Its use in free-living populations requires exceptionally close supervision to ensure that complete samples are collected. It has been used in epidemiological studies where a single day's duplicate has been collected from a number of subjects in order to characterize the group diet rather than individual diets. The composite diet technique is easier to use for assessing group diet characteristics by chemical analysis, but has the disadvantage of relying on food records or recall.

The weighed inventory has been very widely used, and for this reason there are many values in the literature, against which new data can be compared. It is less demanding of both respondent and interviewer than the duplicate diet technique, but because it relies on food consumption tables there is a loss of precision in estimating nutrient intake. The household measures technique is useful where subjects are unused to using scales, or where resources are limited, and it requires a lower level of numeracy than the weighed inventory, but there is a loss of validity owing to variation in portion sizes not reflected in the descriptions. *See* Food Composition Tables

Retrospective Surveys of Individuals

In comparison with prospective techniques, retrospective techniques are relatively inexpensive, demanding less time of both respondent and interviewer. They therefore tend to have slightly higher cooperation rates. For foods which are consumed only occasionally (e.g. liver) or about which there may be some stigma (e.g. sweets or alcoholic beverages), and for assessing the intake of nutrients (such as carotene or vitamin B_{12}) which would require many days of recording, there are advantages in using retrospective techniques which ask about the usual frequency of consumption of foods. Retrospective techniques also have the unique advantage of allowing assessment of past diet, although in practice this is most likely to relate to diet over the previous month or, exceptionally, over the past year. Most recalls of diet in the distant past (2 or more years prior to the interview) correlate as strongly with current diet as with the past diet assessed at the time.

Results from retrospective methods, in common with those from prospective methods, are subject to differential misclassification, but for different reasons. Memory and conceptualization skills (the ability to describe quantitatively what was actually eaten) differ in an unsystematic way between individuals. The very young (under 12) and the very old (over 70) are less likely to be able to recall their diets correctly. The number of food items recalled has been shown to correlate with the estimated energy intake, independent of the true level of intake. Apart from the use of repeat 24-h recalls, retrospective methods provide little information on day-to-day variation in diet, which can be useful in determining the likely accuracy of ranking of individuals according to nutrient intake. For the diet history and questionnaires in particular, subjects who do not have regular eating habits will have difficulty in describing 'usual' frequency of consumption or portion size.

The diet history is especially valuable for assessing 'usual' diet, but the nature of the interview may encourage over-reporting, and results from the diet history assessments usually exceed those from weighed inventories, which in normal-weight individuals are probably a good reflection of 'usual' intake. The 24-h recall is very quick, demanding little of respondents' time, but cannot be used to characterize individuals' diets unless repeated over a number of days. In general, because of the absence of a 'training effect', respondents are likely to omit items, and estimates of nutrient intake using 24-h recalls therefore tend to be low in comparison with other techniques (whether prospective or retrospective). Questionnaires are suitable for very large numbers of subjects, partly because their administration can be more readily standardized than other types of dietary assessment, and partly because, for hypotheses relating to specific foods or nutrients, they can be of limited length pertaining to relatively few foods. They can thus have the advantage of brevity while still able to rank subjects with a known degree of validity. Because of the uncertainty regarding the successful completion and validity of assessment of newly designed questionnaires, it is essential that they are properly evaluated against a dietary survey method in which the errors of assessment can be estimated. If they are to be self-completed (e.g. if they are posted to subjects), then literacy and numeracy skills will be needed.

Use of Computers

Computers are used universally to calculate the nutrient content of diets for which no direct chemical analysis is made, but they can also be used directly in the dietary assessment of individuals. Data entry programmes such as UNIDAP (Unilever) have been tailored to allow interviewers to enter patterned food consumption data, thus effectively providing the facility for an interactive diet history. Branching interactive programmes allow for 24-h recall data to be entered directly at interview, and more structured questionnaires have also been devised for interactive use. A technique for combining data entry via a hand-held computer linked to digital electronic weighing scales with an RS232 serial port allows weighed inventory data to be recorded without the need for manual coding of a written record and subsequent computer entry. Scales have also been linked to computers with special keypads bearing symbols instead of letters (FRED and FREDA), allowing respondents to use pictures to indicate the food being consumed; again, weights and codes are recorded automatically. A tape recorder has also been linked to

scales (PETRA), allowing subjects to describe foods orally rather than in writing, a weight being recorded automatically on the tape in association with each item described.

Use of Biological Markers

Given the errors that are inherent in any reporting of diet, there is a need to find objective measures which reflect usual food consumption or nutrient intake. Biochemical measurements of nutrients or related metabolites in blood or urine have long been used to identify nutrient deficiencies or irregularities, but markers of diet which span the whole range of intake are rare. Moreover, collection and storage of appropriate sample material may be a problem in itself (e.g. ensuring completeness of collection of 24-h urine samples). For a fuller discussion of the use of biological markers, readers are referred to Margetts and Nelson (1991).

Bibliography

Bingham SA (1987) The dietary assessment of individuals: methods, accuracy, new techniques and recommendations. *Nutrition Abstracts and Reviews* 57: 705–742.

Cameron ME and Van Staveren WA (1988) *Manual on Methodology for Food Consumption Surveys.* Oxford: Oxford University Press.

Margetts B and Nelson M (1991) *Design Concepts in Nutritional Epidemiology.* Oxford: Oxford University Press.

Nelson M, Dyson PA and Paul AA (1985) Family food purchases and home food consumption: comparison of nutrient contents. *British Journal of Nutrition* 54: 373–387.

Nelson M, Morris JA, Black AE and Cole TJ (1989) Between- and within-subject variation in nutrient intake from infancy to old age: estimating the number of days required to rank dietary intakes with desired precision. *American Journal of Clinical Nutrition* 50: 155–167.

M. Nelson
King's College, London, UK

Surveys of National Food Intake

National surveys of food intake, by definition, should have one important element in common. They are intended to portray the eating practices, and usually the nutrient intake, of the population as a whole and often of defined subgroups or strata of the population. Beyond that, surveys may show substantial differences in purpose and design. Some, such as the US National Health and Nutrition Examination Survey (NHANES), are designed to collect health measures as well as dietary data and are commonly identified as 'nutrition surveys'. Others, such as the US Nationwide Food Consumption Survey (NFCS), also discussed below, are concerned with food use and nutrient intakes without attempt to describe or assess nutritional status. Inevitably, in the design and implementation of a national survey, there must be trade-offs between what is desirable and what is feasible to examine. There are few generic descriptors of national surveys. Each is relatively unique, designed to meet specified individual goals.

Purpose and Design

Unlike the special purpose surveys discussed in the next article, national surveys are seldom undertaken to accomplish only a single goal because they are too expensive. Two US survey series are described to illustrate relationships between purpose and design. The fundamental purposes of the NFCS series of surveys has been 'to measure (i) the food and nutrient content of the diet and the money value of food used by US households and (ii) the nutrient intakes at home and away from home of individuals' (National Research Council, 1984). The data collected are used for many purposes including the following: (1) to assess apparent adequacy of the food supply (and consumption patterns) and to monitor this over time; (2) to identify, and localize in sociodemographic terms, food-related problems; (3) to provide benchmark national data for use as a comparison for smaller, special-purpose surveys; (4) to support analyses related to agricultural production and economic demand as well as socioeconomic analyses of food consumption and factors affecting it; (5) to provide an intake distribution data base for use in food safety considerations (potential exposure) and food additive regulation; (6) to provide background information needed for design of food guides and other educational materials; (7) to monitor the need for food-related consumer programmes managed by the US Department of Agriculture (USDA) and other agencies. In addition, the data sets generated are used by industry in the design and marketing of food products and the time trend data (collected across sequential surveys) are used in studies attempting to link changes in (national) health profiles with changes in food consumption.

The goal of NHANES was stated as follows: 'to develop information on the total prevalence of a disease condition or physical state; to provide descriptive or normative information; and to provide information on the interrelationships of health and nutrition variables within population groups'. To this should be added 'to measure the health and nutritional status of the US population and specific subgroups and to monitor changes in health and nutritional status over time'. Many of the actual uses of NHANES data overlap described uses of NFCS data, yet the two are very different in fundamental purpose and design. The NFCS is basically a food survey with much associated household economic and sociodemographic information; the

NHANES is fundamentally a health survey with associated dietary information. Because of the presence of dietary, biochemical and clinical data at the level of individuals, in the NHANES data sets, it finds use in many epidemiological studies. Perhaps because the NHANES survey is seen as serving the needs of other users, whereas the primary user of the NFCS is the USDA itself, the NHANES data sets have been released in formats that facilitate use by others and find application in many epidemiological and other analyses conducted across the USA. While summary reports of the NFCS are widely used, actual secondary use of the data sets is probably more restricted. Both surveys now find extensive use in nutrition monitoring activities at the federal level in the USA.

The specified goals of the NHANES and the NFCS heavily influence their design and implementation, so heavily that it was deemed very undesirable, it not impossible, to attempt to combine them (National Research Council, 1984). The NFCS started as a household survey and collected extensive information about the household. The NHANES started as a health examination and focused on the individual, collecting much less sociodemographic information. More important, logistical considerations demand that the NHANES, with its clinical component, be designed in a manner that permitted the establishment and relocation of a physical facility (actually achieved with trailer units). A stratified multistage probability cluster sampling design was adopted. By comparison, the NFCS is much less demanding in terms of physical facilities; data are collected by interviews and records in the home. The design adopted is a stratified probability sample. Both surveys are intended to provide estimates (after application of appropriate weighting factors) that are representative of the non-institutionalized US population (contiguous states) or for subgroups of that population (differing between the two surveys).

Both surveys are designed to sample broad geographic regions and time (season). As might be expected, this is easier to accomplish with the FNCS than the NHANES. While seasonal differences in nutrient intake, but not specific food use, are now small in North America, the importance of sampling time as well as the population is illustrated in extreme form in Fig. 1, taken from studies in The Gambia. Clearly, if only one part of the year were examined, a very biased estimate of intake might be obtained. Such patterns, although not usually this extreme, can be seen in many agrarian populations of developing countries.

History

The first USDA food consumption survey of national scope was conducted in 1936–1937. Since then, surveys have been undertaken at roughly 10-year intervals.

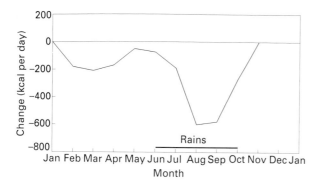

Fig. 1 An extreme example of seasonality in total food intake: seasonal changes in energy intake in Gambian women. In estimating 'usual intake' this mandates the appropriate sampling of time as well as people. (Based on Lawrence and Prentice, as presented by Ferro-Luzzi *et al.*, 1987.)

Household food use data were collected from the beginning; individual food intake assessment began in the 1965–1966 survey. Recently, the USDA initiated a different form of individual food use survey, the Continuing Survey of Food Intake by Individuals (CSFII) in which the same individuals (women and young children only) were asked to contribute a single day of data six times at equal intervals during a year. The first NHANES survey was implemented between 1976 and 1980.

The USDA surveys are perhaps the longest-standing series in the world, although many countries have conducted national surveys of one type of another on a nonrecurring basis. The pressures of World War II gave major incentive for examination of the adequacy of food supplies and their distribution within populations. In the postwar period, a series of surveys were undertaken in developing countries under the aegis of the US Interdepartmental Committee on Nutrition for National Defense/National Development (ICNND). Initially targeted toward military populations, the surveys soon expanded to include the civilian population. That series of surveys provided invaluable experience in the design and implementation of nutrition surveys in less developed settings and became the forerunner of many national surveys since conducted.

Full nutrition or food surveys of the type discussed above are not the only valuable source of information about food supplies used by governments in planning. Regular collection, reporting and analysis of 'food balance sheet' data, intended to estimate per capita disappearance of food for human consumption at the retail level, now characterizes most countries. In Canada, for example, such statistics go back to 1935 and are regularly used in trend analyses and in a range of economic analyses and projections. These data have been justifiably criticized when used as estimates of per capita intake. Close study of the per capita disappearance data and food consumption data collected in the same time-frame suggest that, in countries such as the USA, Canada and the UK, the disappearance data may give estimates that are 50% or more above estimates of energy intake based on consumption data. Recent comparisons, performed by and for the Food and Agriculture Organization (FAO), have suggested that the two types of estimates may be in much closer agreement in developing countries. Many possible sources of the discrepancies in industrialized countries have been suggested. At least one – food wastage between the retail and individual consumption levels – is certainly a factor. Less clear is the problem of identification of commodities as they move through the food processing and food distribution chains (diversion to nonhuman uses, possibility of multiple counting, etc.) For trend analysis a potentially serious problem is the periodic (necessary) updating of the system of collecting and collating data within countries; such changes can result in methodology-driven differences in derived per capita estimates. While such per capita data are very useful in monitoring national and international trends (and have been used in 'international epidemiology'), a major limitation is that they provide no information on distribution of food within the populations. In connection with its world food surveys, the FAO has taken an indirect, and much criticized, approach wherein distributions of energy intakes to the household level have been modelled on reported relationships between household income and food purchase, using actual or assumed information about income distribution. Many countries also collect, on an ongoing basis, information about food expenditure patterns. In Canada, this is done in target cities rather than attempting to represent the country as a whole. Such studies are primarily intended to support economic analyses but they also provide important information about trends in food acquisition.

Data Limitations and Analyses

As indicated in the opening paragraph, national surveys, by definition, are intended to yield estimates applicable to the population as a whole or to defined subgroups. They are designed to be representative. A serious potential problem in any large survey is nonresponse bias, i.e. the danger that those who declined to participate are different from those who did participate and hence that the resultant national estimates are biased. In the 1987–1988 NFCS survey the design goals were a 74% response rate for households and an 85% response rate for individuals within households (i.e. a 63% response rate at the level of individuals potentially included). Limited information about nonrespondents was to be collected so that bias might be assessed. In the actual survey, the individual response rate (as a percentage of individuals in occupied target households) has been estimated as only 33%, and information about nonresponders is not available (US General Accounting Office Report RCED91-117, *Nutrition Monitoring: Mismanagement of Nutrition Survey has Resulted in Questionable Data*). The USDA has had to issue a cautionary statement warning users about possible or probable biases in the data. While the data are still usable for some purposes, the primary purposes of the national survey have certainly been compromised. Problems of nonresponse are not unique to the NFCS. In the Canadian national survey (Nutrition Canada), conducted in 1970–1972, the overall response rate was estimated to be 46% (of selected individuals actually attending the clinics). However, it varied appreciably among various design strata: lower for men than women; lower for those aged under 20 than over 20 years; lowest for those living in urban centres and highest for those in rural areas.

Setting aside the sampling issues, one may direct attention to limitations imposed by the nature of the data collected. Mention has already been made of the difference in ancillary data collected in the NFCS and NHANES surveys, and the obvious effect that has on usage of the data.

Data from dietary surveys may be examined in terms of foods and food use patterns, involving no data transformations other than groupings. Customarily, the food use information is also transformed to estimates of energy and nutrient intake. Any limitations of the coding system and of the food composition data base will in turn have an impact on the utility of the computed nutrient intakes.

With either foods or nutrients, analyses begin with an explicit question. The question may require only the estimation of mean or median intakes for predefined population groups (design strata of the population). More often, the objectives of the survey require the posing of questions that relate to the distribution of intakes among individuals. In the area of food safety, interest may lie in estimation of the upper centiles of usage of particular foods, alone or in combination (as a measure of possible exposure to a foodborne material). In most nutritional assessments interest is directed toward the proportion of intakes falling below estimated requirements, although interest is increasingly also focusing upon the prevalence of higher than desirable intakes (e.g. for dietary fat).

A very serious issue in distributional analyses is inflation of the distribution because of the presence of a random error in the estimate of individuals' usual intakes. This is illustrated in Fig. 2. The random error arises primarily, but not exclusively, from within-person or day-to-day variation in reported intakes of individuals. Random error in reporting and random error in

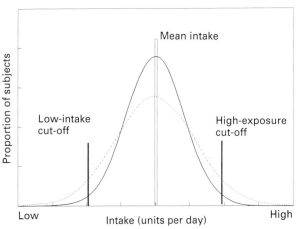

Fig. 2 Impact of random error in distribution analyses. —— The distribution of true usual intakes of the individuals in the population group; – – – the distribution that might be seen with 1-day intake data. Note that the group mean is unaffected (unbiased) but, because of the inflation of the distribution, the estimated prevalence of high or low intakes (areas under the curves beyond the portrayed cut-offs) are clearly biased. Distributions are simulated.

the food composition data base also contribute. If there is no systematic bias in the reporting of food intake (see below), one might expect that the group mean would be unbiased and the random error term only affects the confidence bounds on that mean. In contrast, it is readily apparent from Fig. 2 that the presence of appreciable random error will lead to important biases in the estimation of prevalence of either low or high intakes. The preferred approach to avoiding this problem is to increase the number of days of data collected for each individual (*see* previous article). This may not be feasible within the logistical and cost constraints of the survey. In the absence of major skewing in the intake data, there are statistical approaches that can be applied to reduce the effect of this random error. However, those approaches require that there must be at least a statistically adequate sample of replicated observations so that the error term can be estimated, using analysis of variance techniques. The current NHANES survey, in common with its predecessors, collects a single day's intake data for each participant. So that the error term can be estimated and used in subsequent analyses, NHANES is also collecting a second day of intake data for a sample of participants. The NFCS surveys collect 3 days' data by a mixture of recall and record methods. Nutrition Canada collected a single day's data. While some argue that food frequency and/or diet history methods could overcome the problem of day-to-day variation, there remains much scepticism about the magnitude and nature of errors that may be inherent in data collected by those methods. They have not found generalized application in national surveys although they have been used.

The foregoing relates to random error. Over the years, many have suggested that certain types of individuals tend to systematically over- or underreport their actual intakes. Unless such individuals are randomly distributed in the population or population group under examination, there will be biases in the group mean and in any distributional estimates. Recently, Mertz has suggested that the national surveys conducted by the USDA suffer such a bias and that reported energy intakes are underestimates of true population mean intakes.

Another issue of nutritional data analysis and interpretation relates more to the mode of analysis than the nature and properties of the data. The oft-stated goal is to assess adequacy of the food supply or pattern of food use. This involves comparison of estimated intakes with some sort of reference to desirable intake. Estimates of human energy or nutrient requirements are frequently the intended comparator. James and Schofield (1990), on behalf of the FAO, published a manual addressing the estimation of per capita energy needs to be used in comparisons with estimates of per capita energy intakes. While suggesting avenues around problems of existing approaches and providing an interpretation of the FAO/WHO/UNU (1985) report on energy requirements, the approach outlined is *not* appropriate for nutrient assessments. The fundamental reason is that while we believe that, in the presence of adequate food supplies, there is a general regulation of energy balance such that chronic intake and chronic expenditure (requirement) correlate strongly, this is not the case for nutrients. For nutrients, the intake and requirement distributions are likely to be essentially independent of one another unless both relate to a third variable (see FAO/WHO/UNU, 1985).

For nutrient assessment, a 'probability approach' has been described (National Research Council, 1986; FAO/WHO/UNU, 1985) (*see* next article). FAO and World Health Organization (WHO) reports on estimated requirements for protein, thiamin, riboflavin, nicotinic acid, folate, vitamin A and iron (and the soon-to-be-published report on copper, selenium and zinc) provide sufficient information to permit implementation of this approach. Most national reports on nutrient needs have failed to include the requisite information. The approach, portrayed in Fig. 3, although criticized on grounds of statistical imprecision (or implied overprecision), is far superior to its usual alternative, the counting of individuals below some relatively arbitrary percentage of the 'recommended dietary intake – at least if the goal is to estimate the prevalence of intakes inadequate to meet the individuals' own needs. An even greater error in interpretation of national surveys has been to compare group mean intakes directly with the 'recommended intake' as presented in most requirement reports. While that is the approach used (appropriately)

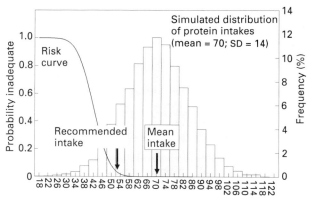

Fig. 3 The probability assessment of reported intakes. The probability that a given level is inadequate for a randomly selected individual is portrayed by the solid line on the left. The curve is the cumulative distribution of requirements. The probability of inadequacy multiplied by frequency of persons, summed across all intervals of intake portrayed in the figure, yields an estimate of the expected prevalence of individuals with intakes inadequate to meet their own needs (but does not identify which individuals have inadequate intakes). (Based on FAO/WHO/UNU, 1985.)

for energy, where the published figures represent group mean requirements and correlation between intake and requirement is expected, it is wrong for nutrients, where the published figures usually represent an estimate of the upper range of requirements of individuals and independence of intake and requirement distributions is believed to hold. An interesting contrast in interpretation of the same data set is to be found in reports describing the findings of Nutrition Canada. The first national report attempted to interpret the 1-day intakes categorized as falling into low-, moderate- or high-risk intervals. The second series of regional reports compared group mean intakes with the published recommended intakes and largely ignored the distribution of intakes. As might be expected, the two sets of interpretations left the reader with quite different images of the likely adequacy of existing dietary intakes in Canada. In retrospect, both were incorrect, in opposite directions, and the true picture lies between those extremes. *See* Dietary Requirements of Adults; Food Composition Tables; Dietary Reference Values

National survey data are sometimes analysed in relation to recommended patterns of food use. Usually this is carried out only at the level of group mean intakes. Distribution analyses would present problems analogous to the assessment of nutrient intake – does the food intake recorded for an individual represent his or her 'usual intake' pattern? As one moves from large aggregated groupings of foods toward single, irregularly

Surveys of National Food Intake

used food items, the problem of within-person variation in intake is exacerbated.

It is critical that the inevitable limitations of dietary data collected in national surveys be recognized during data analysis and interpretation. It is desirable, of course, that surveys be designed to minimize, or at least estimate, the inherent errors. The existence of limitations must not be allowed to distract attention from the important uses of national survey data.

Bibliography

Beaton GH (1985) Nutritional assessment of observed nutrient intake: an interpretation of recent requirement reports. In: Draper HH (ed.) *Advances in Nutrition Research*, vol. 7, pp 101–128. New York: Plenum Press.

Bureau of Nutritional Sciences (1975) *Nutrition Canada – Regional Reports*. Ottawa: Health and Welfare Canada.

FAO/WHO/UNU (1985) *Energy and Protein Requirements: Report of a Joint FAO/WHO/UNU Expert Consultation*. *World Health Organization Technical Report Series* 724.

Ferro-Luzzi A, Pastore G and Sette S (1987) Seasonality in energy metabolism. In: Scurch B and Scrimshaw NS (eds) *Chronic Energy Deficiency: Consequences and Related Issues*, pp 37–58. Lausanne: Nestlé Foundation.

James WPT and Schofield EC (1990) *Human Energy Requirements: A Manual for Planners and Nutritionists*. Oxford: Oxford University Press.

Life Sciences Research Office (1986) *Guidelines for the Use of Dietary Intake Data*. Bethesda, Maryland: Federation of American Societies for Experimental Biology (FASEB).

Life Sciences Research Office (1988) *Estimation of Exposure to Substances in the Food Supply*. Bethesda, Maryland: FASEB.

Life Sciences Research Office (1989) *Nutrition Monitoring in the United States: An Update Report on Nutrition Monitoring*. Bethesda, Maryland: FASEB.

Liu K (1989) Consideration of and compensation for intra-individual variability in nutrient intakes. In: Kohlmeier L and Helsing E (eds) *Epidemiology, Nutrition and Health*, pp 87–98. London: Smith–Gordon–Nishimura.

Mackerras D (1991) *Interpreting Dietary Data*. Highgate Hill, Queensland: Xyris Software.

National Research Council (1984) *National Survey Data on Food Consumption: Uses and Recommendations*. Washington, DC: National Academy Press.

National Research Council (1986) *Nutrient Adequacy: Assessment Using Food Consumption Surveys*. Washington, DC: National Academy Press.

Rand WH, Windham CT, Wyse BW and Young VR (eds) (1987) *Food Composition Data: A User's Perspective*. Tokyo: The United Nations University.

Sabry ZI (1973) *Nutrition Canada: National Survey*. Ottawa: Information Canada.

Willett W (1990) *Nutritional Epidemiology*. Monographs in Epidemiology and Biostatistics, vol. 15. New York: Oxford University Press.

G. H. Beaton
University of Toronto, Toronto, Canada

Surveys of Food Intakes in Groups and Individuals

Studies of food intake by individuals or groups are usually undertaken for a narrowly defined purpose. In the case of individuals, intake assessments are undertaken most often in connection with dietary counselling, monitoring compliance with a prescribed dietary regime, and, sometimes, as a part of a risk assessment programme. The potential purposes of group surveys are more diverse. The study might be a mininational survey intended to collect supplementary information about a population group not adequately represented in a national survey (in which case approaches and considerations would parallel those discussed in the preceding article). More often, group surveys are undertaken as a part of a research study or as a component of programme monitoring and evaluation. The precise purpose of a given study dictates the important elements of design and choice of methodology of food intake data collection. The fact that small numbers of persons (down to the level of a single individual) are involved has an important bearing on the impact of error terms. What may be acceptable in the connotation of a national survey might destroy the utility of a study of an assessment of intake of a particular individual. When compared with the discussion of national surveys, the reader will quickly recognize the increasing impact of error terms as one moves from the very large descriptive national survey through the group research study to assessment of an individual's intake.

Group Studies

Epidemiological Studies

The most common research application of group food intake surveys is in the area of nutritional epidemiology, where the investigator may wish to examine the hypothesized association between intake of a food or class of foods, a nutrient or other chemical present in foods, with the occurrence of a specified health condition. Such surveys may involve large numbers in subjects, but they differ from national surveys in at least three critically important features: (1) in national surveys sampling is designed to represent the population; in epidemiological studies there is seldom an intent to represent a national population, rather the design usually involves intentional sampling of a defined group holding characteristics of interest to the investigator; (2) in epidemiological studies the investigator is usually interested in a predefined aspect of diet; hence the dietary methodology may be selected or modified to optimize the capture of this information, potentially at the expense of other dietary information, an approach that would be unacceptable for a national survey of food intake; (3) in a national survey one is interested in estimating the *mean or median* intake and the *distribution* of usual intakes in the population or population subgroup; a reliable estimate of the usual intake of each individual is not needed. In epidemiological studies one wishes to relate intake and health status at the level of the individual; one is interested in estimating usual intakes of each individual. Fortunately, for many epidemiological applications, it may be sufficient to adequately rank the usual intakes of individuals without actually having valid estimates of true intake. These considerations have an important bearing on the choice of dietary methodology. *See* Epidemiology

Many epidemiologists have adopted food frequency or diet history methodologies, sometimes selectively abbreviated, to obtain semiquantitative information about usual usage of the foods of particular interest (e.g. sources of vitamin A and carotenoids in a cancer epidemiology study). There are at least two apparent advantages in this choice, one theoretical and one logistical: (1) the frequency questionnaire is assumed to circumvent the problems of day-to-day variation in intake by asking about usual eating practices (see discussion of this source of error under *Studies of Food Intake in Individuals*, below); (2) a frequency questionnaire is more easily administered than a record, recall or diet history and can be coupled with disease history and demographic questionnaires (the whole package may be self-administered and returned by mail). There is a potential or real disadvantage: food frequency and diet history approaches are *perceived* to provide less precise quantitative information about intake of the whole range of foods than daily recalls and records of actual consumption. Thus there may be a trade-off of errors involved in the selection of methodologies.

There are other potential disadvantages to the food frequency instrument applied in epidemiological investigations. It seems clear that, in common with all other dietary methodologies, there is an error term attached to the data collected. This may be the equivalent of 'random error' in records and recalls, although of much smaller magnitude. The disadvantage arises from the fact that the investigator has only a single measure of intake; there is not an opportunity, within a study, to estimate the error term and apply it in analyses and interpretations. Epidemiological studies are concerned with associations between intakes and health conditions in individuals as estimated by regression, correlation or analogous statistical techniques. The presence of 'random' error in the variables under examination attenuates the coefficients in statistical analyses (masks true associations). Drawing on the theory of errors in measurement, approaches have been described by which analyses might be adjusted, or at least by which the

analyst can estimate what the association might have been were there no error. To adopt this strategy, the error term must be estimable. Therein lies the potential disadvantage of the food frequency method (and the diet history method). The food frequency methods appear to generate their own sets of errors and, in the end, may yield nutrient data that have little advantage over a 3- or 4-day intake estimate. For large epidemiological studies, involving geographically dispersed subjects, logistical feasibility must be an overwhelming consideration in the selection of dietary methodology. In this context, feasibility includes consideration of respondent burden. The food frequency method often carries overwhelming logistical advantages for epidemiological studies – advantages that far outweigh the potential or real disadvantages mentioned above.

Evaluation and Monitoring of Interventions

When the objective of a special-purpose survey is to evaluate or monitor an intervention programme, there could be interest in a specific dimension of food intake, allowing adoption of a specifically designed and targeted food intake methodology. Often, the investigator may wish to estimate intakes of many foods, patterns of food use, or multiple nutrient intakes. If so, he or she may elect to adopt records or multiple recalls as a preferred method. Depending upon planned analyses, the investigator may be more interested in group behaviour than in individual response. This too will affect choice of methodology based on judgements about which types of errors are more acceptable.

Conclusion

Because group surveys are usually undertaken for very specific purposes, it is often feasible and desirable to design and implement methodologies that optimize capture of information about the dietary variable(s) of interest. The obverse of this is that the danger in *post hoc* use of these specialized data bases for other purposes is much greater than that which exists in secondary uses of national survey data bases.

Studies of Food Intake in Individuals

The worst case scenario is presented first. This arises when the goal of investigation is an attempt to evaluate the apparent adequacy of dietary intake for the particular individual (without assessment of health condition of the individual). This involves estimation of the individual's 'usual' intake of one or more nutrients and comparison of this with his or her requirements for

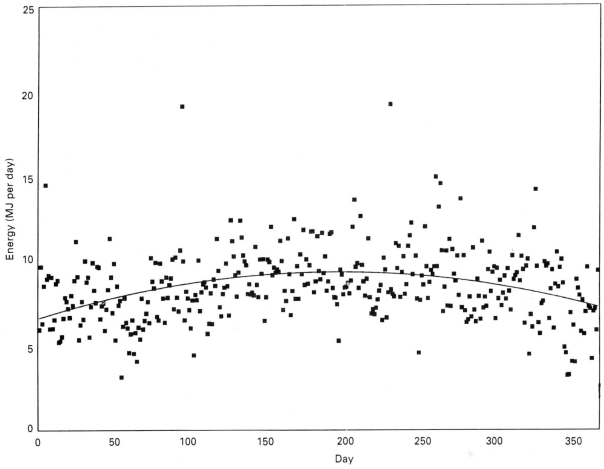

Fig. 1 Long-term pattern within the day-to-day variation of energy intake in a single subject who reported intake for 365 consecutive days. From Tarasuk V and Beaton GH (1991a). Data from the Beltsville One Year Study of Dietary Intake (Mertz W and Kelsay JL, 1984).

those nutrients. In this situation, three very serious issues must be addressed.

The most obvious problem is that associated with day-to-day variation in reported intake. We know that the coefficient of variation (CV) of day-to-day variation is in the order of 15–25% for most nutrients. Vitamin A, dietary cholesterol and fatty acid ratios have notoriously high variances. Consider the conservative estimate of a CV of 15%. For a single day's intake, this translates to suggest that the individual's true intake lies within $\pm 30\%$ of the estimate (95% confidence interval). With 7 days of data, the true intake might lie within ± 11–12% and with 14 days of data the confidence interval might be $\pm 8\%$. It has been suggested that for dietary cholesterol, 4 weeks or more of data might be required to bring the confidence bounds down to about $\pm 10\%$. To make matters worse, it is generally assumed that day-to-day variation in reported intake is a random phenomenon and that its magnitude is comparable across individuals. Both of these assumptions have recently been shown to be wrong. The magnitude of day-to-day variation is a characteristic of the individual. The

confidence bounds on an estimate of intake based on a fixed numbers of days of data will vary between individuals. Furthermore, a part of the variation is not random. It has long been recognized that day of the week and other social patterns exert effects on food intake of individuals. Any individuals exhibit long-term patterns within their day-to-day variation. The reported energy intakes of one such individual collected across 365 sequential days is portrayed in Fig. 1. An implication of this patterning of variation is that, in order to correctly estimate an individual's true 'usual' intake, one must define the time-frame of 'usual' and then sample the population of days in that time-frame, rather than simply worrying about the number of days of data to be collected. Since dietary assessments of individuals usually have to be completed in relatively short periods of time, it is seldom feasible to collect many days of data and it is rarely possible to sample time as suggested above. Instead one must accept that there are inherent errors, perhaps substantial, in the estimates of the individual's 'usual' intake and, furthermore, given the work of Tarasuk and Beaton, these errors are likely to be

Surveys of Food Intakes in Groups and Individuals

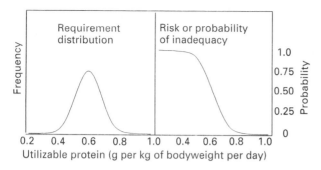

Fig. 2 The probability approach to assessment of observed intake. The estimated distribution of protein requirements of young adult men is portrayed on the left (based on FAO/WHO/UNU, 1985). The probability or risk curve, portraying the likelihood that a particular level of intake is inadequate to meet the actual (but unknown) requirement of a randomly selected individual, is shown on the right. See text for explanation.

underestimated if data are collected over a finite period of time (mean intakes may appear more reliable than they really are). It is not clear that diet history methods can overcome this problem, although they may attenuate it. *See* Energy, Energy Expenditure and Energy Balance

A second issue in the assessment of the nutrient intake of a particular individual is that, for nutrients such as iron and zinc, we must take into account the effect of concurrent consumption of enhancers and inhibitors of absorption or utilization. While our understanding of these effects is increasing, and algorithms to factor them into estimation of utilizable nutrient intake are appearing, the state of the art is such that we must face appreciable errors at the level of the particular individual no matter what method of dietary data collection is adopted. *See* Bioavailability of Nutrients

The third issue, this time relating to data analysis and interpretation rather than to a limitation of the intake estimate itself, arises in the comparison of intake with requirement. While individuals have specific requirements, these differ between seemingly similar individuals (described by age, gender, body size and composition, physical activity, etc.). At best we can describe the distribution of requirements that associates with individuals in the specified class. There can never be a way of classifying the dietary intake of an individual as being 'adequate' or 'inadequate' unless his or her intake falls well above or well below the range of requirements. If the observed intake falls within the range, we can only offer a probability statement. This is illustrated for protein in Fig. 2. Consider the estimated utilizable protein intake of an adult man. If that intake were 0·1 g per kg of bodyweight per day, it is almost certain that it would be inadequate. Very few individuals would be expected to have requirements that low (see requirement

distribution in Fig. 2). If the intake were 1·5 g per kg of bodyweight per day, one might feel comfortable in asserting that it was almost certainly adequate; very few, if any individuals are expected to have a requirement that high. However, if the intake were 0·6 g per kg of bodyweight per day, the mean requirement estimate, then it would be expected that about 50% of individuals have higher needs and 50% have lower needs. For the individual under examination, there would be about a 50:50 chance that the intake is adequate. These are probability statements. The approach can be formalized by the preparation of a probability, or risk, curve (see Fig. 2) describing the proportion of individuals expected to have requirements above any specified level of intake. Given that individuals are likely to match intake to requirement to some degree, the true probability of inadequacy at a given level of intake is probably lower than this theoretical curve suggests. The 'probability approach' is applicable to nutrients but not to energy. *See* Dietary Reference Values

Consider again the discussion of 'random' error terms. If a single day of intake data were under consideration, then the estimate of usual protein intake might have confidence bounds of ±30% or more. The estimated intake of 0·6 g per kg of bodyweight per day might reflect a true intake lying between 0·4 and 0·8 g per kg per day. This would span the whole requirement distribution. Thus one would be left suggesting that the true probability of inadequacy was somewhere between 1 and 0 (certainly inadequate and certainly adequate) – not a very useful assessment!

What may be particularly difficult to understand is that while these issues may appear insurmountable in investigation of the particular individual, they become less important as one moves to groups and, more particularly, to population assessments. Many of the errors discussed above behave like random error terms. As such they tend to cancel each other as group sizes increase, or, if estimated, they can be taken into account in analyses. The probability assessment of observed intake, which was seriously questioned in application to the particular individual, has clear merit when applied in population or large group assessments (see preceding article). It is at the level of the particular individual or small group that the full weight of the limitations of dietary data are felt.

From the above it follows logically that if evaluation of nutrient intake of the particular individual is very problematic, one must ask whether or not it is worth doing. Much simpler dietary methodologies can suffice to provide general descriptions of current food use patterns, even though these may be more qualitative than quantitative. For many counselling applications, or for monitoring compliance with a prescribed dietary regime, these may suffice and are almost certainly more acceptable to the patient. The professional must assess the likely error term associated with finally derived estimates and decide whether such estimates are useful for the required purpose. If not, the analyst should consider different strategies of accomplishing the objective without relying on detailed dietary assessment.

Bias in Food Intake Estimates

The foregoing discussions have focused upon 'random' error. As noted, as the numbers of individuals studied increases, there are statistical approaches that can reduce the impact of random error. Such is not usually the case with bias. It remains with the data at all levels of analysis. The only real exception is the very rare situation in which there is known systematic bias affecting all reported intakes to the same degree (or that can be accurately estimated from other information collected). If the bias is known, the intake data can be adjusted. The epidemiologist may not even need to adjust the data since the presence of uniform bias would not be expected to affect *detection* of associations; it would have an impact on the *description* of those associations in quantitative terms. Uniform bias would be very unusual. The more typical problem is the suspicion, or knowledge, that certain types of people provide consistent under- or overestimates of their intake. This is believed to occur in overweight subjects. It may also occur in persons who perceive that it is to their advantage to report better or worse intakes than actually exist, or who simply wish to impress the interviewer. To the analyst the serious danger here is that bias will move with a health or economic variable of interest; there will be serious confounding of analyses.

In analysis and interpretation of dietary data, bias in reporting or recording intake may be randomly distributed among individuals. For some purposes of group and population examinations, this may be tolerable. However, in examination of the individual, bias in reporting leads to an unavoidable error in analysis.

Bias in estimated nutrient intakes can arise in the process of computing nutrient intakes rather than in reporting and recording food intake. A systematic error in the food composition table is an obvious potential source of such bias. A specific example of this, in the Canadian setting, was a shift in consumer preferences toward leaner cuts of meat and an associated alteration of meat grading standards. Until the food composition data bases caught up with this change in the composition of foods actually being consumed, there was a bias of overestimation of fat intake for anyone reporting the consumption of the affected meats. It is an ongoing task of the food analyst to monitor the marketplace and ensure that the food composition data bases reflect foods currently available and used. Another vivid example is found in the estimation of selenium intake in

countries depending heavily on imported wheat. Depending upon the source of that wheat, the selenium content can vary quite extensively. The consumer is not aware of the source of the wheat that he or she eats; the food composition tables may or may not be in phase with then-current import practices. *See* Food Composition Tables

This leads to a final comment on possible sources of error in dietary data. Food composition data bases evolve with time. Individual centres are likely to add new composition data obtained from a variety of sources. A net result is that data bases tend to evolve away from one another. This has been demonstrated repeatedly in North America and Europe. By sending identical test records of food intake to multiple centres for coding and computation of nutrient intakes, estimates of the intercentre error associated with coding and food composition data bases can be obtained. These are sometimes quite alarming, particularly for 'new interest' food components that centres may have added independently to their own data bases.

Conclusion

There are serious limitations associated with the estimation of food and nutrient intakes in individuals. As one moves to larger groups, some of these limitations diminish in importance. Certainly, they have not precluded important advances in fields such as nutritional epidemiology. However, at the level of the particular individual, they call into serious question the merit of attempting detailed dietary assessments. There is a need for vigilance in the collection, analysis, and particularly the interpretation of dietary data. There is a continuing need for improvement of dietary data collection methods and for the development and implementation of approaches that can provide useful estimates of the error terms in dietary methods, in particular the food frequency and diet history methods, in which the nature and magnitude of inherent errors remain uncertain. Limitations of data collected in a study of individuals or groups must be considered in the context of the defined purpose and selected methodology of the particular study. When there is a mismatch between purpose and methodology, data quality is likely to suffer and limitations on interpretation are likely to increase.

Bibliography

Beaton GH (1985) Nutritional assessment of observed dietary intake: an interpretation of recent requirement reports. In: Draper HH (ed.) *Advances in Nutrition Research*, vol. 7, pp 101–128. New York: Plenum Press.

FAO/WHO/UNU (1985) *Energy and Protein Requirements:*

Report of a Joint FAO/WHO/UNU Expert Consultation. World Health Organization Technical Report Series 724.

Life Sciences Research Office (1986) Guidelines for Use of Dietary Intake Data. Bethesda, Maryland: Federation of American Societies for Experimental Biology.

Liu K (1989) Consideration of and compensation for intra-individual variability in nutrient intakes. In: Kohlmeier L and Helsing E (eds) Epidemiology, Nutrition and Health, pp 87–98. London: Smith–Gordon–Nishimura.

Mackerras D (1991) Interpreting Dietary Data. Highgate Hill, Queensland: Xyris Software.

Mertz W and Kelsay JL (1984) Rationale and design of the Beltsville one-year dietary intake study. American Journal of Clinical Nutrition 40: 1323–1326.

National Research Council (1986) Nutrient Adequacy: Assessment Using Food Consumption Surveys. Washington, DC: National Academy Press.

Rand WH, Windham CT, Wyse BW and Young VR (eds) (1987) Food Composition Data: A User's Perspective. Tokyo: The United Nations University.

Tarasuk V and Beaton GH (1991a) The nature and individuality of within-subject variation in energy intake. American Journal of Clinical Nutrition 55: 464–470.

Tarasuk V and Beaton GH (1991b) Statistical estimation of dietary parameters: implications of patterns in within-subject variation – a case study of sampling strategies. American Journal of Clinical Nutrition in press.

Willett W (1990) Nutritional Epidemiology. Monographs in Epidemiology and Biostatistics, vol. 15. New York: Oxford University Press.

G. H. Beaton
University of Toronto, Toronto, Canada

DIETETIC FOODS – TYPES AND USES

Dietetic foods or foods for particular nutritional uses include products for dietary management for the following people: those with specific metabolic disorders, e.g. diabetics; those who are unable to digest or absorb nutrients from a normal diet; those who have special dietary requirements, e.g. sportspersons; and those whose food intake requires special compositional standards, e.g. babies.

Legislation, Controls and Claims

The Food and Agricultural Organization (FAO) and World Health Organization (WHO) have, via the Codex Alimentarius Commission, been working for many years upon defining standards for the various groups of dietetic foods. In addition, local regulations and recommendations apply in many countries throughout the world. In the USA, the Code of Federal Regulations (CFR) details standards for foods for special dietary uses, which include foods for infants, diabetics, weight reduction or control, as well as hypoallergenic and low-sodium foods. The European Society of Paediatric Gastroenterology and Nutrition (ESPGAN) is also recognized for setting compositional standards for foods for infants and young children. From May 1991, dietetic foods have been controlled by an EEC Council directive relating to foodstuffs for particular nutritional uses (PARNUTS), reference 89/389/EC, on the provision that they fulfil one of three nutritional requirements, stated as follows:

(i) of certain categories of persons whose digestive processes or metabolism are disturbed; or

(ii) of certain categories of persons who are in a physiological condition and who are, therefore, unable to obtain special benefit from controlled consumption of certain substances in foodstuffs; or

(iii) of infants or young children in good health.

This directive lays down general guidelines for the complete category of foods, labelling and introduction of new groups of foods onto the market. With regard to labelling, presentation and advertising, they must not attribute properties for the prevention, treatment or cure of human disease to such products, or imply such properties. It also classifies groups of foods for which specific provisions will be laid down by specific directives, and includes the following:

1. Infant formulae and follow-on foods.
2. Baby foods.
3. Low-energy and energy-reduced foods intended for weight control.
4. Dietary foods for special medical purposes.
5. Low-sodium foods including low-sodium or sodium-free dietary salts.
6. Gluten-free foods.
7. Foods intended to meet expenditure of intense muscular effort, especially for sportspersons.
8. Foods intended for persons suffering from carbohydrate metabolic disorders (diabetics).
9. Food supplements.

At the time of writing, some directives have been completed whilst others are still in the draft working party stage.

In addition to the PARNUTS and specific directives

contained within it, other EEC directives cover provisions such as nutrient substances which may be used in their manufacture, additives for technological purposes, flavours, and colours, as well as purity criteria for all these substances. As with all other foodstuffs, dietetic foods are controlled by general food legislation relating to labelling, claims, weights and measures, hygiene of manufacturing premises and procedures, etc., except where these are overridden, either by the PARNUTS and/or a specific directive.

Infant Formulae and Follow-on Foods

Infant formulae are intended for infants for the first year of life, when their mother is either unable or unwilling to breast-feed them, but may be replaced, partially or totally, by follow-on formulae from 4 months onwards when the introduction of weaning foods commences. Since infant formulae constitutes the only source of nutrition, the compositional standard is defined, as are the ingredients which may be used to supply the nutrients and technological additives. Purity criteria with respect to microbiological quality and defined levels of chemical contaminants is also a requirement. EEC legislation defines a clear code for labelling, advertising, and any claims which may be made for various products. Follow-on foods which are formulated to complement weaning foods also have strict compositional standards and purity criteria. *See* Infant Foods, Milk Formulas

The range of formulae available includes milk- and soya-protein based products as dry powders to be reconstituted with water, or in a liquid, ready-to-feed form. These may contain only lactose as the carbohydrate source or may be lactose-free. Other claims may be made for adapted-protein, low-sodium, added-iron and sucrose-free formulae.

Weaning Foods and Baby Foods

Infants are usually weaned between 4 and 6 months as baby's feeding behaviour progresses from sucking to biting and chewing. An EEC working party draft directive proposes dividing weaning foods into two categories for setting of compositional standards. These reflect the types of foods which are currently available in the EEC market and include the following:

1. Processed cereal-based products, which are subdivided into simple cereals, cereals with an added high-protein food, pasta, and rusks and biscuits.
2. Baby foods, which are primarily intended for use during the usual infant weaning period and for progressive adaptation of infants and young children to ordinary food. Baby foods constitute a very diverse category

of products, comprising complete or incomplete meals, soups, desserts, puddings, vegetable juices, fruit juices and nectars. They may be presented as ready-to-use in jars or cans, or be in a dried form and require reconstitution. *See* Infant Foods, Weaning Foods

Foods are formulated to meet the particular needs for the different stages of weaning. Those recommended for early introduction are of a smooth texture and bland flavour, not too dissimilar from milk; as weaning progresses, stronger and more varied flavours with a wider range of textures to encourage chewing, are available. Strict in-house compositional standards of these foods are imposed; babies are not exposed to unsuitable levels of sodium or refined sugars, and they receive a balanced diet with respect to vitamin and mineral content. In addition, microbiological standards are very high.

The European Commission intends to detail compositional standards with respect to protein, carbohydrate, fat, and some vitamins and minerals, as well as labelling standards.

Slimming Foods

There are a variety of slimming foods on the market, including the following:

1. Portion control foods for which the manufacturer calculates and declares the energy content of a complete food as a convenience to the consumer.
2. Energy-reduced foods, which have a minimum of 25% energy reduction of the normal food, or low-energy foods, which have a maximum of 50 kcal (210 kJ) per 100 g or 100 ml of product.
3. Products which are a sole source of nutrition and are, at the time of publication, classified as very-low-calorie diets (VLCDs) at 400–800 kcal (1680–3360 kJ) per day, and low-calorie diets (LCDs) which contain 800–1200 kcal (3360–5040 kJ) per day. Complete diets below 400 kcal per day are not, at present, classified as foodstuffs and may be taken only under strict medical supervision.

Energy-reduced or low-energy foods, as well as meeting the definition as above, should have the nutritional equivalence for vitamins and minerals as the comparable normal food, and the proposed compositional standards for LCDs are as follows:

1. Proteins, minimum 20–50 g at 100% of the WHO/FAO quality reference.
2. Lipids, maximum 30% of total energy.
3. Linoleic acid, minimum 4·5 g.
4. Vitamins and minerals, to 100% of the Recommended (RDA), as detailed in the EEC labelling directive. *See* Obesity, Treatment; Slimming, Slimming Diets

Foods for Special Medical Purposes

The growing awareness of the unique nutritional requirements for certain medical conditions has resulted in the formulation of foods either by specialized industries or within the hospital, following consultation with the medical profession. Two distinct types are recognized: enteral nutrition, in which foods are administered via the gastrointestinal (GI) tract, either orally or by means of a tube into the stomach or intestine; and parenteral nutrition, in which foods are administered intravenously. The latter is used to provide nutritional support in situations where enteral feeding is not possible, e.g. when the GI tract is unable to absorb nutrients, or complete bowel rest is required. It is more expensive and has more complications than enteral feeding, and the support equipment requires more skill to administer.

Enteral nutrition is of benefit to the following patients:

1. Those with an intact GI tract who are unable to maintain a satisfactory nutritional status on a normal diet. This may include postoperative patients, those with central nervous system or psychiatric disorders, burns or stroke victims, and comatose patients.
2. Those patients with a disease or abnormality of the GI tract which impedes digestion and absorption of nutrients.
3. Patients with limited oral access to the GI tract, owing to facial or oesophageal injuries, disease, or obstruction of the upper GI tract.
4. People who, either because of an inborn metabolic disorder such as phenylketonuria (a disorder in which the amino acid phenylalanine cannot be metabolized), or because of individual organ failures, have specific requirements. *See* Inborn Errors of Metabolism

The products, which are always at the recommendation of the medical profession, are generally divided into two classes, either nutritionally complete or incomplete.

Nutritionally Complete Foods

There are two main types which are generally available in powders or liquid ready-to-use forms:

1. General-purpose formulae are manufactured from normal food ingredients.
2. Defined formulae are manufactured from more specialized ingredients; for example, proteins may be hydrolysed to various degrees in order to reduce the chain length and thus aid digestibility, or simple sugars may replace complex carbohydrates.

Nutritionally Incomplete Formulae

1. Modules or supplemental formulae, usually in the form of a single source of a particular nutrient (protein, fat or carbohydrate), may be used to supplement the patient's diet when specialized nutritional needs are recognized by the health care professional.
2. Specialized products are formulated for specific metabolic conditions or diseases, or for the patients with specific organ failure or nutritional requirements. These are not nutritionally complete for the general population, but are usually appropriately balanced for the specific condition.

In addition to those receiving complete nutritional formulae under medical supervision, there are groups of normal healthy people who may temporarily lose the desire to eat normal foods, e.g. the elderly or those convalescing from minor illness; these people purchase nutritionally complete foods which are freely available in shops and supermarkets. *See* Food Intolerance, Elimination Diets

Low-sodium Foods

Processed foods with a low, or reduced, sodium content were originally developed for patients with kidney disorders, hypertension, and other medical conditions which require reduced sodium intake. Various studies have shown that the average salt intake is 10 times that required for physiological needs to maintain optimum muscle and nerve activity, as well as normal blood pressure. Sodium chloride has been traditionally added to food as a preserving agent, as well as a flavour enhancer. The latter property, which increases the palatability of foodstuffs, may be achieved by the use of sodium-free salt substitutes, herbs and spices.

At the time of publication, the EEC draft directive recommended two categories of food:

1. Very-low sodium: the sodium content should not exceed 40 mg per 100 g or 100 ml in the ready-to-eat product.
2. Low-sodium: the sodium content should not exceed 120 mg per 100 g or 100 ml of the ready-to-eat product.

The directive also lists salt substitutes with maximum addition levels where applicable, and these have to be declared on the food label. *See* Hypertension, Hypertension and Diet; Sodium, Physiology

Gluten-free Foods

Gluten-free foods are required for the dietary management of people with coeliac disease, the causative agent being the gluten content of cereals such as wheat, rye, barley and oats. Most of the symptoms result from malabsorption of nutrients from the intestine caused by damage to the cell wall. *See* Coeliac Disease

One of the problems which many sufferers of the

disease face is the necessity to avoid all foods containing cereals and, in order to maintain dietary choice, they require reliable gluten-free raw materials. The food industry is particularly suited to the manufacture of foods for gluten-free diets, to act as substitutes for cereal-based foods, utilizing rice and maize flour. Vitamins and minerals are usually added to the equivalent level with regard to the foods they are replacing. The products available include bakery goods and raw materials for baking, and pasta, as well as foods which are naturally free from gluten. Freedom from gluten is a requirement for foods for infants, and some manufacturers provide gluten-free foods for babies and young children.

For labelling purposes, gluten-free means that the total nitrogen content of the gluten-containing cereal grain ingredient does not exceed 0·05 g per 100 g, i.e. 0·3% protein of the product. In addition, a food may be labelled 'gluten-free by nature' to show that it is naturally free from gluten and is suitable for use in a gluten-free diet. A logo may be used for ease of identification.

Foods for Intense Performance – Sports Food

To maintain enhanced physical fitness, coupled with intense performance, and the stresses that this places on the body, means that sportspersons have special nutritional requirements beyond those adequate for normal levels of activity. Initially, products were designed for body building and weight training, but as appreciation for the different needs for the nature of the sport has been recognized, so products formulated for other activities, such as track and field athletics, have become available. *See* Exercise, Metabolic Requirements

In view of the variety of foodstuffs currently available on the market, a working party for EEC legislation proposes to classify these as follows:

1. Food products specially formulated to supply energy. Emphasis has been placed on the type and amount of the carbohydrate used, since scientific research has shown that it can have a significant effect on the storage and utilization of glycogen in the body. These products are also required to supply other energy-producing nutrients, such as fat and protein, in the correct ratio. In addition to direct meal replacements, supplements are also available as carbohydrate concentrates sold in powder form, usually with added vitamins and minerals, energy bars and instant-energy drinks.
2. Food products, tablets, capsules and hydration beverages with a defined content of minerals, trace elements, vitamins, and other substances with nutritional affects, or combinations of these, supporting the physiological performance.

3. Food products with a defined content of protein and/or amino acids, especially formulated for intense muscular effort. Products in this group include high-protein powders, concentrates, protein-enriched foods as bars, muesli, or special beverages, and single or multiple amino acid supplements which are available in tablet or capsule form.
4. A combination of the products as detailed above.

Food for Diabetics

In healthy people, glycaemia rises during meals and returns to a fasting level at around 0·8 g per litre of blood at the end of the postprandial period. In the untreated diabetic, glycaemia remains chronically higher than normal. There are two types of diabetes:

1. Low or no insulin secretion or insulin-dependent diabetes; patients are under medical supervision aimed at controlling insulin supply, so that the diet is not a major concern as long as carbohydrates are supplied at a regular interval.
2. Normal or exaggerated secretion, but accompanied by a resistance of tissues to insulin which is controlled by the diet and not insulin. Foods formulated for this type of diabetic allow them to receive a normal daily supply of carbohydrates (50–60% of the energy intake), which require as little insulin as possible, in order to limit the effects of insulin insufficiency.

At the time of publication, two options were being discussed with regard to an EEC directive on nutritional requirements and compositional standards for foods and diabetics:

For control of carbohydrate which limits the addition of d-glucose, invert sugar, disaccharides, maltodextrins, or glucose syrup, to 6% in ready-to-use products, and then only if necessary for technical reasons, or from natural sources.
Declaration of glycaemic index, which allows the consumer to evaluate the repercussions of a food on the glycaemia in comparison to a reference product. To qualify, the glycaemic index of the food must be reduced by one third in comparison to that of the corresponding normal food, with at least 20% of the energy provided by carbohydrates.

For both options, the total energy and fat content should be no more than those of comparable normal foods. The choice is very wide and includes confectionery, bakery products, dairy products, desserts and puddings, fruit juices, soft drinks and beer, sauces and salad dressings, sweeteners, and tablets and pills rich in soluble fibre for diet supplementation. *See* Glucose, Glucose Tolerance and the Glycaemic Index

Food Supplements

At the time of going to press, the EEC was considering the inclusion of supplements in the group of generally recognized dietetic foods, provided that these were not marketed with a medical claim and thus covered by the pharmaceutical product legislation. Under consideration were single vitamin and mineral supplements, multivitamin and/or mineral supplements.

Special Ingredients

To support the diverse needs of the dietetic food industry, many raw material suppliers manufacture special ingredients. These include basic nutrients such as single minerals, vitamins, amino acids, fatty acids and sugars, as well as specially treated food ingredients. The latter include proteins, hydrolysed to varying degrees, to aid digestibility or reduce allergenicity, or tailored to a specific amino acid profile; tailored fats with a specific fatty acid profile which may be a balanced blend of fats, a special fraction such as medium-chain triglycerides, or a randomized or co-randomized fat blend, and carbohydrates which may be simple or complex oligosaccharides and may or may not be partially hydrolysed. The formulation of dietetic foods also needs special technological additives as process aids, thickeners, emulsifiers, stabilisers, etc., to improve shelf life and palatability.

Bibliography

Code of Federal Regulations (parts 100–169) (1990) Washington: Office of the Federal Register of National Archives and Records Administration.

Codex Alimentarius Commission, Joint FAO/WHO Food Standards Programme. (1981) *Infant Formula* CAC 72; (1987) *Follow-up Formula* CAC 156; (1981) *Canned Baby Foods* CAC 73; (1981) *Processed Cereal Based Foods for Infants and Children* CAC 74; (1981) *Gluten Free Foods* CAC 118; (1981) *Foods with Low Sodium Content* CAC 53; (1985) *Labelling of and Claims for Prepackaged Foods for Special Dietary Uses* CAC 146. Rome: Food and Agriculture Organization; Geneva: World Health Organization.

EEC Council (1989) Directive on the Approximation of the Laws of Member States Relating to Foodstuffs Intended for Particular Nutritional Uses. *Official Journal of The European Communities* 30.6.89 No. L186/27.

Elaine Underwood
Wyeth Laboratories, Havant, UK

DIETETICS

In this article the terms 'dietetics' and 'dietitian' are defined together with a brief history of the evolution of the profession. The education and role of the dietitian in therapeutic and preventative dietetics is described.

Definition and History of Dietetics

Dietetics is defined as 'the scientific study and regulation of food intake and preparation'. It has also been broadly described as 'the application of the science of nutrition to the human being in health and disease'.

However, the term dietitian, used to describe a practitioner of dietetics, was first used long before the science of nutrition had become an accepted discipline. In 1899, in the USA, the dietitian was described as a person working in a hospital who provided nutritious meals to patients, and the earliest dietitians were primarily home economists. The profession of dietetics and the role of the dietitian have expanded greatly during the twentieth century and no longer involve simply the provision of food. It is recognized that the practice of dietetics requires a wide range of knowledge and skills and in the USA, the UK, Australia, Canada, New Zealand, South Africa and many other countries the training and registration of dietitians has been well established.

The profession of dietetics is relatively new and was first formalized in the USA when, in 1917, the American Dietetic Association (ADA) was founded. In the UK, the first dietitians were nurses and the first dietetic department was started in the Royal Infirmary, Edinburgh, in 1924. Several of the pioneers of British dietetics were able to visit the USA during the 1920s and study the work of established dietetic departments in hospitals there and after several abortive attempts the British Dietetic Association (BDA) was established in 1936. Other countries followed and in 1991 there were 29 dietetic associations throughout the world registered with the International Committee of Dietetic Associations (ICDA). The ICDA organizes an international conference for dietitians every 4 years and is affiliated to the International Union of Nutritional Sciences (IUNS).

Dietetic Qualifications

Although the term 'dietitian' means different things in different countries it is now accepted in most that the practice of dietetics requires a wide range of knowledge and skills. In countries where dietitians are recognized as a distinct profession and must be registered in order to practise, a prescribed programme of training must be undertaken. This usually comprises a degree course at an educational institution, including or followed by a period of practical training in a hospital dietetics department. Undergraduate programmes include coverage of basic and applied sciences (biology, chemistry, biochemistry, physiology, nutrition, microbiology) as well as social sciences (psychology and sociology) and management and communications techniques. In addition, as dietetics is concerned with feeding people, a knowledge of food composition, food preparation and food habits is essential. To this basic foundation is added a knowledge of medicine, pathology and the therapeutic uses of dietary treatment. During the practical part of the training the students learn to apply the theory to individuals or groups of people in various situations. In order to become a registered practitioner the students must demonstrate that they have good theoretical knowledge and are competent practically.

The registration body for dietitians varies from country to country: in the USA, the ADA is responsible for initial and continuing registration, whereas in the UK dietitians are registered by the Dietitians Board of the Council for Professions Supplementary to Medicine (CPSM) who also monitor all training courses. The registration body produces a statement of conduct which delineates the role and responsibilities of the registrant. Registration in one country does not necessarily mean that a person will be accepted as a dietitian elsewhere in the world as qualifications are at different levels. The registration body will usually therefore also examine other countries' qualifications and decide whether they are equivalent.

The Role of the Dietitian

The first dietitians worked only in hospitals and at present the hospital service and clinical dietetics still claim a large majority of practitioners. However, other areas of work are becoming increasingly important. Dietitians work with different groups in the community and in industry to improve the general health of the population through health education. They act as advisers to food companies, retail and wholesale suppliers of food and to companies producing special dietary products. Increasingly, they are also becoming involved in freelance work, in journalism and in private

Table 1. Examples of therapeutic diets that alleviate symptoms

Symptom	Condition	Diet
Nausea	Gall bladder disease	Low-fat
	Renal disease	Low-protein
Dysphagia	Disease of mouth or oesophagus	Semisolid
Weight loss	Trauma, carcinoma, severe burns	High energy
Constipation	Diverticular disease and others	High-fibre
Diarrhoea	Pancreatic insufficiency	Low-fat
	Lactose intolerance	Lactose-free

practice. Whatever aspect of work a dietitian chooses one of the primary roles will be that of an educator, whether this be with individuals or to groups of people. The ability to communicate is therefore an essential attribute for the profession. *See* Nutrition Education

Dietetics in Hospitals

In the USA and countries which follow the US model, dietitians in hospitals work in either administrative or clinical (therapeutic) areas. Administrative dietitians are involved with the management of food services for patients and staff. They are responsible for food production and quality control in the delivery of the hospital meal service. They are also often responsible for budgeting and staffing of the dietary departments and usually relate to the other administrators and managers but not to the medical staff. The clinical dietitian is the person who has direct contact with the doctors and paramedical staff concerned with patient care.

In the UK the practice of dietetics developed along a different route, and dietitians do not have overall responsibility for the food service. However, there is usually close liaison between the dietitian and catering manager to ensure the provision of nutritionally sound selective menus. The dietitian will also be consulted in matters of policy such as the implications of changes in food preparation systems or the introduction of 'healthy eating' policies.

Clinical or Therapeutic Dietetics

The term 'therapeutic dietetics' has been used in the past to describe the work of the dietitian in his or her direct dealings with patients who require 'special diets' for various reasons, as outlined in Tables 1 and 2. In the past, the role of the therapeutic dietitian was to calculate, teach and facilitate compliance to dietary

Table 2. Examples of therapeutic diets used to correct disturbances in physiological or metabolic function

Condition	Cause	Diet
Uraemia	Renal failure	Low-protein, low-phosphate
Oedema	Heart failure, liver or renal diseases	Low-salt or low-sodium
Failure of absorption	Pancreatic disease, gall bladder disease	Low-fat and medium-chain triglyceride (MCT)
Reduced glucose tolerance	Diabetes mellitus	Control energy: low-fat, high-complex-carbohydrate
Villous atrophy	Coeliac disease	Gluten-free

regimens prescribed by medical or surgical practitioners for specific disorders. These functions are still important but, increasingly, the dietitian is becoming involved in the assessment and nutritional support of patients not traditionally seen as requiring a therapeutic diet. Feeding patients who are nutritionally compromised because of trauma, surgery or cancer has become an important part of the workload of many dietetic departments and the dietitian has had to learn quickly and apply this knowledge in parallel with the rapid evolution of alternative methods of nutritional support, such as enteral and parenteral feeding.

Clinical dietitians are increasingly involved in decisions about nutritional support and the appropriateness of particular therapeutic regimens, and in many institutions they are responsible for prescribing the patient's diet in consultation with the physician or surgeon, who recognizes the dietitian as the expert. (However, in the UK at least, the medical practitioner is ultimately responsible for the patient and for any therapeutic regimen, including dietary treatment.)

As new advances occur in clinical practice, the dietitian must be aware of these, and many dietitians are now involved both in research into the development of new treatments and in evaluating current practice. There has been a rapid increase in the numbers of dietetic practitioners with research qualifications and dietitians are increasingly initiating their own projects, working alongside experienced investigators rather than acting as technicians in other people's projects, as sometimes happened in the past. These advances are contributing in some part to a re-evaluation of dietetic practice and result in a need for dietitians to set priorities in their work.

As dietetics has developed it has become more specialized and this has resulted in the formation of practice groups within the dietetic associations. These groups have become a forum where advances in practice

in particular areas can be shared and are often a focus for continuing education, both formally (by running courses) and informally.

Some of the more specialist roles in which dietitians are working are described below.

Paediatric Dietetics

The paediatric dietitian has a unique role in that she has to combine the metabolic requirements of the disease process or condition with the normal nutritional requirements for growth and development. With the advances in early diagnosis of many complex metabolic disorders, children may require complicated diets which are very different from those of the rest of the family, which need constant modification as the child grows, and which may be lifelong. The dietitian is responsible for modifying the diet where necessary to take account of the patient's metabolic requirements, any feeding difficulties, whether mechanical or physiological, and the patient's food preferences as he or she grows. The dietitian is an essential part of the support system for children with inborn errors such as phenylketonuria and cystic fibrosis, conditions such as renal disease, food allergy, diabetes and many others, having access to the information about special foods and products of which the carer might be unaware or have difficulty in locating.

The paediatric dietitian also has an important role as an educator, often teaching the child's parent initially, and later the child him/herself, how to cope with the constraints of the special diet both at home and in school. As is the case with adult patients, the dietitian will often be able to put families in touch with support groups where newly diagnosed patients or parents will be helped by others with first-hand experience of the problems of the disease and its treatment. *See* Children, Nutritional Requirements; Infants, Nutritional Requirements

Renal Dietetics

Renal dietitians are usually attached to specialized renal units and are an integral part of the team involved in the treatment of people suffering from varying degrees of renal impairment. In the USA, there is a legal requirement related to funding of patient care which states that a qualified dietitian must be part of the professional team which develops short- and long-term care plans for renal patients. The dietitian, together with the nephrologist, has responsibility for nutritional assessment, the diet prescription and for monitoring response to treatment. A thorough knowledge of physiology, the processes involved in kidney disease, and an ability to understand and interpret patients' biochemical data are essential for the renal dietitian.

In addition, the dietitian will devise individualized dietary plans, taking into account other ongoing disease processes, and will teach the patient and family, and monitor dietary compliance.

Patients with renal disease may be managed conservatively before dialysis, by haemodialysis, peritoneal dialysis or by transplantation. Each of these stages requires different dietary treatment. the dietitian will deal with a variety of patients at different stages of the disease and with different needs with respect to diet, and will also have to teach the patient how to cope with the changes in diet which follow as he or she changes from one treatment to another.

Nutritional Support

Nutritional support of patients who are unable to feed themselves adequately by the normal oral route is a growing area of dietetic practice. Nutritional support may vary from simply advising on and providing supplements for the patient who cannot sustain an appropriate oral intake, to designing and advising on complete parenteral nutrition regimens for the unconscious patient in intensive care. Between these two extremes will be patients who need enteral feeds to provide complete or supplementary nutrition for a variety of reasons.

Patients requiring nutritional support may be acutely ill or may require long-term feeding, sometimes at home. The dietitian must be able to assess the nutritional requirements of each individual and design appropriate feeding regimens under all circumstances and will be closely involved in the monitoring of the patient's progress.

Diabetes Care and Education

The role of the dietitian in the treatment of diabetes mellitus has always been an important one. Traditionally, the dietitian was often the person who spent most time with the patient and it was often left to him or her to explain the details of the disorder. The dietary treatment of diabetes has undergone a radical change over the last decade. The basis of treatment for all patients, whether young and insulin-dependent or older and non-insulin-dependent, is now a diet low in fat, in which at least 50% of the energy is provided by complex carbohydrates. Many established diabetics find the change of emphasis away from the old regimen (which advised a low carbohydrate intake) confusing, and the dietitian's role in re-educating younger diabetics in this position is very important.

Other Areas of Specialization

There are many other areas of clinical dietetics in which individuals may specialize, including oncology, liver disease, gastroenterology, eating disorders, gerontology, care of the patient who is HIV-positive or has acquired immune deficiency syndrome (AIDS), care of the mentally ill or mentally handicapped. Many of the activities in these areas and those described in the sections above are not confined to the hospital but require input from the dietitian in the community.

The Dietitian in the Community

In the UK, there has been a huge increase in the number of dietitians working in the community in the last decade. At the time of writing, the community service in most areas is still the responsibility of the dietetic manager of a hospital or group of hospitals and hence there is close liaison between the hospital and community services. The community dietitian may do some therapeutic work but his or her main role is more to contribute to public health. Many of these dietitians work by educating other professional groups, such as doctors, nurses, health visitors and midwives, who will then pass the specific knowledge on to the individual or groups of patients. Prevention of diseases which may be diet-related has recently become a much more important issue, and dietitians are working with schools, health education departments and industry to try to educate the public towards consuming a healthier diet. The role of the community or public health dietitian therefore differs from that of his or her clinical counterpart in that he or she works mainly with groups rather than individuals and does not treat specific diseases.

Dietitians also work as advisors in government departments and are therefore involved in planning nutrition policies for the country as a whole.

Dietitians in Research and Education

The advances in medical and nutritional knowledge over the last 30 years have led to an increase in the numbers of dietitians employed in research. Some are employed in research institutes and others on various nutritionally orientated projects in hospital departments. Many more are carrying out research as part of their regular duties. Involvement in research has led to registration for higher degrees and the number of dietitians with masters' degrees or doctorates is now considerable in countries such as the USA, UK, Canada and Australia.

Research is also seen as an important part of the role of those dietitians employed in universities and colleges to teach dietetic and other students. In the UK and other countries, there is a requirement that each dietetic training course has registered dietitians on the staff and in many cases these people also work in hospital dietetics or other fields in order to keep up-to-date with current practices.

Dietitians are also involved in the education of many other professional groups, e.g. medical students, nurses and home economists.

Bibliography

Bateman EC (1986) *A History of the British Dietetic Association 1936–1986*. Sunderland: Edward Thompson.

Chernoff R (1983) The dietitian in the hospital setting. In: Schneider HA, Anderson CE and Coursin DB (eds) *Nutritional Support in Medical Practice*. Philadelphia: Harper and Row.

Weigley ES (1979) Professionalism and the dietitian. *Journal of the American Dietetic Association* 74: 317.

Patricia A. Judd
King's College, London, UK

DIGESTIVE AND ABSORPTIVE PHYSIOLOGY

The functions of digestion and absorption are primal, and fundamental to the existence and health of the human species. The anatomical apparatus responsible for these functions is also vulnerable to disease and dysfunction. The second most common complaint in the general medical practice of adults is that of gastrointestinal manifestations.

In order to understand the role of digestion and absorption in terms of food and nutrition, one must consider the evolution of species. Life evolved progressively from single-celled organisms in the so-called 'primaeval soup' to more complex organisms, with more specific molecular needs and without the capacity to synthesize all of the molecules required by their metabolism. As exogenous nutrients became essential, it was necessary for organisms to develop strategies and mechanisms to harvest and scavenge elemental and organic substances from the environment.

The alimentary tract is an expression of this evolutionary adaptation to the need for capturing exogenous nutrients. Its complexity and peculiarities reflect the specific habitat, nutritional requirements and dietary opportunities of all species from the planaria to the primate. In the metamorphosis from plant-eating caterpillar to nectar-sucking butterfly, and from land-dwelling salamander to aquatic newt, the alimentary tract is transformed to suit the consequent nutritional and dietary changes within the same lifetime.

Of course, not even the absorptive function is specific for nutrients. The majority of drugs and medicinal compounds enter the body across the gut. The stomach and intestine manifest a selective permeability, transport and metabolism for pharmacological agents, and the study of pharmacokinetic provides insights into gut function with respect to nutrients.

Alimentary Tract Physiology

The apparatus in which the processes of digestion and absorption take place is called the alimentary tract. No consideration of the topic would be complete, however, without considering both the exocrine glands that secrete substances into the lumen of the tract and the endocrine glands and cells that secrete bloodborne hormones which regulate the processes. At the most essential level, the function of the alimentary tract of any organism is to extract the necessary nutrients from the environment, in terms of the foods and beverages that the host consumes.

In general terms, absorption in the alimentary tract should be selective, excluding those compounds that are harmful, or simply not useful to the internal milieu of the body. The system must propel the food to the digestive cavities and the nutrients to the absorptive surfaces while moving the residue along for excretion from the body. Appropriate conditions of fluidity, pH and ionic concentration must be maintained. The whole processes of absorption and digestion must be *regulated* in two domains: (1) they need to be turned on (initiated) and turned off (terminated) in appropriate relation to meals; and (2) they need to be blended and balanced in concert with one another. The major molecular species in the process are proteins and polypeptides. These serve as enzyme for digestion, transport proteins in absorption, and circulating hormones in regulation.

The nutrients are classified as follows: (1) water; (2) macronutrients (proteins and amino acids, fats, carbohydrates, and ethanol); (3) micronutrients (minerals, vitamins, and vitamin-like substances). Both comparative physiology and clinical gastroenterology have identified a series of functions for an alimentary tract: (1)

motility; (2) *secretion*; (3) *digestion*; (4) *absorption*; (5) *host defence*.

In a more global sense, the alimentary tract must maintain its own health and function. Not only do pathogens from without and disorders from within constitute hazards, but the instrinsic functional elements themselves (e.g. acid, proteolytic enzymes and secreted fluids) pose the threat of self-damage and autodisruption of the alimentary tract. The modulations of the lifespan changes – development, senescence, and even pregnancy and lactation – modify the structure and function of the alimentary tract.

Physiological Functions of the Alimentary Tract

Motility

Motility is the capacity to propel luminal contents either in a downward direction (usual) or in a retrograde manner, derived from the coordinated contraction and relaxation of the musculature of the hollow viscera and the contractile organs and ducts (gall bladder, bile duct, pancreatic duct).

Secretion

Secretion is the emission into the luminal areas of the tract from exocrine glands or from mucosal cells, transudative (aqueous) or exudative (proteinaceous) fluids with various electrolytic composition. The contents generally contain, as their functional elements, digestive enzymes, emulsifiers (bile acids) or modifiers of pH (hydrochloric acid, bicarbonate).

Digestion

Digestion is the catalytic hydrolysis of organic molecules into progressively smaller and more elemental units mediated by enzymes. The enzymes can be either of host origin, or produced and released by the bacterial flora of the gut and the colon.

Absorption

Absorption is the set of processes for taking elemental units such as organic molecules or elements (drugs, nutrients or non-nutritive components of the diet) into the mucosal cells and through, or between and around, the enterocytes and into the internal circulation (lymph, bloodstream) of the body.

Host Defence

Host defence is the series of measures, including physical barriers, motility, immune and phagocytic elements, which prevent unwanted or harmful (toxic, infectious, allergenic) agents from entering the organism or damaging the function or structure of the alimentary tract tissues and organs.

Functional Anatomy of the Alimentary Tract

Gross Anatomy

The alimentary tract is the tubular barrier between the external environment and the internal metabolism of the body. It begins in the mouth and continues sequentially through the pharynx, oesophagus, stomach, small intestine (divided into the duodenum, jejunum and ileum), the large bowel and, finally, the rectum and anus. The small intestine is convoluted and folded to increase the absorptive surface. Exocrine secretions are provided by the liver (bile) and pancreas (bicarbonate, digestive enzymes), and the gall bladder provides a storage reservoir. *See* Bile; Gall Bladder; Liver, Nutritional Management of Liver and Biliary Disorders; Liver, Enterohepatic Circulation

Cellular Anatomy

The lining cells of the alimentary tract generally have one of two functions – secretion or absorption; most cells can perform both. The cell is covered by the mucosal membrane which is specialized for bidirectional flow of water and molecules. The cytoplasm is specialized for protein synthesis and packaging of proteins for export. Other proteins, such as metallothionein and ferritin provide storage for nutrients within the cell. Adjacent cells are connected by tight junctions, which in recent years have been shown to be not-so-tight, and many nutrients bypass the cellular interstitium in reaching the bloodstream. Cells at all levels of the tract have a rapid turnover rate, being desquamated and replaced by cells moving up from the mucosal crypts. *See* Cells

Gut Hormones and Hormones that Influence Alimentary Tract Function

The cells lining the gut, and other cells, produce hormonal substances, peptide chains of various sizes and brief half-lives. They travel through the bloodstream to reach the target tissue which can be secretory glands, secretory ducts, nerves or smooth muscles. Their roles are regulatory, either to turn on a function, such as secretion or motility, or to suppress the respective functions. Gastrin from the distal stomach stimulates gastric acid secretion by the same organ in response to intraluminal protein, amino acids, or calcium. Its release is inhibited by gastric acidity. Secretin is produced by the gut in response to acidity, and cholecystokinin-pancreatin is produced in response to fats or amino acids. The former acts to promote bicarbonate secretion by the pancreatic duct cells, and the latter acts to stimulate pancreatic digestive enzyme secretion by the glandular cells of the pancreas. It also stimulates contraction of the gall bladder to deliver bile into the proximal small intestine. Motilin, a peptide from the upper gut, is believed to initiate the neuromuscular events of peristalsis. *See* Hormones, Gut Hormones

Gastrointestinal Handling of Macronutrients

Digestion of Proteins and Absorption of Oligopeptides and Amino Acids

The terms 'proteolysis' and 'proteolytic enzymes' refer to the digestion of proteins by hydrolysing the peptide bonds that unite adjacent or cross-linked amino acids. Certain proteins, such as secretory immunoglobulin A (IgA) and gastric intrinsic factor, are resistant to intraluminal digestion. Most are susceptible to successive attack by acid hydrolysis, gastric pepsin and the family of proteases of pancreatic origin, some of which split amino acids from the carboxy-terminal or the amino-terminal ends of peptide chains (exopeptidases), while others attack specific peptide linkages within the chain (endopeptidases). A related class of enzymes are nucleotidases, which hydrolyse the deoxyribonucleic acid (DNA) and ribonucleic acid (RNA) that are found in the cellular elements of foods. *See* Protein, Digestion and Absorption of Protein and Nitrogen Balance

There are transport mechanisms for the distinct classes of amino acids (neutral, basic, acidic) and for specific classes of two- or three-amino-acid oligopeptides. The former mechanism is sodium-dependent and active, with the energy-dependent step at the mucosal membrane; the latter is mediated by specific membrane transport proteins and involves proton cotransport. Once inside the cell, peptides are hydrolysed to their constituent amino acids. Some of the absorbed protein is used within the mucosa for the synthetic needs of the epithelial cells. A non-energy-dependent transport system on the baso-lateral surface of the cell transports the amino acids from the cytoplasm to the capillary bloodstream.

About half of the protein digested and absorbed daily originates in luminal secretions or exfoliated lining cells, while the other half comes from proteins ingested in the diet. Certain proteins, such as gastric intrinsic factor and secretory IgA, are resistant to intraluminal hydrolysis.

Digestion of Triglycerides and other Fatty Acid Esters and Absorption of Fatty Acids

The handling of fats has three important considerations: (1) the luminal content of the gut is largely aqueous, and lipids have an inherent incompatibility of phase that needs to be addressed; (2) up to half of dietary energy can be in the form of fats; (3) the adverse functional consequences of substantial fat maldigestion or malabsorption (steatorrhoea). In the healthy gut, even large loads of fat are digested and absorbed with an efficiency of over 90%. *See* Fats, Digestion, Absorption and Transport

The body overcomes the incompatibility problem ('oil and water do not mix') of lipids in the aqueous milieu of the digestive juices by emulsification of the solid fat particles, first by physical dissociation in the stomach and then by the detergent action of bile salts. Dietary fat is generally in the form of triglycerides, i.e. is three fatty acids attached to the trialcohol, glycerol. The fatty acids can be composed of short chains (4 to 9 carbons), medium chains (10 to 15 carbons) or long chains (16 or more carbons). Enzymes from the class of lipases hydrolyse triglycerides to release free fatty acids, monoglycerides, and free glycerol. Lingual lipase from glands in the back of the tongue is active against the short- and medium-chain fatty acids. These are important in infants on a breastmilk diet. Pancreatic lipase is responsible for the bulk of fatty acid liberation. This enzyme functions at neutral to alkali pH and works in conjunction with a polypeptide known as colipase, required for the attachment of the hydrolytic enzyme to the hydrophobic fat. Additional hydrolysis of less common dietary lipid forms – phospholipids, cholesterol esters – is effected by phospholipases and cholesterol esterases.

The final step of the disaggregation and preparation of the fats for absorption is their incorporation with bile salts to form mixed micelles, cylindrical aggregates of bile salts and fatty acids or monoglycerides. These can approach the mucosal cells. In the enterocyte, fatty acids are re-esterified to triglycerides and released into the lymph as chylomicrons.

Digestion of Complex Carbohydrates and Polysaccharides, and Absorption of Simple Sugars

Rarely does dietary carbohydrate come in the form of simple sugars. The majority comes as starch or fibre, with glycogen, sucrose and lactose contributing lesser amounts. All must be hydrolysed to their constituent monosaccharides for absorption. The failure to remove carbohydrates from the gut lumen leads to fermentation in the colon and the generation of the bloating, gaseousness and diarrhoea of carbohydrate gastrointestinal intolerance. *See* Carbohydrates, Digestion, Absorption and Metabolism

Starch is digested by amylase, an insignificant amount of which is secreted by salivary glands, and the majority of which is of pancreatic origin. Starch is reduced to glucose, to maltose and to oligosaccharides of glucose (maltotriose; dextrins). The brush border of the enterocytes contains disaccharidases and oligosaccharidases which release; (1) glucose from starch derivatives; (2) fructose and glucose from sucrose; and (3) galactose and glucose from lactose. *See* Carbohydrates, Metabolism of Sugars

The uptake of liberated monosaccharides proceeds by two mechanisms. When the intraluminal concentrations of these sugars is vastly superior to that in the plasma, they move down the concentration gradient by simple diffusion. In lower intraintestinal concentrations, specific transport processes take over; these act at the basolateral and serosal surfaces to move the monsaccharides from the cytoplasm to the bloodstream. For fructose, this is a carrier-mediated mechanism which does not require energy. A common, active (Na^+)-ATPase-dependent mechanism (Na^+, sodium ion; ATP, adenosine triphosphate) is involved with the uptake of glucose and galactose.

Absorption of Ethanol

Ethanol is an alcohol of finite, dose-dependent and relatively mild toxicity, which can enter into the energy metabolism of the organism and provide the equivalent of 29·7 kJ (7·1 kcal) of energy per gram. It passes by passive diffusion down the concentration gradient into the capillary circulation from the distal stomach through the upper small intestine. *See* Alcohol, Metabolism, Toxicology and Beneficial Effects

Gastrointestinal Handling of Micronutrients

The most common nutritional deficiencies known to humans are those of micronutrients: minerals and vitamins. Although the micronutrients are thought of and discussed as if they were isolated chemical entities, in practice a great deal of processing of food is required to free the nutrients from their matrices, and regulation of body stores of vitamins and minerals is often effected at the intestinal level. The entry of iron and zinc into the body is controlled homeostatically by the gut, as is the fractional conversion of provitamin A carotenoids to active vitamin A.

Absorption of Elemental Nutrients (Minerals)

The primary extracellular-fluid electrolytes (sodium, chloride) and intracellular electrolyte (potassium; K) are virtually completely absorbed in the upper small intestine by diffusion. Active absorption of sodium can also occur as a consequence of the numerous, energy-dependent absorptive processes involving (Na^+ or K^+)-ATPase coupling, such as the absorption of glucose and neutral amino acids against a concentration gradient. In these energy-related uptake processes, chloride also moves into the body to conserve electroneutrality. Lithium is a minor constituent of the diet, but it is assumed that this mineral is handled in a manner closely similar to chemically related sodium. *See* Potassium, Physiology; Sodium, Physiology

Calcium is absorbed by both a passive mechanism, at intraluminal concentrations of more than 10 mmol l^{-1} and by an active mechanism at lower concentrations. Passive absorption can occur along the entire length of the intestine, including the colon. Lactose and other sugars enhance calcium uptake by this mechanism. The predominant site of active absorption is the duodenum. Vitamin D, in the form of the metabolite 1,25-dihydroxyvitamin D, plays a role as a hormonal regulator of nuclear messenger RNA synthesis concerning transport proteins for calcium within the cell. Calcium is released at the serosal membrane of the cell through an energy-dependent mechanism involving calcium-ATPase. Phosphorus, in the form of phosphate, follows an uptake, translocation and excretion scheme similar to that described for calcium. *See* Calcium, Physiology; Cholecalciferol, Physiology

Magnesium can be absorbed through the small intestine. In a dietary context, the fractional absorption is from 20% to 30% of intake. A carrier-mediated system operates at low concentration, and absorption occurs by simple diffusion at higher concentrations. Movement of water into cells influences the uptake of magnesium by the passive mechanism. *See* Magnesium

Iron is found in the diet (1) in a unique organic form, as a component of the haem moiety of haemoglobin in red cells and myoglobin in muscle in foods of flesh origin, and (2) as an inorganic (nonhaem) iron in the ferrous (divalent) or ferric (trivalent) form. Iron in storage tissues, such as liver, is essentially in an inorganic form, clustered on ferritin. Iron of plant origin is also inorganic. Absorption of inorganic iron is usually less than 10%, and is influenced by luminal pH, the valency of the ion, and binding and chelating agents. Nonhaem iron uptake is homeostatically regulated by host iron reserves. Haem iron is taken into the cell as part of the intact haem moiety. It is much more efficient and not influenced by the host iron status. *See* Iron, Physiology

Zinc can be absorbed from foods with an efficiency of up to 40%. Its uptake is regulated by host zinc nutriture. Zinc is absorbed throughout the length of the small intestine, with a carrier-mediated, energy-dependent mechanism for low concentrations, and simple diffusion at higher levels. Zinc enters the alimentary tract both from the diet and from secretions. Pancreatic juice is exceptionally rich in zinc, and an active enteropancreatic recycling of the metal is present. *See* Zinc, Physiology

Copper is absorbed in the stomach and small intestine. Estimates of fractional absorptions of up to 90% have been reported. Copper can be absorbed in the ionic form and in association with L(−) amino acids. Quantities of copper enter the gut in the bile, but it is bound to pigments in such a manner that it does not become available for reabsorption. There is no enterohepatic recycling of copper. *See* Copper, Physiology

Selenium is found in the natural diet in the form of seleno amino acids, in selenomethionein in plants and selenocysteine in foods of animal origin. Supplements have been created with various inorganic forms of selenium salts, such as selenite. Selenium absorption is not regulated by host selenium status, and efficiencies range from 50% for inorganic forms to over 90% for organic forms. The latter absorptive mechanism is linked to the uptake of the parent amino acids. *See* Selenium, Physiology

The efficiency of manganese and chromium absorption is poor. In young animals, manganese is almost unabsorbable. In adult humans, manganese absorption is estimated to be in the order of less than 15%. Chromic (trivalent) chromium absorption is 0·5–1%. Whether or not chromium in organic complexes in foods is substantially better absorbed has not been definitively resolved. *See* Chromium, Physiology

Absorption of Vitamins

Fat-soluble Vitamins

In general, fat-soluble vitamins share many features of the absorptive pathways for lipids. The more polar vitamers, however, often behave more like water-soluble vitamins. Dietary vitamin A is found in two principal forms in the diet: as retinyl esters (preformed vitamin) and as provitamin A carotenoids. Retinol is released in the gut, absorbed like fatty acids, then re-esterified in the enterocyte and released in chylomicrons into the lymph. The efficiency of absorption can reach 70% and the process is not regulated by host nutriture. Carotenes have two possible destinies. If the organism has suboptimal hepatic retinol reserves, carotenes are hydrolysed by cleavage enzymes to retinaldehyde. If the host is replete, the carotenes that are absorbed remain intact and enter the body in the chylomicron fraction. *See* Retinol, Physiology

Vitamin D can be synthesized in the skin through the action of ultraviolet light. In foods, ergosterols from light-exposed milk and cholecalciferol from animal tissues are the major forms. Synthetic varieties of 25-hydroxy- and 1,25-dihydroxycholecalciferols are also available in medicinal forms. The natural varieties are

absorbed as lipids and packaged in chylomicrons. The more polar forms are taken up directly in the portal circulation.

Vitamin E is represented primarily as α-tocopherol in the diet. Tocopherols are absorbed to the extent of 50%. Tocopherols are packaged into chylomicrons in a free form, re-equilibrated into other lipoproteins, and stored in adipose tissue. *See* Tocopherols, Physiology

Vitamin K in the diet comes from plants in the form of phylloquinones, which are absorbed via the lymphatic system. The colonic flora produces menaquinones, which are absorbed to a variable extent by mechanisms not well understood.

Water-soluble Vitamins

The water-soluble vitamins vary from vitamin C with molecular weight (M_r) 256 Da to vitamin B_{12} with a M_r of 1357 Da. Although their absorption from vitamin supplements is highly efficient, in foods they are most often not free, but are in their coenzyme forms, i.e. bound to proteins.

Thiamin is present in foods as thiamin pyrophosphate (TPP). This is hydrolysed nonspecifically to the free vitamin, which is taken up largely in the jejunum. At low concentrations uptake is carrier-mediated, whereas diffusion operates at higher concentrations. The thiamin is rephosphorylated to TPP prior to release into the bloodstream. *See* Thiamin, Physiology

Riboflavin in foods is found primarily in the coenzyme forms, flavin adenine dinucleotide (FAD) and flavin mononucleotide (FMN), but it is liberated nonspecifically during luminal passage. Riboflavin has both an energy-dependent and diffusional uptake mechanism. That which is not required for the needs of the enterocyte is released into the circulation. *See* Riboflavin, Physiology

Niacin comprises the vitamers nicotinic acid and nicotinamide, represented in foods in the cofactor form, nicotinamide adenine dinucleotide (NAD). Intestinal uptake and release into the bloodstream primarily involves the nicotinamide form. *See* Niacin, Physiology

Vitamin B_6 is composed of three vitamers: pyridoxine (PN), pyridoxal (PL) and pyridoxamine (PA). In food the aldehyde and the amine are phosphorylated as PLP and PNP, and the alcohol (PN) is often linked to glucose. In the lumen the vitamers are released by nonspecific hydrolysis. All three forms are absorbed in the jejunum by diffusion and released into the portal circulation in the nonphosphorylated form. *See* Vitamin B_6, Properties and Determination

The majority of bioton in the diet is bound to protein via a peptide linkage with the ε-amino group of lysine. Some is liberated in the lumen by a pancreatic enzyme, and the rest shares the uptake pathway for lysine and small oligopeptides. Biotin absorption is regulated by the biotin status of the host. The vitamin can be taken up from the colon, consistent with a nutritional role for the biotin of bacterial origin synthesized in the large bowel. *See* Biotin, Physiology

Pantothenic acid is derived from coenzyme A (CoA) in tissues of animal origin. It is released from CoA in the intestinal lumen, absorbed by a saturable, energy-dependent mechanism, and released into the circulation as the free acid. *See* Pantothenic Acid, Physiology

Folic acid in foods is found in the polyglutamate form with up to six glutamic acid units linked to the terminal glutamate of the basic vitamin. These glutamic acid units are released by brush border hydrolyases. A more acidic luminal pH favours a neutral electric charge to the glutamic acid and easier traversal of the mucosal membrane. A surface receptor assists in the internalization of the folic acid which is metabolized to the 5-methyl tetrahydrofolic acid form and released into the circulation. *See* Folic Acid, Physiology

The absorption of vitamin B_{12} (cyanocobalamin) of food origin is the most complex for any vitamin. The vitamin is bound to specific proteins (R-proteins) in foods. The action of acid and pepsin releases vitamin B_{12} in the stomach, to be firmly bound by gastric intrinsic factor (IF). Absorption takes place exclusively in the distal ileum, mediated by cellular receptors for the IF–vitamin B_{12} complex which releases the vitamin through the intervention of trypsin in the presence of ionic calcium. Within the ileal cell the vitamin is combined with transcobalamin II and released into the portal circulation. *See* Cobalamins, Physiology

Vitamin C is absorbed in the small intestine both by an energy-dependent mechanism at low concentrations and by simple diffusion at higher concentrations. Net efficiency of absorption is 80–90%. *See* Ascorbic Acid, Physiology

Colonic Salvage of Nondigested and Nonabsorbed Residue

Although the majority of nutrient absorption occurs at the level of the upper small intestine, the colon still plays a role in absorption. It is a major site for the recovery of water and electrolytes that flow through the ileocaecal valve. Limited amounts of magnesium, calcium and zinc are known to be absorbed at the level of the large bowel. The most significant absorptive function of the large intestine, however, may be the salvage of nondigested or nonabsorbed carbohydrate. The colon is normally inhabited by anaerobic and facultative microbial flora. Bacterial enzymes are capable of hydrolysing the covalent bonds of starch, lactose, cellulose, hemicellulose, and the oligosaccharides of beans. Normally, up to 6% of dietary starch is not digested during a typical meal. The fermentation of the carbohydrates liberates carbon

dioxide and hydrogen, with the production of short-chain fatty acids (SCFAs; propionate, butyrate, acetate). The SCFAs are absorbed and can be used for energy metabolism. *See* Colon, Structure and Function; Fatty Acids, Metabolism; Microflora of the Intestine, Role and Effects; Starch, Resistant Starch

Developmental and Senescent Changes in Gastrointestinal Structure and Function

The organs and tissues of the alimentary tract and their functions evolve in a developmental way over the lifespan. Both the nutritional requirements and the gastrointestinal function of the newborn infant are geared to the contents of human milk. As hepatic secretion is immature, pancreatic lipase, which is activated by bile salts, is less active. *Lingual* lipase, from the sublingual glands, initiates the digestion of milk triglycerides in the first years of life. Human milk contains 7% lactose by weight, and the activity of intestinal lactase is increased in early infancy. Conversely, since milk contains no starch, amylase secretion is delayed until the third or fourth month of life. *See* Infants, Nutritional Requirements

Pregnancy is a situation in which a woman is required to provide nutrients to the fetus in addition to her own needs for energy metabolism, work, and augmented tissue. There is evidence of progesterone-induced changes in gut function that increase the efficiency of absorption of minerals such as calcium and zinc, and increased lactase function of the intestine.

It is not resolved whether normal senescence is a developmental or degenerative process. Ageing in humans is associated with decreased motility, a decreased mesenteric blood flow, a lower volume of secretions, and a decreased absorptive surface area. Most notable among the secretory effects is a relative decrease in gastric acid secretion. The consequence of the hypochlorhydria would be a decreased absorptive efficiency for iron and vitamin B_{12}. The combination of slower motility would increase contact time with the absorptive surface, compensating in part for the loss of area. Although there is an age-related decrease in secretions, there is also an age- and activity-related diminution in energy requirements and food intake. The secretory deficit for pancreatic juice and bile does not begin to approach the 90% reduction which is critical for symptomatic maldigestion. *See* Ageing – Nutritional Aspects

Bibliography

Alpers DH (1989) Digestion and absorption of carbohydrates and proteins. In: Johnson LR (ed.) *Physiology of the Gastrointestinal Tract*, pp 1469–1487. New York: Raven Press.

Carey MC, Small DM and Bliss CM (1983) Lipid digestion and absorption. *Annual Review of Physiology* 45: 651–678.

Gray GM (1989) Carbohydrate malabsorption. In: Johnson LR (ed.) *Physiology of the Gastrointestinal Tract*, pp 1063–1072. New York: Raven Press.

Solomons NW and Rosenberg IH (eds) (1984) *Absorption and Malabsorption of Mineral Nutrients*. New York: Alan R Liss.

Walsh JH (1987) Gastrointestinal hormones. In: Johnson LR (ed.) *Physiology of the Gastrointestinal Tract*, pp 181–253. New York: Raven Press.

Noel W. Solomons
Hospital de Ojos y Oidos, Guatemala City, Guatemala

DISEASES

Contents

Diseases of Affluence

Concept

The heart of the proposition is that wealth has become as strongly associated with disease as poverty; and that many of the diseases of the affluent are related to their life style, of which diet is a part. In poverty the nutritionally related diseases are a consequence of deficiencies and, in extreme cases, of starvation. In affluence the nutritionally related diseases result from excesses of particular nutrients and may be further aggravated by specific nutrient imbalances, as well as by the environment and life styles of the populations in the industrialized nations where these diseases are dominant.

There is, however, an anomaly. Within the affluent and industrialized nations, the victims of the 'diseases of affluence' are not only the rich but also the poor.

Morbidity or death from the abuse of alcohol, tobacco or drugs, which are also major health problems in affluent societies, are not included in this review. *See* Alcohol, Metabolism, Toxicology and Beneficial Effects, Smoking, Diet and Health

Scientific Basis of the Concept

The opportunity provided by the creation of the World Health Organization (WHO) within the United Nations (UN) has made possible the study of the aetiology of disease on a comparative basis internationally between continents, subcontinents and nations, and between ethnic and socioeconomic groups as they occur throughout the world. *See* World Health Organization

Such studies are essentially statistical: accumulating data, identifying similarities, assessing the probability of causal relationships between identified associations and postulating a hypothesis to explain the observations that have been acquired.

This method of statistical study, combined with a profound knowledge of human physiology and biochemistry, is the *modus operandi* of the epidemiologist, but it is contrary to the experience of the laboratory scientist, who expects demonstrable proof of causality through intervention. *See* Epidemiology

The near impossibility of intervention in human studies, and the failure of many to understand the philosophical difference in approach between epidemiologists and laboratory-based experimental scientists has not only led to sterile arguments but also, in the UK, may have delayed the introduction and implementation of preventive measures.

Currently Recognized Diseases of Affluence

Life-shortening

Two groups of diseases are associated with premature death in the developed countries: cardiovascular diseases and cancers. In the UK it has been reported by the Department of Health that, in 1988, these diseases accounted for approximately half of the years of life lost up to the age of 65 (44% in men and 52% in women).

Cardiovascular diseases Coronary heart disease (CHD) has been recognized as a public health problem in North America and in Europe since the early part of the century; by the 1950s it was recognized by WHO to be the single major cause of adult death. The classical studies of Ancel Keys began at that time and the involvement of diet in the aetiology of CHD is now beyond dispute. *See* Coronary Heart Disease, Intervention Studies

Cerebrovascular disease (stroke) The strong correlation between stroke and diastolic blood pressure (risk increases 10-fold over a range of 40 mmHg) has resulted in more recent studies concentrating on blood pressure. Here, the increase with age appears to be a characteristic of advanced societies rather than of developed versus developing countries. The causes of high blood pressure are multifactorial and include diets that are common in Western-style societies. *See* Hypertension, Hypertension and Diet

Cancers There are many aetiologies characterizing the wide variety of situations in which cancers occur. Cancers particularly associated with the 'Westernized' world and with the dietary habits prevailing there include the following: lung; gastric; endocrine-related – prostate, breast and ovary; endometrium; colon – distal and rectal. Other cancers occur in affluent societies and also in developing countries. *See* Cancer, Epidemiology

Increasing Morbidity

Obesity Whilst not conventionally classified as a disease, obesity is so strongly associated with diseases that increase morbidity as well as with those that shorten life, that it would be misleading to omit this dominant characteristic of the 'affluent societies'. *See* Obesity, Aetiology and Assessment

Dental caries Attention has been drawn to the high incidence of dental decay in children aged 11–12 years in Westernized societies and the correlation with the high consumption of sugar in these societies. *See* Dental Disease, Aetiology of Dental Caries

Non-Insulin-Dependent Diabetes Mellitus (NIDDM) A chronic metabolic disorder, NIDDM is characterized by an inability to utilize glucose. Its onset is typically in middle age in overweight individuals. Whilst not exclusively a disease of 'Westernized societies', it is dominant in these societies which are also characterized by overweight and obesity.

Evidence for Links with Diet

In 1926, in one of the earliest publications on diet and health, Sir Robert McCarrison propounded two principles concerning food and health derived from his classical comparative studies of populations from north and south India. These were (1) the importance of eating from a wide range of foods, and (2) the vital role in these of essential nutrients. During the following 25 years the identities of the essential nutrients were established and their function in preventing the onset of the acute, but reversible nutritional disorders which then prevailed was elucidated. In the current decade a new role has been postulated for many of these micronutrients in the prevention of some of the chronic diseases of affluent societies. This will be discussed later in this article, in the section on prevention.

It was not until the second half of this century that the first of McCarrison's principles was examined internationally and in depth, and it is from these studies that the current concepts of diet and health in relation to macronutrients and chronic disease have developed.

It is not surprising, from the broad scope of McCarrison's two principles, that the many different diseases of affluence are associated with the same macro- and micronutrients. Consequently this section is organized, not by disease, but by nutrient.

Correlation with Chronic Disease

The evidence is mainly dependent on multivariant analysis, including national, international and migratory studies. However, it is not always possible to quantify the contribution of a particular nutrient because of interactions, both between nutrients and with nondietary components, including genetic, environmental and behavioural.

Nevertheless, it is possible to indicate that associations between classes of nutrients and particular diseases are probable, and also to make positive recommendations with statistical confidence on the classes of foods that are desirable.

Complex Carbohydrates

Dietary Fibre from Cereals

Professor Dennis Burkitt and the late Dr Hugh Trowell proposed that, in Westernized societies, the decline in the consumption of dietary fibre from cereals was related to the rise there of the diseases of affluence. *See* Dietary Fibre, Fibre and Disease Prevention

Wholewheat flour was once a major part of the diet, and Trowell's data demonstrate the extent of the change in consumption over two centuries (Table 1). Moreover, the lower intakes of cereal dietary fibre (measured as crude fibre at that time) in the current century correspond with the rise in the incidence of disorders of the bowel, including cancers.

A Report in 1981 of the Royal College of Physicians of London, UK, concluded that there was a link between a deficiency of dietary fibre and diseases of the large bowel, including irritable bowel syndrome, constipation, diverticulitis, and colonic cancer.

Subsequent research has resulted in the chemical fractionation of Trowell's 'dietary fibre' and the more precise term 'nonstarch polysaccharide' (NSP) has been proposed and endorsed in the UK by the Department of Health in its *Report on Dietary Reference Values.*

Diseases of Affluence

Table 1. Consumption of wheat flour in England and Wales

	Year		
	1770	1870	1970
Preparation	Light sifting	Moderate sifting	70–72% Extracted
Crude fibre content (g per 100 g of wheat)	1·25	0·35	0·10
Consumption of wheat (g per day)	500	375	200
Crude fibre intake (g per day)	6·25	1·30	0·20

Burkitt DP and Trowell HC (1975)

Correlations of NSP with disease

Negative correlations, i.e. the more NSP consumed the lower the incidence of disease, have been reported for cancers of the lung, prostate, bladder, rectum, oral cavity, stomach, cervix and oesophagus, and also for diverticular disease, haemorrhoids, constipation and gallstones.

Lipids

The Seven Countries study, published in 1980, confirmed the views that had been developing since 1945, that there was a positive correlation between CHD and the consumption of fat. Specifically, a correlation of 0·84 was found in men, between age-adjusted deaths in the 10-year period and the consumption of saturated fatty acids. Comparable data were obtained within one country, Italy, where 14 regions were compared. In all cases the correlations for women were weaker.

In much of the earlier data the positive correlation of CHD with plasma cholesterol led to some confusion, plasma cholesterol being an indicator and consequence of the ingestion of fat, dietary cholesterol not being a direct cause. In the past decade the situation has been clarified. Cholesterol is carried in the plasma in association with lipoprotein in two main forms: high-density lipoprotein (HDL)-cholesterol and low-density lipoprotein (LDL)-cholesterol. The HDL form appears to be beneficial in respect of vulnerability to CHD, whereas the LDL form is strongly correlated with premature incidence of CHD. *See* Cholesterol, Role of Cholesterol in Heart Disease; Hyperlipidaemia; Lipoproteins

The incidence of CHD is not related directly or solely to the amounts of saturated fatty acids consumed, but to an interaction of the following dietary factors, although their effects may be modified in any one individual by

Table 2. Bodyweight and mortality ratios from coronary heart disease in males and females aged between 40 and 49 years

Weight index	Mortality ratio		Notes
	Male	Female	
90–109	1·00	1·00	Average
110–119	1·34	1·59	Mild overweight
120–129	1·67	2·71	Overweight
130–139	1·93	2·71	Obese

Royal College of Physicians of London (1983) Obesity *Journal of the Royal College of Physicians* 17: 3–58.

nondietary factors including genetic susceptibility, smoking, exercise and stress:

- The percentage of dietary energy obtained from saturated fatty acids.
- The ratio of polyunsaturated to saturated fatty acids (P:S ratio).
- Concentration of plasma LDL-cholesterol
- A significant, but as yet unquantified amount of dietary monounsaturated fatty acid.

Dietary Energy

Obesity, at least in part, is a consequence of overconsumption of energy and is a confounding issue in most diseases of affluence. The impact of bodyweight on mortality ratios from CHD (Table 2) was reported by the Royal College of Physicians of London in 1983 and the results of subsequent research enhance rather than reduce the significance of their findings.

Salt

The correlation with stroke is indirect. The incidence of stroke is positively correlated with diastolic blood pressure, which is correlated with the consumption of salt. The WHO data support the following statements:

1. Sustained difference of 7·5 mmHg in diastolic blood pressure confers up to a 44% difference in risk of stroke (from nine major international studies).
2. There is no increase in diastolic blood pressure with age when intakes of salt are less than 3 g per day (from the Intersalt study of 52 centres in 32 countries). *See* Sodium, Physiology

Prevalence

There follows a summary of the mortality from these diseases of affluence in the UK (from national statistics) and internationally (from WHO statistics).

Diseases of Affluence

Table 3. Classification of body mass

| | Body Mass Index | |
	Male	Female
Acceptable	20·1–25·0	18·7–23·8
Overweight	25·1–29·9	23·9–28·5
Obese	30·0 and over	28·6 and over

Table 4. Trends in body mass index, expressed as a percentage of the total UK population

| | Male | | Female | |
	1980	1986–1987	1980	1986–1987
Acceptable	51	49	54	52
Overweight	33	37	24	24
Obese	6	8	8	12
Underweight	10	6	14	12

Coronary Heart Disease

In the seven Countries study, published in 1980, the death rate from CHD per 100 000 ranged from 144 in Japan to 1202 in east Finland. In 1982 the rate in the UK was 370.

Stroke

The death rate for stroke in the UK is low. In 1978, for example, it was only 112 per 100 000, whereas in Japan it was the major cause of death from circulatory disorders. Nevertheless, in rural populations amongst tribal societies the condition is almost unknown.

Cancers

Deaths per 100 000 between the ages of 55 and 64 from all neoplasms in 1988 ranged from 340 in Japan to 470 in the UK. Deaths from breast cancer were 22 in Japan and 104 in the UK. In all cases, deaths from these causes in other European countries and in the USA and Australia were intermediate between those of Japan and the UK.

Obesity

Because of the interaction of bodyweight with the major diseases of affluence, it is appropriate to consider overweight, and particularly obesity, as a disease of affluence itself.

The internationally accepted measure of obesity is based on the body mass index (BMI). This is the body mass, m (in kg), divided by the square of the height, h^2 (in m), i.e. $m/(h^2)$. Using this measure, body mass is classified as shown in Table 3.

Recently published data in the UK (1990) indicate the trends in bodyweight during the past decade shown in Table 4.

Consequences for Populations

Populations consist of aggregates of individuals and their health is determined by the interaction of four sets of circumstances: genetic, environmental, personal habit and diet. This section is concerned with only one of these, namely diet, but it must be borne in mind that the effects described may be modified by one or more of the other influencing factors.

Occurrence and Distribution

Unless there is evidence to the contrary, it is customary to assume that the frequency of consumption of a food or nutrient within a population will be distributed in accordance with the 'normal' distribution curve. Hence there will be equal numbers of abstainers and excessive consumers, and the majority will be spread evenly on either side of the median. It is simplest to assume that the median is coincident with both the mean and the mode. In other words, the arithmetical average coincides with that point where there are equal numbers consuming less and more, and with the highest consumption. It is this model which is used in the subsequent discussion.

Risk

It is implicit in the previous discussion that certain habits, and specifically dietary ones, will increase the risk of the incidence of a chronic disease. In practice this will be translated into a certain number of individuals who will develop the disease. In terms of their occurrence within a population, they will be at one end of the distribution curve, and it is conventional to consider that those at the most risk are to the right of the median.

It is a problem for those concerned with public health to define 'acceptable risk' and, conventionally, this will be taken to be at the median of the distribution of the population. Those to the right of this median will be at increased risk, those to the left at decreased risk.

Whilst an undesirable diet is an important risk factor in predicting premature death, it is not the only one, and it should be noted that when total risk is being assessed, the individual factors are not additive – they must be multiplied.

Impact of Premature Death

In Westernized societies the infant mortality is low, at 8·4 per 100 000 in the UK and spreading between 6·8 and 13·1 per 100 000 in western Europe. There is also an increased expectation of life for those over the age of 65. In the UK population, for example, there is the highest proportion ever of centenarians. A consequence is a distortion of the age–population–distribution curve in which the numbers of young and old are disproportionately large compared with the numbers of middle-aged individuals. There is a further distortion in favour of the longer survival of females compared with males. The economic and social implications of these distortions from a 'normal' distribution are considerable.

Prevention

The writers of the preface to the discussion paper, *Proposals for Nutritional Guidelines for Health Education in Britain* (NACNE, 1983), drew attention to two major theoretical issues of great practical importance:

> The first is whether in mass disease with exceedingly high incidence such as dental caries or coronary heart disease efforts should be made to rectify the manifest dietary defects of the populations as a whole, or whether such efforts should be limited to those individuals who can be shown to be at specifically high risk ... The second is the dilemma that in public education clear and specific, quantitative messages are now manifestly desirable instead of the general admonitions to reduce this, or increase that, which have so often been ineffectual in the past.

It is clear from the earlier discussion of the quantitative significance of a 'normal' distribution that the greatest numbers lie around the median, and that risk is decreased if the median is moved to the left. It follows that the greatest impact on the health of a population will be made by policies which have an impact on the total numbers who are most at risk. Of course, a secondary objective of counselling those individuals at most risk is not precluded by a population approach. This rationale is now accepted in virtually all Westernized societies and the population recommendations recently published by the WHO are summarized in Table 5. *See* Nutrition Education

The impact of these recommendations on the populations of an industrialized nation such as the UK is illustrated in Table 6, which shows the average nutrient intakes of British adults (aged 16–24 years) during the period 1986–1987, reported by the Office of Population Censuses and Surveys (OPCS). *See* National Nutrition Policies

Micronutrients

Two recently proposed hypotheses have renewed scientific interest in certain micronutrients. The first concerns

Table 5. Limits for average intakes for populations

Nutrient	Lower limit	Upper limit
Total energy	Sufficient to maintain in adults a BMI of 20–22	
As percentage of total energy		
Total fat	15	30
Saturated fatty acids	0	10
Polyunsaturated fatty acids	3	7
Total carbohydrates	55	75
Complex carbohydrates	50	70
Free sugars	0	10
Protein	10	15
As absolute amounts (g per day)		
Total dietary fibre	27	40
Nonstarch polysaccharides	16	24
Salt	Not defined	6
Dietary cholesterol	0	0·3

BMI, body mass index.

Table 6. Nutrient intakes of British adults

	Mean	Lower 2·5 percentile	Upper 2·5 percentile
Total energy (kcal)			
Male	2450	1330	3620
Female	1680	800	2580
As percentage of total energy			
Total fat			
Male	37·6	26·6	47·1
Female	39·2	28·3	48·6
Saturated fatty acids			
Male	15·4	9·6	21·7
Female	16·5	10·4	22·9
Polyunsaturated fatty acids			
Male	0·7	0·4	1·3
Female	0·7	0·4	1·4
Total carbohydrate			
Male	41·6	29·1	53·8
Female	43·0	30·3	55·5
Protein			
Male	14·1	9·4	19·9
Female	15·2	10·4	23·4
As absolute amounts (g per day)			
Total dietary fibre			
Male	24·9	10·3	44·8
Female	18·6	7·5	33·5
Salt			
Male	8·8	4·0	14·6
Female	6·1	3·0	9·7
Dietary cholesterol			
Male	0·4	0·2	0·7
Female	0·3	0·1	0·5

the possible relation between essential and polyunsaturated fatty acids (EFAs and PUFAs) in reducing the risk of CHD. The first two fatty acids listed below are essential and the rest are formed in the body but, because their rate of formation may not always be adequate, they are sometimes included as EFAs:

- Linoleic acid (C18:2 n−6)
- α-Linolenic acid (C18:3 n−3)
- Arachidonic acid (C20:4 n−6)
- Eicosapentaenoic acid (C20:5 n−3)
- Docosapentaenoic acid (C22:5 n−3)
- Docosahexanoic acid (C22:6 n−3)

The 'Multiple Risk Factor Intervention Trial' research group have recently demonstrated support for the hypothesis that these fatty acids, and especially those found in fish oils (C20:5, C22:5, and C22:6), protect against cardiovascular disease. *See* Fatty Acids, Metabolism; Fatty Acids, Gamma Linolenic Acid; Fish Oils, Dietary Importance

The second, and more recent, hypothesis relates to the possibility that certain cancers arise from an excessive activity of 'free radicals', resulting from the oxidation of metabolites, and that vitamins with an antioxidant activity might reduce the risk.

Antioxidant Vitamins

The antioxidant vitamins are carotene and vitamins C and E; the group also includes the trace mineral selenium because of its interaction with vitamin E. Their possible role in the 'antioxidant' theory and the validity of the hypothesis itself is currently being tested through six intervention trials, sponsored in whole or in part by F Hoffmann–La Roche from a coordinating centre in Basle and involving multicentre studies as well as studies located in Duisburg, Helsinki, London and Nottingham. *See* Antioxidants, Natural Antioxidants

The incidence of both cancers and coronary vascular diseases are being studied through placebo-controlled and double-blind studies in major clinical centres. The total number of individuals is 46 000.

Health Education

The challenge facing health education workers is to reach communities. There are fewer problems on a one-to-one basis; in such circumstances there is generally a history of illness and the 'patient' is anxious to avoid a repetition.

Concepts

Educationists recognize two approaches:

1. Health communication aiming to induce behaviour change.
2. Community organization for health.

Underlying the first is diffusion theory, whilst the second depends on concepts of community self-development.

Approach

It is necessary to assess the following before initiating a community programme:

1. Critical mass: a minimum of 15% of the community must be sympathetic to the proposed programme at the outset.
2. Structural obstacles.
3. Natural rhythm: cyclic activities or external factors which may influence behaviour in the community, such as national campaigns.
4. Marketing.
5. Cost–benefit awareness.

Implementation

Six key steps are recommended by health professionals:

1. Become proficient in the use of effective mediated and face-to-face teaching methods.
2. Establish a sound and ethical content of instruction.
3. Collaborate with local forces in programme development.
4. Use communication pathways that are natural to the system.
5. Activate opinion leaders to accelerate diffusion and the adoption of transformation.
6. Assist in community transformation.

Examples of Successful Community Studies

Examples of large-scale multifactorial community studies that have been completed and have resulted in a change in the desired direction of the behaviour of the communities with respect to health are listed in Table 7.

Table 7. Examples of successful community studies

Location	Number of individuals	Period
Stamford, USA	350 000	1980–1986
North Karelia, Finland	435 000	1972–1980
North Coast Project, Australia	70 000	1977–1980
Swiss National Research Programme	224 000	1979–
Heidelberg, FRG	30 000	1980–
South Africa Study	16 000	1980–

Bibliography

Boyden S (1987) *Western Civilization in Biological Perspective: Patterns in Biohistory*. Oxford: Clarendon Press.

Burkitt DP and Trowell HC (eds) (1975) *Refined Carbohydrate Foods and Disease*. London: Academic Press.

Department of Health (1991) *Dietary Reference Values for Food Energy and Nutrients for the United Kingdom*. Report on Health and Social Subjects 41. London: HMSO.

Glass RL (ed.) (1982) The First International Conference on the Declining Prevalence of Dental Caries. *Journal of Dental Research* 61: 1304–1383.

Gregory J, Foster K, Tyler H and Wiseman M (1990). *The Dietary and Nutritional Survey of British Adults*. London: Her Majesty's Stationery Office (HMSO).

Holland B, Welch AA, Unwin ID *et al.* (1991) *McCance and Widdowson's: The Composition of Foods* 5th edn. Cambridge: Royal Society of Chemistry.

Holland WW, Detels R and Knox G (ed.) (1985) *Oxford Textbook of Public Health*, vol. 3. Oxford: Oxford University Press.

James WPT and Schofield EC (1990) *Human Energy Requirements*. Oxford: Oxford University Press.

Keys A (1980) *Seven Countries: A Multivariate Analysis of Death and Coronary Heart Disease*. Cambridge, Massachusetts: Harvard University Press.

NACNE (1983) *Proposals for Nutritional Guidelines for Health Education in Britain*. London: The Health Education Council.

Simopoulos AP, Kifer RR, Martin RE and Barlow SM (eds) (1990) *Proceedings of the 2nd International Conference on the Health Effects of omega-3 Polyunsaturated Fatty Acids in Seafoods*, Washington, DC. London: Karger.

Weisburger JH (1991) Nutritional approach to cancer prevention with emphasis on vitamins, antioxidants, and carotenoids. *American Journal of Clinical Nutrition* 53(supplement): 226s–237s.

WHO Study Group (1990) Diet, nutrition, and the prevention of chronic diseases. *World Health Organization Technical Report Series* 797.

Derek H. Shrimpton
Cambridge, UK

Diseases Transmitted by Food

The presence of microorganisms in food is not necessarily an indicator of hazard to the consumer. Except for a few sterilized products, every mouthful of food contains some innocuous yeast, mould, bacteria, or other microflora. Most food becomes potentially hazardous to the consumer only when the principles of sanitation and hygiene are violated. If food has been subjected to conditions that could allow growth of infectious or toxigenic agents, it may become the vehicle for transmission of disease in humans, either by the proliferation of the microorganisms in the host or as a result of preformed toxin following multiplication in the food. A number of diseases require a sufficient number of infective cells to be present in the food before ingestion in order to proliferate successfully in the gastrointestinal tract against many competing and inhibiting microorganisms and to produce characteristic symptoms. Others require only a few initial cells from which rapid proliferation to toxigenic levels can proceed in the gastrointestinal tract. In addition, the degree of virulence and severity of toxic effects is affected by factors which are related to the host, the food, and the bacterial environment.

There are five sources of bacteria causing foodborne diseases: (1) faecal matter (either with a normal microflora, or infected) and/or urine of infected humans or animals; (2) nasal and throat discharges of sick individuals or asymptomatic carriers; (3) infection or natural carriage of toxigenic microorganisms on body surfaces of food handlers; (4) infected soil, mud, surface waters, dust; (5) sea water and marine materials. One or more of these sources may contribute to food contamination. The Joint World Health Organization (WHO) and Food and Agriculture Organization (FAO) Expert Committee has noted that even in developed countries foodborne diseases are the second largest cause of morbidity. In most of these diseases, the food serves only as a vehicle of transmission – the final link in the chain of infection. The role of food here is significant, since the product may not only permit the survival of the pathogen, but also provide a suitable medium for the rapid proliferation of the microorganism, and the production of toxin, as in the case of exotoxin-producing organisms. Thus the degree to which these parameters are made possible by the contaminated food product may determine the final infectiveness of these products, the severity of the symptoms, and the extent of the outbreak or epidemic. *See* Food Poisoning, Statistics

Occurrence of Corynebacteriaceae and Streptococcaceae

The genus *Corynebacterium* was created essentially for the diphtheria bacillus and a few other animal pathogenic species. However, over many years other nonsporing, irregularly staining, Gram-positive species, both aerobic and anaerobic, were assigned to the genus. Now well-defined on the basis of chemical criteria, the genus *Corynebacterium* consists of 16 species, including 6 human pathogens: *C. diphtheriae*, *C. pseudotuberculosis*, *C. xerosis*, *C. minutissimus*, *C. mycetoides* and *C. ulcerans*. Among the species of *Corynebacterium* only *C. diphtheriae*, the causative agent of diphtheria, and *C. ulcerans* are transmitted by food, including raw milk. In temperate climates the diphtheria bacilli colonize the mucous membranes of the fauces, pharynx and trachea. These forms of the infection are called, respectively, faucal, pharyngeal, laryngeal, and tracheal diphtheria. In moist tropical areas colonization often occurs on the mucous membranes of the skin and results in cutaneous diphtheria. Three cultural types of *C. diphtheriae* are recognized, described as gravis, intermedius and mitis. Each of the cultural types contains numerous serological types and phage types. Thus *C. diphtheriae* have the potential to accommodate to the defences of the human host against invasiveness, much as in the case of group A streptococci and *Streptococcus pneumoniae*. Most strains produce a highly lethal exotoxin which is the cause of death in diphtheria, and the toxin produced by all three cultural types is identical. The exotoxin from *C. ulcerans* is distinct chemically from the diphtheria toxin(s), but the pharmacological impact is similar.

The genus *Streptococcus* consists of a heterogeneous group of Gram-positive, nonmotile and nonsporulating bacteria with a broad significance in medicine and industry. They are traditionally separated from other genera on the basis of their mode of cell division and the major products of glucose fermentation, although the validity of these criteria is perhaps debatable. Because of the diversity of the streptococci, several attempts have been made over the years to organize the organisms into broad groups. The designation of four main divisions (pyogenic, viridous, lactic and enterococcus) by Sherman in 1937 proved to be useful, at least for descriptive purposes. A recent numerical study of streptococci revealed 28 reasonably distinct phenons. In Bergey's system, the genus is divided into six groups designated pyogenic, oral, enterococci, lactic, anaerobic and other streptococci. *Streptococcus pneumoniae* was included in the pyogenic group. A recent trend in streptococcal taxonomy has been towards the more extensive application of numerical, chemotaxonomic and genetic techniques, with less emphasis on serological criteria for classification. However, serology remains important for identification and typing of some major pathogens.

The nomenclature of the streptococci is still based largely on serogroup identification of cell wall components (Lancefield serogroup). The antigens known as group-specific antigens, also called C-substances, are either polysaccharides (as in groups A, B, C, E, F and G), which are associated with the cell wall, or teichoic acids (groups D and N) situated in the region between the cell membrane and the inner surface of the cell wall. In addition to the major group antigens, a number of type-specific antigens (such as M, T and R antigens of *s. pyogenes*) are also recognized. Such antigens are commonly proteins, although polysaccharide types also occur, as in group F.

Streptococci are responsible for a large number of important diseases of humans and animals. Some strains are essential in industrial and dairy processes while others are indicators of pollution. The pyogenic group are the major pathogens, but many of the other species are commonly involved in disease processes, often as opportunistic pathogens. Much of the available evidence about toxins and pathogenic mechanisms is related to *S. pyogenes*, which produces haemolysins (streptolysins O and S), erythrogenic toxin, pyrogenic exotoxin, streptokinase, nucleae, proteinase, hyaluronidase and nicotinamide adenine dinucleotide (NAD)-ase, in addition to other extracellular products. However, despite the variety of cell-associated and extracellular products produced by streptococci, no clear scheme of pathogenesis has been defined.

From the standpoint of human health, by far the most important streptococci are two major species that cause severe infections: *S. pyogenes* and *S. pneumoniae*. Some of the other medically important streptococci are as follows: *S. agalactiae*, aetiological agent of neonatal disease; *Enterococcus* (see below) *faecalis*, a major cause of endocarditis; *S. zooepidemicus*, which has been linked with fatalities associated with raw milk ingestion; *S. mutans* and *S. sanguis*, which are involved in dental caries. The streptococci are widely distributed in nature and are frequently part of the endogenous microbial flora, particularly of the mouth, nasopharynx and intestinal tract; they are also part of the normal flora of the genitourinary tract and the skin of humans and animals. Approximately 5–15% of humans carry *S. pyogenes* or *S. agalactiae* in the nasopharynx, and the carrier rate of *S. pneumoniae* in the normal human nasopharynx is even higher, ranging from 20% to 40%. Although the primary habitat of the group D streptococci (now classified in the genus *Enterococcus*) is the human and animal gastrointestinal tract, they have also been isolated in large numbers from cheese, milk and meat, as well as from vegetables, other plants and insects, indicating the widespread distribution of streptococci.

Mechanism of Entry into Food and Transmission to Humans

Corynebacterium diphtheriae has no known host other than humans. Animals such as cows may be infected but, in general, human carriers play a definite role in the spread of diphtheria, transmitting the organism to food products. Whenever a food source of the infection is incriminated, it is generally raw milk or milk products, such as ice cream. However, at the present time, pasteurization has profoundly diminished the role of milk in the epidemiology of diphtheria, especially in developed countries such as the UK and the USA.

Although most streptococcal diseases are spread by direct or indirect human contact, numerous outbreaks of a serious and explosive nature have been transmitted by food, particularly via raw milk and other dairy products, or by human carriers involved in the preparation of food. In the dairy-associated cases, the source of infection was usually the mastitic udder of the cow which supplied the milk. Presumably, the udders of these cows were infected by milkers and farmers who were suffering from β-haemolytic streptococcal infection such as septic sore throat. The source of another outbreak of group A streptococcal infection was ham believed to have been contaminated by a human carrier in the pre-eruptive stage of scarlet fever. In this outbreak, the ham, prepared by the carrier and another woman, was allowed to stand for several hours at room temperature before being served. Thus the streptococci were allowed ample time to multiply. Other foods have also been incriminated as vehicles of reported outbreaks. These include creamed eggs, egg salad, potato salad, shrimp salad, rice pudding, custard, cold cuts and tuna salad. In general, almost all foods associated with β-haemolytic streptococcal outbreaks are those prepared by hand from basic cold ingredients and served without preliminary heating or cooking, i.e. salads of all types. *See* Milk, Processing of Liquid Milk

Although group B streptococci (*S. agalactiae*) are transmitted mostly through other routes, it has been reported that neonatal infection may be transmitted through the mother's milk. Presumably, the contamination is transmitted to the nipple by the mother's hand. On the other hand, the infant contaminated with group B streptococci during birth may harbour the organisms in the throat and nose, and the child may then contaminate the mother's nipple or the milk inside the mammary gland by negative pressure during suckling. The bacteria, having proliferated in large numbers in the milk, may then be ingested by the child and produce a serious infection.

Foods may also contain other streptococci, both from the oral group and the enterococci. The route of their transmission to food is direct or indirect faecal contamination.

Fate on Processing and Storage

Corynebacterium diphtheriae can withstand dry conditions for at least 5 weeks and frozen storage for at least 5 days. It can be killed by heating for 10 min at 58°C and by treatment with a disinfectant. Thus pasteurization, wherever it is practised properly, has certainly eliminated the occurrence of *C. diphtheriae* in food. Nevertheless, post-pasteurization contamination of milk has been known to occur. *See* Pasteurization, Principles

The pyogenic streptococci generally grow within the temperature range 20–40°C, with an optimum of about 37°C. Most of the enterococci (group D streptococci) grow at 45°C, but also at 10°C. The enterococci can tolerate a high salt concentration (6·5% sodium chloride; NaCl) and will grow at pH 9·6. Most streptococci are killed by heating at 55°C for 30 min, but the enterococci survive at 60°C for 30 min. Furthermore,

some strains of enterococci (*Enterococcus faecalis*) as well as some β-haemolytic streptococci are able to survive at even higher temperatures, e.g. 71·7°C for 15–16 s. Fortunately, these strains, in contrast to non-heat-resistant *S. pyogenes*, are not pathogens. A remarkable characteristic of enterococci is their ability to recover from thermal injury and to transmit this trait to succeeding generations. The sublethal injury of enterococcal cells may thus lead to selection of organisms with greater salt tolerance and heat resistance. In semipreserved, processed, and heat-treated, nonsterile foods, the enterococci, along with spore-formers, are very often the only surviving organisms. Enterococci may proliferate to very large numbers in foods held in the mesophilic range, particularly between 10°C and 45°C. If a canned food, particularly one of neutral pH, becomes contaminated from unchlorinated cooling water, or is underprocessed, then enterococci may survive at 37°C for at least 30 days. Their growth may continue unrestricted for 60 days at 22–37°C.

Pathogenicity, Symptoms and Characteristics

Diphtheria is an acute, highly contagious and, in many cases, very severe and fatal infection. The symptoms develop gradually following an incubation period of 1–10 days. The symptoms may begin initially with moderate fever (38·9°C), mild sore throat, malaise and fatigue. A membranous layer or formation, which is either white, yellowish, or greenish-yellow tinged with grey, develops in the throat. This membrane, which is diagnostic of diphtheria, may develop first on one tonsil, then spread to the other tonsil and other structures of the throat, parts of the palate and nasal passages. As the disease advances complications involving the cardiovascular systems, nervous system (paralysis of various muscles) and respiratory system soon develop.

Streptococci vary widely in pathogenic potential. As previously described, *S. pneumoniae* and, to a lesser extent, *S. pyogenes* are part of the normal human nasopharyngeal flora. Their numbers are usually limited by competition from the nasopharyngeal microbial ecosystem and by nonspecific host defence mechanisms, but failure of these mechanisms can result in disease. More commonly, disease can result from acquisition of a new strain, following alteration of the normal flora. *Streptococcus pyogenes* causes inflammatory purulent lesions with resulting tissue damage directly at the portal of entry, often the upper respiratory tract; alternatively, it may affect the skin. In general, however, streptococcal isolates from the pharynx and respiratory tract do not cause skin infections. Invasion of other parts of the respiratory tract results in infections of the middle ear (otitis media), sinuses (sinusitis), or lungs (pneumonia).

In addition, meningitis can occur by direct extension of infection from the middle ear or sinuses to the meninges or by way of bloodstream invasion from a pulmonary focus. Bacteraemia can also result in damage to bones (osteomyelitis) or joints (arthritis).

Streptococcus pyogenes is the leading cause of bacterial pharyngitis and tonsillitis. The disease most often caused by these bacteria is commonly called septic sore throat or 'strep throat'. From reports of foodborne outbreaks of septic sore throat, the incubation period ranges from 12 to 108 h. Another group A streptococcal disease is scarlet fever, which has an incubation period between 1 and 6 days, and commonly 2 to 3 days. Both diseases are characterized by fever (37·8–40°C), headache and sore throat, manifested by pain on swallowing. The other symptoms are chills, malaise, prostration, nausea, vomiting, hoarseness, diarrhoea, anorexia, syncope, incapacitating muscular weakness, nasal symptoms, earache and epistaxis. Pharyngeal exudate, tender, enlarged cervical lymph nodes, oedema of the uvula, and swollen tonsils and posterior oropharynx are also seen together in patients. In addition, the characteristic erythematous skin rash with red specks or puncta (punctate erythema), and strawberry or raspberry tongue are striking symptoms of scarlet fever. Although scarlet fever was formerly very disabling and fatal, especially following such toxic complication as myocarditis, it is now little more than streptococcal pharyngitis accompanied by a rash. Similarly, erysipelas, a form of cellulitis accompanied by fever and systemic toxicity, is less common today. Group A streptococcal infections can also result in sinusitis, otitis, mastoiditis, pneumonia, arthritis or bone infections, and, more infrequently, meningitis or endocarditis; infections of the skin can be superficial (impetigo) or deep (cellulitis). *Streptococcus pneumoniae* is the leading cause of bacterial pneumonia in adults. This organism is also the most common cause of sinusitis, acute bacterial otitis media, and conjunctivitis beyond early childhood. Dissemination from the respiratory focus results in serious disease: outpatient bacteraemia in children; meningitis; occasionally, acute septic arthritis and bone infections in patients with sickle cell disease; more rarely, peritonitis or endocarditis.

Recently, the pathogenic potential for humans of some of the non-group-A streptococci has been clarified. Group B streptococci, a major cause of bovine mastitis, are also a leading cause of neonatal septicaemia and meningitis and, thus, account for significant mortality. They have also been associated with pneumonia in elderly patients, as well as with adult urogenital infections, meningitis, bacteraemia and endocarditis. Streptococci of groups C and G are associated with mild as well as severe human diseases, such as mild upper respiratory tract infection, and endocarditis. Enterococci (group D streptococci) are important aetiological agents in enteritis and are associated with urinary tract infections, bacteraemia, and endocarditis, and in some causes of disseminated infection. The toxic dose in enteritis involves a large number of organisms. The incubation period is from 2 to 36 h; average 6–12 h. The symptoms may last 3 to 4 days and include nausea, abdominal pain (colic), diarrhoea and vomiting. Although there have been many claims of the involvement of foods heavily contaminated with enterococci in foodborne disease, the majority of authors have failed to induce experimental disease in humans. Aside from possibly being associated with foodborne disease, the enterococci occasionally become 'opportunistic pathogens'. It is not uncommon, for example, to find them as the causative organism in cases of urinary infections, neonatal meningitis, endocarditis, septicaemia, etc.

Group F streptococci are associated with abscess formation and purulent disease. Group R streptococci – well-documented causes of meningitis and septicaemia in pigs – also pose a serious health hazard to workers in the pork industry. The diverse group of organisms classified as viridans streptococci and oral streptococci includes important aetiological agents of subacute bacterial endocarditis. Dental manipulation and dental disease are the most common predisposing factors in subacute bacterial endocarditis. *Streptococcus mutans* and *S. sanguis* are responsible for the formation of dental plaque, the dense adhesive microbial mass which colonizes teeth and is linked to caries and other human oral disease. Finally, anaerobic streptococci are linked to a wide variety of serious infections of the female genital tract, as well as brain, pulmonary, and abdominal abscesses. *See* Dental Disease, Aetiology of Dental Caries; Pork

Detection in Foods

Routine examination of foods for haemolytic streptococci is unwarranted, except perhaps for raw milk and canned meats. However, special epidemiological investigations of disease outbreaks may require extensive sampling and analysis of suspect foods. Detection of pyogenic β-haemolytic streptococci in food in any quantity should be cause for serious concern. The other haemolytic streptococci are of considerably less significance to human health, but their presence may indicate inadequate thermal processing of food, or subsequent contamination by carriers. The enterococci, however, survive milk pasteurization.

No satisfactory selective medium exists for the quantitative estimation of haemolytic streptococci in foods, particularly when they are present as a minority percentage of the overall flora. Nevertheless, horse blood agar serves reasonably well for examining raw milk or similar dairy foods in which the predominant flora is most likely to be streptococci and other lactic acid bacteria that characteristically produce punctiform colonies. Haemolytic streptococci numbering as few as 1% of the flora can generally be detected and enumerated in milk. Blood agar also serves well to isolate causative organisms, including streptococci, from local abscesses and other suppurative material in raw meats.

Numerous attempts have been made to devise selective or differential media for the quantitative determination of group D streptococci in food. At least 30 such media have been used with varying degrees of success. However, two common plating media employed for enumerating the enterococci in foods are Parker's crystal-violet azide blood agar and KF-Streptococcus agar. The KF-agar appears to be more selective and differential than Parker's medium. The enterococcus colonies are recognized by their characteristic size and coloration. Confirmation tests are performed on isolated cultures. In addition, proof that the cultures belong to serological group D can be obtained by preparing extracts and testing with group D serum.

Prevention and Hygiene Education

The primary sources of all corynebacterium and streptococcus infections are human carriers and patients. However, it should be emphasized that there appears to be no relationship between the carrier rates in a community and the outbreak of disease. In addition, although patients recovering from a bout of the infection may still harbour the organism in their upper and lower respiratory tract, the individuals may or may not be infectious. The original infecting organisms may die off or lose their virulence while still in the patient's respiratory tract. Nevertheless, prevention of infection, when transmitted via food, first entails the prevention of those with active infection from handling or preparing food. Second, these pathogenic strains (in particular, corynebacteria and group A streptococci) organisms are highly heat-sensitive, and almost all foods associated with outbreaks are those prepared by hand from basic cold ingredients and served without preliminary heating or cooking, i.e. raw milk and salads. It therefore behoves those responsible for food preparation to recognize the hazard associated with human carriers. These individuals should not be involved in food preparation, particularly of cold foods, which should be kept refrigerated until consumed. In addition, all food handlers should be scrupulously clean in their personal habits and be provided with clean lavatories and facilities for washing their hands with running water after use. Hands should be washed before and between handling of different cold foods. Preventive measures against diseases caused by corynebacterium and streptococcus are similar to those suggested for other pathogens. However, special care must be exercised to ensure that organisms are not allowed to multiply rapidly to pathogenic levels. Prompt consumption or refrigeration below 4°C after cooking, and heating of suspected food above 65°C for at least 30 min (or a shorter period at higher temperatures) before consumption would ensure killing of all corynebacteria and group A streptococci, or reduction of the number of enterococci (group D streptococci) to a safe level. The usual methods of food preservation also ensure food safety with respect to possible enterococcal pathogens.

Identification, isolation, and antibiotic treatment of cases and active carriers, identification of diphtheria-susceptible individuals (using the Schick test) and active immunization programmes (DPT vaccine) are means that have been employed to eradicate diphtheria. In countries where no immunization is undertaken, diphtheria remains a severe and highly fatal disease, especially for children.

Bibliography

Baron S (ed.) (1986) *Medical Microbiology* 2nd edn. Menlo Park, California: Addison-Wesley.

Christie AB (ed.) (1980) *Infectious Diseases: Epidemiology and Clinical Practice* 3rd edn. Edinburgh: Churchill Livingstone.

Elliott RP (ed.) (1978) *Microorganisms in Foods. 1. Their Significance and Methods of Enumeration* 2nd edn. Toronto: University of Toronto Press.

Holt JG (ed.) (1986) *Bergey's Manual of Systematic Bacteriology*, vol. 1 and 2. Baltimore: Williams and Wilkins.

Roberts TA and Skinner FA (eds) (1983) *Food Microbiology: Advances and Prospects*. Orlando: Academic Press.

WHO (1983) Food safety. The role of food in the epidemiology of acute enteric infections and intoxications. *Weekly Epidemiological Record* 58(31): 241–243.

R. Cichon
University of Agriculture and Technology, Olsztyn, Poland
D. N. Salter
Agricultural and Food Research Council – Institute for Grassland and Environmental Research, Shinfield, UK

DISINFECTANTS

See Cleaning Procedures in the Factory

DISTILLED BEVERAGE SPIRITS

See Individual Spirits

DISTRIBUTION

See Retailing of Food in the UK and Transport Logistics of Food

DOWN'S SYNDROME – NUTRITIONAL ASPECTS

Down's syndrome is the commonest genetic cause, and most frequently occurring form of mental handicap. It is named after Dr John Langdon Down, who, whilst working in London in 1866, remarked on the similarity of the physical features of some people with mental handicap. As these physical features were characteristic of people of the Mongol race, he used the terms 'Mongoloid' or 'Mongol'. These are now no longer used and have been replaced by the term 'Down's syndrome'.

Cause

There are three causes of Down's syndrome, all involving an excess of all or part of chromosome 21:

1. *Trisomy 21* accounts for about 95% of cases. Abnormality arises from nondisjunction of the chromosome during meiosis, i.e. ova or sperm are formed containing two number 21 chromosomes instead of one, and fertilization therefore leads to cells with three number 21 chromosome.

2. *Mosaic* accounts for about 2–5% of cases. A proportion of body cells are normal, whilst some have trisomy 21. Clinical features are between Down's syndrome and non-Down's syndrome.

3. *Translocation* accounts for about 2–5% of cases. All or part of the extra chromosome 21 is attached to another, often chromosome 14. Clinical features are similar to those of trisomy 21.

In texts, all types of Down's syndrome are usually referred to as trisomy 21, unless otherwise specified.

Incidence

The overall occurrence in most countries is 1 in 700–1000 births. The incidence of having a child with Down's syndrome increases with maternal age. It is postulated that this is a result of the hormonal changes in women which occur as they age. Various studies show an incidence of approximately 1 in 1500 births if a woman is aged 20–24, rising to 1 in 400 births by the age of 35. By the age of 40 the incidence has risen to about 1 in 100 births and up to 1 in 35–50 births if a woman bears children well into her 40s. Although the incidence of having a child with Down's syndrome rises with maternal age, most children are born to women aged under 35. Thus the majority of babies with Down's syndrome are born to women aged under 35.

Clinical Features

Intellectual ability may vary from near normal to an intelligence quotient (IQ) of less than 20 (profound handicap). The many associated physical features have no correlation to the degree of mental handicap.

As a result of the physical features, Down's syndrome is one of the few causes of mental handicap recognizable at birth. These features include a small round head, a small nose with poorly developed bridge, eyes which slope downwards and inwards, and small ears which may have poorly developed lobes. In the mouth, the palate may be high and arched, and the tongue may protrude. Fingers and toes may be shorter than usual; the palm of the hand is square and a 'four-finger line', or Simian crease, occurs in about 30–40% of cases. Mouth breathing is common and there is a tendency to chest infections and respiratory problems. The skin in childhood through to early adulthood is soft and supple but begins to lose its elasticity and appears dry and wrinkled usually by the mid-30s. Hair often becomes sparse with age.

Congenital abnormalities of internal organs include disorders of the digestive tract in up to 5% of births, including atresia of the upper part of the digestive tract and Hirschsprung's disease (incidence of 1 in 5000 births, however occurence is greater in Down's syndrome), both of which necessitate abdominal surgery. Cardiac abnormalities may occur in about 50% of births, which may also require surgery.

Senile degenerative brain disease, with associated dementia of the Alzheimer's type, is very common and often occurs at an earlier age than in the rest of the population.

Life Expectancy

Life expectancy has increased dramatically over the past 50 years as a result of improved paediatric care, advances in the treatment of cardiac defects, the advent of antibiotics, and other medical developments. Even so, up to 50% of children die before their fifth birthday,

due mainly to one or more of the following: cardiac abnormalities; complications of the abdominal disorders; respiratory problems. This results in a lower incidence of these features in adults than in newborns or children.

In later life, the problems associated with dementia, compounded with the clinical features of Down's syndrome, may contribute to shortened life expectancy.

The average life expectancy, if a child lives to its its first birthday, has risen during this century from 9 to 35 years. People with Down's syndrome may now live to be well over 60 years of age.

Nutritional Status

Various nutritional problems can occur, many resulting from the clinical features.

As babies with Down's syndrome are more prone to infection, particularly chest infections, breast-feeding is recommended because of the antibodies present in breast milk, but mothers may prefer to bottle-feed. The baby may tire easily when sucking; if so, small frequent feeds are recommended. *See* Infants, Breast- and Bottle-feeding

The rooting reflex and the tongue-thrusting action required for sucking, which are present at birth and are used when feeding from a breast or bottle, need to diminish before spoon feeding can commence. These actions may be maintained longer than normal in babies with Down's syndrome and, as a consequence, weaning may be delayed. If such a delay occurs and adequate nourishment cannot be given, some babies may temporarily fail to gain weight, until they can take adequate solids from a spoon.

If a protruding tongue and/or high palate are present, the infant may have an initial difficulty in sucking but this is normally overcome as he or she matures. In the child and adult with such problems, there may be difficulty in biting on and controlling foods of a very firm texture, and some foods may need to be finely chopped before being placed in the mouth. All too often, and sometimes unnecessarily, foods of too soft a texture, having been overcooked or mashed with nutrient-poor liquids, are offered. This results in nutrient loss, mainly of the water-soluble vitamins, particularly in fruits and vegetables. Some softer foods are higher in food energy than those of a firmer texture, e.g. milk pudding or chocolate-based items rather than fresh fruit, and this may be one of the contributing factors in obesity.

For the infant with a congenital abnormality of the abdominal tract, surgery is required as soon as it becomes apparent. Atresia, which is complete obstruction of the small intestine resulting from defective development in the fetus, will require immediate bowel resection. Possible subsequent surgery may result in further loss of intestinal length, leading to problems of malabsorption. For infants with Hirschprung's disease, in which ganglion cells are absent in the bowel wall, resulting in a form of megacolon, bowel resection is needed, often with a temporary colostomy. Long-term bowel control may be imperfect for some years. Infants, children and adults with bowel resection may need dietary modifications and possible nutritional supplements, depending on the extent of the surgery. *See* Colon, Diseases and Disorders

It is important that any person with Down's syndrome who has loose bowel function or diarrhoea, whether or not they have undergone bowel surgery, is investigated for possible food intolerance, e.g. coeliac disease, lactose intolerance, etc. Poor bowel control may not be fully investigated if it is thought to be due to the mental handicap or as a result of surgery, rather than a food sensitivity or intolerance. *See* Coeliac Disease; Food Intolerance, Types

For the infant with severe congenital cardiac abnormalities, the nutritional status can be severely compromised. Such infants tire extremely easily and may be exhausted after only a few mouthfuls; they will need to be offered small, frequent, high-energy feeds. Even this may not provide adequate nutrition and the infant may fail to thrive, in which case total or supplementary enteral feeding may need to be initiated.

For all children up to the age of 5, the UK Down's Syndrome Association, along with the Paediatric Group of the British Dietetic Association, recommend multivitamin supplements as per the recommendation for most children. As children with Down's syndrome may have problems with feeding, they should receive B vitamins in addition to the routinely used vitamins A, D and C supplement. As with all vitamin preparations, it is dangerous to exceed the stated dose.

Vitamin and Mineral Supplementation and Requirements

In addition to the routine use of multivitamins in early childhood, interest in the possibility of using megavitamin therapy as a treatment for reducing the degree of mental handicap in children with Down's syndrome was stimulated by the publication of the results of a study by Harrell *et al.* (1981). The hypothesis investigated was that retardation is a genetotrophic disease, i.e. one in which the genetic pattern requires an augmented supply of adequate specific nutrients to ameliorate the disease. In the controlled partial double-blind study of 16 children with a mental handicap, IQ gains were found after daily supplementation of relatively large doses of 11 vitamins and moderate doses of 8 minerals (see Table 1). The 8-month supplemented group showed a significant increase in IQ after 4 months and a further increase after 8 months. The second group showed no

change in IQ during the 4-month placebo period but a significant increase after a subsequent 4-month period of supplementation. The children with Down's syndrome in the study made the greatest improvement in IQ and showed physical changes towards normal. *See* Health Foods, Dietary Supplements

However, similar follow-up studies of people with Down's syndrome have not supported Harrell's findings, and various criticisms of the study's methodology and conclusions have been made. These subsequent studies have clearly indicated no significant change in IQ or appearance between treated and untreated groups, although no study has exactly replicated Harrell's. Variables have included not giving thyroid hormone supplement to subjects as Harrell did, or using hospital-based adults with Down's syndrome rather than home-based children. Nevertheless, parents in some studies chose to continue the vitamin supplementation for their children with Down's syndrome in spite of failure of the studies to demonstrate their efficacy. Such a response may reflect a stubborn optimism, or positive expectations for improvement, or of attributing normal developmental changes to the magical power of vitamins.

No studies reported negative side-effects from the administration of such large doses of vitamins, with the exception of transient skin flushing in one, and slight elevations of some liver functions in another. Yet the toxic and dangerous effects of vitamin megadoses (vitamins A, D, E and B_6) are increasingly recognized. The large dose of vitamin A which Harrell suggested leads to considerable anxiety because of the potential danger of liver toxicity. Other doses are also very high (Table 1).

Other vitamins have been studied separately, and some papers suggest that people with Down's syndrome are prone to suffer specific vitamin deficiencies (vitamins A, E, B_1, B_6 and C) and shortages of some minerals and trace elements (calcium, copper, manganese and zinc), either because of poor gut absorption or because of poor tissue utilization. Reduced intestinal absorption in Down's syndrome has been found using the xylose absorption test (the amount of xylose present in the urine for 5 h after an oral xylose dose is proportional to that absorbed through the intestinal wall). However, these deficiencies have not been consistently confirmed or documented. Although there have been conflicting results in investigations of serum vitamin A levels and vitamin A absorption in Down's syndrome, some studies show dermatological symptoms suggestive of hypovitaminosis A in people with Down's syndrome with normal or high serum vitamin A levels. It has been suggested there may be impairment of vitamin A utilization at its site of action. *See* Hypovitaminosis A and also individual vitamins, metals and minerals

Despite conflicting and controversial studies, pres-

Table 1. Daily dose of supplementary vitamins, according to Harrell *et al.* (1981), compared to UK (1979) and World Health Organization (WHO) Recommended Daily Intakes (RDIs) and UK (1991) Reference Nutrient Intakes (RNIs) for vitamins

Vitamin	Harrell's dose	UK RDI (1979) (0–17 years)	WHO RDI (approximate for childhood)	UK RNI (1991) (0–17 years)
Vitamin A				
(iu)	15 000	1000–2500	1000	1165–2331
(μg)	4500	300–750	300	350–700
Vitamin D				
(iu)	300	Up to 400	400	Up to 360
(μg)	7·5	Up to 10	10	Up to 8·5
Vitamin B				
Thiamin, B_1 (mg)	300	0·3–1·2	0·5–0·9	0·2–1·1
Riboflavin, B_2 (mg)	200	0·4–1·7	0·8–1·3	0·4–1·3
Nicotinic acid, B_3 (mg)	750	5·0–19·0	9·0–14·5	3·0–18·0
Pyridoxine, B_6 (mg)	350	—[a]	1·1–1·25	0·2–1·5
Cobalamin, B_{12} (μg)	1000	—[a]	0·9–1·5	0·3–1·5
Vitamin C (ascorbic acid) (mg)	1500	20·0–30·0	20	25·0–40·0
Vitamin E (α-tocopherol)				
(iu)	600	—[a]	5·0–12·0	(above 4·47 adult female / above 5·96 adult male)[b,c]
(mg)	402	—[a]	3·3–8·0	(above 3 adult female / above 4 adult male)[b,c]

[a] No RDI.
Both the UK 1979 and 1991 figures are quoted as the 1979 figures applied at the time of Harrell's and subsequent studies.
[b] Safe intake for adults.
[c] No safe intake given for children, but for infants 0·4 mg per g polyunsaturated fatty acids.
iu (international unit), biological activity of a vitamin.

sure from parents to try vitamin and mineral therapy to help their children with Down's syndrome to reach their highest potential is increasing. Dangers of excessive dosage and dependency can be emphasized, but from a position of uncertainty about the real interrelationship between Down's syndrome and vitamins, this therapy cannot be condemned outright.

Body Mass

Children and adults with Down's syndrome are thought of as being typically short in stature and obese. Often their shortness of stature and body proportions, which may include shorter than expected leg length, give the impression of having a greater body mass index (BMI) than is actually the case. Body mass index is calculated as weight (kg) divided by height (m) squared. (In adults if BMI < 20 then person is underweight, if BMI = 20–25 this is acceptable bodyweight, if BMI = 25–30 then person is overweight and if BMI > 30 then person is obese.)

Although there is a tendency to obesity, many people with Down's syndrome are of average weight and may even be underweight. Few middle-aged or elderly people with Down's syndrome are overweight; many experi-

ence weight loss as they age and invariably become underweight. *See* Obesity, Aetiology and Assessment

Children with Down's syndrome are often shorter than their peer group. In adolescence the growth spurt may be smaller than average, often ceasing earlier, resulting in short adult height.

Obesity, if it is present, can arise for a variety of reasons including the following: the use of softer, high-energy foods; parents and carers may inadvertently provide a diet that gives an excessive energy intake; food is used as a reward, treat or palliative measure; low activity levels (many people with Down's syndrome have placid, nonenergetic personalities); restriction in activity due to cardiac problems; hypothyroidism. Most people with Down's syndrome, if obese, respond well to a reduction in energy intake and, where possible, an increase in energy expenditure. For many people with a mental handicap, any weight-reducing programme can often be included in teaching and life skills lessons, looking at healthy foods and healthy meal plans, with games, incentives and praise being given, rather than using a strict weight-reducing programme in isolation.

People with Down's syndrome may be underweight and have a BMI of less than 20. Reasons for this include the following: difficulty in chewing and swallowing; tiredness when eating and drinking due to cardiac problems, so that inadequate energy is consumed at meal times; excessive energy needs (particularly if someone has high activity levels, whether or not this is structured exercise); loss of interest in food, often associated with ageing; dementia, which leads to (1) an increase in energy expenditure, (2) inability to follow through the thought process involved in preparing, cooking and eating food, with accompanying poor nutritional status, and (3) lack of interest in eating; hyperthyroidism. For those who are underweight, small frequent meals and snacks are necessary, with possible nutritional supplementation.

Babies, children and adults with cardiac abnormalities need careful monitoring of their nutritional intake and of any weight gain or loss. Nutritional supplementation may be necessary but for those who can achieve adequate nutrition, care must be taken to prevent obesity as excess weight is detrimental to cardiac function.

Thyroid Function

Studies that have looked at the thyroid status of people with Down's syndrome show an increase in the incidence of thyroid disease, which varies with the age, sex, numbers studied and how they were selected. Two recent studies in the UK, each looking at over 100 adults, male and female, both found hypothyroidism in over 7% of subjects, as compared with less than 1% in the general population. The incidence of hyperthyroidism was over 1%, as compared with less than 0·1% in the general population. Both studies found high levels of thyroid microsomal antibodies in about 30% of subjects, whether or not they had overt hypothyroidism. These antibodies may later cause damage to the thyroid gland by the autoimmune process causing hypothyroidism. Other studies quote even greater figures. Hypothyroidism in people with Down's syndrome may be under diagnosed as some of the clinical features of both may be similar, e.g. obesity, dry skin, alopecia, placidness, apathy and forgetfuless, the latter having an increased incidence in people as they age. Hyperthyroidism, if it occurs, leads to agitation, excitability and weight loss. Recent studies suggest a need for regular monitoring of people with Down's syndrome for thyroid status. *See* Thyroid Diseases

Premature Ageing, and Theories concerning Antioxidant and Selenium Requirements

People with Down's syndrome have the physical appearance of accelerated ageing. In addition, many show signs of accelerated ageing in brain tissue by

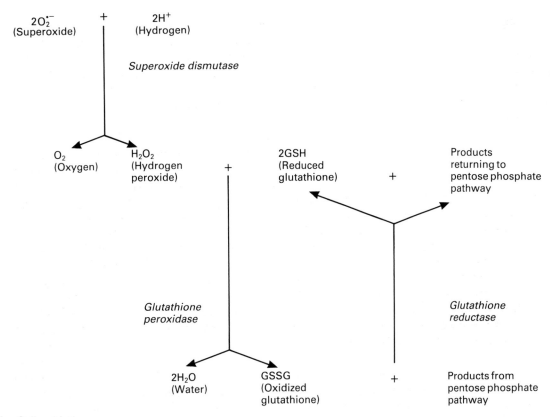

Fig. 1 Cell oxidation.

exhibiting dementia of the Alzheimer type at an earlier age than average. Many studies have looked at the ageing process in people with Down's syndrome. Sylvester (1984) looked at the incidence of senile plaques and tangles in the brains of people with Down's syndrome and compared them to a control group, consisting of people who had a mental handicap but not Down's syndrome. For the people with Down's syndrome, senile changes were present in 95% of those who died between the ages of 30 and 39, and 100% for those who died aged over 50. In the control group, there were senile changes in only 27·9% who died over the age of 60. Many other studies have shown both physiological and psychological accelerated ageing processes. *See* Ageing – Nutritional Aspects

To look at ageing, it is necessary to look at cell oxidation (Fig. 1). Superoxide dismutase is a copper- and zinc-containing enzyme which forms oxygen (O_2) and hydrogen peroxide (H_2O_2) from superoxide (O_2^-) and hydrogen ions ($2H^+$). In the next stage of the enzyme pathway, the H_2O_2 combines with reduced glutathione (GSH) and is converted by the selenium-containing enzyme, glutathione peroxidase, to form water (H_2O) and oxidized glutathione (GSSG).

In Down's syndrome this process is unbalanced. Superoxide dismutase is dosage controlled by chromosome 21. There is thus an over-production of this enzyme by 50% and, as a result, H_2O_2 production is increased; studies suggest that there is not a compensatory increase in glutathione peroxidase in some body cells such as the brain cells. Without this increase in glutathione peroxidase, excess H_2O_2 will accumulate.

Hydrogen peroxide leads to lipid peroxidation in the cells and cell ageing; an excess will lead to an accelerated ageing process. Vitamin E (α-tocopherol) is an antioxidant; it is membrane-soluble and protects against lipid peroxidation in the cells. From various studies the hypothesis has emerged that vitamin E helps to slow down the ageing process in people with Down's syndrome, particularly in cells of the brain. Another hypothesis is that there is an increase in selenium requirements so as to facilitate glutathione peroxidase production. *See* Antioxidants, Role of Antioxidant Nutrients in Defence Systems; Selenium, Physiology

Other studies concentrate on the physical aspects of ageing, and possible implications with this metabolic pathway.

All aspects of ageing in people with Down's syndrome, whether physiological or psychological, have been and are still the subjects of ongoing research, the results of which basically agree in general principles but may contradict each other in fine detail.

Recent evidence is also beginning to emerge about abnormalities in chromosome 21 in some cases of familial Alzheimer's disease (FAD). Any concrete link between FAD and Down's syndrome, particularly with recent advances in genetic studies, will lead to exciting research possibilities and, it is hoped, to a reduction in the incidence of dementia.

Bibliography

Dinani S and Carpenter S (1990) Down's syndrome and thyroid disorder. *Journal of Mental Deficiency Research* 34: 187–193.

Emslie-Smith D, Paterson CR, Scratcherd T and Read N (eds) (1988) *BDS – Textbook of Physiology* 11th edn. London: Churchill Livingstone.

Foreman PJ and Ward J (1986) Treatment approaches in Down's syndrome. *Australia and New Zealand Journal of Developmental Disabilities* 12(2): 111–121.

Harrell RF, Capp RH, Davis DR, Peerless J and Ravitz L (1981) Can nutritional supplements help mentally retarded children? An exploratory study. *Proceedings of the National Academy of Sciences of the USA* 78(1): 574–578.

Heaton-Ward WA and Wiley Y (1984) *Mental Handicap* 5th edn. Bristol: John Wright and Sons.

Hogg J, Sebba J and Lambe L (eds) (1990) *Profound Retardation and Multiple Impairment*, vol. 3. London: Chapman and Hall.

Jackson CVE, Holland AJ, Williams CA, Dickerson JWT (1988) Vitamin E and Alzheimer's disease in subjects with Down's syndrome. *Journal of Mental Deficiency Research* 32: 479–484.

Kinnell HG, Gibbs N, Teale JD and Smith J (1987) Thyroid dysfunction in institutionalised Down's syndrome adults. *Psychological Medicine* 17: 387–392.

Smith GF (ed.) (1985) Molecular structure of the number 21 chromosome and Down's syndrome. *Annals of the New York Academy of Sciences* 450.

Sylvester P (1984) Nutritional aspects of Down's syndrome with special reference to the nervous system. *British Journal of Psychiatry* 145: 115–120.

Various pamphlets, including *Children with Down's Syndrome and Vitamins* (by Clayden G) and *Healthy Eating for your Child* (written by Antcliff E, in association with the Paediatric Group of the British Dietetic Association). Available from Down's Association (UK) 155, Mitcham Road, London SW17 9PG.

Williams CA, Quinn H, Wright E *et al.* (1985) Xylose absorption in Down's syndrome. *Journal of Mental Deficiency Research* 29: 173–177.

Philippa Hewitt
Borocourt Hospital, Reading, UK
Dorothy Smith
Southmead Hospital, Bristol, UK